J. HALL
1259 IRONWOOD
WILLIAMSTON MI
48895

517-655-3780

Two-dimensional echocardiography
Clinical-pathological correlations in
adult and congenital heart disease

Two-dimensional echocardiography
Clinical-pathological correlations in adult and congenital heart disease

Arthur D. Hagan
M.D., F.A.C.C.
Professor of Medicine and
Adjunct Professor of Medical
Biophysics and Computing,
University of Utah School
of Medicine; Chief of
Cardiology, LDS Hospital,
Salt Lake City, Utah

Thomas G. DiSessa
M.D., F.A.C.C.
Assistant Professor of
Pediatrics and Director,
Pediatric Echocardiography
Laboratory, University of
California, Los Angeles
(UCLA) School of Medicine,
Los Angeles, California

Colin M. Bloor
M.D., F.A.C.C.
Professor, Department of
Pathology, University of
California, San Diego School
of Medicine, La Jolla,
California

H. B. Calleja
M.D., F.A.C.C.
Head, Department of
Cardiology, Philippine Heart
Center for Asia, Quezon
City, Philippines

Little, Brown and Company
Boston/Toronto

Copyright © 1983 by Arthur D. Hagan, M.D., Thomas G. DiSessa, M.D., Colin M. Bloor, M.D., and H. B. Calleja, M.D.

First Edition

All rights reserved. No part of this book may be reproduced in any form or by any electronic or mechanical means, including information storage and retrieval systems, without permission in writing from the publisher, except by a reviewer who may quote brief passages in a review.

Library of Congress Catalog Card No. 82-83675

ISBN 0-316-33781-1

Printed in the United States of America

HAL

To my parents, Roscoe and Catherine; my wife, Linda; and my children, Doug, Kim, and Brett, who have given me inspiration and perseverance while demonstrating love and understanding

A. D. H.

My enduring gratitude is extended to my parents, Rose and Fred, whose love, patience, and guidance have always fostered my best efforts. The devotion and understanding of my wife, Patricia, and my children, Thomas, John, and Peter, were indispensable in creating the milieu that allowed preparation of this book

T. G. D.

Contents

Preface	xiii
Abbreviations	xv

1
Normal cross-sectional anatomy: two-dimensional echocardiographic imaging and measurement techniques

	1
Approach to the patient having a two-dimensional echocardiographic examination	1
Two-dimensional imaging systems	4
Two-dimensional echocardiographic imaging techniques	22
Echocardiographic measurements: M-mode and two-dimensional images	41

2
Rheumatic valvular disease

	47
Normal mitral valve	47
Clinical manifestations of rheumatic mitral disease	50
Rheumatic tricuspid disease	69

3
Nonrheumatic mitral valve disease

	83
Pathophysiology of mitral regurgitation	83
Mitral valve prolapse	83
Mitral annulus calcification	96
Ruptured chordae tendineae	98
Papillary muscle dysfunction	102
Congenital mitral regurgitation	106

4
Diseases of the aortic valve and aorta

	111
Normal anatomy and physiology of the aortic valve	111
Imaging techniques of aortic valve and aorta	111
Aortic valve disease	115
Membranous subvalvular and supravalvular aortic stenosis	128
Aortic regurgitation	128
Diseases of the aorta	134

5
Infective endocarditis — 145
Clinical features — 145
Aortic valve vegetations — 147
Mitral valve vegetations — 151
Tricuspid valve vegetations — 153
Pulmonic valve vegetations — 158

6
Coronary artery disease — 163
Clinical indications — 163
Two-dimensional imaging techniques — 170
Use of pharmacologic agents to evaluate regional myocardial function and reversible ischemia by echocardiography — 180
Evaluation of uncomplicated myocardial infarction and global left ventricular performance by echocardiography — 181
Quantitation of infarct size and/or ischemia — 186
Complications of myocardial infarction — 189
Postoperative assessment of patients following coronary artery bypass graft — 214
Examination of coronary arteries — 214

7
Left ventricular function — 227
Left ventricular cavity size, wall thickness, and mass — 227
Left ventricular wall stress — 230
Left ventricular volumes and performance — 232
Echocardiographic and Doppler estimates of cardiac output — 238
Influence of cardiovascular drugs and exercise on left ventricular function — 240
Left ventricular diastolic filling and compliance — 241
Interdependence of the right and left ventricles — 243

8
Diseases of the right heart — 251
Normal criteria for dimensions of right heart structures — 251
Imaging techniques of right heart structures — 252

Right ventricular function and pulmonary hypertension	254
Right ventricular volume overload	257
Interatrial septum, inferior vena cava, and superior vena cava	268
Pulmonic valve and tricuspid valve	269

9
Cardiomyopathies — 287

Hypertrophic cardiomyopathy	287
Hypertrophic cardiomyopathy in association with other cardiac disorders	320
Hypertension and miscellaneous forms of hypertrophic cardiomyopathies	321
Cardiomyopathy of hypothyroidism	322
Cardiac abnormalities in scleroderma	323
Congestive cardiomyopathy	323
Restrictive or infiltrative cardiomyopathy	328
Endomyocardial fibrosis	330

10
Pericardial diseases — 341

Normal anatomy and function of the pericardium	341
Role of the pericardium in diastolic properties of the ventricles	341
Relationship of the pericardium to the pathophysiology of cardiac failure	342
Pericardial effusion and primary left ventricular disease	343
Pericardial thickening and constrictive pericarditis	347

11
Cardiac tumors and masses — 363

Left atrial tumors and masses	363
Left ventricular tumors and masses	370
Right atrial tumors, masses, and benign structures	374
Right ventricular tumors	375
Extracardiac tumors	390

12
Prosthetic valves — 395

13
Interventional echocardiography — 421

Contrast echocardiography — 421

Pharmacologic and physiologic maneuvers — 429

Exercise echocardiography — 432

Echophonocardiography — 434

Esophageal echocardiography — 434

Intraoperative echocardiography — 438

14
Acyanotic congenital heart disease with left-to-right shunt — 443

Atrial septal defect: secundum type — 443

Atrial septal defect: primum type — 447

Ventricular septal defect — 451

Complete endocardial cushion defect — 456

Patent ductus arteriosus — 462

15
Congenital valvular, subvalvular, and supravalvular lesions — 467

Ebstein's anomaly — 467

Isolated infundibular stenosis — 469

Valvular pulmonic stenosis — 470

Left ventricular inflow tract obstruction — 473

Discrete subaortic stenosis — 477

Congenital aortic stenosis — 481

Supravalvular aortic stenosis — 485

Coarctation of the aorta — 488

16
Cyanotic congenital heart disease — 493

Tetralogy of Fallot — 493

Transposition of the great arteries — 496

Congenitally corrected transposition of the great arteries — 500

Truncus arteriosus — 508

Double-outlet right ventricle — 511

Single ventricle — 518

Tricuspid atresia	519
Total anomalous pulmonary venous return	524

17
Echocardiographic assessment of postoperative congenital heart disease — 529

Tetralogy of Fallot	529
Ventricular septal defect	531
Atrial septal defect: secundum type	533
Atrial septal defect: primum type	534
Complete endocardial cushion defect	538
Transposition of the great arteries	538
Double-outlet right ventricle	543
Truncus arteriosus	544
Valvular pulmonic stenosis	545
Discrete subaortic stenosis	546
Valvular aortic stenosis	547
Appendix	551
Index	557

Preface

During the past seven years the growth and clinical application of two-dimensional echocardiography has been enormous. New advances in technology have afforded marked improvement in the available instrumentation during the past three years. The status of echocardiography has changed significantly with the addition of real-time, two-dimensional sector imaging to existing M-mode echocardiography. Not only has the image quality of 2-D echo been improving, but M-mode information is now better because of newer integrated systems. Two-dimensional echocardiography has become an integral part of the diagnosis and management of patients with acquired and congenital heart diseases.

The primary purpose of this book is to discuss the role of two-dimensional echocardiography in the many clinical settings of congenital and adult heart diseases. A further emphasis is placed on correlating normal and abnormal cardiac anatomy as viewed in the various tomographic planes of 2-D echo with corresponding anatomic sections of numerous hearts. The cross-sectional anatomy and pathophysiology are better understood with this type of clinical, echocardiographic, and pathological correlation. Considerable attention is also devoted to discussing the various imaging techniques for the different diseases.

The text and figures are primarily from the Cardiology Division of the LDS Hospital in Salt Lake City with important contributions from the Cardiology Department of the Philippine Heart Center for Asia in Manila. Most of the figures in the four chapters on congenital heart disease are from the Pediatrics Department of the University of California, Los Angeles (UCLA). Most of the anatomic sections are from the Department of Pathology at the University of California, San Diego.

I am particularly indebted to five individuals without whom this book could never have been completed: photographer Leroy "Bud" Lewis; Richard Strickland and Judy Wong, who assisted in preparation and illustration of the figures; and Gaye Rhodes and Karen Gross, who did the typing and provided vital editorial assistance. I also wish to express my gratitude to Monica Noble, Vicki Collins, Richard Strickland, Linda Hagan, Barbara Sternlight, and John Leighton for their technical assistance in performing many of the echocardiographic examinations illustrated in the text.

A. D. H.
T. G. D.

Abbreviations

A, Ant	Anterior
AAo	Ascending aorta
AL, AML	Anterior mitral leaflet
Ao	Aorta
Ap	Left atrial appendage
ASD	Atrial septal defect
AS	Anterior portion of interventricular septum
AV	Aortic valve
CS	Coronary sinus
DAo	Descending aorta
EDD, ED	End-diastolic dimension
ESD, ES	End-systolic dimension
EN	Endocardium
EP	Epicardium
I, Inf	Inferior
IVC	Inferior vena cava
IVS, VS, S	Interventricular septum
L, Lt	Left
LA	Left atrium
LV	Left ventricle
LVO, LVOT	Left ventricular outflow tract
MAn	Mitral annulus
MB	Moderator band
MPA, PA	Main pulmonary artery
MV	Mitral valve
MVO	Mitral valve orifice
NC, N	Noncoronary cusp of aortic valve
P, Post	Posterior
PE	Pericardial effusion
PL, PML	Posterior mitral leaflet
PM	Papillary muscle(s)
PS	Posterior portion of interventricular septum
PW	Posterior wall of left ventricle
R, Rt	Right
RA	Right atrium
RV	Right ventricle
RVO, RVOT	Right ventricular outflow tract
SL, STL	Septal leaflet of tricuspid valve
Sup	Superior
SVC	Superior vena cava
TAn	Tricuspid annulus
TAo	Transverse aorta
TV	Tricuspid valve
VSD	Ventricular septal defect

Two-dimensional echocardiography
Clinical-pathological correlations in
adult and congenital heart disease

Normal cross-sectional anatomy: Two-dimensional echocardiographic imaging and measurement techniques

Echocardiography, which consists of both M-mode and two-dimensional cardiac imaging, is a safe, noninvasive, easily repeatable diagnostic examination that provides reliable and valuable information about the structure and function of the heart. Diagnostic ultrasound has achieved broad application in medicine as its reliability, contribution to patient care, and cost-effectiveness have been increasingly recognized. During the past two decades M-mode echocardiography has gained increasing popularity and clinical application. However, this method provides a one-dimensional or "ice pick" view of the heart which represents a major limitation of the technique. During the past few years two-dimensional or real-time, cross-sectional imaging of the heart has been perfected that overcomes many of the limitations of the one-dimensional technique. Two-dimensional imaging provides a spatial orientation of cardiac structures and the opportunity to image the heart from multiple transducer positions over the left precordium, apical area, subcostal region, and suprasternal notch location. The combination of these two imaging techniques in the same system has afforded opportunities to provide more information about cardiac structures and function than either of the systems can give by itself.

Approach to the patient having a two-dimensional echocardiographic examination. A patient who is referred for an echocardiographic examination usually benefits from having a combined study consisting of both M-mode and two-dimensional imaging. There are, however, occasional clinical circumstances in which either M-mode or two-dimensional imaging by itself is adequate.

When the patient arrives in the laboratory certain necessary clinical information must be obtained by the echocardiographer before proceeding with the examination. Because a nonphysician-echocardiographer has as much responsibility for obtaining this clinical information as a physician-echocardiographer, it is obvious that allied health personnel performing echocardiographic examinations must learn additional skills with respect to interviewing and examining patients. In reality these technicians or technologists function as specialized cardiovascular physician assistants with additional technical ability to operate the echocardiographic equipment.

After the initial demographic information is obtained from the patient, the first important question to be asked is why the patient was referred to the laboratory for the study. At that point a cardiovascular history must be obtained, including not only significant information with respect to the present illness but also valuable past medical history. Cardiac physical examination as well as notation of certain key information available from the electrocardiogram and chest x-ray may be important (Fig. 1-1).

It is particularly important for the echocardiographer to be aware of the cardiac physical findings and the present cardiovascular history as well as pertinent past

1. Normal cross-sectional anatomy

```
Date ___/___/___   File # _____   Tech _____   Tape #         Count to
                                                   [       ]      [   -   ]
Patient's name _____  Hosp # _____       [       ]      [   -   ]
[ ] Male  [ ] Female  Height _____  Weight _____ BSA _____ DOB ___ RM # ___
Referring doctor _____   Reason for referral _____
[ ] M-Mode  [ ] 2-D  [ ] Combined  [ ] Contrast  [ ] Portable  [ ] Serial  [ ] Protocol _____
Study quality:  [ ] Excellent      [ ] Satisfactory     [ ] Poor

PRESENT ILLNESS
Chest pain              Dyspnea                    [ ] Fatigue      [ ] Palpitations
Duration _____        Duration _____           [ ] Cough        [ ] Fever
[ ] Ischemia            [ ] Exertional  [ ] Nocturnal  [ ] Edema    [ ] Cyanosis
[ ] Pleural/Pericardial [ ] Orthopnea              [ ] Syncope      [ ] Dizzy/
[ ] Atypical                                       [ ] Other CNS    [ ] Lightheaded


Medications:  [ ] Digitalis    [ ] Antiarrhythmics _____
[ ] Diuretics/Antihypertensives _____           AHA Class: _____

PAST HISTORY
[ ] Hypertension × _____ years     [ ] Myocardial infarction: dates _____
[ ] Heart failure _____
[ ] RF  [ ] Known murmur: Duration _____    [ ] Cardiomyopathy _____
[ ] Endocarditis  [ ] Pericarditis _____    [ ] Pulmonary disease _____
[ ] Other _____
[ ] Cardiac surgery: dates _____            [ ] CABG × ___  [ ] Valve:type ___

ECG:  Rhythm:  [ ] Sinus    [ ] Atrial fib.   DX: _____

EXAMINATION
Blood pressure _____/_____  Heart rate _____   Heart sounds: _____
                                    [ ] S3  [ ] S4  Other _____
Murmurs: Systolic _____           Diastolic _____
```

Fig. 1-1. Page 1 of the 2-D echo interpretation forms used in our laboratories.

medical history and previous cardiac surgery. This information is necessary so that the echocardiographer can direct the examination and imaging techniques along clinically relevant lines. The electrocardiogram is not only important for timing purposes in analyzing the echocardiogram but is significant in that certain arrhythmias or conduction defects may cause motion abnormalities that can be confused with other types of cardiac abnormalities if the electrocardiogram is unknown. Under certain circumstances chest x-ray information is important, particularly when the cardiac position is unusual or there is evidence of other mediastinal or pulmonary masses in proximity or compressing the heart. Knowledge of pleural effusions on chest x-rays may be beneficial in performing and interpreting an echocardiographic examination. If there is superior displacement of the left hemidiaphragm, this may realign the position of the heart, making it necessary to perform two-dimensional imaging from unusual transducer positions.

PERSONNEL. Echocardiography, particularly two-dimensional cardiac imaging, is operator-dependent and requires immediate "on-line" interpretative evaluation in order to obtain comprehensive and technically adequate studies. Unless the type and significance of the abnormal structures, motion, and function are recognized, adequate views and complete anatomy will not be recorded and the study will be incomplete or inadequate for diagnostic purposes. For that reason, either a nonphysician- or physician-echocardiographer must have certain background knowledge as well as certain essential clinical facts about the patient being studied:

1. A thorough background and understanding of cardiac anatomy as well as hemodynamics and pathophysiology of acquired and congenital heart diseases
2. The understanding and ability to conceptualize three-dimensional spatial relationships of the various cardiac structures as they are being viewed in a two-dimensional perspective from the various transducer locations
3. A thorough understanding of all the numerous transducer positions and the minimum number of tomographic images required for a comprehensive examination as well as of additional views to the standard positions in order to optimize the imaging information obtainable on any given cardiac abnormality
4. The ability to perform cardiac auscultation and interpret abnormal cardiac findings
5. A working knowledge of electrocardiography, phonocardiography, and cardiopulmonary hemodynamics to facilitate their correlation with the anatomical and functional findings of the echocardiogram
6. The ability to perform certain diagnostic interventions (contrast studies, maneuvers, exercise, or administration of drugs) to complement the imaging information
7. A thorough understanding of the physical and technical principles of the ultrasonic instrumentation being utilized

The necessary resources for an M-mode echocardiographic examination were reported on by the Inter-Society Commission for Heart Disease Resources in 1975 [1] and updated by the Commission in a report entitled *Optimal Resources for Ultrasonic Examination of the Heart* in 1982 [2].

Allied health personnel who are ideally suited to obtain further specialized training in two-dimensional imaging are those individuals who have spent a minimum of two years of formal training in a related field such as performing other types of noninvasive cardiac procedures or working in cardiac catheterization laboratories. (Physician assistants and registered nurses also have excellent background training for this field.) Having started with that type of allied health background, most technologists, physician assistants, or nurses will require an additional year of specialized training in performing two-dimensional imaging in order to perform high-quality work in an independent fashion. It should be emphasized, however, that these echocardiographers should still be working under the supervision of a qualified physician; this is even more important when acutely ill patients are being imaged and the examination is technically difficult. Complete knowledge of the clinical situation in a hemodynamically unstable patient is very important. Because it is frequently necessary to image acutely ill patients at the bedside, the echocardiographer must understand nursing procedures and be able to work with other personnel in the overall care of the patient in acute care units. Furthermore, it is important to recognize that certain high-risk cardiac patients may be examined in the echocardiography laboratory; therefore adequate support facilities and knowledge of cardiopulmonary resuscitation are also required of the echocardiographer.

The American College of Cardiology in conjunction with the American Society of Echocardiography and other allied health and professional organizations applied to the American Medical Association for recognition of the field "cardiovascular technology"; this application was approved in December, 1981. The cosponsoring organizations are currently working on essentials of training, curriculum, and plans for certification and accreditation of echocardiographers (cardiac sonographers).

Two-dimensional imaging systems. Several approaches have been employed during the past few years in the development of real-time, two-dimensional ultrasonic scanning. The principal techniques employed include:

1. Mechanical scanners employing an oscillating transducer
2. Linear-array scanners using multiple crystals
3. Phased-array scanners that electronically sweep the beam through the target

The original design of the mechanical scanner consisted of a transducer reciprocating continuously through a 30-degree sector at a rate of 15 cycles per second. Each complete cycle resulted in generating two separate 30-degree sectors providing 30 separate frames per second [3].

In addition to mechanical scanners utilizing an oscillating single crystal transducer, some of the mechanical scanners now utilize multiple rotating crystals with the capability of imaging wide angles of 80 to 90 degrees.

Multiscan echocardiography consists of a transducer containing 20 adjacent piezoelectric elements in a linear array [4]. Rapid electronic switching from one element to the next and appropriate display of the resultant images produces a continuous two-dimensional image of the cardiac structures. The multiscan transducer head is relatively large and measures approximately 8 cm in length. Each crystal is pulsed sequentially and the image displayed as a series of single line reflections. This large transducer size, the low line density, and the wide beam size result in overall poor resolution with discontinuity of the images from the underlying ribs; this scanner is generally not satisfactory for clinical purposes.

The electronic steering of the ultrasonic beam by phased-array excitation has been the most recent development in real-time, two-dimensional imaging of the heart. The transducers with the phased-array systems vary in frequency from 2.25 to 3.5 MHz. Some systems employ an external acoustic lens for focusing the ultrasound beam while others have attempted to employ dynamic focusing with the use of computer steering of the beam [5]. A marker on the handle of the transducer indicates the orientation of the sector beam. An 80- to 90-degree sector image of the heart is obtained with a scan rate varying from 25 to 60 frames per second depending upon the depth scale and type of equipment utilized.

Resolution is the ability to distinguish two closely spaced objects as separate entities rather than as parts of a single larger structure. Resolution of two-dimensional imaging systems can be measured in three directions: along the axis of the ultrasonic beam (axial resolution), within the scanning arc (azimuthal resolution), and perpendicular to the plane of the scanning arc (lateral resolution). Axial resolution is usually the best in the two-dimensional systems and probably approaches 1 mm. However, azimuthal and lateral resolutions are not as accurate and vary between manufacturers. Azimuthal resolution determines how well structures located at the same depth in the scanning arc are separated, and lateral resolution determines how well structures that lie outside the plane of the scanning arc are excluded from the image. Azimuthal and lateral resolution for certain echocardiographic systems which have been tested appear to be 2–3 mm [6]. Furthermore the azimuthal and lateral resolution may diminish at greater depths. When a rotary system was evaluated and the line density increased by reducing the sector angle, a slight improvement in the azimuthal resolution occurred; however, the lateral resolution was not affected [6]. The phased-array system utilizing a 2.4 MHz transducer was noted to have the same azimuthal resolution of the system as did a mechanical scanner utilizing a 3.5 MHz transducer. Latson and associates [6] recommended the higher frequency transducer and lowest possible gain setting to optimize resolution. The degree of resolution has significant clinical implications; for example, the ability to visualize a ventricular septal defect would not be possible unless the hole were larger than 3 mm in most systems. Bierman and colleagues [7] were able to identify ventricular septal defects in the 1–2 mm diameter range by employing a 5 MHz, short-focused transducer. They reported a beam width of the crystal to be 1 to 2 mm at 3.8 cm between -6 db and -20 db. The useful zone (i.e., lateral resolution two times the minimum beam width) extended from 2.5 to 7.5 cm from the crystal and the axial resolution was 0.5 cm at -20 db. Most of the echocardiographic systems tested underestimated the size of a myocardial defect by 1.0 to 2.5 mm [7]. This problem is secondary to the fact that limited resolution results in some "smearing" of the image. Because the smearing effect is exaggerated by high gain settings, it is recommended that the lowest possible gain be used when measurements are made from a two-dimensional image. Latson's study did not reveal important differences in the resolution ability of three basic types of ultrasonic equipment tested: one electronic phased-array, one mechanical rotary, and the two mechanical oscillating sector scanners. The results, however, did confirm the superior resolution of higher frequency transducers in a given system.

Helak and associates [8] evaluated the reliability of 2-D echo images of short axis slices of human hearts post mortem using two phased-array and two mechanical systems. Two phased-array and one mechanical system compared favorably in determining by planimetry the total myocardial and left ventricular cavity areas and showed excellent correlation with the actual anatomy.

The digital scan processor, available on some phased-array systems providing variable persistence of the image data and greater flexibility in gray-scale processing, has improved the quality of clinical studies. Simultaneous M-mode recordings together with two-dimensional tomographic imaging has further enhanced the overall capability of echocardiographic data gathering. Transducer design and small contact surface area with the skin are important since all precordial and apical images must be obtained between the narrow intercostal spaces. The development of higher frequency transducers together with new focusing techniques should lead to further improvement in resolution.

The M-mode and two-dimensional echocardiographic data are recorded on two formats, paper strip-chart recorders and videotape recorders respectively. Manufacturers are currently using either one-half inch or three-fourths inch videocassette recorders. Some of the instrumentation is equipped to record the M-mode data on videotape instead of or in addition to paper recorders.

TRANSDUCER POSITIONS: 2-D ECHO TERMINOLOGY AND IMAGE DISPLAY. The American Society of Echocardiography has attempted to standardize the nomenclature for transducer locations and two-dimensional echocardiographic imaging planes [9]. All views can be categorized into three orthogonal planes (Fig. 1-2). These planes are the long axis, short axis, and four-chamber views. The long axis

6   1. Normal cross-sectional anatomy

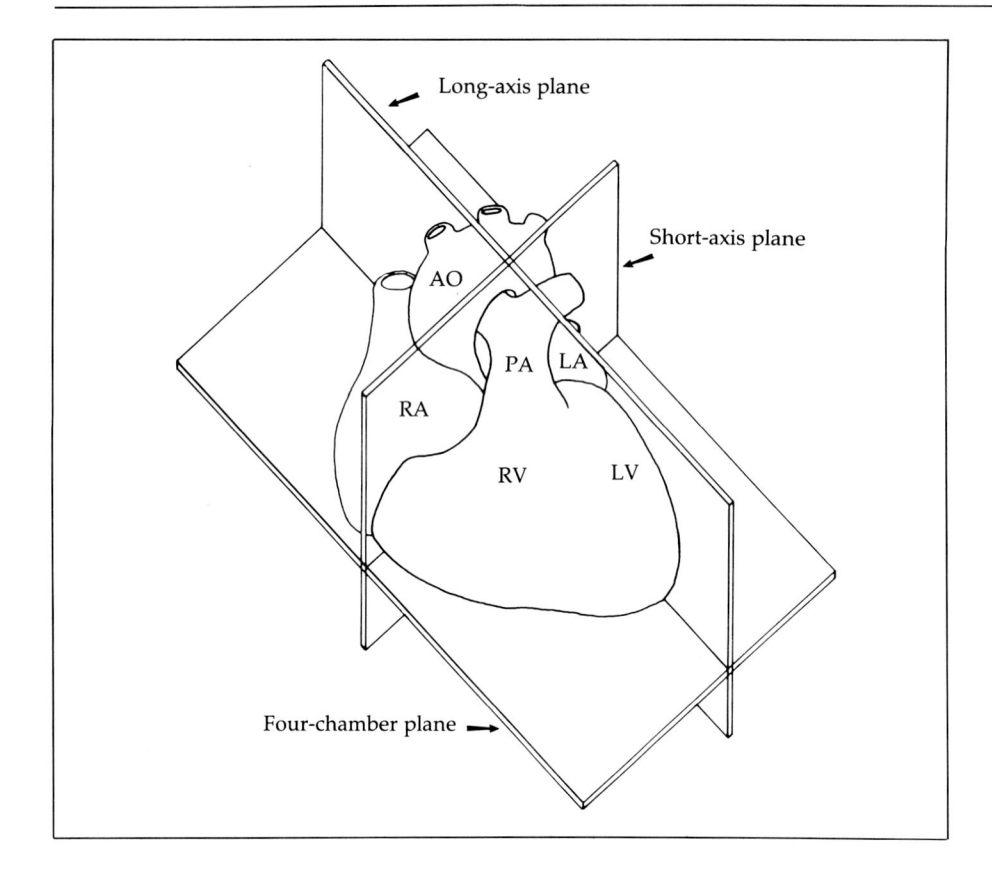

Fig. 1-2. All 2-D echo-imaging planes of the heart are adapted from three fundamental tomographic planes; the long axis, short axis, and 4-chamber planes. The long axis and short axis planes are oriented in reference to the left ventricle. PA = pulmonary artery.

plane is the tomographic plane that transects the heart parallel to the long axis in the left ventricle. The short axis plane is obtained by rotating the sector 90 degrees and transecting the heart perpendicular to the plane of the long axis. When the beam is directed *superiorly* toward the base of the heart, it is designated "short axis at the base"; when angled *inferiorly* toward the left ventricle, the heart is transected in short axis tomographic planes from the atrioventricular sulcus to the left ventricular apex. The plane that transects the heart approximately parallel to the dorsal and ventral surfaces of the body is referred to as the four-chamber plane. The four-chamber plane is obtained with the transducer position either over the apex of the left ventricle or in the subcostal position. The American Society of Echocardiography recognizes that modifications may be introduced and that the three orthogonal planes can vary according to the structures being examined. Furthermore they recommend that any examination within 45 degrees of a basic plane be identified with that plane. Thus there are multiple views within each examination plane.

Table 1-1 lists the various two-dimensional echocardiographic views categorized according to the location of the transducer, the tomographic plane of the sector beam, and the cardiac structures being viewed.

The Committee on Nomenclature and Standards in Two-Dimensional Echocardiography of the American Society of Echocardiography recommends the following terminology and image orientation: The transducer location should be identified and precede identification of the imaging planes. The three orthogonal planes

Table 1-1. Transducer positions and 19 standard two-dimensional echocardiographic views

Parasternal/precordial position
    Long axis plane
        Left ventricular long axis
        Right ventricular inflow (right ventricular/right atrial)
        Right ventricular outflow (sub-pulmonic)
    Short axis plane
        Short axis at the base
        Short axis at the base directed toward the pulmonary artery
        Left ventricular short axis at the mitral valve
        Left ventricular short axis at the chordae tendineae
        Left ventricular short axis at the papillary muscles
        Left ventricular short axis at the apex
Apical position
    4-Chamber plane
        4-Chamber without aortic valve
        4-Chamber with aortic valve
    Long axis plane
        Apical long axis with aortic valve and aorta
        Apical long axis view without aortic valve
Subcostal position
    4-Chamber plane
        4-Chamber directed toward ventricles
        4-Chamber directed toward atria and interatrial septum
        Inferior vena cava and right atrium
    Short axis plane
        Left ventricular short axis and right ventricular outflow tract
Suprasternal notch position
    Long axis of the aorta
    Short axis of the aorta

employed for tomographic imaging by two-dimensional echocardiography are not based strictly on the sagittal, transverse, and coronal planes commonly employed by the anatomist to describe body orientation but rather on the manner in which the two-dimensional echocardiographic imaging planes transect the heart. These imaging planes are illustrated in Figure 1-3. The imaging plane that transects the heart perpendicular to the dorsal and ventral surfaces of the body and parallel to the long axis of the heart is referred to as the long axis plane. The plane that transects the heart perpendicular to the dorsal and ventral surfaces of the body but perpendicular to the long axis of the heart will be referred to as the short axis plane. The plane that transects the heart approximately parallel to the dorsal and ventral surfaces of the body will be referred to as the four-chamber plane. For example, if the transducer is positioned in the left parasternal region and oriented so that the imaging plane transects the heart parallel to the long axis of the left ventricle, the Committee recommends that the resulting image be referred to as a parasternal long axis view. Accordingly if the transducer is placed in the apical location and oriented to view the four-chamber imaging plane, the Committee recommends that the resultant image be referred to as the apical four-chamber view. The Committee also attempted to adopt standards that are compatible with image orientation most commonly used by clinicians. In addition the group attempted to develop image orientation standards that result from transducer orientations that are consistent from one view to the next and therefore can be easily taught and explained to both the experienced and inexperienced user of two-dimensional imaging equipment. It

8   1. Normal cross-sectional anatomy

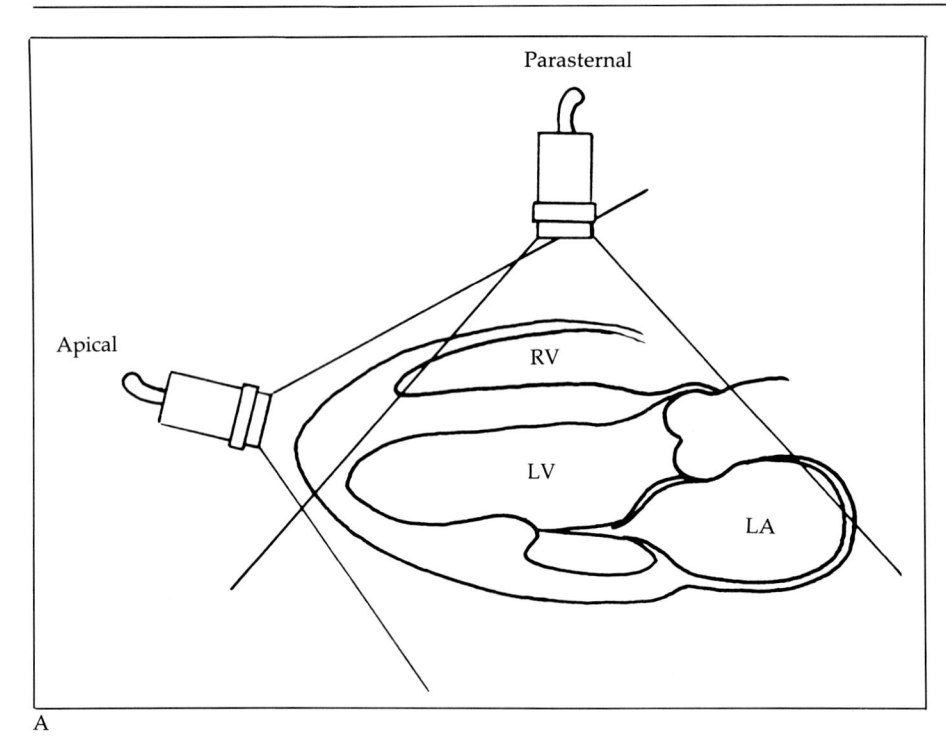

Fig. 1-3A. Long axis view of the left ventrical can be obtained from either parasternal or apical transducer positions. B. Short axis views of the left ventricle can be obtained from either parasternal or subcostal transducer positions. C. Four-chamber views of the heart can be obtained from either apical or subcostal transducer positions. The apex of the left ventricle is usually deleted from view in the subcostal 4-chamber plane.

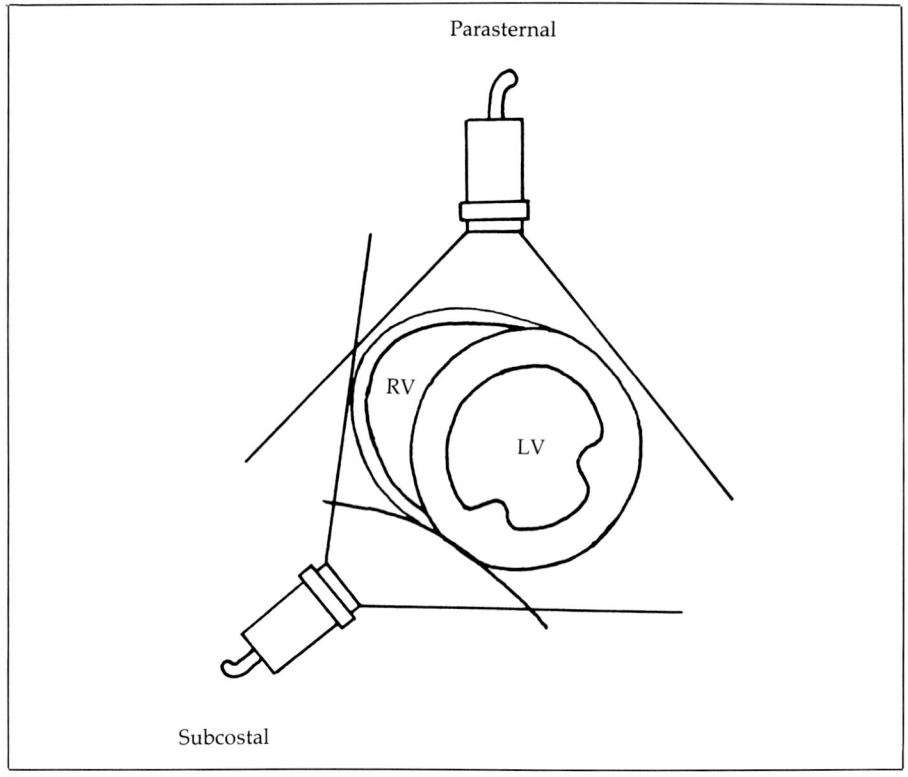

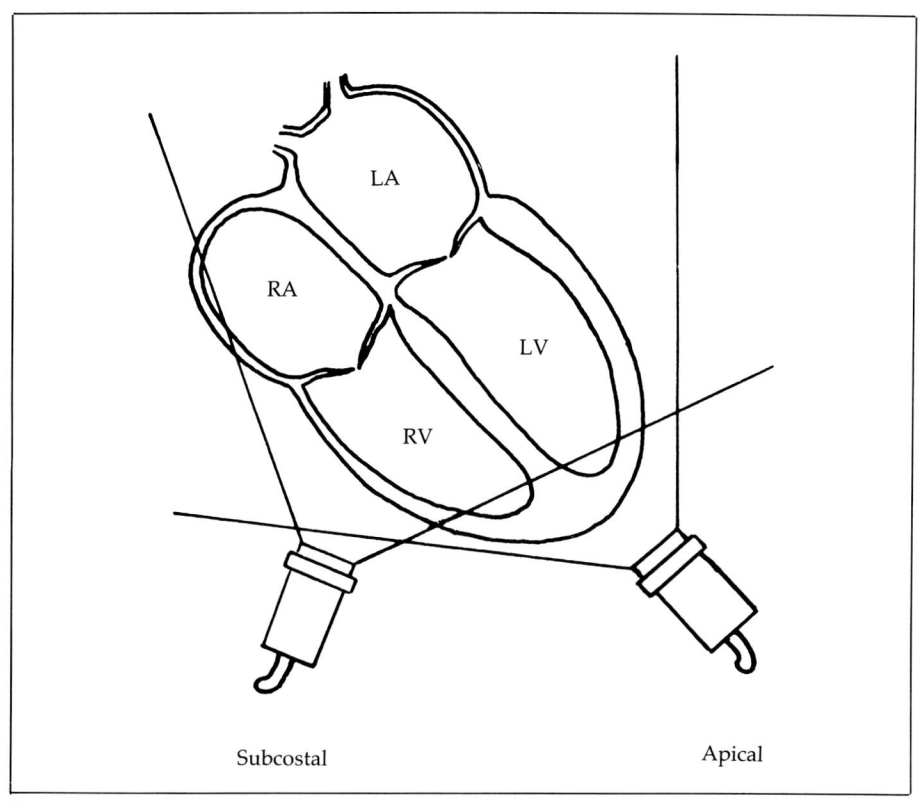

Subcostal   Apical

C

is recommended that an index mark be placed on every 2-D echo transducer. This index mark should be placed on the side of the transducer to indicate the edge of the imaging plane to keep the operator oriented in the direction in which the ultrasound beam is being angled. The index mark should be located on the transducer to indicate the part of the image plane that will appear on the right side of the image display. For example, if the index mark is pointed in the direction of the aorta in a parasternal long axis view, the aorta should appear on the right side of the image display. In viewing the images on the screen, the signals returning from the structures located near the surface of the transducer will appear on the top of the image display. Conversely the ultrasound signals returning from structures located far from the transducer will appear at the bottom of the image display. Some of the equipment is provided with an image inversion switch that enables the operator to reverse the image and show the structures near the surface close to the transducer appearing at the bottom of the image and the more distant structures appearing at the top of the image display. To orient the transducer during the performance of a study, the Committee recommended that the transducer index mark always be pointed either in the direction of the patient's head or to the left side of the patient.

PARASTERNAL TRANSDUCER POSITION. The parasternal left ventricular long axis view demonstrates the aortic valve to the right of the sector image and the apex to the left of the sector (Fig. 1-4). In this view a portion of the right ventricular outflow tract appears anteriorly at the top of the image display and the posterior wall of the left ventricle and left atrium appear at the bottom of the image. The base of the heart, which is superior, is to the right of the image; the apex of the left ventricle, which is inferior, is to the left of the image. The terminology of "base" and "apex" are synonymous with "superior" and "inferior" respectively throughout the book.

The parasternal right ventricular inflow view is obtained by orienting the sector beam through the right atrium, tricuspid valve, and inflow tract of the right ventricle (Fig. 1-5A, B, C). This view is obtained from the same parasternal interspace employed to image the left ventricular long axis; however, the transducer is rotated slightly counterclockwise, and the beam is angled in the plane of the right atrium and the inflow tract of the right ventricle. If the transducer is positioned lower along the left sternal border with the sector oriented through the right ventricular inflow tract the resultant view is a precordial four-chamber (Fig. 1-5D).

The parasternal right ventricular outflow (subpulmonic) view is obtained by rotating the sector beam clockwise from the left ventricular long axis orientation and pointing the beam in a superior leftward direction toward the pulmonic valve (Fig. 1-6). The tomographic plane of the sector beam is oriented in the long axis of the right ventricular outflow tract and main pulmonary artery. A portion of the ventricular septum and anterior mitral leaflet are imaged; however the aortic valve is not seen since the tomographic plane passes slightly to the left of it.

The parasternal short axis views are obtained by rotating the transducer 90 degrees clockwise from the long axis plane of the left ventricle. We routinely attempt to record a minimum of six short axis views from the cardiac base to the left ventricular apex (Fig. 1-7). Usually these views are recorded by varying the angulation of the sector beam superiorly toward the base (Fig. 1-8) and inferiorly toward the apex. However, to image the pulmonary artery, including the bifurcation of the right and left pulmonary arteries, requires leftward angulation of the sector beam

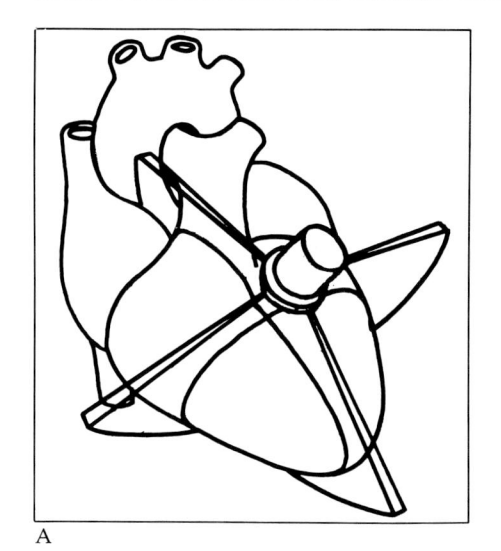

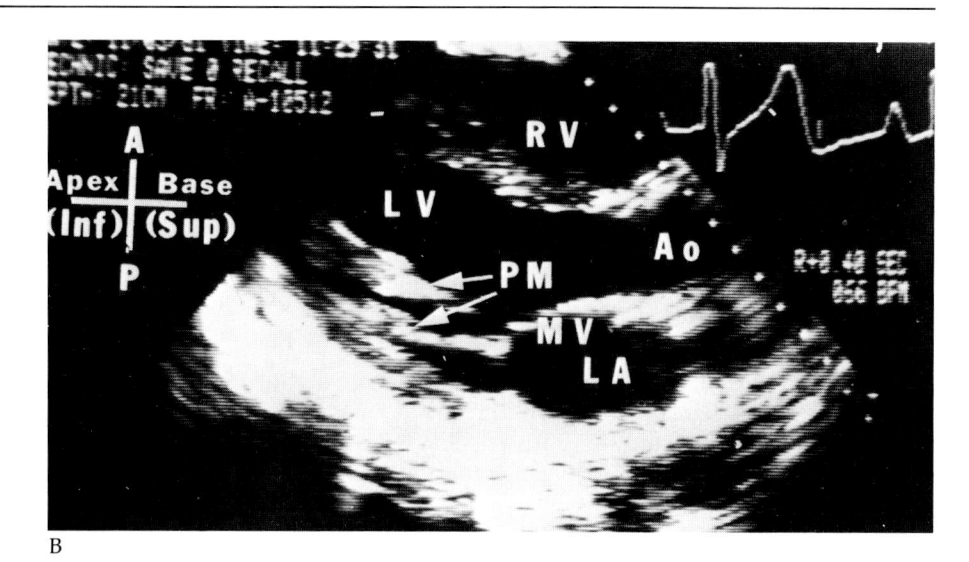

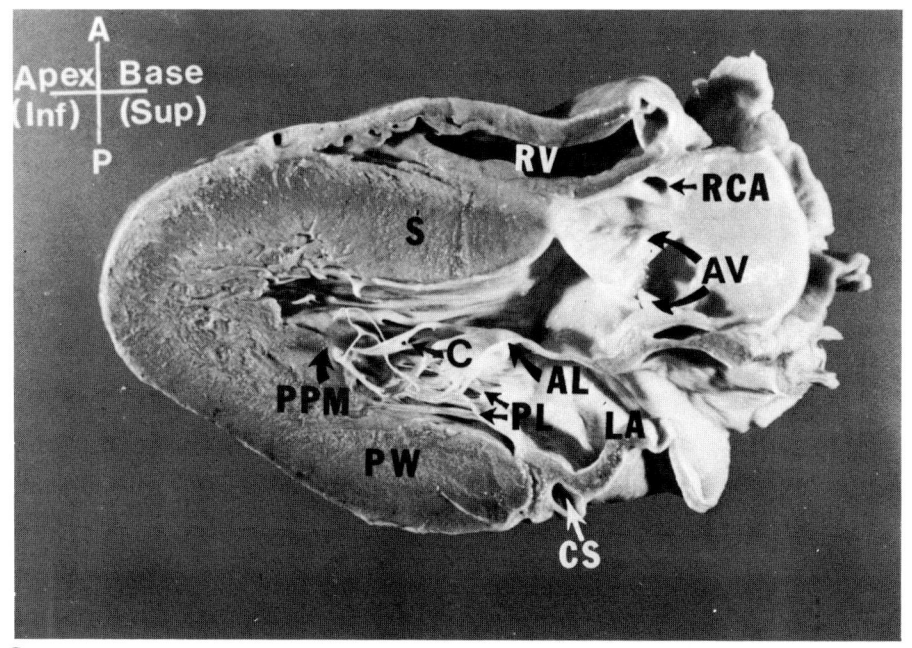

Fig. 1-4A. Diagram showing the orientation of the sector beam and transducer position for both parasternal long axis and short axis planes. B. Parasternal long axis image. Apex of the left ventricle is usually not seen in this view. The calibration scale to the right of the sector image shows dots 1 cm apart. C. View of normal parasternal long axis anatomy. AV = aortic valve leaflets; C = chordae tendineae; PM = posterior medial papillary muscle; PPM = posterior medial papillary muscle; RCA = orifice of right coronary artery.

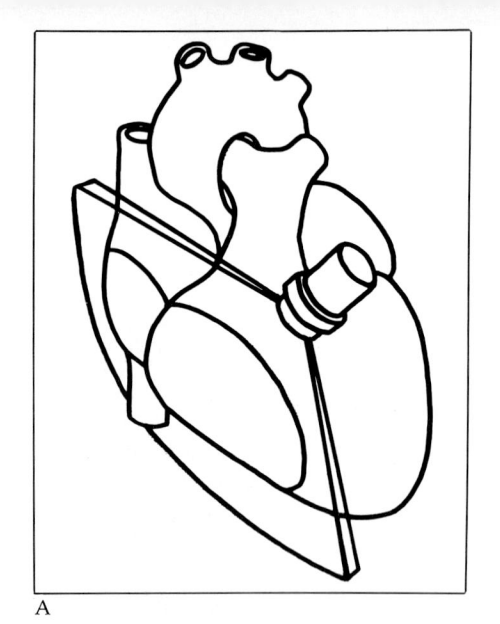

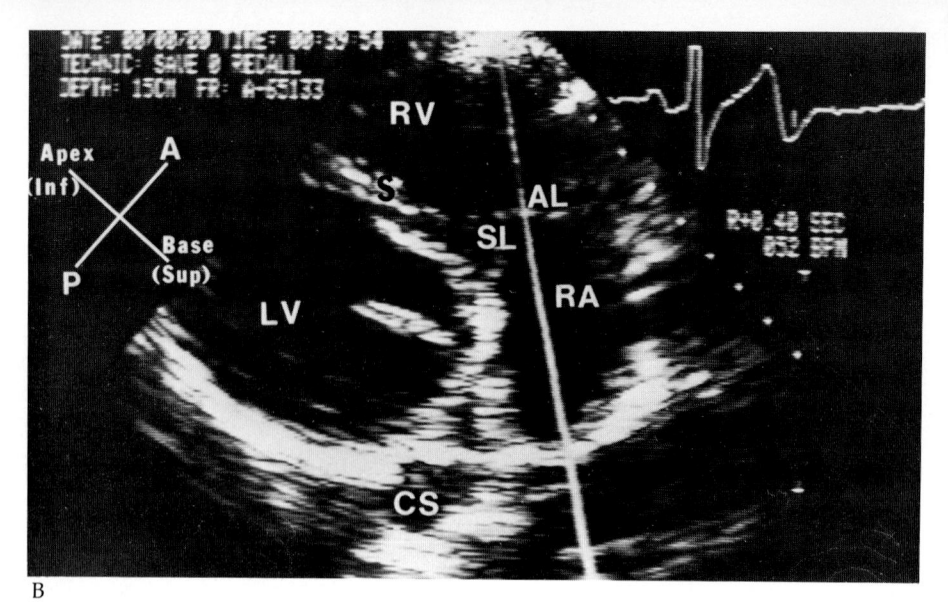

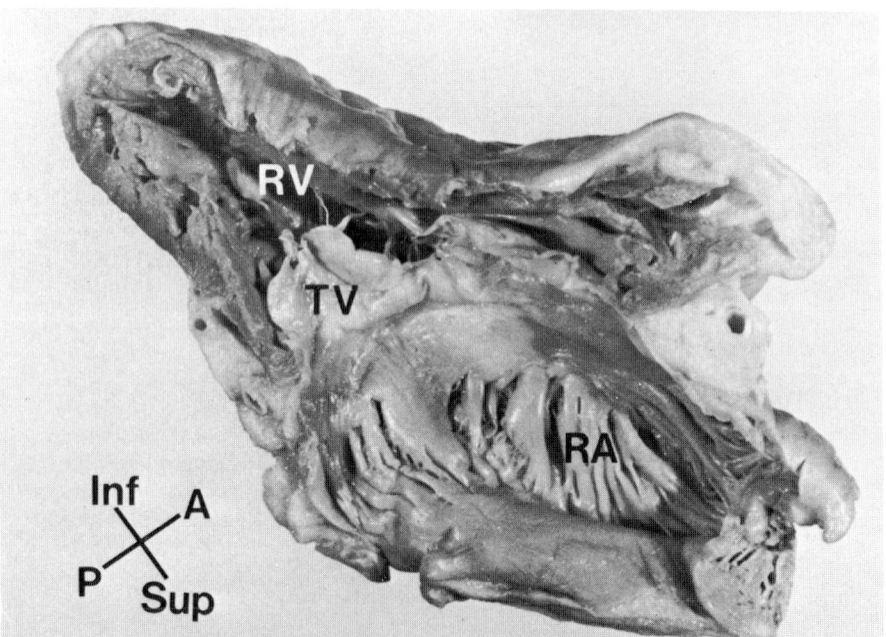

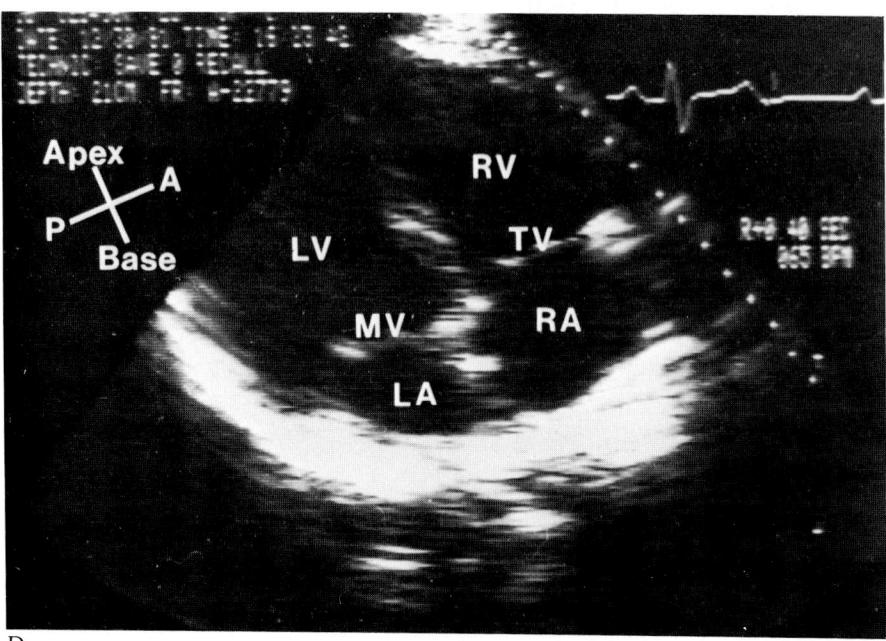

Fig. 1-5A. Diagram showing the orientation of the sector beam and transducer position for the parasternal right ventricular inflow plane. B. Parasternal right ventricular inflow plane. The M-mode cursor is shown intersecting the right ventricle, anterior tricuspid leaflet, and right atrium. C. Anatomic slice showing normal right ventricular inflow anatomy corresponds to tomographic plane in B. D. Precordial 4-chamber or right ventricular inflow image obtained with the transducer in a low left sternal position. AL = anterior tricuspid leaflet.

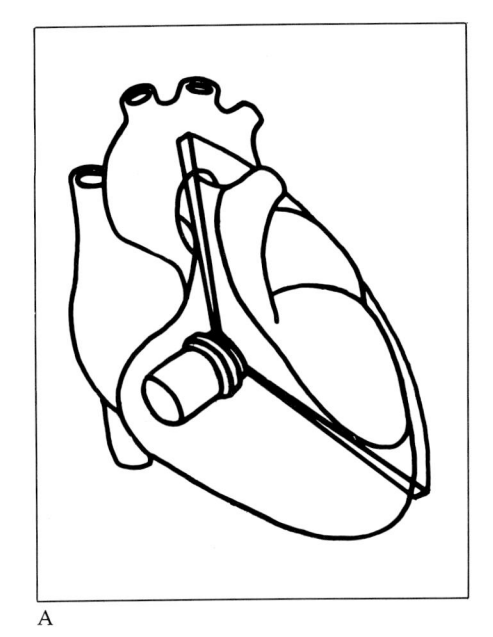

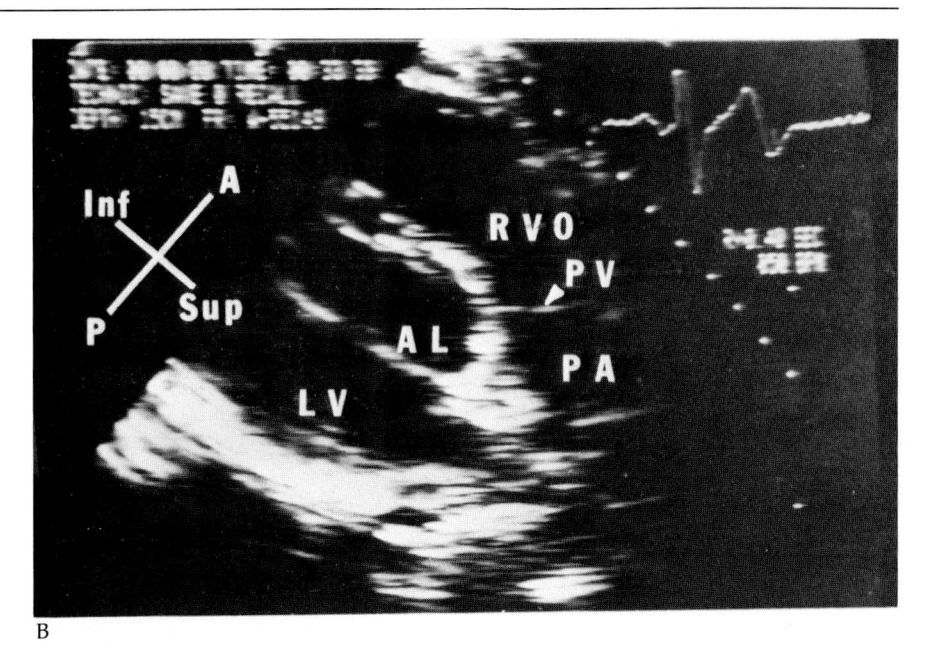

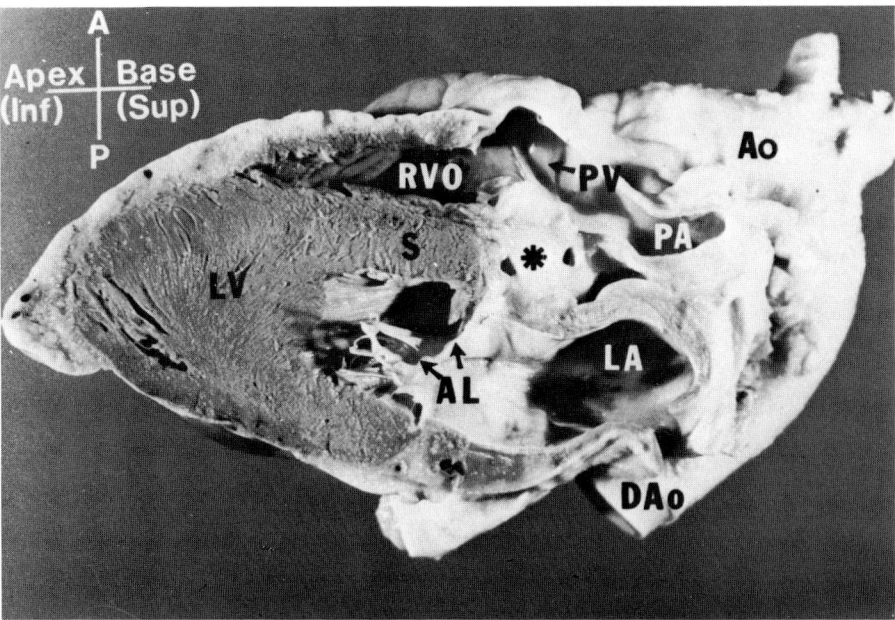

Fig. 1-6A. Diagram showing the orientation of the sector beam and transducer position for the parasternal right ventricular outflow plane. B. Parasternal right ventricular outflow image. C. Normal parasternal right ventricular outflow anatomy in a plane through the supracristal portion of the system below the pulmonic valve. The asterisk marks the location of the aortic valve, which is to the right of the plane of this tomographic slice. PV = pulmonic valve.

14   1. Normal cross-sectional anatomy

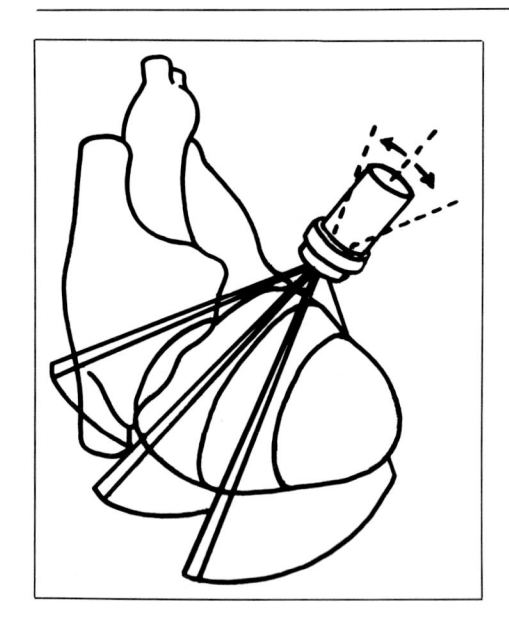

Fig. 1-7. Diagram showing the orientation of multiple short axis planes obtained by angling the transducer from the same parasternal position. The transducer may have to be moved superiorly and inferiorly along the left sternal border to obtain all six short axis views.

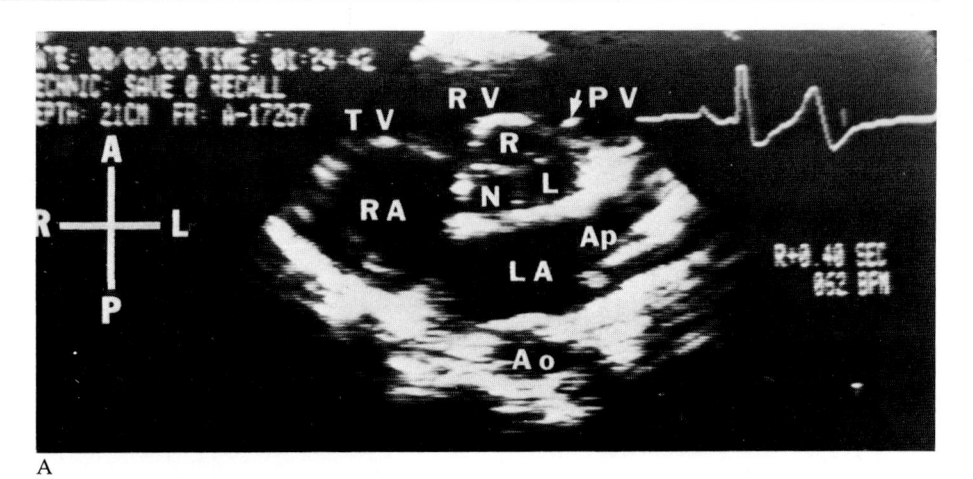

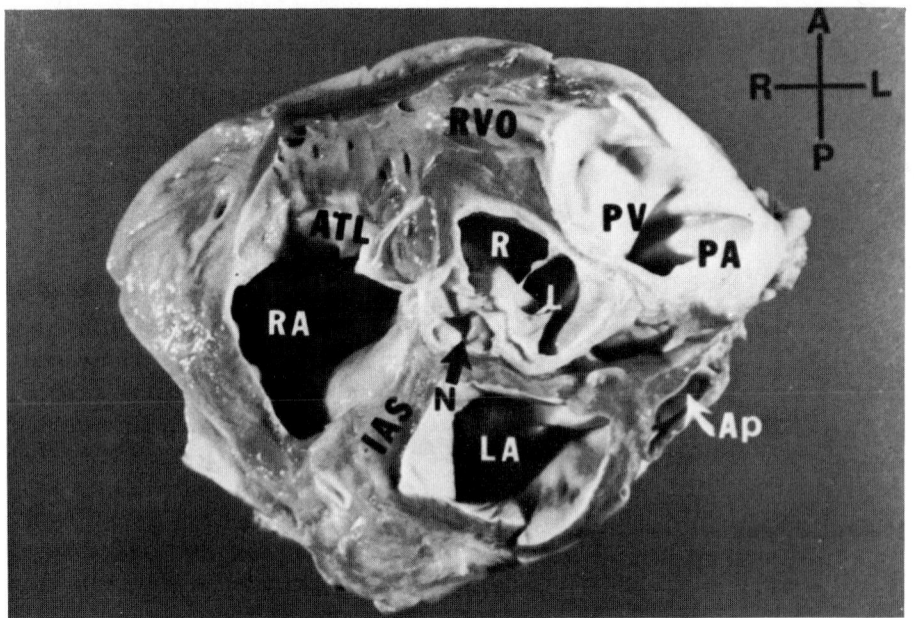

Fig. 1-8A. Parasternal short axis image at the base. B. View of normal parasternal short axis at the base anatomy. Most of the pulmonary artery is not seen in this tomographic plane. Notice the position of the appendage to aorta and pulmonary artery and the corresponding image in A. Ao = descending aorta; ATL = anterior tricuspid leaflet; IAS = interatrial septum; L = left cusp of aortic valve; PA = proximal portion of main pulmonary artery; PV = pulmonic valve; R = right cusp of aortic valve.

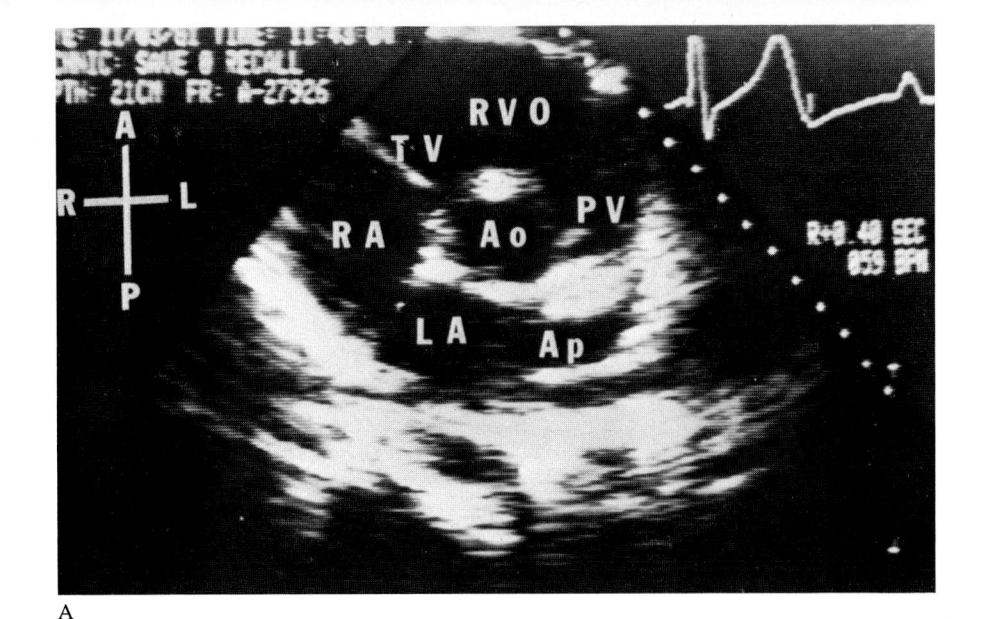

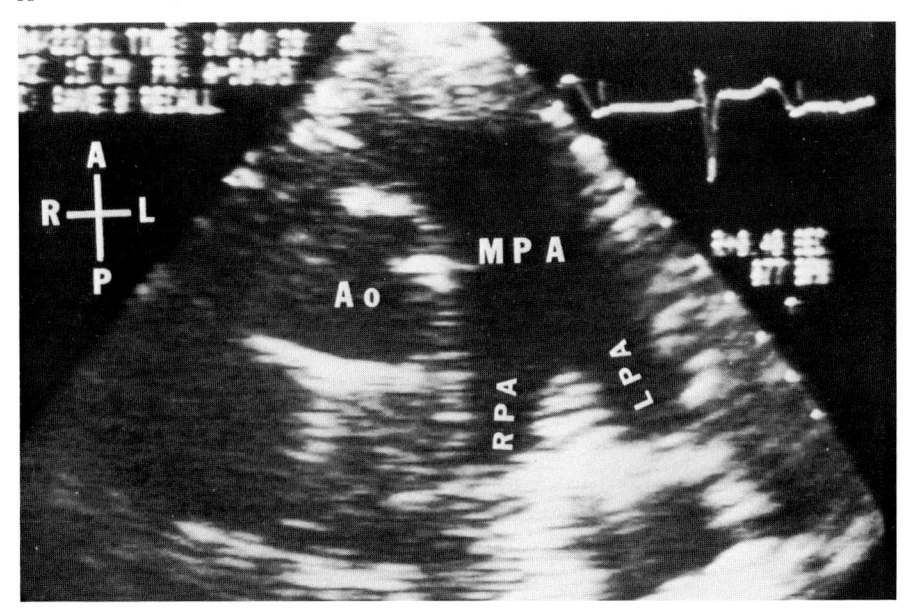

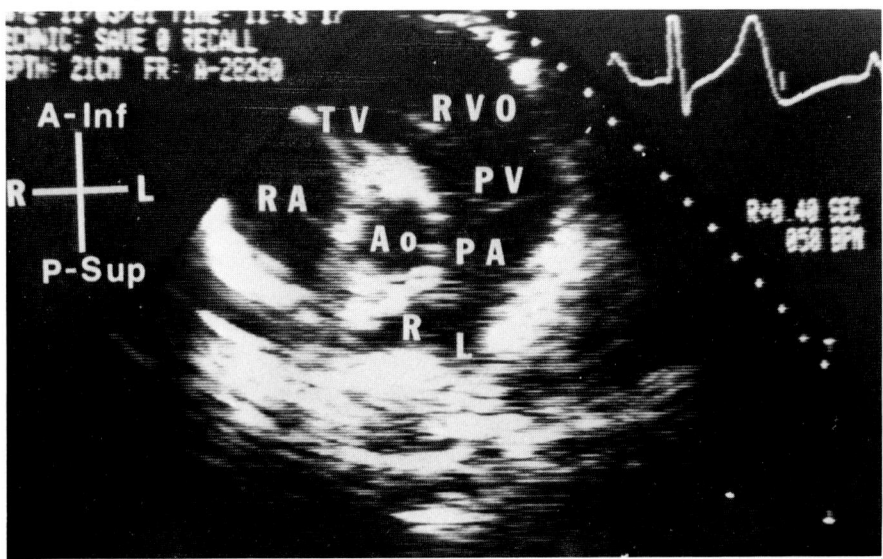

Fig. 1-9A. Parasternal short axis view at the base with minimal lateral (leftward) angulation as evidenced by the deletion of a small portion of the right ventricular inflow tract. The sector beam now includes the lateral wall of the pulmonary artery. B. Parasternal short axis view at the base with significant leftward angulation to identify more of the pulmonary artery, including the bifurcation of right and left pulmonary arteries. This angulation usually deletes the tricuspid valve and most of the right atrium from view and intersects the ascending aorta superiorly to the plane of the aortic valve leaflets. Part of the left atrium is visible but not labelled. C. Parasternal short axis view at the base with the transducer positioned low and more laterally over the precordium. This tomographic plane affords an excellent view of the right ventricular outflow tract (RVO), pulmonic valve (PV), main pulmonary artery, and bifurcation of right (RPA) and left (LPA) pulmonary arteries. Since the sector beam is angled so far superiorly through the ascending aorta (Ao), most of the left atrium is deleted from view. A portion of the tricuspid valve and right atrium are also seen.

16   1. Normal cross-sectional anatomy

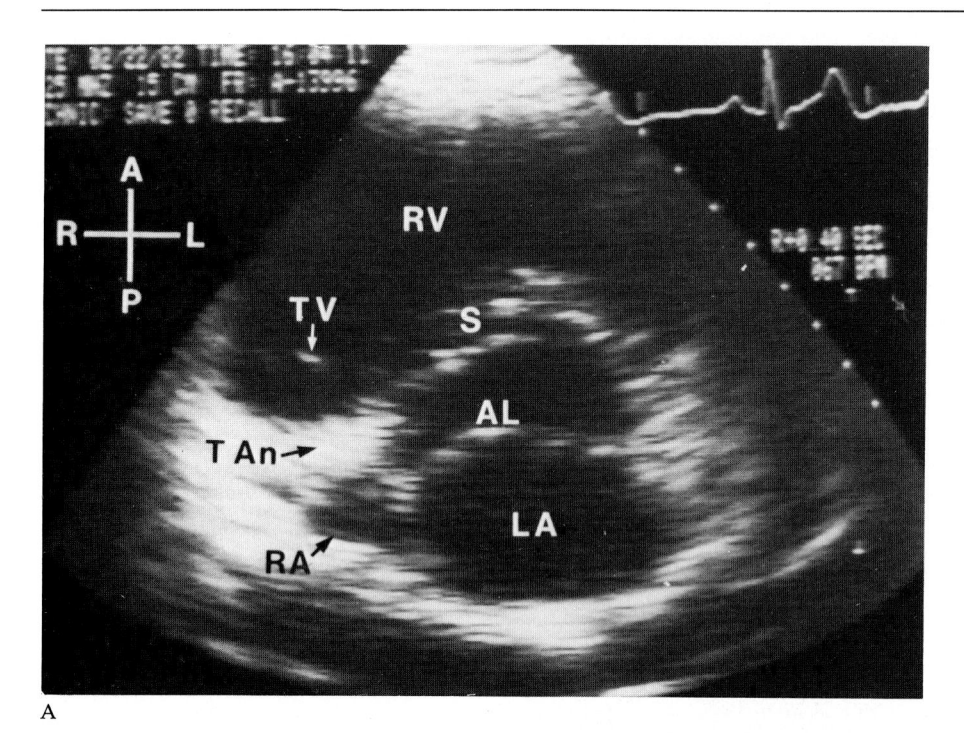

Fig. 1-10A. Parasternal short axis view through the atrioventricular sulcus (groove). B. Normal parasternal short axis anatomy through the atrioventricular sulcus (groove). The left atrial appendage is considerably behind (superior to) the plane of the cut. ATL = anterior tricuspid leaflet.

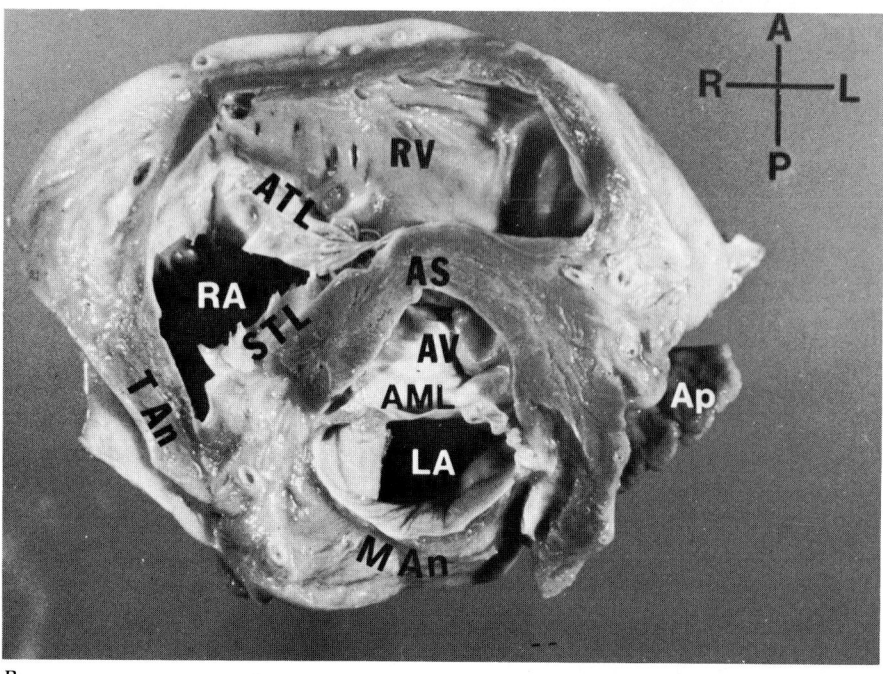

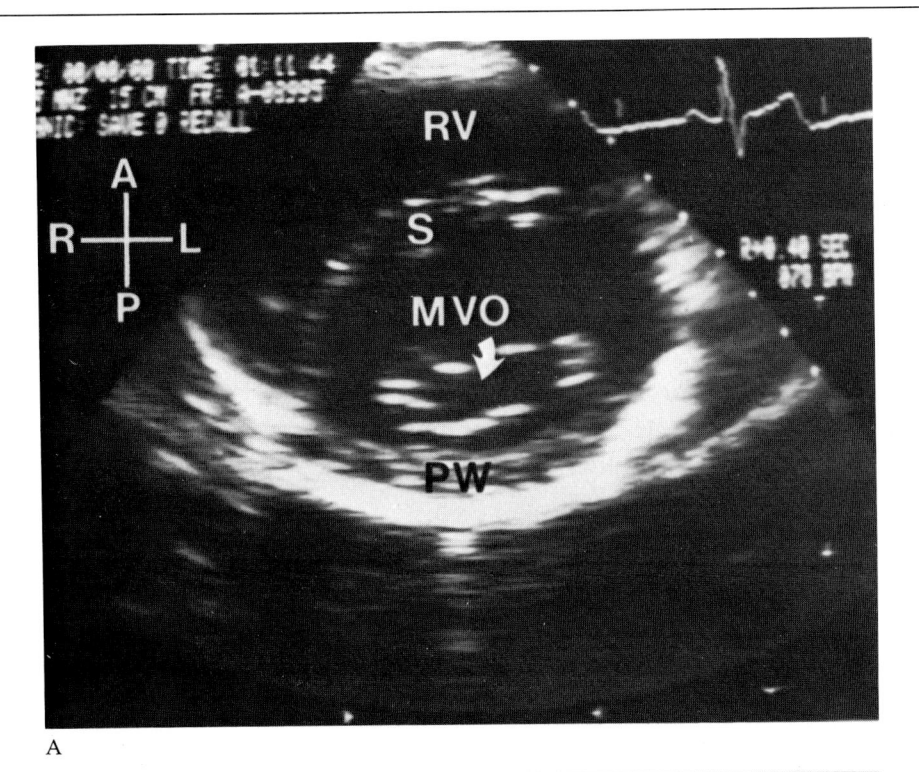

Fig. 1-11A. Parasternal short axis image through the orifice of a normal mitral valve shows the right ventricle, anterior and posterior portions of the interventricular septum, and posterior wall of the left ventricle. Although not labelled, all the parasternal short axis views of the left ventricle demonstrate the lateral wall very well. B. Corresponding normal anatomic short axis slice. Although the three tricuspid leaflets are labelled (ATL = anterior, PTL = posterior, STL = septal), they are situated superiorly to the plane of the cut and in normal subjects are not imaged in this 2-D echo tomographic plane. Other structures corresponding to the echo images include the right ventricle, anterior portion of interventricular septum, posterior portion of interventricular septum, anterior mitral leaflet, left ventricular outflow tract between AS and AML (asterisk), and posterior mitral leaflet. The left atrial appendage can be seen behind (superior to) the plane of the cut.

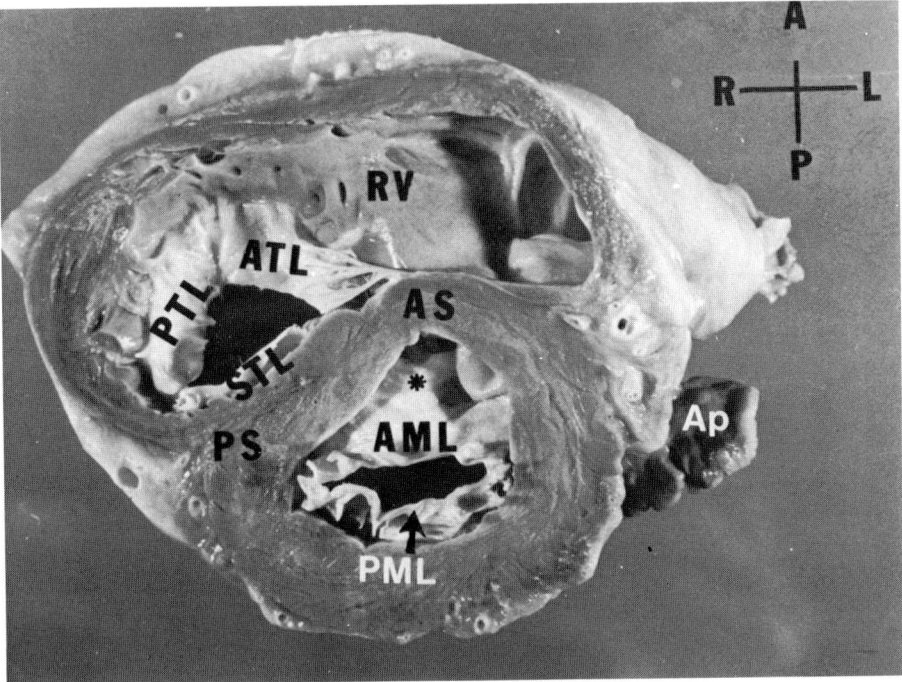

18   1. Normal cross-sectional anatomy

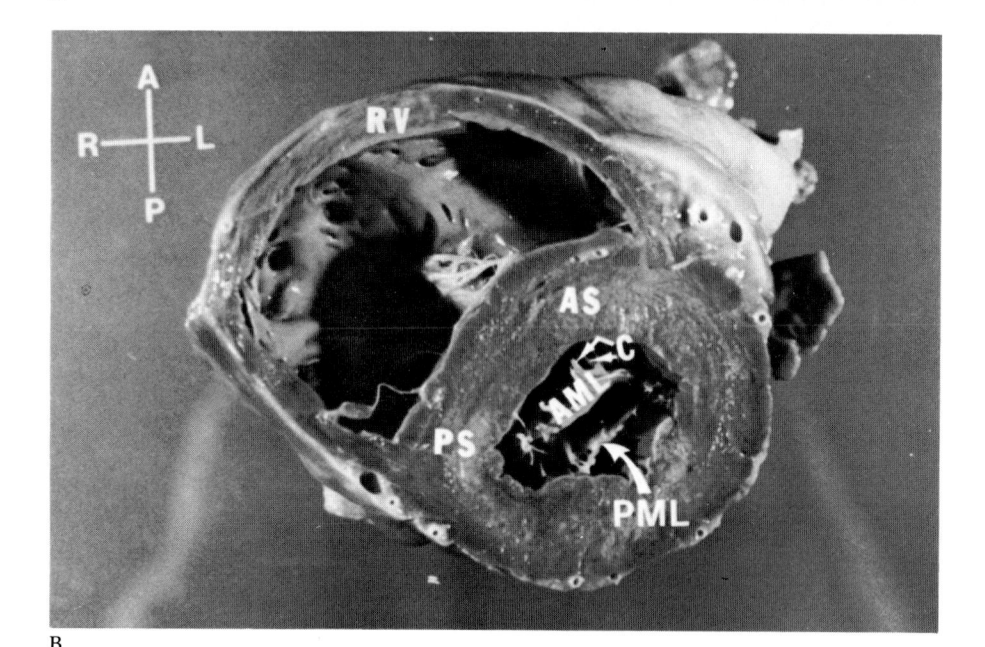

Fig. 1-12A. Parasternal short axis view at the level of the chordae tendineae. Structures identified in this 2-D echo plane include the right ventricle, interventricular septum, chordae tendineae (C), lateral and posterior walls of the left ventricle. The endocardium can be easily seen and the epicardial surface is also well appreciated in real-time motion adjacent to the strong reflectance from the pericardium. B. Parasternal short axis section at the level of the chordae tendineae in a normal heart showing anatomy corresponding to the structures in A. Although the anterior and posterior mitral leaflets are seen, they are behind (superior to) the plane of the cut. RV = anterior wall of the right ventricle.

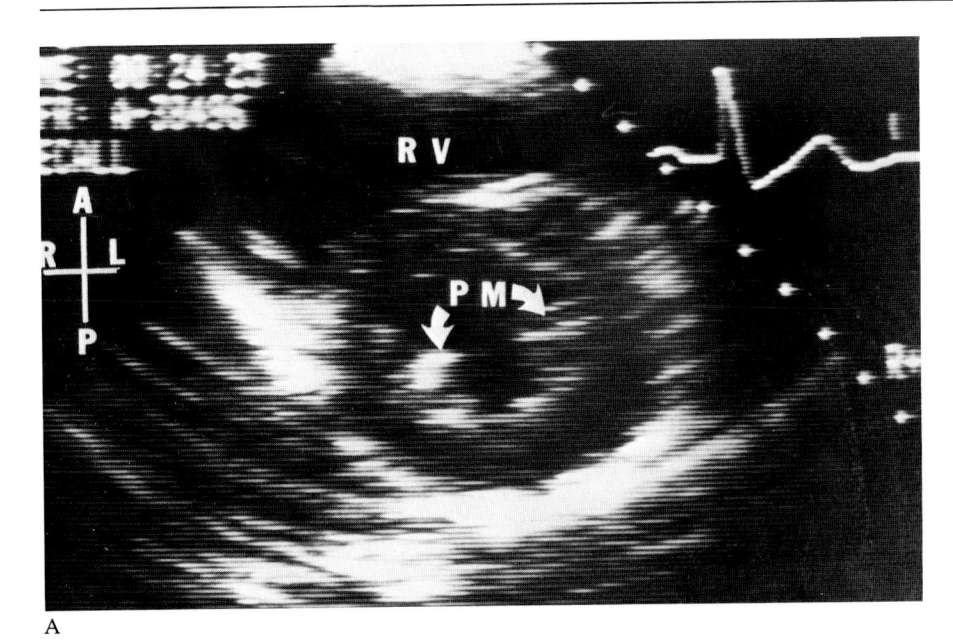

Fig. 1-13A. Parasternal short axis view at the tips of the papillary muscles. Note that the right ventricle is smaller than in the view in Figure 1-12A. B. Parasternal short axis section of a normal heart at the tips of the anterolateral (LPM) and posteromedial (PPM) papillary muscles corresponding to the image in A. Note the prominent trabeculations in the right ventricle; a portion of a papillary muscle and the moderator band are also present.

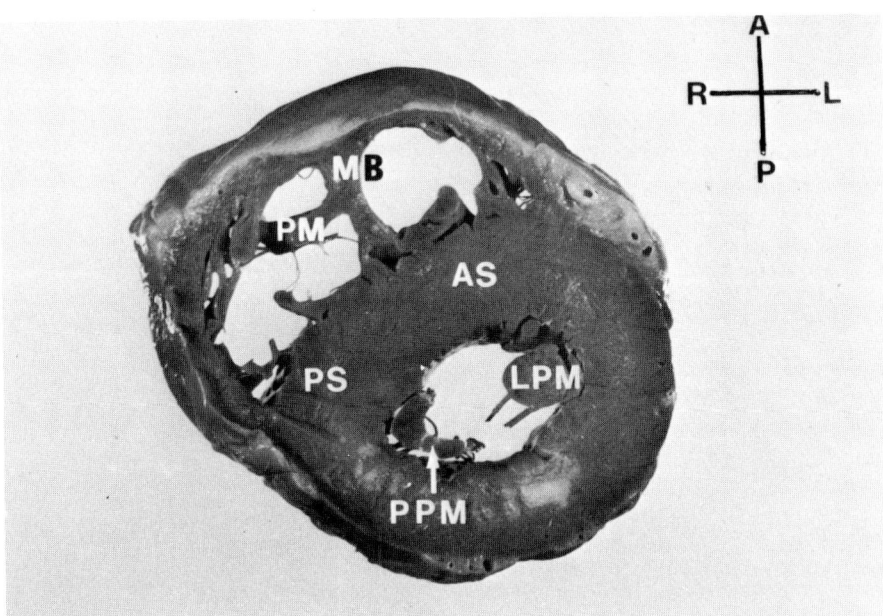

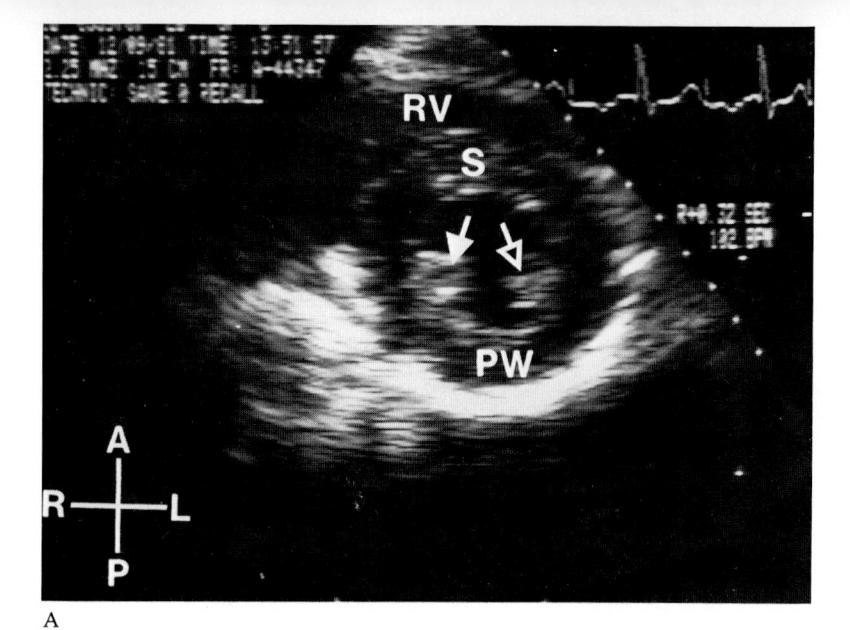

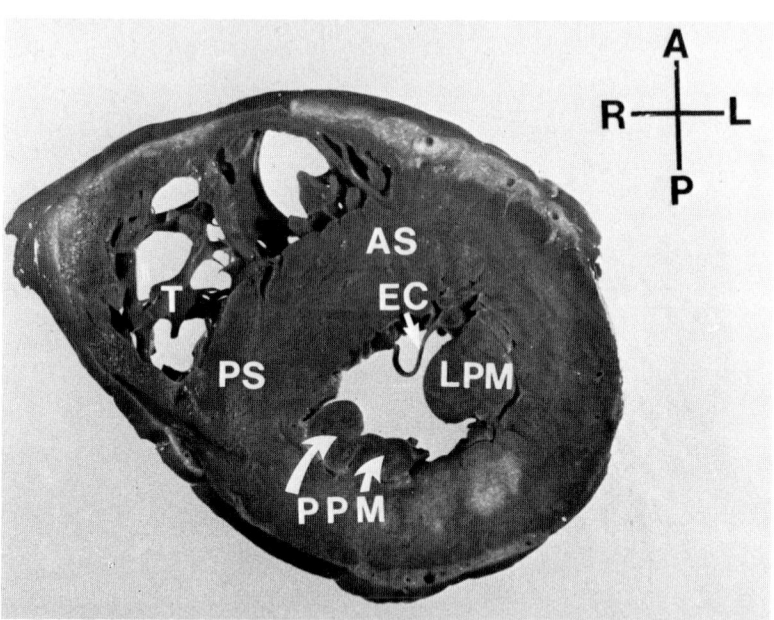

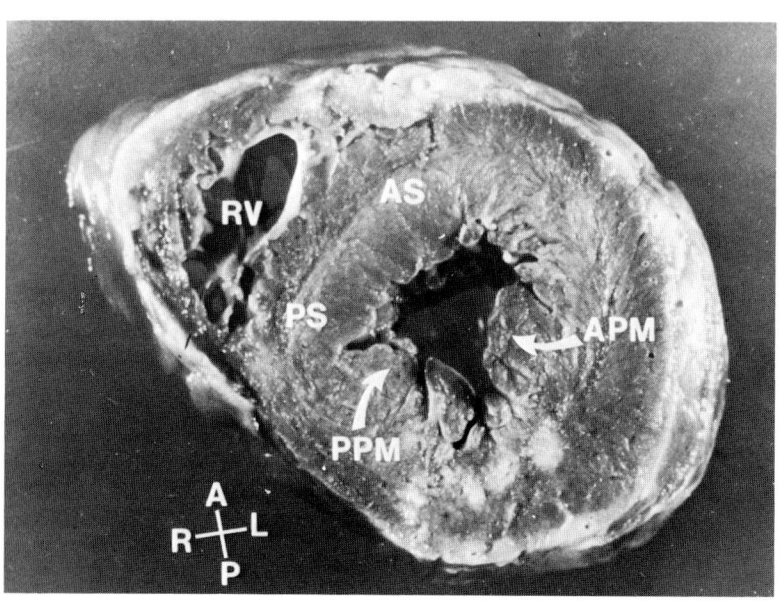

Fig. 1-14A. Parasternal short axis view through the midportions of the papillary muscles, posteromedial (solid arrow) and anterolateral (open arrow). The cavity of the right ventricle is quite small at this level. B. Parasternal short axis section of normal cardiac anatomy at the level of midpapillary muscles. Often the papillary muscles are normally asymmetric with one larger than the other or with dual or multiple heads. Note the small right ventricular cavity and heavy trabeculations (T). Ectopic chordae (EC) or muscle bridging is frequently seen in normal left ventricles. C. This anatomic section is close to the base (origin) of the papillary muscles. Note that the cavity sizes of both right ventricle and left ventricle are quite small. The circumference of the left ventricle is smaller than at the level of the mitral valve. It is difficult to distinguish separate anterior and posterior portions of the interventricular septum since the right ventricle is so small and the length of the septum is quite short at this level. APM = anterolateral papillary muscle; LPM = anterolateral papillary muscle; PPM = posteromedial papillary muscle.

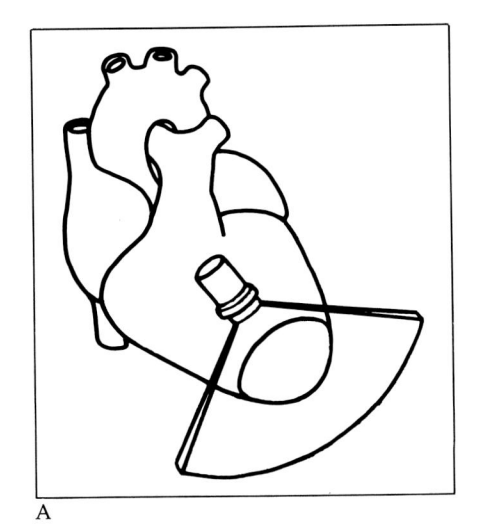

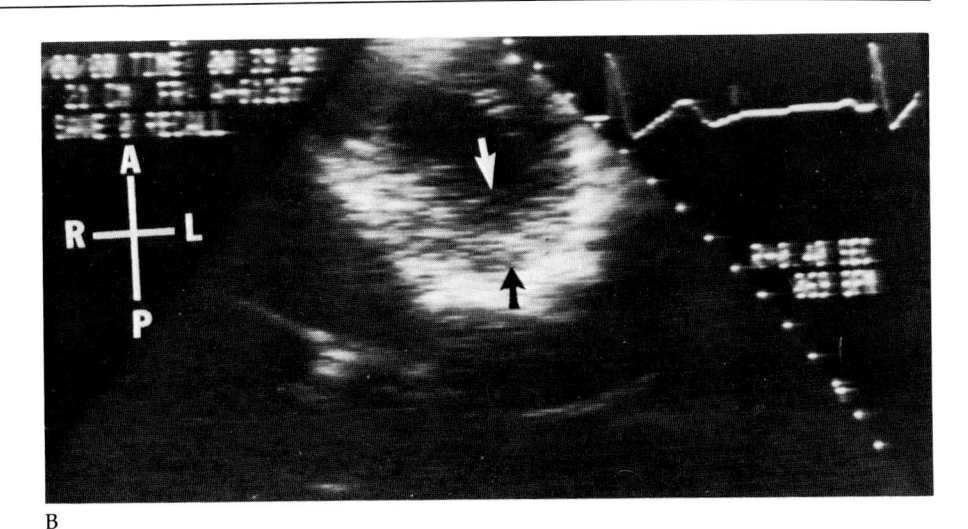

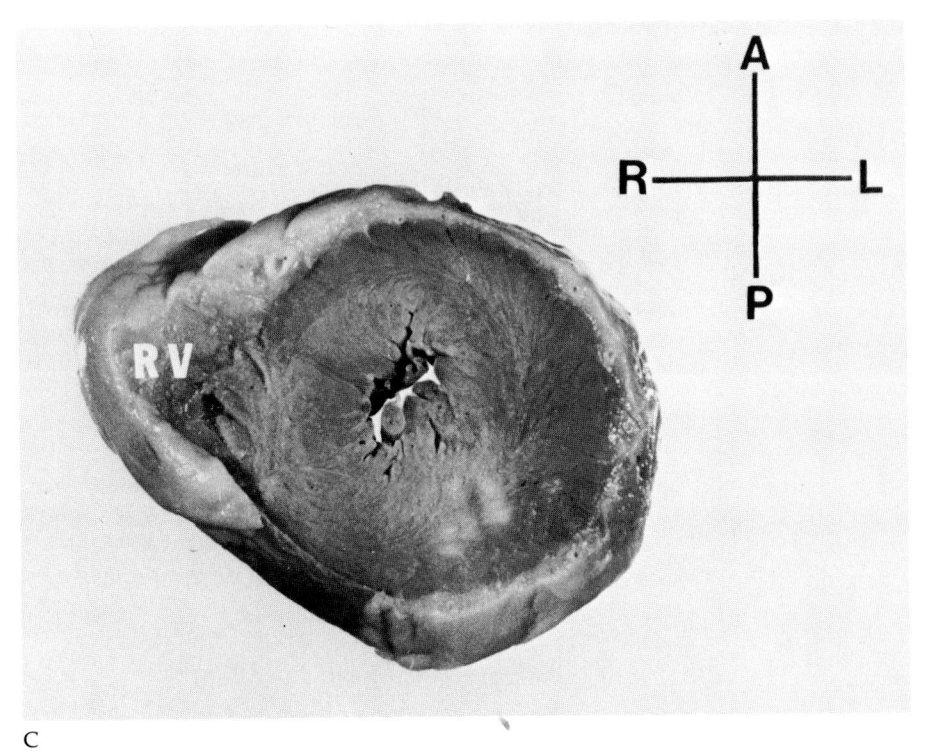

Fig. 1-15A. Diagram showing the sector beam in an apical short axis orientation with the transducer positioned on the left precordium directly anterior to the left ventricular apex. B. Left precordial apical short axis view showing very small left ventricular cavity and thick-appearing, oblique tomographic plane of left ventricular posterior wall (arrows). No right ventricle is present in this view. C. Short axis anatomic section through a normal left ventricular apex at a level distal to the right ventricle and corresponding to the 2-D echo view in B.

(Fig. 1-9). Although these multiple short axis views can often be recorded from the same parasternal interspace (Figs. 1-10 through 1-15), it is frequently necessary to move the transducer into different locations over the left precordium to obtain all the short axis images (see Figs. 1-9C and 1-15). It should be noted that the short axis views of the heart depict the anatomy as seen by the echocardiographer close to the patient's left hip and looking up at the cross-section of the heart through the cardiac apex.

APICAL TRANSDUCER POSITION. The apical four-chamber plane is obtained by positioning the transducer directly over the left ventricular apical impulse and aiming the transducer toward the right shoulder (Fig. 1-16). This view is usually more easily obtained when the patient is positioned in steep left lateral decubitus with slight elevation of the head. If the heart is enlarged several recordings may be necessary for optimal imaging of all four chambers from this position. Depending upon the degree of anterior-posterior tilt of the transducer, the tomographic plane will include or exclude the aortic valve (Fig. 1-17). The right-left orientation of the cardiac chambers is the same as in the parasternal short axis images.

When the transducer is rotated 90 degrees counterclockwise from the apical four-chamber position, the plane of the beam is parallel to the ventricular septum and demonstrates the left ventricle and left atrium in an apical long axis view (Fig. 1-18). Slight angulation of the beam anteriorly will include the aortic valve and proximal portion of the ascending aorta (Fig. 1-19). Posterolateral angulation of the transducer to image an apical oblique view of the left ventricle may be clinically useful as a supplemental plane to the standard apical four- and two-chamber views (Fig. 1-20).

SUBCOSTAL TRANSDUCER POSITION. At least four different tomographic planes should be recorded subcostally. There are two important four-chamber views, one directed primarily toward the ventricles (Fig. 1-21) and the other view directed primarily toward both atria and the interatrial septum (Fig. 1-22). The other two subcostal views include the inferior vena cava with right atrium (Fig. 1-23) and left ventricular short-axis with right ventricular outflow tract and pulmonic valve (Fig. 1-24).

SUPRASTERNAL NOTCH TRANSDUCER POSITION. Tomographic imaging from this position is more difficult than from any of the other locations. Both views, long axis (Fig. 1-25) and short axis (Fig. 1-26) of the aorta are employed clinically to evaluate the ascending and descending aorta, pulmonary artery, and superior vena cava. Usually the cardiac chambers cannot be imaged adequately enough from this position to be of clinical value.

Two-dimensional echocardiographic imaging techniques. The position of the patient in bed is a key factor; it is recommended that the patient be positioned with the head slightly elevated, approximately 10 to 20 degrees, and positioned in left lateral decubitus. It is preferable to have the patient on a thick, firm, foam-rubber mattress approximately 8 inches thick with a "half-moon" cutout on the left side. The patient is then positioned so that the cardiac apex is directly over this cutout, which will enable apical imaging to be accomplished with greater

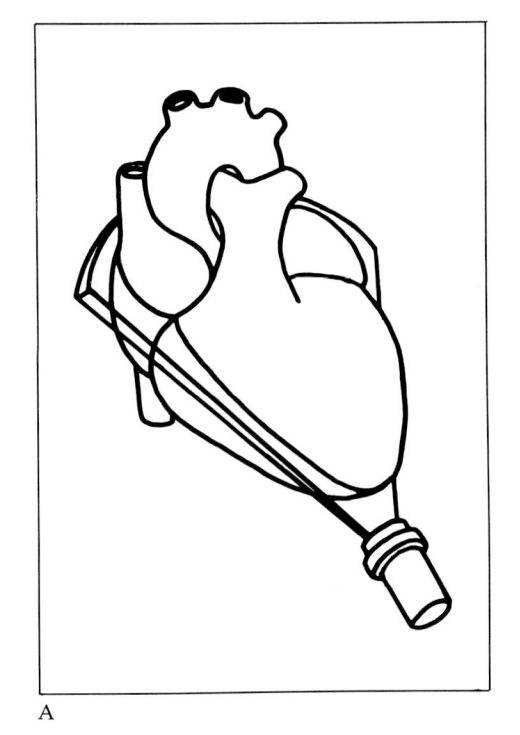

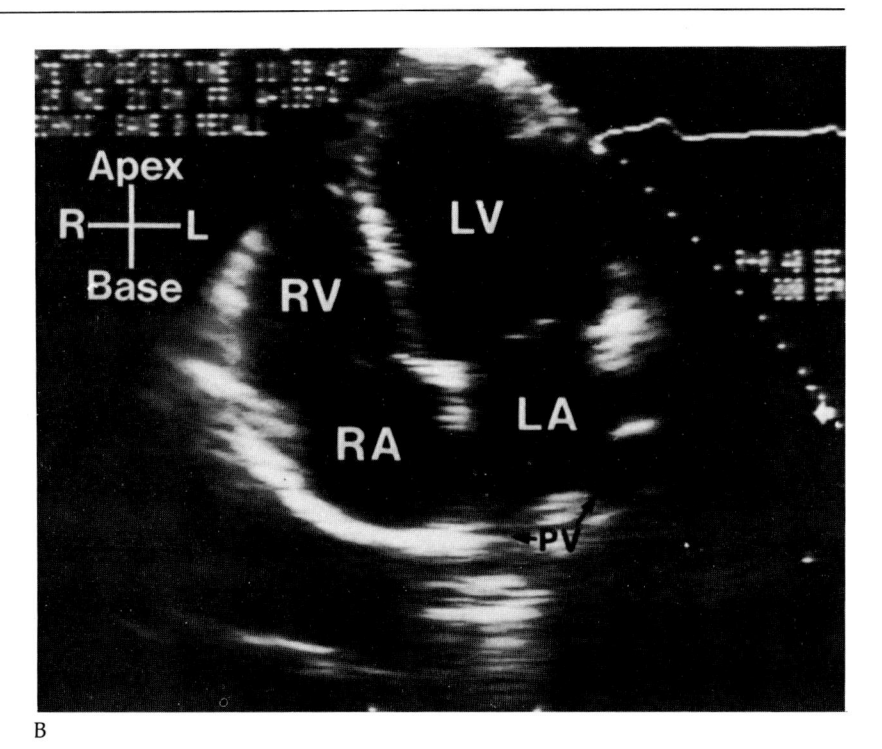

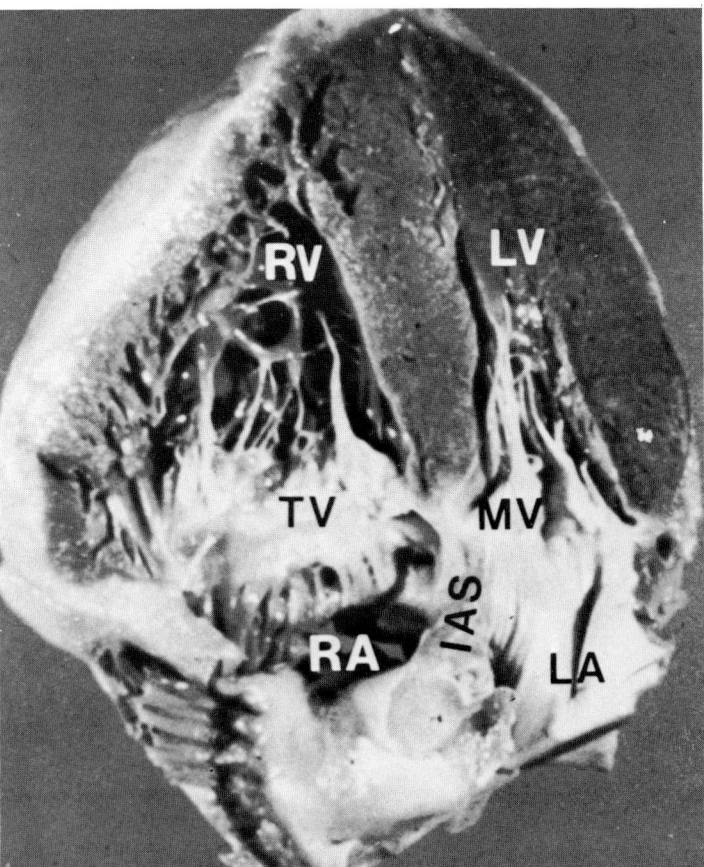

Fig. 1-16A. Diagram showing the sector beam in an apical 4-chamber orientation with the transducer positioned over the left ventricular apex. B. Apical 4-chamber view of a normal heart showing right ventricle, left ventricle, right atrium, left atrium, and pulmonary veins (PV). C. Anatomic section in apical 4-chamber view of a normal heart corresponding with structures shown in B. IAS = interatrial septum.

24   1. Normal cross-sectional anatomy

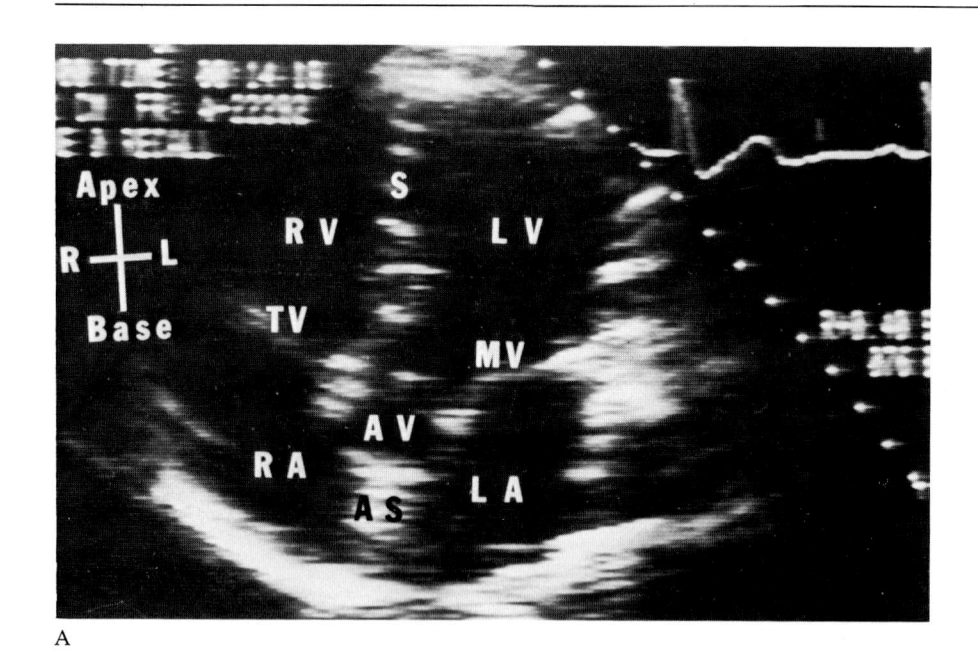

Fig. 1-17A. Apical 4-chamber view including the aortic valve obtained by tilting or angulating the transducer anteriorly showing the right ventricle, left ventricle, interventricular septum, tricuspid valve, mitral valve, aortic valve, right atrium, interatrial septum (AS), and the left atrium. B. Anatomic section of a normal heart in the apical 4-chamber plane anteriorly directed through the aortic valve corresponding to the echocardiographic image in A. PM = anterolateral papillary muscle.

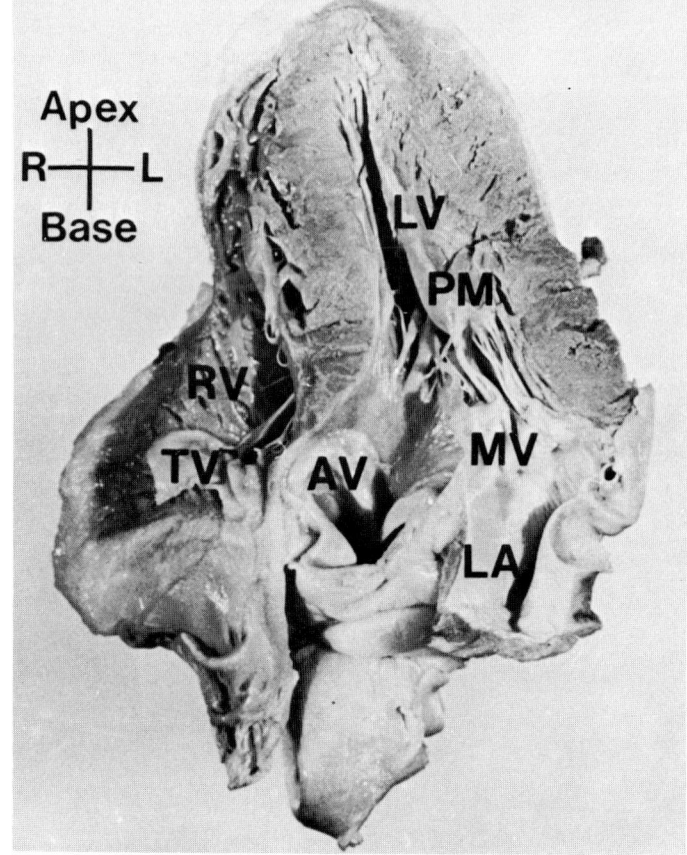

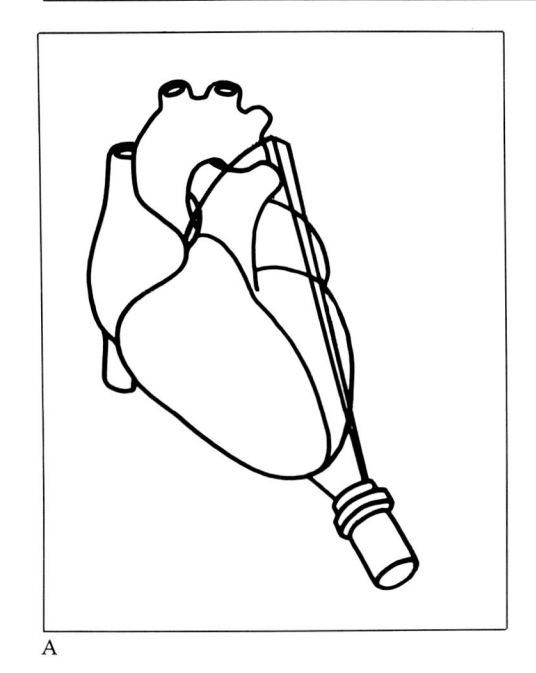

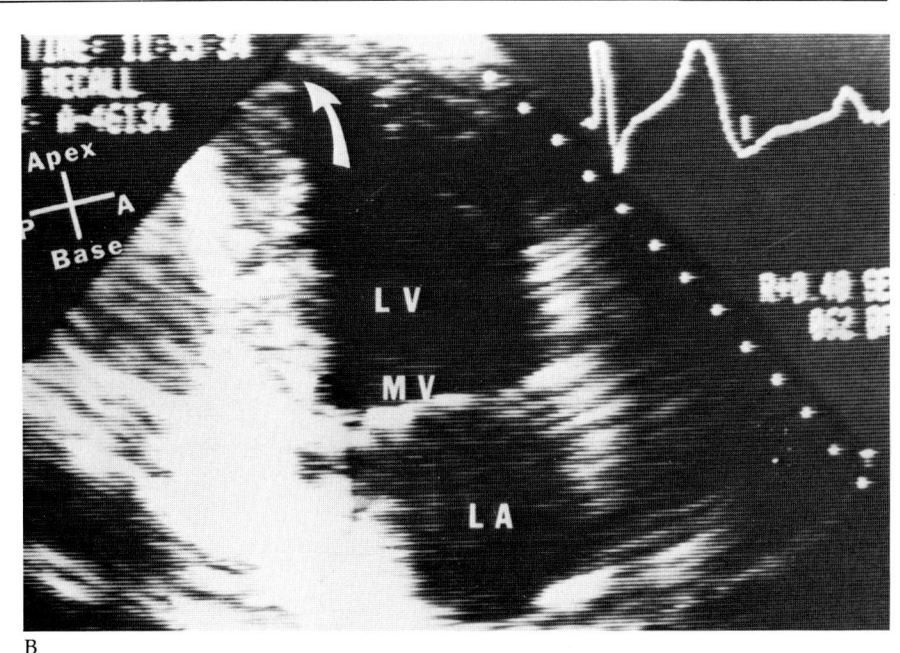

Fig. 1-18A. Diagram showing the sector beam in an apical long axis orientation with the transducer positioned over the left ventricular apex. B. Apical long axis view without the aortic valve showing the true left ventricular apex (arrow) in a normal subject.

26   1. Normal cross-sectional anatomy

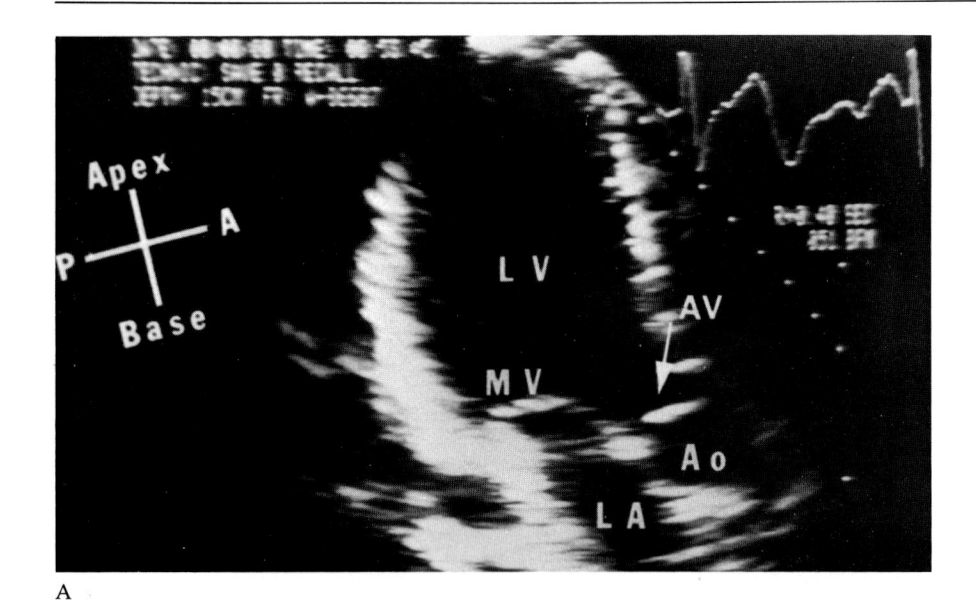

Fig. 1-19A. Apical long axis view including aortic valve and proximal portion of ascending aorta (Ao). Sometimes the true left ventricular apex is deleted in this tomographic plane when tilted anteriorly to include the aortic valve. B. Anatomic section of normal left ventricle in an apical long axis plane through the aortic valve. The posteromedial papillary muscle is routinely seen in this view. Since the section plane is parallel to the interventricular septum, no right heart chambers are seen in this view. The anterolateral wall (AW) and the posteromedial wall of the left ventricle together with the left atrium are seen. C = chordae tendineae.

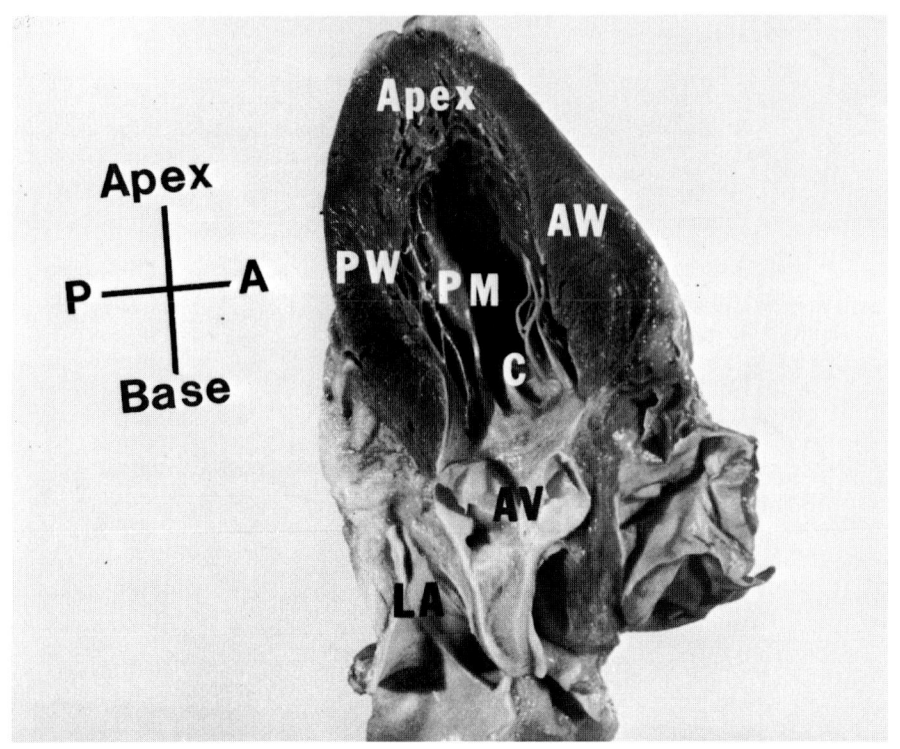

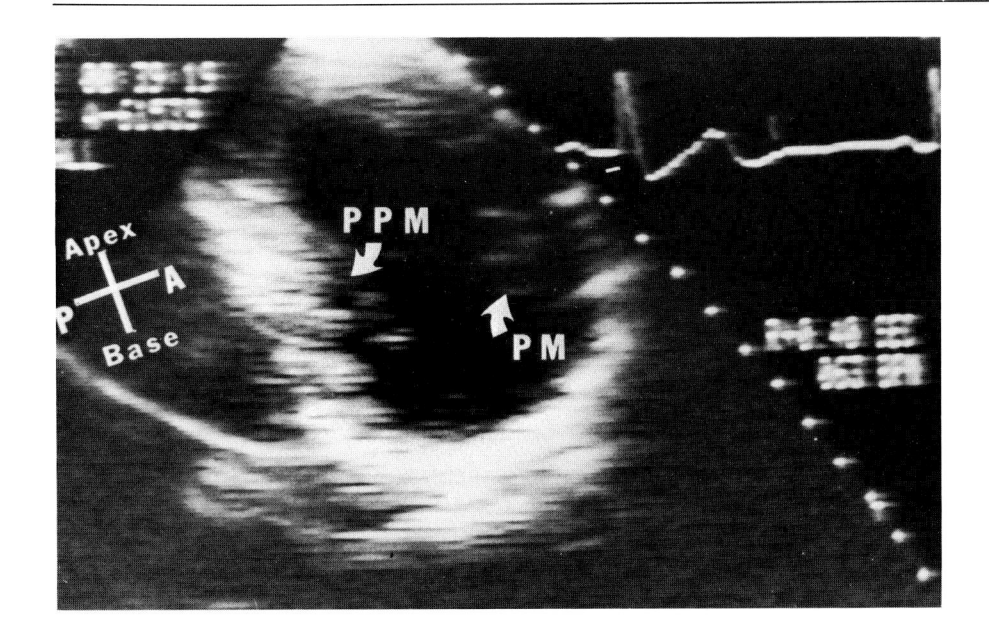

Fig. 1-20. Apical oblique view of the left ventricle showing the posteromedial papillary muscle (PPM) and a small tip of the anterolateral papillary muscle.

28   1. Normal cross-sectional anatomy

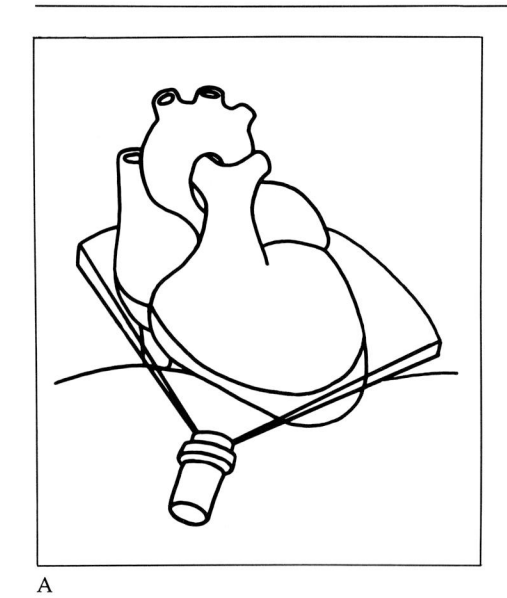

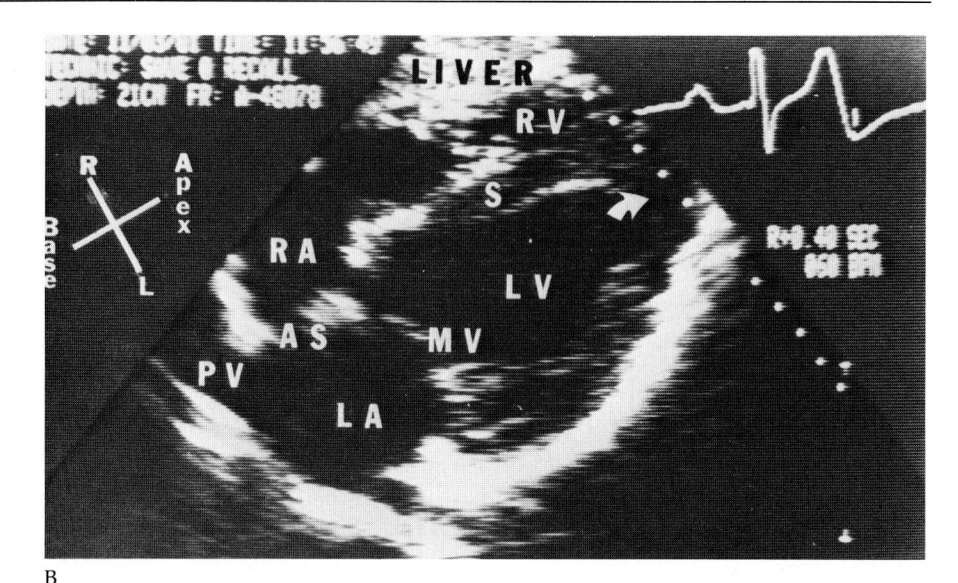

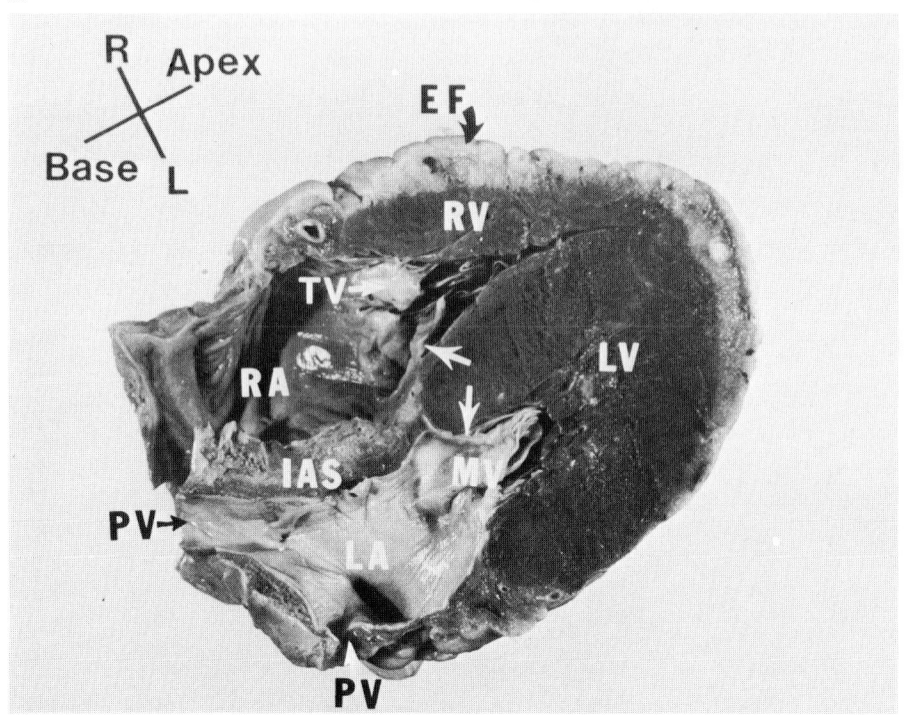

Fig. 1-21A. Diagram showing the sector beam in a subcostal 4-chamber orientation with the transducer positioned in the subcostal (subxiphoid) location below the diaphragm. B. Subcostal 4-chamber view showing normal structures. The left ventricular apex (arrow) is deleted from view in this tomographic plane. C. Anatomic section in the subcostal 4-chamber plane of a normal heart showing corresponding anatomy of structures imaged in B. Often a considerable amount of epicardial fat (EF) is seen on the free wall of the right ventricle. The septal leaflet of the tricuspid valve (upper arrow) always arises more inferiorly (by 2–6 mm) toward the apex than the anterior mitral leaflet (lower arrow). AS = interatrial septum; IAS = interatrial septum; PV = pulmonary veins; RV = right ventricular diaphragmatic free wall; TV = posterior leaflet of tricuspid valve.

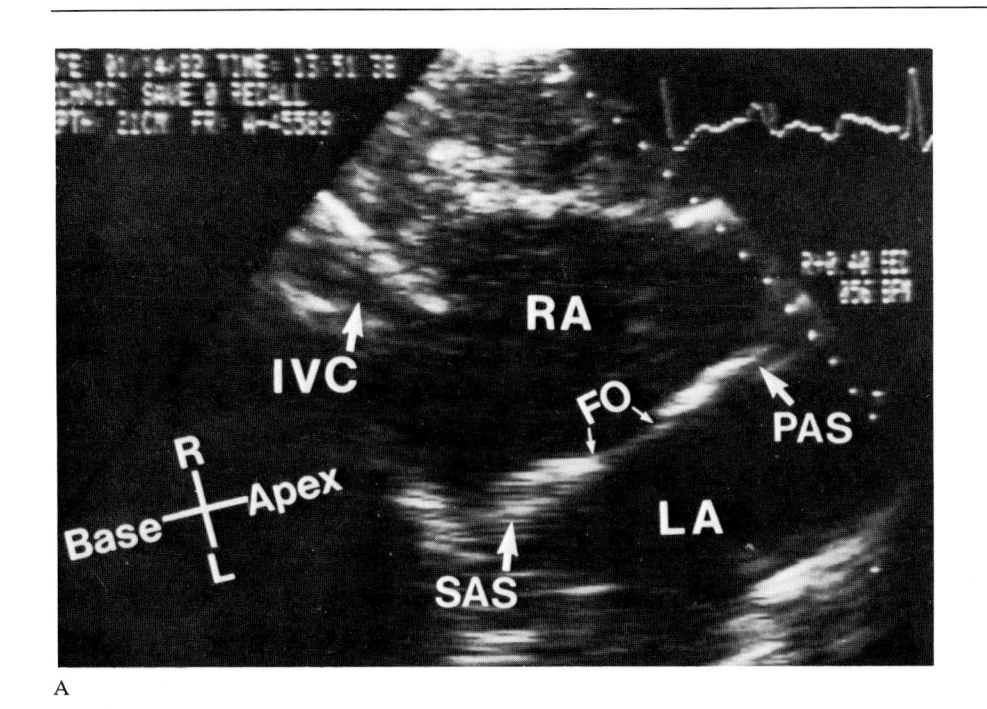

Fig. 1-22A. Subcostal 4-chamber view with sector beam directed toward both right and left atria. In this plane the interatrial septum is perpendicular to the sector beam, enabling visualization of the secundum atrial septum (SAS), foramen ovale (FO), which is anatomically thinner than the surrounding portions of atrial septum, and the primum atrial septum (PAS). A small portion of the inferior vena cava at its junction into the RA can be seen; more complete visualization of the IVC requires counterclockwise rotation and rightward angulation of the sector beam. B. Subcostal view of RA, interatrial septum (IAS), and LA with superior angulation demonstrating entrance of superior vena cava into the RA in a normal infant. The azygous (AZ), left brachiocephalic (LB), and right brachiocephalic (RB) veins entering the SVC are all well visualized. Although the SVC junction with the RA can be visualized in infants from the subcostal transducer position, this anatomic region is better imaged from the suprasternal notch in adults.

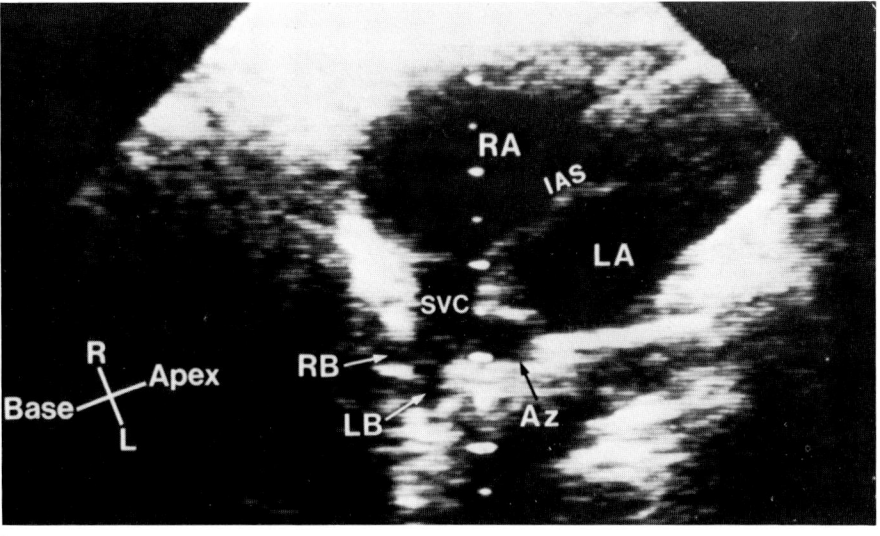

30   1. Normal cross-sectional anatomy

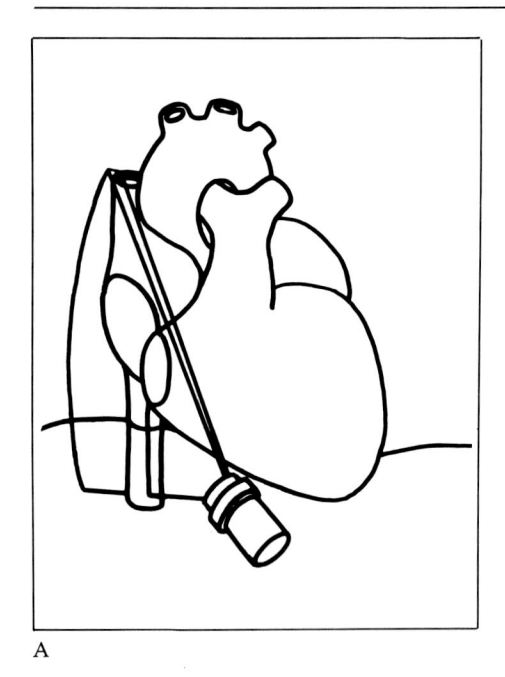

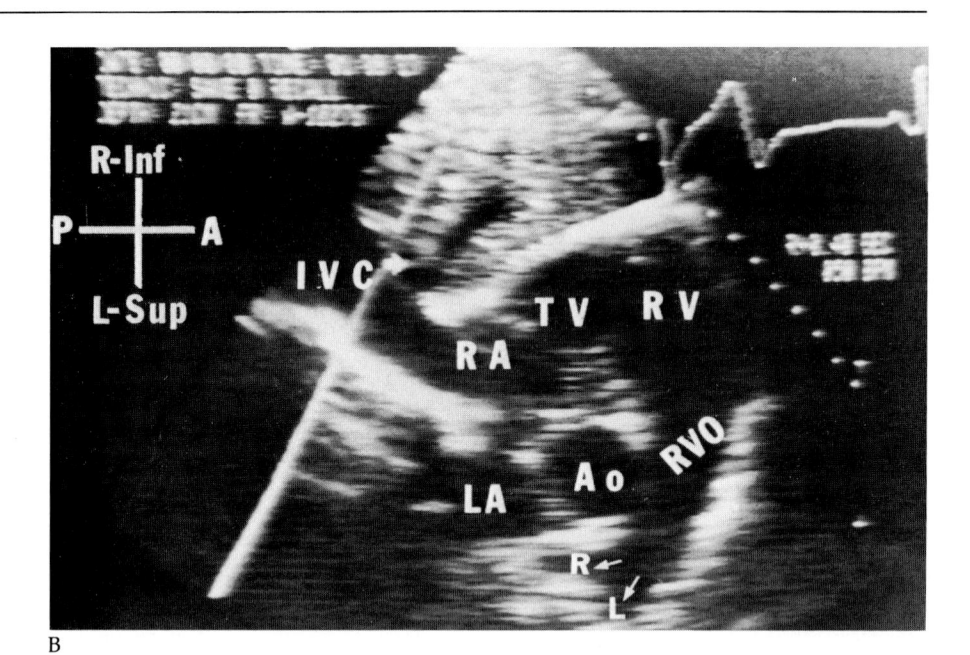

Fig. 1-23A. Diagram showing the sector beam oriented through the inferior vena cava and its junction with the right atrium with the transducer in the subcostal position. B. Subcostal view of the inferior vena cava entering the right atrium together with the tricuspid valve, right ventricle, right ventricular outflow tract (RVO), ascending aorta (Ao), left atrium, and a portion of the pulmonary artery bifurcating into the right and left pulmonary arteries. The white arrow overlying the M-mode cursor, which intersects the IVC, points to a hepatic vein entering the IVC. The sector beam is directed more leftward and superiorly, which enables simultaneous imaging of the pulmonary artery. This image plane is different from that diagramed in A, which is oriented only through the RA and IVC.

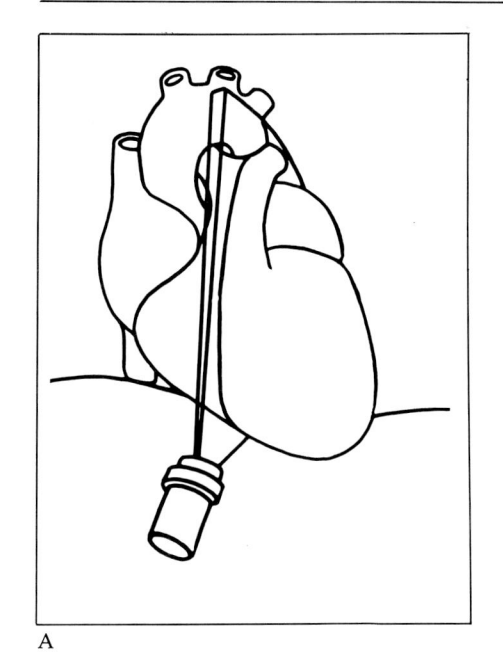

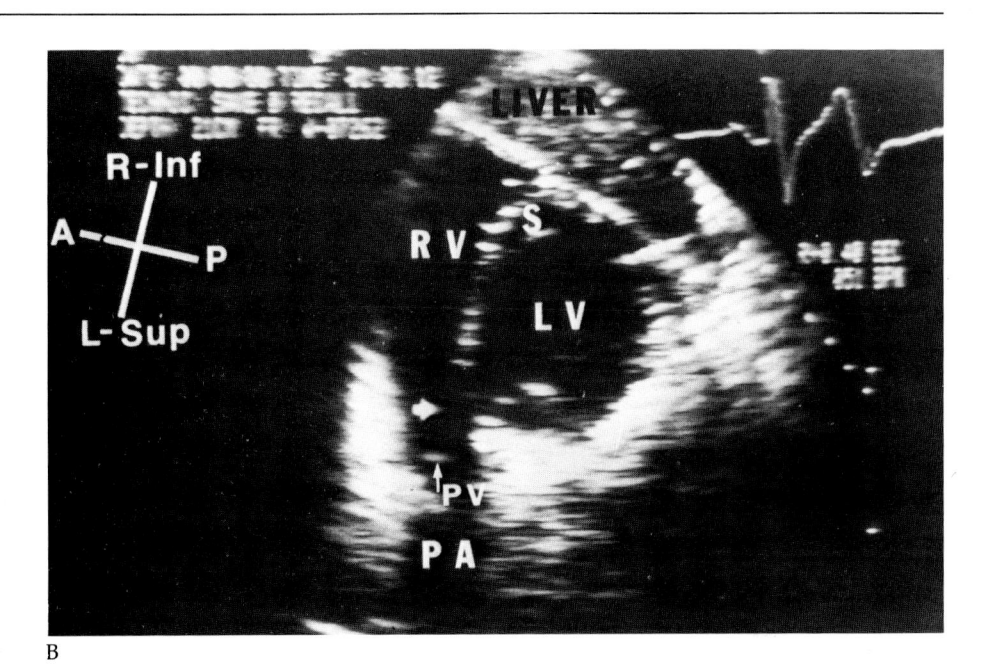

Fig. 1-24A. Diagram showing the sector beam oriented through the left ventricle, right ventricular outflow tract, and pulmonary artery with the transducer in the subcostal position. B. Subcostal short axis view through the left ventricle, right ventricle, right ventricular outflow tract (white arrow), pulmonic valve (PV), and pulmonary artery (PA).

32   1. Normal cross-sectional anatomy

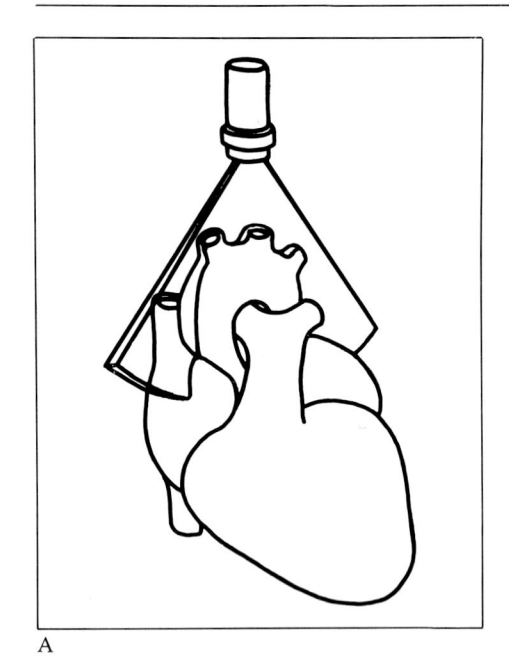

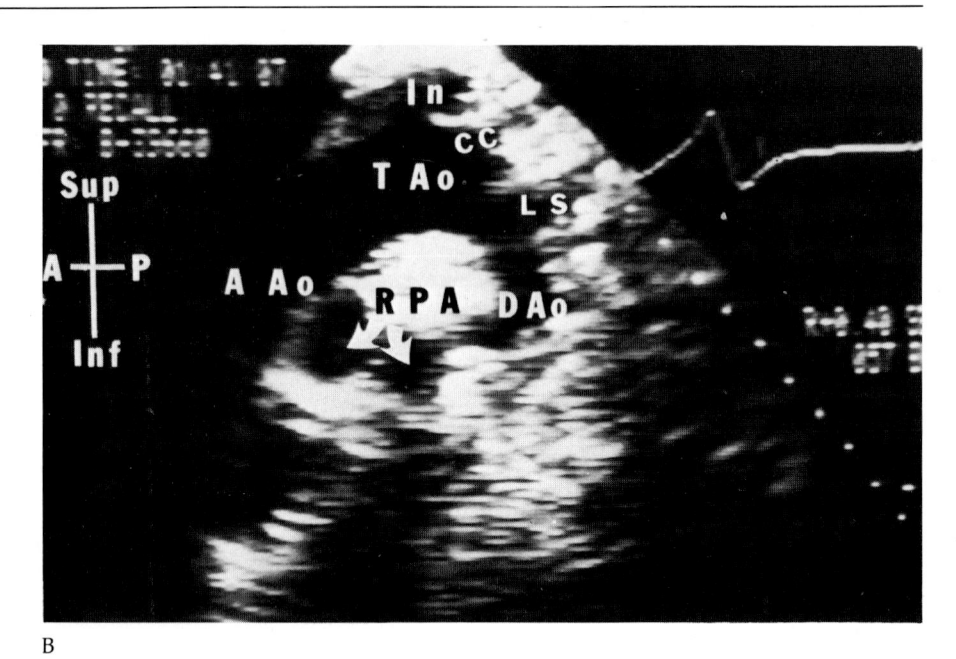

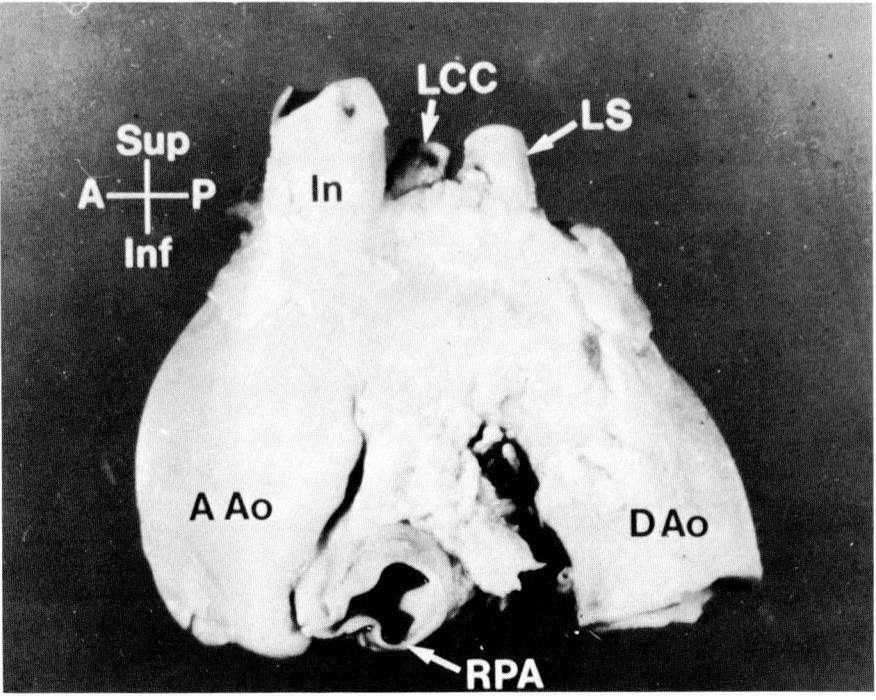

Fig. 1-25A. Diagram showing the sector beam oriented in the long axis of the aorta with the transducer in the suprasternal notch position. B. Suprasternal notch long axis view of the aorta showing ascending aorta, transverse aorta, descending aorta, innominate artery (In), left common carotid artery (CC), left subclavian artery (LS), and right pulmonary artery (RPA). The RPA usually appears as a single, not double, lumen; either the appearance in this normal subject is due to beam obliquity intersecting the RPA or the vessel is bifurcating at the point where the sector beam passes through it. C. Anatomic slice showing normal aorta oriented in suprasternal long axis view corresponding to B. LCC = left common carotid artery.

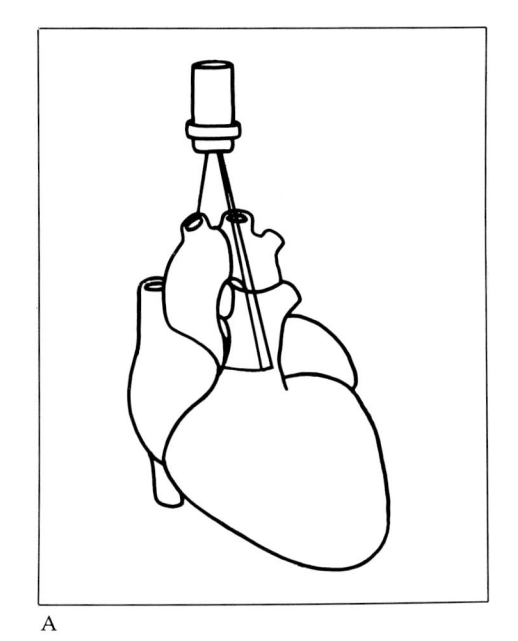

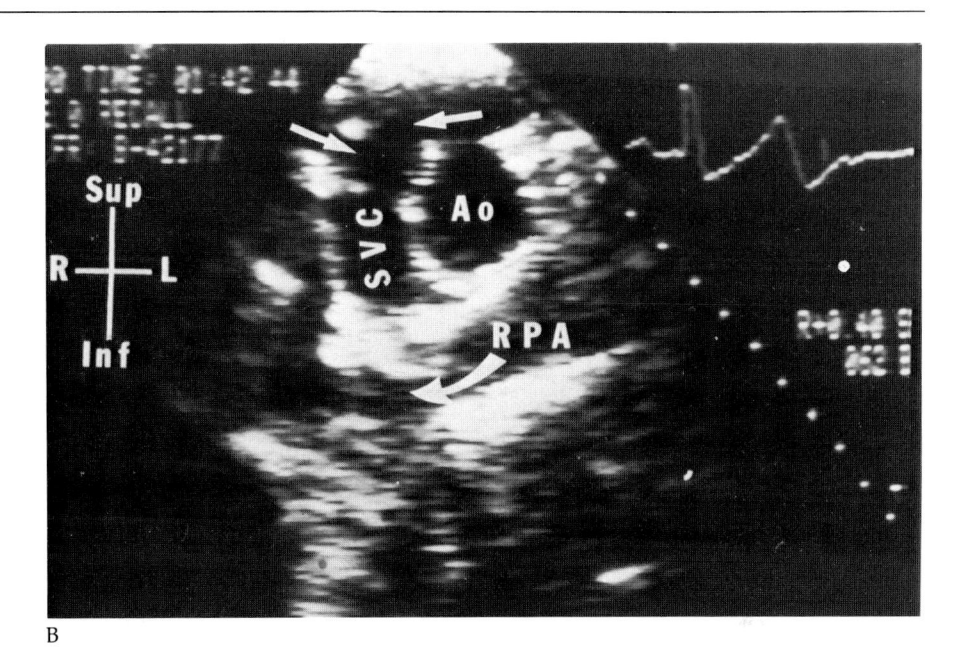

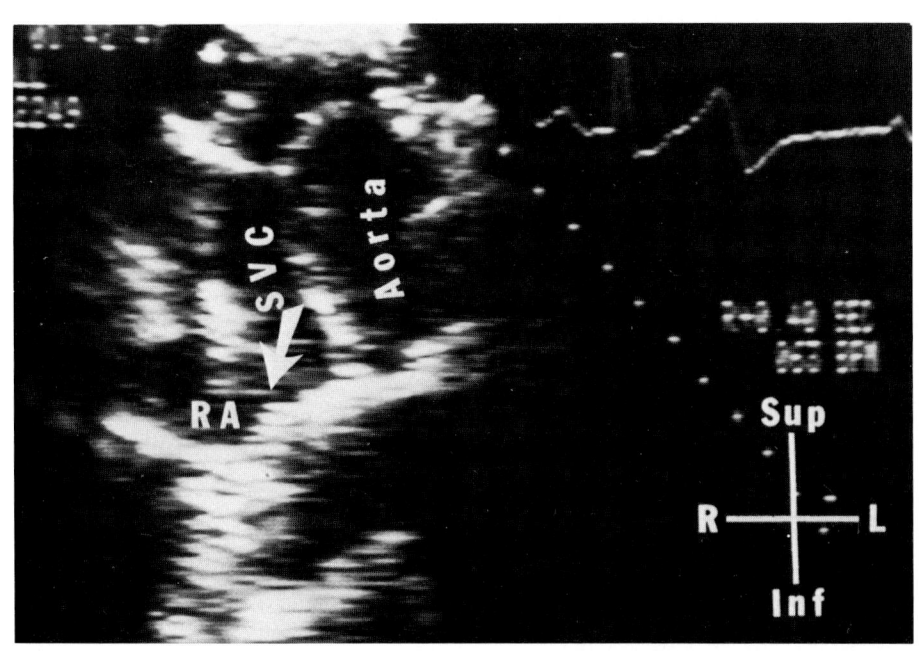

Fig. 1-26A. Diagram showing the sector beam oriented in the short axis of the aorta with the transducer positioned in the suprasternal notch. B. Suprasternal notch short axis view of the ascending aorta (Ao) with the innominate and left subclavian veins (arrows) entering the superior vena cava. An oblique view of the right pulmonary artery (RPA) is also seen. C. Suprasternal notch oblique short axis view of the ascending aorta together with the SVC entering the right atrium in a normal subject.

ease. For portable bedside studies and certain acutely ill patients in acute care units, it may not be possible to position the patient ideally.

It is recommended that the echocardiographer perform the examination from the left side of the bed. When the patient is in a steep left lateral decubitus position, which is preferable for apical imaging, reaching across from the right side of the bed is much more difficult; if the patient is quite large or obese, it is harder for the operator to palpate and impossible to visualize the apical impulse. The examination technique usually involves both hands. The left hand should be used as a stabilizing hand with the forearm and hand resting on the bed and the patient and the right hand being used to angulate and rotate the transducer as well as to operate the controls on the machine. Maintaining stability of the transducer on the chest wall without excessive pressure or loss of image is an important function of the left hand, while the right hand is used to make machine adjustments. In my experience it is more difficult to maintain transducer position, rotation, and angulation with one hand without causing pressure discomfort to the patient's chest.

Although it is usually easier to obtain better imaging from the parasternal windows and apical position while patients are on their left side, the supine position should be used for subcostal imaging. During subcostal imaging the patient is encouraged to relax the abdominal muscles, which is often made easier by flexing the knees and resting the feet on the bed while the head is slightly elevated.

For suprasternal notch imaging the patient should be supine with a pillow or wedge under the shoulders so that the head and neck are slightly hyperextended, providing the operator with better access to the suprasternal and/or supraclavicular spaces.

It is possible to obtain many different tomographic views of the heart. However, it is recommended that a minimum of 17 standard two-dimensional images be obtained together with integrated M-mode recordings for comprehensive anatomical and functional information on each patient. When clinically indicated, two additional suprasternal notch views should be obtained. These standard views and recommended sequence of recordings are as follows:

1. Parasternal left ventricular long axis view together with M-mode recording sweeping from the level of the chordae tendineae (Fig. 1-27) through the mitral valve, aortic valve, and left atrium.
2. Parasternal view of the inflow tract of the right ventricle (RA/RV view). M-mode recording of the tricuspid valve and right atrium is obtained (see Fig. 1-5B).
3. Parasternal right ventricular outflow (subpulmonic) view and M-mode recording through the pulmonic valve (Fig. 1-28).
4. Parasternal short axis view at the base together with M-mode recordings of tricuspid, aortic, and pulmonic valves (Fig. 1-29). Rightward and slightly inferior angulation of the transducer views the right atrium and IVC junction (Fig. 1-30).
5. Parasternal short axis view with direction toward the pulmonary artery and bifurcation of the right and left pulmonary arteries and M-mode recording of the pulmonic valve (Fig. 1-31).
6. Parasternal short axis view at the mitral valve with M-mode recording (Fig. 1-32).
7. Parasternal short axis view at the chordae tendineae together with M-mode

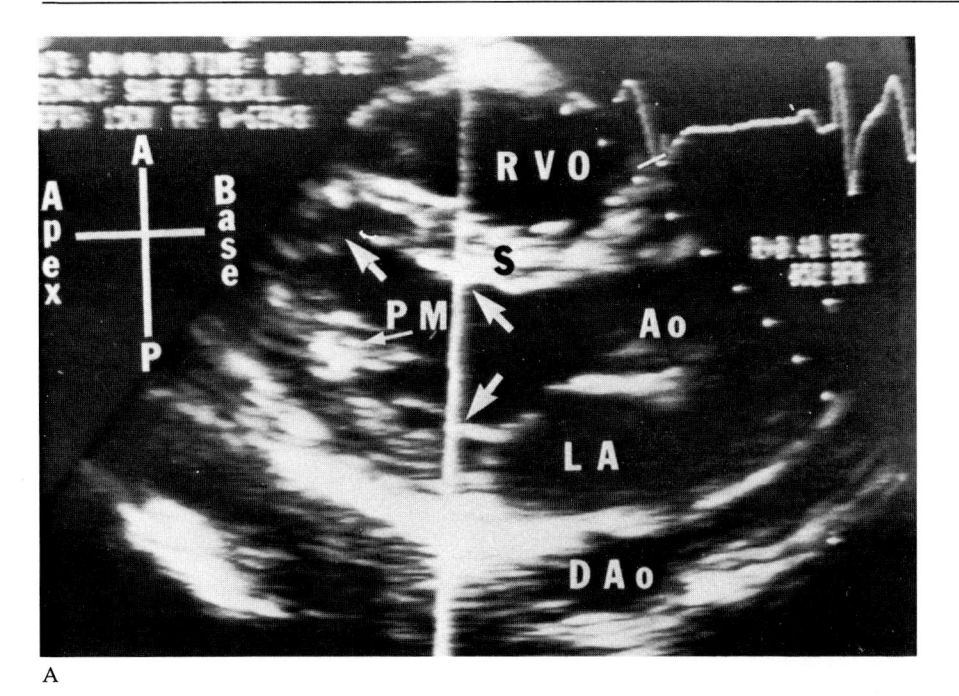

Fig. 1-27A. Parasternal long axis view showing M-mode cursor correctly positioned through the interventricular septum (upper arrow), the chordae tendineae (arrow), and posterior wall. With the proper long axis plane, the apex (arrow at left) can often be visualized at end systole. B. Parasternal long axis view with M-mode cursor through right ventricle, septum, anterior mitral leaflet, posterior mitral leaflet (arrow), and posterior left ventricular wall close to the atrioventricular sulcus. This position of the M-mode cursor is incorrect for recording the left ventricle. C. Oblique parasternal long axis view. The sector beam is not directed correctly, resulting in deletion of the apex (white arrows). Even though the M-mode cursor is directed through the chordae tendineae (C) correctly, the tomographic plane is not through the true long axis, which will cause the M-mode recording of the left ventricle to be a tangent chord rather than a true short axis diameter. Ao = descending aorta; PM = posteromedial papillary muscle.

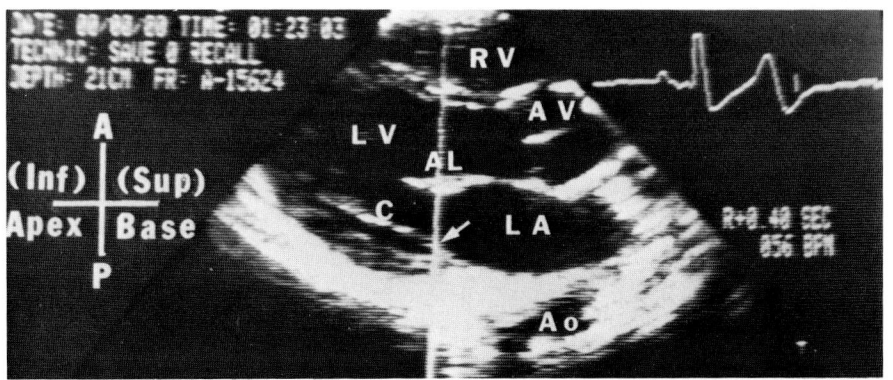

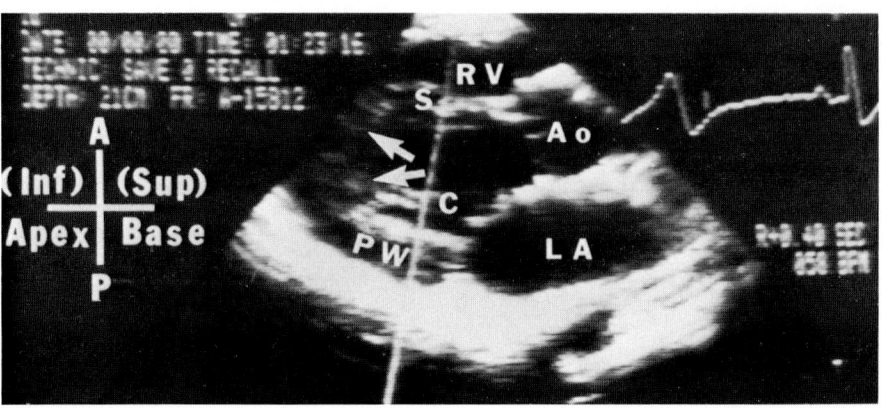

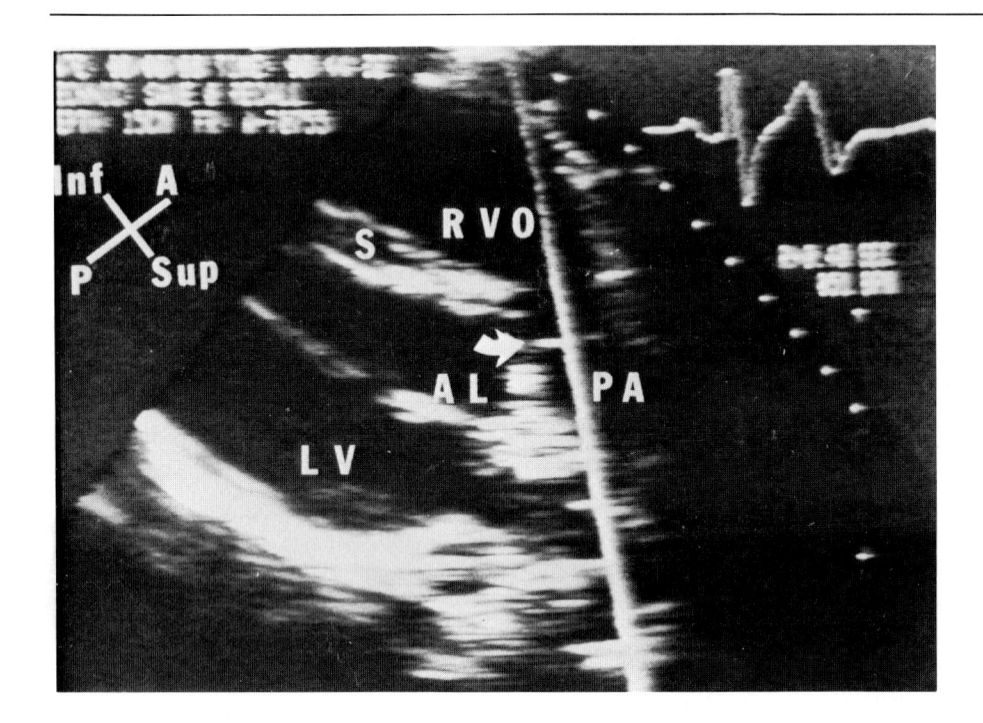

Fig. 1-28. *Parasternal right ventricular outflow (subpulmonic) view with M-mode cursor directed through the pulmonic valve* (white arrow). *The structures and image are otherwise the same as in Figure 1-6B.*

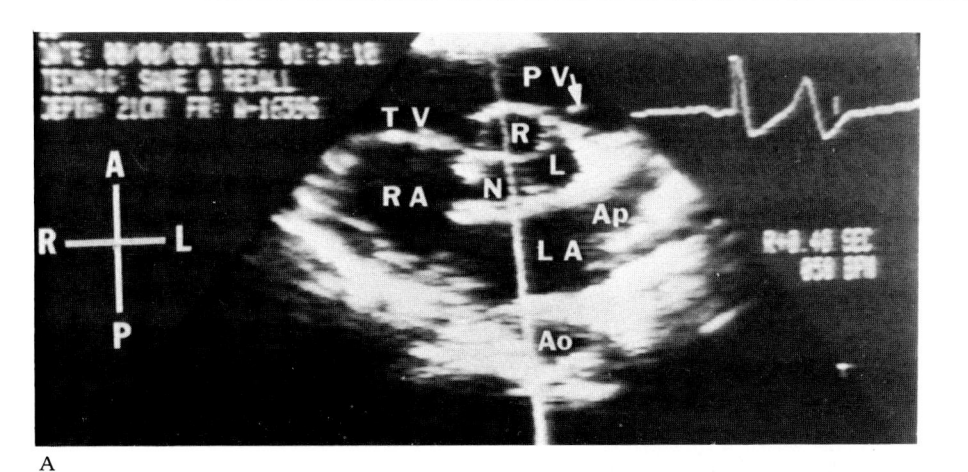

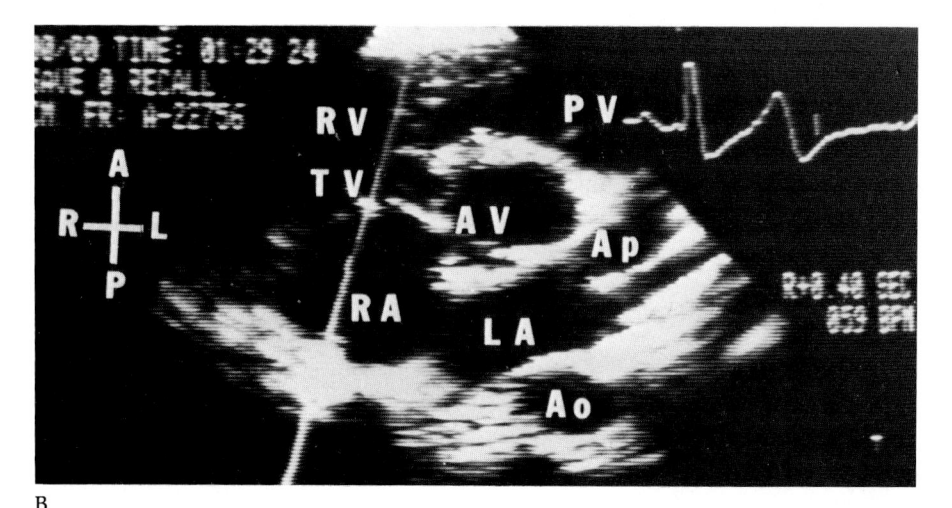

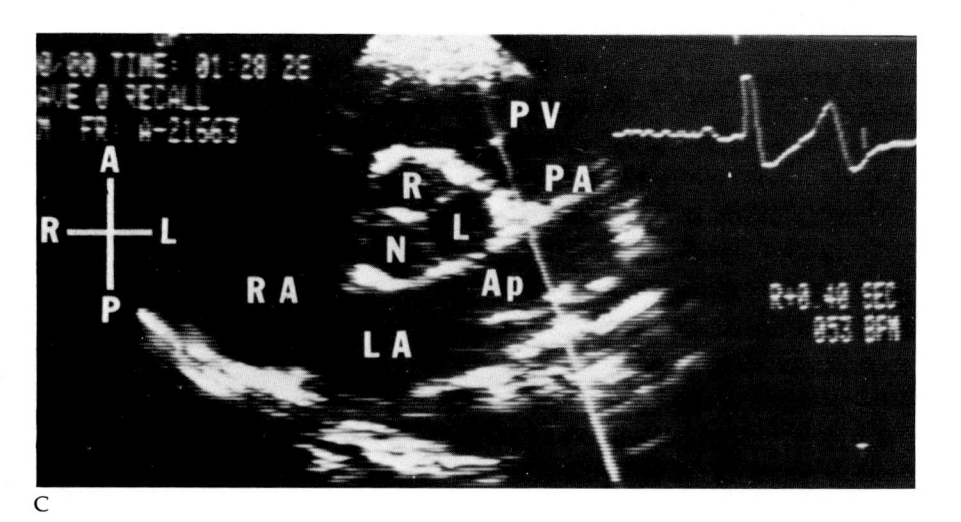

Fig. 1-29A. Parasternal short axis view at the base with M-mode cursor properly directed to obtain good M-mode recording of the aortic valve. B. Same parasternal short axis view at the base as A except that the M-mode cursor is directed through the tricuspid valve. The M-mode view of the tricuspid valve is frequently not as well recorded as in the right ventricular inflow plane. C. The same parasternal short axis view at the base as shown in A and B with a slight leftward or lateral angulation images more of the pulmonary artery. The M-mode cursor is directed through the pulmonic valve. Ao = descending aorta; L = left cusp of aortic valve; PV = pulmonic valve; R = right cusp of aortic valve.

38   1. Normal cross-sectional anatomy

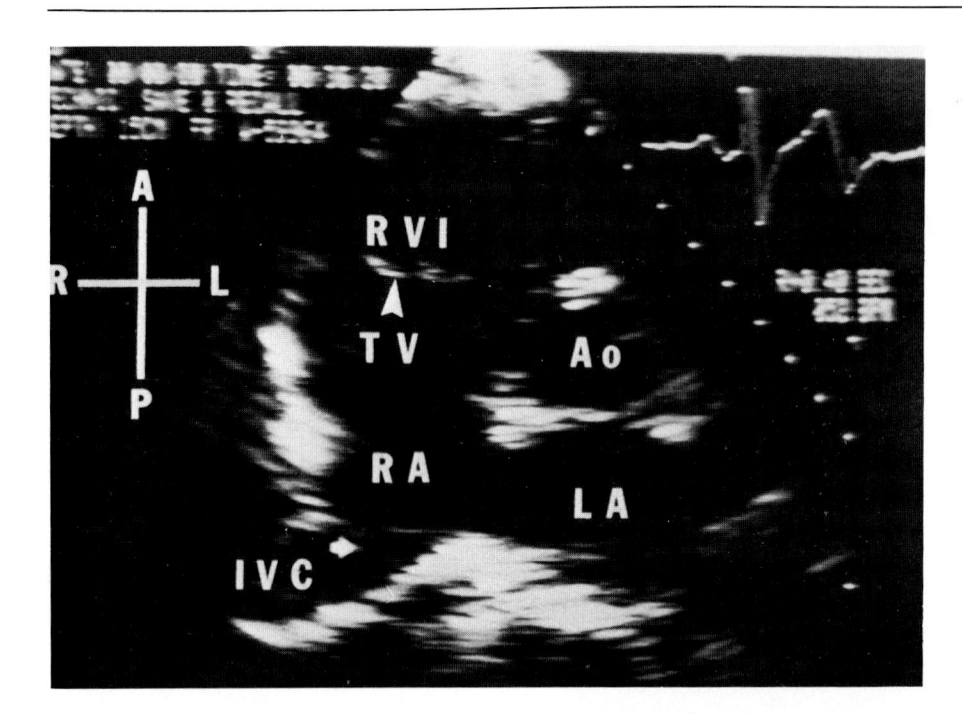

Fig. 1-30. Parasternal short axis view at the base with slight rightward and inferior angulation of the sector provides good visualization of the junction of the right atrium and inferior vena cava. RVI = right ventricular inflow tract.

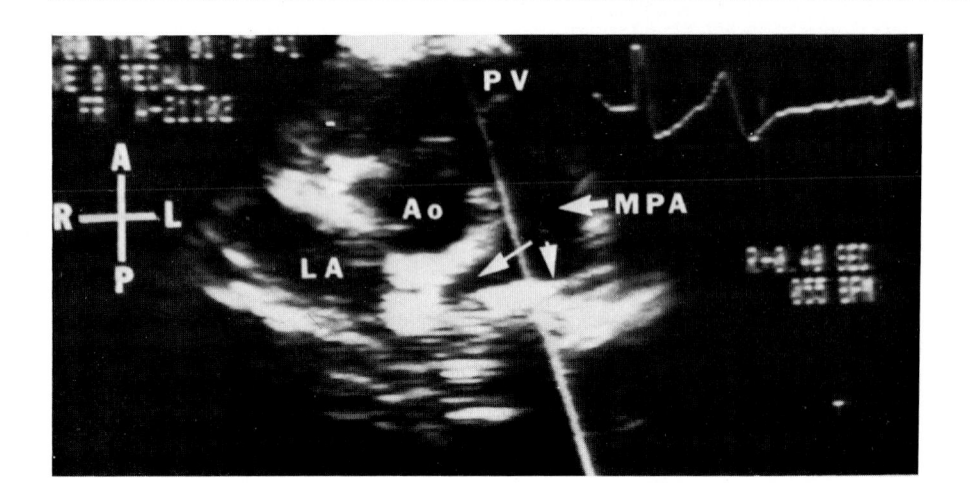

Fig. 1-31. Parasternal short axis view at the base with direction toward the pulmonary artery and bifurcation of right and left pulmonary arteries (arrows). This angulation provides another excellent opportunity to obtain a high-quality M-mode recording of the pulmonic valve (PV).

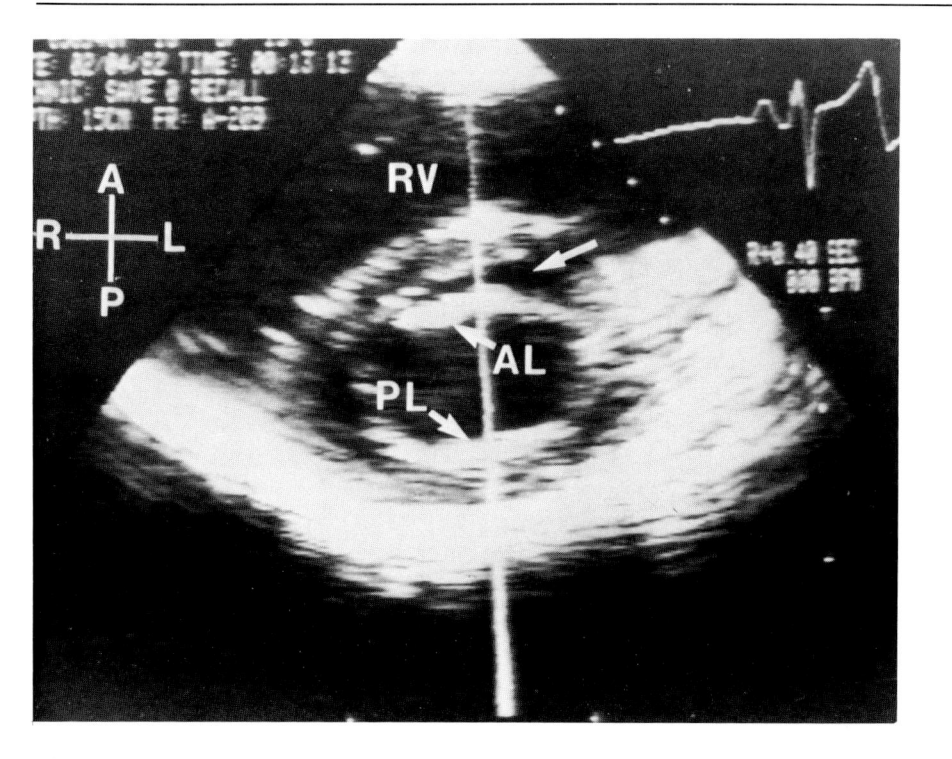

Fig. 1-32. Parasternal short axis view with the M-mode cursor through the anterior and posterior mitral leaflets (arrows) in a normal subject at onset of diastole. The upper arrow points to the left ventricular outflow tract and the proximity of the AL to the ventricular septum. The machine setting is overgained (excessive transmit power), causing both mitral leaflets to appear thickened.

recording with simultaneous two-dimensional imaging to ensure that the M-mode record was obtained with the beam perpendicular through the septum and posterior wall as well as intersecting through the true short axis diameter of the left ventricle (Fig. 1-33).
8. Parasternal short axis views at the papillary muscles (see Figs. 1-13A and 1-14A).
9. Parasternal short axis view at the apex of the left ventricle (see Fig. 1-15B).
10. Apical four-chamber view without the aortic valve (see Fig. 1-16B).
11. Apical four-chamber view with the aortic valve (see Fig. 1-17A).
12. Apical long axis view without aortic valve (see Fig. 1-18B).
13. Apical long axis view with aortic valve and ascending aorta (see Fig. 1-19A).
14. Subcostal four-chamber view directed toward the ventricles with M-mode recording of the free wall of the right ventricle (Fig. 1-34).
15. Subcostal four-chamber view directed toward both atria with emphasis on visualization of the interatrial septum and, if clinically indicated, M-mode recording through the atria and the interatrial septum (see Fig. 1-22A).
16. Subcostal view of the right atrium and inferior vena cava with M-mode recording through the inferior vena cava and noting changes with respiration (Fig. 1-35).
17. Subcostal left ventricular short axis view with right ventricular outflow tract and pulmonic valve; occasionally requires M-mode recording of these structures (see Fig. 1-24B).
18. Suprasternal long axis of the aorta (see Fig. 1-25B).
19. Suprasternal short axis of the transverse aorta (see Figs. 1-26B and 1-26C).

40   1. Normal cross-sectional anatomy

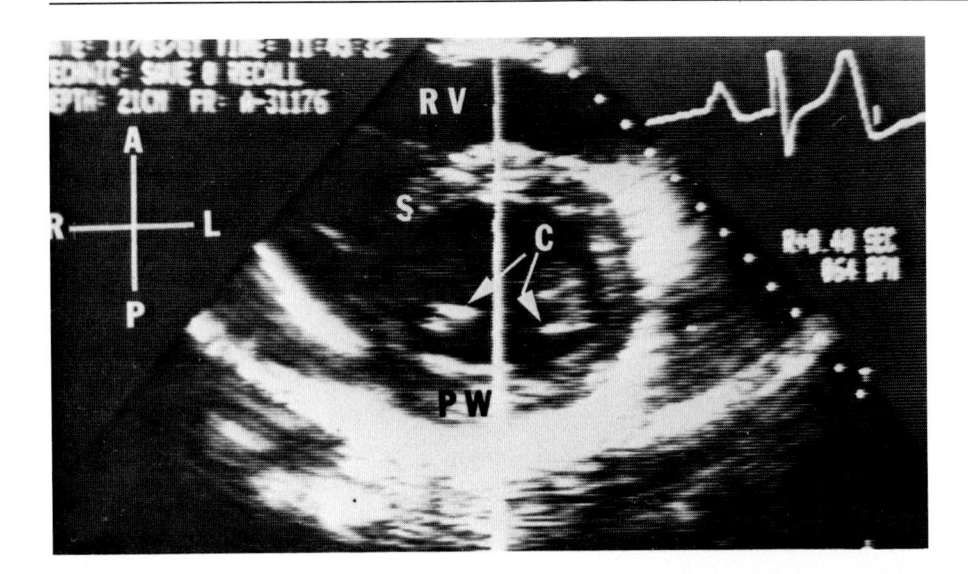

Fig. 1-33. Parasternal short axis view at the level of the chordae tendineae (C) with the M-mode cursor properly directed through the septum and posterior left ventricular wall for accurate M-mode recordings of the left ventricle. Simultaneous 2-D echo imaging ensures better quality control of the M-mode records.

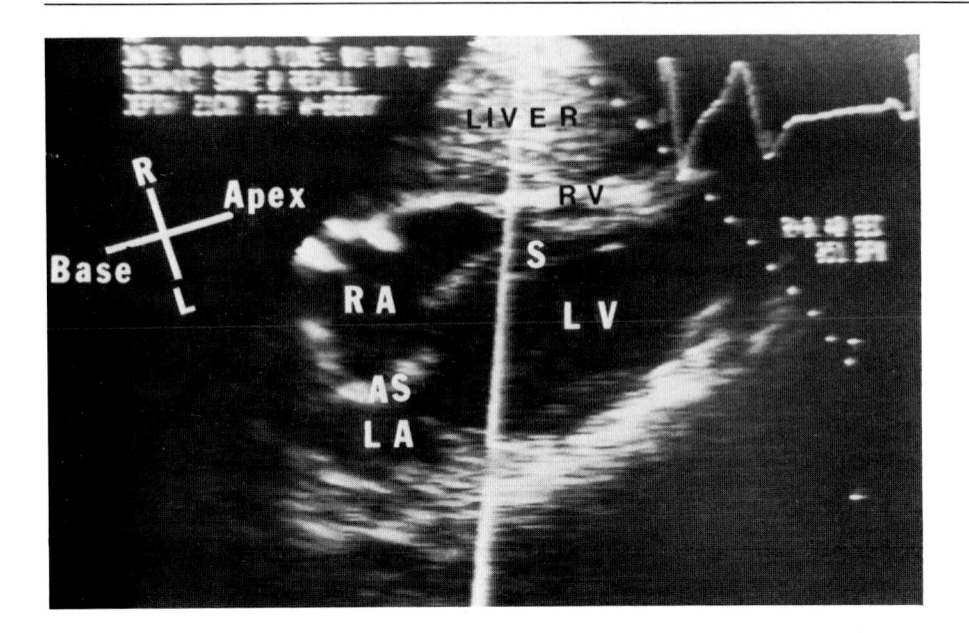

Fig. 1-34. Subcostal 4-chamber view directed toward the ventricles for M-mode recording of cursor intersecting free wall of the right ventricle in a perpendicular manner. This usually provides the best assessment of right ventricular wall thickness. AS = interatrial septum.

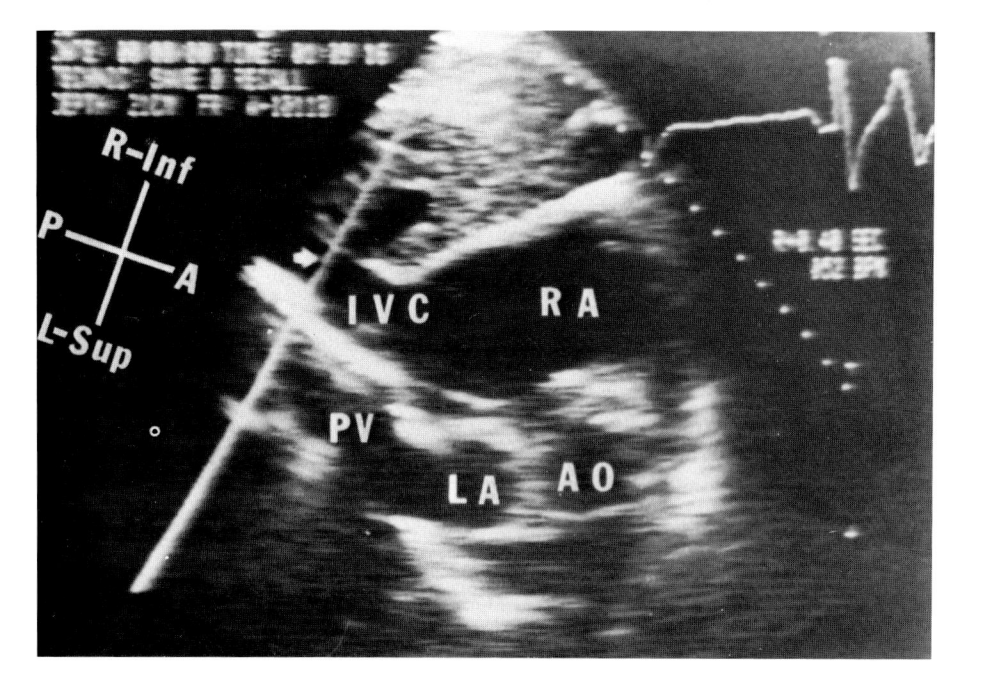

Fig. 1-35. *Subcostal view of the junction of the inferior vena cava and right atrium. The M-mode cursor is directed perpendicularly through the IVC (arrow) at a point just distal to the hepatic vein entering the IVC. The size of the IVC and effects of normal respiration on diameter are measured from the M-mode record. PV = pulmonary vein.*

Echocardiographic measurements: M-mode and two-dimensional images. The reliability of quantitative determinations from 2-D echo images is dependent upon the resolution of the instrumentation utilized, the technical quality of the views recorded, and the skills of the echocardiographer or physician who performs the measurements. In addition, there may be limitations inherent in the operation of the videotape recorder and display on the television monitor, such as the freeze frame stability and precise identification of end systole. Simultaneous recording of a phonocardiogram together with the electrocardiogram will provide a marker (the aortic component of the second heart sound) that can be used by some machines to trigger a freeze frame at end systole. Additional benefit has been realized by transferring the images from the videotape to a videodisc, which provides greater flexibility in the off-line analysis of the data, such as slow-motion forward and reverse as well as a stable, artifact-free still-frame. Accordingly the type of videotape recorder and the method available for off-line measurements can have a significant effect upon the overall reliability of quantitative determinations of 2-D echo images. The technology is evolving quite rapidly with respect not only to the basic instrumentation for obtaining two-dimensional echo data but also to improved methods for manual and automated analyses of the images. A considerable amount of effort has been made and is currently being exerted to quantitate segmental and global functions of the left ventricle with two-dimensional echocardiography (see Chapters 6 and 7). Because of certain limitations that exist in any equipment available to perform 2-D echocardiography, echocardiographers and physicians continue to depend upon M-mode recordings to obtain certain measurements and aid in making clinical interpretations.

We perform both M-mode and two-dimensional recordings simultaneously or in sequence as part of the same examination. Occasionally there is clinical need for only a 2-D study or an M-mode examination without the other in combination;

however, these clinical circumstances account for less than 5 percent of the monthly volume of procedures in our echo laboratories. For that reason we believe it is important to combine measurements and interpretative information from both recordings into a single echocardiographic interpretation. It is important to realize that the quality of M-mode recordings is significantly improved by employing simultaneous 2-D imaging that identifies the precise location and direction of the M-mode beam. With the flexibility of directing the M-mode beam anywhere in the plane of the 2-D sector, the echocardiographer's ability to record chamber size, wall thickness, valve motion, and appearance or motion of other structures is greatly enhanced. This greater capability of M-mode recordings has clinical significance for two important reasons: improved accuracy of measuring left ventricular size, function, and wall thickness by ensuring from the parasternal 2-D short axis view that the M-mode recordings were obtained in the proper location; and more complete recordings of valves and anatomy, made possible by many transducer positions and improved imaging opportunities when coupled with a two-dimensional system.

We recommend obtaining the measurements that potentially have the most clinical relevancy in any given patient. M-mode measurements are employed to complement 2-D measurements, and 2-D imaging is used to improve quality control of the M-mode measurements; the resultant worksheet is a combination of both (Fig. 1-36). Although a single number may be recorded for a chamber dimension or wall thickness, it represents the best estimate from several different 2-D views plus an M-mode recording; in other determinations, no M-mode data is obtainable. Many different 2-D views together with M-mode recordings compose a complete study. All appropriate qualitative and quantitative information should constitute a clinical interpretation. The measurement and calculation worksheet utilized in our laboratories records left heart data followed by right heart information. The dimensions of the left ventricle and wall thickness of both ventricular septum and posterior wall are made at the level of the chordae tendineae in either parasternal long axis or short axis views. The function of the left ventricle is evaluated by global and segmental parameters.

The shape of the left atrium varies from spherical to oblong in appearance; usually the inferior–superior dimension, as measured from either apical four-chamber or long axis views, is slightly greater than the anterior–posterior dimension.

The cavity size of the right ventricle is best evaluated from the apical four-chamber view; however, the free wall thickness is best imaged in the subcostal four-chamber plane. Directing the M-mode cursor perpendicularly through the right ventricular free wall in the subcostal position is usually the best method for determining RV wall thickness. The apical four-chamber plane is also the best single view for evaluating the size of the right atrium. Subcostal imaging of the inferior vena cava with both 2-D and M-mode recordings provides useful information which reflects the functional status of the right ventricle and right atrial pressure. The effects of respiration on the diameter of the IVC should also be observed from the subcostal position.

In order to carefully evaluate the left ventricle it should be divided into segments for careful analysis for segmental dysfunction. Investigators have divided the left ventricle in different ways; we divide it into 15 different segments (Fig. 1-37). After having divided the ventricle into these segments, one should make a

I. LEFT VENTRICLE
   A. DIMENSIONS
      Septum   _____ mm (8–11)
      Posterior wall   _____ mm (8–11)
      LVEDD   _____ mm (<53–58)
      LVESD   _____ mm
   B. FUNCTIONS
     Global
      1. FS   _____ % (30–44)
      2. $V_{\overline{cf}}$ _____ circ/sec (1.0–1.5)
      3. EPSS   _____ mm (<10)
      4. EDV   _____ ml/m^2
      5. ESV   _____ ml/m^2
      6. SV   _____ ml/m^2
      7. EF   _____ % (55–70)
     Segmental
      1. WTPW   _____ % (40–100)
      2. WT$_S$ _____ % (40–100)
      3. Wall motion
         index   _____ (5)

II. LEFT ATRIUM
   A–P dimension   _____ mm (<35–40)
   I–S dimension   _____ mm (<50–55)
   Area   _____ cm^2 (<18)
   LA/AO ratio   _____ (<1.3)

III. VALVES   Normal   Abnormal
   Aortic   [ ]   [ ]
   Mitral   [ ]   [ ]
   Pulmonic   [ ]   [ ]
   Tricuspid   [ ]   [ ]

IV. RIGHT VENTRICLE
   Subcostal view
     Free wall RV   _____ mm (<7)
   Apical 4-chamber
     Max short axis _____ mm (<40–47)
     Area   _____ cm^2 (<30)
     RV/LV diam ratio _____ (<1.0)
     RV/LV area ratio _____ (<.9)

V. PULMONARY ARTERY
   Diameter   _____ mm (<38–42)
   PA/AO ratio   _____ (<1.2)
   RVPEP/RVET   _____ (<0.30)

VI. AORTA
   A–P diameter   _____ mm (<35)

VII. RIGHT ATRIUM
   I–S dimension   _____ mm (<50–55)
   Area   _____ cm^2 (<18)
   RA/LA area ratio _____ (0.8–1.1)

VIII. IVC DIAMETER
   Exhalation   _____ mm (<25)
   Peak inspiration _____ mm

COMMENTS: _____

_____, M.D.

Fig. 1-36. Page 2 of our echocardiographic worksheets showing the measurements obtained.

1. Normal cross-sectional anatomy

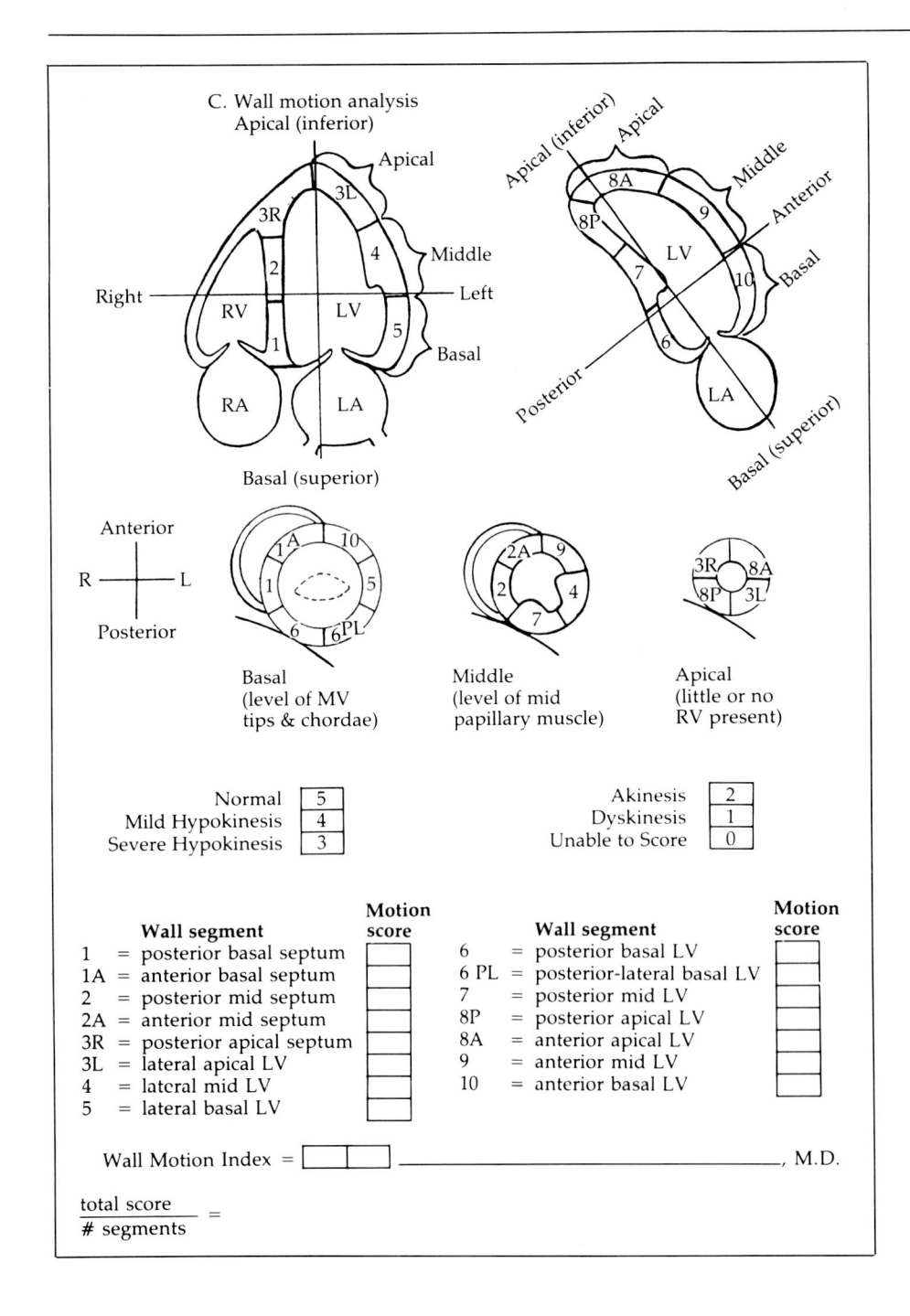

C. Wall motion analysis

Fig. 1-37. Page 3 of our echocardiographic worksheets showing the manner in which the left ventricle is divided into 15 segments.

Basal (level of MV tips & chordae)

Middle (level of mid papillary muscle)

Apical (little or no RV present)

Normal	5
Mild Hypokinesis	4
Severe Hypokinesis	3
Akinesis	2
Dyskinesis	1
Unable to Score	0

Wall segment	Motion score	Wall segment	Motion score
1 = posterior basal septum		6 = posterior basal LV	
1A = anterior basal septum		6 PL = posterior-lateral basal LV	
2 = posterior mid septum		7 = posterior mid LV	
2A = anterior mid septum		8P = posterior apical LV	
3R = posterior apical septum		8A = anterior apical LV	
3L = lateral apical LV		9 = anterior mid LV	
4 = lateral mid LV		10 = anterior basal LV	
5 = lateral basal LV			

Wall Motion Index = ☐☐ _____, M.D.

$\dfrac{\text{total score}}{\text{\# segments}} =$

qualitative evaluation of each of the segments to identify normal, hypokinetic, akinetic, or dyskinetic motion. In doing so, a wall motion index can be derived by dividing the total score by the total number of segments evaluated; there is some predictive value in assessment of wall motion index that correlates with left ventricular performance. Imaging techniques and methods of analyzing these left ventricular segments are discussed in depth in Chapter 6.

References

1. Gramiak R, Fortuin NJ, King BL, Popp RL, Feigenbaum H: Optimal resources for ultrasonic examination of the heart (report of the Intersociety Commission for Heart Disease Resources). *Am J Cardiol* 35:898, 1975
2. Popp RL, Fortuin NJ, Johnson ML, Kisslo JA Jr: Optimal resources for ultrasonic examination of the heart (Echocardiography Study Group special report of the Intersociety Commission for Heart Disease Resources). *Circulation* 65:421A, 1982
3. Griffith JM, Henry WL: A sector scanner for real time two-dimensional echocardiography. *Circulation* 49:1147, 1974
4. Kloster FE, Roelandt JR, ten Cate FJ, Bom N, Hugenholtz PG: Multiscan echocardiography II. Technique and initial clinical results. *Circulation* 48:1075, 1973
5. Morgan CL, Trought WS, Clark WM, VonRamm OT, Thurstone FL: Principles and applications of a dynamically focused phased array real time ultrasound system. *JCU* 6:385, 1978
6. Latson LA, Cheatham JP, Gutgesell HP: Resolution and accuracy in two dimensional echocardiography. *Am J Cardiol* 48:106, 1981
7. Bierman FZ, Fellows K, Williams RG: Prospective identification of ventricular septal defects in infancy using subxiphoid two-dimensional echocardiography. *Circulation* 62:807, 1980
8. Helak JW, Plappert T, Muhammad A, Reichek N: Two dimensional echographic imaging of the left ventricle: Comparison of mechanical and phased array systems in vitro. *Am J Cardiol* 48:728, 1981
9. Henry WL, DeMaria AN, Gramiak R, King DL, Kisslo JA, Popp RL, Sahn DJ, Schiller NB, Tajik A, Teichholz LE, Weyman AE: Report of the American Society of Echocardiography Committee on nomenclature and standards in two-dimensional echocardiography. *Circulation* 62:212, 1980

Rheumatic valvular disease

Echocardiography is the procedure of choice to record the functional anatomy of the cardiac valves. Whereas the rapid sampling rate and resolution of M-mode echocardiography permits excellent recording of motion of individual valves, the spatial orientation of two-dimensional echocardiography provides a more comprehensive opportunity to study the structure, shape, and motion of the valves in real-time during the cardiac cycle in the various disease states. Accordingly, it is not surprising that one of the most important clinical applications of combined M-mode and two-dimensional echocardiography is for the assessment of the patient with valvular heart disease. Since the first clinical application of cardiac ultrasound by Edler in 1955 [1], enormous progress has been made in the reliability of mitral valve assessment. Significant advances have been made from the early days when clinical evaluation of the mitral valve was largely dependent upon determining the diastolic closing velocity of the anterior mitral leaflet, which used to be considered the most important criterion in diagnosing mitral stenosis [2]. During the 1960s when resolution of the mitral valve was quite poor and the only available method of recording the data was the Polaroid photograph, the value of clinical application was quite limited. With the interfacing of continuous strip-chart recording capability with M-mode echocardiography several years ago, the clinical application of this noninvasive technique became more useful and has been utilized on a more widespread basis. In 1972 Duchak and associates [3] emphasized the importance of identifying the posterior mitral leaflet as well as recognizing other cardiac abnormalities that produce changes of the anterior leaflet mimicking the changes of rheumatic mitral disease.

Although the diagnosis of acute rheumatic fever is uncommon in the United States, the manifestations of rheumatic valvular disease in this country are not unusual. It would appear that the occurrence of acute valvulitis that is clinically unrecognized is not uncommon. Rheumatic valvular diseases occur very commonly in countries where rheumatic fever remains uncontrolled or is ineffectively treated. Rheumatic fever has the potential to involve the endocardium, myocardium, or pericardium [4]. Endocardial involvement characteristically involves the valvular endocardium, causing swelling of the leaflets and secondary erosions along the lines of contact of the leaflets with subsequent scarring of these areas. The mitral valve is most commonly involved, followed by the aortic, less frequently the tricuspid, and quite rarely the pulmonic valve. The frequency distribution of valvular involvement may reflect the degree of pressure to which the individual valves are subjected [5]. While rheumatic involvement isolated to the aortic valve is distinctly unusual, the combined involvement of both mitral and aortic valves frequently occurs. Tricuspid valve involvement is quite unusual in the absence of associated mitral and/or aortic valve lesions. The end result of recurrent rheumatic endocarditis is the addition of fibrous tissue with concomitant contracture affecting the valvular leaflets and chordae tendineae.

Normal mitral valve. The anterior leaflet is considerably longer from its annular origin to the tip compared to the posterior leaflet; however, the posterior leaflet composes approximately two thirds of the total circumference of the mitral annulus (Fig. 2-1). The anterior portion of the mitral annulus is somewhat more deficient

48   2. Rheumatic valvular disease

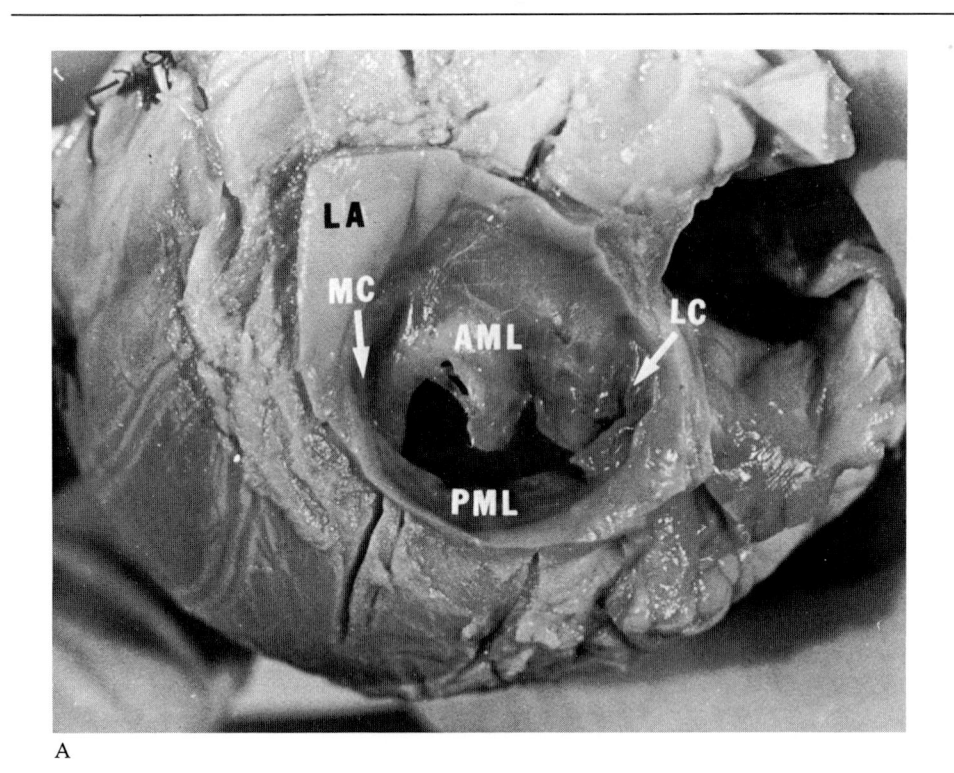

Fig. 2-1A. Normal mitral valve with left atrium removed showing the larger anterior mitral leaflet from its annular origin to leaflet tip and the shorter posterior mitral leaflet. The posterior leaflet usually composes approximately two thirds of the total circumference of the annulus. B. Close-up view of normal AML and PML with the left ventricle open. Normal chordae tendineae (C) and papillary muscles can be seen. MC = medial commissure; LC = lateral commissure.

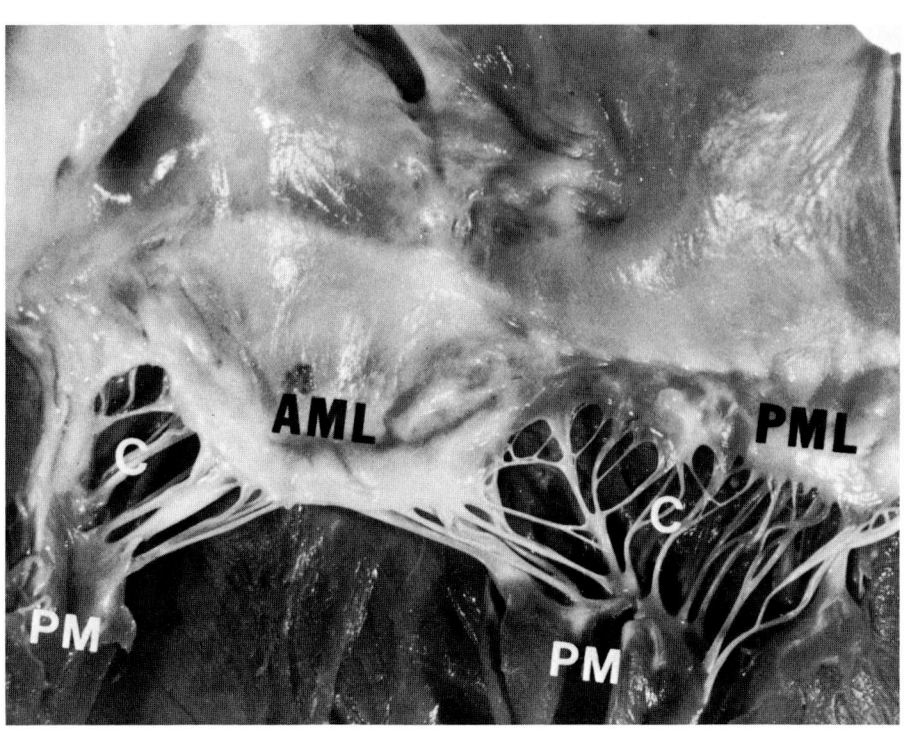

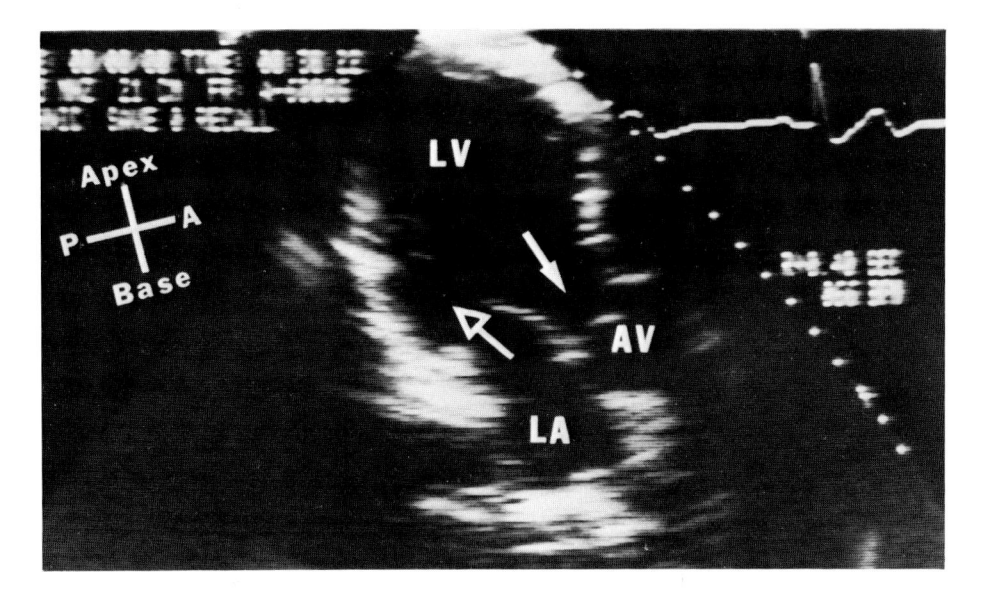

Fig. 2-2. Apical long axis view with aortic valve and the anterior mitral leaflet separating the inflow tract (open arrow) of the left ventricle from the outflow tract (solid arrow).

compared to the better developed portion of the annulus posteriorly where the posterior leaflet is inserted [6, 7]. The anterior leaflet is continuous with the posterior wall of the aortic root. The continuation of the left atrial wall at the atrioventricular sulcus gives rise to the posterior mitral leaflet. The presence of the mitral leaflets permits the division of the left ventricular cavity into inflow and outflow tracts. It is primarily the anterior leaflet that separates the outflow tract anteriorly and superiorly from the inflow tract posteriorly and inferiorly [8] (Fig. 2-2). The normal function of the mitral valve depends upon the following structures and functions: (1) valve leaflets, (2) mitral annulus, (3) chordae tendineae, (4) papillary muscles, (5) atrial and ventricular walls, and (6) sequence of atrioventricular conduction.

The anterior mitral leaflet is considerably larger and more mobile than the posterior leaflet and valve closure occurs more posteriorly and does not occur midway between the anterior and posterior attachments of the leaflets. The normal point of apposition of the two leaflets is not at their free edge but a few millimeters from it. Each leaflet has a rough or appositional zone where the chordae tendineae insert and a clear or free zone, which is more proximal from the free margins and constitutes the body of the leaflets [9, 10]. Histologically this free zone or body of the leaflets is composed of a lamina fibrosa, and the appositional rough zone is made up of a loose network of collagen fibers. Sufficient valve tissue is reserved to ensure competence in closure, since the combined surface area of the two leaflets is considerably larger than that of the mitral ring. Normal systolic closure of the mitral leaflets forms a triangular outline or "chevron" configuration of the inflow tract with the base at the mitral ring and the apex at the opposed mitral leaflets.

The mitral annulus is reduced as much as 34 percent of its maximal diameter with atrial contraction [11]. In the presence of atrial fibrillation this reduction in annular diameter is abolished. Accordingly this decrease of annular size could be an important function of atrial contraction before ventricular systole. Chakorn and colleagues [12] have reported that the excursion of the mitral valve annulus or ring is considerable and contributes significantly to the overall movement of the anterior mitral leaflet. Ormiston and associates [13], by employing two-dimensional echocardiography, noted the maximum diastolic area of the mitral annulus in normal subjects to be 3.8 ± 0.7 cm^2/m^2; the maximum mid-systolic narrowing was reported to be 26 ± 3 percent. These investigators found the maximal annular circumference to be 9.3 ± 0.9 cm and the mean reduction in circumference to be 13 ± 3 percent. The mitral annulus is a pliable, circumferential, fibrous ring that contains two major collagenous structures, the right and left fibrous trigones. The right fibrous trigone, or central fibrous body, lies in the midline of the heart and represents the confluence of fibrous tissue from the mitral valve, tricuspid valve, membranous septum, and posterior aspect of the root of the aorta [14]. Between the trigones ventrally, the anterior leaflet of the mitral valve is in direct fibrous continuity with the posterior wall of the aortic root. Usually there is no thick, fibrous ring in this region, and the annulus is a poorly defined, nonthickened zone that gives attachment to the muscle fibers of the roof of the left atrium. The mitral valve annulus is elliptical in shape.

The mitral apparatus is a complex, finely coordinated mechanism. The annulus has been inaccessible to noninvasive examination until the availability of two-dimensional echocardiography, which may provide new information about the overall function of the annulus in normal and diseased states. The contribution of mitral annular size and dysfunction to mitral regurgitation of dilated cardiomyopathy and hypertrophic cardiomyopathy is still unclear.

Two-dimensional echocardiography is probably the best diagnostic clinical tool available to study the anatomic and functional integrity of the components of the mitral apparatus, namely the mitral annulus, the valve leaflets, the chordae tendineae, the papillary muscles, the posterior left atrial wall, and the left ventricular walls.

Clinical manifestations of rheumatic mitral disease. Mitral stenosis, a very common valvular lesion, occurs predominantly as a sequela of acute rheumatic valvulitis with or without a past history of rheumatic fever. Rarely does it occur on a congenital basis; it has been reported in 0.5 to 4.0 percent of cases of congenital heart disease [15]. Not infrequently in tropical or subtropical countries like India, Indonesia, and the Philippines, mitral stenosis becomes fully developed in adolescence, before the age of 20 years. This type of mitral stenosis has been described as juvenile mitral stenosis. Advanced forms of the disease with severely fibrosed or calcified valves are not uncommon in young adults.

Rheumatic involvement of the mitral valve usually occurs in young people and is three times more common in women than men. With respect to the aortic valve, the opposite is true; rheumatic involvement may occur at any age but is more frequent in middle- and older-age groups with the ratio of men to women being 3:1 [5].

In the United States it commonly takes 20 to 30 years after the initial attack of acute rheumatic fever before progressive narrowing of the mitral valve orifice leads to significant symptoms [4]. The orifice is normally 5 to 8 cm^2 in adults; narrowing of the valve opening is probably insignificant down to approximately 2.5 cm^2. When the valve area is narrowed to 1.5 cm^2 or less, there are usually symptoms

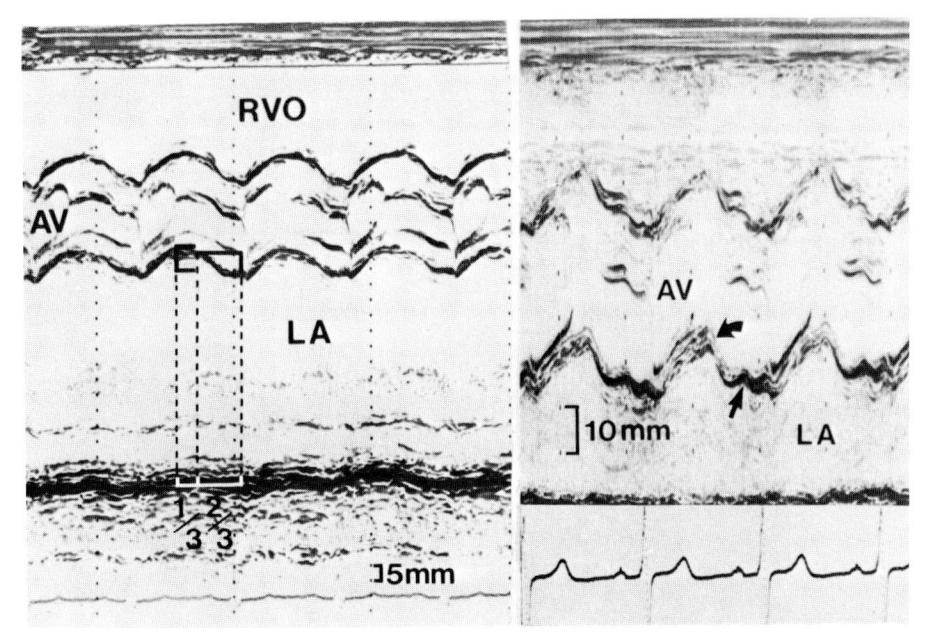

Fig. 2-3. M-mode recordings showing significant mitral stenosis (left panel), abnormal left atrial emptying index (LAEI), and left atrial enlargement. Normal LAEI is recorded in a normal subject (right panel).

significant enough to necessitate surgery. The most common symptoms are exercise limitations due to shortness of breath and fatigue. As the mitral valve becomes progressively stenotic, the left atrial and pulmonary venous pressures continue to rise, with resultant enlargement of the left atrium and eventually development of pulmonary hypertension. With progressive left atrial dilatation these patients will eventually develop atrial fibrillation. Characteristic cardiac physical findings include a loud first heart sound, opening snap, and a diastolic rumble at the apex that terminates with presystolic accentuation of the murmur.

ECHOCARDIOGRAPHIC FEATURES OF MITRAL STENOSIS. The diastolic closing velocity, traditionally measured as the E–F slope on the M-mode echocardiogram, is usually markedly abnormal in the presence of mitral stenosis. This abnormality is readily explained by the slowed ventricular filling with the valve being held open by a persistent pressure gradient between the left atrium and left ventricle caused by the valvular obstruction. Although it is well recognized that the E–F slope alterations in mitral stenosis are partially a function of the degree or severity of stenosis, as an isolated predictive factor this single measurement index is unreliable in determining the severity of the mitral stenosis [16].

The echocardiographic motion of the aortic root reflects to a certain extent left atrial filling and emptying. Strunk and colleagues [17] reported that mitral stenosis has a characteristic pattern of slow left atrial emptying in early diastole with loss of the conduit phase in mid diastole. These investigators believed that the atrial emptying index, defined as the fraction of passive posterior aortic wall motion occurring in the first third of diastole, provided a useful noninvasive quantitation of the severity of mitral stenosis (Fig. 2-3). They also found the atrial emptying index to be useful for evaluating patients with prosthetic mitral valve obstruction and for documenting improvement in left atrial emptying after mitral valve surgery. However, other investigators have reported that the severity of mitral stenosis could not be accurately predicted from abnormalities of aortic root motion [18].

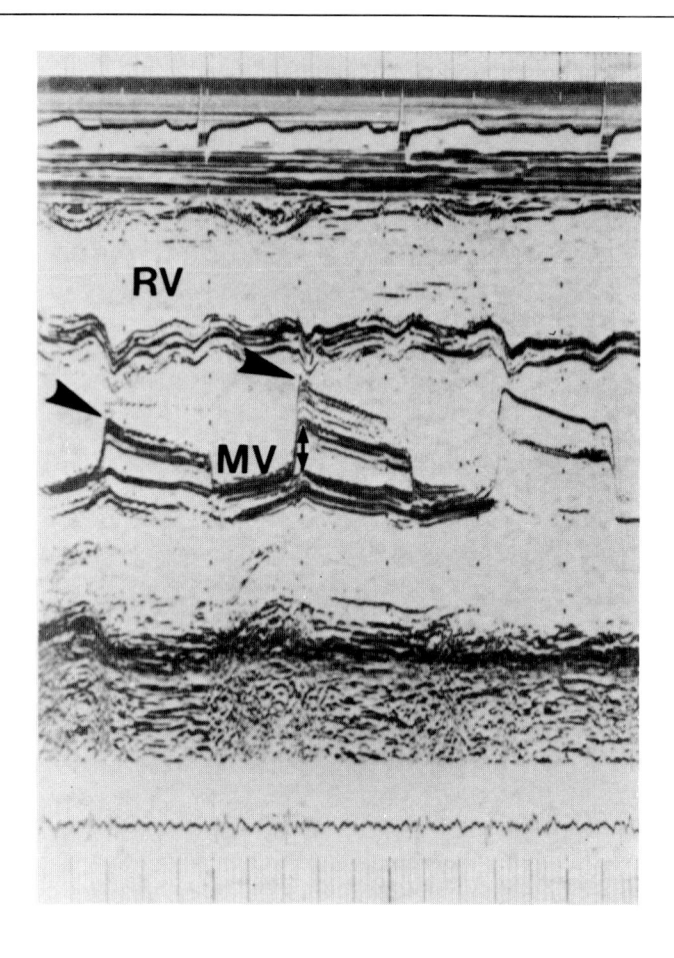

Fig. 2-4. M-mode recording in a patient with mitral stenosis showing abnormal E–F slope, apparent variability in the extent of opening of the anterior mitral leaflet (large arrows), abnormal motion of the posterior mitral leaflet, and reduced separation of anterior and posterior leaflets (small arrow).

Other measurements obtained from the M-mode echocardiogram including the anterior leaflet excursion measured by the D–E amplitude, the separation of the anterior and posterior leaflets, the proximity of the anterior leaflet to the left side of the ventricular septum, and the left atrial size have all been unreliable indicators of the severity of mitral stenosis [17, 19, 20] (Fig. 2-4). A very good correlation has been observed between flow in the first third of diastole and the E–F slope, which indicates that mitral early diastolic closure is primarily a function of ventricular filling [20]. Rarely patients with hypertrophic cardiomyopathy may have inflow obstruction that produces abnormal motion of the anterior mitral leaflet as recorded by M-mode echo as well as apical diastolic murmur with third sound gallop that may simulate an opening snap with resultant mimicking of mitral stenosis [21] (Fig. 2-5). Recognition of normal posterior leaflet motion in such patients has been an important feature in distinguishing between these two conditions. Although it is generally well recognized that the posterior leaflet motion is not only more sensitive but also more specific than anterior leaflet motion in diagnosing rheumatic mitral stenosis, slightly superior positioning of the M-mode transducer along the left sternal border with minimal inferior angulation as the beam intersects the leaflet tips may record the initial diastolic movement of the posterior leaflet in a slightly posterior direction [22]. The limitation of being able to view the abnormal posterior leaflet motion in only a single dimension has been one of the explanations

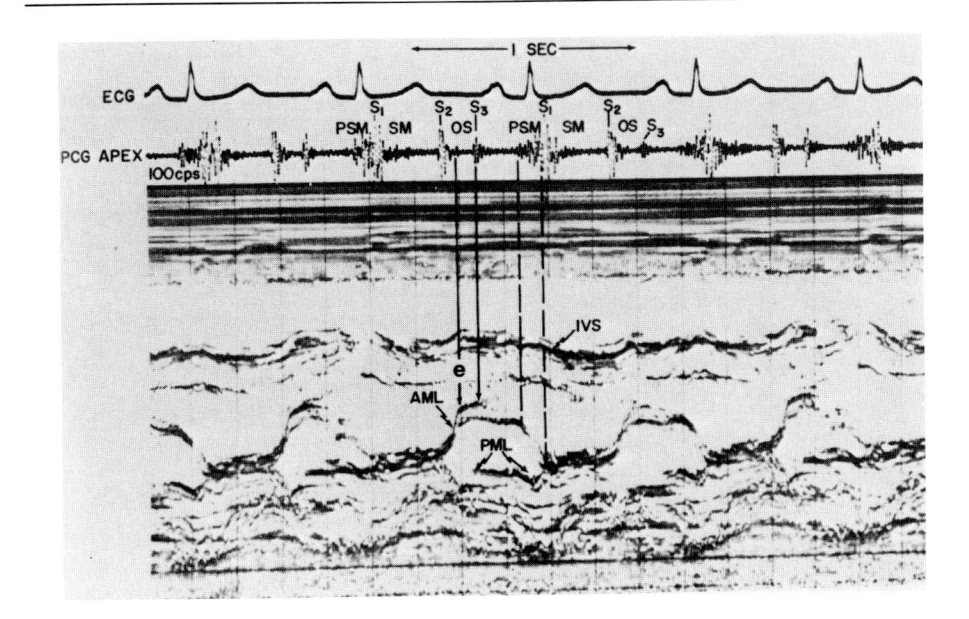

Fig. 2-5. M-mode echocardiogram with simultaneous phonocardiogram showing murmurs and third sound gallop simulating an opening snap and mimicking mitral stenosis. The normal motion of the posterior mitral leaflet excludes the presence of mitral stenosis. E = point of maximal opening of AML at onset of diastole; OS = opening snap; PSM = presystolic murmur; SM = systolic murmur. (From MR Smith et al: Nonobstructive hypertrophic cardiomyopathy mimicking mitral stenosis: Documentation by echocardiography, phonocardiography and intracardiac pressure and sound recordings. Am J Cardiol 35:89, 1975.)

for so-called false negatives or "normal" posterior leaflet movement in the presence of documented mitral stenosis. We have demonstrated that a posterior motion of the posterior leaflet recorded on M-mode in occasional patients with mild mitral stenosis has occurred as a result of this *inferior* motion caused by the pulling effect of the abnormal chordae tendineae on the rheumatic valve. This initial opening movement can be appreciated only with two-dimensional imaging displaying simultaneous anterior–posterior as well as inferior–superior dimensions. Careful observation of the posterior leaflet on the M-mode echocardiogram to detect absent motion or slight anterior movement with atrial contraction is another very sensitive way of identifying truly abnormal movement of the posterior leaflet due to rheumatic mitral disease (Fig. 2-6). In other words, the identification of subtle motion features together with precise phonocardiographic and electrocardiographic timing remains a function of M-mode echocardiography.

Observation of the anterior leaflet excursion and measurement of the E–F slope are quite dependent upon technique and upon the angle of the beam intersecting the mitral valve. Accordingly these quantitative measurements have little clinical significance and may contribute misleading information in the overall M-mode echocardiographic assessment of rheumatic mitral stenosis.

Numerous conditions that cause an abnormal M-mode recording of the mitral valve have been reported in the literature; however, these conditions are unrelated to any intrinsic disease of the valve. These nonindications can be summarized in five general categories [23]:

1. Technical reasons (equipment malfunction or improper transducer placement)
2. Conduction disturbances and arrhythmias (atrial or ventricular arrhythmias, first-degree, second-degree, or third-degree atrioventricular block)
3. Extra-cardiac causes (pericardial effusion or extra-cardiac tumor displacement)
4. Right heart abnormalities (pulmonary hypertension, right ventricular volume overload, Ebstein's malformation)

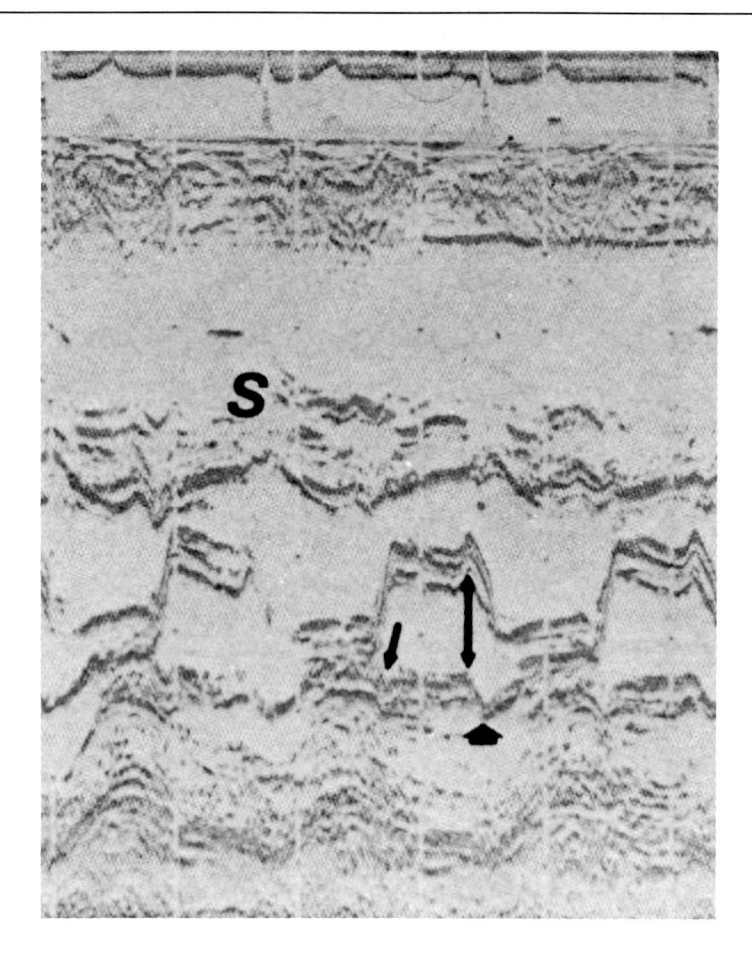

Fig. 2-6. M-mode recording in a patient with mitral stenosis evidenced by abnormal posterior leaflet motion. Double-headed arrow pointing to the "A" wave of anterior leaflet shows the flat posterior leaflet motion; the later posterior motion of the posterior mitral leaflet (wide arrow) is due to annular movement as the mitral valve closes; this delayed motion should not be confused with normal posterior leaflet motion caused by atrial contraction. In addition, the initial opening motion (arrow) of the posterior leaflet is restricted. S = septum. (From AD Hagan: Correlates of M-mode and 2-D echocardiography to evaluate the mitral valve. CVP 8:37, 1980.)

5. Left heart diseases (hypertrophic, hypertensive, or congestive cardiomyopathies; coronary artery disease; aortic valve disease)

It must be remembered that many of the limitations previously discussed with respect to the diagnostic accuracy and reliability of determining severity of rheumatic mitral disease are related to the single-dimensional, M-mode technique used by itself and not in conjunction with other available information. When this technique is incorporated with two-dimensional imaging there is the distinct advantage of obtaining M-mode records with a movable cursor positioned through the structures in the precise location the echocardiographer desires to record. The mitral valve motion is quite easy to record in most patients even without simultaneous two-dimensional, real-time imaging. However, the operator, in attempting to obtain the best quality record, usually directs the beam through the body of the anterior leaflet, where continuous reflectances are obtained as a result of the leaflet's being more perpendicular to the angle of the intersecting echo beam. Very often, however, this does not result in the beam's being directed precisely through the leaflet tips and, furthermore, it may not be possible to distinguish a reflectance coming from a chordal structure or from a leaflet tip without simultaneous imaging with a two-dimensional imaging system. With appropriate parasternal left ventricular long axis imaging, the anterior and posterior mitral leaflets can be profiled to show chordal attachments to the free edge of the leaflets, and by directing the M-mode beam precisely through the leaflet tips the operator can obtain a much more reliable assessment of leaflet tip separation (Fig. 2-7). Furthermore, the qualitative assessment of leaflet thickness of anterior and posterior mitral leaflets can be improved by careful adjustment of gain settings, transducer angulation, and beam rotation to ensure the proper tomographic plane for imaging of the mitral valve. It is also quite easy with 2-D echo to distinguish abnormal reflectances of the mitral annulus from the posterior leaflet.

The area of the mitral valve orifice can be reliably measured by two-dimensional echocardiography; obtaining this measurement is potentially the most accurate method of quantitating mitral stenosis [19, 24–27]. These studies have demonstrated that if proper technique is employed planimetry of the mitral valve orifice from two-dimensional echocardiography correlates closely with those measurements calculated from cardiac catheterization data or measured at the time of surgery. However, the quality and reliability of measurements from the 2-D echo depend heavily on correct technique and operator skill. After obtaining a parasternal short axis image, the operator must angle the transducer precisely through the leaflet tips (Fig. 2-8). To ensure sufficient views of the valve orifice it is important for the operator to sweep from the body of the leaflet inferiorly to the chordae tendineae and back through the leaflet tips while maintaining constant imaging of the medial and lateral commissures and proper gain settings on the equipment. When gain settings are set too low image dropout occurs, contributing to a falsely large valve orifice image. Another technical error that may contribute to underestimating the severity of the stenosis is imaging through the body of the leaflet or through the domed portion rather than through the leaflet tips. If receiver gain settings are too high this will lead to image saturation and a falsely narrowed-appearing orifice [27]. In addition to careful imaging in the parasternal short axis position through the leaflet tips, good parasternal long axis views are helpful to estimate the extent of leaflet tip separation, the relative degree of leaflet thickness, and the amount of anterior leaflet doming. Attention to these details will enable the echocardiographer to determine the exact location for making planimetry measurements in the short axis view.

The noninvasive nature of two-dimensional echocardiography makes it particularly well suited to serial evaluation of re-stenosis in patients who have undergone mitral valve commissurotomies or reconstructive surgery. Heger and associates [28] reported in a long-term follow-up study of mitral commissurotomy that cardiac symptoms were associated with severity of mitral stenosis but did not predict re-stenosis.

In our experience from the Philippine Heart Center for Asia, from a total of 1320 rheumatic heart disease patients between the ages of 14 and 72 years who underwent cardiac catheterization in anticipation for surgery, a total of 241 patients (18%) with isolated pure mitral stenosis were identified [29]. There were 161 females and 80 males in this group. Mitral stenosis plus mitral regurgitation was found in 143 patients (11%) with 98 females and 45 males and a female-to-male ratio of 2:1. Interestingly, mitral stenosis occurred more frequently with aortic regurgitation (194 [15%] with 107 females and 87 males) than with mitral regurgitation. Pure aortic insufficiency was found in 103 (8%) patients with 36 females and 67 males

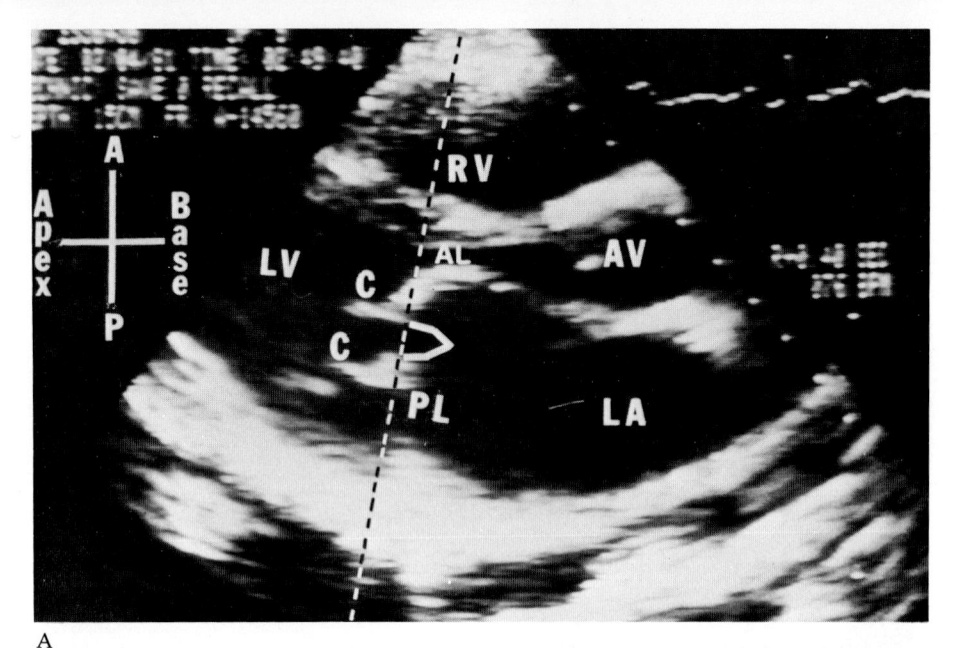

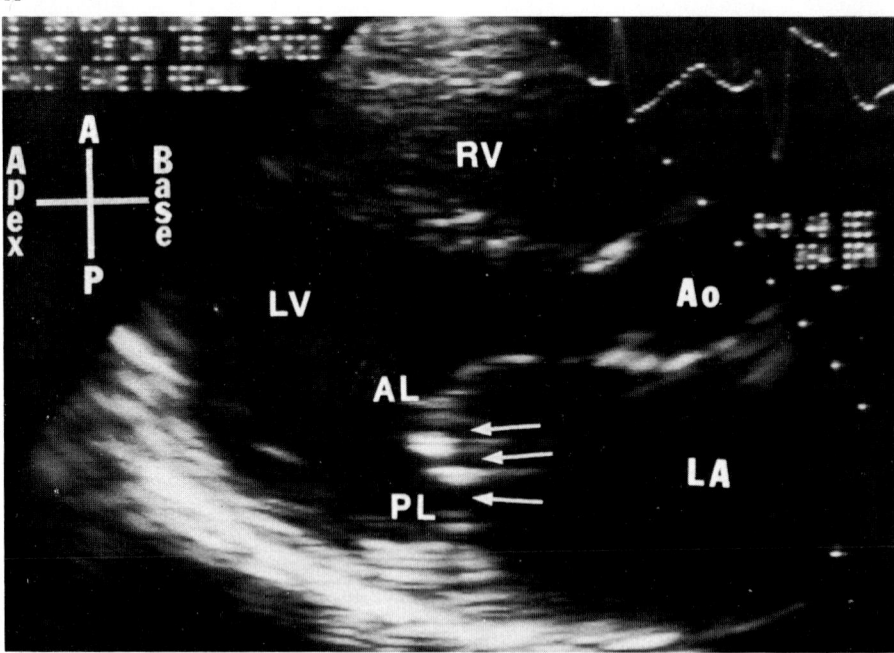

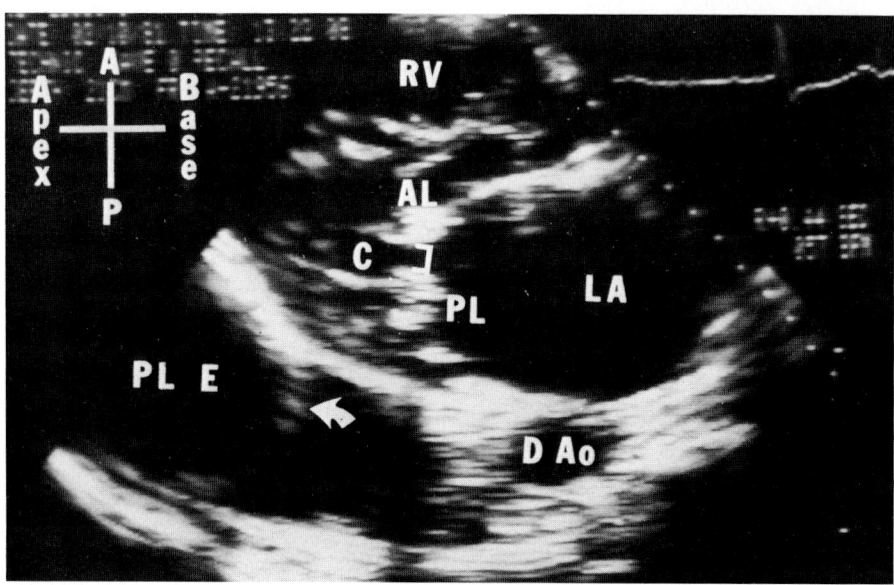

Fig. 2-7A. Parasternal long axis view in a patient with mitral stenosis. The dashed line simulates the correct positioning of an M-mode cursor for proper recording of leaflet separation. The tips of both anterior mitral leaflet and posterior mitral leaflet are thickened. The AL demonstrates considerable doming, commonly seen in rheumatic mitral stenosis in the absence of valve calcification; the proximal portion of the AL is normal in thickness. Depending on the extent of involvement, the chordae tendineae (C) will show varying degrees of thickness in the parasternal and apical long axis imaging views. The extent of leaflet-tip separation (bracket) is beneficial in identifying the true orifice in the parasternal short axis plane of the mitral valve. The left atrium is mildly enlarged. B. Parasternal long axis view in a patient with significant mitral stenosis and doming of the AL. When the separation of the leaflet tips is small, care must be taken to avoid confusing intermittent echo dropout of either AL (top arrow) or PL (bottom arrow) with the actual leaflet tip separation (middle arrow). C. Parasternal long axis view in a patient with severe mitral stenosis, markedly increased thickening of tips of both AL and PL, no apparent doming of AL, and severe restriction of leaflet motion with maximum tip separation measuring only 6 to 7 mm (bracket). There is marked LA enlargement and a large pleural effusion (PL E). Linear echo reflections (arrow) or strands of tissue probably represent pleural adhesions.

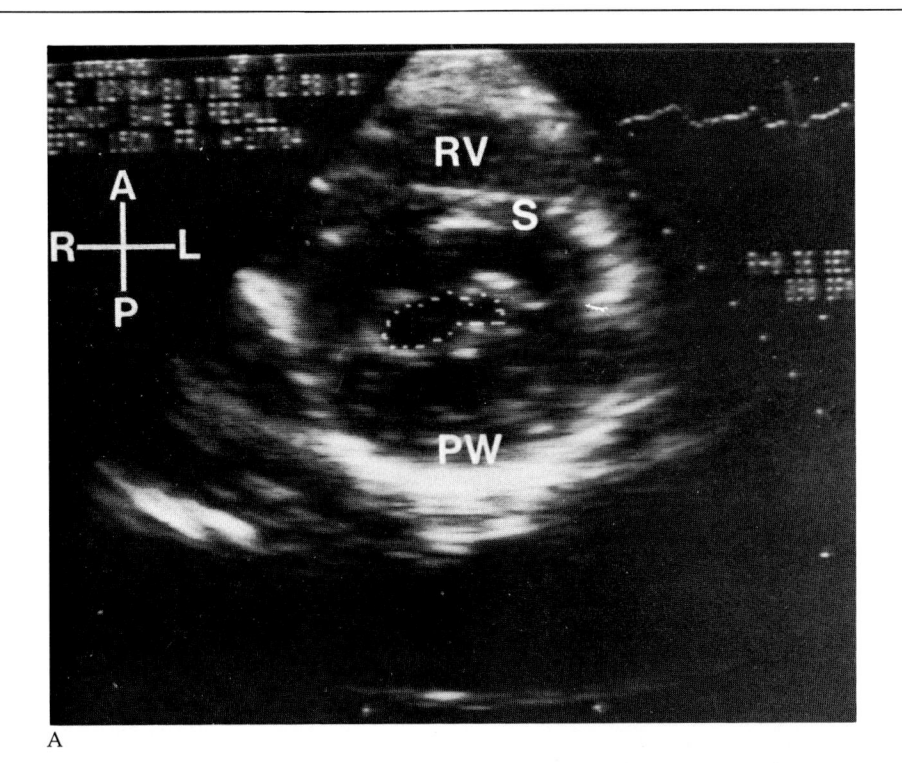

Fig. 2-8A. Parasternal short axis view through the tips of the mitral leaflets demonstrating the technique for determining mitral valve area; the dotted line outlines the valve orifice. Assessment of leaflet tip separation in the parasternal long axis view is helpful as a rough guide to judge whether the parasternal short axis image is precisely through leaflet tips. Planimetry of the valve area is performed at the onset of diastole when the orifice appears the largest. B. Parasternal short axis view during systole in a patient with mitral stenosis showing the thickened leaflet tips coapted (arrow). S = septum.

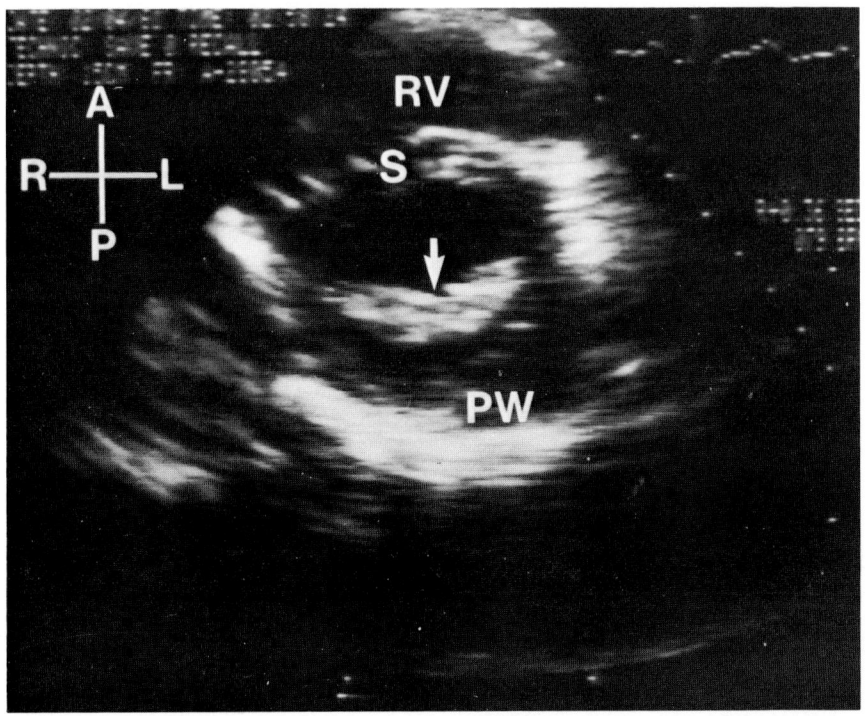

and a reversed sex ratio compared to that for mitral stenosis. A group of 39 patients with mitral stenosis who underwent cardiac catheterization and mitral valve surgery were evaluated to determine the accuracy of assessing mitral valve area by two-dimensional echocardiography compared to measurements obtained at catheterization and surgery. Although the variability in the three different measurement techniques was not statistically significant, the mean value derived by 2-D echo (0.67 cm^2) was closer to that measurement obtained at surgery (0.65 cm^2) than at cardiac catheterization (0.70 cm^2).

A variety of qualitative changes can be assessed with two-dimensional imaging in patients with rheumatic mitral stenosis:

1. Atrialization of the ventricular inflow tract due to ballooning of the anterior and posterior leaflets into the ventricle in diastole
2. Increased thickness of the free margins and leaflet tips compared to the body and more proximal portions of the leaflets
3. Characteristic doming motion of the anterior mitral leaflet associated with the restricted excursion of the leaflet tip
4. Relative fixation of the posterior leaflet that at times is viewed to have little or no diastolic motion, occasionally slight inferior-apical movement, or an anterior movement
5. Increased reflectance due to thickening and fusion of the chordae tendineae
6. Fusion of the commissures contributing to further narrowing of the orifice and reduction of leaflet tip separation
7. Diffuse increased thickness of the leaflets with little or absent doming of the anterior leaflet and presence of calcification
8. Subvalvular fibrosis and/or calcification of the posterior portion of the mitral annulus
9. Enlargement of the left atrium
10. Presence or absence of right heart manifestations of pulmonary hypertension

PATHOLOGICAL FEATURES OF DIFFERENT STAGES AND SEVERITY OF RHEUMATIC VALVULAR DISEASE. In the early phases of rheumatic valvular involvement, the most conspicuous lesion consists of minute translucent nodules (verrucae) located along the lines of closure or contact of leaflets or cusps (Fig. 2-9). They are usually located on the atrial surface of the atrioventricular valves and on the ventricular surface of the aortic and pulmonic valves. These verrucae consist of platelet and fibrin aggregates on exposed collagen or damaged endocardial tissue. Their predilection for lines of closure of leaflets or cusps is related to the fact that endothelial damage is most likely at these sites. Later these nodules develop into opaque red-gray or tawny masses that are firmly adherent to the leaflets. Occasionally they may occur on chordae tendineae of the mitral and tricuspid valves and are usually found on the corpora arantii of the aortic valve cusps. In the early phase of valvular involvement, the atrial surface of the atrioventricular valves may show small vessels, indicating vascularization as part of the inflammatory process. Initially this vascular proliferation consists of thin-walled capillary channels; however, thick-walled muscular elastic vessels may appear after six weeks [15].

In recurrent rheumatic valvulitis the gross changes observed during the acute phase are accentuated. The valve surfaces become thickened and irregular, and grossly visible vascularizations are present. The thickening is most severe in the

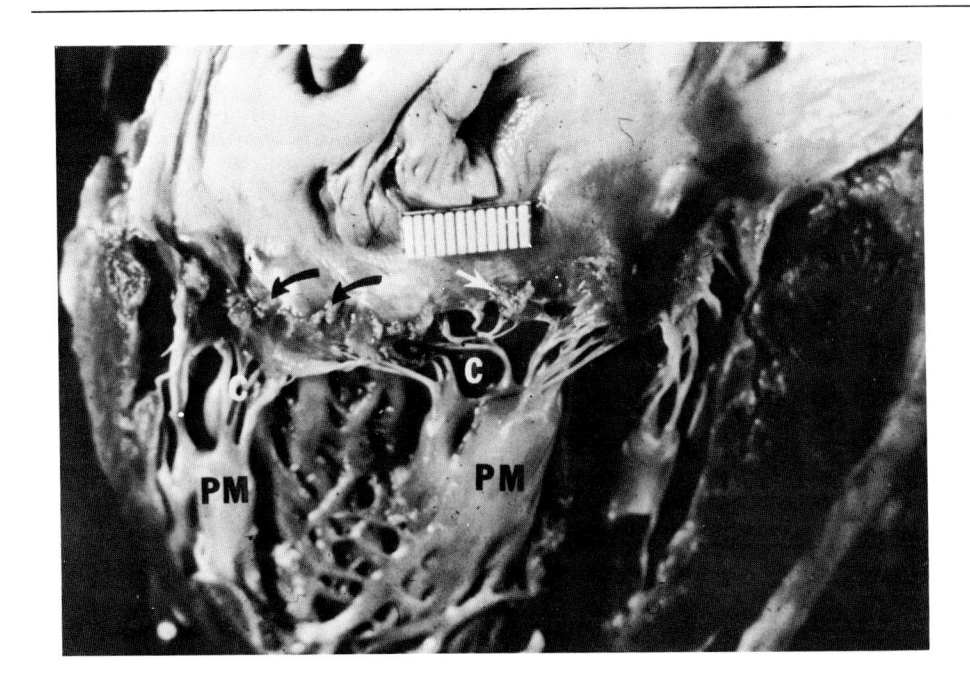

Fig. 2-9. Verrucae lesions (arrows) *due to acute rheumatic valvulitis are located along the margins or tips of the mitral valve. The chordae tendineae* (C) *are normal.*

distal third of the valve leaflets (Fig. 2-10). This thickening of the mitral valve may extend to involve insertions of the chordae tendineae, which become thickened and shortened, thus bringing the papillary muscle closer to the leaflet margins. Adjacent thickened chordae tendineae may also fuse, particularly near their insertion into the leaflet. Newly formed verrucae are superimposed on the ridge of old verrucae at the lines of closure. When the aortic valve is involved in this process, the free margins become rolled and inverted toward the pocket of the sinuses of Valsalva (Fig. 2-11). Adhesions and verrucae may be present on the aortic cusp near the commissure, and the commissures may eventually fuse [5].

In chronic rheumatic valvulitis the changes resemble those described in recurrent valvulitis except that they are at a more advanced stage of thickening and fibrosis (Fig. 2-12). There is a loss of elasticity, narrowing of the valve orifice, and fusion of the commissures, which leads to progressive stenosis of the involved valve. When the involvement is severe, retraction and curling of the margins of the valve leaflets may create a degree of regurgitation in combination with stenosis. When thickening, shortening, and fusion of the chordae tendineae are severe, the papillary muscles may come in direct contact with the margins of the valve leaflets. Fibrous adhesions may extend from the valve leaflets to the ventricular wall. The subvalvular angles are thickened and prominent in the regions of the valve annulus. Eventual calcium deposition frequently occurs, further distorting the valve leaflets. When the aortic valve is involved, calcification is usually present in the region of the corpora arantii and in the commissures that have become fused. Verrucae are less common in chronic valvulitis than in recurrent valvulitis and when present are broad and flat [5].

Mitral stenoses can be grouped anatomically into four types: commissural, cuspal, chordal, and combined. Stenosis may result from thickening, rigidity, and fusion of the commissures alone (31%); from rigidity to the cusp alone (15%); from

60   2. Rheumatic valvular disease

Fig. 2-10A. Recurrent rheumatic mitral valvulitis showing thickened fusion of some of the chordae tendineae (arrows). *B. Recurrent rheumatic valvulitis showing marked thickening of leaflet margin* (solid arrow) *as well as increased thickness and fusion of chordae tendineae* (open arrow).

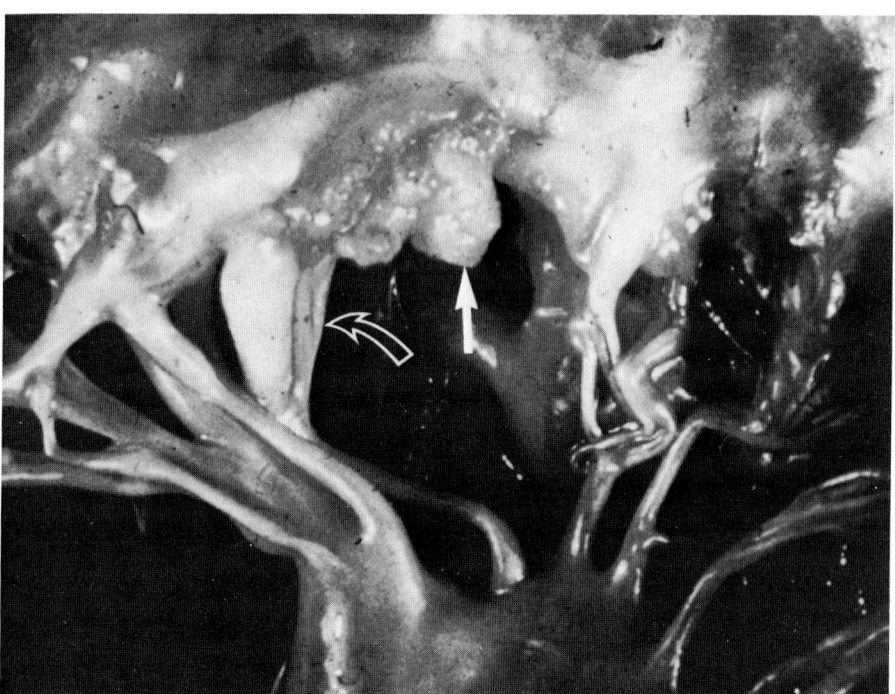

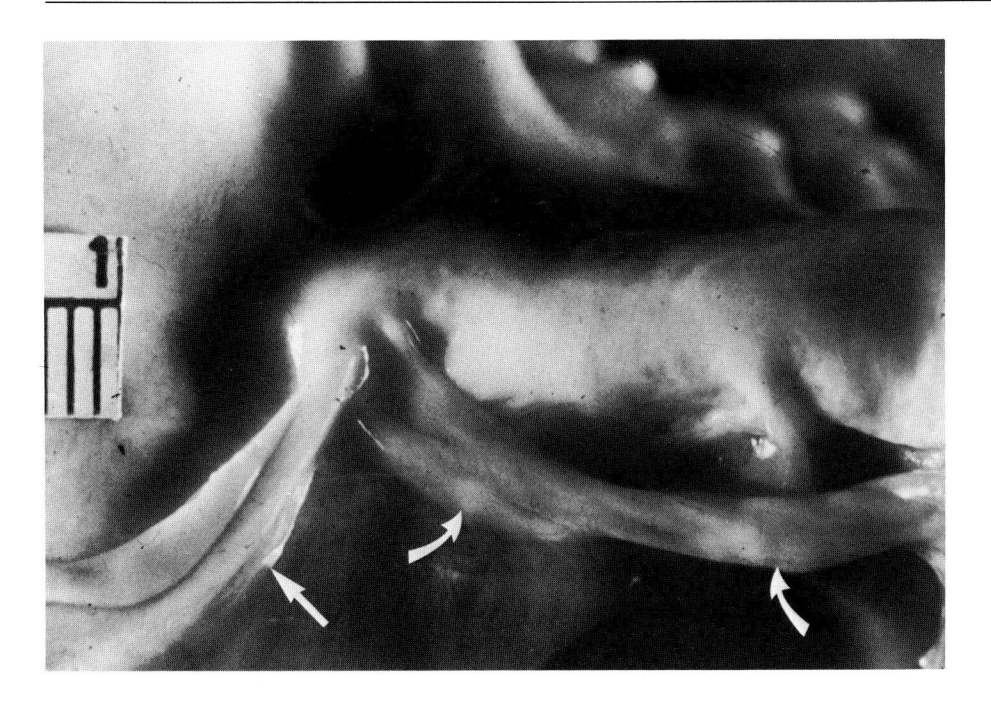

Fig. 2-11. Close-up view of two aortic cusps showing thickened free margins (arrows).

shortening and fusion of the chordae tendineae alone, which restricts the valve orifice (9%); and from combined anatomical features (45%). When viewed from the left atrium, the mitral valve has a characteristic funnel shape, with the walls of the funnel being formed by the fused leaflets and the tapering being caused by the shortened chordae tendineae. The mitral orifice is narrow and commonly appears to be "fishmouthed." In vivo the funnel shape can best be visualized with two-dimensional echocardiographic imaging in the parasternal left ventricular long axis plane; the fishmouth orifice is best seen in the parasternal short axis view with the sector beam directed through the tips of the leaflets. Calcification may involve the annulus or erode the endocardium and become exposed to the blood flow. On rare occasions calcification has eroded through to the posterior wall of the heart. Usually the posterior mitral leaflet is predominantly involved when mitral regurgitation is present. Another feature specifically related to severe mitral regurgitation is focal thickenings of the endocardium or cusplike lesions (accessory valves) along the posterior wall of the left atrium resulting from regurgitant blood flow striking the endocardium at these points (Fig. 2-13) [5].

The variable anatomic findings described above can be imaged with 2-D echocardiography and divided into four different groups reflecting different anatomic features or degrees of severity of rheumatic mitral involvement. In order to establish the severity of the stenosis, the area of the valve orifice must be measured and an evaluation made for the presence or severity of pulmonary hypertension. Given complete imaging, the experienced echocardiographer can describe the mitral involvement as follows:

1. Mitral stenosis with doming of the anterior mitral leaflet but no evidence of significant chordal abnormality or leaflet calcification
2. Mitral stenosis with doming of the anterior mitral leaflet and increased reflectance consistent with thickening of the chordae tendineae and leaflet edges; probably no calcification in the valve

62   2. Rheumatic valvular disease

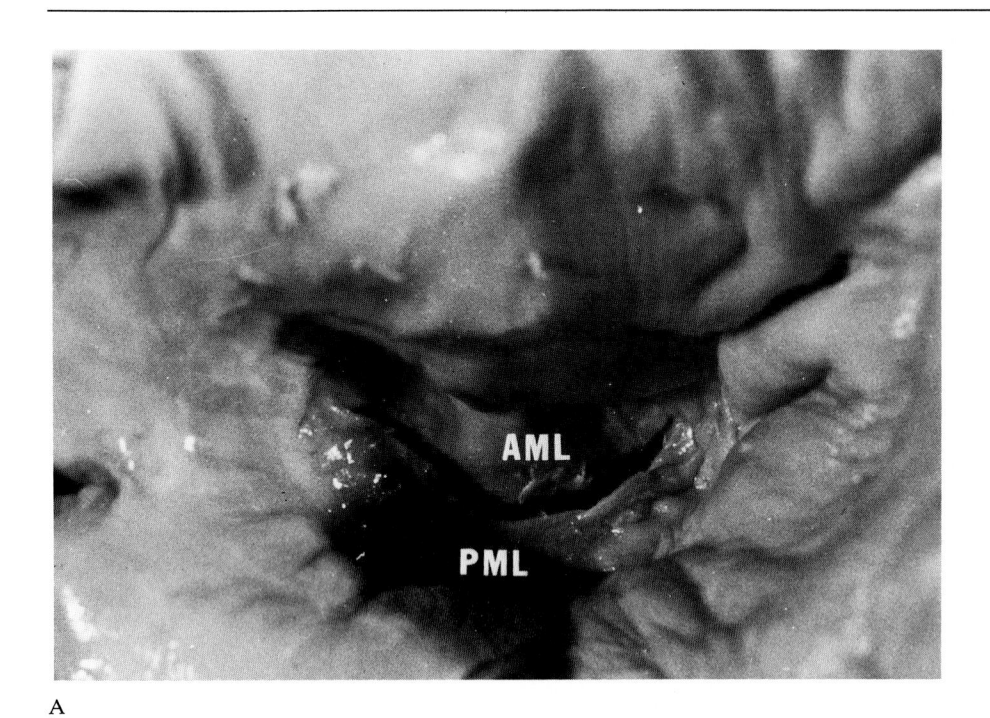

Fig. 2-12A. Chronic rheumatic valvulitis viewed from the left atrium. Both anterior and posterior mitral leaflets are markedly thickened and the commissures are fused. B. Chronic rheumatic valvulitis viewed from the left ventricle showing the mitral valve and marked thickening, fusion, and shortening of chordae tendineae (C).

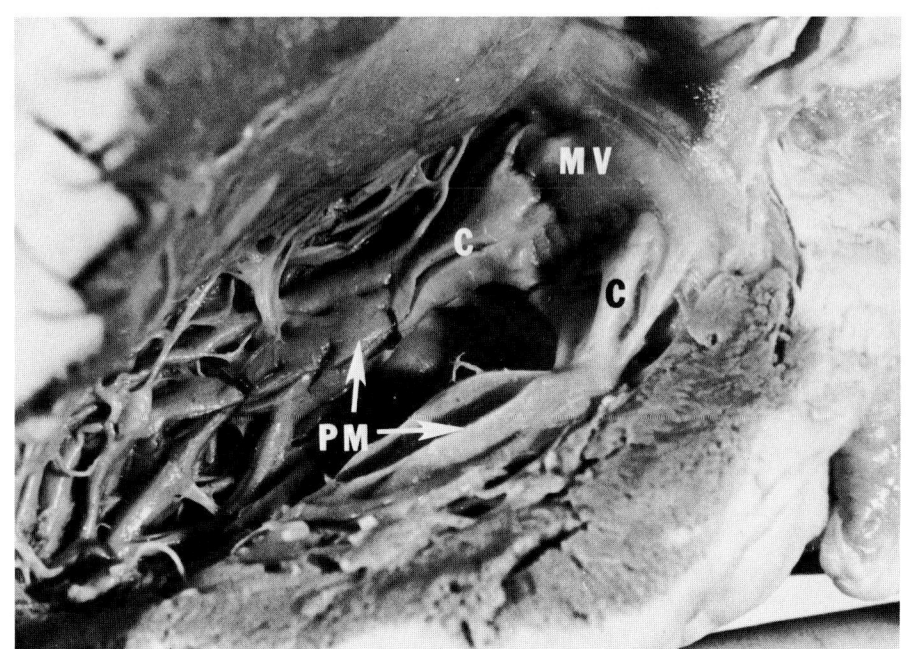

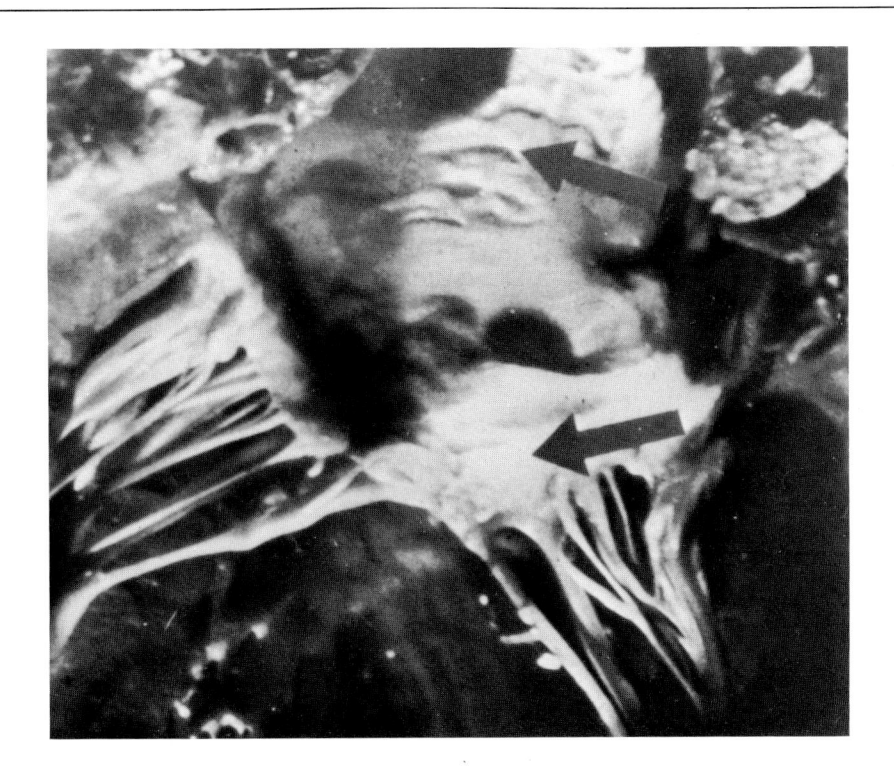

Fig. 2-13. Focal thickenings or cusplike ridges (upper arrow) situated on the posterior wall of the left atrium are caused by the regurgitant blood flow striking the left atrial wall. The lower arrow points to the mitral leaflet.

3. Mitral stenosis with minimal doming of the anterior mitral leaflet, increased thickening of the chordae tendineae and the leaflets; findings consistent with calcification of anterior and/or posterior leaflets
4. Mitral stenosis with severe reduction of anterior leaflet mobility and no apparent doming; marked increase in thickness of chordae and leaflets consistent with prominent calcification and marked deformities of the valve

Interpretative information of rheumatic mitral disease should always include mitral valve area as determined by planimetry of the valve orifice obtained in the parasternal short axis imaging. We recommend obtaining several views of the mitral valve orifice to select the best frames for planimetry as the leaflet tips are separated widest at the onset of diastole. We recommend averaging the areas obtained from 4 to 5 different beats. Another method of estimating valve area (MVA) is to express the area in terms of degree of stenosis:

1. Minimal degree: MVA $\geq$ 2.5 cm^2
2. Mild degree: MVA = 2.0 to 2.4 cm^2
3. Mild-moderate degree: MVA = 1.5 to 1.9 cm^2
4. Moderate degree: MVA = 1.0 to 1.4 cm^2
5. Severe degree: MVA = 0.5 to 0.9 cm^2
6. Extremely severe degree: MVA < 0.5 cm^2

If technically adequate images of the orifice at the leaflet tips are unobtainable, planimetry should not be attempted. When patients have heavy calcification of both leaflets together with marked thickening of the chordae tendineae it is not uncommon to have difficulty in determining the exact mitral orifice because of the highly reflected targets. Under these circumstances it is often academic to attempt planimetry of the orifice because other available information in assessing the patient is adequate to determine the clinical severity of the mitral valve disease (Fig. 2-14).

Two-dimensional echocardiographic imaging is usually not very specific in identifying or quantifying mitral regurgitation in the presence of rheumatic mitral disease. No M-mode or 2-D echo features are sufficiently sensitive or specific to be reliable in identifying or estimating the severity of mitral regurgitation in the presence of rheumatic mitral stenosis. Wann and associates [30] have reported that it is possible to recognize mitral regurgitation in the presence of mitral stenosis by incomplete leaflet closure and resultant separation between the anterior and posterior leaflets observed in the parasternal short axis view. This technique has not been very reliable in our hands in identifying mitral regurgitation because of frequent occurrences of echo dropout that simulate lack of leaflet closure; in this view dropout may be secondary to imaging technique, the rocking motion of the beating heart, and overall gain settings. Other anatomic clues obtained from two-dimensional imaging that suggest the presence of mitral regurgitation in patients with rheumatic mitral stenosis include

1. An obvious flail or prolapsing valve leaflet
2. The unusual occurrence of abnormal leaflet coaptation as observed in the parasternal long axis view with the tip of one leaflet sliding posterosuperiorly to the other leaflet tip (Fig. 2-15A, B, C, D)
3. Greater left atrial enlargement and/or associated findings of pulmonary hypertension with a larger mitral valve area than would be expected to produce such secondary abnormalities with only mitral stenosis
4. Evidence of left ventricular dilatation together with hyperdynamic motion of the left ventricle in the absence of aortic regurgitation
5. Systolic bulging of left atrial posterior wall and/or prominent rightward bulging with or without "fluttering" motion of the interatrial septum (Fig. 2-15E)

Doppler echocardiography is more sensitive for identifying a mild degree of mitral regurgitation than M-mode or 2-D echo in patients with rheumatic valve disease. Of course, the presence of mitral regurgitation should already be known to the echocardiographer from cardiac physical examination previous to the 2-D echo examination. The severity of mitral regurgitation is still best ascertained by left ventricular angiography.

Atrialization of the inflow tract of the left ventricle is the hallmark of mitral stenosis. The mitral valve and chordae tendineae assume a convex, funnel-like position pointing toward the left ventricle. Several factors may contribute to the abnormal convex contour of the valve toward the ventricle during diastole. The chordae tendineae are shortened, the valve orifice is narrowed with the leaflet margins and commissures fused; in addition, the diastolic pressure in the left atrium is elevated, and there may be an associated suction effect of the left ventricle, all of which may play contributing roles. The constant pressure gradient from behind the narrowed mitral orifice and the negative pressure in the left ventricle at the moment of rapid filling in early diastole help to maintain the convexity of the mitral valve. Some studies have stressed the importance of this left ventricular

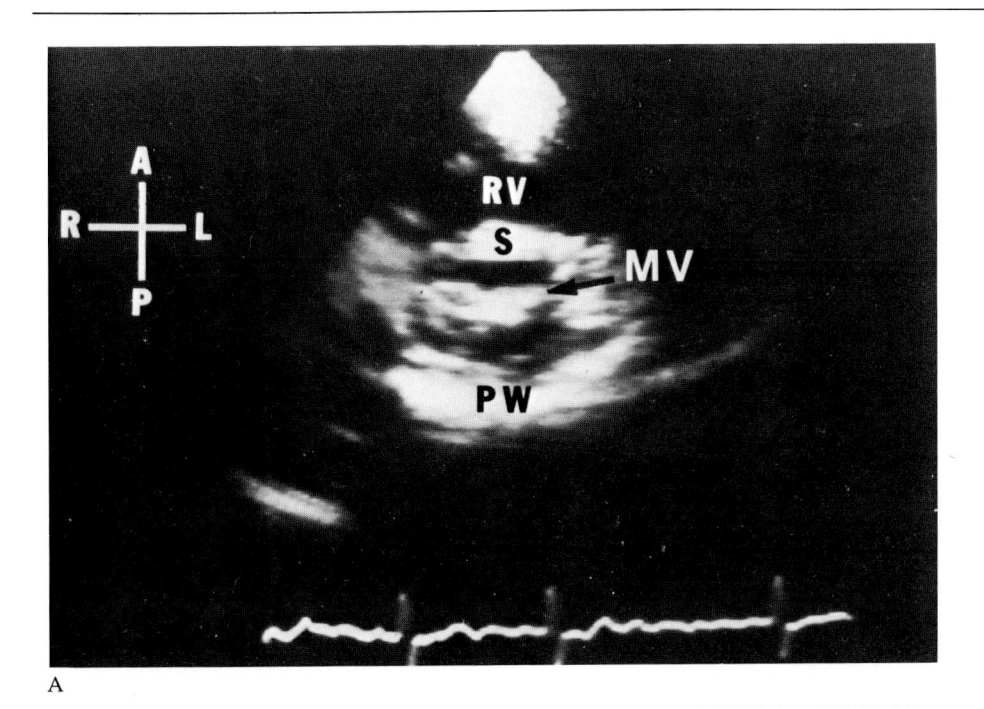

Fig. 2-14A. Parasternal short axis view through the tip of the mitral valve; however, because of marked thickening and calcification the orifice cannot be identified for planimetry. B. Parasternal long axis view showing severely thickened anterior mitral leaflet and left atrial enlargement. PW = posterior wall; S = septum.

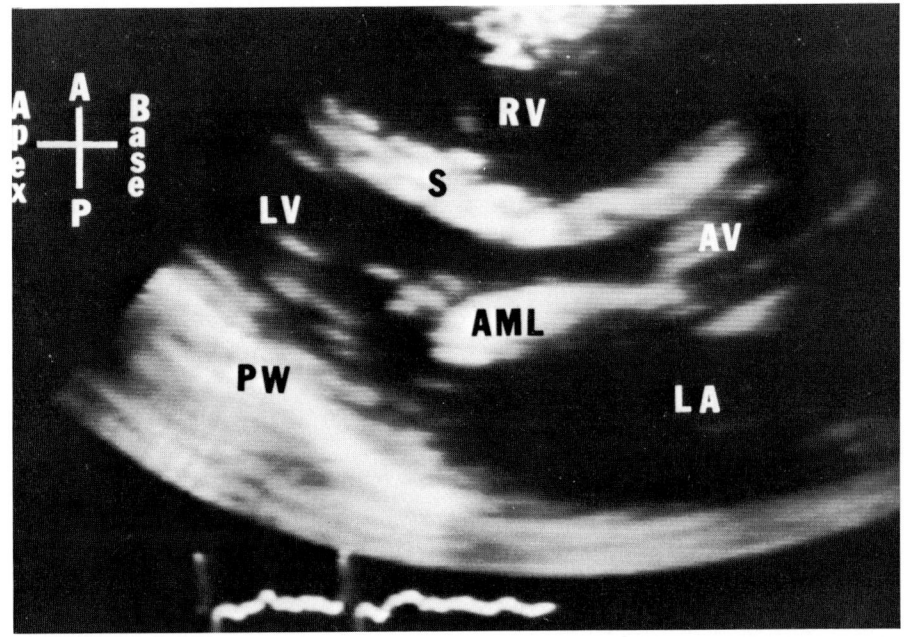

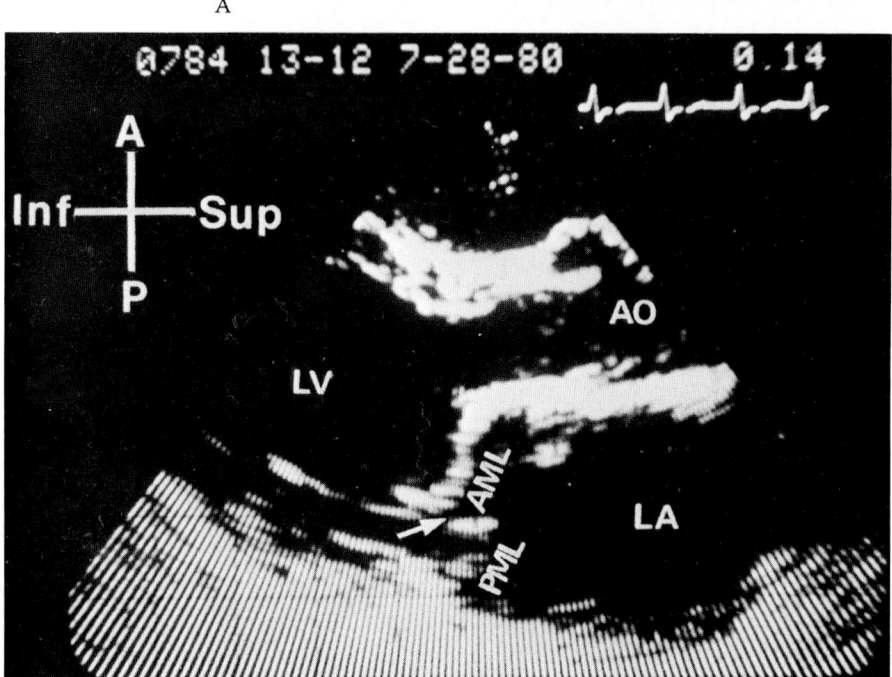

Fig. 2-15A. Parasternal long axis view showing the anterior mitral leaflet sliding past (arrow) the normal coaptation point with the posterior mitral leaflet producing a prolapselike contour. Such a systolic closure abnormality in patients with rheumatic mitral disease is a useful indicator of associated mitral regurgitation. B. Parasternal long axis view in a patient with rheumatic mitral disease and mitral regurgitation showing a more posterosuperior mitral leaflet that contributes to abnormal coaptation of the leaflets (arrow). Left atrial enlargement is present. C. Surgical specimen of mitral valve removed intact at time of valve replacement. Both anterior and posterior mitral leaflets are thickened, and there is mild fusion of the commissures. The leaflets did not coapt normally, causing considerable mitral regurgitation. Because the photograph was taken from the left atrial side, the chordae tendineae are not well visualized. D. Parasternal short axis view through the tips of the mitral leaflets during systole showing a regurgitant orifice (arrow) in a patient with rheumatic mitral disease and mitral regurgitation. E. M-mode recording of the interatrial septum obtained from subcostal position. Both "A" and V waves are easily identified. The V wave (arrow) is abnormally prominent with bulging into right atrium because of mitral regurgitation. Coarse fluttering of the interatrial septum has been observed during systole in patients with flail mitral valve and severe regurgitation. ALC = anterolateral commissure; PMC = posteromedial commissure.

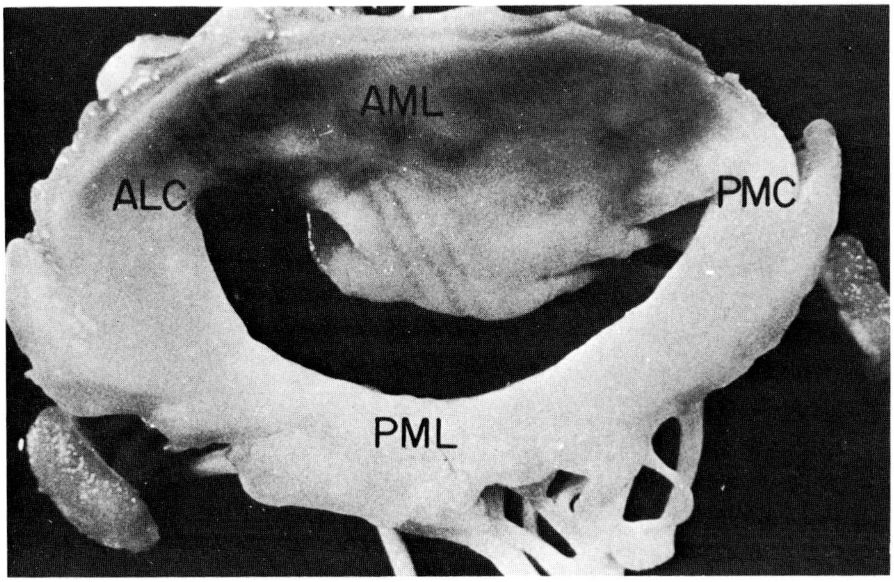

C

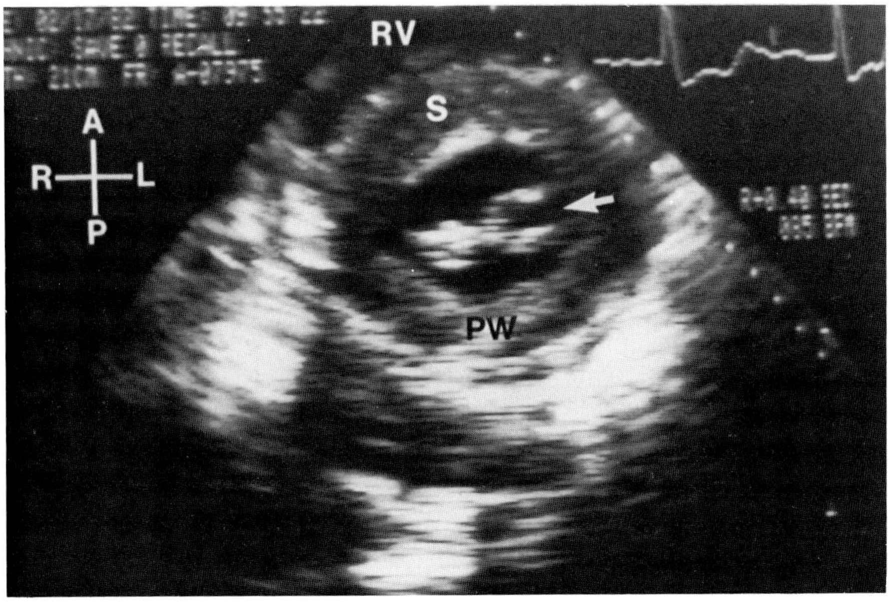

D

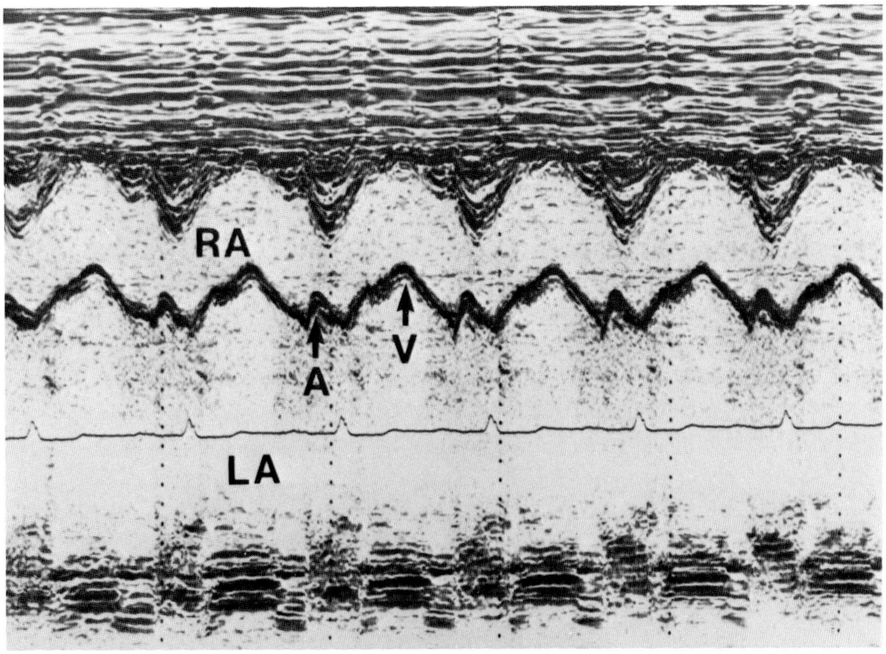

E

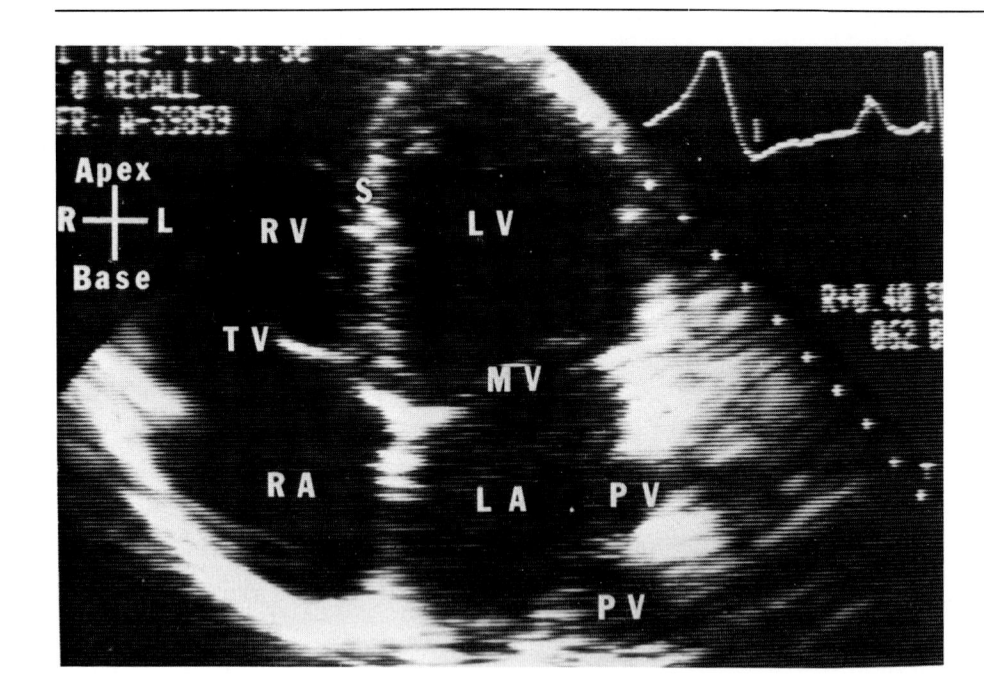

Fig. 2-16. Apical 4-chamber view showing the typical appearance of left atrium, slightly longer in the inferosuperior dimension compared to the right-left dimension. Two or three pulmonary veins (PV) are usually seen entering the LA.

suction effect in driving blood from the left atrium to the left ventricle through a narrow orifice [31, 32]. The role of negative intraventricular diastolic pressure in 55 patients with pure mitral stenosis has been studied in the laboratory by one of the coauthors (H.B.C.). When the mitral valve area was correlated with the negative intraventricular pressure, the negative pressure was found to increase with decreasing valve area.

Depending upon the pliability of the anterior leaflet, varying degrees of systolic bulging or "prolapse" of the body of the leaflet occur. As the anterior leaflet becomes more fibrotic or calcified, diastolic doming is reduced and the systolic bulging or buckling motion is also less apparent or absent. It should be recognized that this motion is simply a manifestation of systolic closure abnormality in the presence of thickened leaflet edges, fused commissures, and a pliable body of the anterior leaflet. This systolic bulging of the body of the anterior leaflet should not be confused with actual prolapse as seen in the presence of myxomatous degeneration of the valve.

Careful visualization of the left atrium in all three dimensions is another important aspect of the 2-D echo examination in a patient with rheumatic mitral disease. Normally the left atrium is somewhat oblong in shape with the anteroposterior and right–left dimensions being approximately equal while the inferosuperior dimension is usually 5 to 15 mm longer than the other two dimensions (Fig. 2-16). In unpublished data involving more than 100 normal subjects we have noted the upper limits of normal in adults to be 40 mm in both the anteroposterior as well as the right–left dimensions. However, depending on the body surface area of adults, the upper limit of normal in the inferosuperior dimension ranges between 40 and 55 mm. The one area of the left atrium that is still difficult to image thoroughly even with two-dimensional imaging is the left atrial appendage. Particular emphasis

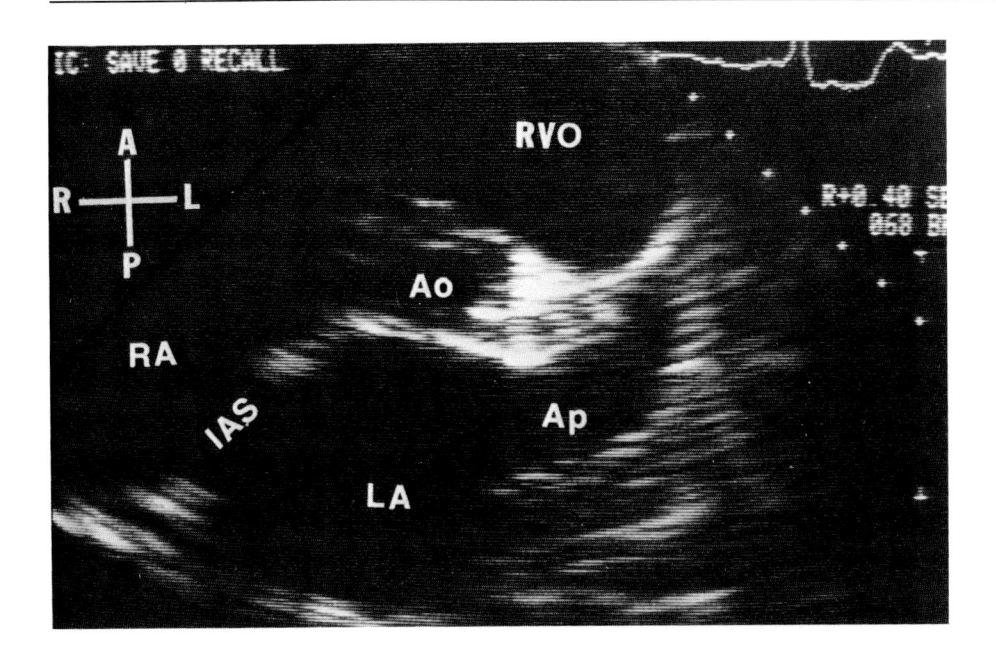

Fig. 2-17. Short axis view at the base with the sector beam directed slightly laterally (leftward) into the left atrial appendage. The patient has rheumatic mitral disease and left atrial enlargement. IAS = interatrial septum.

should be placed on this area, imaging in the parasternal short axis view at the level of the base and with some slight leftward angulation while scanning posteriorly to the aortic annulus near the origin of the right pulmonary artery. The echocardiographer is usually able to image the left atrial appendage; however, it is difficult to determine whether it has been completely visualized. Short axis imaging at the base and good visualization of the left atrial appendage is technically easier when the atrium is dilated in the presence of rheumatic mitral disease (Fig. 2-17). Patients with dilated left atrium and atrial fibrillation are at greater risk for development of left atrial thrombi than those who are in sinus rhythm (Fig. 2-18). Besides atrial fibrillation another contributing factor to the development of left atrial thrombi is reduced cardiac output [33].

Although a limited number of studies have been reported in which 2-D echocardiography was used in the early postoperative period, it appears to be a valuable method not only of assessing adequacy of mitral commissurotomy but also of following patients on a long-term basis for evidence of re-stenosis [29].

The clinical and echocardiographic assessment of rheumatic aortic valve disease will be described in Chapter 4. Pulmonary hypertension secondary to rheumatic mitral disease will be discussed in Chapter 8.

Rheumatic tricuspid disease. The pathological features of rheumatic tricuspid disease are similar to those abnormalities encountered in mitral valve disease, which have been covered earlier in this chapter.

The typical M-mode recording of the tricuspid valve is usually obtained from the anterior tricuspid leaflet (Fig. 2-19). The motion and appearance of the anterior tricuspid leaflet are essentially the same as those recorded from a normal anterior mitral leaflet. It is valuable to employ two-dimensional imaging simultaneously during M-mode recording to ensure that full leaflet excursion of the tricuspid valve

70   2. Rheumatic valvular disease

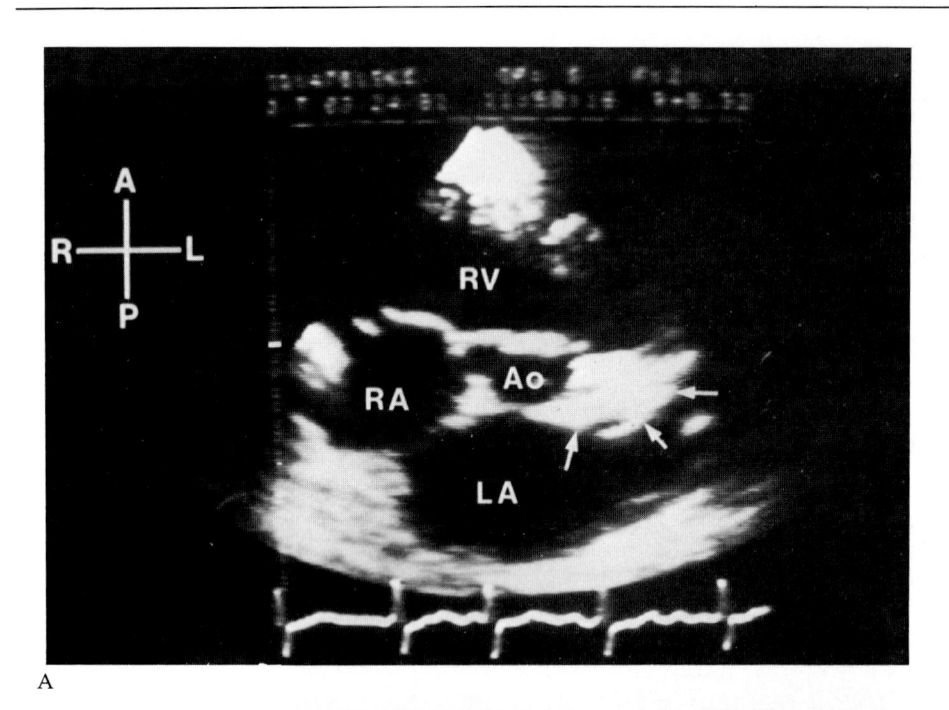

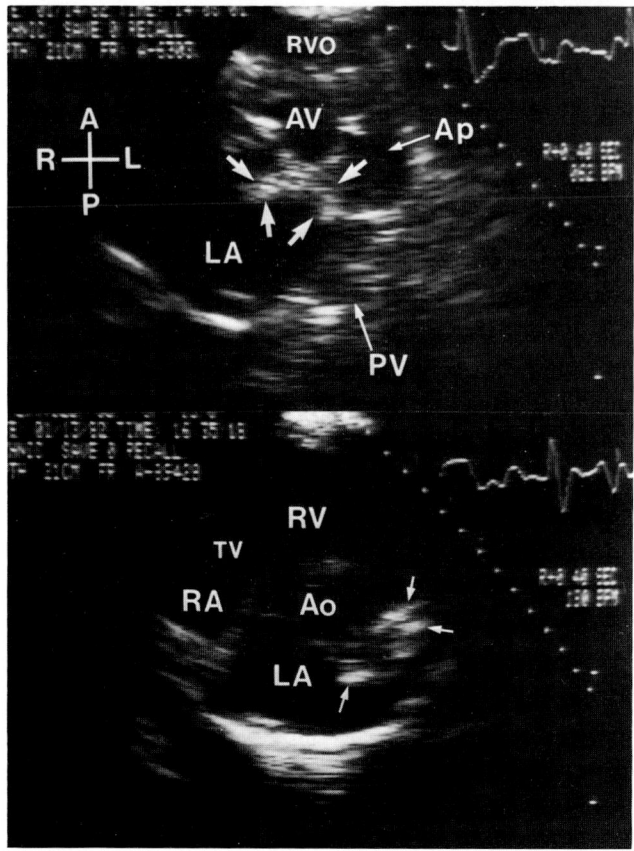

Fig. 2-18A. Parasternal short axis view at the base in an elderly woman with severe mitral stenosis, left atrial enlargement, and a large thrombus (arrows) in the dilated atrial appendage. B. Two different parasternal short axis views at the base in the same patient demonstrating a left atrial thrombus at the opening to the atrial appendage. The upper panel view was obtained with the transducer positioned in the second left intercostal space with lateral angulation showing the thrombus from this angle to appear bilobed (arrows) in configuration. The lower panel shows a slightly different shape of the thrombus (arrows) when the transducer is located at the mid left sternal border and somewhat laterally on the precordium. C. Parasternal oblique long axis view in same patient as in B with the transducer close to left sternal border to show more of the ascending aorta. Orienting the sector beam into an oblique view of the atrial appendage posterior to the aorta reveals yet another tomographic plane of the thrombus (arrows). The sector plane is oblique through the left ventricle showing only a small portion at the base, and mitral valve is not well seen here. The descending aorta posterior to the left atrium is well visualized. D. Parasternal long axis (left panel) and short axis views at the base (right panel) from the same patient with rheumatic mitral disease, atrial fibrillation, left atrial enlargement, and a large thrombus (arrows) adherent to posterior wall of the LA and adjacent to the atrioventricular sulcus near the origin of the posterior mitral leaflet. PV = pulmonic vein.

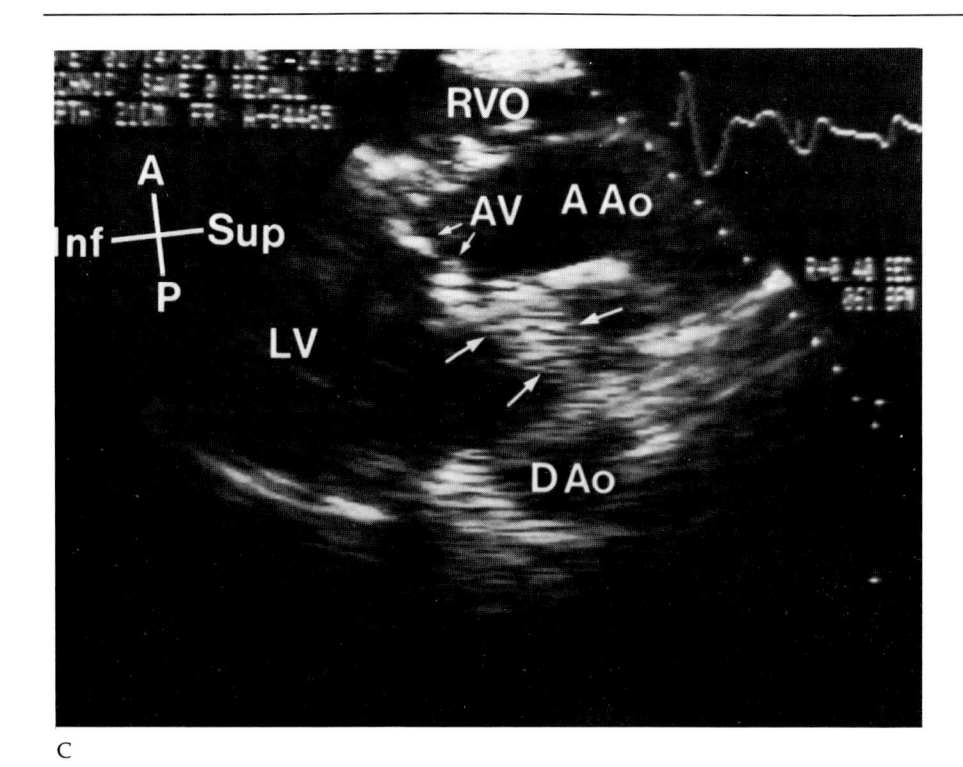

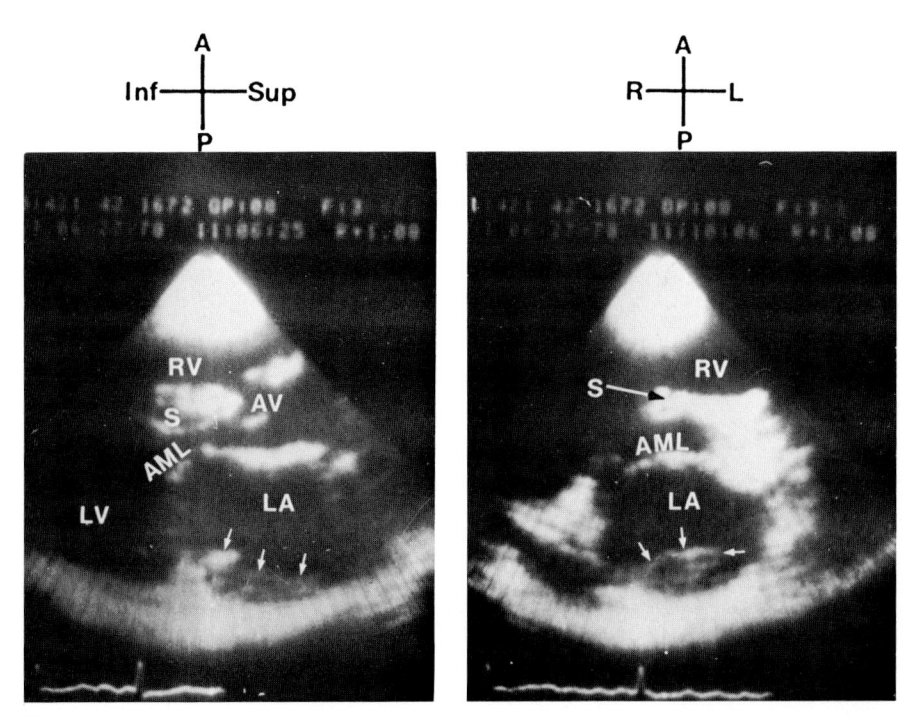

C

D

72   2. Rheumatic valvular disease

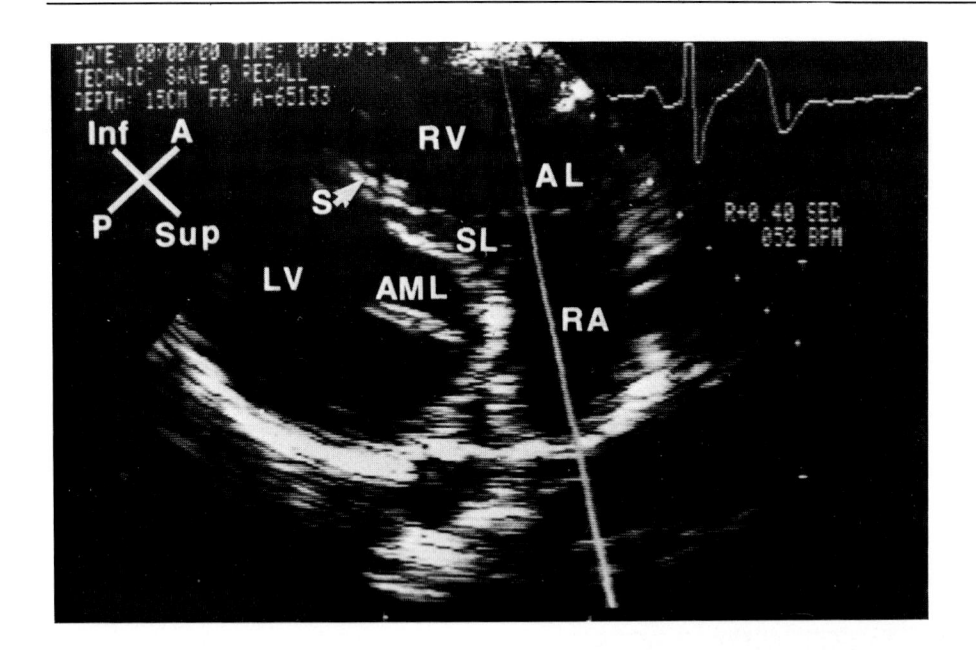

Fig. 2-19. Parasternal right-ventricular inflow view with M-mode cursor intersecting the anterior tricuspid leaflet (AL) in a normal subject. This view is usually preferable to the parasternal short axis view at the base for showing the tricuspid valve motion and obtaining good-quality M-mode recordings.

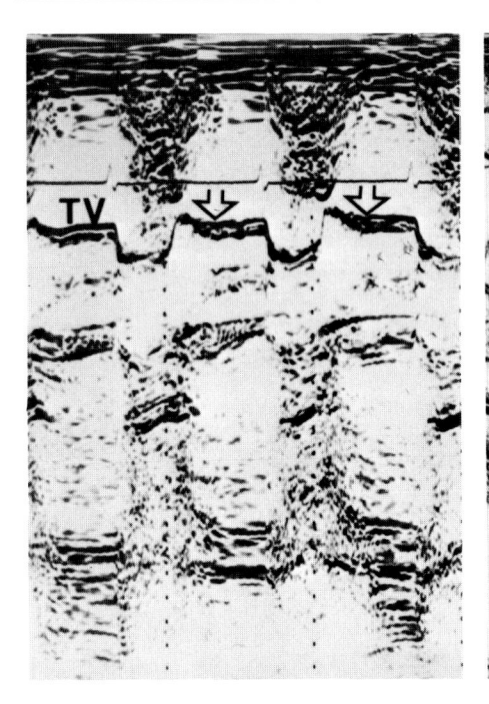

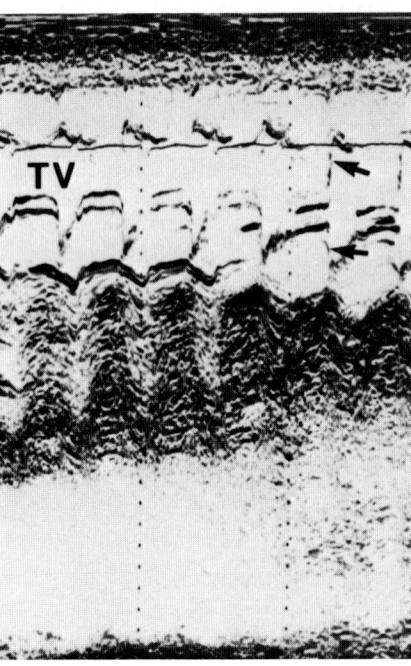

Fig. 2-20. M-mode recordings obtained on different days from a patient with right ventricular enlargement and clinical question of tricuspid stenosis. The left panel shows an improper recording taken very close to the tricuspid annulus with the tricuspid valve motion and thickness simulating tricuspid stenosis (open arrows). Utilizing simultaneous 2-D echo imaging to visualize maximum excursion of the leaflets and directing the M-mode cursor through such a view demonstrates that the tricuspid leaflets are actually entirely normal (right panel). The excursion and thickness of both anterior and septal leaflets (black arrows) are normal.

is being recorded; otherwise the M-mode recordings may simulate tricuspid stenosis, because the structure recorded is a mixture of annulus and proximal portion of the tricuspid leaflet (Fig. 2-20). However, with two-dimensional imaging the tricuspid valve can be adequately evaluated in nearly all subjects. For the most part, isolated M-mode examination to evaluate for presence of tricuspid stenosis or rheumatic tricuspid disease is inadequate without the benefit of two-dimensional imaging.

The tricuspid valve is usually easy to image with 2-D echo employing left parasternal, apical, and subcostal transducer positions. At least two views should be obtained from the parasternal position, namely the short axis at the base and the right ventricular inflow (RA/RV). Furthermore, the apical four-chamber and subcostal four-chamber views are very important for evaluation of the tricuspid valve.

The right ventricular inflow (RA/RV) plane is an excellent view to evaluate the tricuspid valve for presence of tricuspid stenosis. This view is somewhat analogous to the parasternal left ventricular long axis view for evaluation of the mitral valve in that the anterior and septal leaflets are imaged in profile; the ability to distinguish actual from apparent restricted leaflet motion is better here in many patients than in the parasternal short axis view at the base (also a valuable tomographic plane). Visualizing the profile of the tricuspid leaflets allows one to evaluate increased thickening, restricted motion, reduced leaflet separation, abnormal contour, or evidence of calcification (Fig. 2-21). It is important to observe carefully the types of qualitative features that suggest intrinsic abnormality of the leaflets, since the reduced separation of leaflets may be noted in patients with poor right ventricular function similar to the mitral valve motion in the presence of reduced left ventricular performance. No large studies employing two-dimensional echocardiography for the quantitative assessment of tricuspid stenosis have been reported to date.

The anterior tricuspid leaflet is the largest and is well delineated in the right ventricular inflow view. The posterior tricuspid leaflet, like its counterpart in the mitral location, is divided into scallops; the septal leaflet is the smallest and least mobile, with chordal attachments to the papillary muscle as well as to the right side of the interventricular septum. The tricuspid opening, the largest of the four valves, is somewhat triangular in appearance. The circumference of the annulus measures 11.4 ± 1.1 cm in men and 10.8 ± 1.3 cm in women [34]. In addition to the right ventricular inflow plane another excellent view for qualitative assessment of the tricuspid valve is the apical four-chamber position in which, depending upon the tomographic plane, either the anterior or posterior leaflet may be imaged together with the septal leaflet. Because of the anatomic plane of the tricuspid annulus it is usually not possible to image a short axis tomographic plane through the orifice and visualize all three leaflets simultaneously. Therefore, the severity of tricuspid stenosis cannot be planimetered or quantitated as can be done with the mitral valve. There are occasions, however, in the presence of marked right ventricular dilatation when the plane of the tricuspid annulus is shifted leftward and inferiorly, which enables imaging of all three leaflets in the parasternal left ventricular short axis position (Fig. 2-22). We have observed this on several occasions in patients with significant tricuspid regurgitation associated with marked enlargement of both right ventricle and right atrium. However, we have not observed the tricuspid valve in this manner in patients with isolated tricuspid stenosis to determine whether it would be possible to image the valve orifice in such cases.

74   2. Rheumatic valvular disease

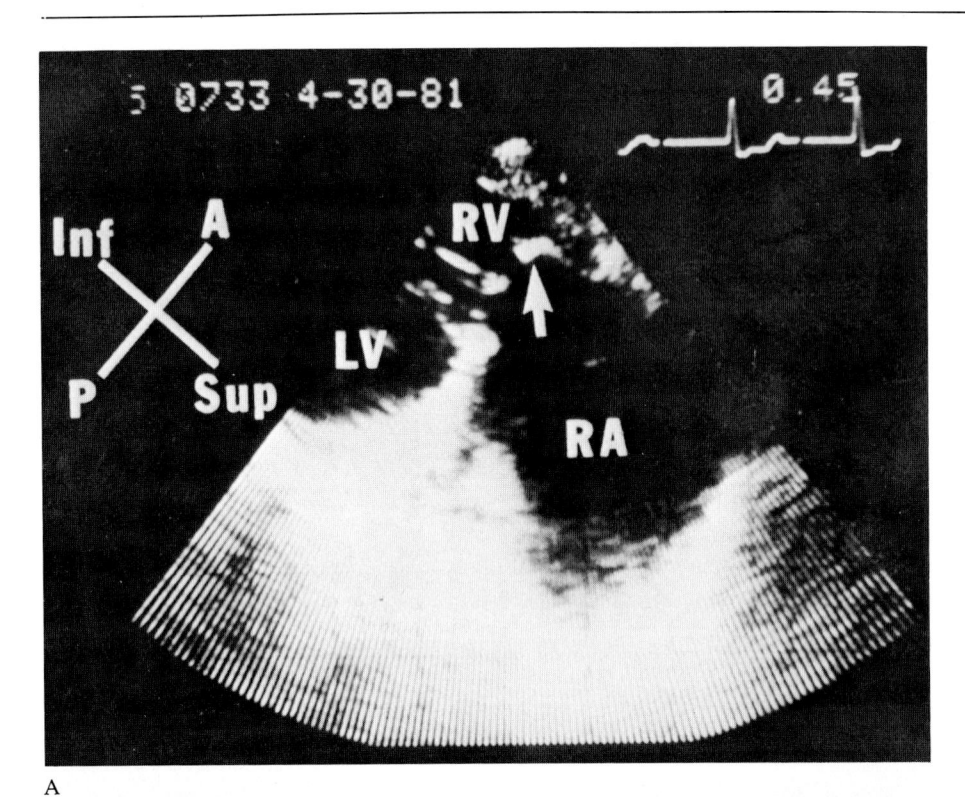

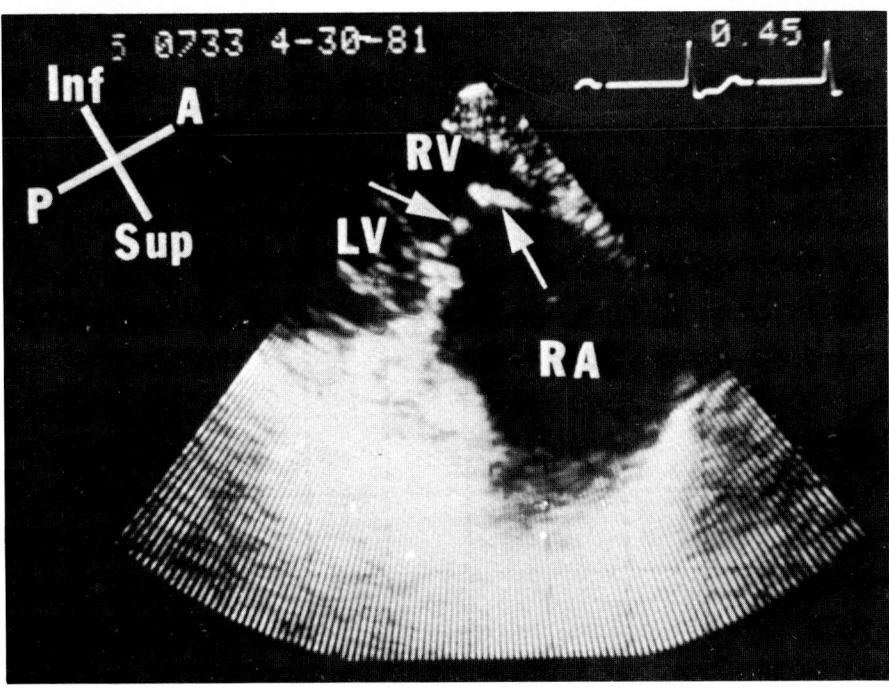

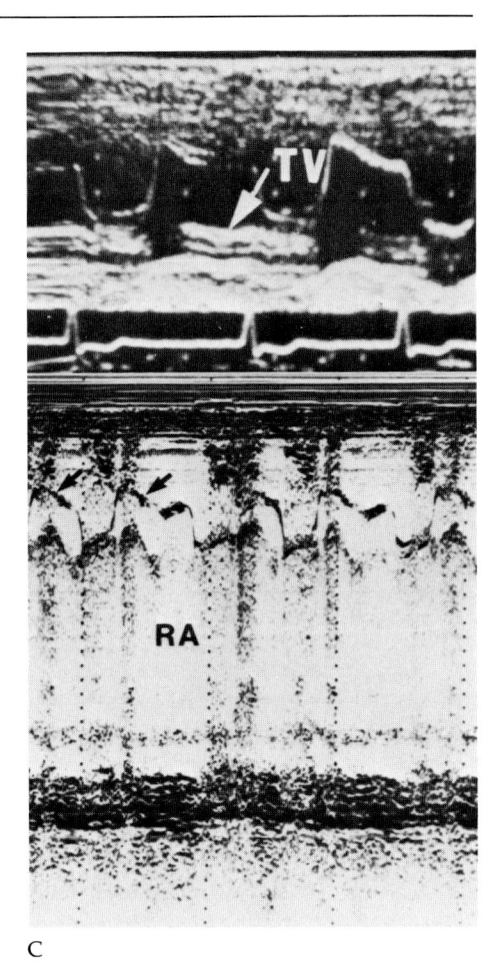

Fig. 2-21A. Parasternal right-ventricular inflow view showing thickened, domed anterior tricuspid leaflet (**arrow**) and large right atrium due to tricuspid stenosis. Right ventricular inflow diameter does not appear enlarged. The reduced mobility of the tricuspid leaflets can be easily appreciated with real-time imaging. B. Parasternal right-ventricular inflow view during diastole in the same patient. Arrows point to the septal and anterior tricuspid leaflets, which are thickened with narrowed separation of leaflets and reduced diastolic motion of both leaflets. The RA is very dilated; scale = 1 cm present along the right margin of the sector. C. M-mode recordings from two patients with tricuspid stenosis. Upper panel shows abnormal tricuspid valve with arrow pointing to thickened, immobile septal leaflet. Lower panel shows tricuspid stenosis in the other patient; arrows point to abnormal diastolic motion of the anterior leaflet. The RA is very large, measuring 75 to 80 mm in this view; scale = 5 mm between dots.

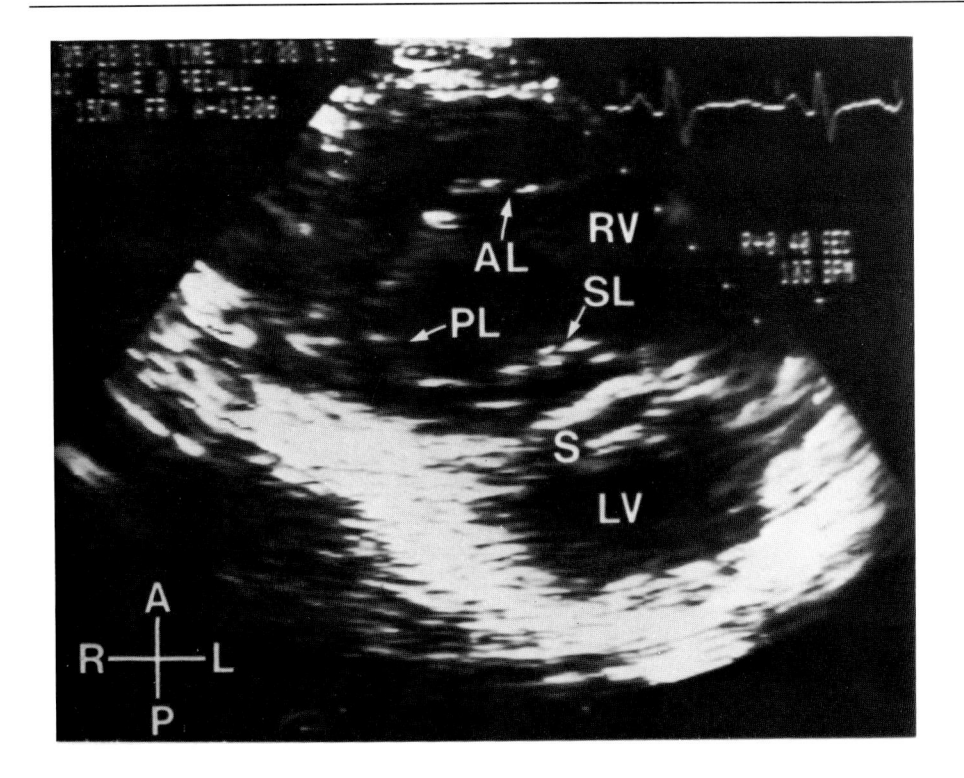

Fig. 2-22. Parasternal short axis of the left ventricle view showing a dilated right ventricle and the orifice of the tricuspid valve outlined by all three leaflets. The interventricular septum is flattened and the LV is small. Scale = 1 cm.

Compared to the mitral valve, the tricuspid valve is anatomically more prone to incompetence [35, 36]. Right ventricular dilatation from any cause may make the tricuspid valve incompetent; functional tricuspid regurgitation commonly accompanies congestive heart failure. When tricuspid stenosis is present tricuspid regurgitation may also be significant. Pulmonary hypertension secondary to rheumatic mitral valve disease commonly leads to tricuspid regurgitation. Accordingly, relief of the pulmonary hypertension following mitral valve surgery is expected to benefit or eliminate the secondary tricuspid regurgitation. However, sometimes the tricuspid disease may persist or even become more obvious after mitral commissurotomy. Mounsey [37] explained this seemingly paradoxical situation by an increase in cardiac output and a frequent onset of atrial fibrillation following mitral valvulotomy. The experience of Simon and associates [38] confirmed the persistence of tricuspid regurgitation following mitral valve surgery and proposed that depressed shortening of the tricuspid annulus during ventricular systole is an important contributing factor to its pathogenesis.

Isolated rheumatic tricuspid disease is infrequent. More commonly the tricuspid valve is involved in either double- or triple-valve disease.

In a catheterized series of 1320 patients studied at the Philippine Heart Center tricuspid regurgitation was found with the following frequency: (1) isolated tricuspid insufficiency, 9 (0.7%); (2) mitral stenosis plus tricuspid insufficiency, 30 (2.3%); (3) mitral regurgitation plus tricuspid insufficiency, 6 (0.5%); (4) mitral stenosis plus mitral regurgitation plus tricuspid insufficiency, 26 (2.0%); (5) aortic insufficiency plus tricuspid insufficiency, 2 (0.2%); (6) mitral stenosis plus aortic insufficiency plus tricuspid insufficiency, 26 (2.0%); (7) mitral regurgitation plus aortic insufficiency plus tricuspid insufficiency, 8 (0.6%); (8) mitral stenosis plus mitral regurgitation plus aortic insufficiency plus tricuspid insufficiency, 41 (3.1%); (9) mitral stenosis plus mitral regurgitation plus aortic insufficiency plus aortic stenosis plus tricuspid insufficiency, 3 (0.2%). A total of 151 patients (11.4%) in the study group had tricuspid regurgitation. These data clearly demonstrate the increased frequency of tricuspid involvement in multivalve lesions as well as primarily in association with mitral valve disease.

In another study at the Philippine Heart Center, an autopsy series of 204 patients with rheumatic valvular disease demonstrated combined mitral-tricuspid disease in 20 (9.8%) and combined mitral-aortic-tricuspid disease in 39 (19.1%) for a total incidence of rheumatic tricuspid valve disease in this series of 28.9 percent. Like mitral stenosis, tricuspid disease is more common in females than males.

The most reliable method for identifying tricuspid regurgitation is to employ contrast echocardiography utilizing combined M-mode and two-dimensional imaging from the subcostal position. In this position the inferior vena cava and hepatic vein are viewed together with a portion of the right atrium; simultaneous two-dimensional imaging ensures adequate filling of the right atrium following bolus injection of a fluid in a peripheral arm vein (Fig. 2-23). The M-mode cursor is directed in a perpendicular fashion through the inferior vena cava 2 to 4 cm distal to the junction of the inferior vena cava and right atrium; simultaneous careful recording of the electrocardiogram permits timing of any reflux of contrast seen in the inferior vena cava (Fig. 2-24). The patient must be properly positioned supine with the knees flexed so that the abdominal muscles can be relaxed; the patient should be carefully instructed so that cooperation can be achieved. Furthermore, breathing must be suspended during the procedure itself, since normal respiration may cause a false positive reflux into the inferior vena cava in the absence of tricuspid regurgitation. It is also important to observe whether reflux is occurring with systole, since it may be possible to see reflux into the inferior vena cava following atrial contraction before ventricular systole, particularly if there is elevated right atrial pressure and vigorous right atrial contraction. The technique for contrast echocardiography is reviewed in Chapter 13.

Persistence of the contrast effect in the right atrium and right ventricle is usually found in the presence of pulmonary hypertension or right ventricular failure; therefore the delay in evacuation of the microbubbles from the right heart structures is not a reliable criterion for the diagnosis of tricuspid regurgitation. Ozaki and colleagues [39] reported false positive findings of tricuspid insufficiency in normal subjects and that contrast echocardiography may demonstrate reflux into the inferior vena cava during mid-to-late diastole or early systole. Furthermore these investigators reported that exhalation exaggerated mild tricuspid insufficiency, whereas respiration appeared to have no effect on severe tricuspid regurgitation.

Unfortunately there has been no infallible test for the diagnosis of tricuspid regurgitation [40, 41]. Right ventricular angiography is not an ideal test because it is invasive, and false positive results may occur because of catheter interference with normal tricuspid valve mechanics. Even intraoperative palpation of the right atrium may be subject to false negatives due to insufficiently widespread palpation; false positive palpation of a thrill in the right atrium can occur from intraoperative manipulation of the heart with resulting distortion and incompetence of the tricuspid valve.

Atrial fibrillation and aberrant ventricular beats are electrocardiographic abnor-

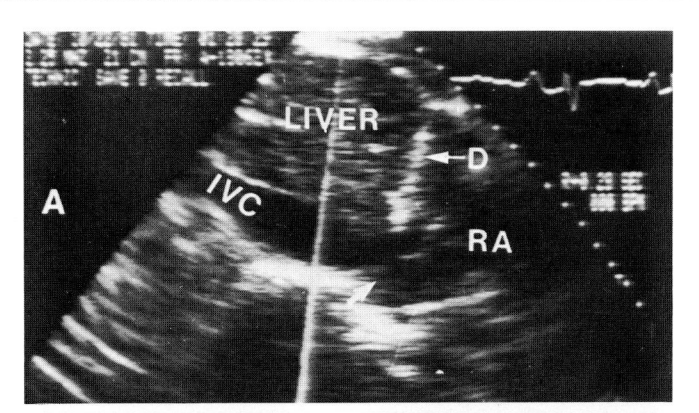

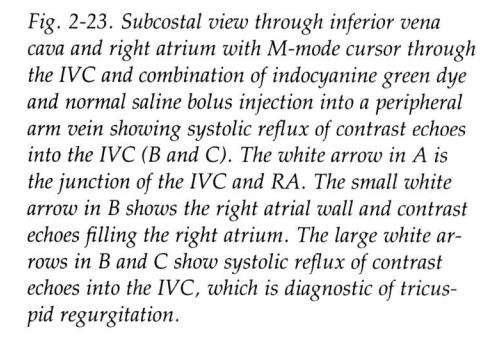

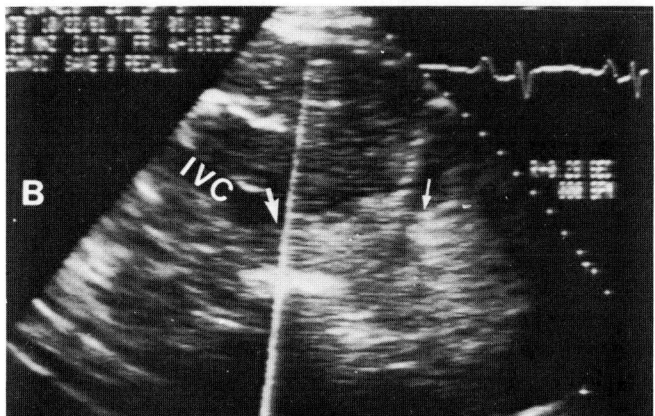

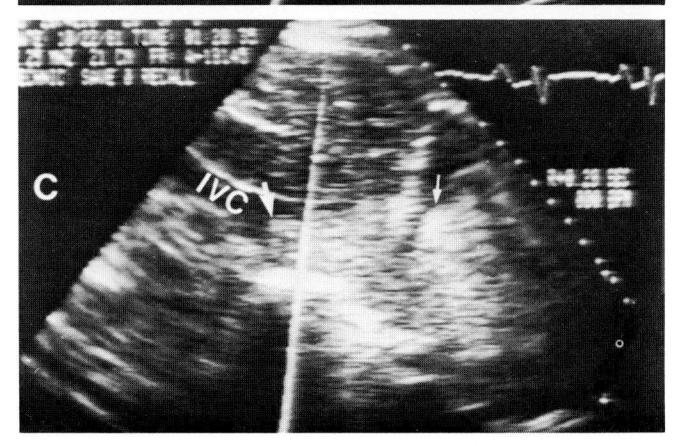

Fig. 2-23. Subcostal view through inferior vena cava and right atrium with M-mode cursor through the IVC and combination of indocyanine green dye and normal saline bolus injection into a peripheral arm vein showing systolic reflux of contrast echoes into the IVC (B and C). The white arrow in A is the junction of the IVC and RA. The small white arrow in B shows the right atrial wall and contrast echoes filling the right atrium. The large white arrows in B and C show systolic reflux of contrast echoes into the IVC, which is diagnostic of tricuspid regurgitation.

78   2. Rheumatic valvular disease

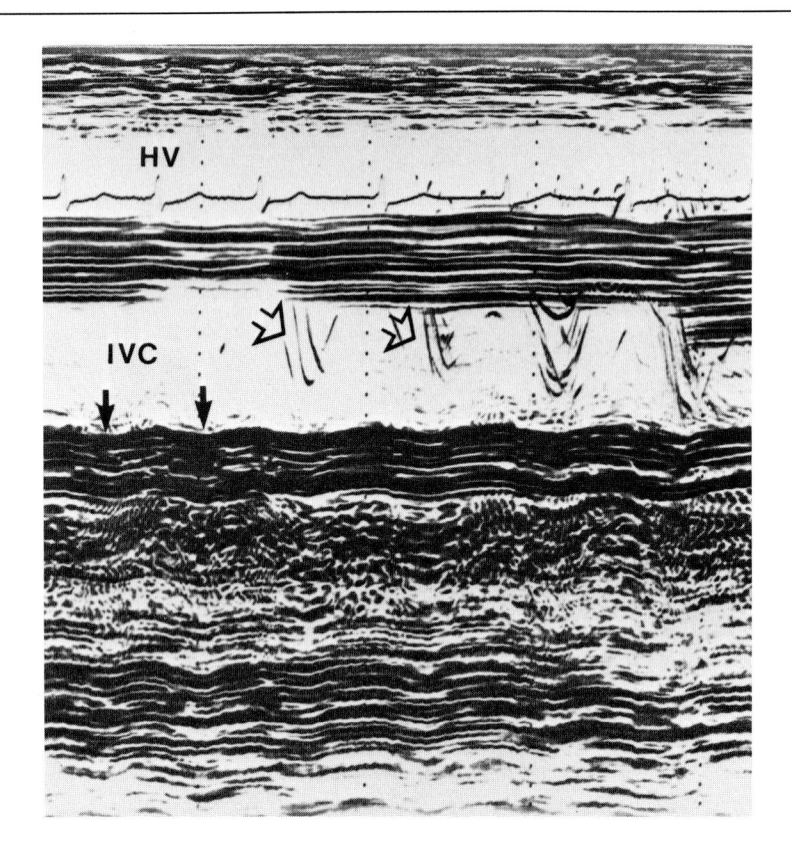

Fig. 2-24. M-mode recording of the inferior vena cava and hepatic vein (HV) *showing systolic reflux of contrast echoes* (open arrows) *due to tricuspid regurgitation. IVC V waves are indicated by solid black arrows.*

malities that may produce reflux into the inferior vena cava and represent additional causes of false positive diagnosis of tricuspid insufficiency. Furthermore patients with constrictive pericarditis have been observed to have contrast appearing in the IVC following atrial contraction and before ventricular systole [42, 43].

Another echocardiographic feature of tricuspid regurgitation is excessive systolic pulsations or prominent V waves seen in either hepatic veins or the inferior vena cava; this finding is best appreciated from M-mode recordings utilizing two-dimensional imaging for proper placement of the M-mode cursor. Abnormal motion and displacement of the interatrial septum toward the left atrium due to tricuspid regurgitation has also been reported [44].

Doppler echocardiography has also been employed to identify the presence of tricuspid regurgitation. A systolic regurgitant jet within the right atrium is one criterion that has been proposed [45]. The degree of regurgitation has not yet been quantitated with Doppler techniques to date. Another Doppler technique was used by Sivaciyan and Ranganathan to examine the jugular venous flow pattern for evidence of retrograde systolic flow; these authors then calculated a ratio of systolic to diastolic flow to semiquantitate the extent of regurgitation [46].

RHEUMATIC PULMONIC VALVE DISEASE. Primary involvement of the pulmonic valve secondary to rheumatic valvular disease is extremely rare and, if present, is usually a manifestation of pulmonary insufficiency secondary to pulmonary hypertension occurring on a functional basis rather than from organic valvular involve-

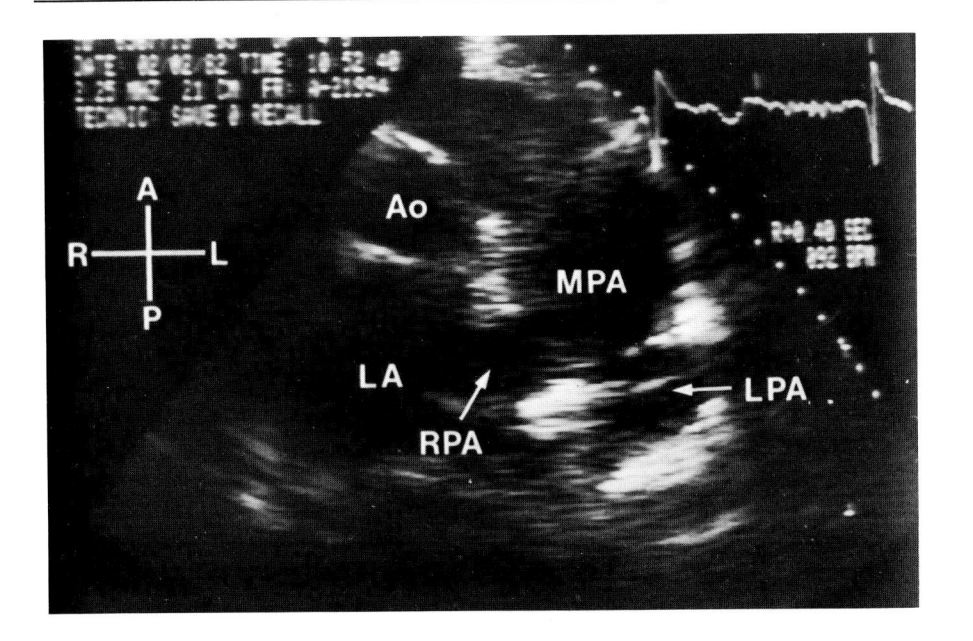

Fig. 2-25. Parasternal short axis at the base view with superior-leftward angulation of the transducer toward the pulmonary artery. The patient has rheumatic mitral disease with secondary pulmonary hypertension and dilatation of the main pulmonary artery (diameter = 48 mm). Both right (RPA) and left (LPA) pulmonary arteries are also prominent in size. The left atrium is enlarged. The aorta is normal size and measures 30 mm in diameter, giving an abnormal PA/Ao ratio of 1.6.

ment. Evaluation of pulmonary insufficiency during cardiac catheterization is difficult because of the catheter's passage through the valve [47].

In the autopsy series of 204 cases of rheumatic valvular disease previously referred to, only one case demonstrated evidence of pulmonic valve involvement. This case demonstrated thickening of the pulmonic valve but the valve was not stenotic in spite of the presence of severe mitral stenosis, aortic insufficiency, and tricuspid insufficiency. Gibson and Wood reported one patient with pulmonic stenosis together with tricuspid stenosis and mitral stenosis [48]. The anatomic features of rheumatic pulmonic stenosis are similar to those described earlier for chronic rheumatic valvulitis.

A rare case of acquired pulmonic stenosis secondary to carcinoid syndrome has been reported [49]. Other causes of acquired pulmonic valve stenosis include atherosclerotic pulmonic valve stenosis, infective endocarditis, and papillary fibroma of the valve.

Most patients with clinically significant mitral stenosis have secondary pulmonary hypertension with dilatation of the pulmonary artery and features of pulmonic valve motion consistent with pulmonary hypertension (Fig. 2-25). The optimal view for two-dimensional imaging of the pulmonary artery is with the transducer in the parasternal position imaging in the short axis through the base but with leftward angulation directed toward the main pulmonary artery. Maneuvering the sector beam in this fashion brings out the lateral wall of the pulmonary artery as well as the bifurcation of the right and left pulmonary arteries; this view enables reasonably accurate measurement of the diameter of the pulmonary artery as well as clear visualization of the pulmonic valve motion. After obtaining this view, the M-mode cursor should be positioned through the pulmonic valve and the M-mode record obtained for more careful evaluation of pulmonic valve motion. The operator should look particularly for evidence of mid-systolic closure, which is usually specific, but not always present, in pulmonary hypertension (Fig. 2-26). This view

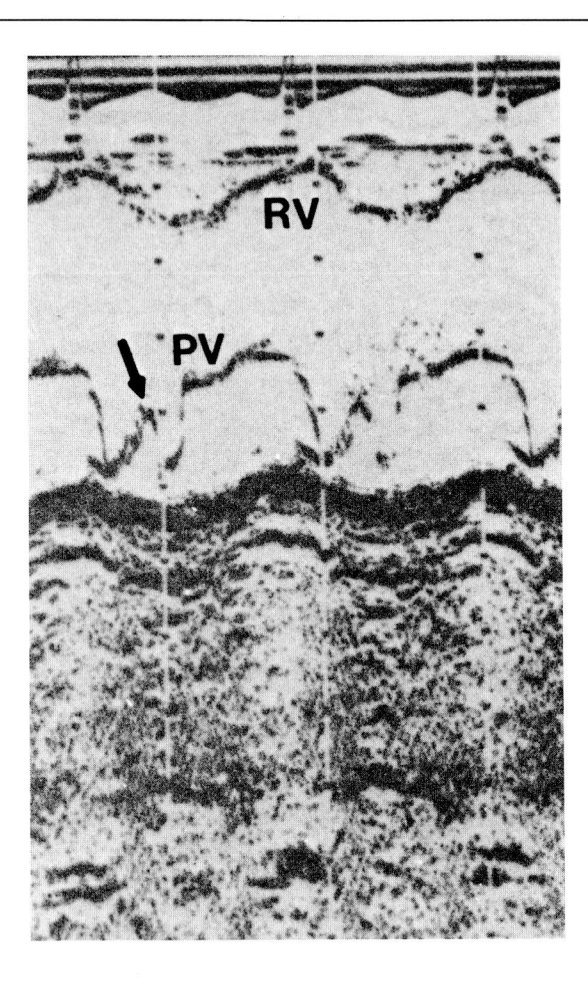

Fig. 2-26. M-mode recording of pulmonic valve (PV) showing abnormal mid-systolic closure (notch) (arrow) due to pulmonary hypertension. Other M-mode patterns (E–F slope and "A" wave) of the pulmonic valve are of limited or no value for diagnosing or excluding pulmonary hypertension.

demonstrates two of the three pulmonic valve leaflets in profile, which enables good visualization of leaflet motion as well as detection of leaflet thickening, doming of the valve, or features of pulmonic stenosis. Another view of the valve can be obtained in the right ventricular outflow (subpulmonic) plane with the transducer in the parasternal position. In addition to these two views, a third opportunity to image the right ventricular outflow tract and pulmonic valve is obtained from the subcostal position with rotation of the transducer into a short axis view of the left ventricle and direction of the beam through the outflow tract of the right ventricle and pulmonic valve simultaneously.

Contrast echocardiography may be of some value for recognizing pulmonary insufficiency because of the abnormally long retention of the contrast effect in the right ventricular outflow track; however, no specific criteria have yet been reported for diagnosis by this technique.

References

1. Edler I: The diagnostic use of ultrasound in heart disease. *Acta Med Scand* 308:32, 1955
2. Segal BL, Likoff W, Kingsley B: Echocardiography: Clinical application in mitral stenosis. *JAMA* 195:161, 1966
3. Duchak JM, Chang S, Feigenbaum H: The posterior mitral valve echo and the echocardiographic diagnosis of mitral stenosis. *Am J Cardiol* 29:628, 1972
4. Hurst JW: *The Heart* (4th ed.). New York: McGraw-Hill, 1978. P 952
5. Bloor CM: *Cardiac Pathology*. Philadelphia: Lippincott, 1978. Pp 237–245
6. Silverman MI, Hurst JW: The mitral complex. *Am Heart J* 76:399, 1968
7. Loop FD: Technique for repair and replacement of the mitral valve. *Surg Clin North Am* 55:1193, 1975
8. Walmsley R: Anatomy of left ventricular outflow tract. *Br Heart J* 41:263, 1979
9. Inoh T, Maeda K, Oda A: Diagnosis and classification of the mitral valve prolapse by the ultrasound cardiotomography and the evaluation of the M-mode technic. *Jpn Circ J* 43:305, 1979
10. Ranganathan N, Lam JHC, Wigle ED, Silver MD: Morphology of the human mitral valve II. The valve leaflet. *Circulation* 41:459, 1970
11. Tsakiris AG: The Physiology of the Mitral Annulus. In D Kalmanson (Ed.), *The Mitral Valve*. London: Edward Arnold, 1976. P 21
12. Chakorn SA, Siggers DC, Wharton CFP, Deuchar DC: Study of normal and abnormal movements of mitral valve ring using reflected ultrasound. *Br Heart J* 34:480, 1972
13. Ormiston JA, Shah PM, Ter C, Wong M: Size and motion of the mitral valve annulus in man. I. A two-dimensional echocardiographic method and findings in normal subjects. *Circulation* 64:113, 1981
14. Titus JL: Anatomy and Pathology of the Mitral Valve. In FH Ellis (Ed.), *Surgery for Acquired Mitral Valve Disease*. Philadelphia: Saunders, 1967. P 53
15. Hudson REB: *Cardiovascular Pathology* (Vol. 2). London: Edward Arnold, 1965. Pp 1959–1962
16. Cope GD, Kisslo JA, Johnson ML, Behar VS: A reassessment of the echocardiogram in mitral stenosis. *Circulation* 52:664, 1975
17. Strunk BL, London EJ, Fitzgerald J, Popp RL, Barry WH: The assessment of mitral stenosis and prosthetic mitral valve obstruction, using the posterior aortic wall echocardiogram. *Circulation* 55:885, 1977
18. Hall RJC, Clarke SE, Brown D: Evaluation of posterior aortic wall echogram in diagnosis of mitral valve disease. *Br Heart J* 41:522, 1979
19. Glover MU, Warren SE, Vieweg WVR, Hagan AD, Ceretto WJ: M-mode and two-dimensional echocardiographic correlation with findings at catheterization and surgery in patients with mitral stenosis. *Am Heart J* 105:98, 1983
20. DeMaria AN, Miller RR, Amsterdam EA, Markson W, Mason DT: Mitral valve early diastolic closing velocity in the echocardiogram: Relation to sequential diastolic flow and ventricular compliance. *Am J Cardiol* 37:693, 1976
21. Smith MR, Agruss NS, Levenson NI, Adolph RJ: Nonobstructive hypertrophic cardiomyopathy mimicking mitral stenosis. Documentation by echocardiography, phonocardiography and intracardiac pressure and sound recordings. *Am J Cardiol* 35:89, 1975
22. Hagan AD: Correlates of M-mode and 2-D echocardiography to evaluate the mitral valve. *CVP* 8:37, 1980
23. Hagan AD: Non-Mitral Diseases Affecting the Mitral Valve Echogram. In DT Mason (Ed.), *Heart Disease* (Vol. 2). New York: Grune and Stratton, 1978. P 45
24. Henry WL, Griffith JM, Michaelis LL, McIntosh CL, Morrow AG, Epstein SE: Measurement of mitral orifice area in patients with mitral valve disease by real-time, two-dimensional echocardiography. *Circulation* 51:827, 1975
25. Nichol PM, Gilbert BW, Kisslo JA: Two-dimensional echocardiographic assessment of mitral stenosis. *Circulation* 55:120, 1977
26. Wann LS, Weyman AE, Feigenbaum H, Dillon JC, Johnston KW, Eggleton RC: Determination of mitral valve area by cross-sectional echocardiography. *Ann Intern Med* 88:337, 1978
27. Martin RP, Rakowski H, Kleiman JH, Beaver W, London E, Popp RL: Reliability and reproducibility of two-dimensional echocardiographic measurement of the stenotic mitral valve orifice area. *Am J Cardiol* 43:560, 1979

28. Heger JJ, Wann LS, Weyman AE, Dillon JC, Feigenbaum H: Long-term changes in mitral valve area after successful mitral commissurotomy. *Circulation* 59:443, 1979
29. Calleja HB: Valvular heart disease—medical and surgical management. *Philippine J Cardiol* 10:1, 1982
30. Wann LS, Feigenbaum H, Weyman AE, Dillon JC: Cross-sectional echocardiographic detection of rheumatic mitral regurgitation. *Am J Cardiol* 41:1258, 1978
31. Roberts WC, Brownlee WG, Jones AA, Luke JL: Suction action of the left ventricle: Demonstration of physiologic principle by a gunshot wound penetrating only the right side of the heart. *Am J Cardiol* 43:1234, 1979
32. Sabbah HN, Anbe DT, Stein PD: Negative intraventricular diastolic pressure in patients with mitral stenosis: Evidence of left ventricular diastolic suction. *Am J Cardiol* 45:562, 1980
33. Sherrid MV, Clark RD, Cohn K: Echocardiographic analysis of left atrial size before and after operation in mitral valve disease. *Am J Cardiol* 43:171, 1979
34. Silver MD, Lam JHC, Ranganathan N, Wigle ED: Morphology of the human tricuspid valve. *Circulation* 43:333, 1971
35. Hollman A: The anatomical appearance in rheumatic tricuspid valve disease. *Br Heart J* 19:211, 1957
36. Lottenbach C, Shillingford J: Functional tricuspid incompetence in relation to the venous pressure. *Br Heart J* 19:395, 1957
37. Mounsey P: Tricuspid incompetence following successful mitral valvotomy. *Br Heart J* 21:123, 1959
38. Simon R, Oelert H, Borst HG, Lichtlen PR: Influence of mitral valve surgery on tricuspid incompetence concomitant with mitral valve disease. *Circulation* 62(Suppl 1):I152, 1980
39. Osaki M, Handa Y, Okabe M, Naito H, Hesaka K, Takahaski T, Sota K, Ohta N: Problem in the diagnosis of tricuspid insufficiency by contrast echocardiography injected into the peripheral vein: On the false positive findings in normal subjects. *J Cardiography* 10:173, 1980
40. Lingamneni R, Cha SD, Maranhao V, Gooch AS, Goldberg H: Tricuspid regurgitation: Clinical and angiographic assessment. *Cath Cardiovasc Diagn* 5:7, 1979
41. Pepine CJ, Nichols WW, Selby JH: Diagnostic tests for tricuspid insufficiency: How good? *Cath Cardiovasc Diagn* 5:1, 1979
42. Meltzer RS, van Hoogenhuyze D, Serruys PW, Haalebos MMP, Hugenholtz PG, Roelandt J: Diagnosis of tricuspid regurgitation by contrast echocardiography. *Circulation* 63:1093, 1981
43. Wise NK, Myers S, Fraker TD, Stewart JA, Kisslo JA: Contrast M-mode ultrasonography of the inferior vena cava. *Circulation* 63:1100, 1981
44. Tei C, Tanaka H, Kashima T, Yoshimura H, Minagoe S, Kanehisa T: Real-time cross-sectional echocardiographic evaluation of the interatrial septum by right atrium-interatrial septum-left atrium direction of ultrasound beam. *Circulation* 60:539, 1979
45. Waggoner AD, Quinones MA, Young JB, Brandon TA, Shah AA, Verani MS, Miller RR: Pulsed Doppler echocardiographic detection of right-sided valve regurgitation. Experimental results and clinical significance. *Am J Cardiol* 47:279, 1981
46. Sivaciyan V, Ranganathan N: Transcutaneous Doppler jugular venous flow velocity recording: Clinical and hemodynamic correlates. *Circulation* 57:930, 1978
47. Baron MG: Angiographic evaluation of valvular insufficiency. *Circulation* 43:599, 1971
48. Gibson R, Wood P: The diagnosis of tricuspid stenosis. *Br Heart J* 17:552, 1965
49. Okada RD, Ewy GA, Copeland JG: Echocardiography and surgery in tricuspid and pulmonary valve stenosis due to carcinoid syndrome. *Cardiovasc Med* 4:871, 1979

Nonrheumatic mitral valve disease

Pathophysiology of mitral regurgitation. The anatomic elements of the mitral valve complex responsible for regurgitation may operate singly or in combination [1]. Anatomic changes that may be responsible for mitral regurgitation include changes in the mitral leaflets, mitral annulus, the commissures, the chordae tendineae, and papillary muscles, and dilatation of the left atrial and/or left ventricular cavities. During the 1950s and 1960s rheumatic etiology was considered to be the most common cause of mitral regurgitation in the United States. However, during the past decade it has been recognized that mitral valve prolapse secondary to myxomatous degeneration represents the most common cause of mitral regurgitation.

Mitral valve prolapse. Evidence has accumulated that myxomatous degeneration is the predominant cause of mitral valve prolapse [2–6]. Myxomatous degeneration has been found in patients with isolated mitral regurgitation, aortic regurgitation, combined mitral and aortic regurgitation, and combined mitral and tricuspid regurgitation [7–11].

A certain degree of confusion surrounds the concept of myxomatous degeneration of cardiac valves. Some investigators report that it is the result of one specific disease process [12]; others characterize it as a nonspecific tissue response to a variety of factors, and it may be an associated finding in congenital heart disease [10]. Still others have reported it to be secondary to syphilitic aortitis and rheumatic heart disease [10, 13], and, finally, some investigators have considered myxomatous degeneration to be a normal aging change [14].

Depending on the criteria employed to define the entity and the population studied, the percentage of subjects with myxomatous degeneration of cardiac valves varies considerably. Furthermore, if mitral valve prolapse is caused by myxomatous degeneration, then as many as 6 percent of healthy adults and 9 to 16 percent of patients undergoing valve replacement in the United States may have this abnormality [9, 10, 13, 15].

In addition to mitral valve prolapse being commonly found in patients with mitral regurgitation, myxomatous degeneration has also been retrospectively identified in other causes of regurgitant lesions, including endocardial friction lesions [16], ruptured chordae tendineae [3, 15, 16], and a higher incidence of bacterial endocarditis [15]. Mitral valve prolapse has been linked to an increased incidence of arrhythmias [17–20], a higher risk of infective endocarditis [21], and a greater chance of sudden death [22, 23].

Rippe and associates [24] defined primary myxomatous degeneration as degeneration of collagen of the pars fibrosa of the valve with basophilic staining in this region caused by the deposition of acid mucopolysaccharides in the absence of severe calcification or fibrosis, and with no macroscopic evidence of rheumatic valvular disease. These investigators emphasized that the key pathological feature that identified this entity as primary myxomatous degeneration involved significant disruption of the pars fibrosa. While the amount of myxomatous material found in the pars spongiosa was also increased in their patients, this latter feature is a

84   3. Nonrheumatic mitral valve disease

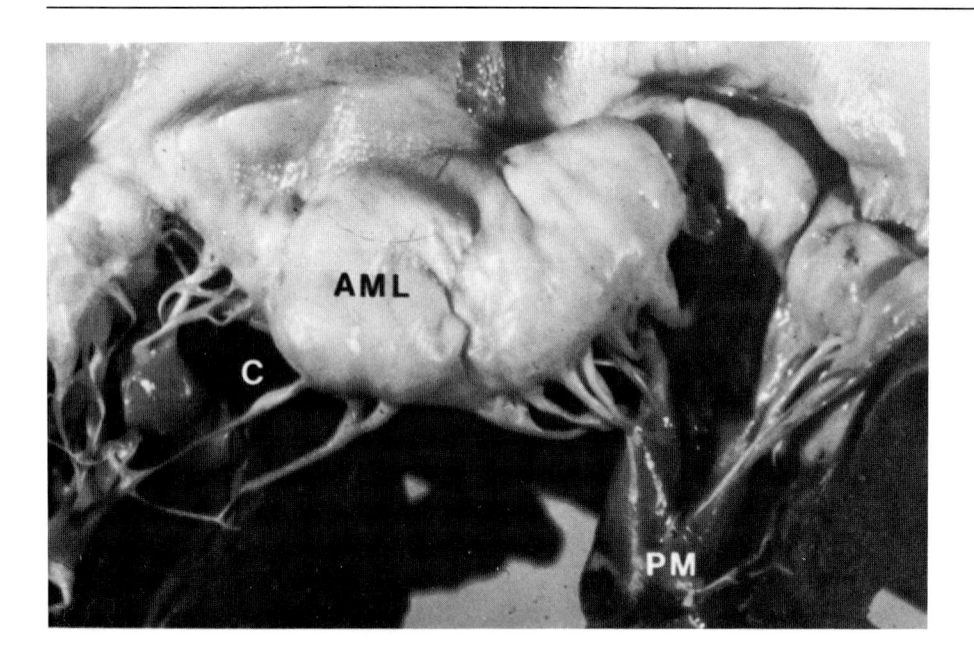

Fig. 3-1. Postmortem view of abnormal mitral valve showing anatomic changes due to myxomatous degeneration. The spongiosa of the anterior mitral leaflet is increased, leading to thickened, redundant valve tissue. The chordae tendineae (C) is thinned and might have spontaneously ruptured. The papillary muscle is normal.

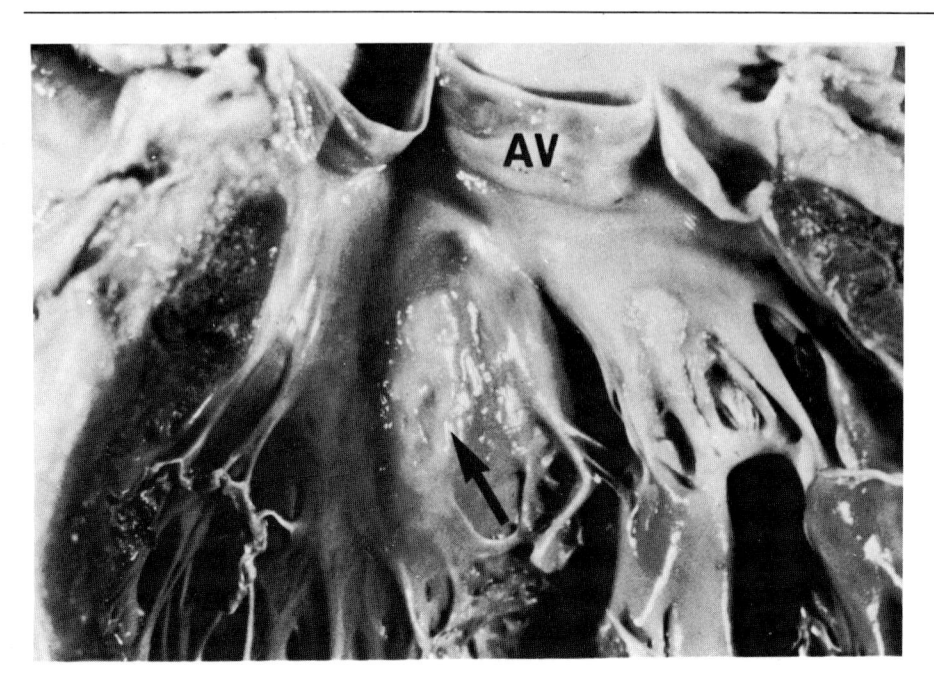

Fig. 3-2. An area of increased thickness forming a plaquelike friction lesion (arrow) appears on the endocardial surface of the interventricular septum. This lesion is located precisely where the anterior mitral leaflet contacted the septum with each diastolic opening.

common pathological finding and may represent a nonspecific response to aging or to a variety of other pathological conditions. These investigators defined a 7 percent incidence of myxomatous degeneration as a major pathological finding but only 3 percent of patients had significant degenerative changes of the pars fibrosa in a group with 499 surgically excised valves. Furthermore, these investigators noted that echocardiography was more helpful than angiography in establishing the diagnosis of either myxomatous degeneration or of mitral valve prolapse in this study.

The normal mitral valve leaflet consists of the fibrosa on the ventricular surface where the chordae tendineae attach and the spongiosa on the atrial side of the leaflet. The spongiosa, which normally contains acid mucopolysaccharide, is increased in patients with mitral valve prolapse. In other types of valvular diseases the fibrosa is increased and replaced by fibrous tissue. The increased spongiosa in mitral valve prolapse encroaches on the fibrosa, inducing collagen dissolution. These changes lead to a "hooding" deformity of the mitral valve with redundant valve tissue, which prolapses during systole (Fig. 3-1). Secondary lesions may also occur, including thickened endocardium of the left atrium with platelet and fibrin deposits, calcium deposits in the leaflet, and friction lesions where elongated chordae tendineae or the anterior mitral leaflet rub against the left ventricular endocardium (Fig. 3-2).

CLINICAL MANIFESTATIONS OF MITRAL VALVE PROLAPSE. PREVALENCE. Mitral prolapse occurs from early childhood to advanced years; however, the usual clinical recognition is more common in the third through fifth decades. Whereas more than two thirds of younger patients are female, the sex distribution appears to be more even in the middle- and older-age groups [9].

The true prevalence of mitral valve prolapse is unknown but varies widely according to the population studied and the diagnostic method employed. Typical auscultatory findings for mitral valve prolapse were present in 1.4 percent of black South African school children [25]; considerably higher incidences of mitral valve prolapse (10–21%) have been reported in presumably healthy young male and female populations [26, 27]. Devereau and associates [23] reported just over 6 percent of echocardiographic examinations among selected populations in their laboratory had mitral valve prolapse. In other studies approximately 5 percent of routine autopsies on patients above 40 years of age showed redundant mitral leaflets [14, 27].

Occasional patients relay a striking family history of atypical heart disease and, rarely, of sudden death. Familial occurrence, although well established, has been uncommon in most large series [2] but may be underestimated because of silent or asymptomatic status. Weiss and associates [28] reported in a study of 74 subjects consisting of 57 first-degree relatives and 17 propositi with mitral valve prolapse that 27 of the 57 first-degree relatives also had mitral valve prolapse. These investigators reported that 53 percent of female and 36 percent of male progeny of propositi were affected. The results of that study indicated that mitral valve prolapse is transmitted in an autosomal-dominant mode with reduced male expressivity and a familial prevalence of 47 percent.

The long-term natural history of individuals with mitral valve prolapse is not fully understood; however, this has been reviewed in part by Appelblatt and colleagues [29]. The major complications consist of sudden death, infective endocarditis, progressive mitral regurgitation, and chordal rupture. The actual risk of sudden death has not yet been established, even in the subgroup with serious ventricular arrhythmias documented during ambulatory electrocardiographic monitoring or exercise stress testing. Despite these complications current evidence suggests that premature mortality among these patients is very uncommon [2, 29, 30]. Aging per se may increase leaflet chordal redundancy in otherwise normal hearts by reducing the annular circumference and left ventricular long axis [9].

SYMPTOMS. While the majority of patients are asymptomatic, others may have symptoms for many years. Fatigue and dyspnea are frequent and often long precede medical recognition of mitral valve prolapse [2, 31]. Palpitations are reported by nearly 50 percent of patients with known mitral valve prolapse [2, 19, 31]. Documented arrhythmias are relatively frequent; however, long-term electrocardiographic monitoring does not necessarily correlate well in a temporal fashion between symptomatic palpitations and recorded arrhythmias [32]. Syncope and presyncope occur in a very small minority of such patients [2, 31].

Atypical chest pain has been noted to occur in one third to one half of patients in referral series and can be insignificant to disabling [2, 19, 25, 31, 33]. Apparently psychological complaints such as anxiety and lassitude seem to bother some patients. Obviously the symptomatic status varies significantly. Individuals in whom the diagnosis is accidentally discovered on routine physical examination are usually asymptomatic whereas many patients seen in referral centers will complain of chest pain, palpitations, fatigue, and dyspnea that may pose significant diagnostic and management problems.

The underlying mechanism of chest pain in patients with mitral valve prolapse has not yet been resolved. Although occlusive coronary disease has no known relationship to chest pain, some patients have S–T segment abnormalities that develop spontaneously or following exercise testing [34]. LeWinter and associates [35] have demonstrated that increasing afterload with phenylephrine infusion reliably induced chest pain in patients with symptomatic prolapse but did not elicit symptoms in those patients without spontaneous chest pain. Increased tension on the papillary muscles or adjacent myocardium has also been proposed as a cause of myocardial ischemia and a mechanism for chest pain in patients with mitral valve prolapse. Rapid atrial pacing has produced chest pain in as many as 40 percent of subjects as well as causing abnormal coronary sinus lactate production in a small number, but with variable electrocardiographic correlation and no relationship at all to left ventricular segmental contraction abnormalities [36].

PHYSICAL EXAMINATION. Auscultatory signs remain the bedside hallmarks of mitral valve prolapse. It is also well known that auscultatory findings are variable and that in certain patients an isolated mid-systolic click may be noted on one examination but that in follow-up reexamination the same patients may be noted to exhibit one or more early, mid-, or late systolic clicks or even bursts of multiple clicks. Multiple clicks are thought to arise from asynchronous prolapse of different areas of redundant leaflet or leaflets [23].

The typical late systolic murmur usually begins with or just following the mid-systolic click and persists up to or slightly beyond the aortic component of the second sound. If no murmur is audible with the patient in the supine position it can often be provoked by simple change of posture, with the patient moving into sudden upright or standing position, or by the administration of amyl nitrite. These postural changes and amyl nitrite inhalation cause reduction in left ventricular volume, which tends to accentuate leaflet-chordae redundancy and hence tends to move the systolic click toward the first heart sound and induce or lengthen the duration of the systolic murmur. An apical holosystolic murmur that may obscure the mid-systolic click is audible in fewer than 10 percent of patients with demonstrated mitral valve prolapse [2]. The frequency of holosystolic murmurs has been reported to increase to as much as 25 percent in older patients, which may be related to the relative shortening of the left ventricular long axis with age [37]. In general, although not always, the earlier the systolic prolapse occurs the earlier the click and the longer the accompanying murmur. In a small proportion of patients a striking systolic "whoop" may be intermittently heard [25]. This murmur is characteristically high-frequency, musical, and widely transmitted. Furthermore, positional changes such as sitting, leaning, or standing up may convert a typical late systolic murmur into a distinctive honking sound.

Positional or pharmacologic interventions that reduce left ventricular volume will tend to induce clicks or, if clicks are present, move them closer toward the first sound, or induce murmurs or change their characteristics. Variations in the onset of prolapse have been shown to be caused by changes in left ventricular end-diastolic volume as well as in the velocity of circumferential fiber shortening in the preprolapse period [38, 39]. Maneuvers and interventions that cause such reduction in left ventricular volume include standing, the Valsalva maneuver, exercise-induced tachycardia, or inhalation of amyl nitrite. Although repeated examinations and use of these maneuvers usually unmask silent disease in the patient with clinical symptoms suggesting mitral valve prolapse, as many as 10 percent of patients with echocardiographic or angiographic mitral valve prolapse remain "silent" to auscultation despite physical and pharmacologic interventions [2, 40]. Occasionally an early diastolic sound resembling an opening snap may be heard in these patients. Epstein and Coulshed [41] postulated that this early diastolic sound may be caused by the sudden termination of the opening movement of the highly mobile mitral leaflets.

ELECTROCARDIOGRAM. Electrocardiographic abnormalities may occur in up to two thirds of patients with mitral valve prolapse; the most typical abnormality is that of nonspecific abnormalities of the T waves [2, 19, 25, 31, 33]. Other electrocardiographic abnormalities noted in patients with mitral valve prolapse include Q–T prolongation, atrial and ventricular arrhythmias, atrioventricular conduction disturbances, and preexcitation. The mechanisms of electrocardiographic abnormalities in mitral prolapse are unknown.

Bharati and associates [42] studied the conduction system in a 45-year-old man with mitral valve prolapse who died suddenly; there was a known past history of recurrent ventricular tachycardia. Pathologically the posterior leaflet was markedly thickened and redundant with typical histologic characteristics of a floppy valve. The annulus was calcified and elongated with the leaflet anchored on the left atrial side (Fig. 3-3). These investigators reported that under normal circumstances the posterior leaflet is found to arise either equally on the ventricular and atrial portions of the annulus or more on the ventricular portion but only very rarely did they encounter the posterior leaflet resting exclusively on the atrial side. Furthermore these authors noted the conduction system to be abnormal, demonstrating marked fatty infiltration in the approaches to the sinoatrial and atrioventricular nodes and interatrial preferential pathways.

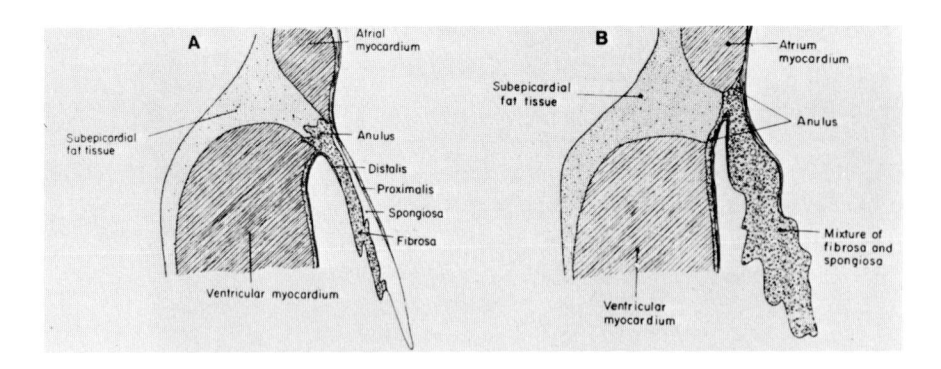

Fig. 3-3A. Diagram of normal poterior mitral leaflet origin at the junction of atrial and ventricular myocardium. B. Myxomatous degeneration of the mitral valve with the posterior mitral leaflet anchored on the left atrial side of the atrioventricular sulcus. It is not known how often this type of abnormal origin of the leaflet occurs in the presence of mitral valve prolapse. (From S Bharati et al: The conduction system in mitral valve prolapse syndrome with sudden death. Am Heart J 101:667, 1981.)

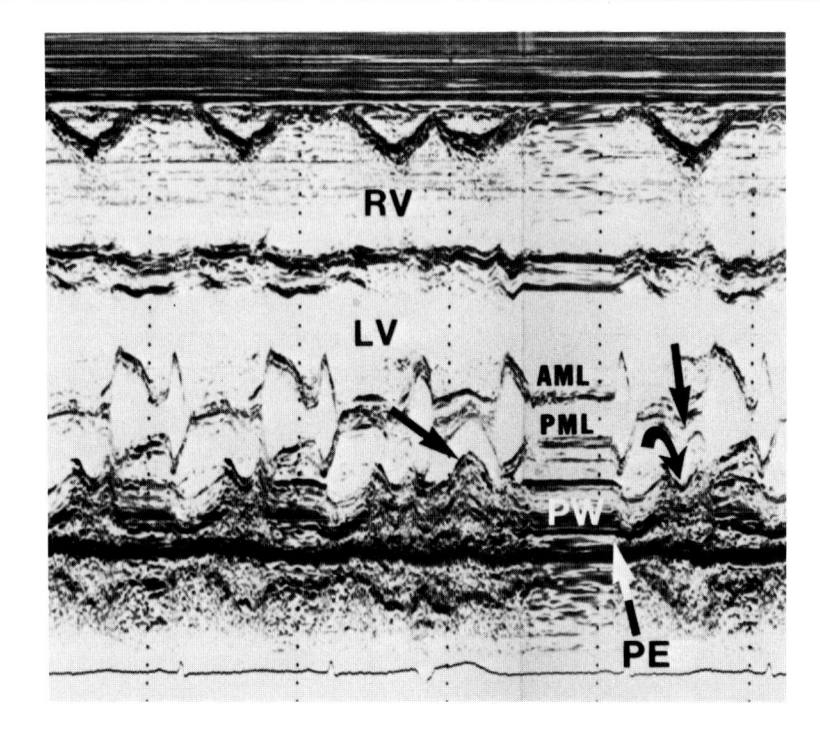

Fig. 3-4. M-mode recording in a 35-year-old patient with mitral valve prolapse and segmental cardiomyopathy demonstrating late systolic retraction of the left ventricular posterobasilar wall (PW) (curved arrow). The posterior wall thickening at the time of a premature extrasystole (straight arrow) does not manifest late systolic retraction. The left ventricular cavity is slightly enlarged. The E-point septal separation of 15 mm is indicative of a reduced ejection fraction. Minimal pericardial effusion is present.

LEFT VENTRICULAR CONTRACTION ABNORMALITIES. Gulotta and associates [34] have noted that the abnormal myocardial contraction features in patients with mitral valve prolapse are sufficiently common to characterize what they call a "segmental cardiomyopathy." Alterations of segmental function might interfere with chordae tendineae and leaflet motion, initiate or aggravate redundancy, and contribute to systolic prolapse. On the other hand, there is ample evidence of patients with mitral valve prolapse who do not have any recognizable abnormalities of left ventricular contractility. Young and associates [43] have reported finding end-systolic retraction of the left ventricular posterior wall in 35 percent of 113 patients with mitral valve prolapse. These investigators postulated that the end-systolic retraction of the left ventricular posterior basilar wall represented premature relaxation of the left ventricle due to pronounced mitral valve prolapse and alteration of left ventricular geometry (Fig. 3-4). D'Cruz and coworkers [44] reported a left ventricular contraction abnormality employing apical imaging with two-dimensional echocardiography and observed motion of the posterior lateral basilar segment of the left ventricle to be diminished and delayed in 11 of 34 patients with typical mitral valve prolapse. This abnormal pattern of left ventricular contraction occurred with equal frequency in patients with holosystolic and late systolic prolapse. However, it was noted more frequently in patients with severe prolapse than in those with mild or moderate prolapse. Finally, a single incidence of improvement in left ventricular contraction abnormalities has been noted following mitral valve replacement [45]. Various hypotheses have been proposed to explain the abnormal patterns of left ventricular contraction, including

1. Diminished regional contractility of the left ventricular posterior-lateral basilar wall or inflow tract with compensatory hyperkinesis of the ventricular septum [46]
2. Lack of normal left ventricular synergy for reasons not yet understood [47]
3. Abnormal momentum or traction of the prolapsing posterior mitral leaflet tending to pull the atrioventricular junction toward the left atrium during late systole [44]

MITRAL VALVE PROLAPSE AND ATRIAL SEPTAL DEFECT. The occurrence of mitral valve prolapse together with ostium secundum atrial septal defect is an observation that remains unexplained. Reduced left ventricular volume associated with left-to-right interatrial shunting may cause otherwise normal mitral leaflets and chordae to be relatively redundant for the chamber size. A high incidence of mitral valve prolapse has been reported in patients with atrial septal defects [2, 48–51]. Since no pathological abnormality of the mitral valve has been demonstrated consistently in patients with atrial septal defect, this high incidence of mitral valve prolapse may be related to the distortion of the left ventricular shape. Schreiber and associates [52] reported that in six of seven patients preoperative mitral valve prolapse either decreased in degree or disappeared following closure of the atrial septal defect. These investigators employed two-dimensional echocardiography to measure the geometry of the closed mitral valve and noted that the mitral valve areas subtended (MVAS) approached 0 or became negative as the overall position of the opposed mitral leaflets became relatively more atrial, therefore contributing to a tendency toward prolapse in the preoperative state (Fig. 3-5). Furthermore these investigators noted that closure of the atrial septal defect not only tended to normalize the left ventricular geometry but also arrested the tendency of the mitral valve to prolapse.

Normal aging results in a reduction in left ventricular volume, mass, annular circumference, and long axis without an appropriate decrease in mitral leaflet area and chordal length [9]. Accordingly, aging per se may result in leaflet-chordal redundancy, which may initiate or aggravate existing mitral valve prolapse.

ANGIOGRAPHIC-ECHOCARDIOGRAPHIC CORRELATIONS. Although the ideal standard does not yet exist for identification of mitral valve prolapse, tomographic imaging with two-dimensional echocardiography from multiple transducer positions to obtain a three-dimensional perspective of mitral valve coaptation is superior to the more limited views of the mitral valve profile from left ventricular angiography. Because of the limitations of M-mode echocardiography with only a single dimensional, "ice pick" view of the mitral leaflets, left ventricular angiog-

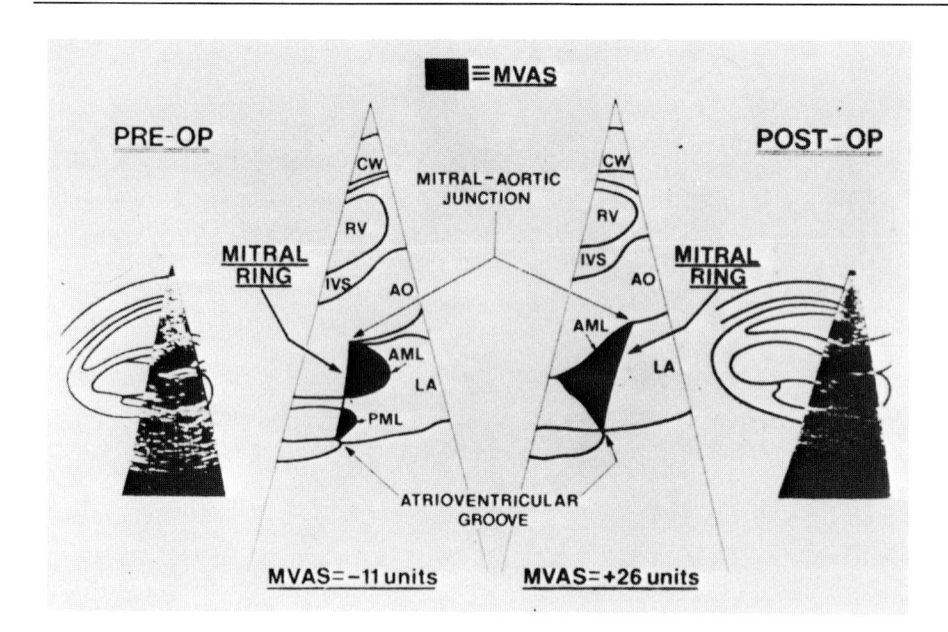

Fig. 3-5. Parasternal long axis views with diagrams showing preoperative and postoperative changes of mitral valve coaptation following surgical closure of an atrial septal defect. Normalization of left ventricular geometry after elimination of the right ventricular volume overload also normalized the mitral valve geometry. (From TL Schreiber et al: Effect of atrial septal defect repair on left ventricular geometry and degree of mitral valve prolapse. Circulation 615:888, 1980, by permission of the American Heart Association, Inc.)

raphy is probably superior to M-mode technique in identification of mitral valve prolapse [53]. Because the anterior mitral leaflet overlaps the posterior leaflet in the right anterior oblique left ventriculogram, prolapse of the former can be hidden and easily missed if this projection alone is used. In contrast, the left anterior oblique projection clearly delineates the anterior leaflet. Although pathological evidence suggests that redundancy of the mitral leaflets and lengthening of the chordae tendineae contribute to the presence of mitral valve prolapse, angiographic evidence of left ventricular wall motion abnormalities and segmental dysfunction demonstrates asynchronous, delayed contraction of the papillary muscles and/or the underlying left ventricular myocardium [19, 34, 46, 47, 54–56]. Leachman and associates [56] reported that the mitral annulus dilated and expanded paradoxically during systole. Grossman and colleagues [54] and Ehlers and coworkers [55] noted in angiographic studies the increased contraction of the mid-ventricular segment, particularly in the inferior wall of patients with prolapsed mitral valve. Scampardonis and associates [47] demonstrated several patterns of wall motion abnormalities in both systole and diastole involving 75 of 87 patients with prolapsed mitral valve. However, the most frequently observed abnormalities consisted of vigorous contraction of the posteroinferior portion and early diastolic relaxation of the anterior wall. Ranganathan and associates [57] noted in a clinical angiographic evaluation of 59 patients with prolapsed mitral valve that the severity of mitral regurgitation was increased in patients with triscallop prolapse and combined mitral leaflet prolapse in contrast to those patients with either single or biscallop prolapse. They also observed that the ST–T wave abnormalities in the inferior leads of the electrocardiogram were more frequently encountered in patients who had isolated posterior leaflet prolapse. Gilbert and associates [58] noted that two-dimensional echocardiographic imaging was significantly better than M-mode echocardiography in identifying mitral valve prolapse in a study of 49 patients undergoing cardiac catheterization. Sahn and colleagues [59] employing two-dimensional echocardiography observed that the prolapsing motion of the mitral valve often occurs in a superior direction as well as a posterior direction; the body of the posterior leaflet may be driven superiorly toward the left atrium while portions of the mitral leaflet near the atrioventricular junction move posteriorly. Morganroth and coworkers [60] reported that the apical four-chamber view was superior to the parasternal left ventricular long axis view for the detection of anterior leaflet prolapse.

ECHOCARDIOGRAPHIC IMAGING TECHNIQUE. In order for two-dimensional echocardiographic imaging to be utilized appropriately to identify or exclude the presence of mitral valve prolapse, good-quality imaging must be obtained in two important views, the parasternal long axis and the apical four-chamber views. Careful attention must be paid in the parasternal long axis imaging to ensure that both anterior and posterior leaflets are seen in optimal profile with good visualization not only of the coaptation point but also of the mitral annulus both anteriorly and posteriorly. In normal patients the coaptation point occurs on the ventricular side of the mitral annulus, whereas in the various types of prolapse conditions the coaptation point is shifted posteriorly and/or superiorly in line with the mitral annulus or superior to that point. Other abnormalities that are commonly observed with respect to abnormal features of the coaptation points include a posterior shifting of the point associated with prolapse of the anterior leaflet (Fig. 3-6) or an anterior shifting of the point associated with prolapse of both leaflets or of the posterior leaflet only (Fig. 3-7). While imaging in the parasternal long axis position the M-mode cursor should be directed through the mitral valve under direct visualization in order to optimize positioning of the cursor to record both leaflets in the specific regions desired. It is our current recommendation that, in the usual patient referred for evaluation of mitral valve prolapse, when the diagnosis can be made from the M-mode recording obtained in this manner there is no need for an additional two-dimensional study to reconfirm what has already been established by M-mode echo. Although it is probably not cost-effective or clinically necessary to perform a two-dimensional examination under such circumstances, an exception to this rule could be made if clinical symptomatology suggests the possibility of systemic emboli or other potential abnormalities that might indicate other structural or functional defects. In our experience the M-mode recording of the mitral valve may be normal when only a portion of the anterior mitral leaflet is prolapsing in a posterior or superior direction and when the prolapsing segment is positioned so that an M-mode beam cannot transect it. The apical four-chamber view is a very important tomographic plane for evaluation of the mitral leaflets; not uncommonly the parasternal left ventricular long axis view will be negative in individuals being evaluated for mitral valve prolapse in whom the prolapse is recognizable only in the apical four-chamber plane (Figs. 3-8A and B). Presumably this is because a portion of a leaflet or scallop that is now being imaged was not seen from the parasternal position. As in the parasternal view it is very important that the mitral annulus be well visualized and the left atrium opened up well in order to obtain clear delineation of the mitral annulus (Fig. 3-9). Although the apical long axis view is a valuable additional view for assessment of the mitral valve, this view rarely adds any additional information for evaluation of prolapse that has not already been obtained from either the parasternal long axis or the apical four-chamber views. The subcostal four-chamber view can also be utilized to identify mitral valve prolapse and may be useful if the apical four-chamber view is technically inadequate. The parasternal

92   3. Nonrheumatic mitral valve disease

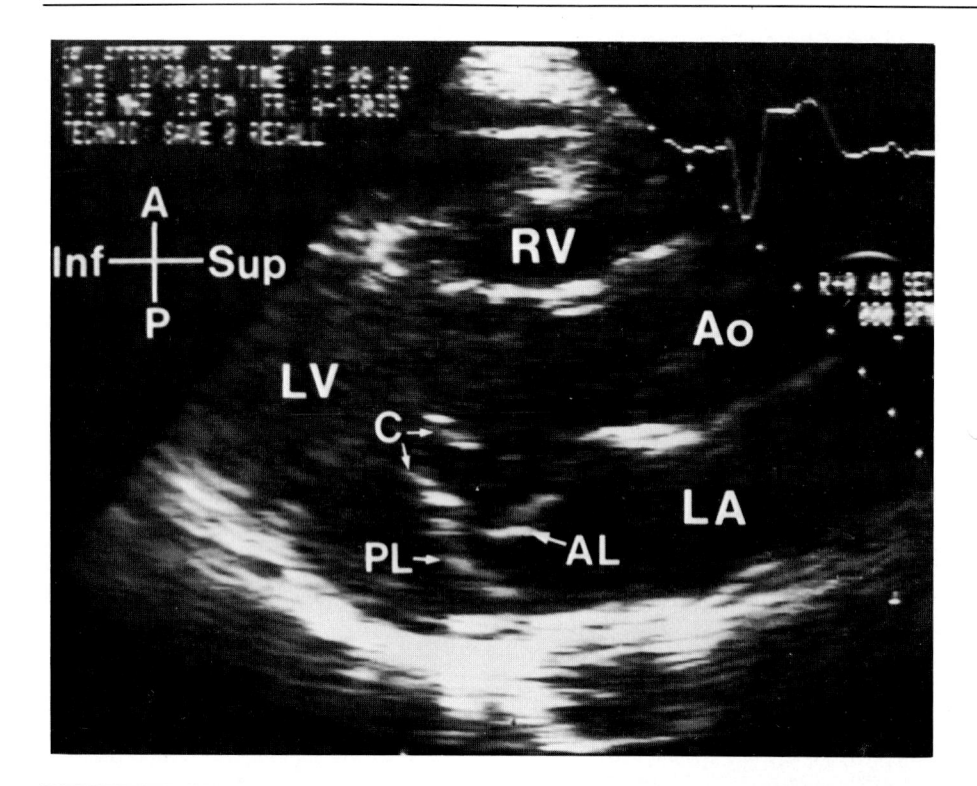

Fig. 3-6. Parasternal long axis view in a patient with mitral valve prolapse. The abnormality is confined to the anterior leaflet, which has moved posteriorly during systole behind the normal coaptation point with the posterior leaflet. C = chordae tendineae.

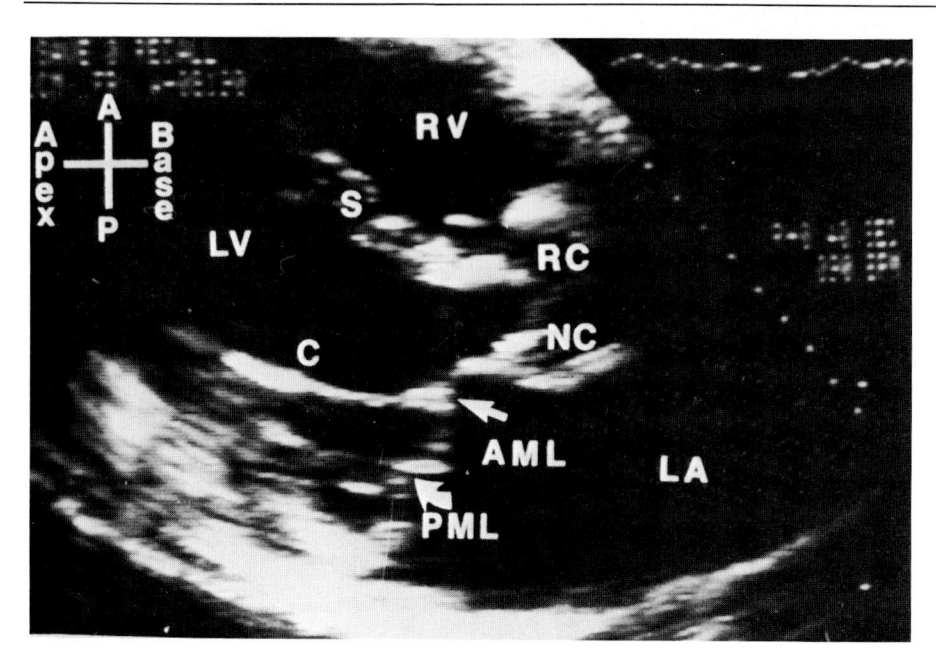

Fig. 3-7. Parasternal long axis view demonstrating prolapse of both anterior mitral leaflet and posterior mitral leaflet. The curved arrow identifies the coaptation point between the leaflets. Prolapse of the AML is distal to the point of attachment of the chordae tendineae (C) (straight arrow). Significant mitral regurgitation is present causing left atrial enlargement (A-P dimension = 60 mm). RC = right cusp of aortic valve.

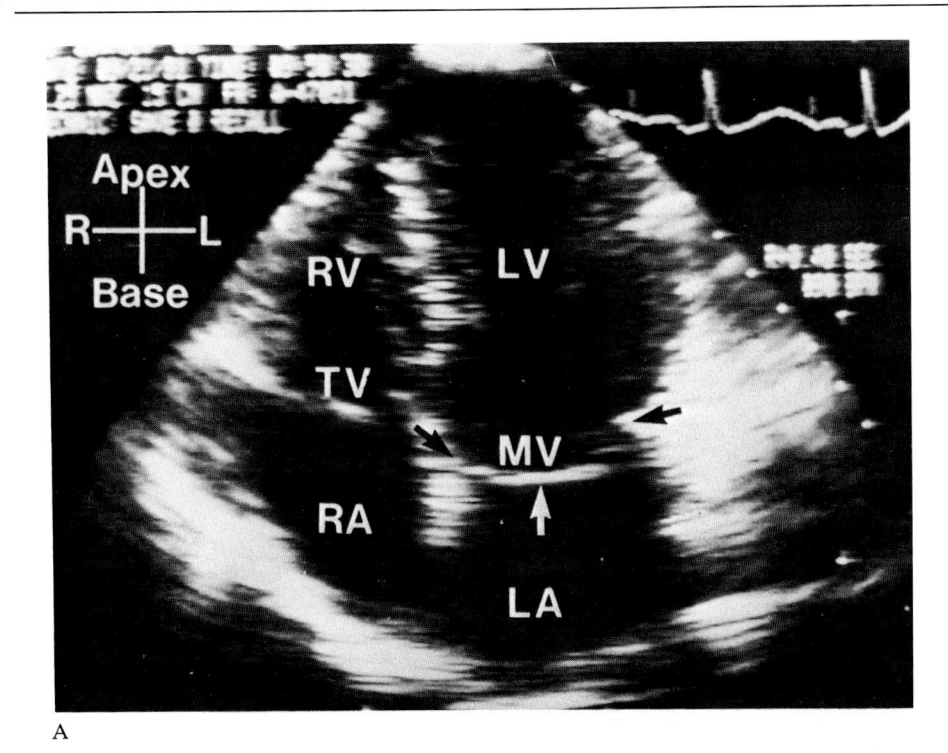

Fig. 3-8A. Apical 4-chamber view showing prolapse superiorly of both anterior and posterior mitral leaflets (white arrow). The mitral valve annulus and origin of each of the two leaflets are identified by black arrows. The tricuspid valve and all 4-chamber sizes are normal. B. Apical 4-chamber view in a patient with mitral valve prolapse affecting only the posterior leaflet and only demonstrable (arrow) in this tomographic plane. Chamber sizes are normal.

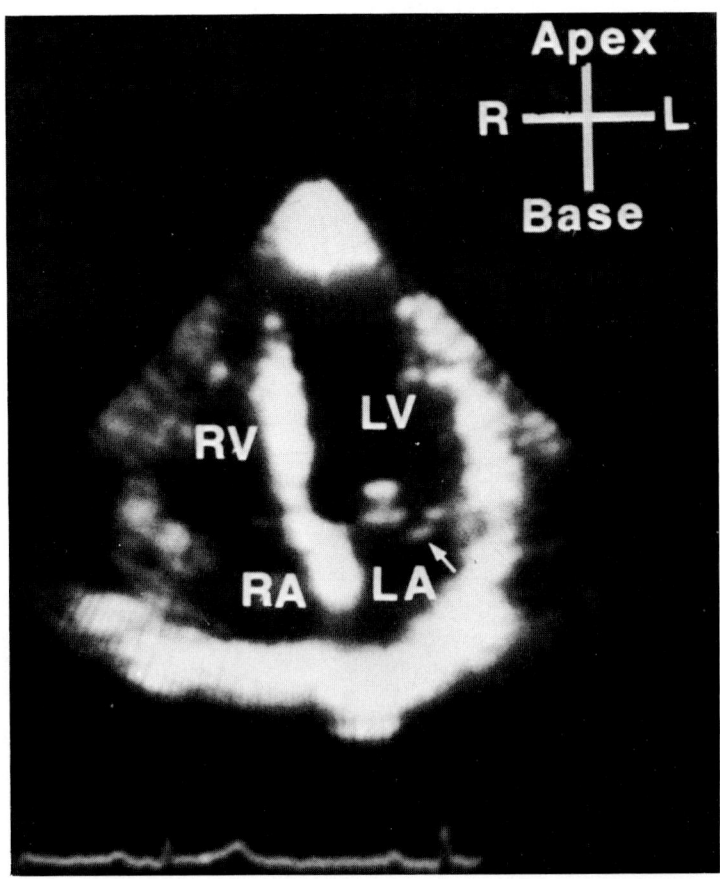

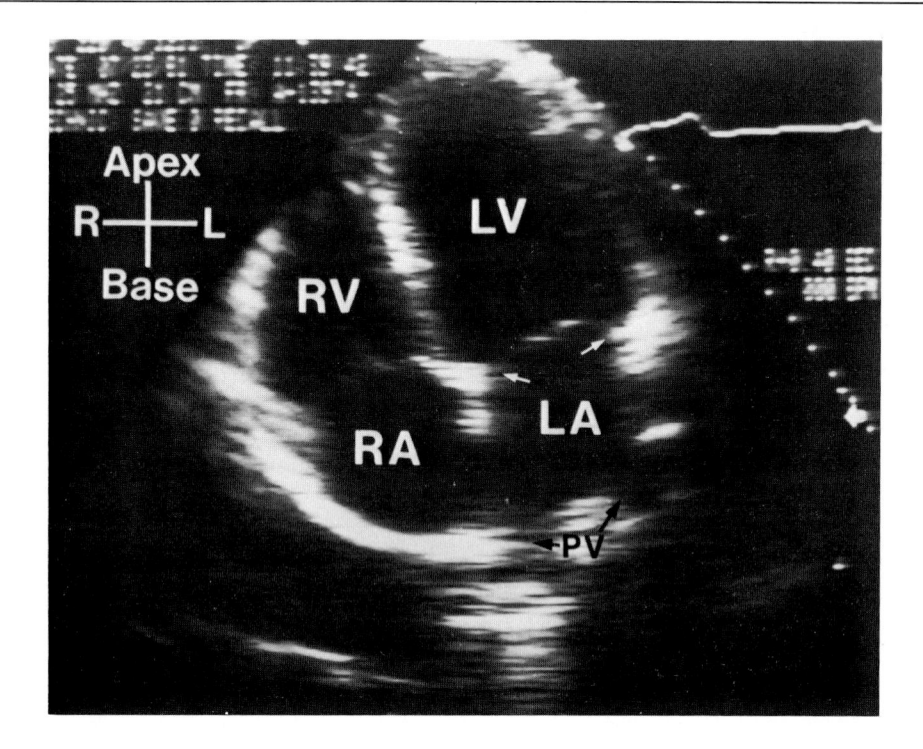

Fig. 3-9. Apical 4-chamber view in normal subject demonstrating mitral coaptation. Curvature of the valve during systole is on the ventricular side of a line between the right and left points (white arrows) of the mitral annulus. Contrast this appearance with the contour of the mitral valve and annulus in a patient with prolapse (Fig. 3-8A). PV = pulmonary vein.

left ventricular short axis view through the level of the mitral valve is of limited clinical usefulness but may demonstrate some redundancy of motion and increased thickness of the leaflets as well as provide an additional opportunity for the M-mode cursor to obtain M-mode recordings of the valve.

In certain borderline cases in which there appears to be a variant of normal systolic closure and the line of coaptation is "straightened" but without definitive prolapse, the echocardiographer should employ physiologic interventions in an effort to induce prolapse. These interventions most commonly include the Valsalva maneuver; if no additional beneficial information is obtained inhalation of amyl nitrite should be employed. Besides evaluating the leaflets for any apparent increased thickness or suggestion of redundancy, the echocardiographer must also know the clinical history, symptomatology, and relevant physical findings in order to determine whether added time and provocative maneuvers should be employed in any given patient.

Whenever a patient is referred to the echo lab because of possible mitral valve prolapse both atrioventricular valves should be evaluated carefully, because 10 to 15 percent of patients with mitral valve prolapse also have prolapse of the tricuspid valve. One of the best views for this evaluation is the apical four-chamber with particular emphasis on tricuspid leaflet coaptation and tricuspid annulus similar to the attention given to the mitral valve in the same view (Fig. 3-10). A second view should also be employed in the assessment of tricuspid systolic coaptation, namely the right ventricular inflow or RA/RV view (Fig. 3-11). A less satisfactory alternative is the parasternal short axis view at the base with attention directed toward the tricuspid valve. Finally the subcostal four-chamber view usually provides an excellent additional means of evaluating the tricuspid valve for evidence of prolapse.

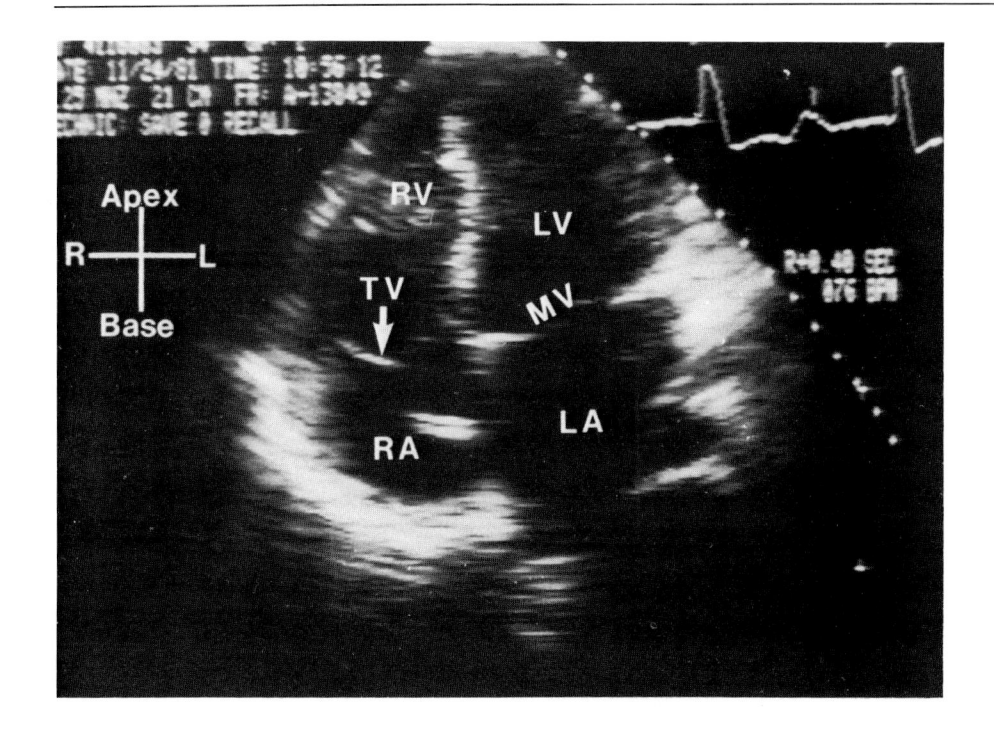

Fig. 3-10. Apical 4-chamber view showing tricuspid valve prolapse (arrow) in the absence of any associated mitral valve prolapse.

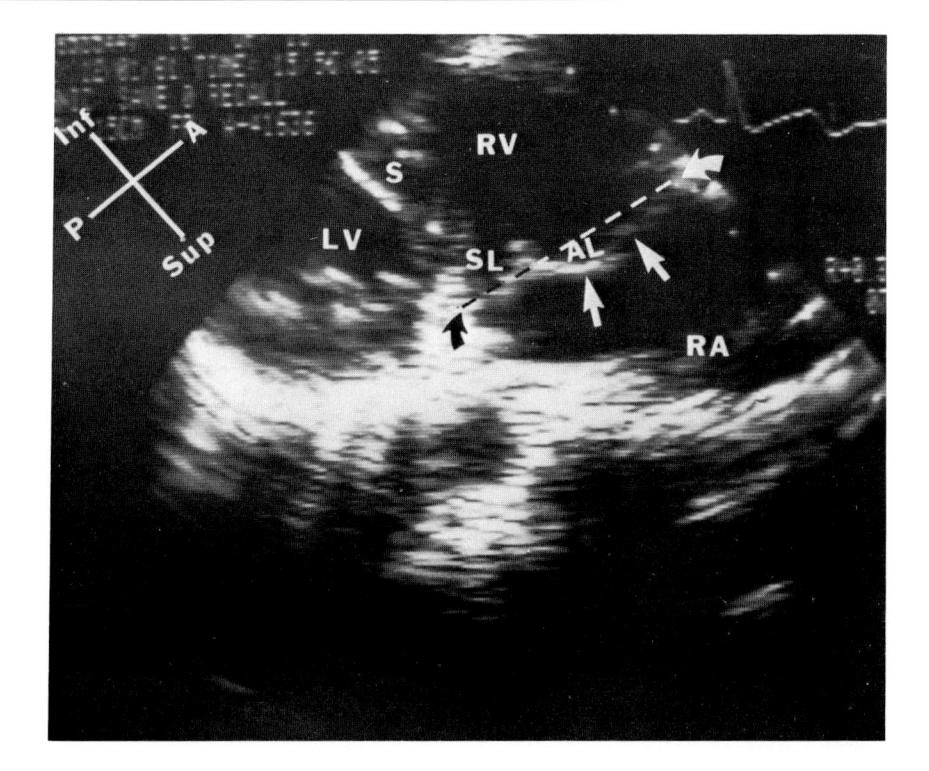

Fig. 3-11. Parasternal right ventricular inflow vein in a patient demonstrating prolapse of the anterior tricuspid leaflet (AL) (straight arrows). The curved arrows identify the tricuspid annulus.

2-D ECHO EVALUATION OF CAUSES OF MITRAL INSUFFICIENCY. Mintz and associates [61] studied 140 patients with mitral regurgitation by two-dimensional echocardiography and noted mitral valve prolapse to be the most common etiology. Two-dimensional echocardiography reliably differentiated mitral insufficiency secondary to valvular disease from that secondary to ventricular or papillary muscle dysfunction.

Kitabatake and associates [62] employed pulsed Doppler technique together with two-dimensional echo to determine the site and direction of regurgitant flow into the left atrium. They found that anterior leaflet prolapse produced a posterior jet in contrast to posterior leaflet prolapse which directed the regurgitant flow in an anterior direction. Accordingly, this difference in direction of regurgitant flow is an important determinant in the radiation of the systolic murmur of mitral regurgitation.

Chandraratna and Aronow [63] reported that dilatation of the mitral annulus occurred only in some patients with a dilated cardiomyopathy, and annular dilatation in those patients was not proportionate to the degree of left ventricular dilatation. Furthermore the annular size did not correlate with the presence or degree of mitral regurgitation. These investigators suggested that when mitral regurgitation occurs in association with left ventricular dilatation the mechanism may be related to loss of sphincteric action of the annulus or malalignment of the papillary muscles and is thus independent of the mitral ring dilatation itself.

Mitral annulus calcification. Calcification of the mitral annulus is a condition frequently encountered in the elderly population and is commonly thought to be clinically silent or benign. However, this is one of the more common causes of mitral regurgitation in this age group. Fulkerson and associates [64], in a review of the clinical features of 80 patients with left ventriculographic evidence of mitral annulus calcification, observed mitral regurgitation in 72. The clinical diagnoses in these 80 patients with calcification of the mitral annulus in decreasing order of frequency included: hypertension (41%), atrial fibrillation (29%), pacemakers (26%), mitral valve prolapse (14%), aortic stenosis (7%), hypertrophic cardiomyopathy (6%), arterial emboli (5%), and endocarditis (4%). Eighty-five percent (68 of 80 patients) had an underlying cardiac disorder associated with either chronically increased left ventricular systolic pressure or abnormal leaflet motion. Twenty-one of these patients eventually required pacemakers for management of symptomatic bradyarrhythmias. Because of the frequent association with serious cardiovascular disease, mitral annulus calcification should not be ignored as a benign marker of the elderly patient. The presence of mitral valve prolapse together with mitral annulus calcification is well known and occurred in 14 percent of the patients in the Fulkerson study [64].

D'Cruz and colleagues [65] pointed out in a study of 82 patients with two-dimensional echocardiography that the calcification was frequently located in the angle between the posterior mitral leaflet and the left ventricular posterior wall rather than in the mitral annulus proper (Fig. 3-12). The anterior mitral cusp is not attached to a true fibrous annulus as is the posterior mitral cusp; therefore the mitral valve ring is deficient anteriorly. When calcification is imaged anteriorly the calcific deposits probably originate on the ventricular surface at the base of the anterior mitral leaflet in the region of the aortic valve annulus (Fig. 3-13), or in the

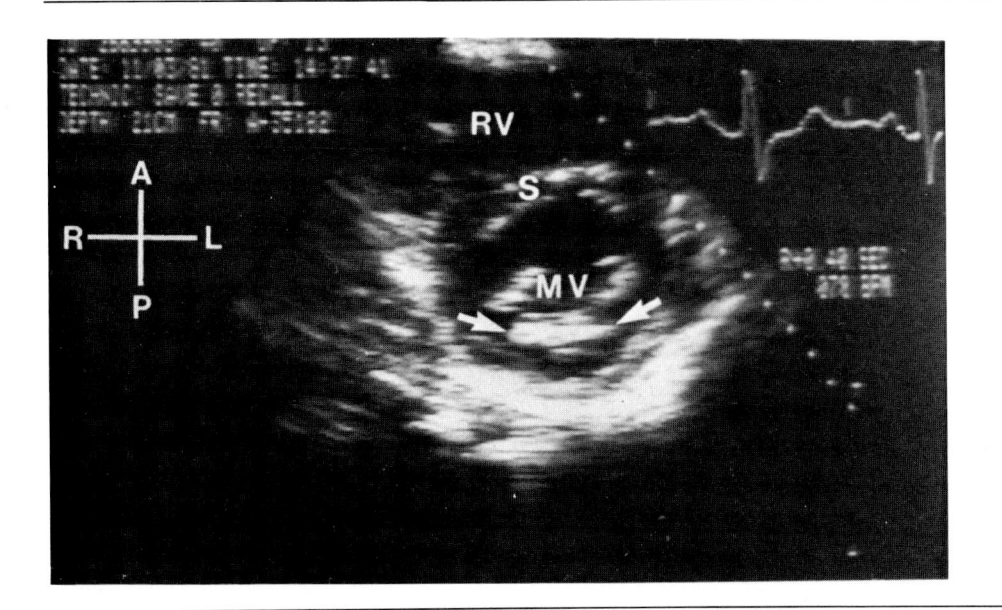

Fig. 3-12. Parasternal short axis view through the left ventricle near the atrioventricular sulcus showing the typical appearance of mitral annulus calcification (white arrows) and located posteriorly to the posterior mitral leaflet and anterior to the endocardium of posterior wall. Mitral valve motion is normal.

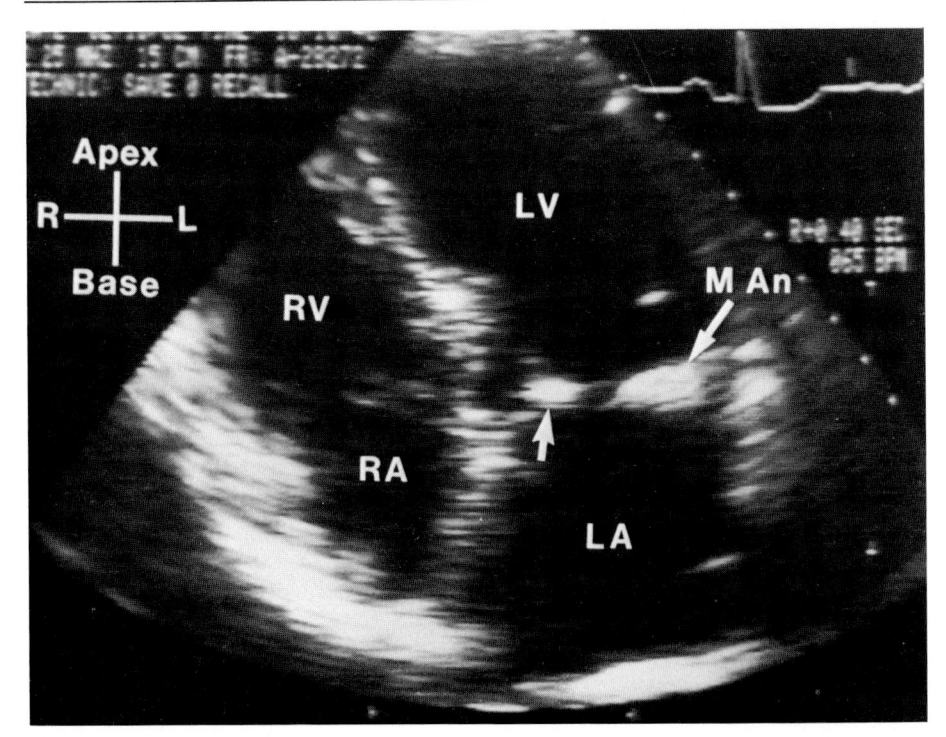

Fig. 3-13. Apical 4-chamber view showing apparent calcification of the proximal portion of the anterior mitral leaflet (arrow), which in other views appears to be confined to the posterior wall of the aortic annulus. The anterior leaflet is probably normal but may appear involved because of the "smearing" effect of the nearby calcium. There is also calcium in the posterior mitral leaflet.

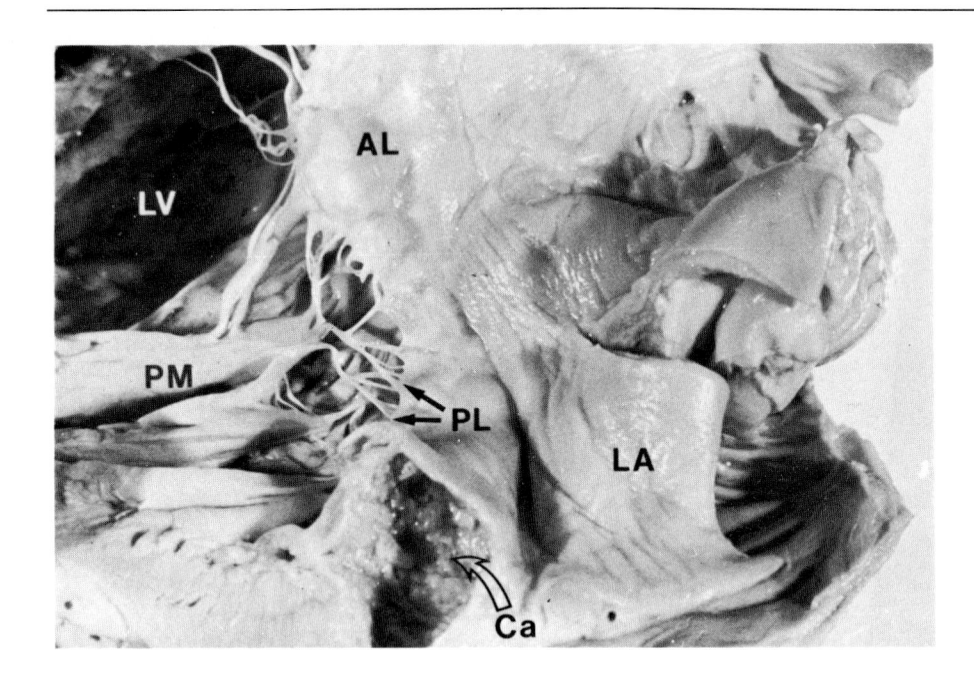

Fig. 3-14. Anatomic section showing heavy calcification (Ca) of the mitral annulus lying beneath the posterior mitral leaflet.

proximal portions of the body of the anterior leaflet rather than in the annulus itself [66]. Although echocardiography is probably more sensitive than fluoroscopy in detecting mitral annulus calcification [67, 68], two-dimensional imaging may be overly sensitive, particularly if the machine settings are somewhat over-gained. Furthermore there may be calcium or fibrosis in the structures immediately adjacent to the annulus; however, because of a "smearing" effect or lack of resolution at that given depth, the abnormal reflectance noted in the adjacent zone may appear to emanate from within the annulus itself.

Annular calcification of the mitral valve consists of calcium deposits ranging in size from a few millimeters to extensive deposits involving the entire valve ring (Fig. 3-14). Such calcification does not produce stenosis and is rarely associated with significant regurgitation. Extension of the calcific deposits may involve the conducting system leading to arrhythmias or complete heart block. The valve leaflets and the chordae tendineae are not involved in the process. In some cases mitral annulus calcification may be accompanied by calcific aortic stenosis, reinforcing the view that calcification of the mitral annulus is a degenerative change associated with aging. Similar calcification of the tricuspid annulus is rare except in association with pulmonary hypertension.

Ruptured chordae tendineae. The reliability of M-mode echocardiographic signs of a flail mitral leaflet have been well accepted and include the following:

1. Systolic echoes within the left atrium
2. Coarse diastolic fluttering of the mitral leaflet
3. Paradoxical or anterior coarse movement of the posterior mitral leaflet (Fig. 3-15A)
4. High-frequency systolic fluttering of the mitral valve in closed position [67–71]

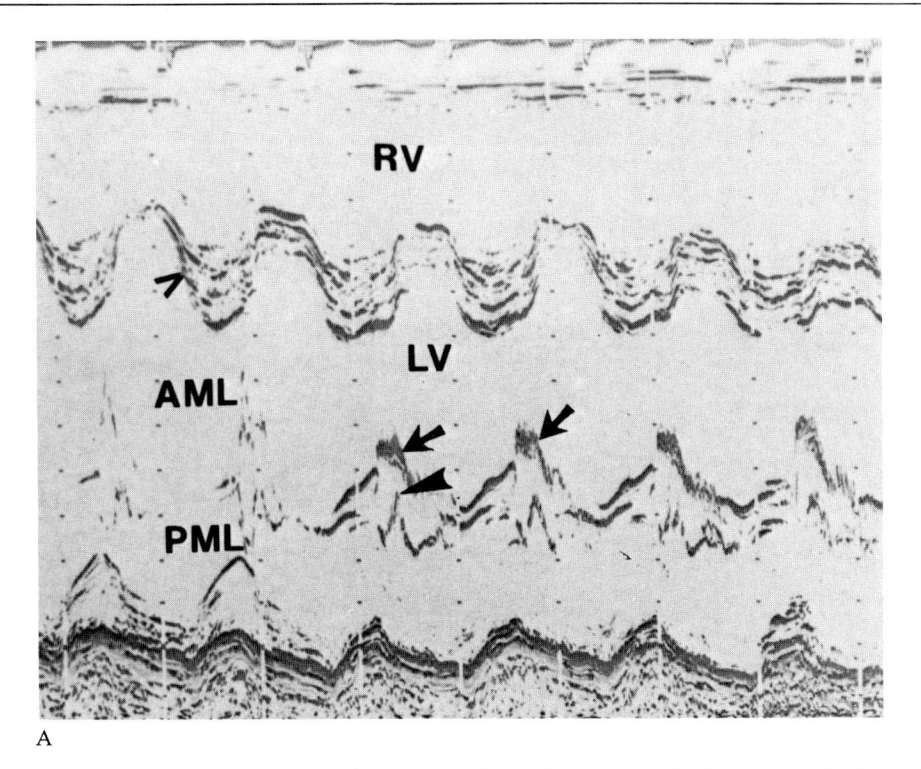

Fig. 3-15A. M-mode recording of a patient with both aortic regurgitation (AR) and mitral regurgitation (MR). The fine, high-frequency fluttering of the anterior mitral leaflet is due to the AR, and the coarse, anterior motion of the posterior mitral leaflet is caused by a flail leaflet, which was confirmed at surgery. The dilatation of the left ventricle and exaggerated septal motion are caused by the volume overloading from both AR and MR. B. M-mode recording of a patient with aortic regurgitation causing high-frequency fluttering of the anterior mitral leaflet (solid arrow) and left ventricular enlargement (end-diastolic dimension = 62 mm). Mitral valve prolapse is also present (curved arrow). The coarse fluttering of the posterior mitral leaflet (open arrows) resembles the motion caused by a flail leaflet (Fig. 3-15A); however, the chordae is not ruptured. The coarse fluttering may be caused by the aortic regurgitation or the mitral valve prolapse or both.

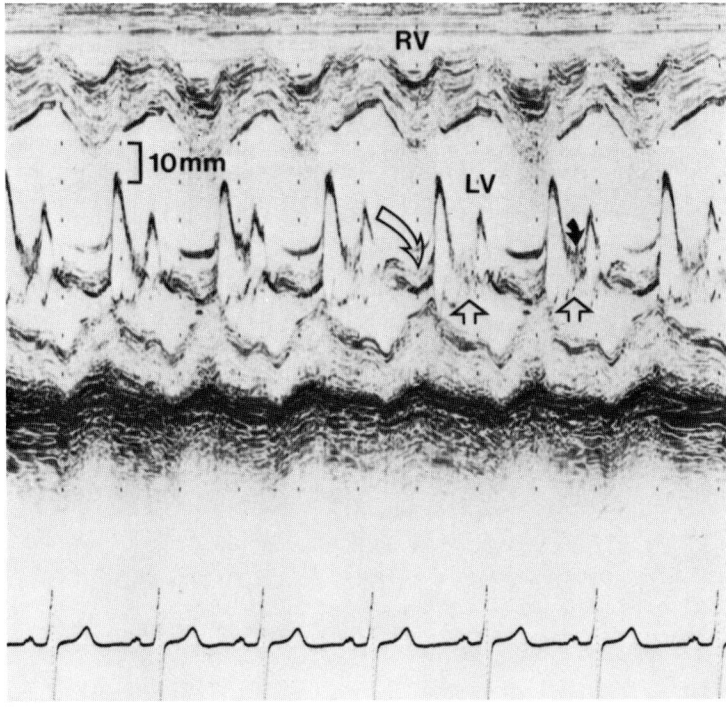

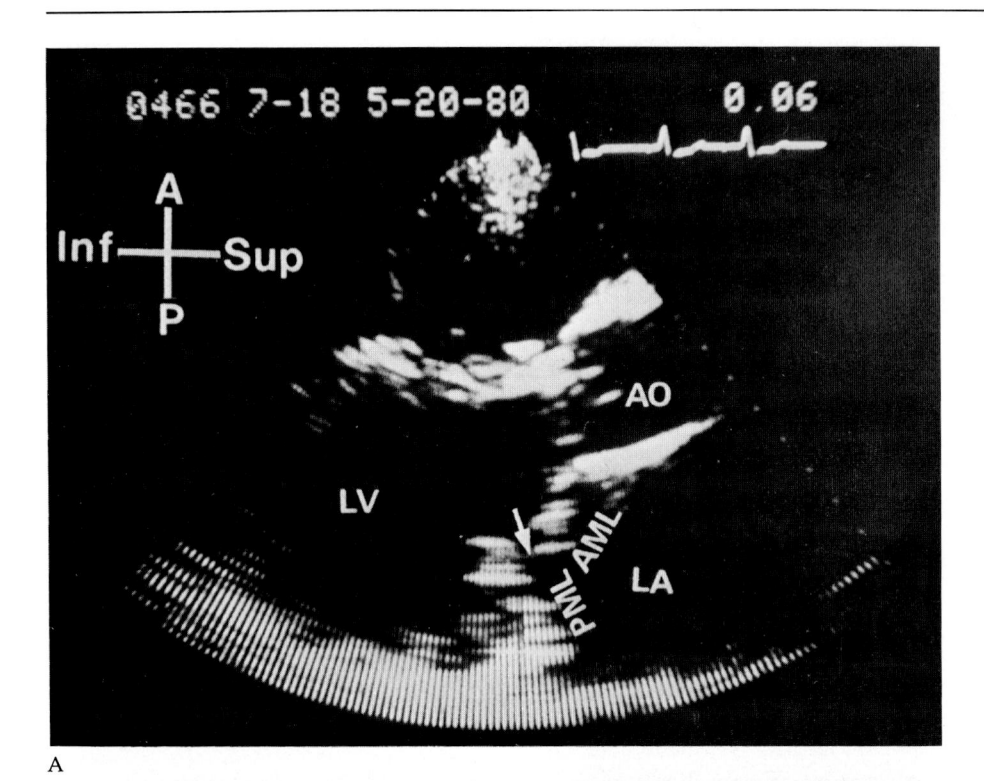

Fig. 3-16A. Parasternal long axis view showing a flail anterior mitral leaflet extending posteriorly and superiorly (arrow) to the point of normal coaptation with the posterior mitral leaflet during systole. Both left ventricle and left atrium are dilated. B. Parasternal long axis view (left panel) showing a flail posterior mitral leaflet and an apical 4-chamber view (right panel) in a different patient with the same diagnosis, namely ruptured chordae tendineae to the posterior mitral leaflet. C. Apical 4-chamber views in an adult with corrected transposition and marked prolapse of the left-sided tricuspid valve (arrows). The prolapse appears to involve primarily the septal leaflet of the tricuspid valve. Prolapse this severe is difficult to distinguish from ruptured chordae. The anatomic right ventricle functions as the systemic ventricle, and the moderator band, a landmark of the right ventricle, is visible in the systolic frame (right panel). The SL always arises more inferiorly than the anterior mitral leaflet and this relationship of the atrioventricular valves identifies the anatomic ventricles. PV = pulmonary vein.

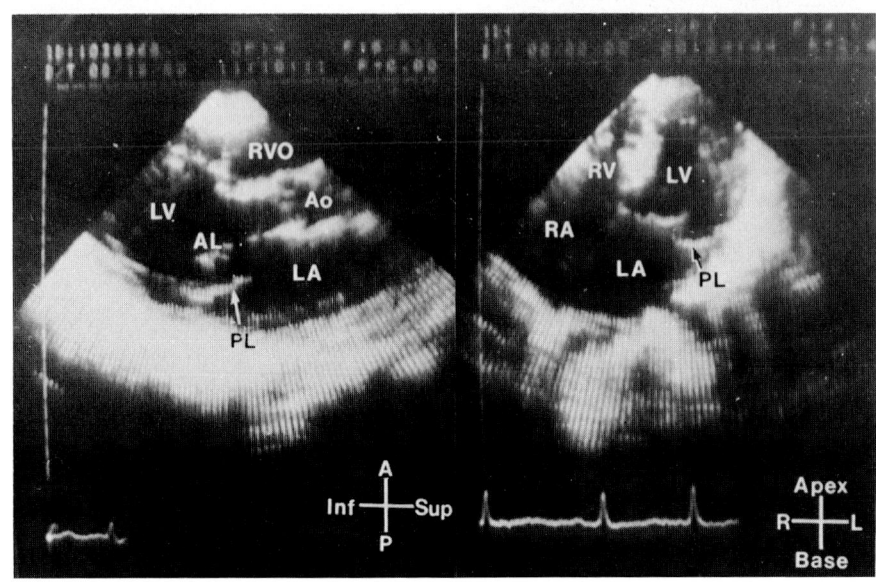

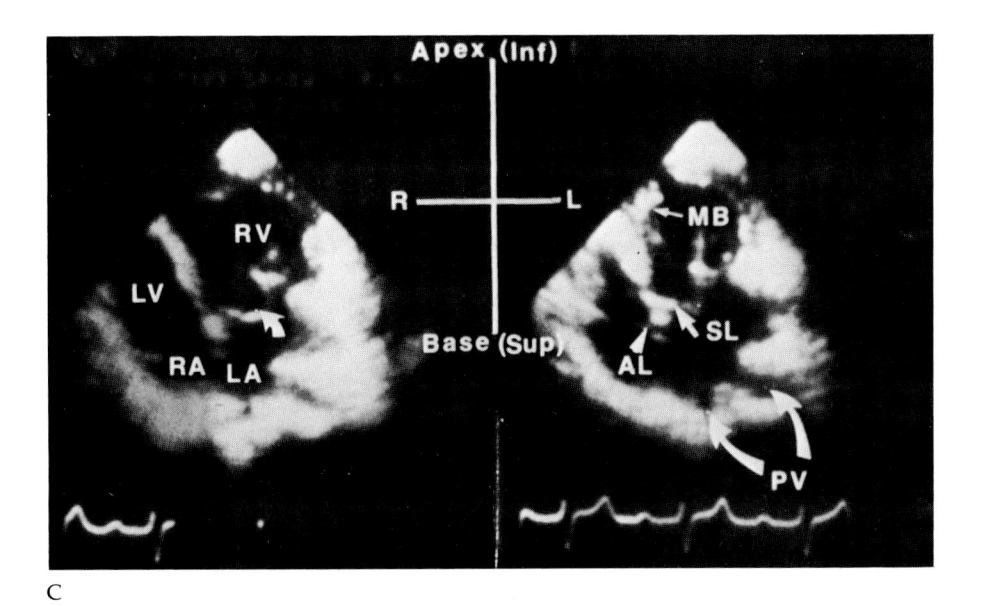

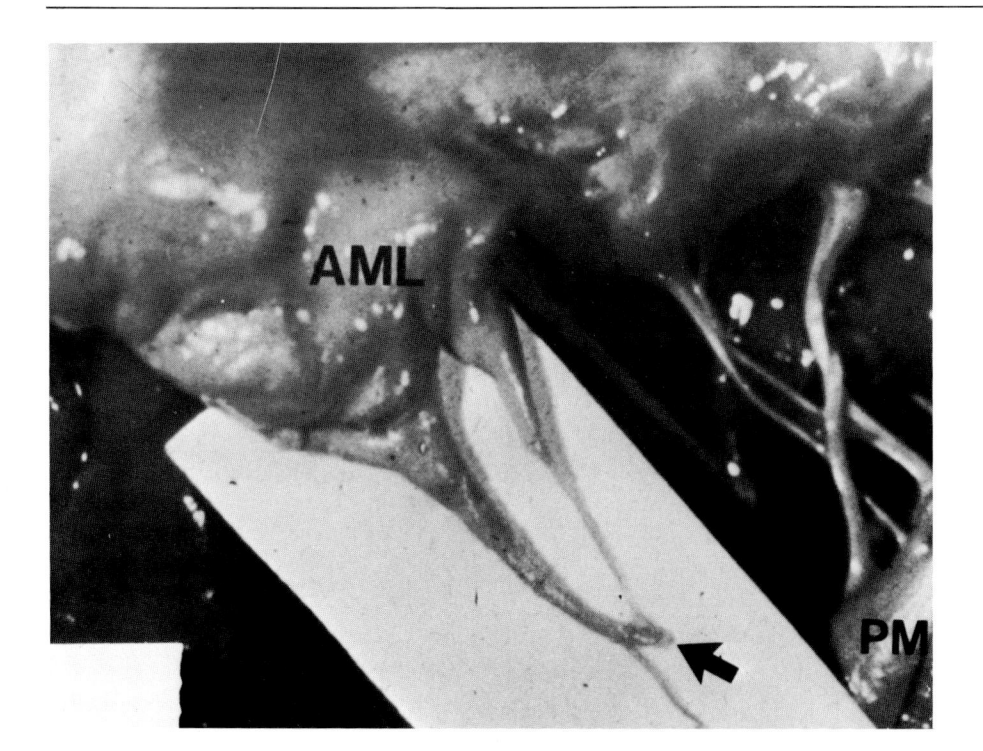

Fig. 3-17. Anatomic features of a thin chordae with spontaneous rupture (arrow).

Two-dimensional echocardiography offers not only added spatial orientation but also more comprehensive imaging of both leaflets and has shown loss of normal systolic mitral leaflet coaptation as well as excessive systolic mitral leaflet motion prolapsing into the left atrium [72, 73]. Although the abnormal motion identified by the M-mode echo is usually diagnostic, the more comprehensive imaging with two-dimensional echo improves the sensitivity of establishing the diagnosis. The two-dimensional imaging views required for evaluating patients for mitral valve prolapse, the parasternal left ventricular long axis and apical four-chamber views, are also the most important here (Fig. 3-16). Additional views that may be of value are the apical long axis and the subcostal four-chamber views. As in simultaneous combined M-mode and two-dimensional imaging technique described for prolapsed valves, the ability to direct the M-mode beam while visualizing the chaotic whipping motion of the flail mitral leaflet can also optimize the M-mode recording by directing it through the more abnormally moving leaflet segments under simultaneous visualization.

The anatomic features of ruptured chordae tendineae consist of rapid tapering of the chordae to thin, threadlike filaments to the point of disruption (Fig. 3-17). Histologic sections of the ruptured chordae show a loss of ground substance, increased mucopolysaccharide deposits, disruption of elastic and collagen fibers, and disarray of the collagen strands that remain. The disruption of the elastic fibers and collagen elements weakens the chordae, leading to eventual rupture.

Although the coarse diastolic fluttering of the mitral leaflet is relatively specific for a flail valve, we have previously reported a 17-year-old with both a systolic and diastolic murmur at the apex, diastolic fluttering of the mitral leaflet, and no evidence of any structural abnormality at the time of cardiac catheterization [74]. Similar coarse fluttering of the posterior mitral leaflet has been observed in a patient with aortic regurgitation and mitral valve prolapse but no ruptured chordae [Fig. 15B].

Tei and associates [75] reported systolic fluttering of the interatrial septum in 5 of 10 patients with ruptured chordae tendineae to the posterior mitral leaflet. They demonstrated that the systolic fluttering of the interatrial septum occurred from a regurgitant jet striking the atrial septum.

Papillary muscle dysfunction. M-mode echocardiography is of little value to the clinician who is attempting to identify the presence of papillary muscle dysfunction. Although two-dimensional imaging does permit visualization of both papillary muscles, specific criteria for identifying papillary muscle dysfunction have not yet been defined. It is not uncommon to image papillary muscles that show an increased reflectance consistent with fibrosis from previous myocardial infarction in one or both zones of myocardium surrounding the papillary muscles. The abnormal reflective pattern together with the abnormal segmental function of the adjoining myocardium suggests an abnormality of papillary muscle and the possibility of papillary muscle dysfunction.

The incidence of fibrosis and calcification of chordae tendineae and papillary muscles in patients with mitral valve prolapse has not yet been determined (Fig. 3-18). Come and Riley [76] reported fibrotic thickening and calcification of mitral valve chordae tendineae and papillary muscles in 17 patients with pathological confirmation in five. These investigators suggested that there was an association

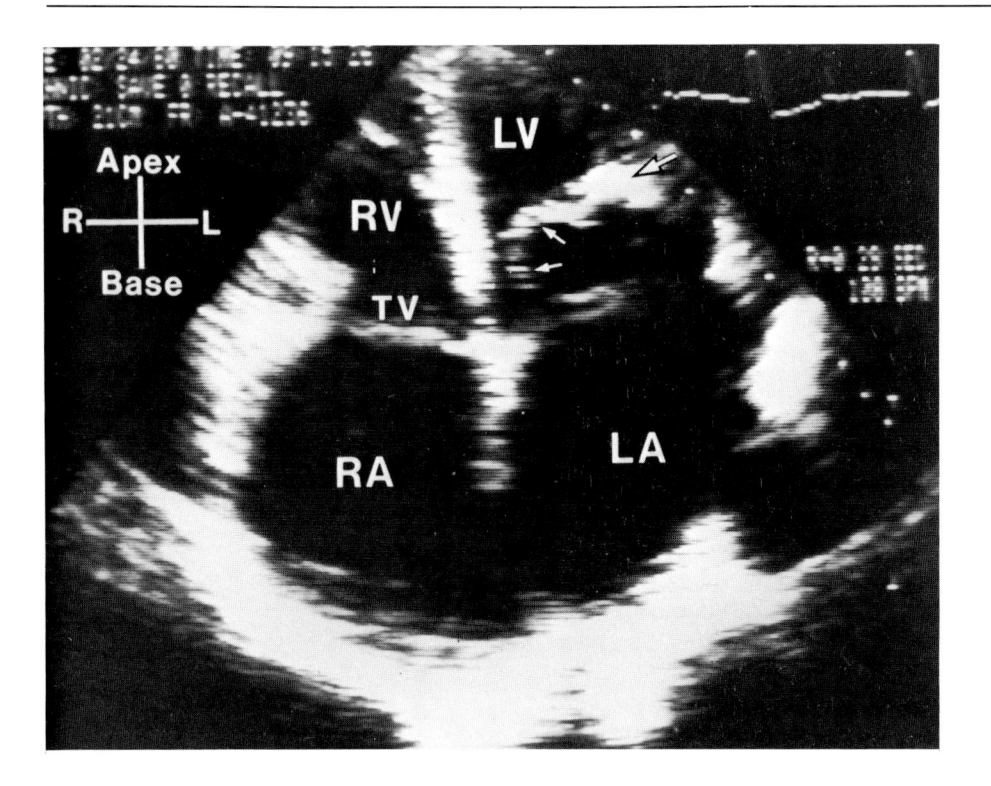

Fig. 3-18. Apical 4-chamber view at onset of systole in a patient with both tricuspid regurgitation and mitral regurgitation due to prolapse, which account for the marked biatrial enlargement. Although mitral valve prolapse is not yet visible at the onset of systole, marked redundancy of the chordae tendineae (small arrows) and increased thickness of the distal chordae at their attachment to the anterolateral papillary muscle can be seen. This increased reflectance of the papillary muscle (open arrow) is probably due to fibrosis and/or calcification also involving the chordae.

between these findings and the presence of mitral regurgitation and congestive heart failure which were present in the majority of these patients.

Ogawa and colleagues [77] reported two abnormal patterns of mitral valve closure in 14 patients with mitral regurgitation in whom the diagnosis was established on clinical grounds of papillary muscle dysfunction. These features were late systolic mitral valve prolapse in three patients with an akinetic inferior-posterior wall together with papillary muscle fibrosis but normal left ventricular cavity size, and displacement of mitral valve coaptation toward the apex of the left ventricle observed in nine patients with ventricular dilatation or ventricular aneurysm.

Thus two-dimensional echocardiography may be useful in identifying structural and functional abnormalities of the papillary muscles, left ventricle, chordae tendineae, and mitral valve that may cause mitral regurgitation secondary to papillary muscle dysfunction (Fig. 3-19).

We have made the observation in our laboratories that if only a single papillary muscle is fibrosed and involved in a region of previous myocardial infarction, there is usually no mitral regurgitation present. This clinical impression is further reinforced by experimental evidence that injury is required to both papillary muscles with left ventricular wall dysfunction for mitral regurgitation to develop [78]. Distortion of the normal spatial relationship of the papillary muscles may result in a loss of normal structural support of the mitral valve [79]. Although coronary artery disease is the most common cause of papillary muscle dysfunction, other causes include cardiomyopathy, any cause of left ventricular dilatation, trauma, endocardial diseases, infiltrative diseases, or inflammatory diseases.

Acute mitral insufficiency with deterioration of left ventricular performance

104   3. Nonrheumatic mitral valve disease

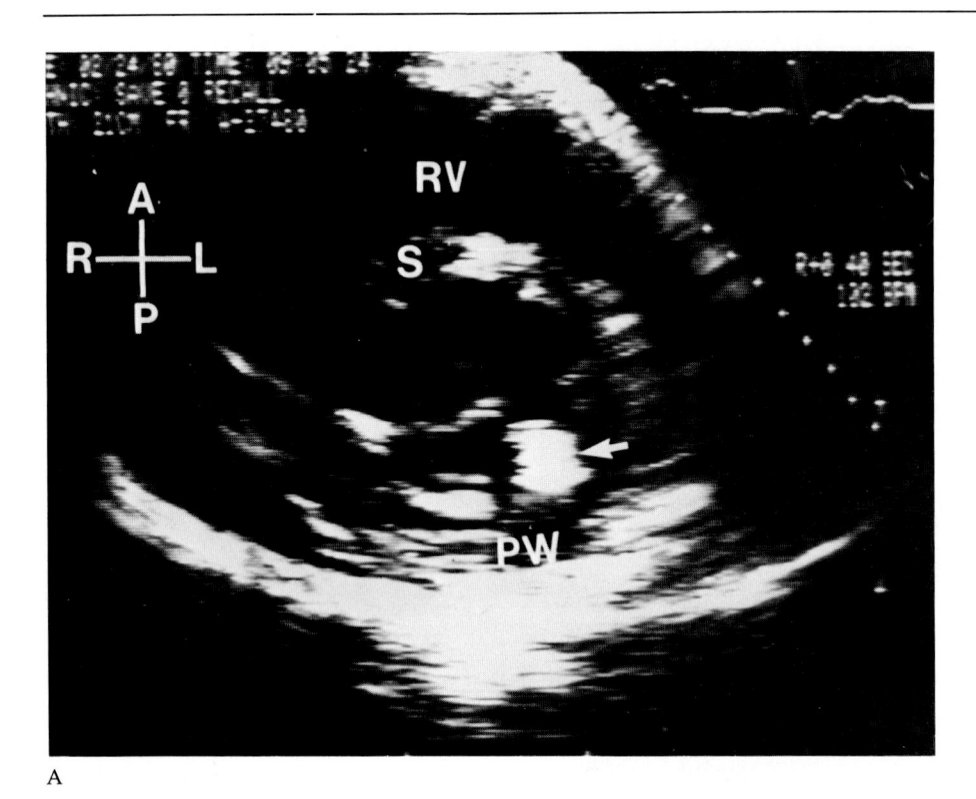

Fig. 3-19A. Parasternal short axis view through the tip of the lateral papillary muscle (arrow), which is fibrosed and/or calcified secondary to coronary artery disease. B. Anatomic short axis section in a patient who died of coronary artery disease. Old posterior myocardial infarction with scarring and fibrosis extends from the posterior septum (open arrow) to the posteromedial papillary muscle (black arrow). Wall thinning and increased reflectances from such zones can be observed in vivo with 2-D echocardiography. AS = anterior septum; RV = right ventricular free wall.

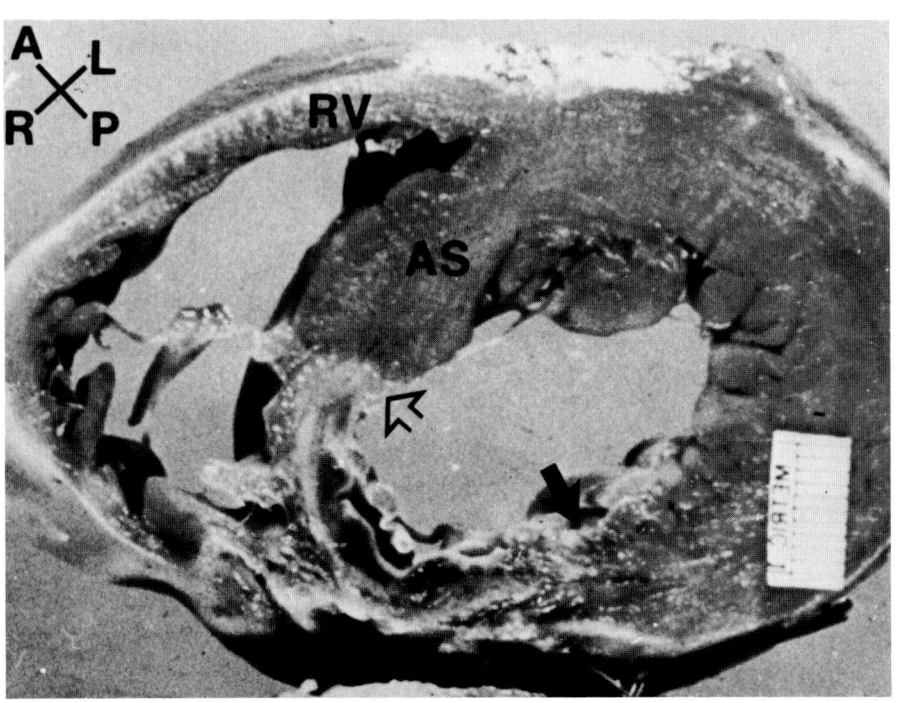

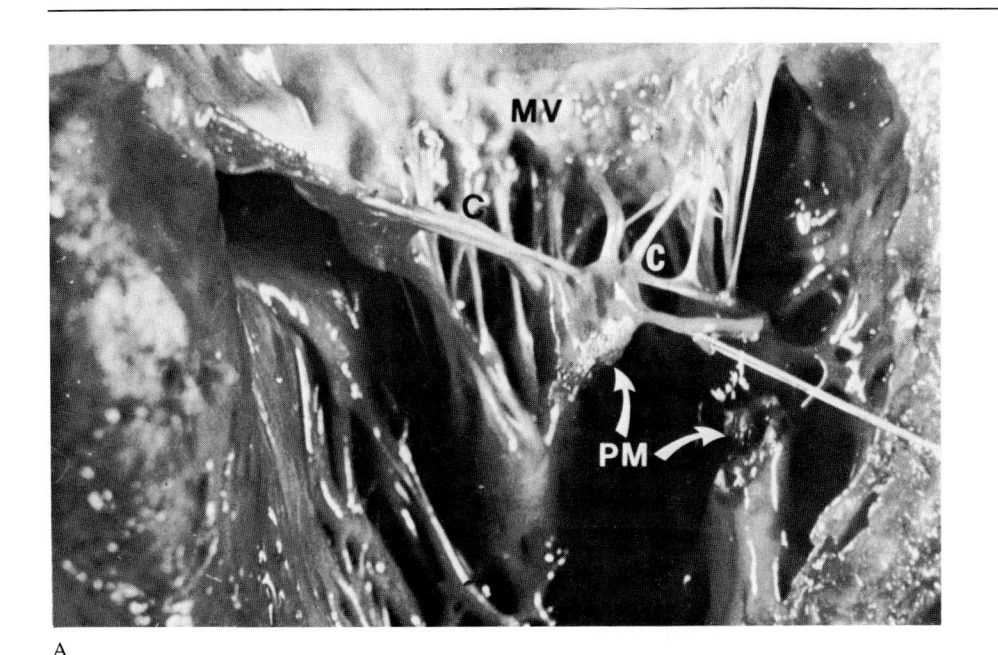

Fig. 3-20A. Postmortem specimen showing a ruptured papillary muscle head resulting in acute severe mitral regurgitation and death. C = chordae tendineae. B. Low parasternal long axis view of ruptured head of the posterior medial papillary muscle. The rupture site (open arrow) and muscle head attached to chordae and anterior mitral leaflet can be seen. C = catheter. (From GS Mintz et al: Two-dimensional echocardiographic identification of surgically correctable complications of acute myocardial infarction. Circulation 64:91, 1981, by permission of the American Heart Association, Inc.)

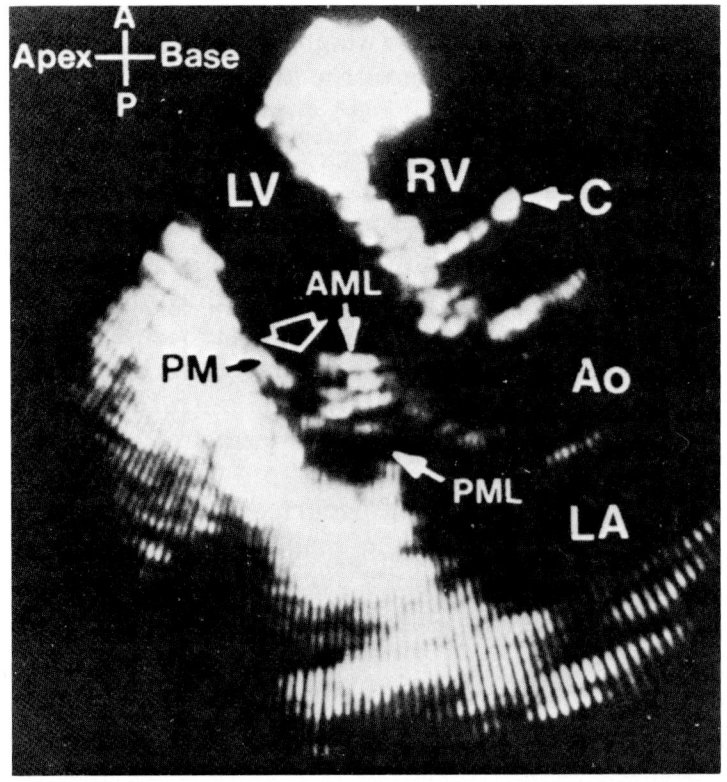

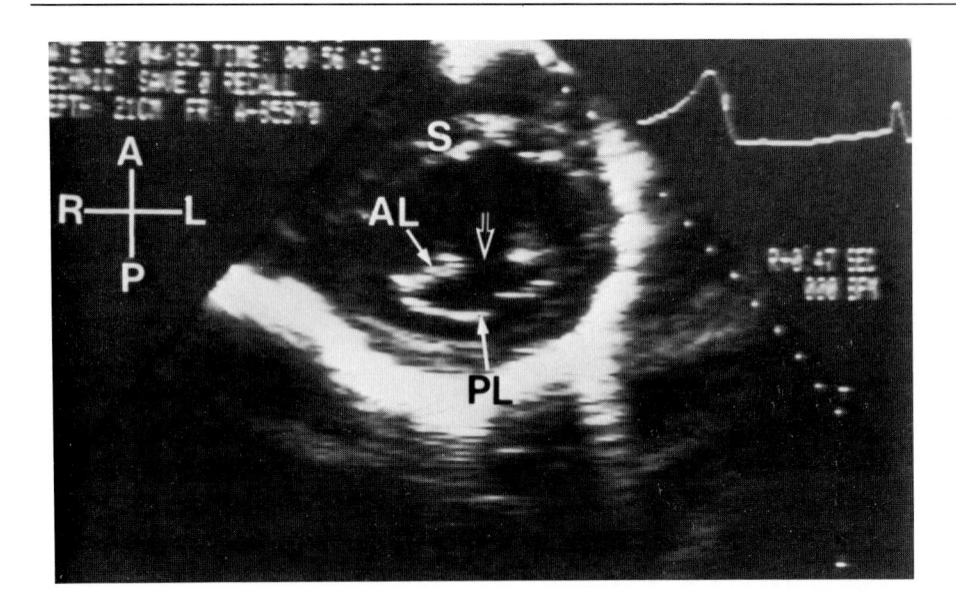

Fig. 3-21. Parasternal short axis view through the mitral valve showing an apparent defect (arrow) of the anterior mitral leaflet simulating a congenital cleft. The patient has normal cardiac anatomy.

can be caused by rupture of a papillary muscle or severe papillary muscle dysfunction complicating myocardial infarction (Fig. 3-20A). Clinical findings may not differentiate between papillary muscle rupture and severe papillary muscle dysfunction [80]. Without surgical intervention a large percentage of patients with rupture of papillary muscle will die within 24 hours. The two-dimensional echocardiographic features of ruptured papillary muscle include [81] (Fig. 3-20B) a mobile mass of echoes attached to normal chordae tendineae in the left ventricle, absent tip of papillary muscle, and severe mitral valve prolapse together with flail motion of the valve.

Congenital mitral regurgitation. Discussion of congenital mitral regurgitation due to cleft of the anterior mitral leaflet is included in Chapter 14. We have found both apical four-chamber and parasternal short axis at the level of mitral valve views valuable in identifying a congenital cleft of the anterior mitral leaflet. It is important to identify the cleft in two views if possible, since echo dropout of one portion of the leaflet without confirmation by a second view may simulate a cleft (Fig. 3-21).

References

1. Levy MJ, Edwards JE: Anatomy of mitral insufficiency. *Prog Cardiovasc Dis* 5:119, 1962
2. Jeresaty RM: Mitral valve prolapse-click syndrome. *Prog Cardiovasc Dis* 15:623, 1973
3. Goodman D, Kimbiris D, Linhart JW: Chordae tendineae rupture complicating the systolic click-late systolic murmur syndrome. *Am J Cardiol* 33:681, 1974
4. Shrivastava S, Guthrie RB, Edwards JE: Prolapse of the mitral valve. *Mod Concepts Cardiovasc Dis* 46:57, 1977
5. Marshall CE, Shappell SD: Sudden death and the ballooning posterior leaflet syndrome: Detailed anatomic and histochemical investigation. *Arch Pathol* 98:134, 1974
6. Trent JK, Adelman AG, Wigle ED, Silver MD: Morphology of a prolapsed posterior mitral valve leaflet. *Am Heart J* 29:222, 1967
7. Pomerance A: Ballooning deformity (mucoid degeneration) of atrioventricular valves. *Br Heart J* 31:343, 1969
8. Gooch AS, Maranhao V, Scampardonis G, Cha SD, Yang SS: Prolapse of both mitral and tricuspid leaflets in systolic murmur-click syndrome. *N Engl J Med* 287:1218, 1972
9. Roberts WC, Perloff JK: Mitral valvular disease: A clinicopathologic survey of the conditions causing the mitral valve to function abnormally. *Ann Intern Med* 77:939, 1972
10. Frable WJ: Mucinous degeneration of the cardiac valves: The "floppy valve" syndrome. *J Thorac Cardiovasc Surg* 58:62, 1969
11. Salomon NW, Stinson EB, Griepp RB, Shumway NB: Surgical treatment of degenerative mitral regurgitation. *Am J Cardiol* 38:463, 1976
12. Read RC, Thal AP, Wendt VE: Symptomatic valvular myxomatous transformation (the floppy valve syndrome): A possible forme fruste of the Marfan syndrome. *Circulation* 32:897, 1965
13. Kern WH, Tucker BL: Myxoid changes in cardiac valves: Pathological, clinical and ultrastructural studies. *Am Heart J* 84:294, 1972
14. Pomerance A: Aging changes in human heart valves. *Br Heart J* 29:222, 1967
15. McKay R, Yacoub MH: Clinical and pathological findings in patients with "floppy" valves treated surgically. *Circulation* 48(Suppl 3):63, 1973
16. Salazar AE, Edwards JE: Friction lesions of ventricular endocardium: Relation to chordae tendineae of mitral valve. *Arch Pathol* 90:364, 1970
17. Procacci PM, Savran SV, Schreiter SL, Bryson AL: Prevalence of clinical mitral-valve prolapse in 1169 young women. *N Engl J Med* 294:1086, 1976
18. DeMaria AN, Amsterdam EA, Vismara LA, Neumann A, Mason DT: Arrhythmias in the mitral valve prolapse syndrome: Prevalence, nature and frequency. *Ann Intern Med* 84:656, 1976
19. Gooch AS, Vicencio F, Maranhao V, Goldberg H: Arrhythmias and left ventricular asynergy in the prolapsing mitral leaflet syndrome. *Am J Cardiol* 29:611, 1972
20. Swartz MH, Teichholz LE, Donoso E: Mitral valve prolapse: A review of associated arrhythmias. *Am J Med* 62:377, 1977
21. Corrigall D, Bolen J, Hancock EW, Popp RL: Mitral valve prolapse and infective endocarditis. *Am J Med* 63:215, 1977
22. Leichtman D, Nelson R, Gobel FL, Alexander CS, Cohn JN: Bradycardia with mitral valve prolapse: A potential mechanism of sudden death. *Ann Intern Med* 85:453, 1976
23. Devereux RB, Perloff JK, Reichek N, Josephson ME: Mitral valve prolapse. *Circulation* 54:3, 1976
24. Rippe J, Fishbein MC, Carabello B, Angoff G, Sloss L, Collins JJ Jr, Alpert JS: Primary myxomatous degeneration of cardiac valves: Clinical, pathological, hemodynamic, and echocardiographic profile. *Br Heart J* 44:621, 1980
25. Barlow JB, Pocock WA: The problem of nonejection systolic clicks and associated mitral systolic murmurs: Emphasis on the billowing mitral leaflet syndrome. *Am Heart J* 90:636, 1975
26. Darsee JR, Mikolich JR, Nicholoff NB, Lesser LE: Prevalence of mitral valve prolapse in presumably healthy young men. *Circulation* 59:619, 1979
27. Hill DG, Davies MJ, Braimbridge MV: The natural history and surgical management of the redundant cusp syndrome (floppy mitral valve). *J Thorac Cardiovasc Surg* 67:519, 1974
28. Weiss AN, Mimbs JW, Ludbrook PA, Sobel BE: Echocardiographic detection of mitral valve prolapse: Exclusion of false positive diagnosis and determination of inheritance. *Circulation* 52:1091, 1975

29. Appelblatt NH, Willis PW, Lenhart JA, Shulman JI, Walton JA Jr: Ten to 40 year follow-up of 69 patients with systolic click with or without late systolic murmur. *Am J Cardiol* 35:119, 1975
30. Barlow JB, Bosman CK, Pocock WA, Marchand P: Late systolic murmurs and non-ejection (mid-late) systolic clicks: An analysis of 90 patients. *Br Heart J* 30:203, 1968
31. Fontana ME, Pence HL, Leighton RF, Wooley CF: The varying clinical spectrum of the systolic click-late systolic murmur syndrome. *Circulation* 41:807, 1970
32. Winkle RA, Lopes MG, Fitzgerald JW, Goodman DJ, Schroeder JS, Harrison DC: Arrhythmias in patients with mitral valve prolapse. *Circulation* 52:73, 1975
33. Sloman G, Wong M, Walker J: Arrhythmias on exercise in patients with abnormalities of the posterior leaflet of the mitral valve. *Am Heart J* 83:312, 1972
34. Gulotta SJ, Gulco L, Padmanabhan V, Miller S: The syndrome of systolic click, murmur, and mitral valve prolapse—a cardiomyopathy? *Circulation* 49:717, 1974
35. LeWinter MM, Hoffman JR, Shell WE, Karliner JS, O'Rourke RA: Phenylephrine-induced atypical chest pain in patients with prolapsing mitral valve leaflets. *Am J Cardiol* 34:12, 1974
36. Khullar SC, Leighton RF: Mitral valve prolapse syndrome (MVPS): Left ventricular function and myocardial metabolism. *Am J Cardiol* 35:149, 1975
37. Reinke R, Higgins C, Gosink B, Leopold G: Significance of mitral valve prolapse. *Circulation* 50(Suppl 3):76, 1974
38. Winkle RA, Goodman DJ, Popp RL: Simultaneous echocardiographic-phonocardiographic recordings at rest and during amyl nitrite administration in patients with mitral valve prolapse. *Circulation* 51:522, 1975
39. Mathey DG, Decoodt PR, Allen HN, Swan HJC: The determinants of onset of mitral valve prolapse in the systolic click-late systolic murmur syndrome. *Circulation* 53:872, 1976
40. Popp RL, Brown OR, Silverman JF, Harrison DC: Echocardiographic abnormalities in the mitral valve prolapse syndrome. *Circulation* 49:428, 1974
41. Epstein EJ, Coulshed N: Phonocardiogram and apex cardiogram in systolic click-late systolic murmur syndrome. *Br Heart J* 35:260, 1973
42. Bharati S, Granston AS, Liebson PR, Loeb HS, Rosen KM, Lev M: The conduction system in mitral valve prolapse syndrome with sudden death. *Am Heart J* 101:667, 1981
43. Young JB, Waggoner AD, Quinones MA, Winters WL, Miller RR: End-systolic retraction of the left ventricular posterior wall: a specific echocardiographic marker of prolapsing mitral valve. *Am J Cardiol* 45:442, 1980
44. D'Cruz IA, Shah S, Hirsch LJ, Goldbarg AN: Cross-sectional echocardiographic visualization of abnormal systolic motion of the left ventricle in mitral valve prolapse. *Cathet Cardiovasc Diagn* 7:35, 1981
45. Cobbs BW, King SB: Mechanism of abnormal ventriculogram (VGM) and ECG associated with prolapsing mitral valve (PMV). *Circulation* 50(Suppl 3):7, 1974
46. Liedtke AJ, Gault JH, Leaman DM, Blumenthal MS: Geometry of left ventricular contraction in the systolic click syndrome: Characterization of a segmental myocardial abnormality. *Circulation* 47:27, 1973
47. Scampardonis G, Yang SS, Maranhao V, Goldberg H, Gooch AS: Left ventricular abnormalities in prolapsed mitral leaflet syndrome: Review of eighty-seven cases. *Circulation* 48:287, 1973
48. Leachman RD, Cokkinos DV, Cooley DA: Association of ostium secundum atrial septal defects with mitral valve prolapse. *Am J Cardiol* 38:167, 1976
49. Betriu A, Wigle D, Felderhof CH, McLoughlin MJ: Prolapse of the posterior leaflet of the mitral valve associated with secundum atrial septal defect. *Am J Cardiol* 35:363, 1975
50. Pocock WA, Barlow JB: An association between the billowing posterior mitral leaflet syndrome and congenital heart disease, particularly atrial septal defect. *Am Heart J* 81:720, 1971
51. Menachemi E, Aintablian A, Hanby RI: Ostium primum atrial septal defect associated with mitral valve prolapse. *NY State J Med* 75:2234, 1975
52. Schreiber TL, Feigenbaum H, Weyman AE: Effect of atrial septal defect repair on left ventricular geometry and degree of mitral valve prolapse. *Circulation* 61:888, 1980
53. Smith ER, Fraser DB, Purdy JW, Anderson RN: Angiographic diagnosis of mitral valve prolapse: Correlation with echocardiography. *Am J Cardiol* 40:165, 1977
54. Grossman H, Fleming RJ, Engle MA, Levin AH, Ehlers KH: Angiocardiography in the apical systolic click syndrome. *Radiology* 91:898, 1968

55. Ehlers KH, Engle MA, Levin AR, Grossman H, Fleming RJ: Left ventricular abnormality with late mitral insufficiency and abnormal electrocardiogram. *Am J Cardiol* 26:333, 1970
56. Leachman RD, De Franceschi A, Zamalloa O: Late systolic murmurs and clicks associated with abnormal mitral valve ring. *Am J Cardiol* 23:679, 1969
57. Ranganathan N, Silver MD, Robinson TI, Wilson JK: Idiopathic prolapsed mitral leaflet syndrome: Angiographic-clinical correlations. *Circulation* 54:707, 1976
58. Gilbert BW, Schatz RA, VonRamm OT, Behar VS, Kisslo JA: Mitral valve prolapse: Two-dimensional echocardiographic and angiographic correlation. *Circulation* 54:716, 1976
59. Sahn DJ, Allen HD, Goldberg SJ, Friedman WF: Mitral valve prolapse in children: A problem defined by real-time cross-sectional echocardiography. *Circulation* 53:651, 1976
60. Morganroth J, Jones RH, Chen CC, Naito M: Two dimensional echocardiography in mitral, aortic and tricuspid valve prolapse. *Am J Cardiol* 46:1164, 1980
61. Mintz GS, Kotler MN, Segal BL, Parry WR: Two dimensional echocardiographic evaluation of patients with mitral insufficiency. *Am J Cardiol* 44:670, 1979
62. Kitabatake A, Matsuo H, Asao M, Tanouchi J, Mishima M, Hayashi T, Abe H: Intra-atrial distribution of mitral valve prolapse visualized by pulsed Doppler technique combined with electronic beam sector scanning echocardiography. *J Cardiography* 10:11, 1980
63. Chandraratna PAN, Aronow WS: Mitral valve ring in normal vs. dilated left ventricle: Cross-sectional echocardiographic study. *Chest* 79:151, 1981
64. Fulkerson PK, Beaver BM, Auseon JC, Graber HL: Calcification of the mitral annulus: Etiology, clinical associations, complications and therapy. *Am J Med* 66:967, 1979
65. D'Cruz I, Panetta F, Cohen H, Glick G: Submitral calcification or sclerosis in elderly patients: M mode and two dimensional echocardiography in "mitral annulus calcification." *Am J Cardiol* 44:31, 1979
66. Walmsley R: Anatomy of human mitral valve in adult cadaver and comparative anatomy of the valve. *Br Heart J* 40:351, 1978
67. Sweatman T, Selzer A, Kamagaki M, Cohn K: Echocardiographic diagnosis of mitral regurgitation due to ruptured chordae tendineae. *Circulation* 46:580, 1972
68. Giles TD, Burch GE, Martinez EC: Value of exploratory "scanning" in the echocardiographic diagnosis of ruptured chordae tendineae. *Circulation* 49:678, 1974
69. Cosby RS, Giddings JA, See JR, Mayo M, Boomershine P: The echocardiogram in non-rheumatic mitral insufficiency. *Chest* 66:642, 1974
70. Meyer JF, Frank MJ, Goldberg S, Cheng TO: Systolic mitral flutter, an echocardiographic clue to the diagnosis of ruptured chordae tendineae. *Am Heart J* 93:3, 1977
71. Humphries WC, Hammer WJ, McDonough MT, Lemole G, McCurdy RR, Spann JF Jr: Echocardiographic equivalents of a flail mitral leaflet. *Am J Cardiol* 40:802, 1977
72. Mintz GS, Kitler MN, Segal BL, Parry WR: Two-dimensional echocardiographic recognition of ruptured chordae tendineae. *Circulation* 57:244, 1978
73. Child JS, Skorton DJ, Taylor RD, Krivokapich J, Abbasi AS, Wong M, Shah PD: M mode and cross sectional echocardiographic features of flail posterior mitral leaflets. *Am J Cardiol* 44:1383, 1979
74. Joswig BC, Pick RA, Vieweg WVR, Hagan AD: Flutter of the mitral valve associated with a diastolic murmur in the absence of disease. *Am Heart J* 97:635, 1979
75. Tei C, Tanaka H, Nakao S, Yoshimura H, Minagoe S, Kashima T, Kanehisa T: Motion of the interatrial septum in acute mitral regurgitation: Clinical and experimental echocardiographic studies. *Circulation* 62:1080, 1980
76. Come PC, Riley MF: M-mode and cross-sectional echocardiographic recognition of fibrosis and calcification of the mitral valve chordae and left ventricular papillary muscles. *Am J Cardiol* 49:461, 1982
77. Ogawa S, Hubbard FE, Mardelli TJ, Dreifus LS: Cross-sectional echocardiographic spectrum of papillary muscle dysfunction. *Am Heart J* 97:312, 1979
78. Mittal AK, Langston M Jr, Cohn KE, Selzer A, Kerth WJ: Combined papillary muscle and left ventricular wall dysfunction as a cause of mitral regurgitation: An experimental study. *Circulation* 44:174, 1971
79. Burch GE, DePasquale NP, Phillips JH: The syndrome of papillary muscle dysfunction. *Am Heart J* 75:399, 1968
80. Cheng TO, Bashour T, Adkins PC: Acute severe mitral regurgitation from papillary muscle dysfunction in acute myocardial infarction. *Circulation* 46:491, 1972
81. Erbel R, Schweizer P, Bardos P, Meyer J: Two-dimensional echocardiographic diagnosis of papillary muscle rupture. *Chest* 79:595, 1981

Diseases of the aortic valve and aorta

Normal anatomy and physiology of the aortic valve. In contrast to the complexity of factors participating in the dynamics of the mitral valve and generation of the first heart sound, the aortic valve opens and closes in response to a simple pressure gradient between the left ventricle and the aorta. Production of a sufficient degree of vortex elements in the sinuses of Valsalva during ejection of blood from the left ventricle keeps the aortic cusp away from the wall of the aorta [1]. Both experimental and clinical data have documented that the aortic valve starts its opening movement with the onset of flow at the same point at which left ventricular pressure exceeds aortic pressure. Aortic valve closure coincides with the trough of the aortic pressure incisura obtained from aortic root pressure recording and the onset of the first high-frequency component of the second heart sound recorded from intracardiac phonocardiography [2–4]. The intensity of the second sound is not related to the amplitude of cusp motion but correlates with the aortic pressure at the time of closure and with peak flow deceleration. Unlike the mitral valve, which may stay open during diastole even with no flow across it, the aortic valve does not stay open unless forward flow is passing through it [5, 6]. In low cardiac output states as well as with premature ventricular beats, when diastolic filling has been significantly compromised the forces applied to the aortic leaflet and the volume of blood passing through the open valve are both reduced; the amount of leaflet separation is reduced, and the open cusps move toward apposition more rapidly under the action of external and internal forces.

The three aortic cusps arise from a fibrous ring of tissue, the aortic annulus (Fig. 4-1). The membranous ventricular septum is continuous with the anterior wall of the root of the aorta. From the right side, the membranous ventricular septum lies beneath the septal leaflet of the tricuspid valve and is in contact with a small segment of the right atrium and the right ventricular outflow tract. In this manner the junction of the right and noncoronary cusps of the aortic valve lie above the membranous septum. The left aortic cusp is oriented to the anterior wall of the left atrium, which is attached to intervalvular septal tissue from below. This "septum" separates the left and posterior aortic cusps from the anterior mitral leaflet, thus forming part of the posterior wall of the left ventricular outflow tract (Fig. 4-2) [7].

Imaging techniques of aortic valve and aorta. Clinically adequate two-dimensional imaging of the aortic valve requires at least two tomographic views, one in a long axis plane and the other in the short axis. The parasternal left ventricular long axis view is valuable because it shows two of the three leaflets in profile, the right cusp being viewed anteriorly and the noncoronary cusp being viewed posteriorly, enabling assessment of leaflet thickness and mobility. This view shows the anteroposterior diameter of the aortic annulus and the proximal portion of the ascending aorta as well. The right and noncoronary sinuses of Valsalva are also viewed in this plane. In addition, the attachments of the membranous portion of the ventricular septum to the anterior aortic root and of the anterior mitral leaflet to the posterior aortic root are well visualized. If technical limitations prevent adequate imaging of the aortic valve in this long axis view, an alternative is

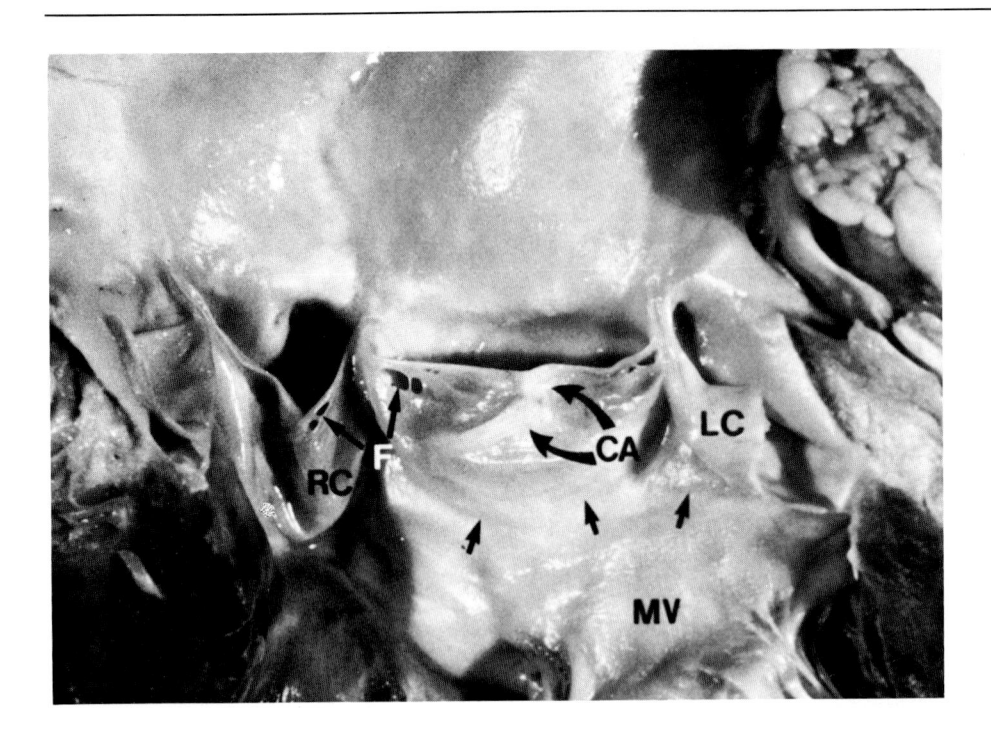

Fig. 4-1. The aortic annulus of this normal postmortem adult heart is opened to show the right cusp (RC), noncoronary cusp containing the corpora arantii (CA), and left cusp (LC), which is divided to expose the anatomy. The corpora arantii, which are normal findings in the center of the aortic cusps at the leaflet edge, are white in appearance and produce a small, localized increase in thickness due to connective tissue. The corpora arantii may generate a slightly more prominent echo reflectance than the surrounding thin cusp tissue and should not be confused with an abnormality. Normal fenestrations (F) may occasionally be seen in the margins of the cusps. The three short black arrows identify the junction of the aortic annulus and the origin of the anterior mitral leaflet.

the apical long axis view with the beam oriented through the aortic valve and ascending aorta. This enables imaging in much the same plane as from the left parasternal region; of course, here the transducer is positioned over the apex and at times actually enables the operator to view a greater extent of the ascending aorta than if it were in the parasternal position. The right and noncoronary aortic leaflets are again visualized but, as in the parasternal long axis view, the left coronary cusp is still not normally imaged from this position.

A very important view to obtain for adequate visualization of the aortic valve is the parasternal short axis view with the beam directed through the base so that the entire aortic annulus is visualized together with all three leaflets. In the closed diastolic position the commissural lines of all three cusps produce reflectances in a Y configuration or "Mercedes-Benz" sign, indicating the presence of the three cusps (Fig. 4-3). The surrounding cross-sectional anatomy seen in this tomographic plane includes the left atrium, interatrial septum, right atrium, tricuspid valve, right ventricular outflow tract, and pulmonic valve. In this position it is possible to image the orifices of both the right coronary and left main coronary arteries. The left main coronary artery is usually easier to image and is visible in most patients with slight lateral angulation toward the pulmonary artery (Fig. 4-4).

A second short axis view at the base should be obtained with the sector beam directed slightly leftward toward the pulmonary artery with the resultant tomographic plane intersecting the ascending aorta above the annulus. With this view, the diameter of the ascending aorta may be measured and compared with that of the pulmonary artery.

There are two opportunities to visualize the aortic valve and aorta from the apical imaging position. In the apical four-chamber position with the transducer angled more anteriorly the aortic valve and annulus are imaged with two of the three leaflets being visible. The apical long axis view, including the aortic valve and

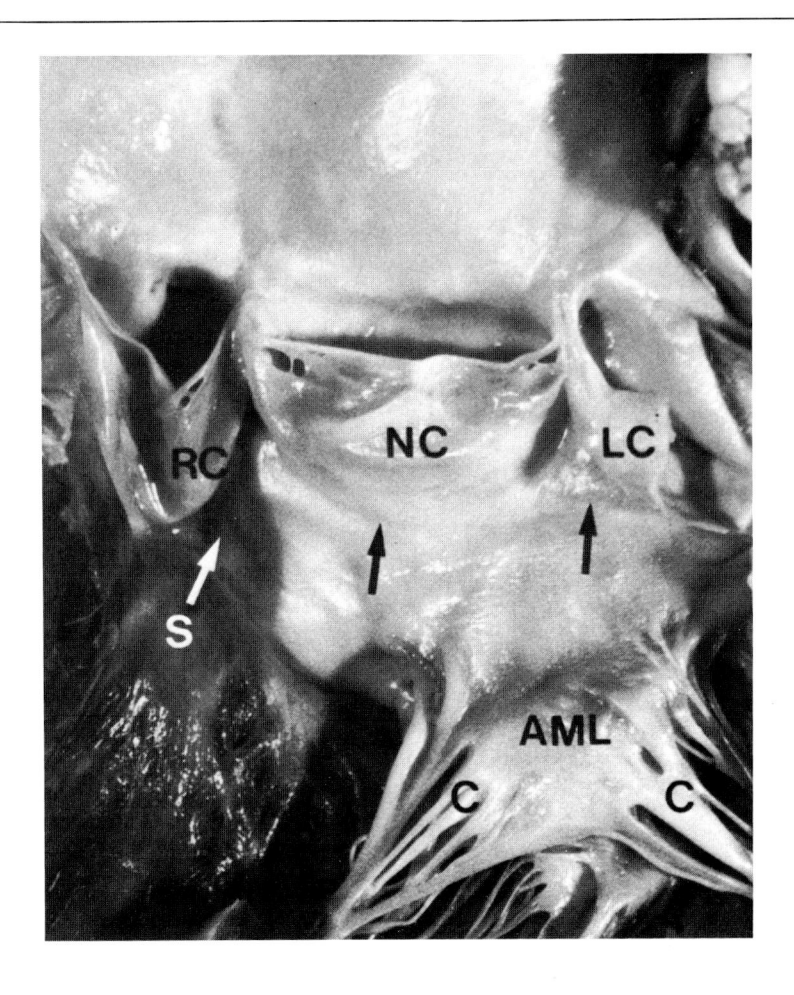

Fig. 4-2. Close-up view of normal anatomic relationships of interventricular septum, anterior mitral leaflet, and the three aortic cusps: right (RC), noncoronary, and left (LC). The three arrows point to the junction of the aortic annulus and the septum anteriorly and the anterior mitral leaflet, which forms part of the posterolateral wall of the left ventricular outflow tract. C = chordae tendineae.

proximal ascending aorta, can be a valuable additional plane, particularly if the parasternal long axis view is inadequate. The aortic valve can also be visualized by placing the transducer in the subcostal position and imaging in the four-chamber view with an anterior angulation similar to the apical four-chamber view.

While imaging the aortic valve with 2-D echo, it is also important to obtain M-mode recordings from the valve. The parasternal long axis view is an ideal angle from which to direct the M-mode cursor through the aortic leaflets with proper positioning to ensure optimal movement and cusp separation on the M-mode record. This view also provides valuable information about the aortic root motion, which is clinically useful in the assessment of left atrial emptying, and about left atrial volume changes, which is useful for evaluation both of the mitral valve and of diastolic filling characteristics of the left ventricle [8–10].

M-mode recordings should be obtained while imaging in the short axis view at the base in order to direct the beam properly through the aortic leaflets and annulus as well as to obtain proper anteroposterior dimension of the left atrium by visually directing the beam through the left atrium. The beam can be directed from a more medial position near the interatrial septum to a more lateral position encompassing a portion of the left atrial appendage to comprehensively scan the anteroposterior

114   4. Diseases of the aortic valve and aorta

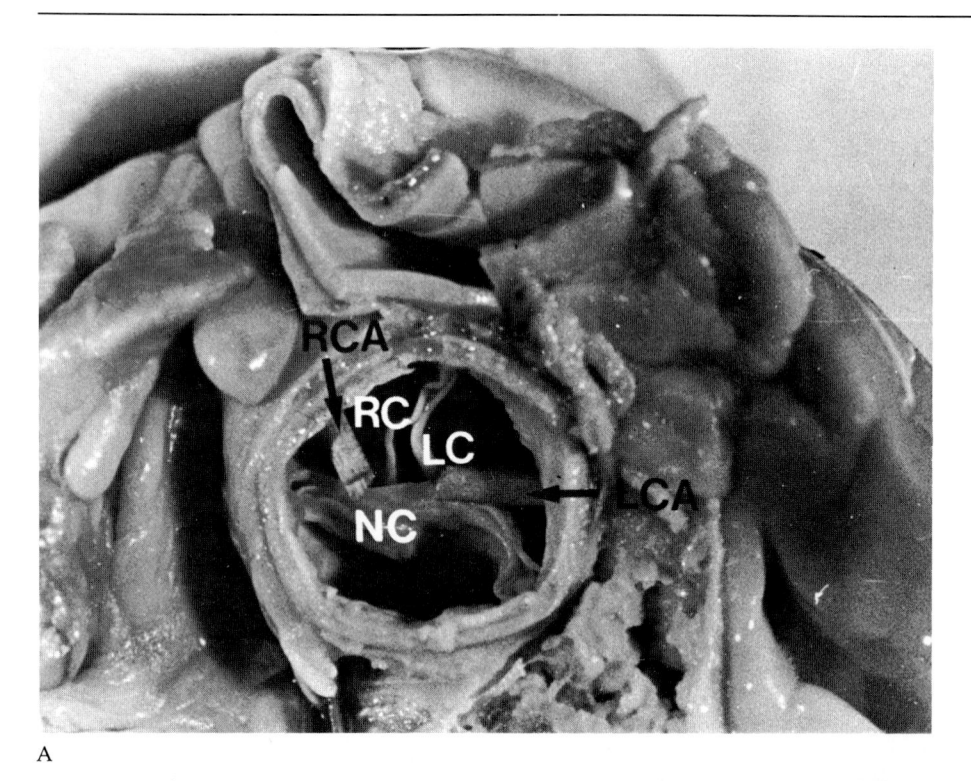

Fig. 4-3A. With ascending aorta removed, a view of the normal right (RC), left (LC), and noncoronary aortic cusps. Small wooden sticks have been placed in the orifices of the right coronary artery (RCA) and the left coronary artery (LCA) for identification purposes since they could not be viewed without cutting or distorting the aortic cusps and annulus. B. Notice the resemblance between the normal anatomy of the aortic cusps (A) and the echo reflectances during diastole of a normal valve. The surrounding structures are seen when the 2-D echo plane is directed in a parasternal short axis view through the aortic annulus. Ao = descending aorta; L = left aortic cusp; R = right aortic cusp; PV = pulmonic valve.

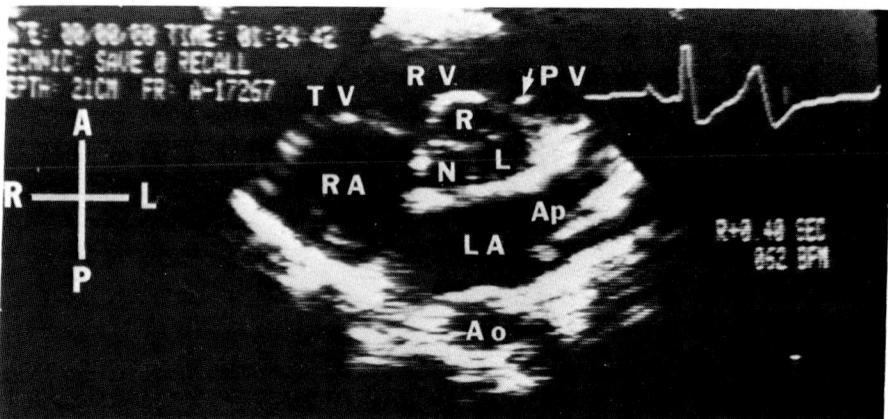

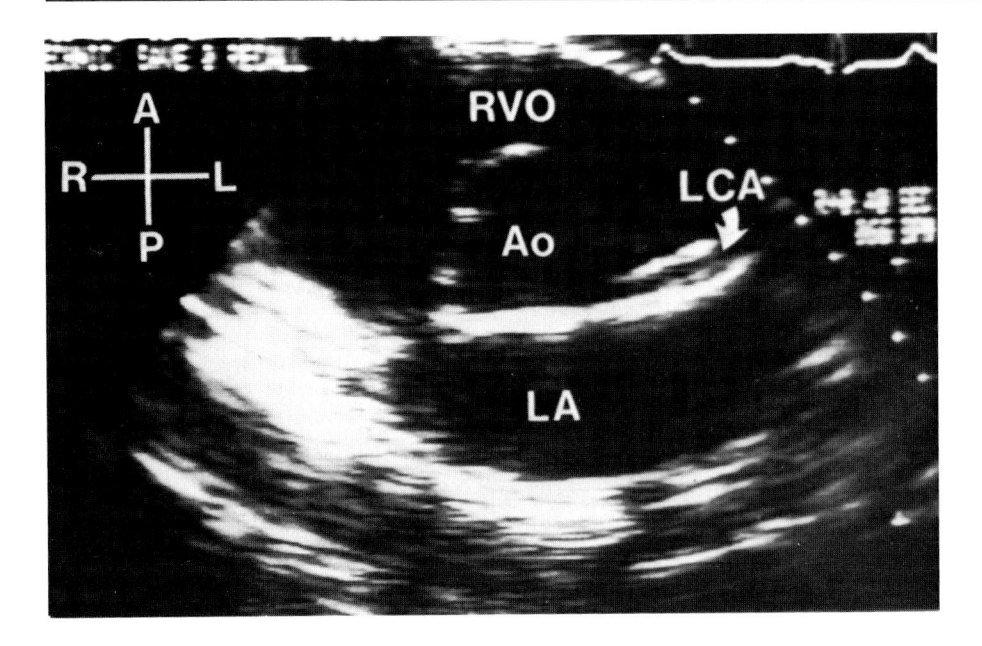

Fig. 4-4. Parasternal short axis view at the base with slight leftward angulation orienting the sector beam in the plane of the left main coronary artery (LCA), causing a portion of the left wall of the aorta to drop out in this image.

diameter of the chamber; the latter may vary as left atrial enlargement occurs. A third opportunity to obtain M-mode recordings of the aortic valve occurs with subcostal imaging when it may be clinically important to obtain a recording of the aortic valve and the traditional parasternal imaging positions have been technically inadequate. Normally there is little if any usable information from the M-mode record obtained in the apical imaging positions because of the parallel nature of the beam intersecting the leaflets and aorta.

Aortic valve disease

CLINICAL PRESENTATION. Aortic stenosis in the characteristic patient is easily recognized by auscultation based on the systolic ejection murmur at the base with referral to the carotid arteries. However, these typical findings are not present in many patients with aortic stenosis; in addition, other organic murmurs may mimic the features of aortic stenosis. Patients with symptoms of chest pain, lightheadedness, or syncope who are noted to have systolic ejection murmurs on physical examination should be evaluated with echocardiography, since unrecognized or underestimated aortic stenosis could be contributing to the patient's symptoms. Loud systolic murmurs over the apex, precordium, and base can be easily confused with mitral regurgitation; or there may be an unknown amount of combined mitral regurgitation and aortic stenosis that requires further echocardiographic evaluation to establish the severity of the valvular lesions. Elderly patients with systolic ejection murmurs are frequently found to have calcification in the aortic leaflets, and it may be very difficult to judge whether the murmurs have clinical significance without further assessment with two-dimensional imaging. It may also be difficult to determine whether a soft systolic ejection murmur with or without ejection sounds heard in a child or young adult is an innocent murmur or is due to a congenitally abnormal aortic valve. Although the question of aortic stenosis may not be relevant in such a patient, it is extremely important to know whether the patient has a normal or abnormal valve because of the potential need for prophylactic treatment for endocarditis. In most patients with known aortic stenosis, regardless of age, combined M-mode and two-dimensional echocardiography provides the most valuable noninvasive method for serial follow-up evaluation to determine whether the aortic stenosis is progressing or if the patient is approaching the need for cardiac catheterization or surgery.

ETIOLOGY OF AORTIC STENOSIS. In discussing the pathogenesis of aortic stenosis, Pomerance [11] emphasizes the relationship of age to the three types of aortic stenosis: congenital, inflammatory, and senile (calcific). A congenitally abnormal valve, typified by a bicuspid aortic valve, is commonly recognized in childhood; however, it may not be clinically diagnosed until much later in adult life after calcification and aortic stenosis have developed. (Congenital aortic stenosis is discussed in greater detail in Chapter 15.) The inflammatory type is represented by those changes seen in rheumatic valvular disease and frequently causes aortic insufficiency alone or together with aortic stenosis. Senile degenerative changes with calcification of the aortic leaflets commonly become manifest after 65 to 70 years of age. Calcification at the base of the cusps and aortic sinuses is typically seen in this senile variety. Calcification in the congenital type of aortic stenosis is easily recognized and distinguished from the senile variety because of the bicuspid or slitlike valve orifice. The bicuspid aortic valve is usually competent, although its motion may be restricted [12]. When calcification or progressive valve changes occur or endocarditis develops in the valve, the bicuspid valve typically becomes stenotic and/or incompetent (Fig. 4-5). Other congenitally abnormal aortic valves have a fused raphe, which may produce reflectances by 2-D echo resembling three leaflets; however, the valve is functionally bicuspid.

When viewed grossly from the aortic side the rheumatic valve has a central triangular or circular opening due to the fusion of the three commissures and the increased thickening of the leaflets caused by fibrosis and calcification (Fig. 4-6).

In a congenitally bicuspid aortic valve, the two cusps are usually of unequal size and an elastic raphe extends from the aortic wall onto the aortic aspect of the larger cusp. This particular feature helps distinguish the congenital lesion from the deformity seen in rheumatic valvulitis, in which a similar raphe from fusion of the commissure shows only valvular tissue elements.

McMillan [13] reported the normal area of the aortic orifice in adults to be 2.6 to 3.5 cm^2. It is generally accepted that a reduction of the valve orifice area to 0.7 cm^2 or less is critical. By this time the pressure gradient between the left ventricle and the aorta usually equals or exceeds 50 mm Hg.

EVALUATION OF AORTIC STENOSIS BY M-MODE ECHOCARDIOGRAPHY. From 1975 to 1980 several investigators reported the clinical value and limitations of M-mode echocardiography in diagnosing and quantitating valvular aortic stenosis [14–23]. The reliability of predicting the severity of aortic stenosis by this method lies in the application of wall stress concepts [24–26]. These studies concluded that left ventricular hypertrophy occurred in response to chronic pressure overload as a compensatory mechanism serving to normalize systolic wall stress and thus preserve pump function of the ventricle. Indices calculated from developed pressures are relatively preload-independent. Fifer and associates [27] reported that the rate

Table 4-1. Comparison of cardiac catheterization findings and M-mode echo in aortic stenosis

Author	Patient group by age range (years)	Constant	LVPSP echo vs cath	AVPSP grad echo vs cath
Bennett [16]	11–70	225		r = 0.87
Glanz [24]	4–17	225		r = 0.89
Johnson [17]	2–22	225	r = 0.89	
Aziz [18]	2–15	225	r = 0.74	
Blackwood [19]	1–19	245	r = 0.83	r = 0.91
Schwartz [20]	2–80	225		r = 0.75
	2–18	225		r = 0.85
	18–80	225		r = 0.79
Hagan [25]	7–89	225	r = 0.87	r = 0.92
Reichek [31]	20–73		r = 0.77	

LVPSP = left ventricular peak systolic pressure; AVPSP grad = aortic valve peak systolic pressure gradient.

of stress development was nearly identical in patients with aortic stenosis and in normal subjects over a wide range of values of developed stress but was significantly lower in patients with cardiomyopathy. These investigators observed that contractile function as characterized by the isovolumic rate of stress development is not necessarily impaired in chronic pressure overload hypertrophy. Gunther and Grossman [28] reported close correlations between circumferential wall stress, ejection fraction, and velocity of fiber shortening in patients with aortic stenosis. Their results indicated that left ventricular wall thickness and geometry are closely correlated with ventricular performance in patients with pressure overload hypertrophy due to aortic stenosis.

Bennett [14] was the first to report the use of M-mode echocardiography to estimate the left ventricular peak systolic pressure by employing the predictive relationship of end-systolic wall thickness to left ventricular dimension in patients with aortic stenosis. The best correlative predictability has been found in studies of pediatric populations in contrast to older age groups [15, 17, 23] (Table 4-1). Swartz and associates [18], in an unselected adult population, has shown poor correlation between M-mode echo predicting left ventricular peak systolic pressure and aortic valve peak systolic gradient when compared with catheterization-determined values.

The aortic valve area cannot be reliably estimated from M-mode echocardiography by measuring the separation between the right aortic cusp anteriorly and the noncoronary cusp posteriorly. When aortic cusp separation is measured, the severity of calcific aortic stenosis is frequently overestimated, while congenital, noncalcific aortic stenosis may be underestimated [29, 30].

METHODOLOGY OF CALCULATING AORTIC VALVE GRADIENT. Because the expected physiologic response in a patient with pure aortic stenosis is concentric hypertrophy of the left ventricle associated with reduction in left ventricular cavity size, the resultant ratio of wall thickness to cavity dimension provides a valuable means of estimating the degree of aortic stenosis in preoperative patients, a ratio that can be determined echocardiographically. Although this methodology is particularly reliable in the pediatric and young adult population, it is also very useful in selected older adults who do not have conditions (listed below) that prevent the expected

118   4. Diseases of the aortic valve and aorta

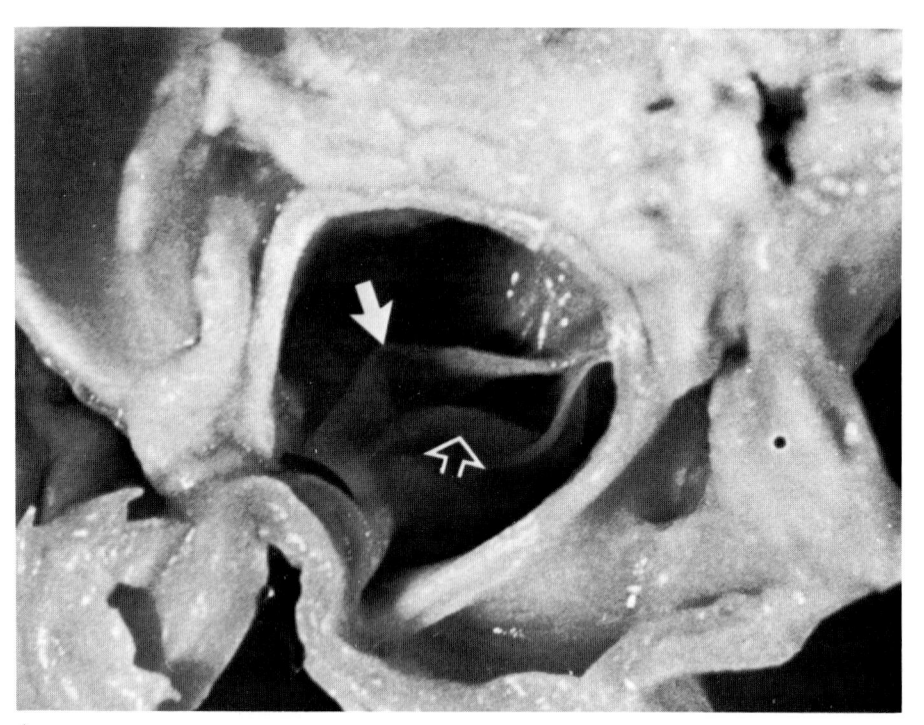

Fig. 4-5A. Close-up view of bicuspid aortic valve with aorta removed. The two leaflets (arrows) have normal thickness with no superimposed calcification. B. Bicuspid aortic valve (short arrows) with marked thickening and calcification (curved arrow). C. Parasternal short axis view of bicuspid aortic valve (arrow) and orifice of left main coronary artery (LCA). There is no associated calcification or obstruction. D. Two parasternal short axis views of the same patient with bicuspid aortic valve and orifice outlined by the small arrows in both upper and lower panels. Both these systolic frames show some increased thickness of the leaflets with a thickened, possibly calcified, raphe anterior (white arrow in both panels).

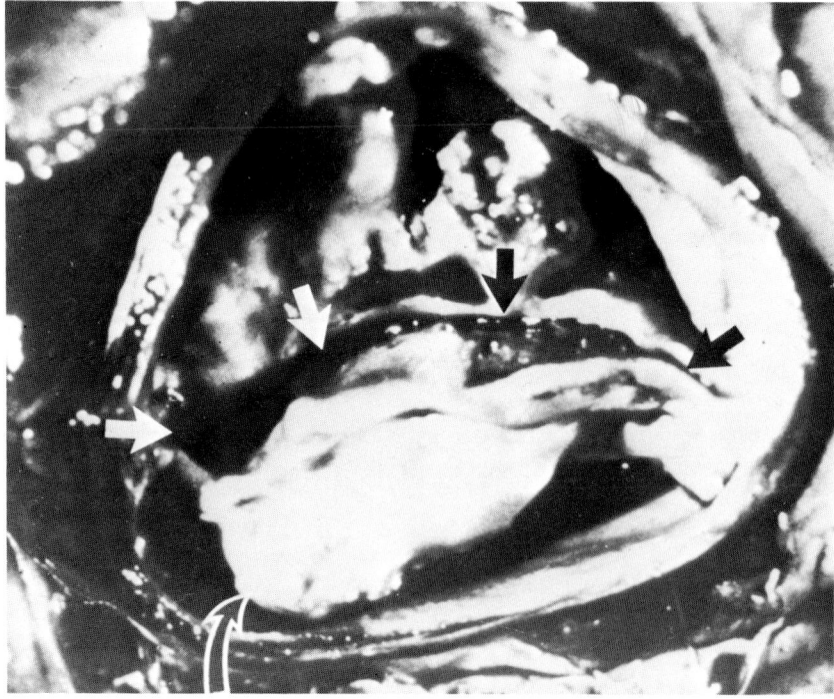

119

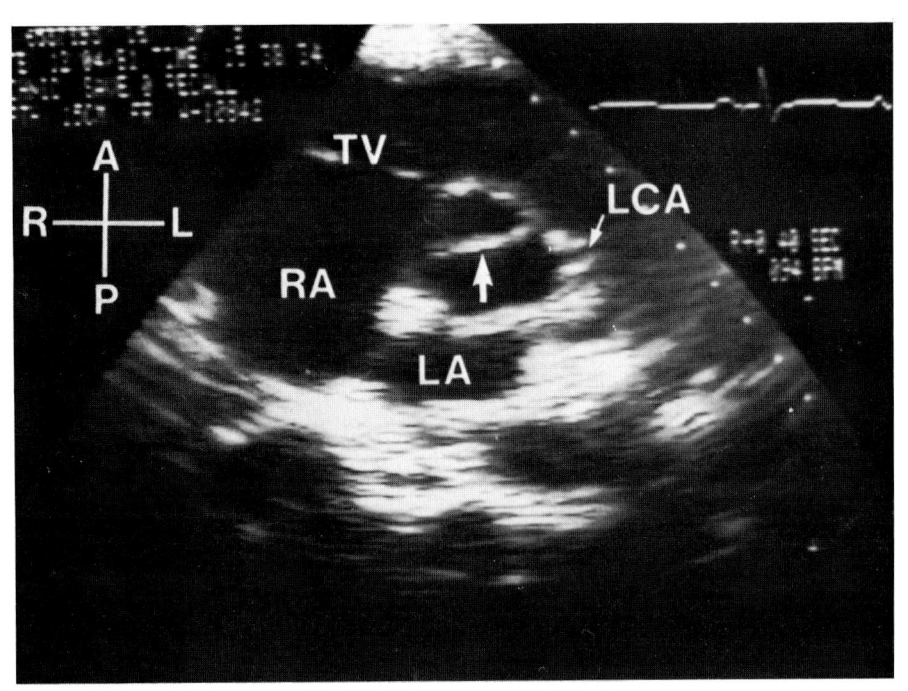

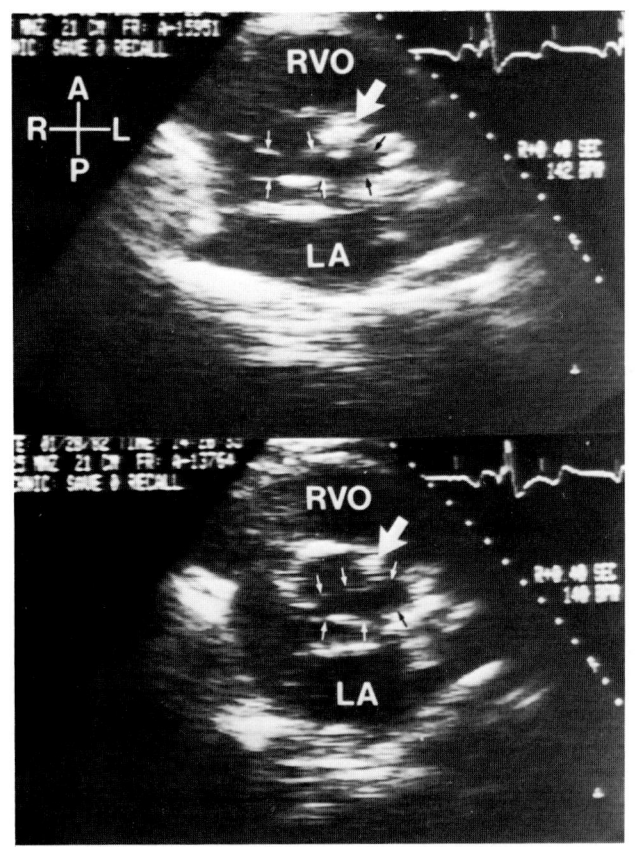

C

D

4. Diseases of the aortic valve and aorta

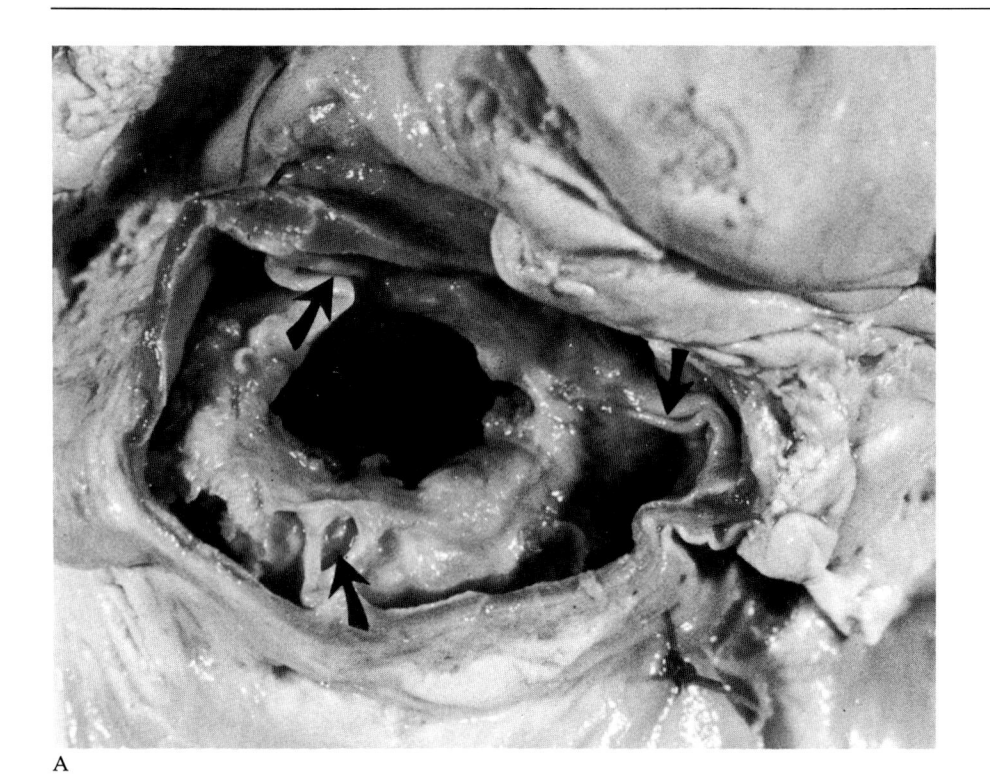

Fig. 4-6A. Anatomic view of a heavily calcified, thickened aortic valve with a circular opening caused by fusion of the three commissures (arrows). B. Three-leaflet aortic valve with calcification of both noncoronary and left (LC) cusps together with partial fusion (middle arrow) of the commissure between LC and NC. C. Parasternal short axis views through a heavily calcified, poorly mobile aortic valve. Both panels recorded during systole show markedly restricted motion of the aortic leaflets with leaflet separation approximately 7 to 9 mm (bracket, top panel). The lower panel shows a small orifice (dots). It is difficult and rarely possible to image the orifice of the aortic valve sufficiently well to measure valve area by planimetry. The large echo-free space posterior and leftward of the outlined orifice in the lower panel is due to echo dropout and should not be confused with the valve orifice. RC = right aortic cusp.

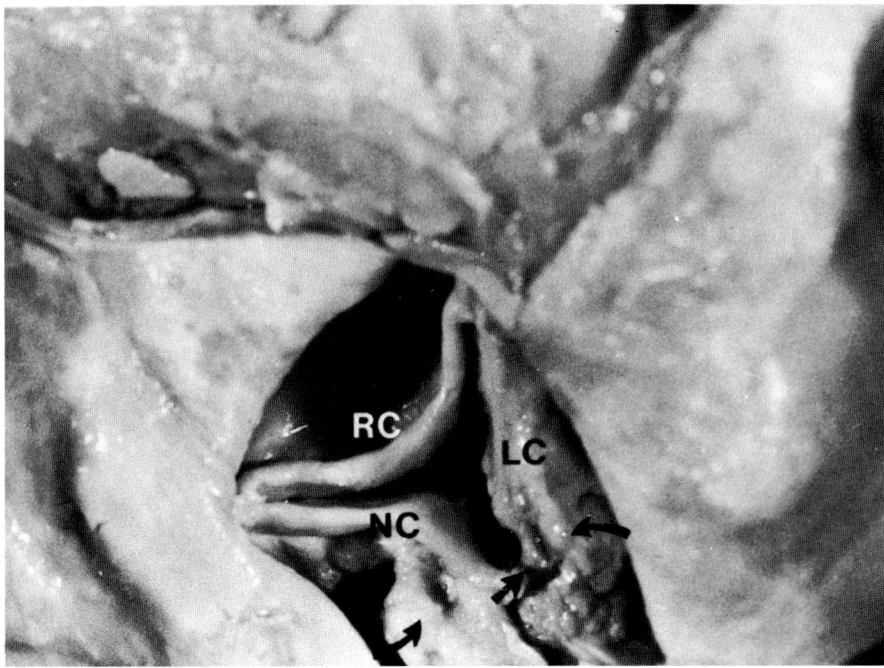

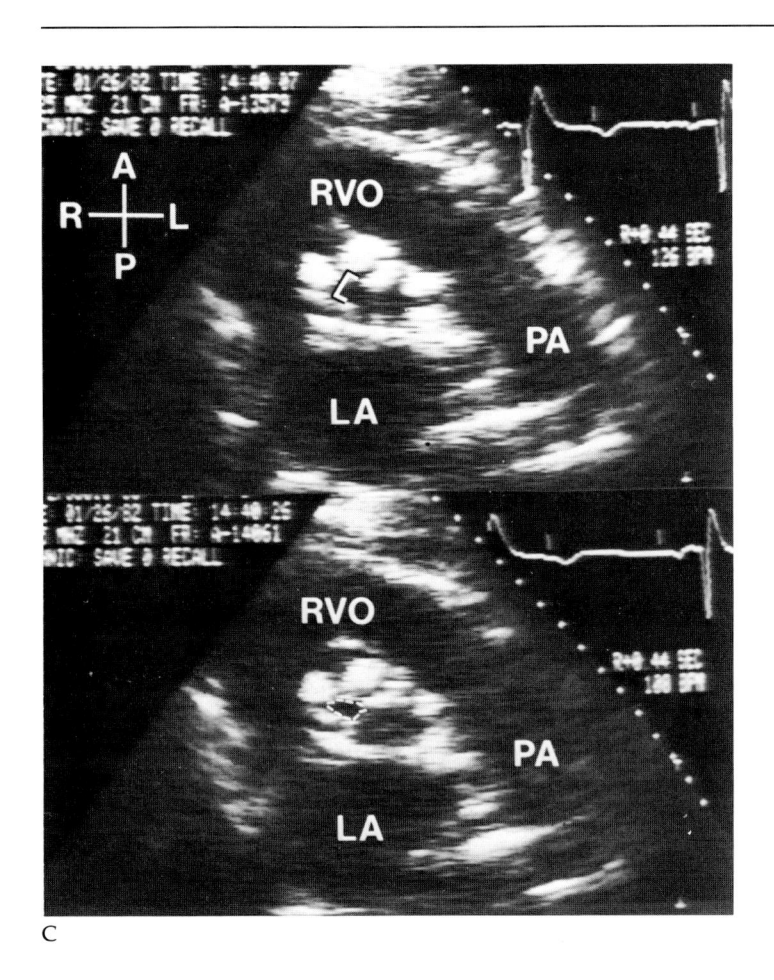

C

4. Diseases of the aortic valve and aorta

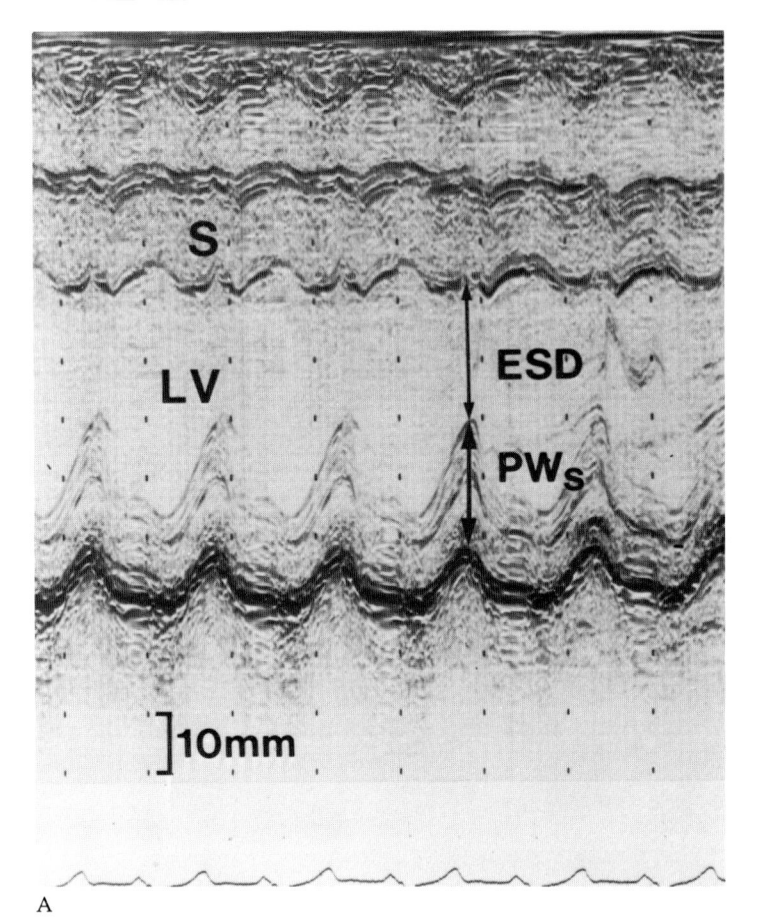

Fig. 4-7A. M-mode recording at the level of the chordae tendineae showing normal left ventricular cavity size and significant hypertrophy of both septum (S) and posterior wall in a patient with aortic stenosis. The arrows depict the end-systolic dimension (24 mm) and the end-systolic posterior wall thickness (PW$_s$) (20 mm) giving an abnormal ratio of 0.83. If one uses a constant for wall stress of 225, the estimated peak left ventricular systolic pressure is 187 mm Hg. Since the patient had a cuff blood pressure of 120/80 when the echocardiogram was performed, the echo estimate of peak systolic gradient across the aortic valve is 67 mm Hg. B. Parasternal short axis view in the same patient showing 2-D echo image at the same level at which the M-mode recording was obtained giving the left ventricular end-systolic dimension and posterior wall thickness (PW$_s$). It is best to record the M-mode from this position for these measurements and to use the simultaneous 2-D image as a quality control check on proper location, beam angle, and correct measurements of the anatomy. Recordings obtained from low left sternal border positions usually cause septal thickness and cavity size to appear larger than they actually are owing to the oblique plane of image of the ventricle.

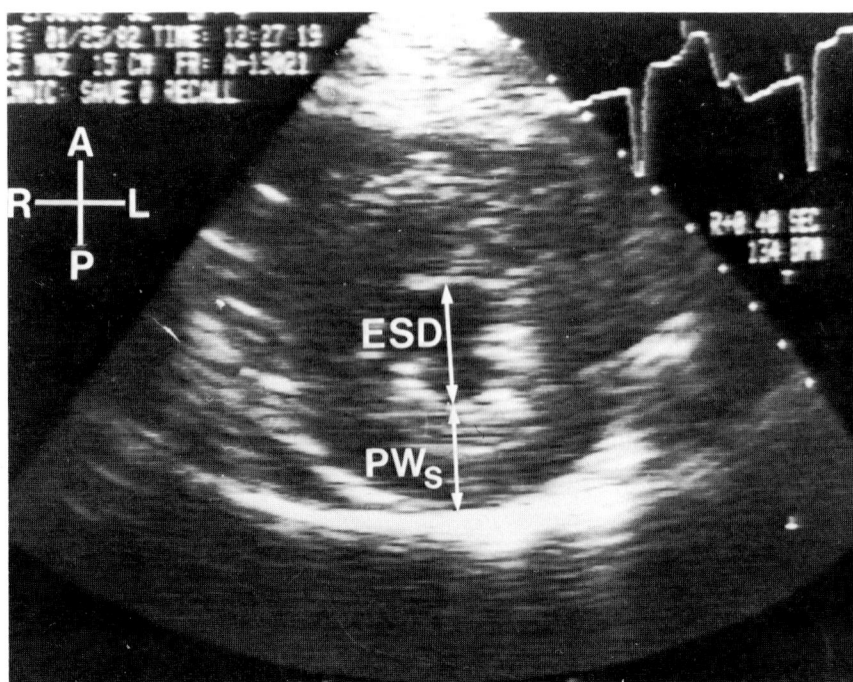

ratio of wall thickness to cavity dimension to occur. The assumption may be made that left ventricular wall stress remains relatively constant in patients with aortic stenosis and progressive left ventricular hypertrophy if the left ventricular cavity has not become dilated or the patient is not in heart failure; then a constant for wall stress (225) multiplied by the ratio of posterior wall thickness at end systole (PW_s) divided by the end-systolic cavity dimension (LVESD) gives the estimated left ventricular peak systolic pressure (LVPSP) (LVPSP = 225 × PW_s/LVESD). The measurement of cuff systolic blood pressure at the time of the examination subtracted from the estimated left ventricular peak systolic pressure equals the estimated peak systolic gradient across the aortic valve (Fig. 4-7).

Certain exclusion factors, if present in any given patient, prevent the reliable use of this formula. This method of estimating the severity of aortic stenosis is unreliable when any of the following conditions is present [23]: (1) Systemic hypertension, (2) dilated left ventricular cavity, (3) left ventricular failure, (4) previous myocardial infarction, (5) coexistent cardiomyopathy, and (6) previous aortic valve surgery.

Some investigators doubt the reliability of estimating a constant for wall stress, since this could lead to significant errors in predicting peak systolic left ventricular pressure [20]. These investigators suggested that because an accurate estimate could not be used for an average wall stress constant, it was more appropriate to utilize the ratio of posterior wall thickness at end systole divided by the end-systolic diameter to estimate the severity of aortic stenosis. The 27 patients in this study were divided into three categories based upon the wall thickness (W_s)-to-cavity dimension (D_s) ratio and the aortic valve area measured at catheterization: first, those patients whose W_s-to-D_s ratio was equal to or less than 0.55 had a mean aortic valve pressure gradient of 37 mm Hg (range 17–42) and mean aortic valve area of 0.83 (0.60 to 1.1) cm^2/m^2; the second category, with a W_s-to-D_s ratio of 0.56 to 0.69, had a mean aortic valve gradient of 47 mm Hg (range 37–80) and mean aortic valve area of 0.68 (0.53–0.85) cm^2/m^2. Finally, the third group, with a ratio equal to or greater than 0.70, had a mean aortic valve gradient of 90 mm Hg (range 60–120) and mean aortic valve area of 0.49 (0.30–0.63) cm^2/m^2. Furthermore, these authors demonstrated that the ratio of systolic left ventricular wall thickness to internal dimension revealed a better correlation with peak left ventricular systolic pressure than did the diastolic wall thickness-to-cavity dimension ratio.

In a later study Reichek and Devereux [31] found that the ratio of diastolic posterior wall thickness to chamber radius correlated better than the end-systolic wall thickness-to-chamber radius ratio with left ventricular systolic pressure. In a series of 81 patients (aortic valve disease in 47, hypertension in 17, and normal subjects in 17), despite the symptoms of heart failure, reduced ejection fraction, or coronary disease, end-diastolic wall thickness ratio (RWT$_D$) correlated well with peak left ventricular systolic pressure (LVSP) ($r = 0.77$). They found 45 of 55 patients with LVSP ⩾140 mm Hg had RWT$_D$ ⩾0.45, while 26 of 26 with LVSP ⩽140 mm Hg had lower values. The RWT$_D$ was ⩾0.50 in 30 of 34 patients with LVSP ⩾180 mm Hg and in 6 of 21 with LVSP 140 to 180 mm Hg. Furthermore, they reported RWT$_D$ correctly indicated LVSP range in 26 of 27 patients with severe aortic stenosis and, combined with echocardiographic evidence of aortic valve calcification, correctly demonstrated the presence or absence of severe aortic stenosis in 99 percent of the patients.

AORTIC STENOSIS EVALUATED BY TWO-DIMENSIONAL ECHOCARDIOGRAPHY. Cross-sectional, two-dimensional echocardiography, by providing improved spatial orientation and more comprehensive imaging of the aortic valve, provides valuable clinical information in the direct assessment of the leaflets in patients with aortic stenosis [14, 24, 32–34]. By imaging in the parasternal left ventricular long axis view, Weyman and colleagues [32] reported an excellent correlation ($r = 0.91$) of the maximum aortic cusp separation to the calculated aortic valve area at catheterization; the cusp separation was then expressed as a percentage of the aortic root diameter to correct for the patient's size. These investigators noted that in 22 normal subjects the maximum aortic cusp separation averaged 72.7 percent (range 63–92%) of the aortic root diameter. In this study the aortic cusp separation averaged 53 percent in patients with mild aortic stenosis and approximately 30 percent in patients with moderate and severe aortic stenosis. DeMaria and associates [33] and Godley and colleagues [34] reported that aortic leaflet separation of 8 mm or less measured from the 2-D echo parasternal long axis view was highly predictive of severe aortic stenosis at 82 and 70 percent, respectively. Godley and associates [34] noted that aortic leaflet separation of 8 to 12 mm had a low predictive value for severity of stenosis. They did, however, observe that greater than 12 mm separation was highly reliable with a predictive value of 96 percent for mild aortic stenosis.

Our experience, together with that of other investigators, has confirmed that two-dimensional echocardiography is a reliable and sensitive method for detecting valvular aortic stenosis and accurately distinguishing patients with aortic stenosis from normal subjects. The specificity of two-dimensional echo is somewhat more limited in differentiating critical from noncritical aortic stenosis; however, the appearance of the leaflet motion and separation together with the degree of left ventricular hypertrophy can usually distinguish those patients having significant or insignificant aortic stenosis.

DIAGNOSIS OF AORTIC STENOSIS WITH DOPPLER ECHOCARDIOGRAPHY. Young and associates [35] have employed pulsed Doppler echocardiography to diagnose and evaluate the severity of aortic stenosis. These investigators evaluated indices indicative of either duration or amplitude of turbulence, amount of frequency dispersion above and below the zero frequency shift baseline, or degree of distortion of the "flow curve" pattern of the analog signal. The overall sensitivity of the technique in 59 patients in detecting valve areas of less than 1.0 cm^2 was 92 percent with a specificity of 87 percent (the predictive values for distinguishing areas less than from those greater than 1.0 cm^2 were 92 and 87%, respectively). These investigators also noted that the presence of aortic insufficiency, increased age, left ventricular dilatation or failure did not appear to alter the results significantly.

POSTOPERATIVE ASSESSMENT OF AORTIC STENOSIS BY ECHOCARDIOGRAPHY. In a postoperative study of 16 patients Gewitz and associates [19] observed that, in contrast to good predictive value preoperatively, postoperative echocardiographic prediction of left ventricular systolic pressure derived from either end-systolic or end-diastolic formulas correlated poorly with postoperative peak left ventricular systolic pressure measured at cardiac catheterization. These investigators noted that left ventricular posterior wall thickness remained significantly hypertrophied for as long as 122 months following surgery for left ventricular outflow obstruction and contributed to postoperative echocardiographic overestimation of peak left ventricular systolic pressure. Furthermore, they noted that left ventricular cavity dimension was not significantly altered postoperatively. It should also be noted that the 16 patients in this study represented a pediatric population with a mean age of 15 years with the interval between operation and the time of the follow-up echocardiographic study ranging from 10 to 122 months with a mean of 36 months. Fifteen of the 16 patients had undergone aortic valvotomy, and only one had received an aortic valve replacement. Eight of the patients had minimal aortic regurgitation, but no patient had aortic regurgitation greater than 1+ on angiography or congestive heart failure.

Henry and colleagues [36] performed echocardiographic and hemodynamic studies in 42 consecutive patients who underwent aortic valve replacement for isolated aortic stenosis. These investigators noted that patients with preoperative left ventricular end-diastolic dimensions greater than 52 mm had a significant decrease in left ventricular internal dimension, wall thickness, and mass after operation. However, wall thickness and mass usually remained abnormal. In contrast, patients without left ventricular dilatation had a slight postoperative increase in left ventricular dimension that accompanied the decrease in wall thickness and, as a result, the patients without left ventricular dilatation had a smaller decrease in left ventricular mass after operation than patients with preoperative dilatation. Among these 42 patients left ventricular dilatation with reduced fractional shortening was observed in approximately 25 percent but was severe in only one patient. These authors also noted at the six-month postoperative study that both left ventricular wall thickness and mass were significantly decreased; however, no further change in these measurements was found between the six-month postoperative study and late postoperative evaluation. The small number of patients who had increased preoperative left ventricular dimensions together with a decrease in systolic function were observed to improve slightly in left ventricular performance following surgery. In other studies employing contrast angiography and radionuclide cineangiographic methods patients with aortic stenosis and low preoperative ejection fraction were noted to improve significantly after operation [37–39].

TECHNIQUES FOR IMAGING AORTIC STENOSIS. Parasternal long axis and parasternal short axis views at the base are essential for evaluating patients with known or suspected aortic stenosis. Both the parasternal long axis view and the apical long axis view with the aortic valve provide profile images of the right and noncoronary cusps. With technically adequate imaging it is usually easy to recognize the presence of increased leaflet thickness and reduced motion. Systolic doming, a feature which is commonly seen in a stenotic, noncalcified bicuspid valve, is best visualized in these two long axis views (Fig. 4-8A, B). The parasternal short axis view at the base is the only plane in which a bicuspid valve can be diagnosed. Occasionally it is possible to see diastolic doming resembling prolapse in these congenitally abnormal valves (Fig. 4-8C).

When calcified aortic leaflets demonstrate reduced cusp separation in the presence of poor left ventricular function, it is very difficult to determine how much of the reduced leaflet motion may be secondary to aortic stenosis and how much may be secondary to reduced left ventricular performance (Fig. 4-9). Accordingly, it may be difficult or even impossible to distinguish whether the aortic stenosis is hemodynamically significant. Accurate planimetry of the aortic valve orifice in the short axis

126   4. Diseases of the aortic valve and aorta

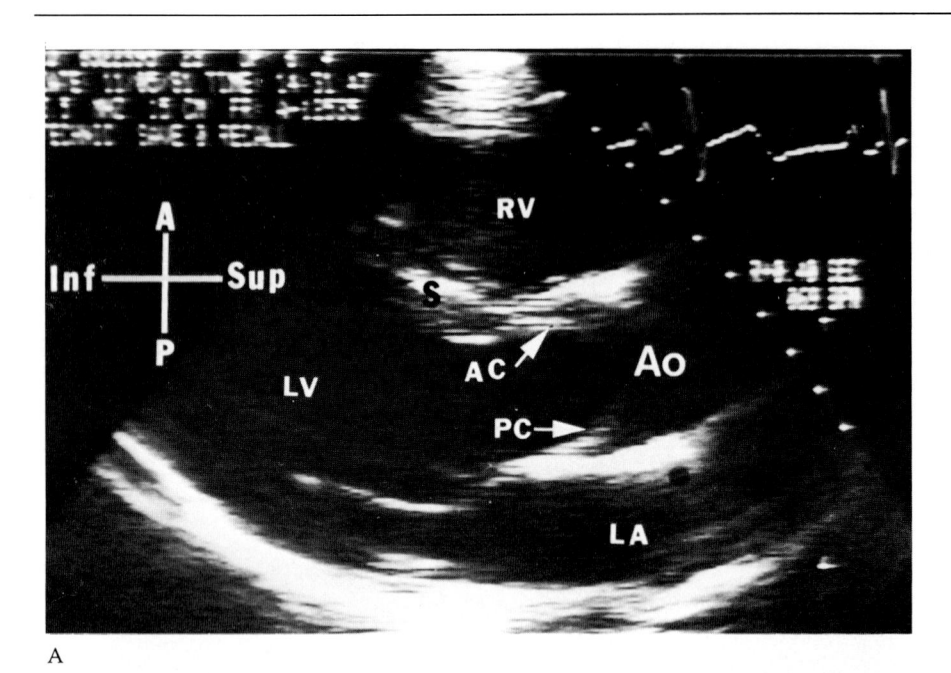

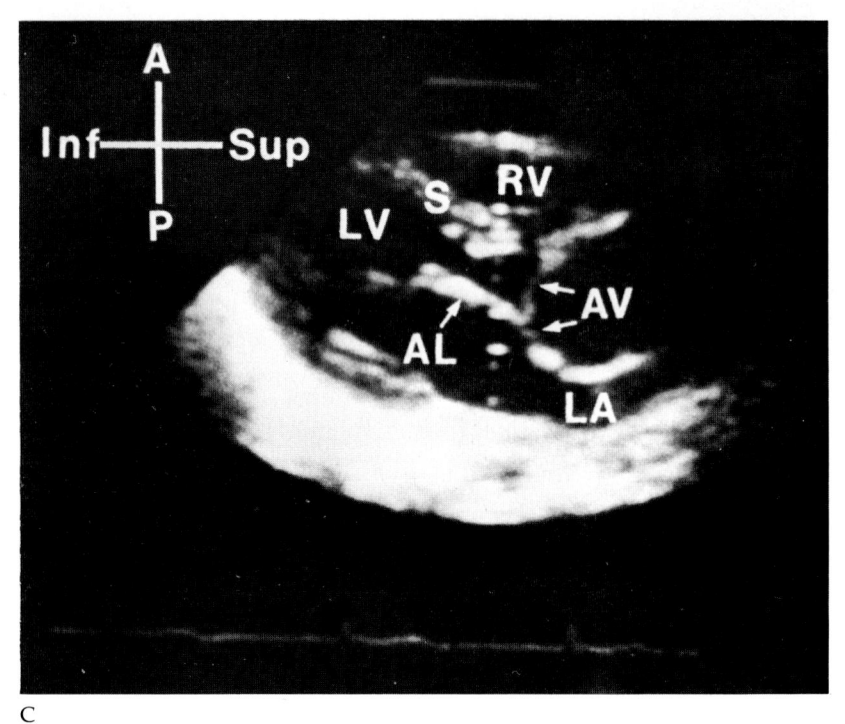

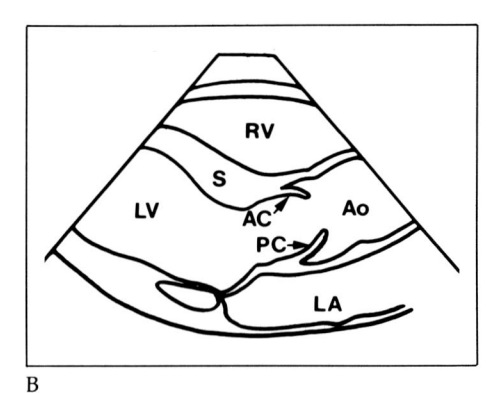

Fig. 4-8A. Parasternal long axis view showing systolic doming of anterior (right) aortic cusp (AC) and posterior (noncoronary) aortic cusp (PC) due to mild congenital aortic stenosis and bicuspid valve. B. Artist's rendering. C. Parasternal long axis view in a child with a bicuspid aortic valve showing diastolic doming or bulging toward the left ventricle when the valve is closed. This diastolic doming contour is occasionally seen in patients with a pliable, noncalcified bicuspid aortic valve and resembles prolapse of the aortic valve; however, the etiology is different.

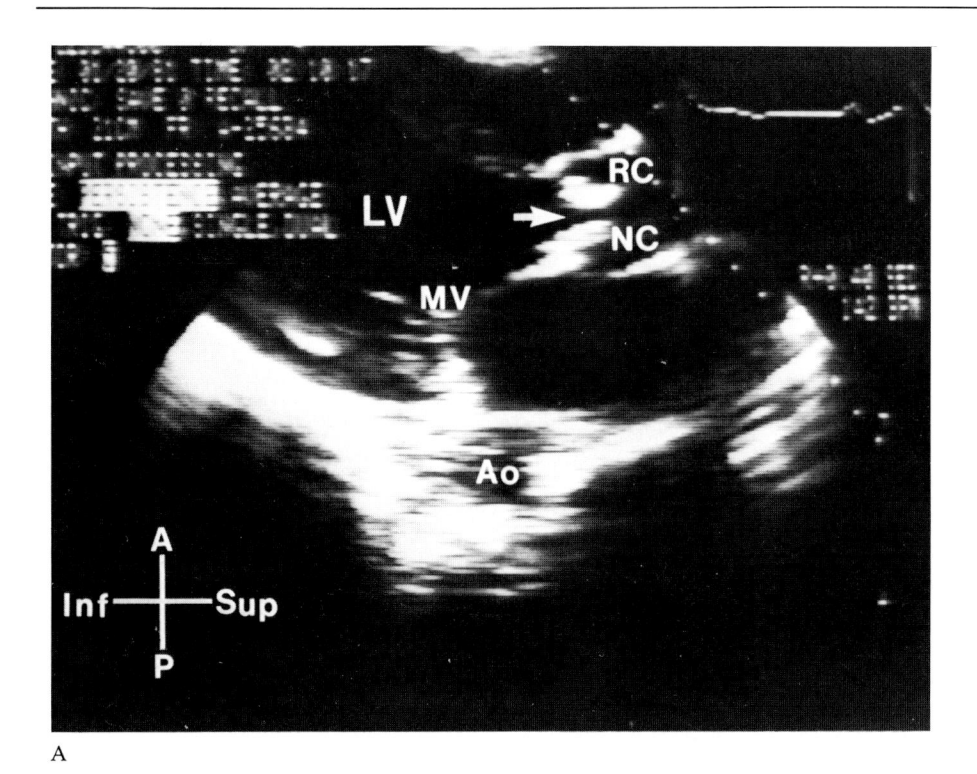

Fig. 4-9A. Parasternal long axis view showing calcified aortic valve with reduced separation (arrow) of the right (RC) and noncoronary aortic cusps. Enlargement and poor function of the left ventricle due to previous myocardial infarctions make it difficult to determine how much of the reduced motion of the aortic leaflets is caused by aortic stenosis and how much by poor left ventricular function. B. Apical long axis view including aortic valve from same patient. This view provides another opportunity to measure leaflet motion of the aortic valve. Ao = descending aorta; PPM = posterior medial papillary muscle.

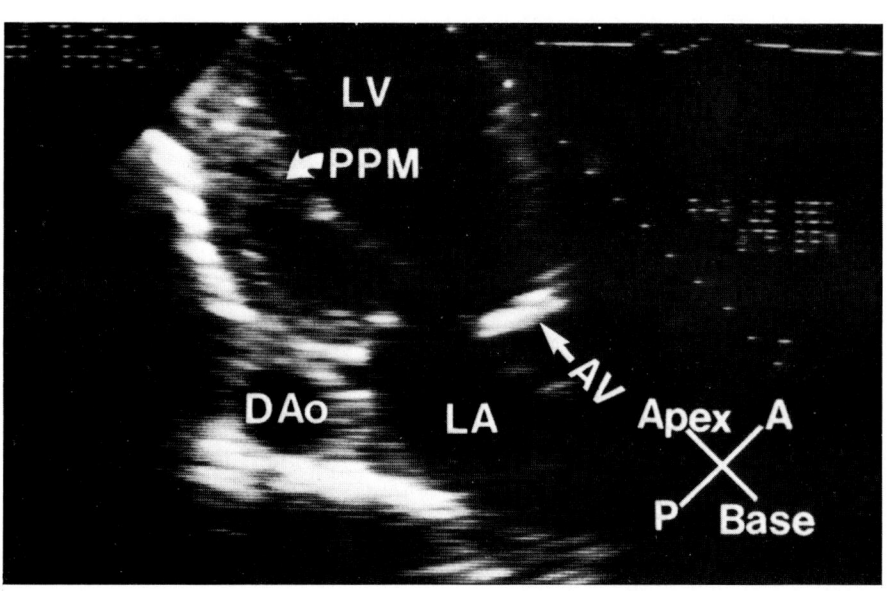

view at the base is rarely possible because of the overall rocking motion of the heart and the related technical difficulty in imaging the leaflets at their tips without loss of a portion of the actual orifice in the image. However, there are occasional exceptions, particularly in persons with poor cardiac function, less cardiac motion, and severely restricted aortic leaflet motion permitting visualization of the true orifice during systole; planimetry of that area is thus possible (Fig. 4-6C, lower panel). Certain clinical conditions may make imaging technically very difficult, and adequate visualization of the aortic valve from parasternal or left precordial windows may not be possible. These conditions include enormous obesity, chronic severe lung disease, severe musculoskeletal deformities, and previous irradiation to the anterior precordium. Under these circumstances valuable qualitative but probably no quantitative information can be obtained by imaging the aortic valve from the apical views as well as from the subcostal planes. The aortic valve can be imaged from both the four-chamber and short axis planes in the subcostal position.

Membranous subvalvular and supravalvular aortic stenosis. Both of these subjects are discussed in greater depth in Chapter 15.

Supravalvular aortic stenosis is an obstructive congenital deformity of the aorta originating just distal to the origin of the coronary artery that may produce either localized or diffuse narrowing of the ascending aorta [40]. The three important two-dimensional imaging views for assessing the ascending aorta for sites of narrowing include the parasternal long axis, the apical long axis with aorta, and the suprasternal notch long axis views of the aorta.

If there is any clinical question about presence of coarctation of the aorta, the descending aorta in the region of the left subclavian artery can be effectively viewed from only one plane, the suprasternal notch long axis view of the aorta.

The echocardiographic features of discrete subaortic stenosis have been well defined and their clinical importance emphasized because of the difficulty that may occur in distinguishing this congenital subvalvular abnormality from aortic valve stenosis itself [41–46]. Although M-mode echocardiography can be valuable in establishing the diagnosis because of the characteristic early systolic closure of the aortic leaflets together with the narrowed left ventricular outflow tract, two-dimensional imaging is usually required in order to visualize the actual membranous obstruction and define its anatomic extent. Although cardiac catheterization is superior for determining the severity of subvalvular obstruction, two-dimensional echocardiography is the procedure of choice for determining the extent of left ventricular hypertrophy as well as for defining the precise anatomy and morphologic spectrum of the lesion causing the subaortic stenosis [45, 46].

Aortic regurgitation. Echocardiography has been a long-standing, valuable tool for the diagnosis of aortic regurgitation as well as for assessing functional abnormalities caused by the insufficiency [47–55].

CLINICAL MANIFESTATIONS AND ETIOLOGY OF AORTIC REGURGITATION. The two most common causes of aortic regurgitation leading to aortic valve replacement are rheumatic and infective endocarditis [55]. In this study, 179 of 200 patients had some degree of aortic regurgitation; it was associated with aortic valve stenosis in 157. With rheumatic etiology accounting for 49 percent and infective endocarditis causing another 22 percent of 189 patients with aortic regurgitation, the third most common etiology was Marfan's syndrome or abnormalities of a similar type, which accounted for the underlying cause of the aortic regurgitation in another 15 patients (8%). The fourth most common cause was a congenital bicuspid valve in another 13 patients (7%) [55]. Other conditions causing isolated pure aortic regurgitation that may lead to aortic valve replacement but that occur very infrequently include the following [55, 56]:

1. Prolapse of the valve from ventricular septal defect
2. Syphilis
3. Aortic dissection
4. Ankylosing spondylitis
5. Subaortic stenosis which may include either discrete membranous or hypertrophic cardiomyopathy forms
6. Trauma
7. Rheumatic arthritis
8. Reiter's syndrome
9. Ehlers-Danlos syndrome
10. Osteogenesis imperfecta
11. Hurler's syndrome

The characteristic features of a decrescendo diastolic blowing murmur at the base and along the left sternal border are sufficiently specific to ensure little difficulty in making the diagnosis at the bedside. In contrast to the systolic ejection murmur of aortic stenosis from several other causes which may mimic aortic stenosis, there are very few conditions that can be confused with aortic insufficiency. Once the typical murmur is heard, echocardiography is not necessary to confirm the diagnosis that has already been established on the basis of the physical findings. There are usually only two reasons for performing an echocardiogram in a patient with aortic regurgitation, first, to determine left ventricular size and function to help estimate the severity of the problem or to continue serial echo examinations for the purpose of selecting the proper time for aortic valve replacement, and second to identify aortic regurgitation by echocardiography in the absence of auscultatory evidence of the murmur. The diagnosis may be difficult to make on auscultation in certain individuals, particularly those who have severe lung disease or who have a large anteroposterior diameter of the chest cage.

MECHANISM OF AUSTIN FLINT MURMUR. In 1886, following the original description of the murmur that bears his name, Austin Flint first postulated the occurrence of early closure of the mitral valve in severe aortic insufficiency [57]. Many years later investigators documented this event with catheterization data by showing that left ventricular pressure exceeds left atrial pressure prior to the onset of mechanical left ventricular systole [58–60]. Botvinick and associates [47] demonstrated echocardiographically that premature closure of the mitral valve is a sensitive and specific indicator for severe acute aortic insufficiency and that this early closure is related to the mechanism of the Austin Flint murmur (Fig. 4-10).

ECHOCARDIOGRAPHIC FINDINGS. The long-standing echocardiographic hallmark of aortic regurgitation is high-frequency oscillations or flutter of the anterior mitral leaflet [61]. Similar diastolic fluttering of the left side of the interventricular septum

130 4. Diseases of the aortic valve and aorta

Fig. 4-10A. M-mode recording showing marked premature closure of the anterior mitral leaflet (short curved arrows) *caused by acute severe aortic regurgitation. The C point arrow marks where normal mitral valve closure should occur. B. A 17-year-old male with chronic (5 years' duration) severe aortic regurgitation following aortic valvotomy for aortic stenosis due to bicuspid aortic valve. Curved arrows pointing to the aortic valve show the increased thickness of the leaflets and an abnormal motion at the onset of systole. The open arrows pointing to the septum show the rapid enlargement of this compliant, volume overloaded left ventricle. Note the marked premature closure of the mitral valve* (black arrows) *due to the severe aortic regurgitation. (Courtesy of John Berg, M.D.)*

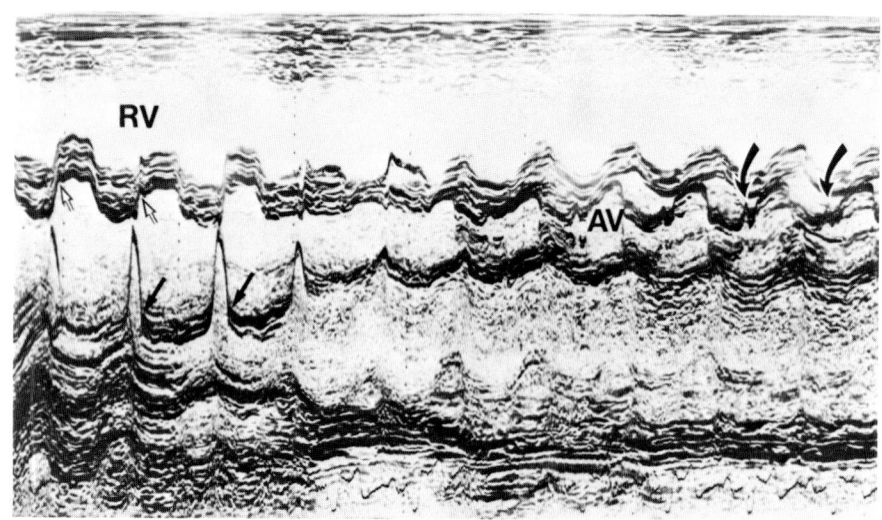

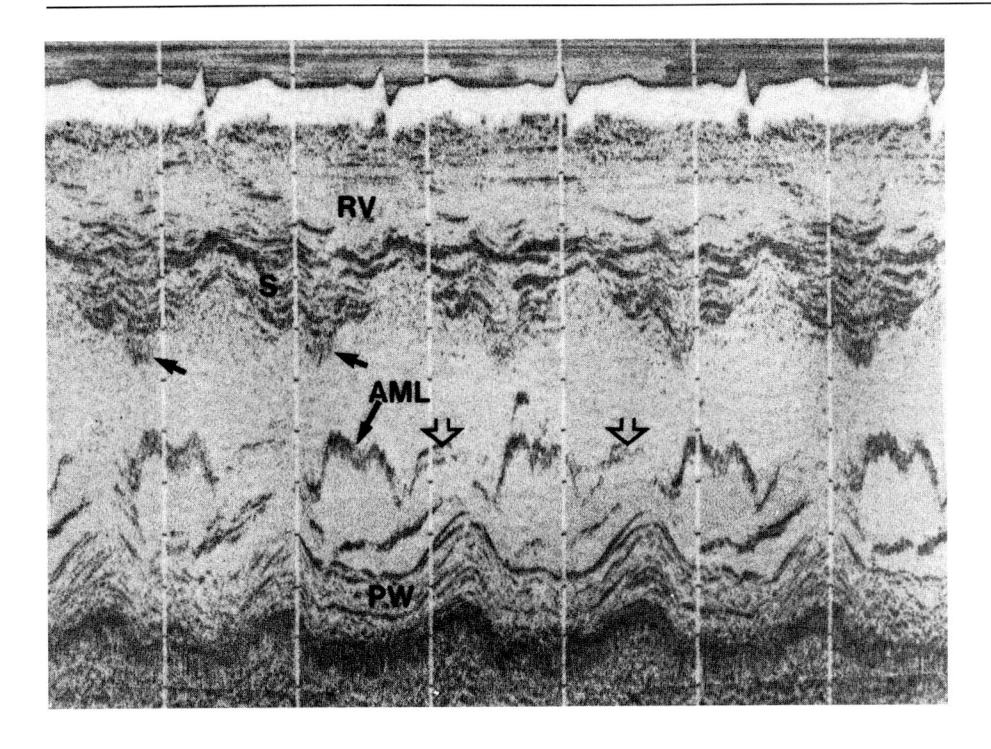

Fig. 4-11. M-mode recording showing mild enlargement of the left ventricle (end-diastolic dimension = 60 mm), fluttering of the left side of the septum (S) at onset of diastole (arrows) and fluttering of the anterior mitral leaflet caused by aortic regurgitation. The open arrows point to systolic anterior motion of the mitral valve and chordae caused by the aortic regurgitation observed in some patients with this condition.

may also be seen in many patients with aortic regurgitation (Fig. 4-11). (This high-frequency flutter has no relationship to the genesis of the Austin Flint murmur.) High-frequency oscillations of the anterior leaflet, although a sensitive indicator for aortic insufficiency, are of no value in estimating the severity or the etiology of the aortic regurgitation. Whenever premature closure of the mitral valve occurs in the presence of aortic insufficiency, first-degree atrioventricular block or loss of sinus rhythm must be ruled out as contributing factors to avoid incorrectly attributing premature closure to severe insufficiency with its more serious implications for treatment [62, 63]. Fluttering of the anterior mitral leaflet simulating aortic regurgitation has rarely been noted in the absence of aortic or mitral valve disease (Fig. 4-12).

The echocardiographic signs of left ventricular volume overload, dilatation of the left ventricle and exaggerated motion of septum and posterior wall, are common findings in aortic regurgitation. These nonspecific signs are similar to what is observed with mitral regurgitation. There is, however, a commonly encountered, nonspecific feature of septal motion seen in patients with aortic regurgitation that is not present in mitral regurgitation consisting of a late systolic notch with anterior septal motion followed by an abrupt posterior diastolic notching, which occurs during the rapid filling phase of the ventricle (Fig. 4-13). The mechanism of this motion has never been adequately explained.

Although it is often not possible to identify the presence of aortic regurgitation with either M-mode or two-dimensional imaging of the aortic leaflets, these views are obviously an important aspect of the overall examination, primarily because of the possible disclosure of abnormal features that could help explain the underlying etiology of the regurgitation. On rare occasions the regurgitant orifice can actually be imaged in the parasternal short axis view during diastole (Fig. 4-14). Since the

132 4. Diseases of the aortic valve and aorta

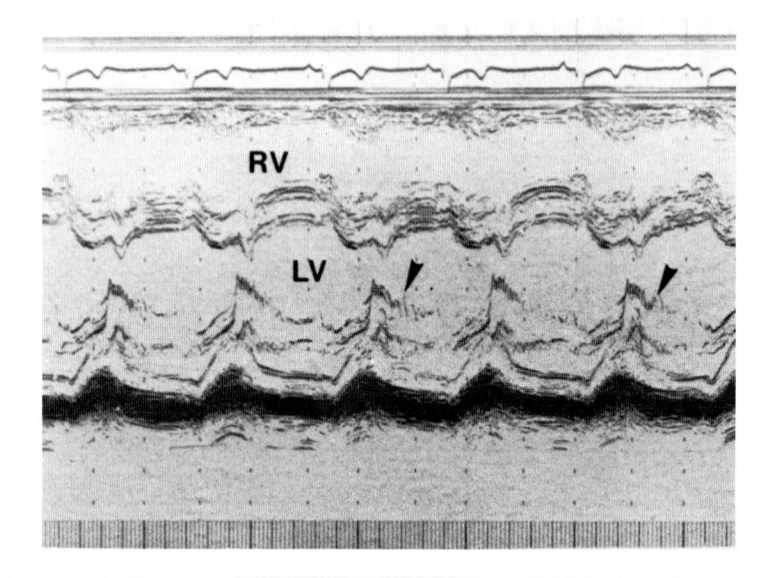

Fig. 4-12. M-mode recording in a young adult with fluttering of the anterior mitral leaflet (arrows) simulating aortic regurgitation. Neither aortic regurgitation nor other evidence of heart disease was found at cardiac catheterization.

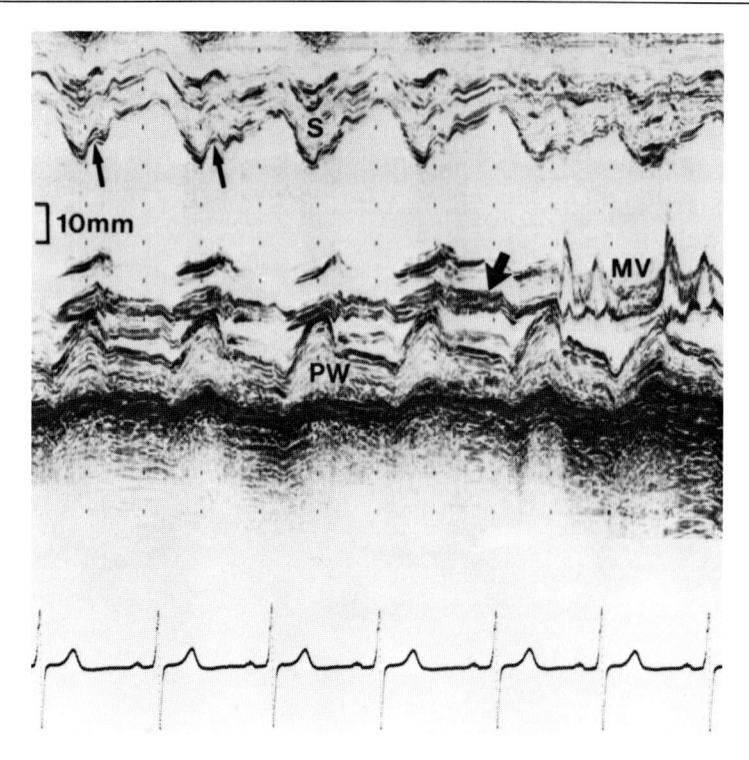

Fig. 4-13. M-mode recording in a patient with aortic regurgitation demonstrating the early diastolic notch of the ventricular septum (S) (arrows), which is very commonly seen in the presence of aortic insufficiency. The left ventricle is enlarged (end-diastolic dimension is 68 mm) and wall thickness is normal. Large arrow points to chordae tendineae, which appear slightly thickened and are fluttering.

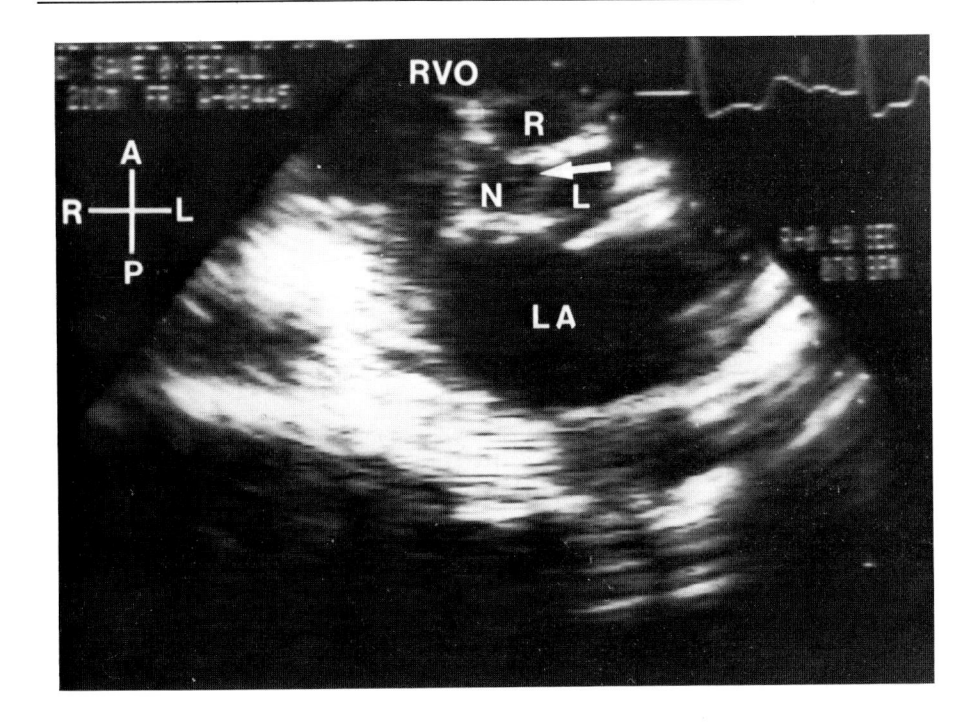

Fig. 4-14. Parasternal short axis view at the base showing the three aortic cusps and a regurgitant orifice (arrow) in a patient with severe aortic regurgitation and no aortic stenosis.

diagnosis, as well as left ventricular size and function measurements, can be determined by M-mode echocardiography, one of the more important clinical applications of two-dimensional imaging in such patients is to more thoroughly image the aortic leaflets together with other cardiac structures to search for the underlying etiology. Useful imaging information of the valve can be obtained when the aortic regurgitation is secondary to rheumatic valvular disease or to a congenitally bicuspid valve. If one of the aortic leaflets is flail or has an attached vegetation this is usually quite easily diagnosed with either M-mode or two-dimensional techniques. Premature opening of the aortic valve has been described in a few patients as an index of a severe form of aortic regurgitation [51, 64].

Although not a common problem, features of prolapse or myxomatous degeneration of the aortic valve have been noted with echocardiography [65–68] (Fig. 4-15). In a group of 50 patients with mitral valve prolapse, Ogawa and colleagues [68] found 12 patients (24%) with redundant, prolapsing aortic leaflets. Eight of these 12 patients had aortic regurgitation.

Pulsed Doppler echocardiography can also be used to detect aortic regurgitation by placing the sample site in the left ventricular outflow tract. Pearlman and associates [69] have suggested that the degree of aortic regurgitation can be quantitated by noting how far into the ventricle the regurgitant jet can be detected. However, the reliability of this observation remains to be confirmed with further investigations.

The management of patients with chronic aortic insufficiency is complicated by a lack of clear-cut guidelines for determining optimal timing of aortic valve replacement; Henry and associates [70] reported that if surgery for these patients is deferred until significant symptoms develop, approximately 50 percent of those surviving the procedure will die within five years, most from congestive heart failure

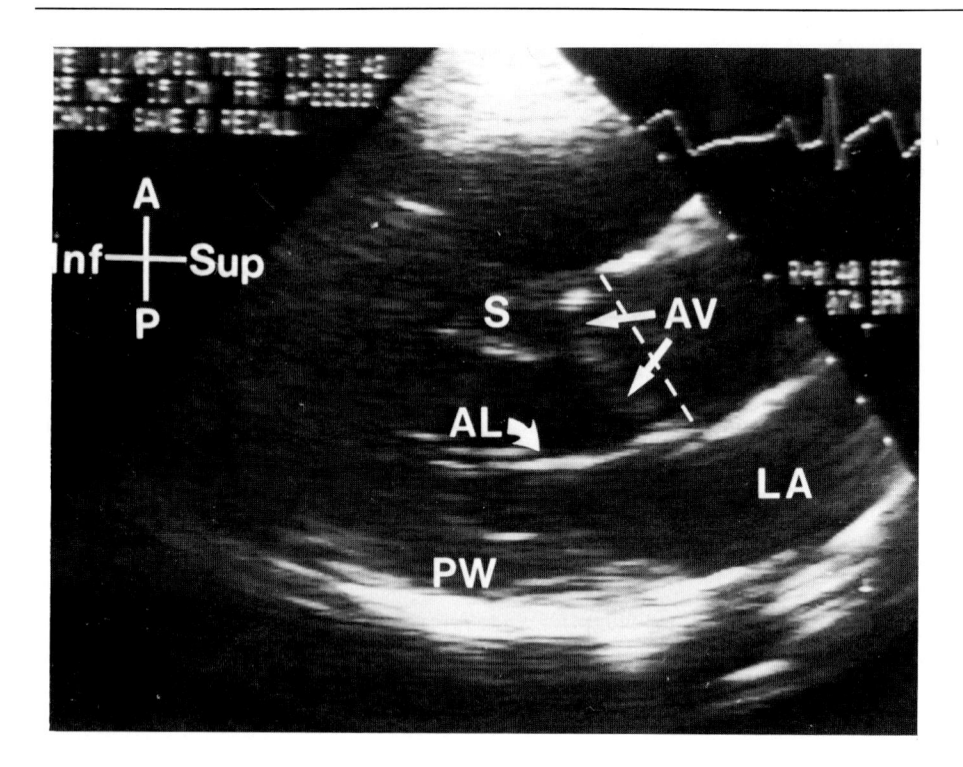

Fig. 4-15. Parasternal long axis view showing prolapse of the aortic valve. The dashed white line marks the aortic annulus and origin of the aortic cusps. Normally the diastolic closure line is on or slightly superior to that line. The right cusp (upper arrow) actually touches the superior aspect of the interventricular septum as a result of this prolapsing motion.

secondary to irreversible myocardial damage. Left ventricular size and function are accurate predictors of late congestive heart failure and poor prognosis following aortic valve replacement. For this reason we agree with other investigators that asymptomatic patients with end-systolic dimensions between 50 and 54 mm should be carefully followed with serial echocardiograms every four to six months, and patients with aortic regurgitation who have an end-systolic dimension greater than 55 mm or percent fractional shortening less than 25 percent, even though without other symptoms, should have aortic valve replacement [54, 71].

Diseases of the aorta. Measurement of the aortic root by M-mode echocardiography is performed in the region of the aortic annulus; therefore, assessment of the ascending aorta for aneurysmal dilatation is usually quite inadequate and incomplete. Published data for the upper limit of normal in adult patients for the aortic root diameter as measured by M-mode echocardiography varies between 33 and 37 mm [72, 73]. Francis and associates [72] noted that in addition to the obvious relationship of aortic diameter to body surface area there was also a significant difference in aortic root diameters between men and women that could not be explained by a difference in body surface area; the mean diameter in 78 normal men averaged 25 mm compared to 22 mm in 81 women. Mintz and associates [74] have established the following normal values for luminal diameter at different levels of the aorta:

16 ± 1.8 mm/m^2 at the level of the aortic valve
13 ± 1.4 mm/m^2 above the level of the sinus of Valsalva
10 ± 1.4 mm/m^2 of the descending aorta

TWO-DIMENSIONAL ECHO IMAGING TECHNIQUES OF THE AORTA. A portion of the ascending aorta is routinely imaged in both the parasternal long axis view and the apical long axis view; however, in order to image the entire ascending aorta, transverse aortic arch, and the superior portion of the descending aorta, suprasternal notch imaging is required (Fig. 4-16). Long axis, short axis, and various oblique views of the aortic arch can be performed from the suprasternal notch transducer position. The patient must be properly positioned in a supine position with a pillow beneath the upper portion of the shoulders; the neck and head are slightly hyperextended, and the subject should look toward the ceiling. A variable amount of the ascending aorta can be imaged from the parasternal long axis plane; directing the sector beam medially toward the aortic valve increases the length of the aorta that can be viewed. An aneurysm of the ascending aorta can usually be diagnosed from this position (Fig. 4-17). Suprasternal notch imaging is technically difficult, and most of the published data utilizing two-dimensional imaging to diagnose dissections and aneurysms have been obtained from various parasternal imaging windows [74–76]. An excellent relationship exists between cineangiographic and two-dimensional echocardiographic measurements of aortic root size [75].

In routine parasternal imaging the descending aorta is visualized posterior to the left atrium and the left ventricle. Care should be taken not to confuse the echo-free space in the atrioventricular groove region caused by the coronary sinus with the descending aorta, the larger structure somewhat more posterior and superior to the atrioventricular groove behind the left atrium.

Sahn and associates [77] have reported the value of two-dimensional imaging from the suprasternal notch position with angiographic correlations in the diagnosis of coarctation of the aorta (Fig. 4-18). Further discussion of the diagnosis of coarctation of the aorta may be found in Chapter 15.

The diagnosis of dissecting aortic aneurysm can be made by M-mode echocardiography; however, the diagnosis is more clearly defined when an aortic intimal flap can be identified. This feature has been noted from parasternal imaging positions as well as from the suprasternal notch [78–82] (Fig. 4-19). The causes of false positive M-mode recordings, such as simultaneous recording of the mitral ring in the posterior aortic wall creating a pattern suggestive of posterior aortic wall dissection or the tangential intersecting of an M-mode beam through a thickened or possibly even normal aortic wall, could also generate a double echo suggesting a false lumen. These causes of false positives are much less a problem with two-dimensional imaging, in which the chief technical difficulty is simply obtaining adequate imaging detail of the ascending and descending aorta.

Iliceto and colleagues [83] have employed a modified apical approach with the transducer positioned near the apex and the plane of the sector beam directed perpendicularly to the sternum; by rotating the beam, the operator can image the descending thoracic aorta in both short and long axis planes.

Echocardiographic features of sinus of Valsalva aneurysms have been described using both M-mode and two-dimensional imaging techniques [84–87] (Fig. 4-20). Rupture of a sinus of Valsalva aneurysm can be suspected clinically when abrupt onset of congestive heart failure is associated with a continuous murmur, evidence of right and left ventricular volume overload and bounding peripheral pulses. Schatz [87] reported the use of two-dimensional echocardiography employing multiple views together with contrast technique as an adjunct to angiography in defining the nature, location, and size of a ruptured sinus of Valsalva aneurysm.

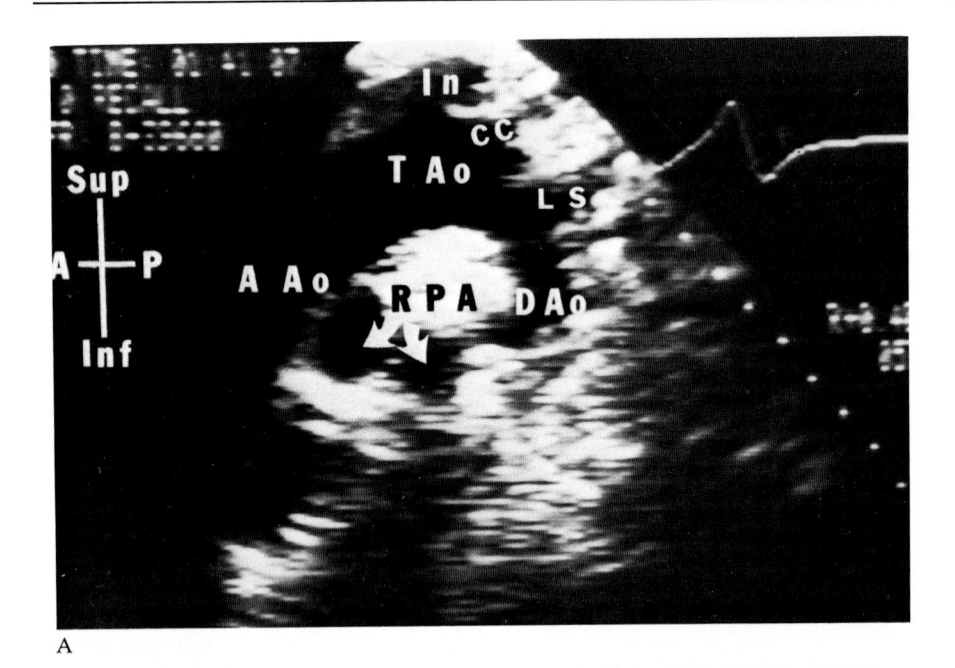

Fig. 4-16A. Suprasternal notch long axis view of a normal adult aorta showing ascending, transverse, and descending portions. The lumen of the right pulmonary artery (RPA) probably appears double because the RPA bifurcates at that point or because it is oblique to the plane of the sector beam. B. Suprasternal notch short axis view in a normal adult showing the superior vena cava, aorta, and right pulmonary artery. CC = left common carotid artery; In = innominate artery; LS = left subclavian artery.

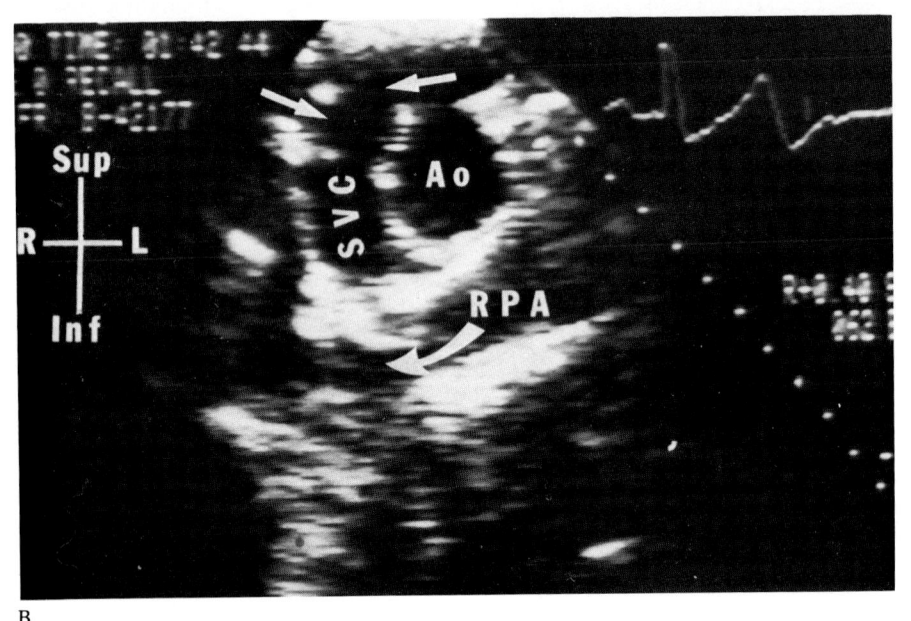

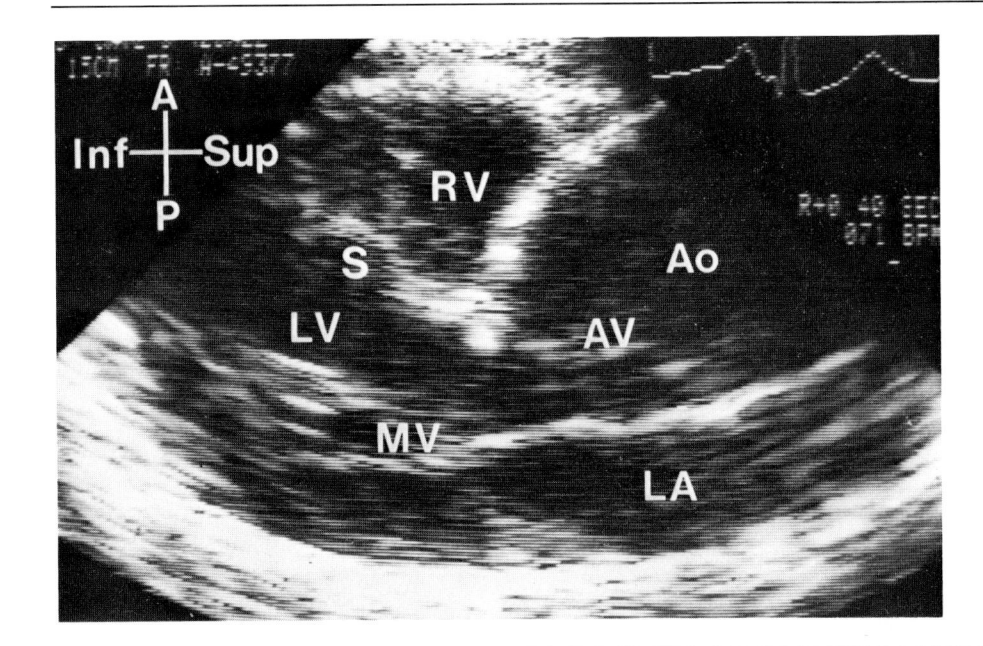

Fig. 4-17. Parasternal long axis view of a patient with a large aneurysm of the ascending aorta. The aortic valve appears normal; there is mild aortic regurgitation but no enlargement of the left ventricle. Other structures are also normal.

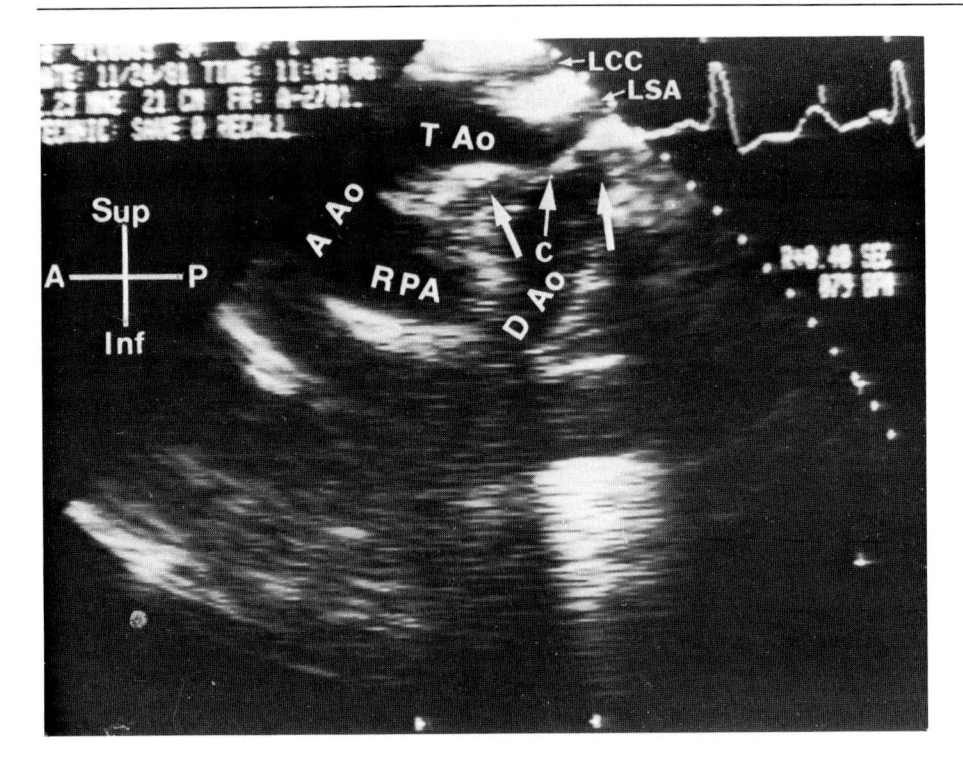

Fig. 4-18. Suprasternal notch long axis view of the aorta showing residual coarctation (C) in a man who had been previously operated on. A graft distal to the coarctation is complicated by a dissection, a portion of which can be seen on either side of the descending aorta just distal to the coarctation (large white arrows). LCC = left common carotid artery; LSA = left subclavian artery; RPA = right pulmonary artery.

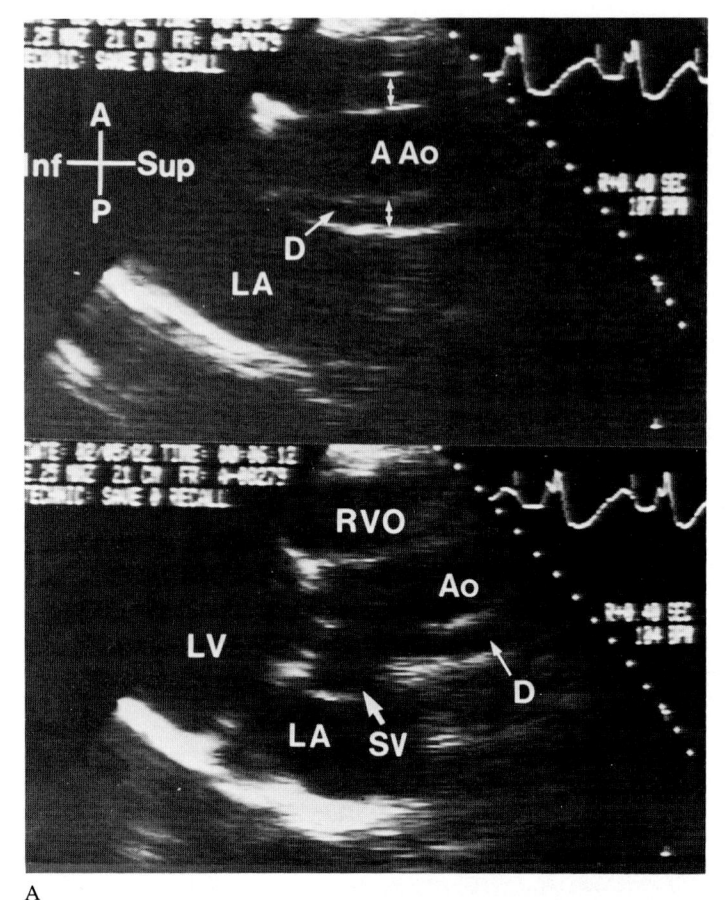

Fig. 4-19A. Parasternal long axis oblique view of the ascending aorta in a patient with dissection (D). Lower panel shows prominent posterior sinus of Valsalva (SV). Upper panel shows the apparent origin of the dissection immediately superior to the sinus of Valsalva and the false lumen anteriorly. B. Parasternal short axis view at the base with leftward angulation showing aortic dissection both anterior and posterior (arrows) in the same patient. LPA = left pulmonary artery; RPA = right pulmonary artery.

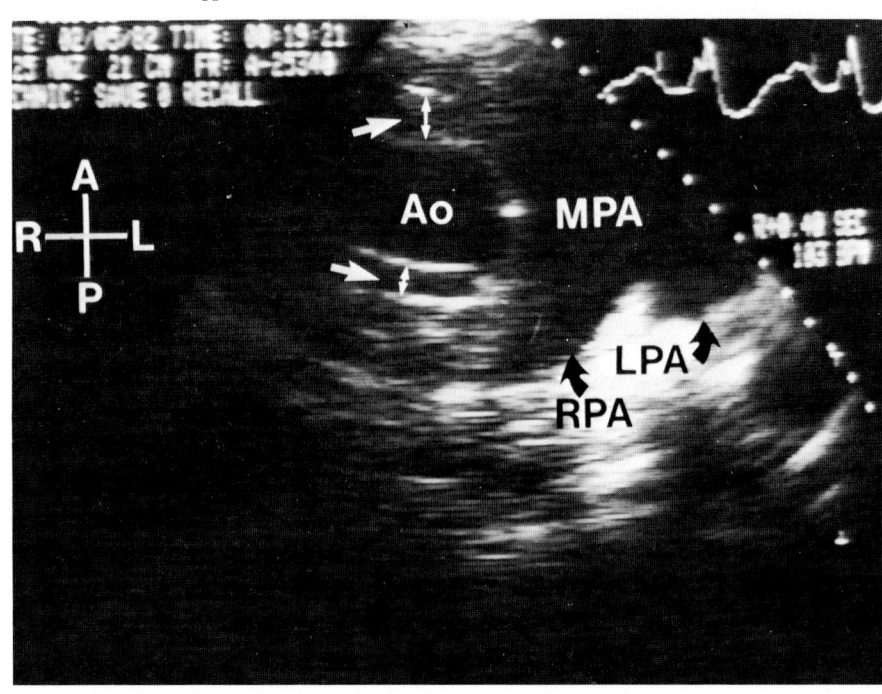

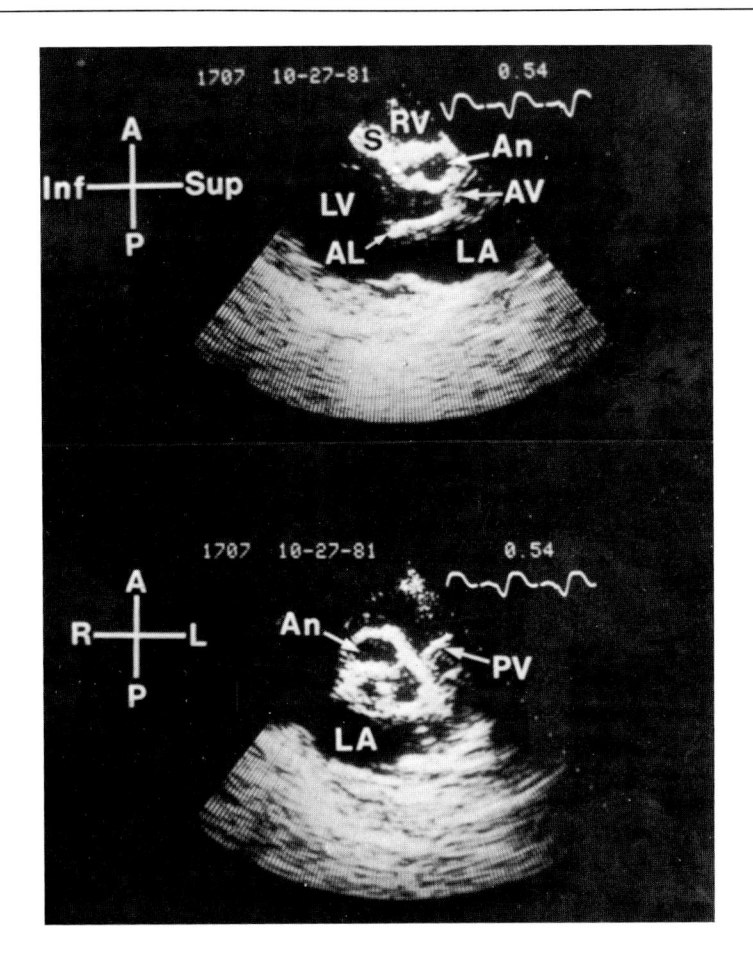

Fig. 4-20. Parasternal long axis (upper panel) and short axis at the base (lower panel) views show an aneurysm (An) of the anterior (right) sinus of Valsalva extending into the superior aspect of the interventricular septum in the upper panel.

References

1. Tsakiris AG, Sturm RE, Wood EH: Experimental studies on the mechanisms of closure of cardiac valves with use of roentgen videodensitometry. *Am J Cardiol* 32:136, 1973
2. Hirshfeld S, Liebman J, Borkat G, Barmuth C: Intracardiac pressure-sound correlates of echographic aortic valve closure. *Circulation* 55:602, 1977
3. Laniado S, Yellin E, Terdiman R, Meytes I, Stadler J: Hemodynamic correlates of the normal aortic valve echogram: A study of sound, flow, and motion. *Circulation* 54:729, 1976
4. Craige E: On the genesis of heart sounds: Contributions made by echocardiographic studies. *Circulation* 53:207, 1976
5. Laniado S, Yellin E, Kotler M, Levy L, Stadler J, Terdiman R: A study of the dynamic relations between the mitral valve echogram and phasic mitral flow. *Circulation* 51:104, 1975
6. Feizi O, Symons C, Yacoub M: Echocardiography of the aortic valve. I. Studies of the normal aortic valve, aortic stenosis, aortic regurgitation, and mixed aortic valve disease. *Br Heart J* 36:341, 1974
7. Walmsley R: Anatomy of left ventricular outflow tract. *Br Heart J* 41:263, 1979
8. Strunk BL, Fitzgerald JW, Lipton M, Popp RL, Barry WH: The posterior aortic wall echocardiogram: Its relationship to left atrial volume change. *Circulation* 54:744, 1976
9. Strunk BL, London EJ, Fitzgerald J, Popp RL, Barry WH: The assessment of mitral stenosis and prosthetic mitral valve obstruction, using the posterior aortic wall echocardiogram. *Circulation* 55:885, 1977
10. Djalaly A, Schiller NB, Poehlmann HW, Arnold S, Gertz EW: Diastolic aortic root motion in left ventricular hypertrophy. *Chest* 79:442, 1981
11. Pomerance A: Pathogenesis of aortic stenosis and its relation to age. *Br Heart J* 34:569, 1972
12. Frank S, Johnson A, Ross J Jr: Natural history of valvular aortic stenosis. *Br Heart J* 35:41, 1973
13. McMillan IKR: Aortic stenosis: A postmortem cinephotographic study of valve action. *Br Heart J* 17:56, 1955
14. Bennett DH, Evans DW, Raj MVJ: Echocardiographic left ventricular dimensions in pressure and volume overload: Their use in assessing aortic stenosis. *Br Heart J* 37:971, 1975
15. Johnson GL, Meyer RA, Schwartz DC, Korfhagen J, Kaplan S: Echocardiographic evaluation of fixed left ventricular outlet obstruction in children: Pre and postoperative assessment of ventricular systolic pressures. *Circulation* 56:299, 1977
16. Aziz KU, vanGrondelle A, Paul MH, Muster AJ: Echocardiographic assessment of the relation between left ventricular wall and cavity dimensions and peak systolic pressure in children with aortic stenosis. *Am J Cardiol* 40:775, 1977
17. Blackwood RA, Bloom KR, Williams CM: Aortic stenosis in children: Experience with echocardiographic prediction of severity. *Circulation* 57:263, 1978
18. Schwartz A, Vignola PA, Walker HJ, King ME, Goldblatt A: Echocardiographic estimation of aortic-valve gradient in aortic stenosis. *Ann Intern Med* 89:329, 1978
19. Gewitz MH, Werner JC, Kleinman CS, Hellenbrand WE, Talner NS: Role of echocardiography in aortic stenosis: Pre- and postoperative studies. *Am J Cardiol* 43:67, 1979
20. Bass JL, Einzig S, Hong CY, Moller JH: Echocardiographic screening to assess the severity of congenital aortic valve stenosis in children. *Am J Cardiol* 44:82, 1979
21. Agulescu SI, Streian C, Mourtada A, Shencoru F: Echocardiographic assessment of aortic stenosis. *Med Interne* 18:371, 1980
22. Glanz S, Hellenbrand WE, Berman MA: Echocardiographic assessment of the severity of aortic stenosis in children and adolescents. *Am J Cardiol* 38:620, 1976
23. Hagan AD, DiSessa TG, Samtoy L, Friedman WF, Vieweg WVR: Reliability of echocardiography in diagnosing and quantitating valvular aortic stenosis. *J Cardiovasc Med* 5:391, 1980
24. Sandler H, Dodge HT: Left ventricular tension and stress in man. *Circ Res* 13:91, 1963
25. Hood WP, Rackley CE, Rolett EL: Wall stress in the normal and hypertrophied human left ventricle. *Am J Cardiol* 22:550, 1968
26. Grossman W, Jones D, McLaurin LP: Wall stress and patterns of hypertrophy in the human left ventricle. *J Clin Invest* 56:56, 1975
27. Fifer MA, Gunther S, Grossman W, Mirsky I, Carabello B, Barry WH: Myocardial contrac-

tile function in aortic stenosis as determined from the rate of stress development during isovolumic systole. *Am J Cardiol* 44:1318, 1979
28. Gunther S, Grossman W: Determinants of ventricular function in pressure-overload hypertrophy in man. *Circulation* 59:679, 1979
29. Weyman AE, Feigenbaum H, Dillon JC, Chang S: Cross-sectional echocardiography in assessing the severity of valvular aortic stenosis. *Circulation* 52:828, 1975
30. Chang S, Clements S, Chang J: Aortic stenosis: Echocardiographic cusp separation and surgical description of aortic valve in 22 patients. *Am J Cardiol* 39:499, 1977
31. Reichek N, Devereux RB: Reliable estimation of peak left ventricular systolic pressure by M-mode echographic-determined end-diastolic relative wall thickness: Identification of severe valvular aortic stenosis in adult patients. *Am Heart J* 103:202, 1982
32. Weyman AE, Feigenbaum H, Hurwitz RA, Girod DA, Dillon JC: Cross-sectional echocardiographic assessment of the severity of aortic stenosis in children. *Circulation* 55:773, 1977
33. DeMaria AN, Bommer W, Joye J, Lee G, Bouteller J, Mason DT: Value and limitations of cross-sectional echocardiography of the aortic valve in the diagnosis and quantification of valvular aortic stenosis. *Circulation* 62:304, 1980
34. Godley RW, Green D, Dillon JC, Rogers EW, Feigenbaum H, Weyman AE: Reliability of two-dimensional echocardiography in assessing the severity of valvular aortic stenosis. *Chest* 79:657, 1981
35. Young JB, Quinones MA, Waggoner AD, Miller RR: Diagnosis and quantification of aortic stenosis with pulsed doppler echocardiography. *Am J Cardiol* 45:987, 1980
36. Henry WL, Bonow RO, Borer JS, Kent KM, Ware JH, Redwood DR, Itscoitz SB, McIntosh CL, Morrow AG, Epstein SE: Evaluation of aortic valve replacement in patients with valvular aortic stenosis. *Circulation* 61:814, 1980
37. Croke RP, Pifarre R, Sullivan H, Gunnar R, Loeb H: Reversal of advanced left ventricular dysfunction following aortic valve replacement for aortic stenosis. *Ann Thorac Surg* 24:38, 1977
38. Smith N, McAnulty JH, Rahimtoola SH: Severe aortic stenosis with impaired left ventricular function and clinical heart failure: Results of valve replacement. *Circulation* 58:255, 1978
39. Borer JS, Bacharach SL, Green MV, Kent KM, Rosing DR, Seides SF, McIntosh CL, Conkle DM, Morrow AG, Epstein SE: Left ventricular function during exercise before and after aortic valve replacement. *Circulation* 56(Suppl III):III-28, 1977
40. Jarcho S: Coarctation of the aorta. *Am J Cardiol* 7:844, 1961
41. Davis RH, Feigenbaum H, Chang S, Konecke LL, Dillon JC: Echocardiographic manifestations of discrete subaortic stenosis. *Am J Cardiol* 33:277, 1974
42. Weyman AE, Feigenbaum H, Hurwitz RA, Girod DA, Dillon JC, Chang S: Localization of left ventricular outflow obstruction by cross-sectional echocardiography. *Am J Med* 60:33, 1976
43. Krueger SK, French JW, Forker AD, Caudill CC, Popp RL: Echocardiography in discrete subaortic stenosis. *Circulation* 59:506, 1979
44. Berry TE, Aziz KU, Paul MH: Echocardiographic assessment of discrete subaortic stenosis in childhood. *Am J Cardiol* 43:957, 1979
45. Wilcox WD, Seward JB, Hagler DJ, Mair DD, Tajik AJ: Discrete subaortic stenosis: Two-dimensional echocardiographic features with angiographic and surgical correlation. *Mayo Clin Proc* 55:425, 1980
46. DiSessa TG, Hagan AD, Isabel-Jones JB, Ti CC, Mercier JC, Friedman WF: Two-dimensional echocardiographic evaluation of discrete subaortic stenosis from the apical long axis view. *Am Heart J* 101:774, 1981
47. Botvinick EH, Schiller NB, Wickramasekaran R, Klausner SC, Gertz E: Echocardiographic demonstration of early mitral valve closure in severe aortic insufficiency: Its clinical implications. *Circulation* 51:836, 1975
48. Chandraratna PAN, Samet P, Robinson MJ, Byrd C: Echocardiography of the "floppy" aortic valve. *Circulation* 52:959, 1975
49. Rolston WA, Hirshfeld DS, Emilson BB, Cheitlin MD: Echocardiographic appearance of ruptured aortic cusp. *Am J Med* 62:133, 1977
50. Srivastava TN, Flowers NC: Echocardiographic features of flail aortic valve. *Chest* 73:90, 1978
51. Pietro DA, Parisi AF, Harrington JJ, Askenazi J: Premature opening of the aortic valve: An index of highly advanced aortic regurgitation. *JCU* 6:170, 1978

52. Schuler G, Peterson KL, Johnson AD, Francis G, Ashburn W, Dennish G, Daily PO, Ross J Jr: Serial noninvasive assessment of left ventricular hypertrophy and function after surgical correction of aortic regurgitation. *Am J Cardiol* 44:585, 1979
53. McDonald IG, Jelinek VM: Serial M-mode echocardiography in severe chronic aortic regurgitation. *Circulation* 62:1291, 1980
54. Kotler MN, Mintz GS, Parry WR, Segal BL: M mode and two dimensional echocardiography in mitral and aortic regurgitation: Pre- and postoperative evaluation of volume overload of the left ventricle. *Am J Cardiol* 46:1144, 1980
55. Roberts WC, Morrow AG, McIntosh CL, Jones M, Epstein SE: Congenitally bicuspid aortic valve causing severe, pure aortic regurgitation without superimposed infective endocarditis. *Am J Cardiol* 47:206, 1981
56. Cawley IS, Morris DC, Silverman BD (Eds.), Valvular Heart Disease. In JW Hurst, *The Heart* (4th ed.). New York: McGraw-Hill, 1978. P. 1022
57. Flint A: On cardiac murmurs. *Am J Med Sci* 91:27, 1886
58. Dodge HT, Sandler H, Evans T: Observations on the hemodynamics of severe aortic insufficiency in man. *Circulation* 22:741, 1960
59. Rees JR, Epstein EJ, Criley JM, Ross RS: Hemodynamic effects of severe aortic regurgitation. *Br Heart J* 26:412, 1964
60. Fortuin NJ, Craige E: On the mechanism of the Austin Flint murmur. *Circulation* 45:558, 1972
61. Pridie RB, Benham R, Oakley CM: Echocardiography of the mitral valve in aortic valve disease. *Br Heart J* 33:296, 1971
62. Hagan AD: Non-mitral Diseases Affecting the Mitral Valve Echogram. In DT Mason (Ed.), *Advances in Heart Disease* (Vol. II). New York: Grune and Stratton, 1978. Pp. 45–69
63. DiSessa TG, Hagan AD: Echocardiographic Manifestations of Normal Sinus Rhythm, Arrhythmias, and Conduction Defects. In A Abbassi (Ed.), *Echocardiographic Interpretation*. Springfield, Ill.: Charles C Thomas, 1981. Pp. 263–278
64. Page A, Layton C: Premature opening of aortic valve in severe aortic regurgitation. *Br Heart J* 37:1101, 1975
65. Shahawy ME, Graybeal R, Pepine CJ, Conti CR: Diagnosis of aortic valvular prolapse by echocardiography. *Chest* 69:411, 1976
66. Rippe J, Fishbein MC, Carabello B, Angoff G, Sloss L, Collins JJ Jr, Alpert JS: Primary myxomatous degeneration of cardiac valves: Clinical, pathological, hemodynamic, and echocardiographic profile. *Br Heart J* 44:621, 1980
67. Morganroth J, Jones RH, Chen CC, Naito M: Two dimensional echocardiography in mitral, aortic and tricuspid valve prolapse: The clinical problem, cardiac nuclear imaging considerations and a proposed standard for diagnosis. *Am J Cardiol* 46:1164, 1980
68. Ogawa S, Hayashi J, Sasaki H, Tani M, Akaishi M, Mitamura H, Sano M, Hoshino T, Handa S, Nakamura Y: Evaluation of combined valvular prolapse syndrome by two-dimensional echocardiography. *Circulation* 65:174, 1982
69. Pearlman AS, Dooley TK, Franklin DW, Weiler T: Detection of regurgitant flow using duplex (two-dimensional/doppler) echocardiography. *Circulation* (Suppl II)60:154, 1979
70. Henry WL, Bonow RO, Borer JS, Ware JH, Kent KM, Redwood DR, McIntosh CL, Morrow AG, Epstein SE: Observations on the optimum time for operative intervention for aortic regurgitation. I. Evaluation of the results of aortic valve replacement in symptomatic patients. *Circulation* 61:471, 1980
71. Henry WL, Bonow RO, Rosing DR, Epstein SE: Observations on the optimum time for operative intervention for aortic regurgitation. II. Serial echocardiographic evaluation of asymptomatic patients. *Circulation* 61:484, 1980
72. Francis GS, Hagan AD, Oury J, O'Rourke RA: Accuracy of echocardiography for assessing aortic root diameter. *Br Heart J* 37:376, 1975
73. Brown OR, DeMots H, Kloster FE, Roberts A, Menashe VD, Beals RK: Aortic root dilatation and mitral valve prolapse in Marfan's Syndrome. *Circulation* 52:651, 1975
74. Mintz GS, Kotler MN, Segal BL, Parry WR: Two dimensional echocardiographic recognition of the descending thoracic aorta. *Am J Cardiol* 44:232, 1979
75. DeMaria AN, Bommer W, Neumann A, Weinert L, Bogren H, Mason DT: Identification and localization of aneurysms of the ascending aorta by cross-sectional echocardiography. *Circulation* 59:755, 1979

76. D'Cruz IA, Jain DP, Hirsch L, Levinsky R, Cohen HC, Glick G: Echocardiographic diagnosis of dilatation of the ascending aorta using right parasternal scanning. *Radiology* 129:465, 1978
77. Sahn DJ, Allen HD, McDonald G, Goldberg SJ: Real-time cross-sectional echocardiographic diagnosis of coarctation of the aorta: A prospective study of echocardiographic-angiographic correlations. *Circulation* 56:762, 1977
78. Krueger SK, Starke H, Forker AD, Eliot RS: Echocardiographic mimics of aortic root dissection. *Chest* 67:441, 1975
79. Brown OR, Popp RL, Kloster FE: Echocardiographic criteria for aortic root dissection. *Am J Cardiol* 36:17, 1975
80. Kasper W, Meinertz T, Kersting F, Lang K, Just H: Diagnosis of dissecting aortic aneurysm with suprasternal echocardiography. *Am J Cardiol* 42:291, 1978
81. Krueger SK, Wilson CS, Weaver WF, Reese HE, Caudill CC, Rourke T: Aortic root dissection: Echocardiographic demonstration of torn internal flap. *JCU* 4:35, 1976
82. Millward DK, Robinson NJ, Craige E: Dissecting aortic aneurysm diagnosed by echocardiography in a patient with rupture of the aneurysm into the right atrium: Rare cause of continuous murmur. *Am J Cardiol* 30:427, 1972
83. Iliceto S, Antonelli G, Biasco G, Quagliara D, Rizzon P: Recognition of the descending aorta by apical two-dimensional echocardiography. In proceedings of the 4th European Congress on Ultrasound in Medicine, Dubrovnik, 1981
84. Rothbaum DA, Dillon JC, Chang S, Feigenbaum H: Echocardiographic manifestation of right sinus of Valsalva aneurysm. *Circulation* 49:768, 1974
85. Wong BYS, Bogart DB, Dunn MI: Echocardiographic features of an aneurysm of the left sinus of Valsalva. *Chest* 73:105, 1978
86. Engel PJ, Held JS, vander Bel-Kahn J, Spitz H: Echocardiographic diagnosis of congenital sinus of Valsalva aneurysm with dissection of the interventricular septum. *Circulation* 63:705, 1981
87. Schatz RA, Schiller NB, Tri TB, Bowen TE, Ports TA, Silverman NH: Two-dimensional echocardiographic diagnosis of a ruptured right sinus of Valsalva aneurysm. *Chest* 79:584, 1981

Infective endocarditis

The development of effective antibiotic therapy together with advances in cardiac surgery has dramatically improved the outlook of patients with infective endocarditis. Although there has been a decrease in mortality as a result, infections with resistant bacterial strains, fungi, and viruses have assumed greater importance [1]. Also, with the widespread use of antibiotics the duration and course of this disease have been so altered that the use of such terms as acute or subacute has become obsolete.

Clinical features. Although no single criterion for the diagnosis of infective endocarditis exists, there is always a high degree of suspicion when a patient who has had congenital heart disease or valvular disease has a fever and is "not doing well." Fever is the most common symptom; additional symptoms include fatigue, malaise, anorexia, headache, night sweats, arthralgias, abdominal pain, and tender fingers and toes. The presence of splenomegaly, hepatomegaly, petechiae, anemia, embolic phenomena, and changing heart murmurs will further support the diagnosis.

Although the fourth decade of life represents the most common age for infective endocarditis, other studies have shown that the disease has become increasingly common in the older age group; the absence of certain physical findings as well as the occasional absence of heart murmur, makes the diagnosis more difficult in the older age group [2–4]. Because of the effectiveness of antibiotic therapy, congestive heart failure secondary to valvular dysfunction has replaced septicemia as the leading cause of death from infective endocarditis. For that reason surgery is currently advocated for the treatment of life-threatening valvular dysfunction even in the face of active endocarditis [5, 6].

Richardson and associates [7] analyzed the medical and surgical treatment of active infective endocarditis in 182 patients over a ten-year period. These investigators noted that heart failure, annular and myocardial abscesses, heart block, and coronary embolism, seen most frequently with staphylococcal and fungal endocarditis, were primary causes of death in native valve endocarditis as well as in prosthetic valve endocarditis.

Ramsey and colleagues [8], in a review of the English literature on endocarditis in drug addicts, concluded that the valves of the left side of the heart are most frequently involved. However, Graham and associates [5] reported that the tricuspid valve is most commonly involved.

In spite of preventive measures, the risk of endocarditis in patients who have undergone prosthetic valve replacement remains significant. In a collaborative study from 26 major cardiovascular centers, Kaplan and associates [9] evaluated 278 patients with documented infective endocarditis and noted that 63 (23%) had had previous cardiovascular surgery and 215 had not. Seventy percent of the 278 patients in this large cooperative study had recognized congenital or acquired heart disease before developing the infection; furthermore, rheumatic heart disease accounted for more than half of the patients with underlying structural heart disease. Of the 63 patients who had been operated on before developing endocarditis, 55 percent had had prosthetic valves inserted. Open-heart surgery is the greatest single predisposing factor for the development of candidal endocarditis [10]. Once vegetations become established in these patients antifungal therapy alone is not sufficient; surgical removal in addition to antifungal therapy is mandatory.

The recognition of a vegetation on a valve leaflet confirms the presence of endocarditis, but the absence of any recognizable vegetation does not exclude the possibility of infective endocarditis. Although the value of echocardiography in detecting valvular vegetations was first described in 1973 [11], other studies have shown that the majority of patients with clinically proven bacterial endocarditis did not have evidence of vegetations on M-mode echocardiography [12].

Heart failure and major peripheral emboli are the most common indications for open heart surgery. However, the size and shape of the vegetation on two-dimensional echocardiography does not accurately predict the need for early valve replacement or the risk of systemic embolization [13, 14].

The management and prognosis of patients with infective endocarditis are significantly influenced by the presence or absence of valve ring abscess. Arnett and Roberts [15], in a study of 95 necropsy patients with active infective endocarditis, reported that ring abscess occurred in nearly one-third (27 of 95 patients), and although common in necropsy patients with active infective endocarditis involving the aortic valve, ring abscess was quite uncommon in patients with endocarditis isolated to any of the other three valves. No significant differences were observed among patients with or without ring abscess when comparing specific organisms. These authors described five clinical clues that suggest the presence of the ring abscess during life: (1) endocarditis involving the aortic valve, (2) presence of valvular regurgitation of recent origin, (3) evidence of pericarditis, (4) evidence of high-degree atrioventricular block, and (5) short duration of symptoms caused by the infective endocarditis resulting in severe debility.

Some investigators have reported that M-mode and two-dimensional echocardiography have a similar ability to detect actual valvular vegetations; however, two-dimensional echocardiography is superior to M-mode method in diagnosing complications of the destructive process [16]. In a study of 58 patients, Martin and associates [17] reported two-dimensional echocardiography to be distinctly superior to M-mode echo for detecting masses secondary to endocarditis. These investigators reported that technically adequate M-mode studies were obtained in 36 of the 43 patients with confirmed endocarditis; only 5 (14%) showed a mass, 12 (33%) showed a nonspecific abnormality, and 19 (53%) showed no mass. Adequate two-dimensional studies were available in 42 of the same 43 cases; 34 (81%) of these studies showed a mass, 7 (17%) had a nonspecific abnormality, and 1 study revealed no mass. Furthermore, these authors noted that two-dimensional studies were particularly helpful in patients with a mass on a prosthetic valve or on the tricuspid valve. Our experience is consistent with the latter group of investigators in that two-dimensional imaging is clearly more valuable in the identification of vegetation than M-mode technique, not only in the actively infected cases but also in judging decrease or increase in the size of the vegetation in serial follow-up studies.

Other noninvasive methods for detecting valvular vegetations in infective endocarditis have been employed besides echocardiography. Wiseman and colleagues [18] reported that 7 of 11 patients with clinical endocarditis had a positive gallium-67 cardiac scan although the specific heart valve was not identifiable. Melvin and associates [19], in a series of 35 documented consecutive episodes of infective endocarditis among 33 patients, studied each subject with M-mode and two-dimensional echocardiography, gallium-67 citrate, and technetium-99m stannous pyrophosphate cardiac scanning to determine the optimal noninvasive method for demonstration of vegetations. These investigators identified vegetations in 17 of 35 (49%) with M-mode echocardiography and in 28 of 35 (80%) with two-dimensional echocardiography; in striking contrast, only 2 (6%) gallium-67 citrate scans were positive and no vegetations were detected with technetium-99 stannous pyrophosphate scanning. These authors noted the superiority of the two-dimensional imaging technique over all other tests for recognizing valvular vegetations, particularly in identifying aortic and tricuspid vegetations.

ECHOCARDIOGRAPHIC FEATURES OF VEGETATIONS. Although careful imaging of all valves with two-dimensional echocardiography is very important in any patient thought to have infective endocarditis, a complementary M-mode recording taken at the time of the two-dimensional examination may be useful. All of the previously described tomographic views should be employed in order to obtain comprehensive imaging for all four valves. A valvular vegetation will have different reflective characteristics in a fresh vegetation and in an old healed one. In general, a fresh or active vegetation on a valve is a localized mass of soft reflectances of similar density to the leaflet's but having an irregular shape and not interfering with the overall motion of the leaflet. Very commonly a portion of the pedunculated vegetation hanging free from the leaflet evinces a conspicuous, chaotic motion apart from the motion of the leaflet itself.

When an M-mode beam directed through the vegetation produces evidence of increased thickness of the leaflet as well as some irregular or "shaggy" appearance on the M-mode recording, the views that portray the leaflet in profile or long axis plane rather than short axis are usually best for demonstrating leaflet vegetation.

The presence or absence of a valve vegetation is more difficult to ascertain when there is obvious preexisting valve disease or prosthetic valves. In rheumatic mitral stenosis and aortic stenosis very abnormal reflectances caused by the thickened, fibrotic, or calcified valve may obscure evidence of a small vegetation. In these situations the most valuable clue for evidence of superimposed vegetation is visualization of a sufficiently large mass or a pedunculated structure with the associated chaotic, flopping motion that characterizes a vegetation. Echoes generated by an old, healed vegetation may simulate calcification of the leaflet because of the dense, hard echoes on the surface of the leaflet.

The diagnosis of vegetations on prosthetic valves represents an even greater challenge. Careful attention must also be given to the annulus in the presence of native valve endocarditis as well as to the sewing ring of any prosthetic valve when infective endocarditis is a clinical consideration. Strom and associates [20] were able to identify a myocardial abscess in only one of five patients with two-dimensional echocardiography. In another study by Stewart and colleagues [21], two patients who had ring abscesses had no evidence of vegetation on 2-D echo. Although individual machines may vary in sensitivity, it is generally accepted that if a vegetation or small, noncalcified mass such as a polyp is larger than 2 to 3 mm in diameter, it should be visualized with two-dimensional echocardiography.

Aortic valve vegetations. Infection of the aortic valve commonly produces significant congestive heart failure or systemic emboli that necessitate valve re-

148 5. Infective endocarditis

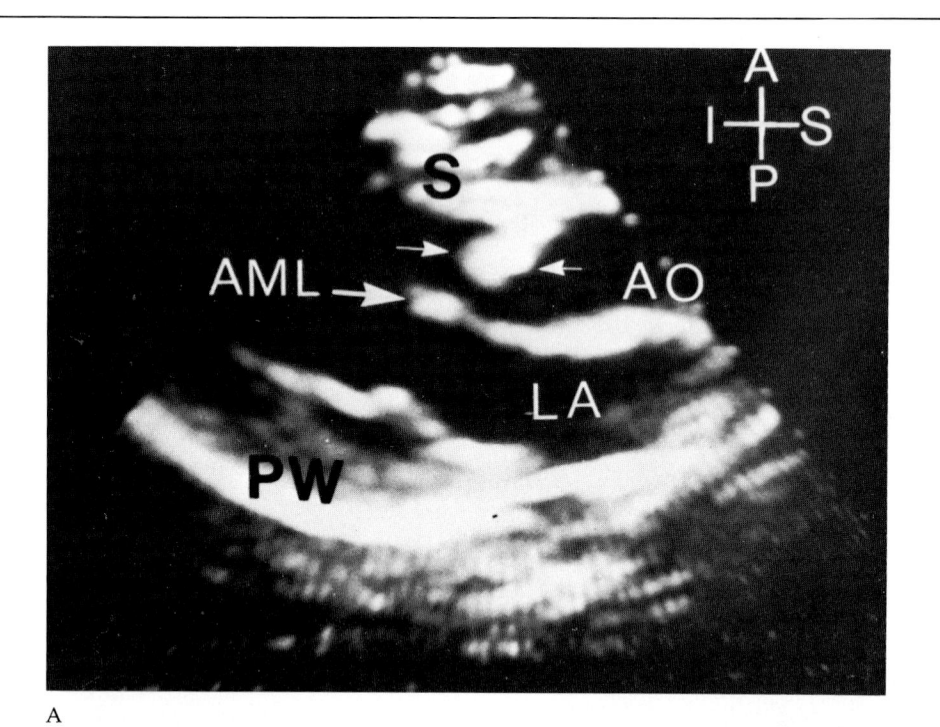

Fig. 5-1A. Parasternal long axis view of aortic vegetation (white arrows) prolapsing into the left ventricular outflow tract during diastole. B. Parasternal short axis view at the base in same patient showing a large vegetation (white arrow) confined to the right side of the aortic annulus suggesting involvement of both right and noncoronary cusps. C. Aortic valve and vegetation in same patient removed at the time of aortic valve replacement. The aortic valve is oriented in the same manner as in B and shows the reliability of 2-D echo localizing the mass lesion.

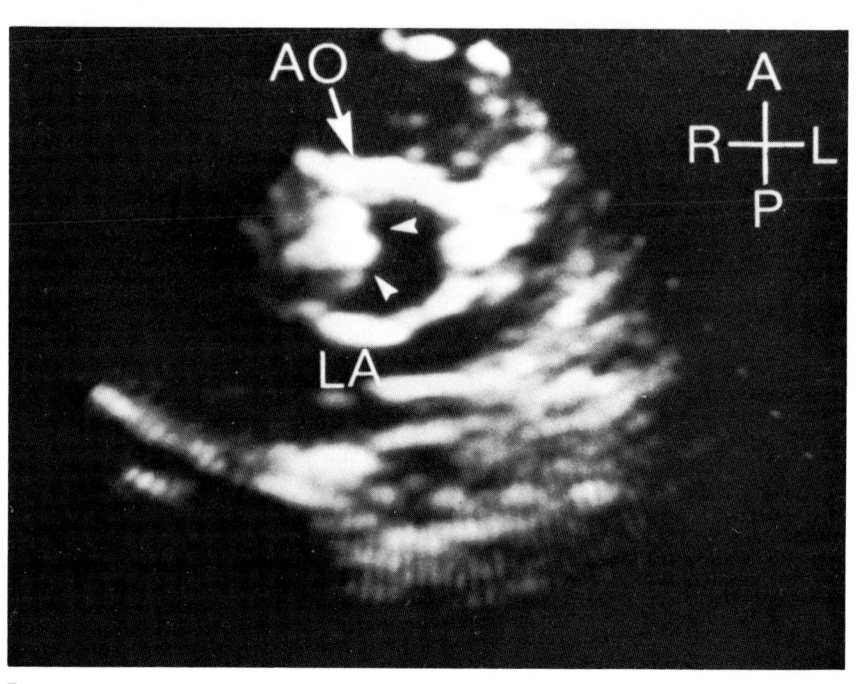

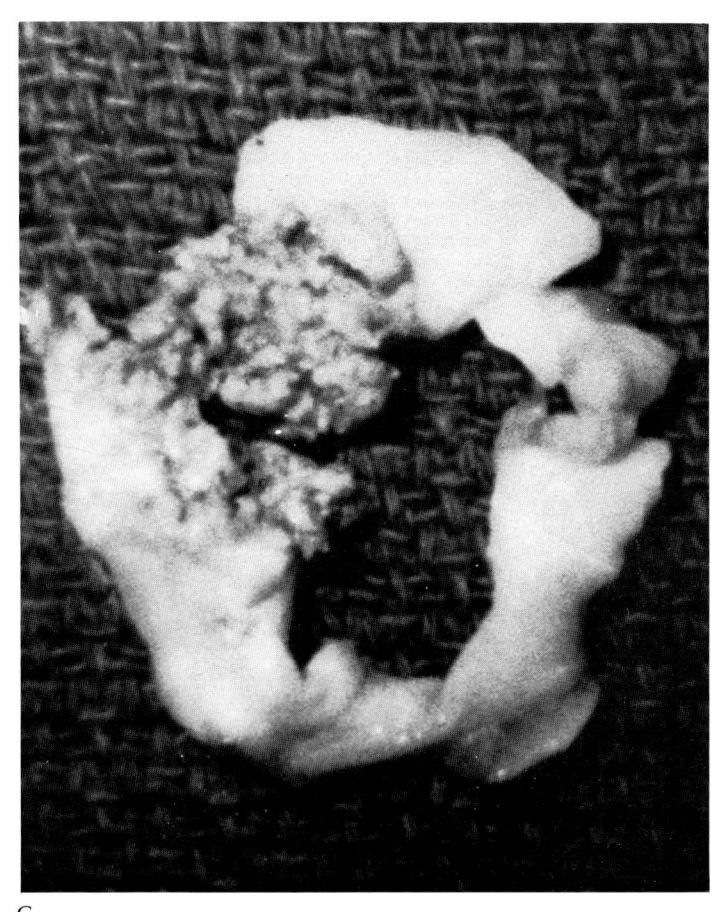

C

placement [22]. There is also a higher mortality in patients with infective endocarditis of the aortic valve when compared to either mitral or tricuspid valve involvement. Patients with demonstrated vegetations attached to the aortic valve have a higher incidence of congestive heart failure and requirement for aortic valve replacement compared to patients with the same diagnosis but no vegetations recognizable on the echocardiogram (Fig. 5-1). Of 46 patients with echocardiographic evidence of aortic valve vegetations reported by different investigators [12, 23–25], 40 (87%) underwent aortic valve replacement or died, whereas of 34 patients without evidence of aortic valve vegetation but with clinical documentation of active infective endocarditis only 4 (12%) underwent aortic valve replacement or died.

Berger and associates [26], in a study involving 14 patients with aortic valve endocarditis, observed three morphologic types of vegetation with two-dimensional echocardiography: global polypoid masses, irregular elongated lesions with chaotic movement, and a chordlike structure. In follow-up 2-D studies performed after completion of treatment in seven patients no change was observed in five, and complete disappearance occurred in two.

It is particularly important to select appropriate gain settings in order to avoid magnification or diminution of the actual size of the vegetations. In the Berger

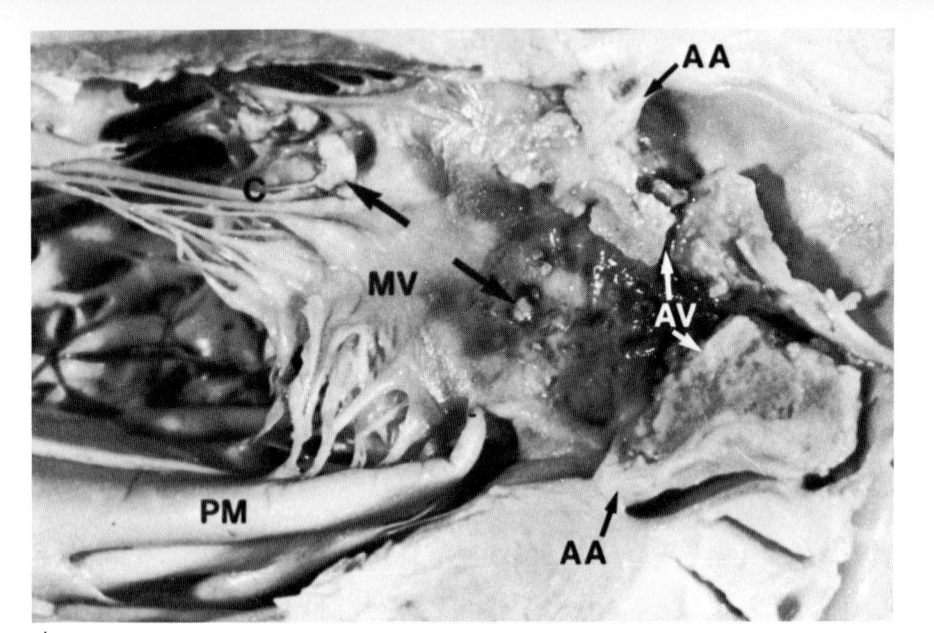

Fig. 5-2A. Autopsy specimen showing large fibrosed, calcified vegetation of the aortic valve, which was obstructive during life. Many smaller vegetations are attached to the mitral valve (black arrows). B. Noninfective thrombotic vegetations (arrows) secondary to carcinoma are attached to the aortic cusps in the region of the corpora arantii. C. Noninfective thrombotic vegetation caused by cancer, attached to the anterior mitral leaflet (arrow). AA = aortic annulus; C = chordae tendineae.

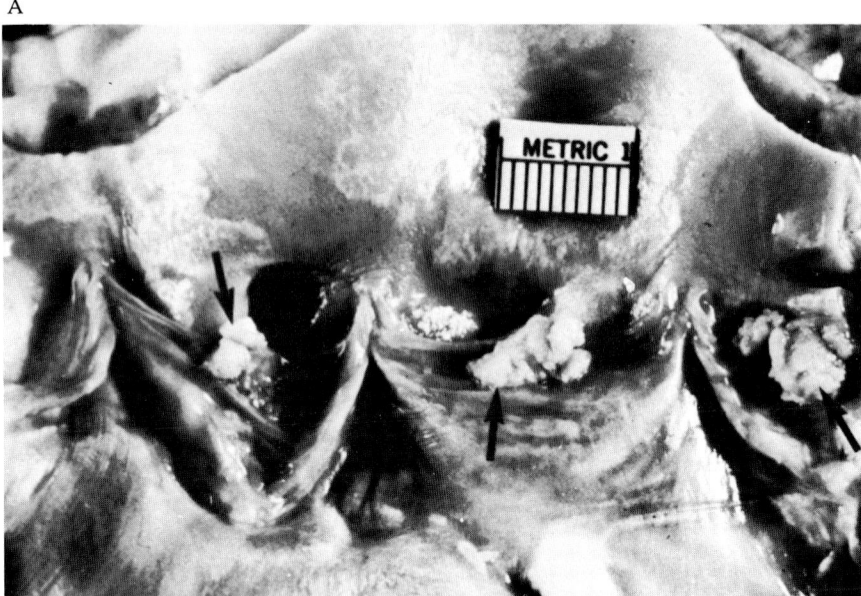

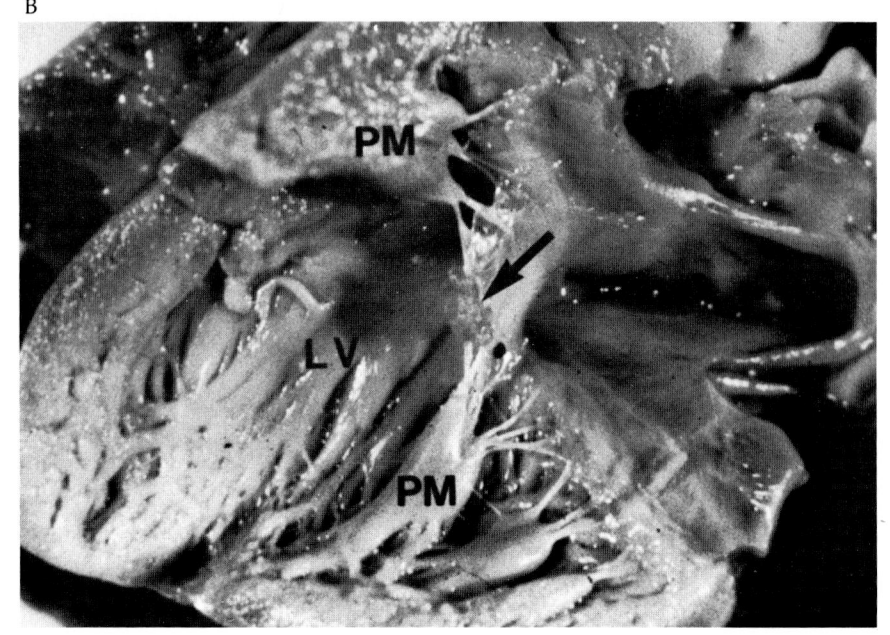

study [26] two-dimensional echocardiography failed to identify vegetations that measured less than 3 mm in diameter on pathological examination. The reflectances from calcification, fibrosis, or myxomatous degenerative changes of leaflets may obscure small underlying vegetations. The echocardiographic features of a ruptured aortic leaflet or flail leaflet may resemble a prolapsing leaflet with attached vegetation [27]. Although these ruptured aortic leaflets may simulate the shaggy echoes generated by a vegetation on M-mode recording, there is much less confusion with two-dimensional imaging.

Some of the vegetations may become very large with erosion and destruction of the aortic leaflets and may even become obstructive in the left ventricular outflow tract (Fig. 5-2A). Noninfective thrombotic vegetations secondary to cancer may be seen on the surface of valve leaflets (Fig. 5-2B, C). In contrast to the vegetations caused by infective endocarditis, these lesions do not cause significant destruction of the underlying leaflet tissue; however, there is risk of systemic embolization.

Pease and associates [28] reported the echocardiographic features in a patient with a large aortic valvular vegetation that contributed to lethal obstruction of the valve although no physical findings of aortic regurgitation had been heard. This patient had a systolic ejection murmur, became acutely hypotensive, and died within 12 hours of admission to the hospital. Postmortem examination disclosed a very large vegetation attached to the noncoronary cusp, which completely filled the aortic outflow tract and caused the lethal obstruction.

Mitral valve vegetations. Sheikh and associates [29] analyzed 99 M-mode echocardiograms in 27 patients during and in follow-up 144 months after healing of active infective endocarditis limited to the mitral valve and noted the following:

1. Little or no change occurred in the echocardiographic size of the vegetations during the first six weeks after institution of antibiotic therapy unless a major systemic embolus occurred.
2. The echocardiographic size of the vegetations did not determine the amount of cardiac damage or dysfunction from the valvular infection.
3. The larger the vegetations the greater was the likelihood of a clinical event compatible with the systemic embolus.
4. The gravest prognostic sign yielded by the echocardiogram was evidence of ruptured chordae tendineae.
5. Once bacteriologic cure was achieved the echocardiogram was of limited value in delineating an active from a healed vegetation.
6. The echocardiographic appearance of the vegetations was not determined by the type of infecting organism.

Mitral valve prolapse, with its added risk of infective endocarditis in affected valves, complicates the clinical recognition of a small vegetation attached to a mitral valve with underlying myxomatous degeneration (Fig. 5-3). Although no large study has been reported employing two-dimensional echocardiography to assess the reliability of detecting valvular vegetations in patients with mitral valve prolapse, Chandraratna and Langevin have shown that only M-mode echocardiography has significant limitations in distinguishing the increased thickness due to the prolapsed valve from similar echoes caused by a vegetation [30]. In a study of 85 patients with mitral valve prolapse, these investigators reported that 40 percent had "shaggy" echoes resembling those seen in valvular vegetations.

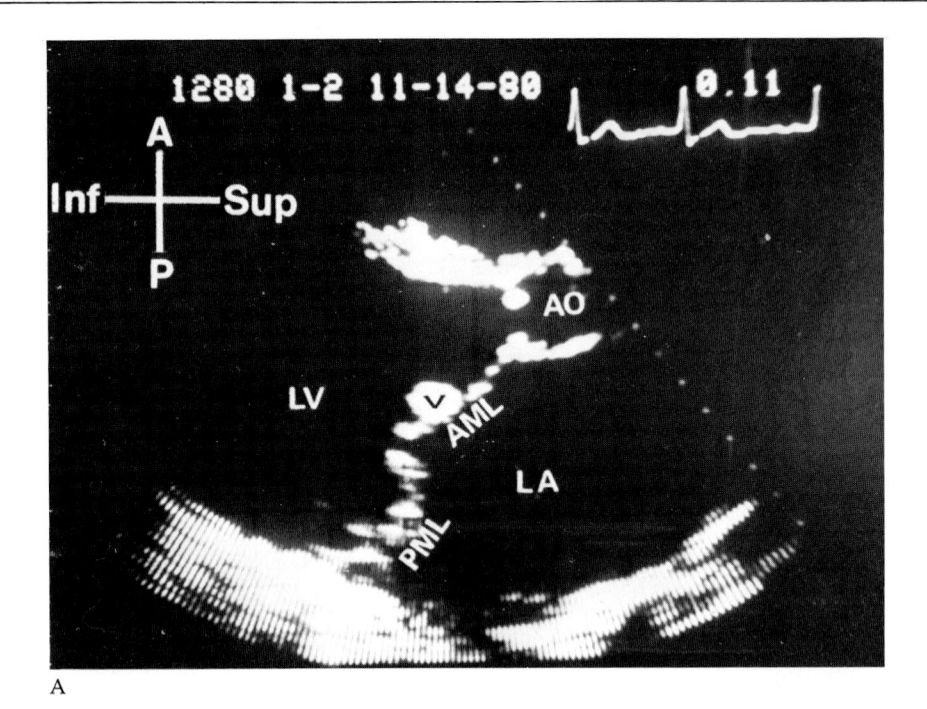

Fig. 5-3A. Parasternal long axis view in patient with prolapse of the posterior mitral leaflet, vegetation (V) attached to the anterior mitral leaflet, and left atrial enlargement due to mitral regurgitation. B. Apical 4-chamber view showing thickened mitral valve caused by myxomatous degeneration. It is very difficult to determine whether the prominent reflectance of the anterior mitral leaflet (white arrows) is due to the underlying valve disease or to a vegetation attached to the leaflet in the absence of any discrete mass or pedunculated structure giving a conspicuous motion. The right atrium is markedly enlarged.

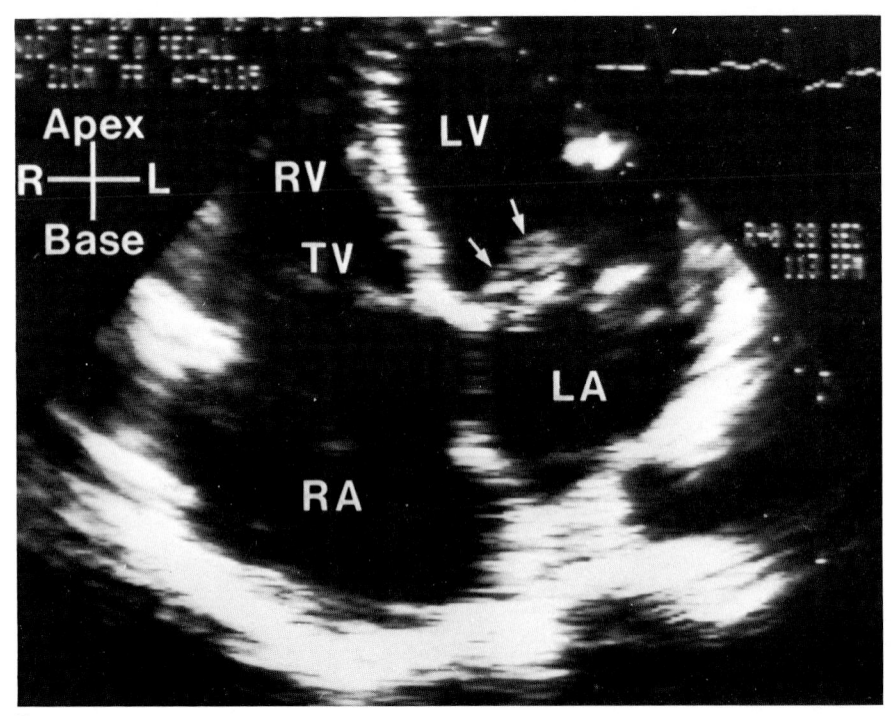

The known higher incidence of mitral annular calcification in the elderly suggests an underlying etiology for development of bacterial endocarditis; if there are some suggestive clinical findings in these patients the index of suspicion must be higher for the presence of infective endocarditis [31].

Large vegetations of the mitral valve have been reported to cause intermittent mitral valve obstruction with resultant pulmonary edema and have been confused with left atrial myxomas [32, 33] (Fig. 5-4A, B). The destructive process can be quite severe, with systemic embolization of leaflet fragments and vegetation that may cause sudden death (Fig. 5-4C).

Bacterial endocarditis in the neonatal period is rare and when present is often not diagnosed until after death [34]. We have seen two infants under the age of 1 year with infective endocarditis, a 9-month-old male with overwhelming *Salmonella* infection and vegetation of the anterior mitral leaflet as well as an additional lesion on the anterior wall of the left ventricular outflow tract. Another 1-year-old infant was diagnosed by 2-D echo as having a large vegetation of the tricuspid valve and embolization to the pulmonary artery, with resultant death secondary to catheter passage through the tricuspid valve at cardiac catheterization. Bender and associates [35] reported a case of a 3-week-old infant with acute staphylococcal endocarditis in which the diagnosis was made from the M-mode echocardiogram; the infant did not survive. At autopsy a large (1 cm) vegetation was found attached and eroding through the posterior mitral leaflet without underlying evidence of congenital heart disease.

Tricuspid valve vegetations. The ability to diagnose infective endocarditis affecting either the tricuspid or pulmonic valves has been significantly improved with the advent of two-dimensional echocardiography. M-mode echo recording of right heart structures in the absence of two-dimensional imaging is very inadequate. The incidence of right-sided infective endocarditis has increased significantly in recent years, particularly in persons with a history of intravenous drug abuse [36–38] (Fig. 5-5). Berger and associates [39], in a study of 12 narcotic addicts with right-sided infective endocarditis, were able to demonstrate vegetations in 10 patients (9 tricuspid and 1 pulmonic) with two-dimensional echocardiography; however, the M-mode echocardiogram was positive in only 6. Of the 10 patients with vegetations in this study, 7 had follow-up echocardiographic examinations after completion of therapy; the vegetation appeared unchanged in 3, diminished in size in 3, and was no longer visualized in 1. No patient required valve replacement. Both M-mode and two-dimensional echocardiographic features in right-sided endocarditis have been well described [39–44] (Figs. 5-6, 5-7).

Necropsy studies have demonstrated that vegetations on the tricuspid valve tend to be larger than those on other cardiac valves [44, 45]. The rupture of tricuspid valve chordae tendineae is uncommon, whereas mitral chordal rupture in infective endocarditis is frequent. It is not fully understood why vegetations tend to be larger on the tricuspid valve; however, the low incidence of chordal rupture on the tricuspid valve may delay development of significant tricuspid regurgitation and allow the right-sided vegetations to grow larger before significant dysfunction occurs [44] (Fig. 5-8). Tricuspid endocarditis often involves previously normal valves, another aspect of the disease that makes it distinctly different from endocarditis affecting either the aortic or mitral valves.

154   5. Infective endocarditis

Fig. 5-4A. Apical 4-chamber views in the same patient during diastole (left panel) *and systole* (right panel) *showing a large vegetation* (Veg) *attached to the posterior mitral leaflet at the junction of the mitral annulus. B. Parasternal long axis view showing a large vegetation* (v) *attached to the posterior mitral leaflet and annulus that is obstructive to flow through the mitral orifice. A second vegetation is attached to the chordae tendineae. C. Close-up view of vegetation* (arrows) *attached to the mitral valve with secondary erosion and destruction of the leaflet.* C = *chordae tendineae.*

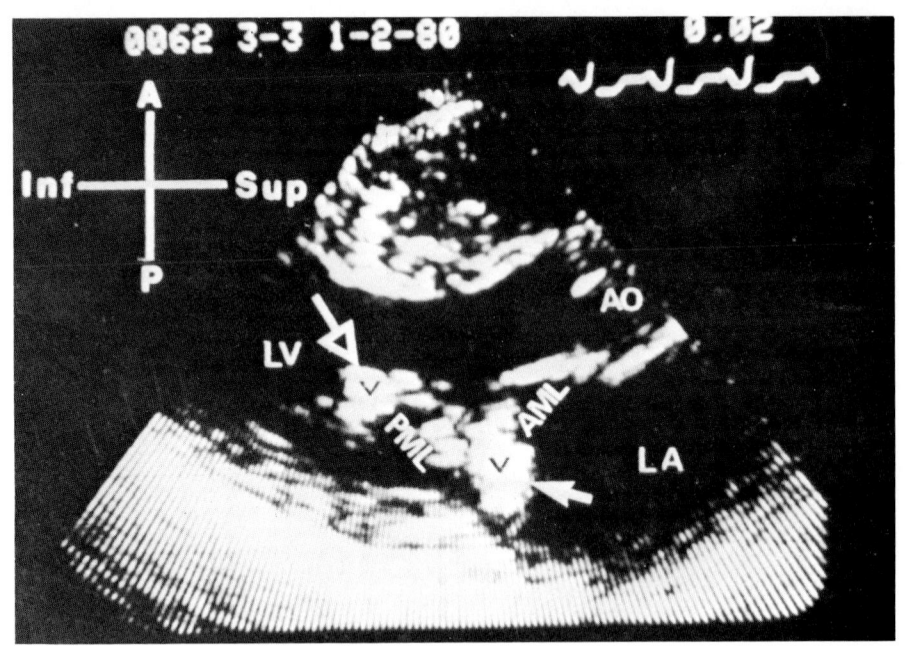

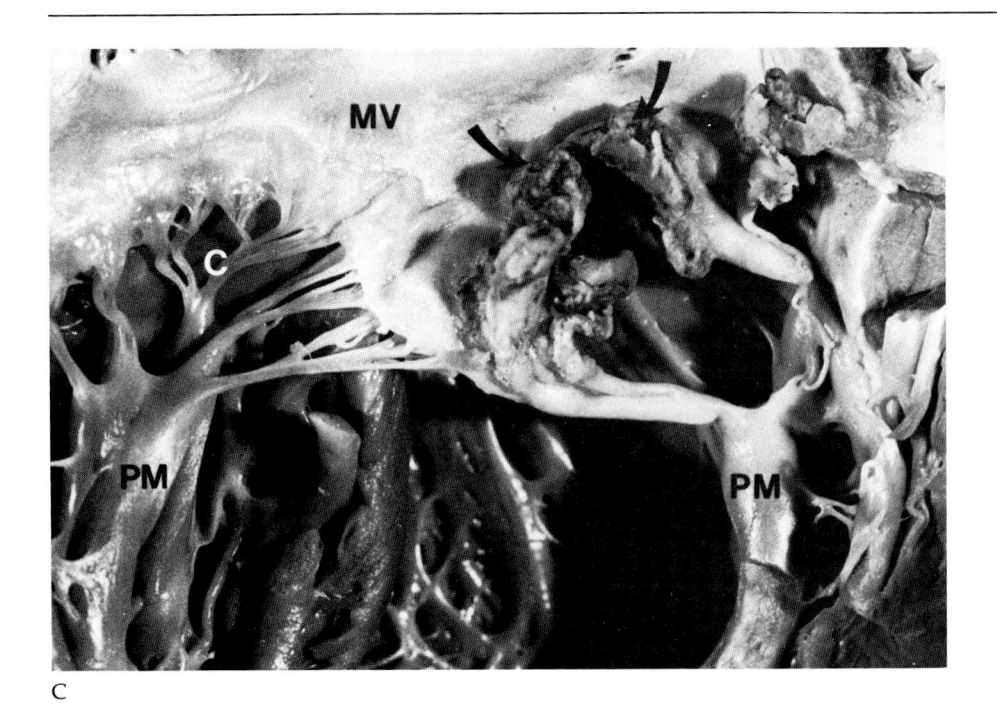

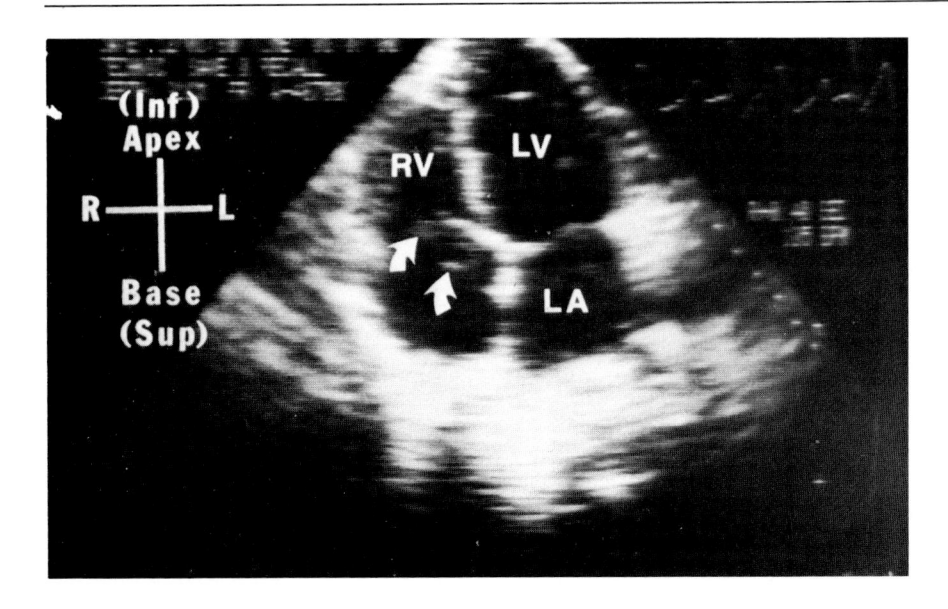

Fig. 5-5. Apical 4-chamber view of a young adult with drug abuse infective endocarditis showing vegetation (arrows) attached to the tricuspid valve. All chamber sizes are normal.

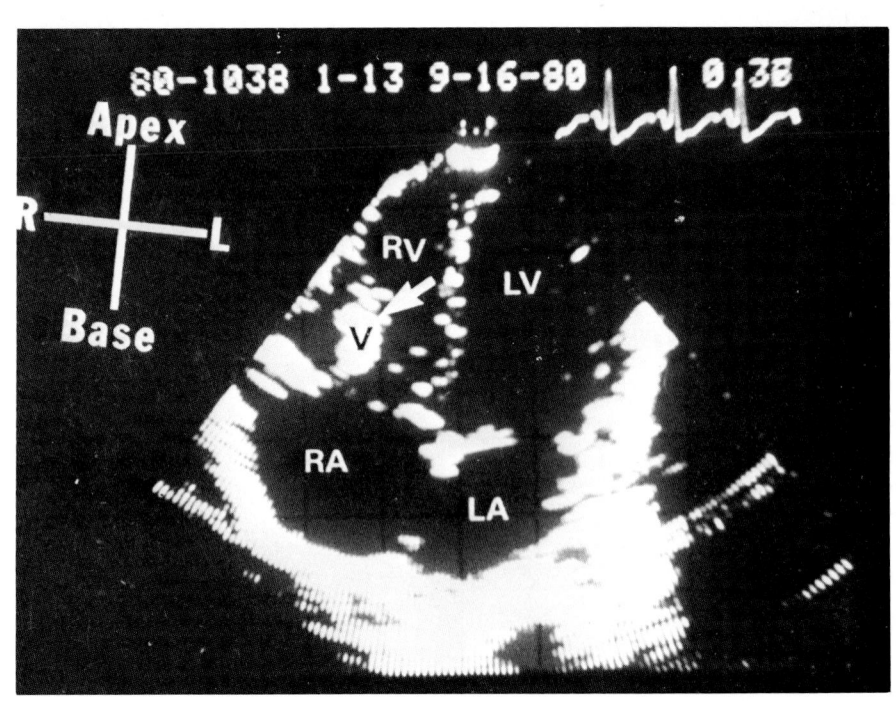

156   5. Infective endocarditis

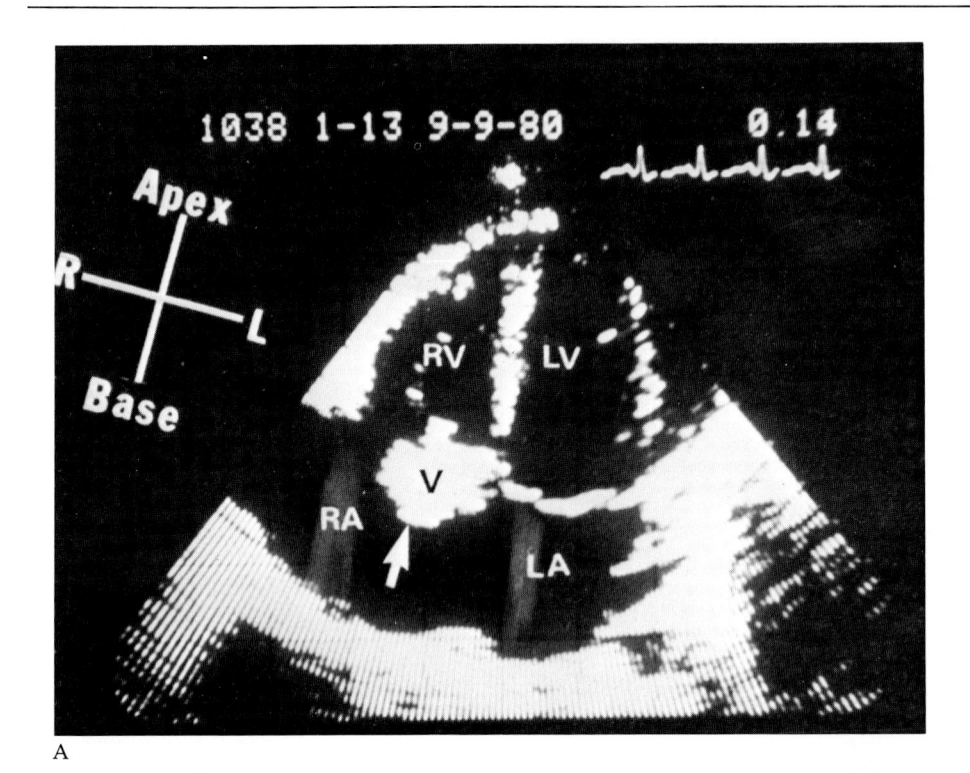

Fig. 5-6A. Apical 4-chamber view showing a large vegetation (V) of the tricuspid valve. B. Apical 4-chamber view in the same patient showing the vegetation in the right ventricle during diastole. Right atrial enlargement secondary to tricuspid regurgitation is present.

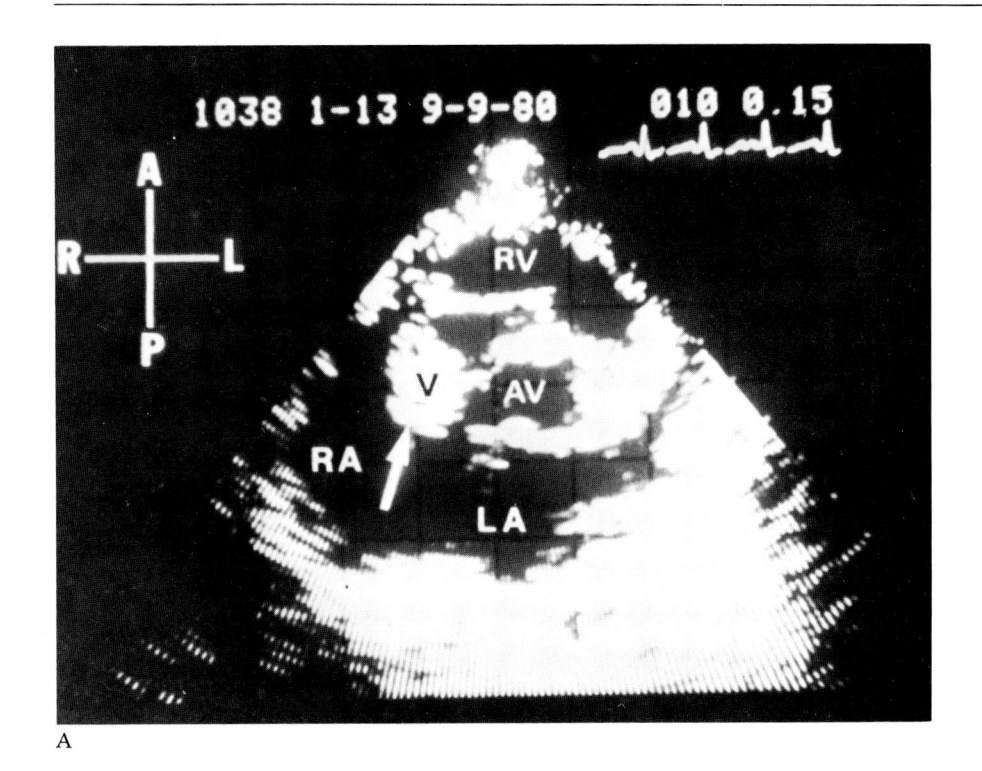

Fig. 5-7A. Parasternal short axis view at the base during systole with a large vegetation (V) of the tricuspid valve prolapsed into the right atrium. B. Parasternal short axis view at the base during diastole in the same patient showing the tricuspid valve vegetation within the right ventricle. The right atrium is enlarged.

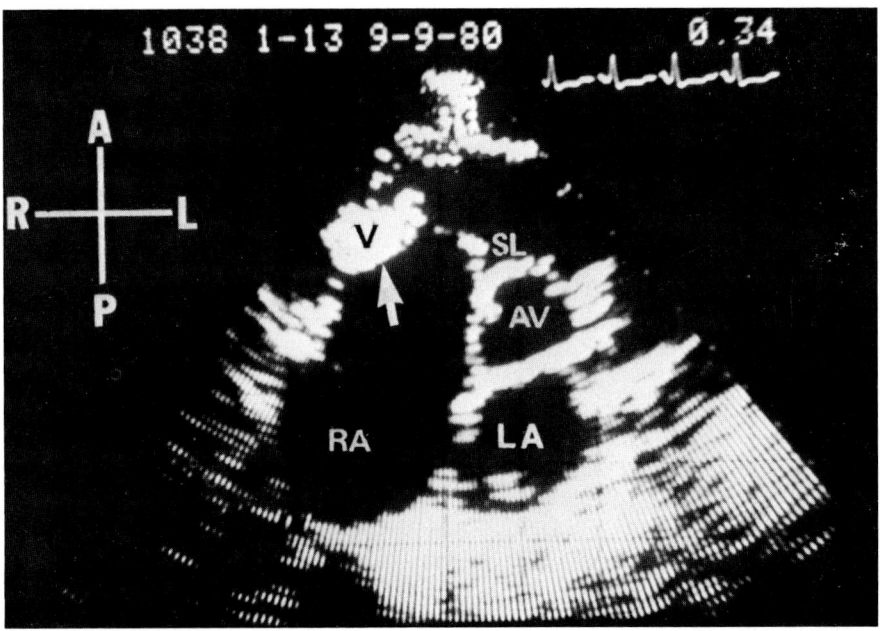

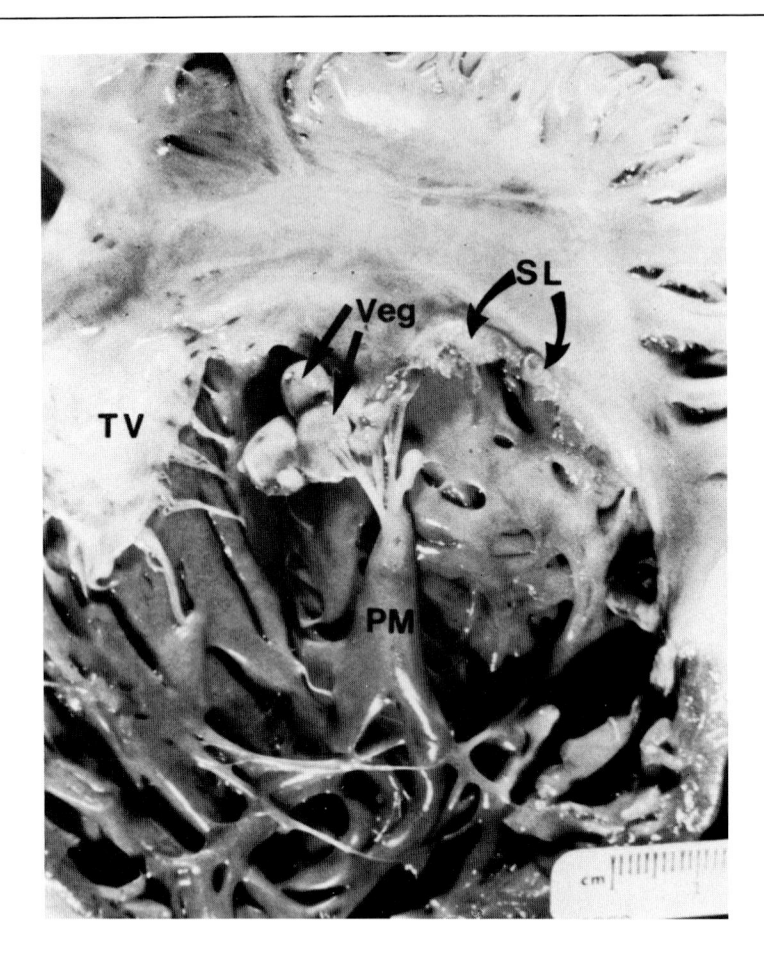

Fig. 5-8. Postmortem view of vegetations (Veg) of the tricuspid valve with nearly total destruction and absence of the septal leaflet.

The presence of tricuspid valve vegetation can interfere with leaflet motion causing delayed tricuspid valve closure, thus causing an abnormally wide and variable splitting of the first heart sound [46]. Combined phonocardiography and echocardiography is useful in determining the origin of wide-splitting first sound and may be helpful in evaluating other causes of abnormal systolic and diastolic sounds.

Pulmonic valve vegetations. The incidence of right-sided endocarditis has increased significantly in recent years, particularly among narcotic addicts. Although several studies have shown the increased frequency of tricuspid valve involvement, pulmonic valve involvement is still thought to be quite rare [36, 44, 47]. Kramer and colleagues [48] reported an unusual case of fatal recurring acute *Pseudomonas* endocarditis in a narcotic addict in whom pulmonic valve vegetations were detected by echocardiography. This patient was found at autopsy to have bulky vegetations on all four valves. Dzindzio and associates [43] reported an interesting clinical course in a 23-year-old male with isolated gonococcal pulmonary valvular endocarditis. In a classic paper on gonococcal endocarditis published in 1922, Thayer [49] reported a high frequency of right heart involvement. In his series

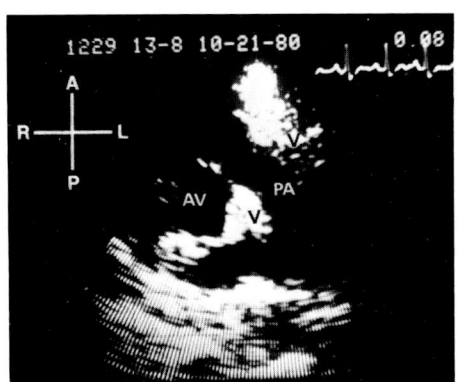

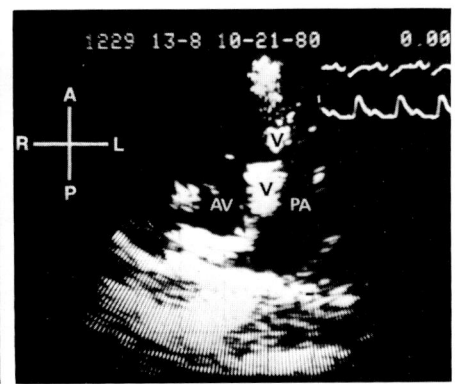

Fig. 5-9. Parasternal short axis views directed toward the pulmonary artery (PA) and pulmonic valve in systole (left panel) and in diastole (right panel) of a patient with vegetations (V) on both anterior and posterior leaflets of the pulmonic valve.

the pulmonic valve was involved in 25 percent of the cases of gonococcal endocarditis; the diagnosis of valvular involvement was made in each case by autopsy examination. Stone [50] reported 112 cases of gonococcal endocarditis and found pulmonic valve involvement in 18 cases (16%). It is obvious that gonococcal involvement of the pulmonic valve was common before the advent of penicillin; however, the incidence since then appears to have dropped markedly, and gonococcal endocarditis is now quite rare.

During a one-year experience (H.B.C.) at the Philippine Heart Center when 18 cases of infective endocarditis were diagnosed, six of these were right-sided vegetations, three tricuspid and three pulmonary. One of the patients with tricuspid endocarditis died from overwhelming *Klebsiella* infection; the other two responded well to antibiotic therapy but had negative blood cultures and none of the three was a narcotics addict. The three patients who had pulmonic valve vegetations all had isolated ventricular septal defects. A *Klebsiella* infection developed in one of these patients two months following patch closure of the ventricular septal defect and vegetation was present on the posterior leaflet of the pulmonic valve. One patient had a staphylococcal endocarditis and the third patient had negative blood cultures. Large vegetations were present on both anterior and posterior pulmonary leaflets (Fig. 5-9).

Right-sided endocarditis secondary to instrumentation or pacemaker implantation is quite rare [51–53]. Pace and colleagues [54] have reported that Swan-Ganz catheterization increases the incidence of aseptic thrombotic endocarditis. The first case of septic endocarditis secondary to a pulmonary artery catheter was reported by Greene and associates [55]. Ehrie and coworkers [51] reported six consecutive burn patients who died with septic or aseptic endocarditis after being monitored with an indwelling pulmonary artery catheter. In two of those six patients right-sided staphylococcal endocarditis was the anatomic cause of death; in the remaining four the lesions were aseptic, thrombotic vegetations involving primarily the right atrium, tricuspid valve, right ventricle, and pulmonic valve.

References

1. Thapar MK, Rao PS, Feldman D, Linde LM: Infective endocarditis: A review. I. Incidence, etiology, pathology and clinical features. *Paediatrician* 7:65, 1978
2. Anderson HJ, Staffurth JS: Subacute bacterial endocarditis in the elderly. *Lancet* 2:1055, 1955
3. Weinstein L, Rubin RH: Infective endocarditis—1973. *Prog Cardiovasc Dis* 16:239, 1973
4. Thell R, Martin FH, Edwards JE: Bacterial endocarditis in subjects 60 years of age and older. *Circulation* 51:174, 1975
5. Graham DY, Reul GJ, Martin R, Morton J, Kennedy JH: Infective endocarditis in drug addicts: Experiences with medical and surgical treatment. *Circulation* 47(Suppl III):III-37, 1973
6. Crosby IK, Carrell R, Reed WA: Operative management of valvular complications of bacterial endocarditis. *J Thorac Cardiovasc Surg* 64:235, 1972
7. Richardson JV, Karp RB, Kirklin JW, Dismukes WE: Treatment of infective endocarditis: A 10-year comparative analysis. *Circulation* 58:589, 1978
8. Ramsey RG, Gunnar RM, Tobin JR: Endocarditis in the drug addict. *Am J Cardiol* 25:608, 1970
9. Kaplan EL, Rich H, Gersony W, Manning J: A collaborative study of infective endocarditis in the 1970s: Emphasis on infections in patients who have undergone cardiovascular surgery. *Circulation* 59:327, 1979
10. Seelig MS, Speth CP, Kozinn PJ, Taschdjian CL, Toni EF, Goldberg P: Patterns of *Candida* endocarditis following cardiac surgery: Importance of early diagnosis and therapy (an analysis of 91 cases). *Prog Cardiovasc Dis* 17:125, 1974
11. Dillon JC, Feigenbaum H, Konecke LL, Davis RH, Chang S: Echocardiographic manifestations of valvular vegetations. *Am Heart J* 86:698, 1973
12. Wann LS, Dillon JC, Weyman AE, Feigenbaum H: Echocardiography in bacterial endocarditis. *N Engl J Med* 295:135, 1976
13. Wann LS, Hallam CC, Dillon JC, Weyman AE, Feigenbaum H: Comparison of M-mode and cross-sectional echocardiography in infective endocarditis. *Circulation* 60:728, 1979
14. Seward J: Personal communication, 1981
15. Arnett EN, Roberts WC: Valve ring abscess in active infective endocarditis: Frequency, location, and clues to clinical diagnosis from the study of 95 necropsy patients. *Circulation* 54:140, 1976
16. Mintz GS, Kotler MN, Segal BL, Parry WR: Comparison of two-dimensional and M-mode echocardiography in the evaluation of patients with infective endocarditis. *Am J Cardiol* 43:738, 1979
17. Martin RP, Meltzer RS, Chia BL, Stinson EB, Rakowski H, Popp RL: Clinical utility of two dimensional echocardiography in infective endocarditis. *Am J Cardiol* 46:379, 1980
18. Wiseman J, Rouleau J, Rigo P, Strauss HW, Pitt B: Gallium-67 myocardial imaging for the detection of bacterial endocarditis. *Radiology* 120:135, 1976
19. Melvin ET, Berger M, Lutzker LG, Goldberg E, Mildvan D: Noninvasive methods for detection of valve vegetations in infective endocarditis. *Am J Cardiol* 47:271, 1981
20. Strom J, Becker R, Davis R, Matsumoto M, Frishman W, Sonnenblick EH, Frater RW: Echocardiographic and surgical correlations in bacterial endocarditis. *Circulation* 62(Suppl I)I-164, 1980
21. Stewart JA, Silimperi D, Harris P, Wise NK, Fraker TD, Kisslo JA: Echocardiographic documentation of vegetative lesions in infective endocarditis: Clinical implications. *Circulation* 61:374, 1980
22. Sheikh MU, Covarrubias EA, Ali N, Sheikh NM, Lee WR, Roberts WC: M-mode echocardiographic observations in active bacterial endocarditis limited to the aortic valve. *Am Heart J* 102:66, 1981
23. Roy P, Tajik AJ, Giuliani ER, Schattenberg TT, Gau GT, Frye RL: Spectrum of echocardiographic findings in bacterial endocarditis. *Circulation* 53:474, 1976
24. Mintz GS, Kotler MN, Segal BL, Parry WR: Survival of patients with aortic valve endocarditis: The prognostic implications of the echocardiogram. *Arch Intern Med* 139:862, 1979
25. Pratt C, Whitcomb C, Neumann A, Mason DT, Amsterdam EA, DeMaria AN: Relationship of vegetations on echogram to the clinical course and systemic emboli in bacterial endocarditis. *Am J Cardiol* 41:384, 1978

26. Berger M, Gallerstein PE, Benhuri P, Balla R, Goldberg E: Evaluation of aortic valve endocarditis by two-dimensional echocardiography. *Chest* 80:61, 1981
27. Das G, Lee CC, Weissler AM: Echocardiographic manifestations of ruptured aortic valvular leaflets in the absence of valvular vegetations. *Chest* 72:464, 1977
28. Pease HF, Matsumoto S, Cacchione RJ, Richards KL, Leach JK: Lethal obstruction of aortic valvular vegetation: Echocardiographic studies of endocarditis without apparent aortic regurgitation. *Chest* 73:658, 1978
29. Sheikh MU, Covarrubias EA, Ali N, Lee WR, Sheikh NM, Roberts WC: M-mode echocardiographic observations during and after healing of active bacterial endocarditis limited to the mitral valve. *Am Heart J* 101:37, 1981
30. Chandraratna PAN, Langevin E: Limitations of the echocardiogram in diagnosing valvular vegetations in patients with mitral valve prolapse. *Circulation* 56:436, 1977
31. Mambo NC, Silver MD, Brunsdon DF: Bacterial endocarditis of the mitral valve associated with annular calcification. *Can Med Assoc J* 119:323, 1978
32. Prasquier R, Gibert C, Witchitz S, Valere P, Beaufils P, Vachon F: Acute mitral valve obstruction during infective endocarditis. *Br Med J* 1:9, 1978
33. Pasternak RC, Cannom DS, Cohen LS: Echocardiographic diagnosis of large fungal verruca attached to mitral valve. *Br Heart J* 38:1209, 1976
34. Johnson DH, Rosenthal A, Nadas AS: Bacterial endocarditis in children under two years of age. *Am J Dis Child* 129:183, 1975
35. Bender RL, Jaffe RB, McCarthy D, Ruttenberg HD: Echocardiographic diagnosis of bacterial endocarditis of the mitral valve in a neonate. *Am J Dis Child* 131:746, 1977
36. Cherubin CE, Baden M, Kavaler F, Lerner S, Kline W: Infective endocarditis in narcotic addicts. *Ann Intern Med* 69:1091, 1968
37. Roberts WC, Buchbinder NA: Right-sided valvular infective endocarditis: A clinicopathologic study of twelve necropsy patients. *Am J Med* 53:7, 1972
38. El-Khatib MR, Wilson FM, Lerner AM: Characteristics of bacterial endocarditis in heroin addicts in Detroit. *Am J Med Sci* 271:197, 1976
39. Berger M, Delfin LA, Jelveh M, Goldberg E: Two-dimensional echocardiographic findings in right-sided infective endocarditis. *Circulation* 61:855, 1980
40. Kisslo J, VonRamm OT, Haney R, Jones R, Juk SS, Behar VS: Echocardiographic evaluation of tricuspid valve endocarditis. An M-mode and two-dimensional study. *Am J Cardiol* 38:502, 1976
41. Crawford FA, Wechsler AS, Kisslo JA: Tricuspid endocarditis in a drug addict: Detection of tricuspid vegetations by two-dimensional echocardiography. *Chest* 74:473, 1978
42. Sheikh MU, Ali N, Covarrubias E, Fox LM, Morjaria M, Dejo J: Right-sided infective endocarditis: An echocardiographic study. *Am J Med* 66:283, 1979
43. Dzindzio BS, Meyer L, Osterholm R, Hopeman A, Woltjen J, Forker AD: Isolated gonococcal pulmonary valve endocarditis: Diagnosis by echocardiography. *Circulation* 59:1319, 1979
44. Andy JJ, Sheikh MU, Ali N, Barnes BO, Fox LM, Carry CL, Roberts WC: Echocardiographic observations in opiate addicts with active infective endocarditis: Frequency of involvement of the various valves and comparison of echocardiographic features of right- and left-sided cardiac valve endocarditis. *Am J Cardiol* 40:17, 1977
45. Arnett EN, Roberts WC: Active infective endocarditis: A clinicopathologic analysis of 137 necropsy patients. *Curr Probl Cardiol* 1:2, 1976
46. Mintz GS, Kotler MN, Parry WR: Wide splitting of the first heart sound secondary to tricuspid valve endocarditis: A phonocardiographic-echocardiographic study. *Am J Med* 66:523, 1979
47. Conway N: Endocarditis in heroin addicts. *Br Heart J* 31:543, 1969
48. Kramer NE, Gill SS, Patel R, Towne WD: Pulmonary valve vegetations detected with echocardiography. *Am J Cardiol* 39:1064, 1977
49. Thayer WS: On the cardiac complications of gonorrhea. *Johns Hopkins Hospital Bull* 33:361, 1922
50. Stone E: Gonorrheal endocarditis. *J Urol* 31:869, 1934
51. Ehrie M, Morgan AP, Moore FD, O'Connor NE: Endocarditis with the indwelling balloon-tipped pulmonary artery catheter in burn patients. *J Trauma* 18:664, 1978
52. Ward C, Naik DR, Johnstone MC: Tricuspid endocarditis complicating pacemaker implantation demonstrated by echocardiography. *Br J Radiol* 52:501, 1979

53. Chan W, Ikram H: Echocardiographic demonstration of tricuspid valvulitis and right atrial thrombus complicating an infected artificial pacemaker: A case report. *Angiology* 29(7):559, 1978
54. Pace NL, Horton W: Indwelling pulmonary artery catheters: Their relationship to aseptic thrombotic endocardial vegetations. *JAMA* 233:893, 1975
55. Greene JF, Fitzwater JE, Clemmer TP: Septic endocarditis and indwelling pulmonary artery catheters. *JAMA* 233:891, 1975

Coronary artery disease

An enormous number of clinical applications of echocardiography for patients with coronary artery disease have been described in the literature. Initially M-mode echocardiography was used to identify segmental wall motion abnormality indicative of ischemic heart disease. However, the method had significant limitations because M-mode technique did not lend itself to complete visualization of the ventricle, thus restricting functional assessment of the left ventricle [1–8]. Although techniques employing multiple intercostal positions over the left precordium to identify myocardial scarring and segmental wall motion abnormalities have produced reasonably accurate results [1, 9, 10], the technical difficulties encountered in satisfactory imaging of many patients with coronary disease from these positions, and hence the unreliability of obtaining complete evaluation of wall motion abnormalities or function, have held back clinical acceptance of this diagnostic method.

One of the most significant clinical applications of two-dimensional echocardiography has been in patients with coronary artery disease. The use of two-dimensional imaging for estimation of ventricular volume and detection of wall motion abnormalities has been very promising. It is limited by compromised image quality or incomplete imaging of all segments of the left ventricle in some patients with ischemic heart disease [11], but because it supplies cross-sectional information about the ventricular chamber and wall thickness simultaneously, this technique lends itself to the anatomic localization of changes in regional performance that accompany ischemic heart disease. It permits simultaneous evaluation of regional dynamic changes in left ventricular circumference, wall thickness, and motion characteristics that give practical information in patients with chronic ischemic disease or acute myocardial infarction.

Clinical indications. The clinical indications for performing two-dimensional echocardiography in patients with known or suspected coronary artery disease can be summarized in three categories: chest pain evaluation, determination of left ventricular performance or evaluation of heart failure, and evaluation of acute myocardial infarction, associated complications, and changes of chronic ischemic heart disease.

The evaluation of patients with chest pain should be done in the context of routine outpatient clinical assessment as opposed to inpatient evaluation in the setting of an acute intensive care or coronary care setting. Chest pain should be categorized as that which is atypical and very unlikely to be due to coronary artery disease, and that which is typically ischemic in etiology (usually determined by history).

In patients with atypical pain two-dimensional echocardiography is primarily justified when the history, physical findings, or other studies suggest the possibility that the discomfort is being caused by pericardial disease, cardiomyopathies, or mitral valve prolapse. All these conditions cause various types of chest pain that may be confused with coronary artery disease or may be found in conjunction with coronary disease. The specific anatomic and functional abnormalities associated with these conditions make two-dimensional echocardiography an ideal diagnostic tool. For example, it is often very difficult to diagnose constrictive pericarditis before the disease has advanced to a significant stage; with echocardiography it is

164   6. Coronary artery disease

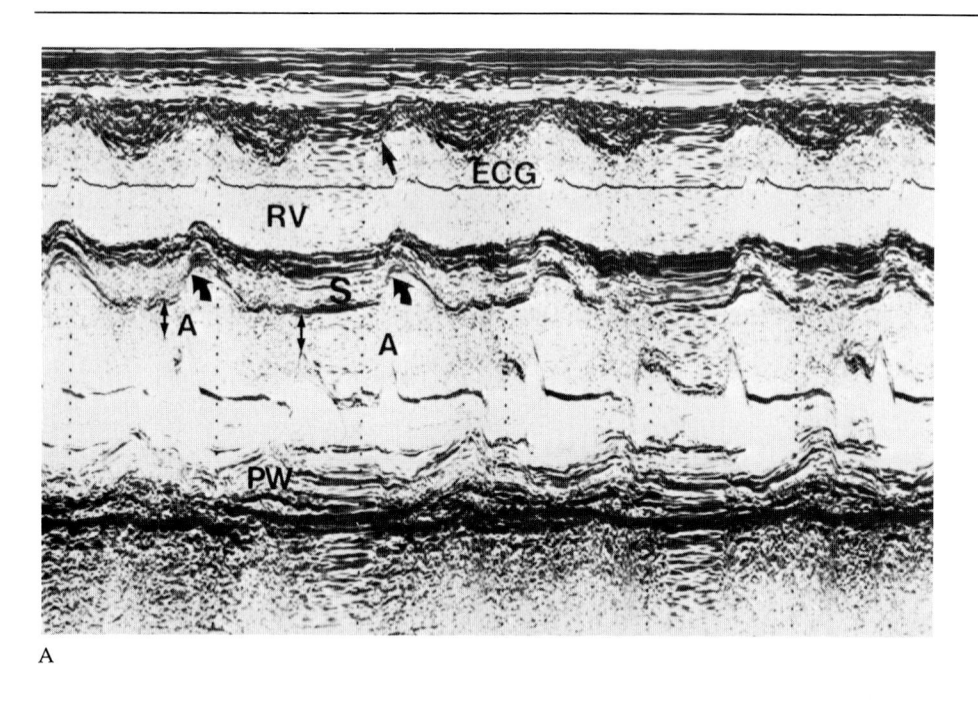

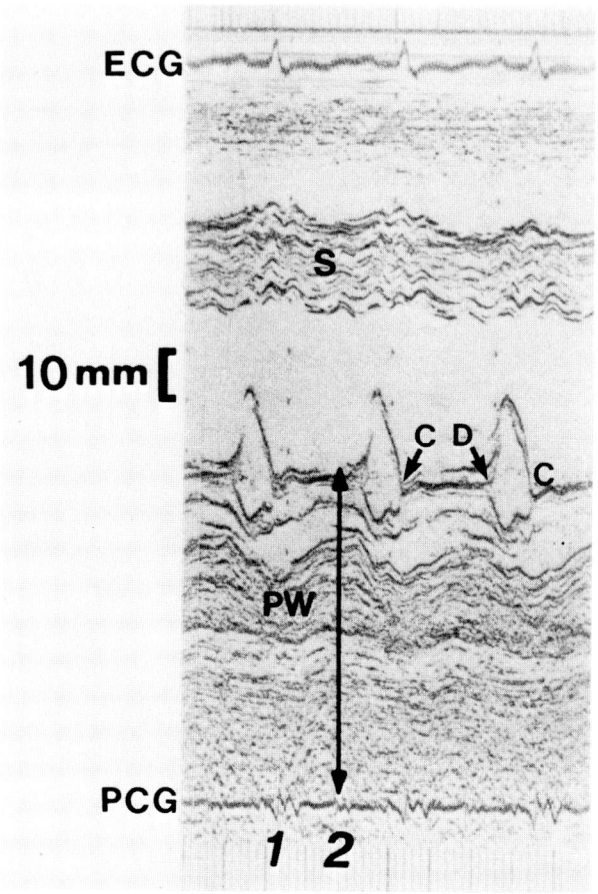

Fig. 6-1A. M-mode recording of left ventricle in patient with normal percent fractional shortening and borderline E point-septal separation (double-headed arrows) of 10 mm. There is abnormal diastolic filling due to reduced compliance and no significant increase in left ventricular dimension during diastole until atrial contraction. Large "A" waves (curved arrows) are present in septal (S) motion. Right ventricular wall thickness (arrow) is increased. B. M-mode recording obtained from an adult with long-standing systemic hypertension, left ventricular hypertrophy, left ventricular failure, and marked delay in opening of the mitral valve. Delayed mitral opening with resultant shortening of diastolic filling period further compromises overall left ventricular performance. S_2-mitral opening interval can be seen following the long arrow marking the second heart sound. Mitral closure (C) is normal. The mitral valve is closed twice as long as the valve is open. First (1) and second (2) heart sounds can be seen on the accompanying phonocardiogram. C. M-mode recording of aortic valve and left atrium in a normal subject (left panel) and in a patient with left ventricular hypertrophy and reduced compliance with slowed rate of diastolic filling (right panel). The rate of left atrial emptying is reflected by the slope of the posterior aortic root in early diastole (curved arrows); that slope is quite flat in the right panel showing that LA emptying, hence left ventricular filling, are both reduced and little change in LA size occurs until atrial contraction (straight arrows). A = mitral valve "A" wave; D = point of mitral valve opening.

C

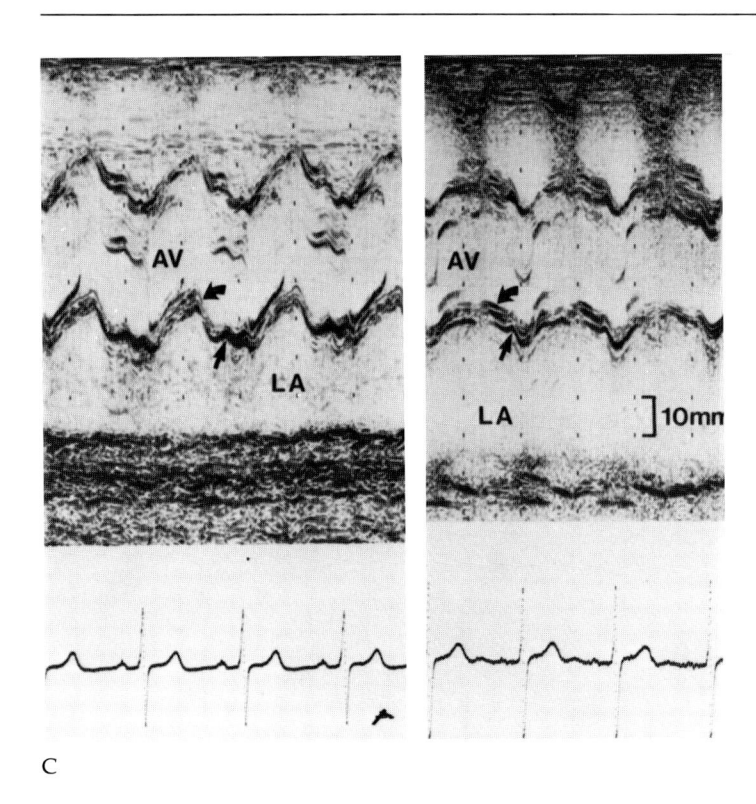

not uncommon to find an otherwise clinically unsuspected pericardial effusion. In another example, hypertrophic forms of cardiomyopathy as well as early forms of congestive cardiomyopathies and infiltrative cardiomyopathies may have no abnormal physical findings and might go unrecognized if two-dimensional echocardiography is not performed. Mitral valve prolapse in patients who have atypical chest pain in the absence of physical findings indicative of the disease is occasionally found with the aid of 2-D echo.

Patients with a history of typical ischemic chest pain in the absence of previous myocardial infarction can be expected to have a normal resting echocardiographic examination. However, we have encountered occasional patients with no history of an infarction or evidence of an infarction on a resting electrocardiogram who have segmental wall motion abnormalities on the two-dimensional echo study indicating the presence of coronary artery disease. More commonly, however, the resting 2-D echo study will be negative in such patients and is usually not clinically helpful unless it is performed in conjunction with exercise or some intervention that will induce wall motion abnormalities. Although there are some technical difficulties associated with performing exercise echocardiography and satisfactory studies cannot be obtained in all patients, this type of interventional echocardiography appears to be a sensitive method of detecting wall motion abnormalities during exercise-induced ischemia and may be applicable in patients in whom exercise electrocardiography is equivocal or in whom the functional significance of a coronary arterial lesion is uncertain [12–18].

Bishop and associates [19] have recently reported the clinical usefulness of echocardiography in the detection or exclusion of acute myocardial infarction in patients admitted to the coronary care unit. Additional investigative data are needed in this area to determine whether it is cost-effective to obtain two-dimensional echocardiograms at the time of admission in order to identify certain patients not having ischemic pain with a view to their earlier discharge from the coronary care unit. Furthermore, it is not yet established whether certain anatomic or functional information obtainable by 2-D echo during the first 24 hours of acute infarction can or should influence treatment or prognosis. Gibson and associates [20] have reported the value of early two-dimensional echocardiography in patients with acute myocardial infarction in order to predict those patients who will have hemodynamic deterioration and later complications.

The determination of left ventricular function as well as better quantitative definition in those patients with known heart failure who have coronary artery disease is another important application of two-dimensional echocardiography. When there is a question about left ventricular performance it is necessary to determine systolic function as well as diastolic filling characteristics. The diastolic filling pattern can be best evaluated by M-mode echocardiography, which provides clinically useful information about the diastolic motion of the left ventricle, mitral valve, and aortic root (an index of left atrial emptying). This pattern is clinically important because some patients may have abnormal diastolic filling in the absence of significant systolic dysfunction (Fig. 6-1A). Other patients with heart failure may have reduced systolic function further compromised because of poor diastolic filling or a noncompliant left ventricle (Fig. 6-1B, C).

The systolic function or left ventricular ejection phase indices are divided into two categories (see Chapter 7) [21–25]:

1. Global indices
   a. Volume dependent (ejection fraction, stroke volume)
   b. Circumferential (mean circumferential fiber shortening rate, percent fractional shortening)
   c. E point septal separation, wall motion index
2. Segmental indices
   a. Quantitative (percent wall thickening, normalized velocity of septum or posterior wall)
   b. Qualitative (hypokinesis, akinesis, dyskinesis)

The third important area of clinical usefulness of 2-D echocardiography consists of evaluating patients with acute myocardial infarction. The estimates of infarct size, presence of mural thrombi, and quantitative left ventricular function indices may or may not have clinical significance in the treatment of patients during their early hospitalization if the patient's course is progressing in an uncomplicated fashion. However, there may be value in obtaining two-dimensional echo studies in conjunction with submaximal exercise testing and ambulatory arrhythmia monitoring in these patients at the time of discharge in an effort to identify ischemic zones remote from the infarction and to quantitate infarct size. Although still somewhat speculative, there is evidence that two-dimensional echocardiography can be employed to estimate infarct size, a factor with well-known prognostic significance in identifying patients at high risk for future life-threatening events [26–31].

The principal reason for performing two-dimensional echocardiography in pa-

Wall motion analysis

Basal (level of MV tips & chordae)
Middle (level of mid papillary muscle)
Apical (little or no RV present)

Normal	5	Akinesis	2
Mild Hypokinesis	4	Dyskinesis	1
Severe Hypokinesis	3	Unable to Score	0

Wall segment	Motion score		Wall segment	Motion score
1 = posterior basal septum		6	= posterior basal LV	
1A = anterior basal septum		6 PL	= posterior-lateral basal LV	
2 = posterior mid septum		7	= posterior mid LV	
2A = anterior mid septum		8P	= posterior apical LV	
3R = posterior apical septum		8A	= anterior apical LV	
3L = lateral apical LV		9	= anterior mid LV	
4 = lateral mid LV		10	= anterior basal LV	
5 = lateral basal LV				

Wall Motion Index = [ ] _____, M.D.

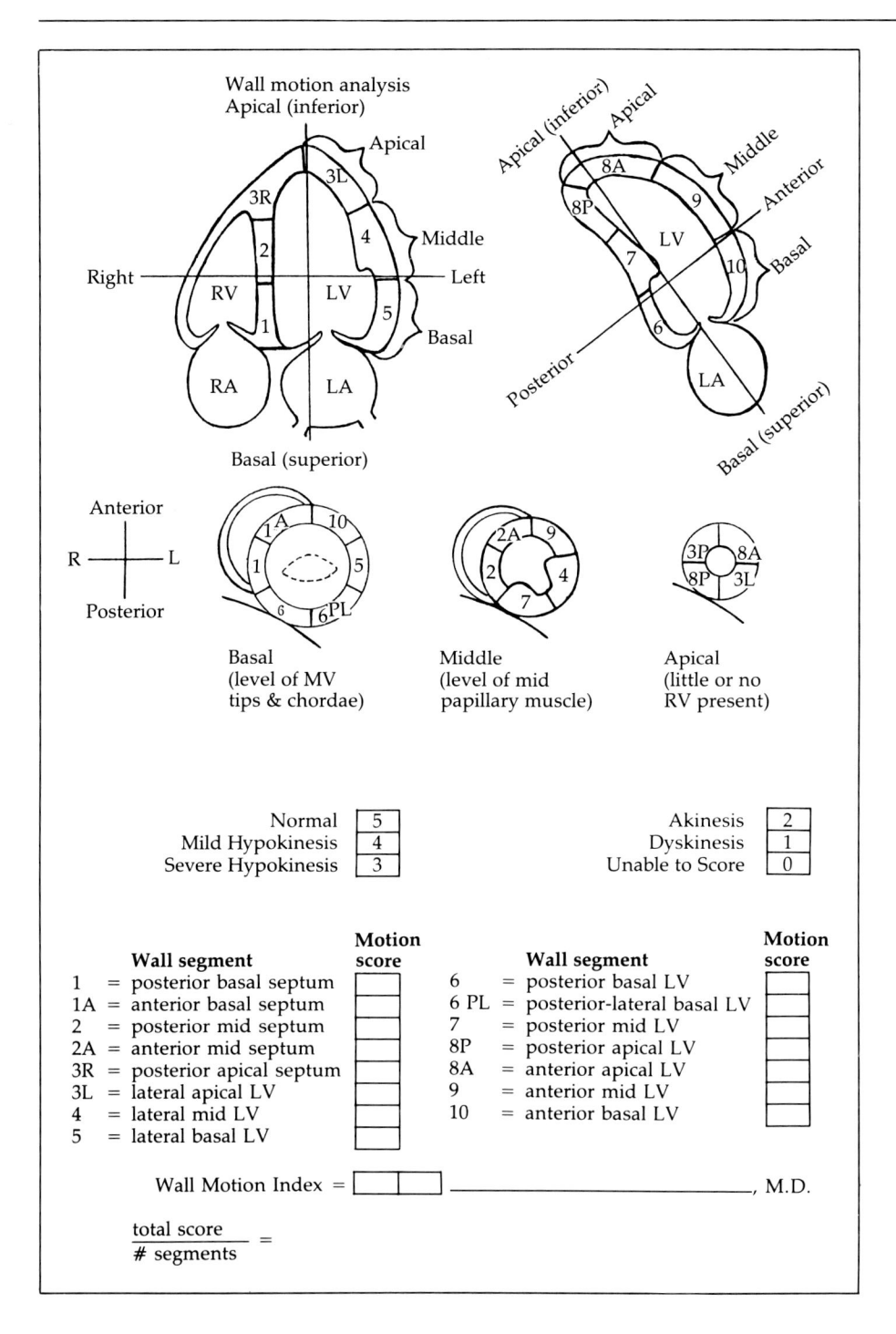

$$\frac{\text{total score}}{\text{\# segments}} =$$

Fig. 6-2. The left ventricle is divided into equal thirds (apical, middle, and basal) from the apex to the atrioventricular sulcus respectively. The interventricular septum should be divided into anterior and posterior portions because of different coronary artery distribution. At the level of the papillary muscles the right ventricle encompasses approximately two-fifths of the circumference of the left ventricle; the extent of the right ventricle and the location of both papillary muscles result in five equal segments being a logical division of the medial one-third of the left ventricle. Since the circumference at the base is larger, the basal third is divided into six equal segments of 60° each.

168   6. Coronary artery disease

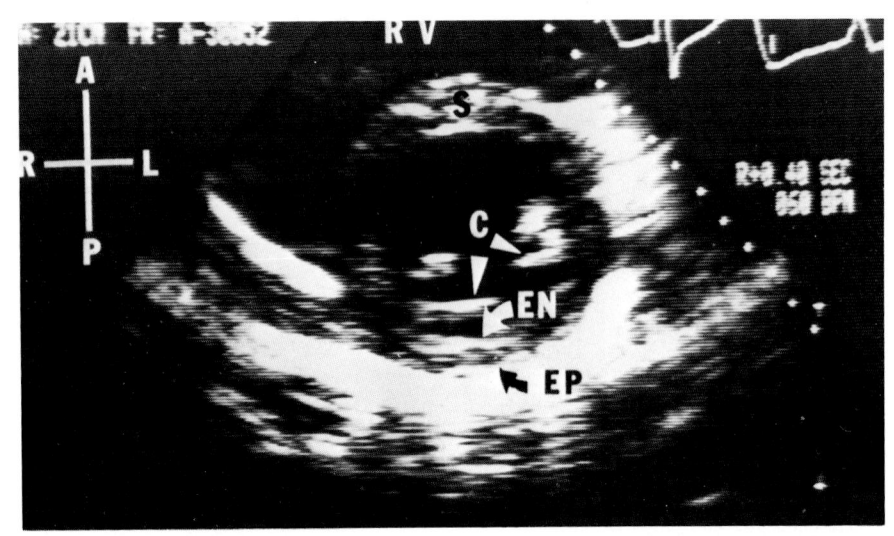

Fig. 6-3A. Parasternal short axis view at the level of the chordae tendineae (C). B. Parasternal short axis view at the level of the papillary muscles (arrows). C. Apical 4-chamber view showing normal left ventricle, right ventricle, right atrium, left atrium, and pulmonary veins (PV). D. Apical long axis view showing normal left ventricle, mitral valve, and left atrium. Arrow points to the apex. No right heart chambers are visible in this tomographic plane.

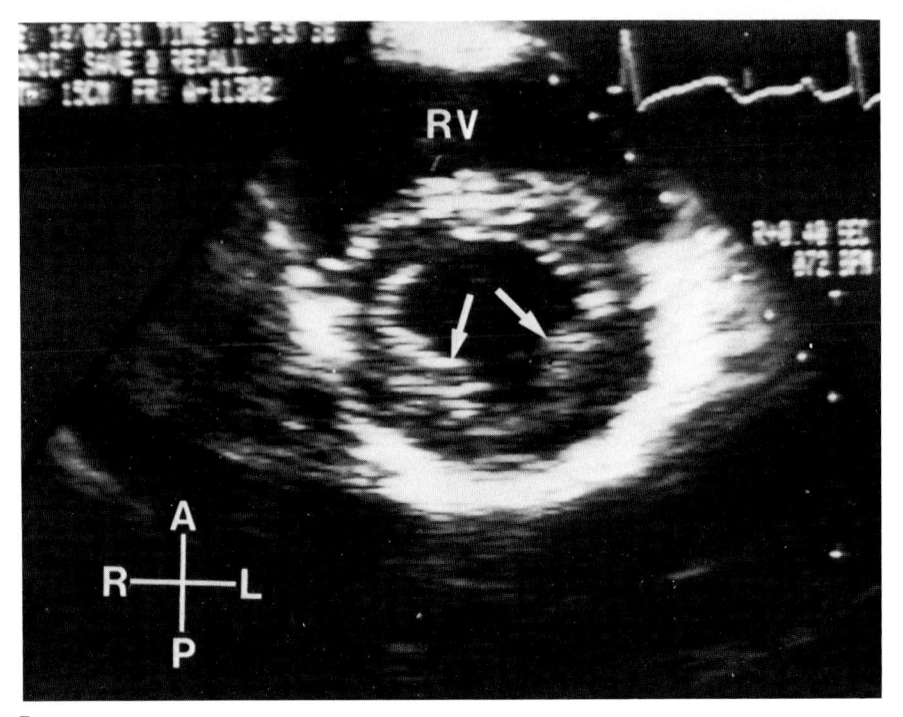

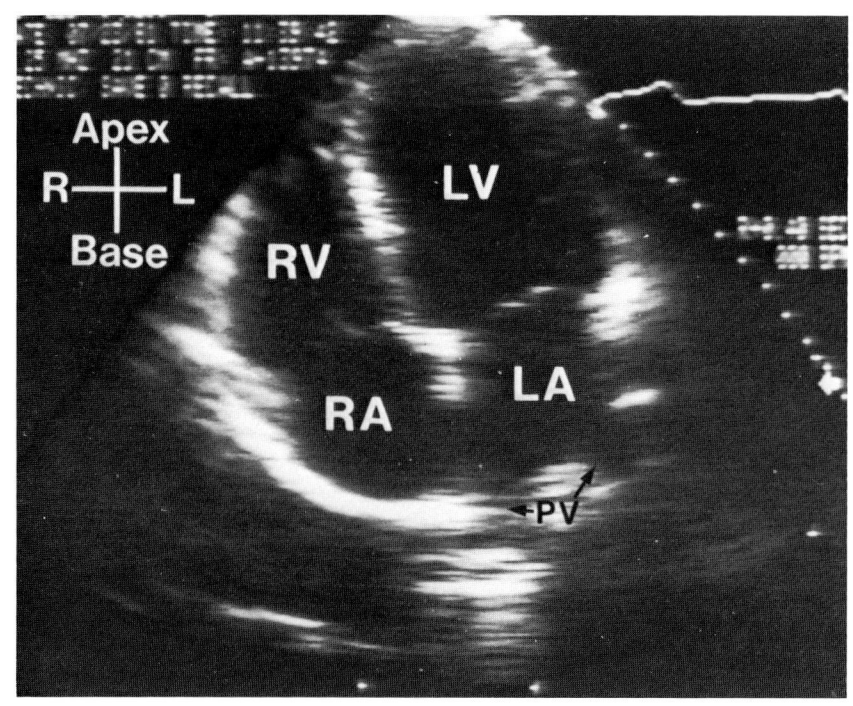

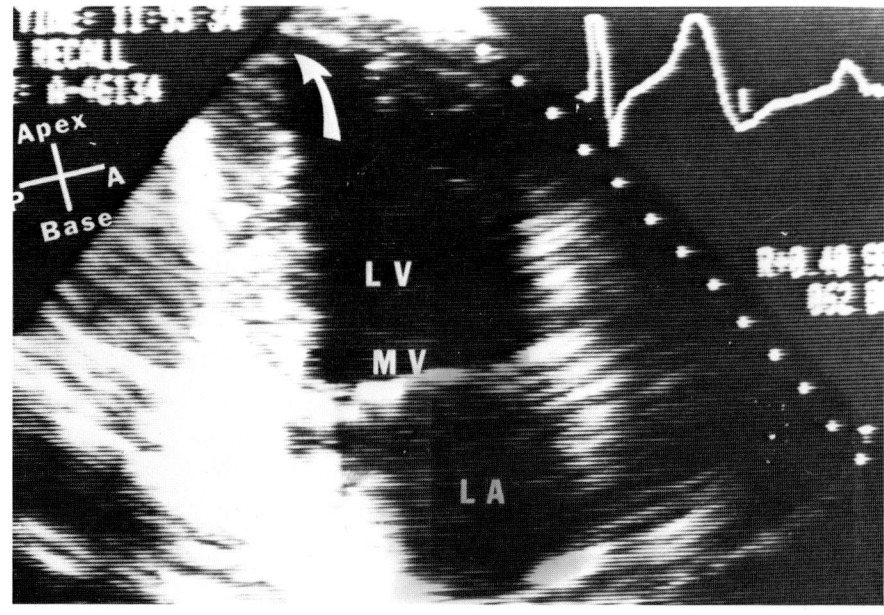

C

D

tients with complicated myocardial infarction is to provide anatomic and functional information about why the patient is in shock, hypotension, or heart failure. Furthermore, providing structural information to explain the etiology and relative significance of murmurs in such patients may be very useful.

Two-dimensional imaging techniques. If two-dimensional echocardiography is to be clinically useful in patients with coronary artery disease the echocardiographer must pay particular attention to comprehensive imaging of all segments of the left ventricle. Investigators have employed a variety of methods to divide the left ventricle as well as varied terminology to describe the different anatomic regions of the heart [26, 27, 32–34]. Although no standard terminology or method of dividing the left ventricle has yet been adopted, we divide the ventricle into 15 segments (Fig. 6-2). In order to obtain complete two-dimensional views of all 15 segments, multiple views must be obtained from the left parasternal and apical transducer positions. The minimal views necessary include parasternal short axis views at the levels of the chordae tendineae and the papillary muscles, and the apical four-chamber and long axis views (Fig. 6-3). With slight variation of transducer angle and rotation from these two positions, all segments of the left ventricle can be imaged twice. Additional important views that often provide third or fourth views of the same segment, thus improving the overall evaluation, include the parasternal long axis, parasternal right ventricular inflow, precordial or low parasternal apical short axis, apical short axis, subcostal four-chamber, and subcostal short axis. All these tomographic planes provide information about different areas of the left ventricle that complement the standard left ventricular views. If all possible views of the left ventricle from the variety of parasternal, left precordial, apical, and subcostal transducer positions are obtained, the left ventricle should be imaged in its entirety. Proper attention to technique, patient positioning, machine settings, and patient cooperation should ensure adequate imaging of the left ventricle in more than 90 percent of patients. Furthermore, we recommend that while imaging in the parasternal short axis view at the level of chordae tendineae an M-mode cursor be directed through the left ventricle and oriented in a perpendicular fashion to image the septum and posterior wall in order to accurately judge wall thickness and systolic thickening as well as to accurately measure the end-diastolic and end-systolic dimensions. With simultaneous two-dimensional imaging the M-mode recordings can be obtained in the proper location to ensure accuracy of wall thickness and cavity dimension measurements. If adequate M-mode recordings cannot be obtained from the standard positions, as occasionally happens in certain difficult situations, cavity dimensions and wall thickness may have to be determined from either the apical or subcostal views.

EXERCISE-INDUCED WALL MOTION ABNORMALITIES. Zwehl and associates [18] conducted a quantitative two-dimensional echocardiographic study in normal subjects performing bicycle exercise in a supine position. Standardized two-dimensional echocardiographic short axis and apical views of the left ventricle were analyzed to derive left ventricular sectional areas and length. Variability of left ventricular short axis area measurements ranged from 2.9 to 8.3 percent in this study. Left ventricular volume reconstruction employed a simplified formula (volume = $\frac{5}{6}$ area × length) with a single papillary muscle level short axis area and left ventricular length. These investigators observed changes in left ventricular function from rest to exercise consisting of a significant reduction in end-systolic volume, no significant change in end-diastolic volume, and increased ejection fraction. Other investigators have demonstrated that, although technically feasible, it is not necessarily easy to accomplish exercise echocardiography in coronary disease patients [12, 14, 15]. Mason and colleagues [12] reported that in a normal group mean systolic thickening of the septum increased in 22 segments from 56 percent at rest to 77 percent with exercise; in contrast, in 22 wall segments supplied by stenotic vessels in patients, the corresponding value fell during peak exercise from 59 to 35 percent. These investigators noted similar findings in evaluating left ventricular posterior wall segments; in normal subjects, wall thickening increased from 89 to 115 percent but fell during peak exercise from 75 to 54 percent in patients who had abnormally perfused segments. They also found that the percent fractional shortening increased with exercise in the normal subjects from 38 to 44 percent but fell in the patients during peak exercise from 35 to 28 percent. Morganroth and associates [32] were able to obtain technically satisfactory two-dimensional echocardiographic examinations during supine bicycle exercise in 43 of 55 (78%) patients. Although these investigators found new regional wall motion abnormalities induced with exercise to be highly specific for the presence of significant coronary artery disease, the overall sensitivity of the examination was less than that of the treadmill test. In a study involving 27 normal adult subjects who underwent hand grip and supine and upright bicycle exercise, Crawford and associates [15] employed M-mode echocardiography to assess left ventricular size and performance. These investigators concluded that end-diastolic left ventricular size is maintained during isometric exercise and moderate dynamic exercise even in the upright position, and that isometric exercise leads to a mild decrease in left ventricular shortening whereas dynamic exercise results in marked increases in shortening; this difference may be related to the relatively greater increase in blood pressure than in heart rate during isometric exercise.

Mitamura and coworkers [16] concluded that two-dimensional echocardiography combined with handgrip exercise has high specificity (94%) but low sensitivity (65%) in detecting coronary artery disease. These investigators reported that it was possible to diagnose multivessel disease in 12 of 13 patients (predictability of 92%). They also observed that isometric exercise-induced akinesia viewed by 2-D echo reflected coronary artery stenosis of greater than 90 percent in 16 of 18 segments (89%).

Maurer and Nanda [35] reported that exercise-induced thallium perfusion defects showed good correlation with exercise-induced asynergy detected by two-dimensional echo. They were able to obtain adequate images in 41 of 48 patients; exercise-induced wall motion abnormalities were detected in 19 of 23 patients with significant coronary artery disease but no prior myocardial infarction as well as in all five patients with known previous infarction.

Exercise 2-D echo has more potential than exercise M-mode studies; however, there are technical problems in performing dynamic exercise echocardiography, and satisfactory studies can be obtained in only 75 to 80 percent of subjects. Results suggest that the sensitivity is probably less than that of either the maximal treadmill exercise test or exercise perfusion radionuclide studies. For these reasons exercise echocardiography is not yet employed on a large scale for clinical evaluation and, except for specialized circumstances, it does not yet have widespread clinical acceptance for screening purposes; it probably does not offer enough additional information to justify the additional cost.

DISTINGUISHING ISCHEMIA FROM INFARCTION BY TWO-DIMENSIONAL ECHOCARDIOGRAPHY. Numerous experimental and clinical studies have demonstrated that segmental wall motion abnormalities are sensitive and specific markers of ischemia or infarction [9, 12, 19, 24, 26–29, 31–33, 36–41]. Noninvasive techniques employing fluoroscopic, electromagnetic, echocardiographic, and nuclear imaging methods now make evaluation of segmental wall motion widely applicable in the clinical setting.

Horowitz and colleagues [41], in a study of 80 patients with acute chest pain syndrome, performed portable two-dimensional echocardiography within 12 hours of admission to the intensive care unit. They found regional wall motion abnormalities in 31 of 33 (94%) patients with acute myocardial infarctions. These investigators also found that when an initial 2-D echo examination showed no regional wall motion abnormality, patients did not develop an acute myocardial infarction or clinical complication during the hospital course.

Investigators have shown that both clinical and hemodynamic measurements of left ventricular function correlate well with the area and magnitude of segmental dysfunction [42]. Segmental wall motion abnormalities have been found in areas without electrocardiographic evidence of infarction; thus ischemic wall motion abnormalities cannot be generally inferred from electrocardiographic analysis [43]. Serial studies after acute myocardial infarction have demonstrated improvement of wall motion in regions with and without infarction demonstrated by electrocardiography [43]. Two reasons have been given; peripheral ischemic (reversible) zones in the margin of the infarction improved and/or areas with less than transmural infarction may show improvement with follow-up studies.

Pichler [36] reported that the site and extent of wall motion abnormalities are closely related to hemodynamic complications (left ventricular failure, hypotension, shock) following acute myocardial infarction. Furthermore, he observed that patients with inferior infarction and concomitant precordial S–T segment depression demonstrated more severe regional dysfunction than patients with inferior myocardial infarction without precordial S–T segment depression. Accordingly, reciprocal S–T segment depression may actually indicate the presence of regional myocardial ischemia. Segmental wall motion abnormalities may be detected at the onset of myocardial infarction by echocardiography before the development of typical electrocardiographic abnormalities. Simultaneous electrocardiographic and segmental wall motion studies reveal that the extent of wall motion abnormalities frequently exceeds those shown by the electrocardiogram and involves zones remote from the site of the infarction [36]. These data are consistent with the concept that the area of acute myocardial infarction is surrounded by an even larger zone of jeopardized tissue. Wyatt and colleagues [44] observed depression of regional function in areas remote from acute ischemia in animals subjected to coronary occlusion.

Radionuclide ventriculography has confirmed that close correlation between ejection fraction and regional wall motion exists in humans but has suggested that neither measurement correlates well with creatine kinase MB fraction (CK-MB) estimates of infarct size. In noting the minimal correlation between enzymatic estimate of infarct size and the extent and severity of left ventricular wall motion

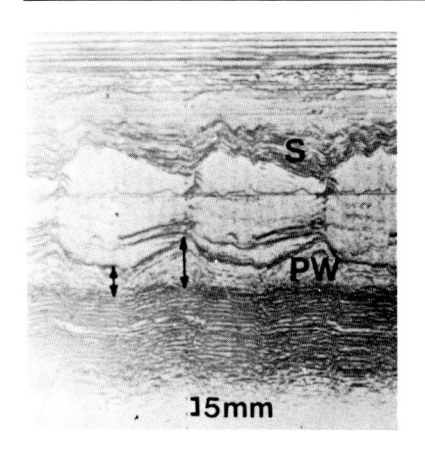

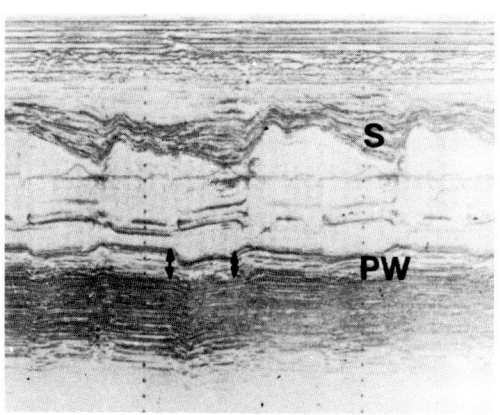

Fig. 6-4. M-mode recordings obtained from a closed-chest pig showing normal segmental thickening of the posterior wall of the left ventricle (left panel). The recording in the right panel was obtained from the same pig 15 seconds after occluding the circumflex coronary artery and demonstrates the rapidity with which akinesis and systolic thinning occurs in the region perfused by the circumflex coronary artery. Thickening of the interventricular septum remains normal.

abnormality, Pichler [36] explains this discrepancy on the basis of the following factors:

1. CK-MB isoenzyme activity measures infarcted myocardium while wall motion abnormalities indicate both infarcted and ischemic muscle.
2. Additional infarction of the right ventricle causes an increase in CK-MB isoenzyme activity out of proportion to left ventricular wall motion abnormality.
3. Difference in muscle mass gives rise to different infarct size with the same extent of segmental wall motion abnormality.
4. Previous "silent" myocardial infarction may cause a more pronounced ventricular dysfunction owing to scar tissue.

Kerber and associates [37, 38] observed in dog studies that acute occlusion of the left anterior descending coronary artery caused a reduction in systolic velocity, excursion, and thickening of both the involved ischemic and adjacent nonischemic region of the septum. Furthermore, these investigators noted that when myocardial ischemia was produced in a portion of the ventricle remote from the septum, the septal velocity and excursion increased.

Other investigators have characterized regional myocardial dysfunction due to acute ischemia in experimental studies using implanted ultrasonic dimension gauges (sonomicrometry) to measure wall thickening [45–47]. Furthermore, it is possible to detect by echocardiography acute changes in regional myocardial function in closed-chest animals subjected to brief coronary artery occlusions [46] (Fig. 6-4). Although quantitation of wall thickness and percent wall thickening differed in echocardiography and sonomicrometry, a close correlation was observed in the ability of both techniques to detect acute myocardial ischemia [45].

Angiographic and anatomic studies have shown that chronic ischemia without infarction may be a frequent cause of ventricular asynergy [48–50]. Patients with coronary artery disease have been shown to have abnormal motion in regions of the left ventricle that appear grossly and histologically normal at surgery, postmortem examination, or in myocardial biopsy specimens. In some cases normally perfused areas adjacent to ischemic zones may also move abnormally owing to the mechanical effect of asynergy in the adjacent ischemic segment [50, 51]. Additional evidence that chronic ischemia causes left ventricular asynergy at rest is provided by ventriculographic [52] and echocardiographic [53] studies showing that in some cases the motion can be improved by nitroglycerin or revascularization surgery.

Abnormal wall motion as viewed by M-mode and two-dimensional echocardiography in patients with coronary artery disease may be caused by ischemic, viable myocardium; scarred or partially fibrotic myocardium; or normal myocardium adjacent to areas that are dyskinetic as a result of ischemia or fibrosis.

In summary, measurement of regional wall motion could quantify the extent of myocardial ischemia and infarction and, if accurately performed, provide a clinically valuable method for assessing the severity of damage from an infarction, determining the prognosis, and evaluating the effects of interventions designed to limit myocardial necrosis. The three most commonly used techniques to measure segmental wall motion are angiography, radionuclide ventriculography, and echocardiography. All three techniques have certain common problems. During the cardiac cycle the heart rotates on its long axis and changes its position within the thorax. The geometric center of the left ventricle changes between systole and diastole [54, 55]. Although in a normal heart these geometric factors are small and probably insignificant, in a left ventricle with significant localized contraction abnormalities they may be large as a result of hypercontraction of one area and hypocontraction of other segments [56]. Cardiac movement during respiration presents more of a problem for radionuclide studies than it does for contrast ventriculograms or echocardiograms, which can be recorded during a fixed phase of respiration.

With the onset of myocardial ischemia, major mechanical abnormalities in wall thickening occur almost immediately; however, the relationship between these abnormalities in mechanical function and the decrease in coronary blood flow is not linear [57]. After a coronary occlusion that lasts only seconds mechanical function promptly returns to normal. However, when myocardial ischemia persists for several minutes or longer myocardial function may not return to normal for many hours or days [58]. Several investigative techniques have shown that segments of myocardium adjacent to but not actually involved in an infarction or ischemic process may display major contraction abnormalities [37, 44]. This "adjacent nonischemia dyskinesis" may in part be the result of a tethering effect, which helps explain the findings in several studies that the extent of wall motion abnormalities detected by two-dimensional echocardiography tends to overestimate infarct size measured pathologically [29, 59, 60].

Some studies have shown that the point in systole at which peak shortening occurs varies in different segments of the ventricle [61]. Ischemia or infarction tends to exaggerate this temporal dyssynergy. The number of segments that can be adequately evaluated depends upon the special resolution of the technique being applied. Accordingly, several fundamental problems remain that limit the usefulness of any technique using segmental wall motion abnormalities to define the size of an infarction or ischemic zone [56]. Two-dimensional echocardiography does have advantages over either angiographic or radionuclide methods with respect to the tomographic imaging and capability for direct measurement of wall thickness throughout the cardiac cycle as well as the absence of radiation or other biologic hazards.

A problem yet to be resolved is that of defining what is "abnormal" with respect to segmental ventricular function. The absence of systolic thickening (akinesis) or systolic thinning or paradoxical expansion (dyskinesis) are clearly abnormal. However, the difficulty arises when one attempts to define the lower limits of normal for segmental thickening—when is something normal and when does something reflect actual hypokinesis? The precise lower limit has not been well delineated, and there appears to be significant variability of degree of thickening and endocardial motion of closely adjacent segments. Franklin and associates [62] found a more than fivefold variation in maximum movement of individual endocardial targets toward a left ventricular centroid and a 35 percent variation in wall thickening along the individual ventricular radii. This marked spatial heterogeneity of thickening and motion may in part be explained by intrathoracic cardiac rotational and translational motion and in part by temporal asynergy [56]. The significant question remains—does hypokinesis in a given segment reflect ischemia, infarction, or abnormal movement of a normal segment due to adjacent mechanical factors? Lieberman and associates [29] did not find a close correlation between the transmural extent of infarction and the severity of impairment of systolic thickening. The findings of these investigators seem to support the thesis that a threshold phenomenon exists: When less than 20 percent of a transmural segment was infarcted (a subendocardial infarction), the segment showed reduced systolic thickening, whereas systolic thinning was seen at all levels of transmural infarction when infarction exceeded 20 percent. They found that segmental systolic thinning did not worsen as the extent of transmural infarction increased from 20 to 100 percent.

Other technical problems relate specifically to echocardiography; for example, what is the actual orientation of any tomographic section? The use of internal markers such as the mitral valve and papillary muscle are helpful in localizing segments in the base and midportions of the ventricle; however, there are no landmarks that can be used within the apex itself. Therefore, when comparing pathological slices to tomographic sections in the region between the papillary muscle and the true apex it is difficult to be certain that the sections are actually the same. Another problem is that long axis and short axis views cannot be obtained simultaneously. Long axis planes must be obtained from the apex in either the apical long axis or apical four-chamber views; short axis sections, on the other hand, must be obtained with the transducer in parasternal positions. Another important prerequisite is to obtain good endocardial and epicardial recordings. This can usually be done quite effectively using two-dimensional imaging to position the M-mode cursor to ensure proper intersecting of the septum, posterior wall, and cavity of the left ventricle. However, precise definition of the endocardial surface, when viewed from the apical long axis positions, frequently results in echo dropout of endocardial reflectances; hence the assessment of wall thickening is potentially less accurate in these areas than in parasternal short axis views.

WALL MOTION INDEX AND PREDICTION OF CORONARY ARTERY DISEASE BY ECHOCARDIOGRAPHY. The wall motion index is calculated simply by adding the values for each segment and dividing by the number of segments visualized (see Fig. 6-2). No score is assigned if a given segment is not adequately imaged; therefore a zero score for any segment does not influence the overall index. The score of the wall motion index does have some reasonably accurate predictive power for left ventricular global function [63]. Assessment of the reliability of two-dimensional echocardiography in evaluating wall motion abnormalities is difficult because there is no firm standard for comparison. Studies have been performed which show that two-dimensional echocardiography compares favorably with angiography; however, it is well recognized that even biplane angiography has significant limitations for accurately identifying wall motion abnormalities and distinguishing ischemia from infarction [33, 63, 64].

Wyatt and associates [65] employed multiple short axis sections of the left ventricle in dogs to quantify the extent of myocardial dyssynergy during ischemia and infarction. Radial wall motion was analyzed by superimposition of end-diastolic and end-systolic images. Dyssynergy was defined as dyskinesis, akinesis, or extreme hypokinesis. The reproducibility of these measurements was found acceptable with a difference of 7.8 percent between two observers. These investigators compared the extent of left ventricular dyssynergy as measured by two-dimensional echocardiography with that estimated by myocardial force gauge mapping and found good agreement ($r = 0.89$). Although both of these techniques can estimate the extent of left ventricular dyssynergy, they measure different components of segmental function. Two-dimensional echocardiography measures radial wall motion at the endocardial surface, whereas the force gauges record myocardial force development tangential to the surface of the left ventricle. In another study by Meltzer and colleagues [28], the extent of left ventricular wall motion measured by 2-D echo correlated well with infarct size as estimated by technetium pyrophosphate ($r = 0.82$). An important difference exists in the methodology of the Wyatt and Meltzer studies; the former employed histochemical staining to delineate infarct size, whereas Meltzer used radionuclide imaging. It is therefore unclear whether the two techniques measure the same indices of myocardial ischemic injury.

Eaton and associates [66] performed serial two-dimensional echocardiographic examinations in 28 patients during the first two weeks following documented transmural myocardial infarction and observed that eight patients developed segmental or regional expansion with disproportionate dilatation and transmural thinning in the infarcted zone, first noted at approximately day 7 following the acute infarction.

Myocardial regions as defined by any system of nomenclature will never correlate precisely with coronary blood flow because the patterns of coronary distribution are so highly variable. As a result of this variability any given myocardial region may receive its blood supply from the branches of two independent major epicardial arteries. Although the geographic areas of ischemic myocardial injury may generally be approximated by a systematic selection of myocardial regions, one should never assume that the correlation between such regions and coronary distribution is absolute. Edwards and associates [34] have divided the myocardial regions into fourteen segments distributed among a basal third, a mid third, and an apical third according to the common patterns of coronary arterial distribution to each of these segments.

REGIONAL ABNORMALITIES. A regional analysis at autopsy of 102 normal hearts from adults was reported by Bizarro [67], DeSonza [68], and Edwards and colleagues [34] (Table 6-1). Edwards and associates [34] have also demonstrated that each of the three levels (basal, mid, apical) accounts for approximately one-third of the base-to-apex length of the left ventricle in the normal heart. In addition, these investigators found that in either hypertrophied or dilated hearts the relative base length de-

Table 6-1. *Regional analysis at autopsy of 102 normal hearts from adults**

Levels of left ventricle	Segments of ventricular septum and left ventricular free wall					Total (by levels)
	Anterior septum	Anterior left ventricle	Lateral left ventricle	Inferior left ventricle	Inferior septum	
Basal	13.5 ± 0.82 9.0	12.5 ± 1.7 8.4	12.6 ± 1.5 8.4	11.8 ± 1.3 7.9	12.9 ± 0.71 8.7	63.3 ± 6.0 42.5
Mid	10.9 ± 0.66 7.3	10.5 ± 1.3 7.1	11.3 ± 1.2 7.6	10.3 ± 1.1 6.9	10.9 ± 0.64 7.3	53.9 ± 4.9 36.1
Apical	5.8 ± 0.40 3.9	6.5 ± 0.87 4.3	7.7 ± 1.0 5.2	6.4 ± 0.82 4.3	5.5 ± 0.36 3.7	31.9 ± 3.5 21.4
Total (by segments)	30.2 ± 1.9 20.2	29.5 ± 3.9 19.8	31.6 ± 3.7 21.2	28.5 ± 3.2 19.1	29.3 ± 1.7 19.7	149.1 ± 14.4 100.0

*For each region, the top row indicates the regional mass (g) ± standard deviation, and the bottom row represents the percent contribution of that region to total left ventricular mass. (Data were extrapolated by Dr. Robert C. Bahn.)
Source: From WD Edwards et al, Standardized nomenclature and anatomic basis for regional tomographic analysis of the heart. *Mayo Clin Proc* 56:479, 1981.

creased by roughly 5 percent, whereas the midlevel length increased by about 5 percent.

We divide the left ventricle into segments in the same manner described by Edwards and coworkers [34] except that the basal third is divided into six segments rather than five (Fig. 6-5A). The anatomic segments are divided and labeled in the same manner as shown in the diagrams in Figure 6-2 (Fig. 6-5).

Regional analysis of the left ventricular walls is useful for the determination of infarct location and size. Although the feasibility of regional tomographic analysis with 2-D echo to assess infarct size has been determined, the ability to accurately delineate infarct size and distinguish between transmural, subendocardial, and acute or chronic ischemic changes remains to be documented. Clinical-pathological correlative studies are essential to validate the tomographic assessment of the heart in this fashion. Pathological studies represent the only acceptable gold standard since neither angiography nor other currently available imaging methods are satisfactory standards of reference. The pathologist must be willing to make tomographic sections of the heart and the clinician must be willing to work closely with him or her in order to firmly establish the validity of the clinical diagnosis of cardiac disease by such 2-D echo methods of analysis.

Vieweg and associates [69] reviewed the distribution and severity of left ventricular wall motion abnormalities according to age and coronary arterial pattern in 500 patients with coronary artery disease and angina pectoris. These investigators found that 40 percent of patients with coronary artery disease and angina pectoris had normal left ventricular wall motion, and left ventricular wall motion abnormalities in the remaining 60 percent of patients were divided evenly among three categories: anterior dyssynergy alone, posterior dyssynergy alone, and combined anterior and posterior dyssynergy. They found no difference in incidence of wall motion abnormalities in patients from the third to the eighth decade of life. The severity of coronary artery disease and the degree of left ventricular dysfunction determine the clinical presentation and natural history of patients with ischemic heart disease [70, 71].

Kolibash and associates [72] studied the relationship of septal motion and myocardial perfusion in patients with obstructive lesions of the left anterior de-

178   6. Coronary artery disease

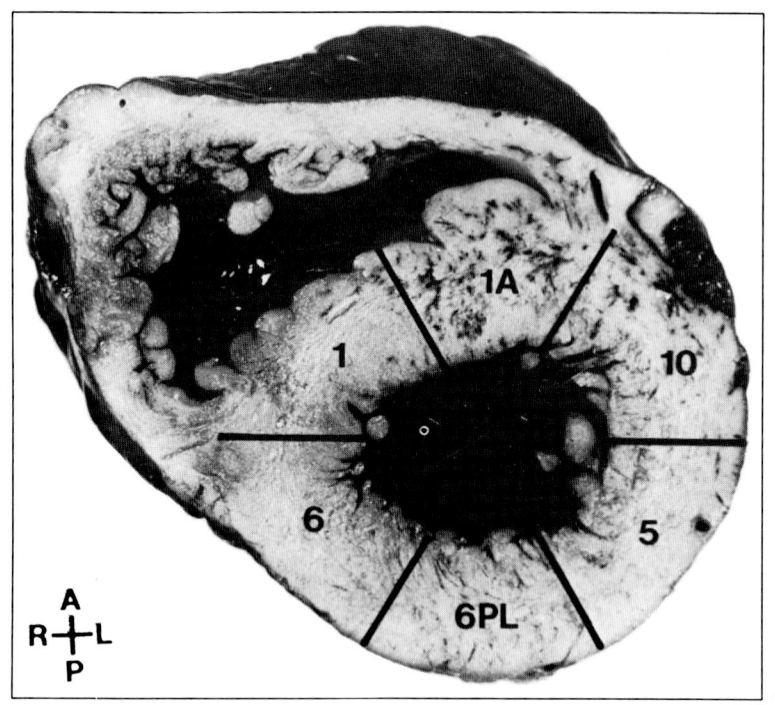

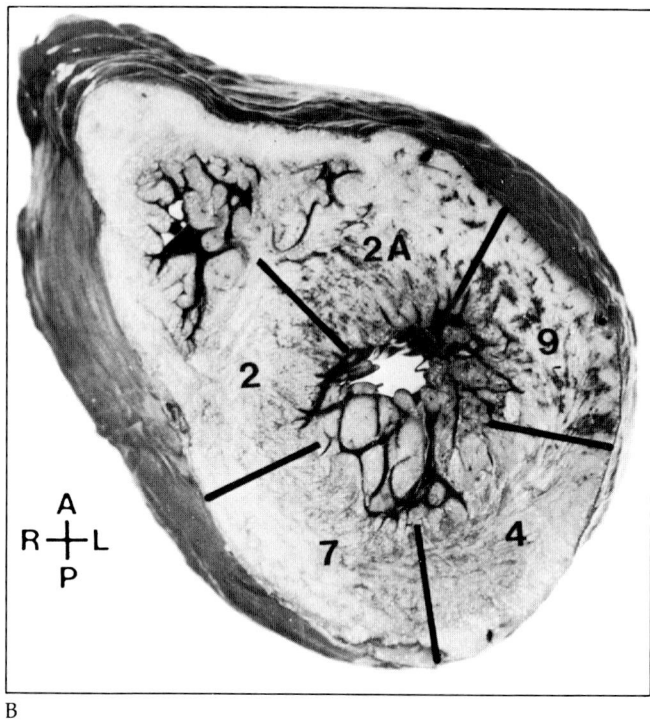

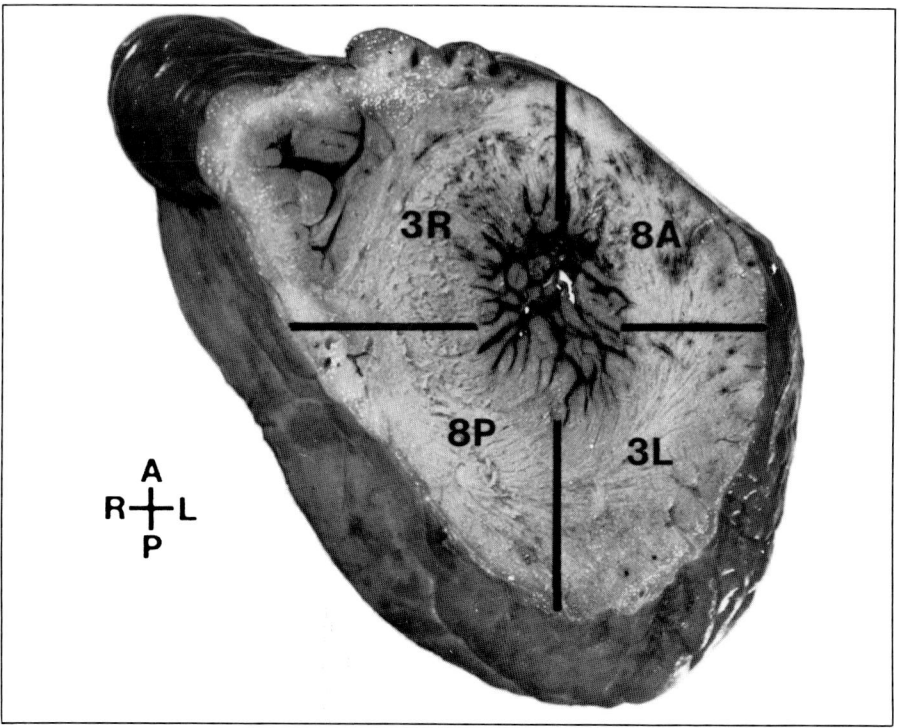

Fig. 6-5A. Basal third of the left ventricle as viewed from the apex of a normal heart. The numbers on each of the segments coincide with the numbers on the diagram of Fig. 6-2. 1A = anterior portion of the septum; 6PL = posterolateral segment of the left ventricle. B. Middle third of the ventricle as viewed from the apex showing the papillary muscles and the left ventricle divided into five equal segments. 2A = anterior portion of midinterventricular septum. C. Apical third of the ventricle as viewed from the apex showing the four anatomic segments. 3R = posterior apical septum; 3L = lateral apical LV; 8A = anterior apical LV; 8P = posterior apical LV.

scending coronary artery and noted that in those with severe stenosis the presence of abnormal septal motion strongly suggested absent septal perfusion and most likely infarction. These investigators reported that normal echocardiographic septal motion implied that resting septal perfusion was normal. These findings indicated that in patients with coronary artery disease abnormal motion of the interventricular septum on echocardiography usually indicates abnormal myocardial blood flow to the septum as detected by selective scintigraphy.

Our observation is in agreement with a study performed acutely in dogs by Kerber and associates [37], in which they observed that segmental dyskinesis correlated with impaired myocardial perfusion as determined by the use of radioactive microspheres. These investigators found 18 of 25 subjects with high-grade left anterior descending lesions to have anterior hypokinesis. However, only half of these subjects had abnormal septal motion and septal perfusion defects. The investigators postulated two explanations for this discrepancy: either the anterior wall was infarcted but not the septum; or collaterals had reestablished perfusion to the septum but not to the anterior wall.

The usefulness of the M-mode echocardiogram in predicting the location of the left anterior descending lesion is controversial [73–75]. Kolibash [72] showed no relationship between abnormal septal motion imaged by echocardiography and the location of the disease proximal to the first septal perforator; this was in agreement with another study by Gordon and Kerber [75]. In the Kolibash study the presence of a perfusion defect rather than the location of left anterior descending artery lesions was best related to echocardiographic septal motion. Although no study has yet been reported correlating wall motion abnormalities identified by two-dimensional echocardiography with coronary arteriographic lesions, our experience has indicated that the location of septal akinesis is a good predictor of how proximal or distal the occlusion of the left anterior descending artery lesion will be in patients with acute myocardial infarction.

Perfusion defects and areas of abnormal contractility do not uniformly indicate areas of fibrosis. Hamilton [76] described perfusion defects in several patients with preinfarction angina but without evidence of infarction.

Contraction abnormalities detected by 2-D echo may not always be the result of a myocardial infarction. Abnormal motion of the posterior left ventricular free wall has been recorded during episodes of angina [7]. In another study by Widlansky and associates [77] of a patient with Prinzmetal's angina, abnormal echocardiographic septal motion was recorded only during an episode of chest pain together with marked S–T segment elevation.

Dortimer and associates [78] studied 48 patients with chronic angina but no prior history of myocardial infarction to determine whether the anatomic sites of coronary artery disease could be predicted accurately by M-mode echocardiographic measurements of septal and posterior wall motion during an angina-free interval. These investigators reported that 28 of 35 patients (80%) with disease of the left anterior descending coronary artery had diminished interventricular septal motion and 14 of 27 patients (52%) with disease of posterior vessels had diminished posterior wall motion on the echocardiogram. Although contrast ventriculography is normally accepted as the reference with which noninvasive techniques are compared, Dortimer and colleagues [78] observed 10 false positives when septal motion abnormalities on the echocardiogram were employed to predict corresponding abnormal ventriculographic systolic motion; however, five of these 10 patients had disease of the left anterior descending artery. Thus the echocardiogram detected five cases of septal motion abnormalities with left anterior descending artery disease that the ventriculogram had shown to be normal.

Use of pharmacologic agents to evaluate regional myocardial function and reversible ischemia by echocardiography. Echocardiography has been found useful in detecting changes in global ventricular function induced by nitroglycerin in both normal patients and those with coronary artery disease [79, 80]. Nitroglycerin ventriculography has been demonstrated to be a valuable means of differentiating reversible and irreversible asynergy [81, 82]. Morrison and colleagues [83] reported the use of M-mode echocardiography in the determination of reversible posterior wall asynergy following administration of sublingual nitroglycerin in patients with coronary disease. Hardarson and Wright [84] studied the effects of sublingual nitroglycerin on cardiac performance in eight patients with coronary artery disease and symmetrical left ventricular contraction and noted an increase in both ejection fraction and mean velocity of circumferential fiber shortening and a decrease in wall stress. Goldstein and associates [85] reported the effects of glyceryl trinitrate on echocardiographic left ventricular dimensions during exercise in the upright position in normal subjects and in patients with coronary artery disease. They considered the end-systolic dimension an index of regional performance rather than an estimate of overall left ventricular performance. They noted that during exercise the end-diastolic dimension increased both in normal subjects as well as in patients; however, the end-systolic dimension fell progressively with exercise in the normal subjects but changed inconsistently in the patients. In patients with hypokinesis of the left ventricle administration of glyceryl trinitrate was noted to significantly improve regional contractile performance.

Komer and associates [86] studied the effects of nitroglycerin on regional left ventricular performance in open-chest dogs during acute myocardial ischemia. They observed during transient occlusion of the left anterior descending coronary artery both end-diastolic thinning and marked reduction of systolic thickening in the central ischemic zone. Similar changes to a lesser degree were noted in the border zone. They concluded that nitroglycerin did not improve regional myocardial performance in the acutely ischemic canine myocardium. Kerber and associates [87] observed similar findings in evaluating nitroglycerin and nitroprusside on regional myocardial function in the presence of acute ischemia in open-chest dogs. These investigators observed that the posterior wall stress index nearly doubled after coronary occlusion but was then substantially lowered to control levels by both nitroglycerin and nitroprusside. These effects should be beneficial because the lowering of wall stress and the resultant reduction of myocardial oxygen demand is a major mechanism for reduction of myocardial injury after coronary artery occlusion [88]. Both drugs were found to reduce the ischemic "wall stress index" (ventricular pressure × ventricular diameter/wall thickness) by almost 50 percent. Thus both nitroglycerin and nitroprusside were equally beneficial in this model of acute myocardial ischemia.

Kerber and associates [89] reported that inotropic agents have two opposing effects on the dyskinesis of acutely ischemic myocardium observed in open-chest anesthetized dogs, increased aneurysmal bulging during isometric contraction but improved wall velocity during ventricular ejection. The latter contributes to the drug-induced improvement in overall ventricular performance and also indicates that acutely ischemic myocardium retains the capacity to respond to pharmacologic stimuli. Accordingly, ischemic myocardium retains the capacity to respond to pharmacologic stimulation for at least a few hours following the onset of acute ischemia; the resultant changes in motion of the ischemic area are achieved only by increasing local oxygen demand, and ultimately this tends to increase infarct size [90].

Interventions that may alter infarct size have been shown experimentally to affect segmental cardiac wall motion [91, 92]. Kerber and associates [93] studied the effect of intraaortic balloon counterpulsation on the motion and perfusion of ischemic left ventricular posterior myocardium in 30 open-chest dogs, employing echocardiography to evaluate motion and radioactive microspheres to determine perfusion. Circumflex coronary artery ligation produced acute aneurysmal bulging during isovolumic contraction and diminished ischemic wall velocity during systolic ejection. During the balloon counterpulsation there was no change in perfusion in the ischemic area and very little change in wall motion. These investigators further noted that neither norepinephrine nor nitroprusside, when added during the time balloon counterpulsation was being performed, contributed to any further improvement in the response of the dyskinesis during the ischemic period. These authors concluded that intraaortic balloon counterpulsation had little effect on ischemic dyskinesis, probably owing to its failure to improve perfusion of the acutely ischemic myocardium.

Investigators have used quantitative methods to evaluate regional left ventricular function with two-dimensional echocardiography, but there is no systematic evaluation of the merits and limitations of the different methods of measurement [94, 95]. Moynihan and associates [96] evaluated different approaches to the quantification of regional left ventricular function from two-dimensional echocardiographic images for their ability to optimize interobserver reproducibility in a heterogeneous patient population and to minimize the variability of regional function observed in a homogeneous normal population. Area, hemiaxis, and perimeter measurements were examined as were the effect of the degree of image subdivision into halves, quadrants, or octants. Each approach was also tested using both a fixed and a floating frame of reference for the definition of a regional axis system. These authors found that the area method was consistently superior to either linear method in optimizing both reproducibility and variability. Furthermore, they noted that the floating access system yielded the same variability as the fixed system for short axis sections at the mitral valve level but slightly less variability for papillary muscle level section. These investigators noted that the reproducibility of 7 percent for the areas of the two-dimensional echo outlines was similar to that reported in angiographic studies where reproducibility varies 5 to 10 percent for volumes [97].

Evaluation of uncomplicated myocardial infarction and global left ventricular performance by echocardiography. Although electrocardiography is excellent in detecting the presence of acute transmural myocardial infarction, many studies have shown that it is significantly less reliable in identifying less than transmural infarctions or in pinpointing the exact anatomic location of the infarct [98–100]. Sullivan and colleagues [98] reported electrocardiography to be reliable in distinguishing between infarcts involving the anterior wall and those involving the posterior wall but unreliable in separating the various subdivisions of anterior and posterior wall infarcts. Furthermore, these investigators reported the extent of fibrosis to be accurately predicted by electrocardiogram in only 26 percent; in 70 percent the myocardial infarction was more extensive at necropsy than predicted by electrocardiogram. These findings were similar to those reported by Vieweg and associates in a study of 245 patients in which the electrocardiogram was found to be quite insensitive in predicting the presence of left ventricular wall motion abnormalities [100]. These investigators found the sensitivity of the electrocardiogram in detecting angiographic anterior wall motion abnormalities to be only 32 percent and the specificity to be 98 percent. Similarly, when electrocardiographic criteria for inferior and true posterior myocardial infarction were combined into posterior myocardial infarction the sensitivity of the electrocardiogram in predicting wall motion abnormalities was 40 percent and the specificity was 94 percent.

Two-dimensional echocardiography has been used to observe sequential changes after acute myocardial infarction [66, 101]. Postmortem studies have shown that among patients dying within 30 days of acute infarction as many as 72 percent show histologic evidence of regional thinning and dilatation of the infarcted area beginning within one week of acute infarction [102]. This process generally occurs without histologic evidence of infarct extension after the acute event and has been termed "infarct expansion." Pathologic evidence suggests that infarct expansion results from intramyocardial rupture of necrotic muscle fibers and appears to be of much greater hemodynamic and prognostic importance than actual infarct extension [102, 103]. Eaton and associates [66] reported the value of two-dimensional echocardiography in detecting infarct expansion within the first two weeks following acute infarction in 28 patients. Eight of these patients showed gross infarct expansion by echocardiography beginning within three to seven days following the acute infarction. These patients could not be separated from the patients without significant expansion by the usual clinical indicators of the extended infarction. However, a very important difference was evident; the eight-week mortality in the patients with infarct expansion was 50 percent, whereas no deaths occurred in patients in whom no infarct expansion was shown by serial two-dimensional echocardiographic examination. In addition, all the surviving patients in whom infarct expansion had been demonstrated by echocardiography continued to have congestive heart failure following discharge from the hospital. Parisi and associates [104] reported the use of two-dimensional echocardiography for systematic study of regional wall motion abnormalities in patients with remote and acute myocardial infarctions. These authors suggested that the technique has the potential not only for identifying the presence of wall motion abnormalities but also for quantifying their extent on a global basis and the possibility of assessing their reversibility. Accordingly, this may have treatment implications, inasmuch as the unusually thinned, echo-dense noncontractile region that is most likely to be composed of scar tissue is unlikely to have its function restored by saphenous vein bypass surgery, whereas a poorly contracting area of myocardium of normal diastolic thickness may indeed recover its function after blood supply is restored. The potential of echocardiography in this regard will have to be determined by future clinical studies.

Left ventricular wall thickness is a determinant of chamber compliance in patients with chronic heart disease, and diastolic wall thickness has been shown to correlate with diastolic compliance in acute studies in canine hearts [105]. Gaasch and Bernard [106] observed that within five minutes of coronary ligation in anesthetized dogs wall thickness decreased and during reperfusion (reactive hyperemia) the wall thickness was greater than in controls. They also reported that increased coronary blood flow produced by intracoronary nitroglycerin resulted in transient increase in wall thickness. These investigators suggested that the observed direct relationship between coronary blood flow and wall thickness suggests a dynamic role for coronary blood flow in calculations of left ventricular mass, diastolic wall stress, and myocardial stiffness constants. They observed that calculations of left ventricular mass vary only by approximately 10 percent when wall thickness is measured during control and ischemic states. However, calculations for left ventricular mass may vary by as much as 30 percent if made during ischemia, compared to calculation during reactive hyperemia.

In the absence of segmental disease there is excellent correlation between the percent increase in wall thickness throughout systole and the overall ventricular performance [107]. These correlations provide a firm basis for the use of wall thickness measurements as indices of ventricular performance in clinical echocardiography.

Gueret and associates [108] employed two-dimensional echocardiographic analysis of global and regional left ventricular function in seven closed-chest dogs to study the effects of nitroprusside in ischemic heart failure. A Simpson reconstruction using five echocardiographic short axis sections was used for assessment of left ventricular volumes. Regional function in short axis cross sections at different levels of the ventricle was expressed as sectional systolic fractional area of change. Each short axis section was subdivided into eight 45-degree segments and segmental fractional area change was automatically calculated by computer. Nitroprusside reduced global diastolic and end-systolic volumes and increased ejection fraction. Differential responses to nitroprusside were observed with two-dimensional echo in various zones of the left ventricle. Normal contraction prevailed in all segments at the mitral valve level, which was above the site of coronary occlusion. In the midpapillary muscle level section, nitroprusside significantly enhanced function of segments that were within the left anterior descending arterial supply zone. In contrast, however, segments in the severely ischemic dysfunctioning zone at the low papillary muscle level did not respond to the vasodilator. This experimental study demonstrates that standardized two-dimensional echocardiography is capable of quantitating serial measurements of cardiac function during interventions. The effects of treatment on the function of regionally ischemic myocardium may be complex and depend on the underlying state of the myocardium. In the case of nitroprusside's effects on contraction in the midpapillary muscle section, Gueret noted that it was difficult to ascertain whether the improved regional wall motion represented recovery by direct alleviation of ischemic injury or reflected indirect effects of a lower mechanical load of the left ventricle. The latter would tend to increase inward wall motion. However, the response of this section to nitroprusside infusion indicates that from a functional standpoint the myocardium is still viable and represents a region where various interventions may be tested for their differential effects on mechanical performance (Fig. 6-6).

Wyatt and colleagues [109] have demonstrated that left ventricular volume can be accurately quantified in vitro by two-dimensional echocardiography. They calculated area, length, and diameter measurements from short and long axis images of the left ventricle and calculated volume by seven different mathematical models. The models using short axis area and long axis length gave higher correlation

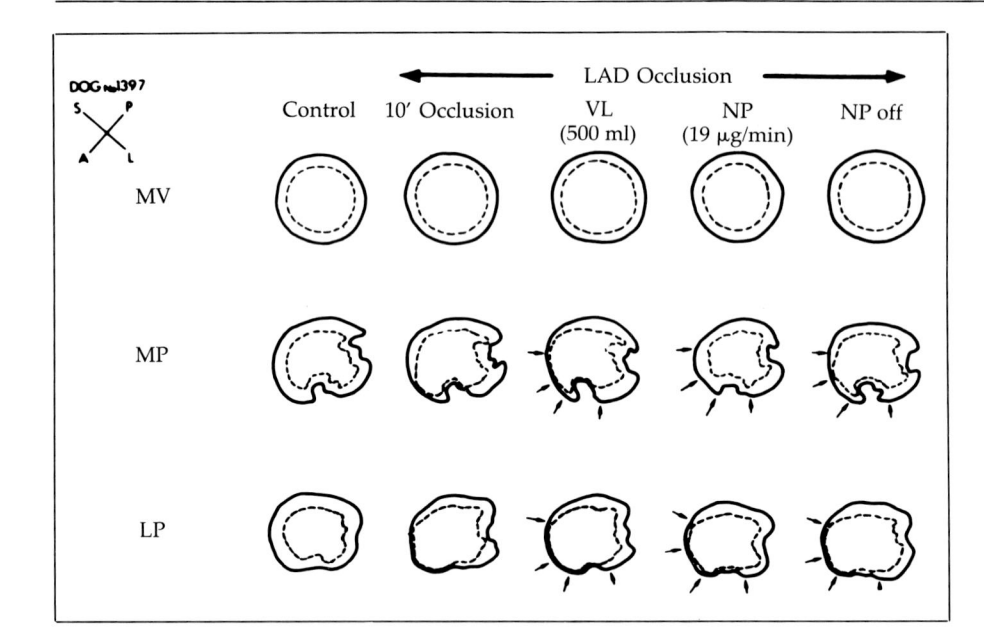

Fig. 6-6. The effects of nitroprusside (NP) infusion and contraction in the midpapillary muscle section (MP) following occlusion of the left anterior descending (LAD) coronary artery suggests that the myocardium in that region is still viable in contrast to lack of improvement in the akinetic zone of the low papillary muscle section (LP). Volume (VL) loading with 500 ml had no effect on the wall motion abnormality in the MP section. MV = mitral valve level. (From P Gueret et al.: Differential effects of nitroprusside on ischemia and nonischemic myocardial segments demonstrated by computer-assisted two dimensional echocardiography. Am J Cardiol 48:59, 1981.)

coefficients ($r = 0.982$ and $r = 0.969$) and lower mean errors (10–20%) than standard formulas previously used with M-mode echocardiography and angiography. Other clinical studies have shown that two-dimensional echocardiography is a reliable method for obtaining left ventricular volume and ejection fraction determination in patients with coronary artery disease [110–113]. Although the ability to derive accurate volume and ejection fraction determinations has been repeatedly demonstrated by investigators with two-dimensional echocardiography, the reliability of the technique is very dependent upon the meticulous imaging detail of obtaining either multiple parasternal short axis images or of both apical four-chamber and long axis views. In certain patients who are especially difficult to image it may not be possible to obtain all the necessary views or to obtain adequate imaging of the endocardium in order to derive volumes and ejection fraction information. The skill of the echocardiographer and the quality of images obtainable from the 2-D echo imaging system obviously weigh heavily upon the overall reliability of obtaining complete imaging of the left ventricle. In some of the earlier models of two-dimensional echocardiographic equipment visualization of the entire left ventricle could be obtained in only 60 percent of patients [64].

Quinones and colleagues [114] have recommended a different method of determining ejection fraction with 2-D echo by using the parasternal long axis, apical four-chamber, and apical long axis views. End-diastolic and end-systolic measurements of the left ventricular short axis at the base and midcavity in the parasternal long axis view and at the basal, middle, and apical thirds of the cavity in the apical views are made, from which an averaged minor axis at end diastole and at end systole is calculated. These investigators concluded that ejection fraction can be determined accurately with 2-D echo in patients with or without dyssynergy by this simple technique, which eliminates the need for planimetry or computer assistance.

Other methods clinically valuable in deriving global function of the left ventricle that do not require volume determinations include E point-septal separation,

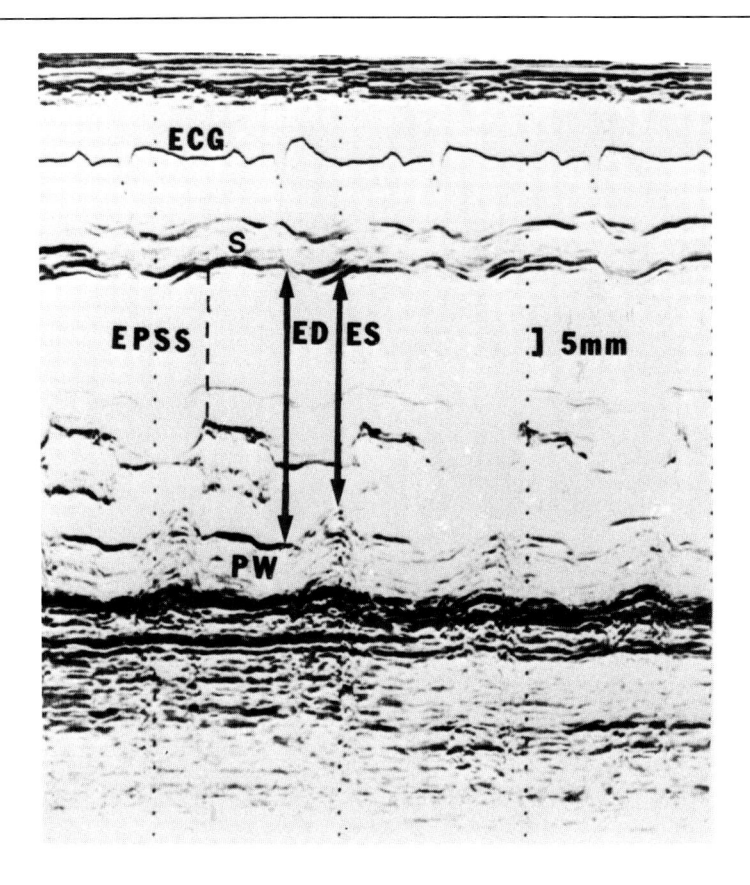

Fig. 6-7. M-mode recording of a patient with previous anterior myocardial infarction showing mild left ventricular dilatation and marked increase in E point-septal separation (EPSS) of 33 mm, which is indicative of marked reduction of the ejection fraction.

percent fractional shortening, mean circumferential fiber shortening rate, and wall motion index. The mitral E point-septal separation, which can be measured from either M-mode or two-dimensional recordings, is a very useful, easily obtainable measurement of global left ventricular function that has been shown to correlate very well with ejection fraction but does not correlate with left ventricular size [23, 115–117]. The specificity for an abnormal E point-septal separation predicting a reduced ejection fraction is approximately 90 percent, whereas the sensitivity has been reported to vary between 65 and 85 percent (Fig. 6-7).

Systolic dimensional changes for percent fractional shortening (%FS) are another easily measurable index of global function. Mean circumferential fiber shortening rate ($\overline{Vcf}$) is calculated in the same manner except that ejection time (ET) must be known.

$$\%FS = \frac{EDD - ESD}{EDD} \quad (1)$$

$$\overline{Vcf} = \frac{EDD - ESD}{ET \times EDD} \quad (2)$$

Beeder and associates [118] have shown there is a predictive relationship between segmental abnormalities and global left ventricular function in coronary artery disease.

Quantitation of infarct size and/or ischemia. Because of incomplete visualization of the left ventricle the clinical application of M-mode echocardiography in attempting to estimate the extent of ischemic muscle or infarct size has been sufficiently limited not to have gained widespread acceptance. Although the diagnosis of coronary artery disease or recognition of previous infarction can often be made from M-mode technique, usually not enough additional information is provided to be cost-justified in most ischemic heart disease patients. Two-dimensional echocardiography offers a significantly better method not only to identify the presence of ischemic or infarcted muscle but also to make quantitative estimates of the degree of damage [27, 28, 59, 60, 65, 96, 119] (Fig. 6-8).

Although a variety of techniques has been employed in attempting to quantitate the extent of ischemic or infarcted muscle, a popular method has been to merely divide the left ventricle into various segments (Fig. 6-2). By employing multiple transducer positions in the parasternal, apical, and subcostal positions tomographic imaging of all these segments of the left ventricle can be viewed repeatedly. For that reason it is possible to make quantitative assessments of segmental wall motion of these respective zones. Although only four diagrams are depicted in Figure 6-2, all other views are employed in a clinical, qualitative assessment in order to optimize visualization of the entire left ventricle.

In addition to evaluating the size of infarctions or zones of ischemia, quantitative methods can be used to assess the effects of diagnostic or treatment interventions on segmental and global function. Accordingly, these same techniques can be applied to determine left ventricular mass and the size of myocardial aneurysms. There are several problems to be faced when any quantitative method is applied to 2-D echo images; the most significant one is the inability to obtain good definition of the endocardium and epicardium in all the parasternal short axis and apical long axis views that are needed. The identification and resolution of these structures is quite variable and is influenced by the type of equipment used, the body size, and certain patient variables and, very importantly, the expertise of the echocardiographer. The border recognition of endocardium and epicardium is usually better in the parasternal short axis views than in the apical long axis views; however, the apex is usually not imaged satisfactorily from a parasternal transducer position. Timing of end diastole and end systole is critical; whereas ECG gating through the R wave satisfactorily identifies end diastole, end systole cannot be reliably identified from the electrocardiogram. A simultaneous phonocardiogram is needed in order to gate the freeze framing of end systole from the aortic closure component of the second heart sound. Other potential problems include variability in measurements secondary to intraobserver and interobserver variance as well as beat-to-beat variance (a significant problem if the patient is in atrial fibrillation since measurement of several different beats for averaging is time consuming). Another practical problem in attempting to quantitate ischemic areas or to measure the size of an infarct or aneurysm is the need for a computer to analyze wall contours, perform data reduction, and present results in a clinically usable format. Still another problem is the lack of proper standards of reference in relating the tomographic segments of the left ventricle as viewed by 2-D echo with the actual anatomy; furthermore, proper standards have not yet been established for defining normal criteria (thresholds) of segmental function for this diagnostic technique. Finally, the computer must be able to define a reference point (fixed versus floating versus hybrid system) within the left ventricular cavity in order to make the necessary measure-

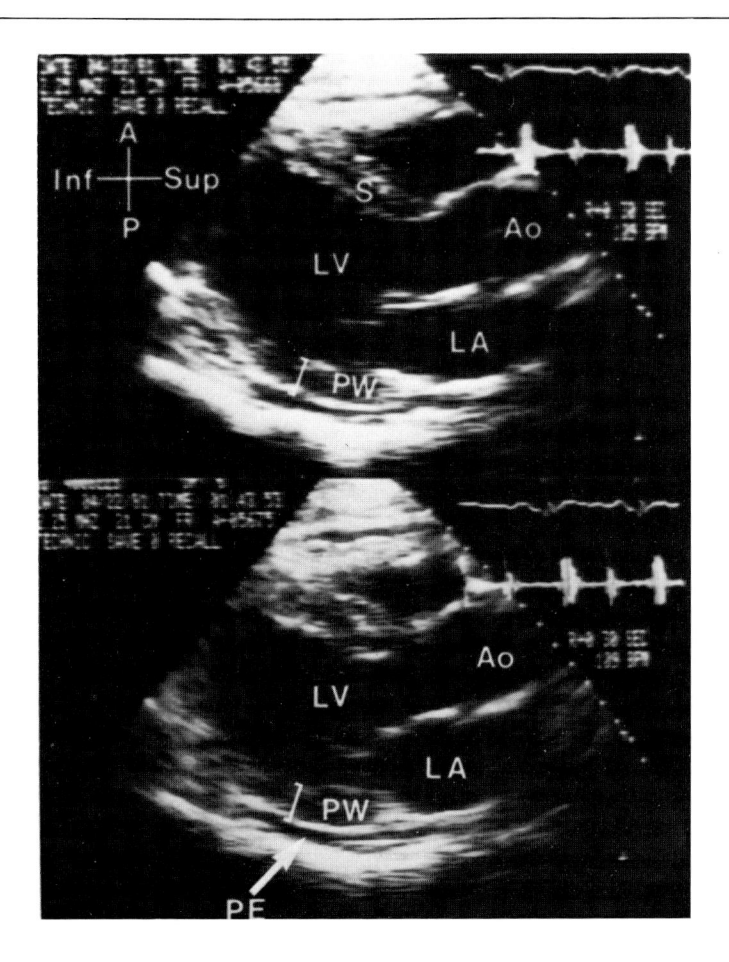

Fig. 6-8. Parasternal long axis views showing end diastole (upper panel) and end systole (lower panel) of a patient with a posterior myocardial infarction and no systolic thickening of the posterior wall. The left ventricle is mildly enlarged (end-diastolic dimension = 60 mm). A small pericardial effusion is present. A phonocardiogram showing S_1 and S_2 is present in upper right corner; freeze frame images for end systole are obtained by triggering on the aortic closure component of the second heart sound.

ments. Two additional movements of the heart may influence these quantitative efforts, namely a rotation of the left ventricle with each systole and a rocking motion caused by the shifting movement of the beating heart in the thorax.

We use four views (two parasternal and two apical) to obtain quantitative analysis of segmental and global function of the left ventricle. The endocardium and epicardium are identified manually by utilizing a computer light-pen system to quantitate segmental wall motion abnormalities in all 15 segments. Figure 6-9 demonstrates systolic and diastolic images from two of these four views in a patient with a posteromedial myocardial infarction. For demonstration purposes only the endocardial border is identified. The following parameters are determined: ejection fraction, percent fractional shortening, percent segmental area change, percent hemi-axis shortening, and percent wall thickening. Such quantitative methods enable more reliable assessment of left ventricular abnormalities following treatment interventions and for serial follow-up studies.

188   6. Coronary artery disease

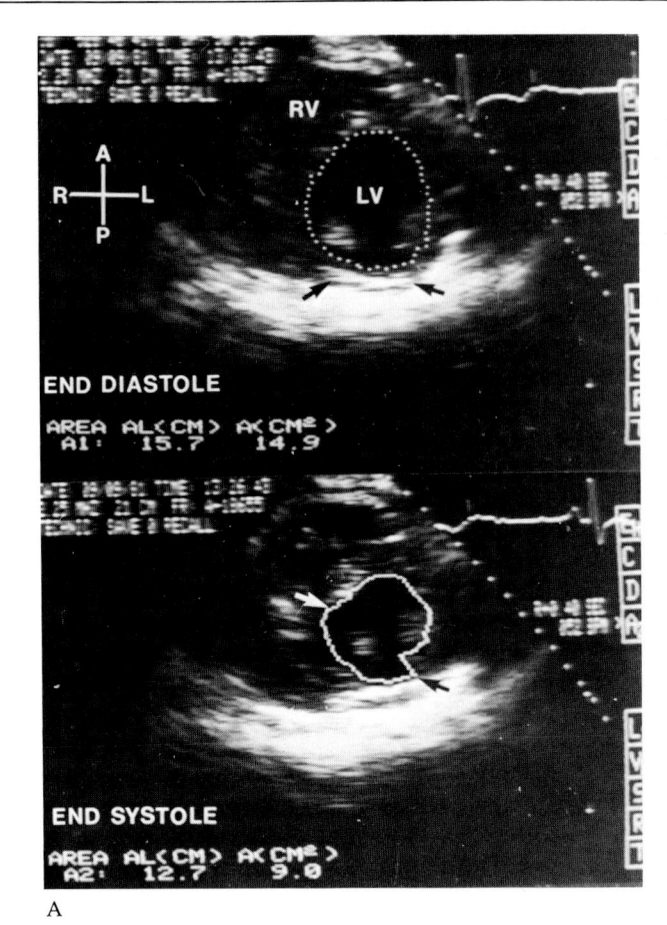

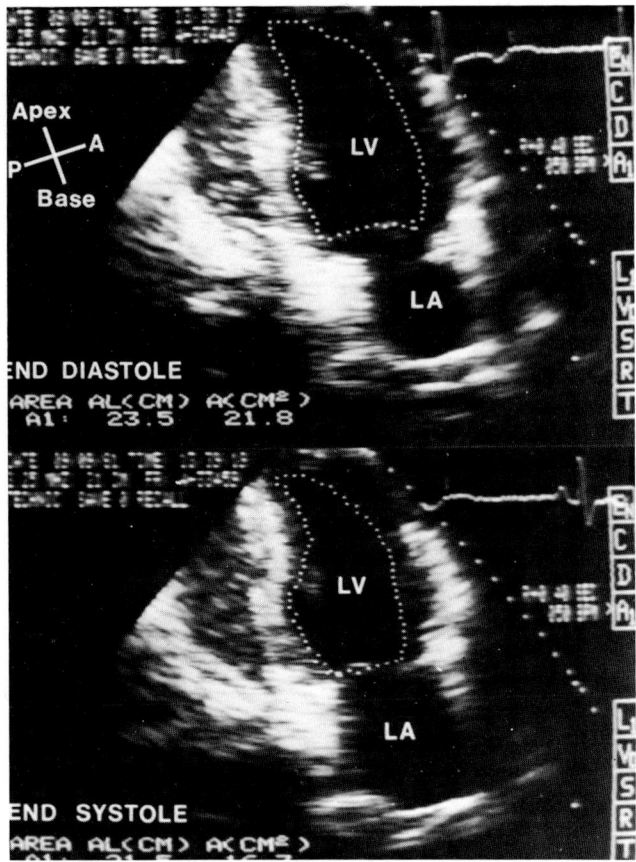

Fig. 6-9A. Parasternal short axis views at the tips of the papillary muscles in diastole (upper panel) and systole (lower panel). Scar from an old posterior (inferior) myocardial infarction is in localized area of increased reflectance (arrows) in the upper panel. The margins of the posteromedial infarct zone are identified by the arrows during systole (lower panel). The white arrow points to the posterior portion of the septum, which is also included in the infarction area. B. Apical long axis views in diastole (upper panel) and systole (lower panel) of the same patient as in A. The akinetic region extends from the posteromedial papillary muscle to the atrioventricular sulcus; the left ventricular apex contracts normally.

Complications of myocardial infarction

VENTRICULAR ANEURYSM. Ventricular aneurysm, which usually involves the apex, is one of the most common complications of myocardial infarction. Since it is usually not possible to image the left ventricular apex by M-mode echocardiography, the diagnosis of aneurysm is rarely made by M-mode echocardiography. Because of the ability to image tomographically through the apex of the left ventricle from various transducer positions, two-dimensional echocardiography is well suited for the recognition of left ventricular aneurysms [120–122] (Fig. 6-10). Aneurysms may involve any segment of the left ventricle (Fig. 6-11). Aneurysms in the posterobasilar region must be distinguished from false or pseudoaneurysms (Fig. 6-12).

Two-dimensional echocardiography provides a better quantitative method than was ever possible with M-mode techniques to judge the amount of normal muscle in patients with aneurysms [121, 122]. Several studies have demonstrated that two-dimensional echocardiographic technique can reliably assess the amount of remaining normal muscle and thus predict the surgical outcome of aneurysmectomy [123]. Other studies have shown that the amount of functional residual myocardium is very important in predicting a favorable surgical outcome [124, 125].

Accordingly, two-dimensional echocardiography has become an extremely important diagnostic tool for both detection and overall evaluation of patients with ventricular aneurysms. Watson and associates [126] proposed a hemispheral ejection fraction to predict those patients likely to benefit from surgical intervention. Lee and associates [127] used the spherical model to calculate excess and angiographic ejection fraction, which was combined with a coronary jeopardy score to stratify patients into high- and low-risk groups. Both of these methods are derived from the right anterior oblique angiographic view alone and therefore do not account for residual myocardium in the interventricular septum and posterolateral wall.

Barrett and associates [122] showed that the index of residual myocardium as determined by two-dimensional echocardiography reliably predicted the six-month mortality of patients with aneurysm, thus identifying a high-risk group of patients in whom aggressive management should be considered. These investigators further showed that aneurysmectomy can be successful in patients with as little as 42 percent of the myocardium contracting normally.

PSEUDOANEURYSM. False or pseudoaneurysm of the left ventricle is a rare form of aneurysm that develops following rupture of a recently infarcted segment of the myocardial wall with perforation through the endocardium and myocardium forming a localized hemopericardium confined by adherent parietal pericardium. Pathologically there is a small, narrow channel connecting the ventricle with a large sac consisting of clot and fibrinous pericardial tissue without any myocardial elements [128]. Clinically both true and false aneurysms may be complicated by systemic emboli, arrhythmias, and congestive heart failure. However, pseudoaneurysms are distinguished from true ventricular aneurysms by their marked tendency for rupture [129, 130]. Clinical features may also include an abnormal bifid precordial impulse and an apical systolic murmur, which may mimic mitral regurgitation [131–133].

Two-dimensional echocardiography is ideally suited to delineating the gross anatomic features of a pseudoaneurysm [134–136]. The 2-D characteristics of false

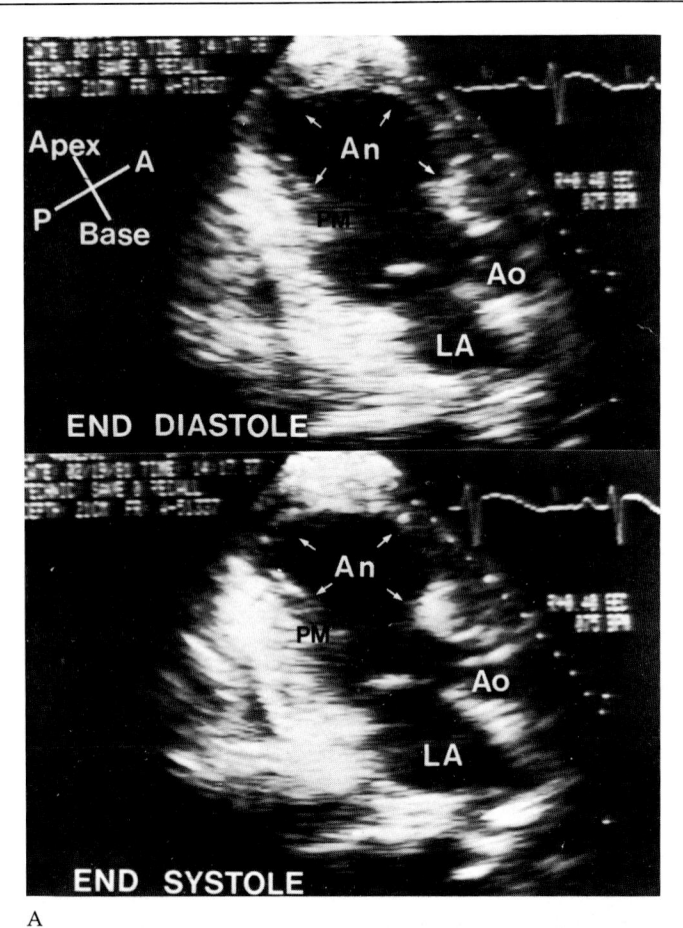

Fig. 6-10A. Apical long axis views showing a large apical aneurysm (An) in diastole (upper panel) and systole (lower panel). B. Apical 4-chamber view showing a very large apical aneurysm with a scarred, thin left ventricular apical wall. C. Apical 4-chamber section of same anatomy as shown in B. Left ventricle is markedly dilated with extensive scarring and wall thinning (arrow) of the apex. PM = posteromedial papillary muscle.

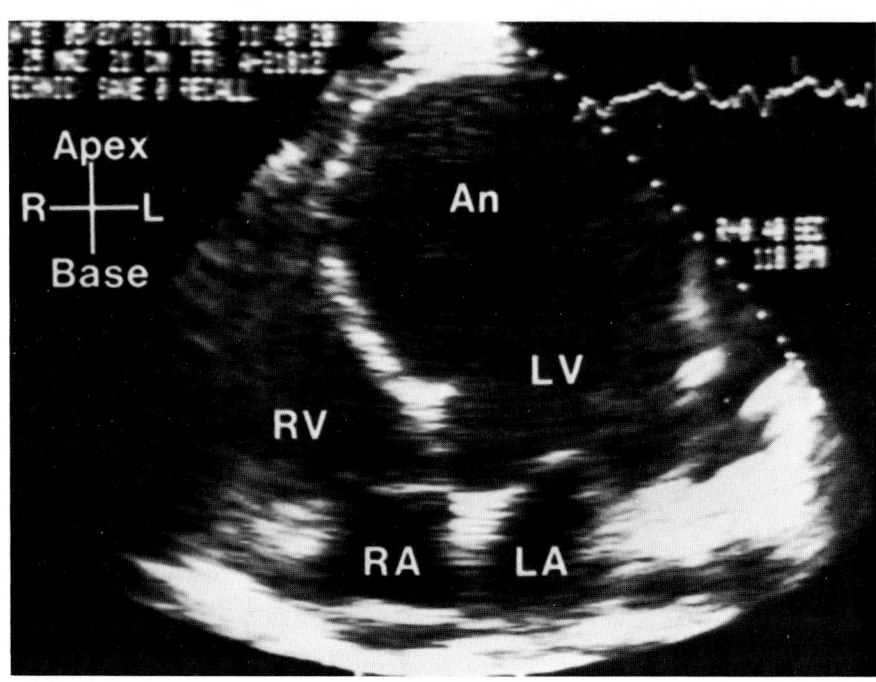

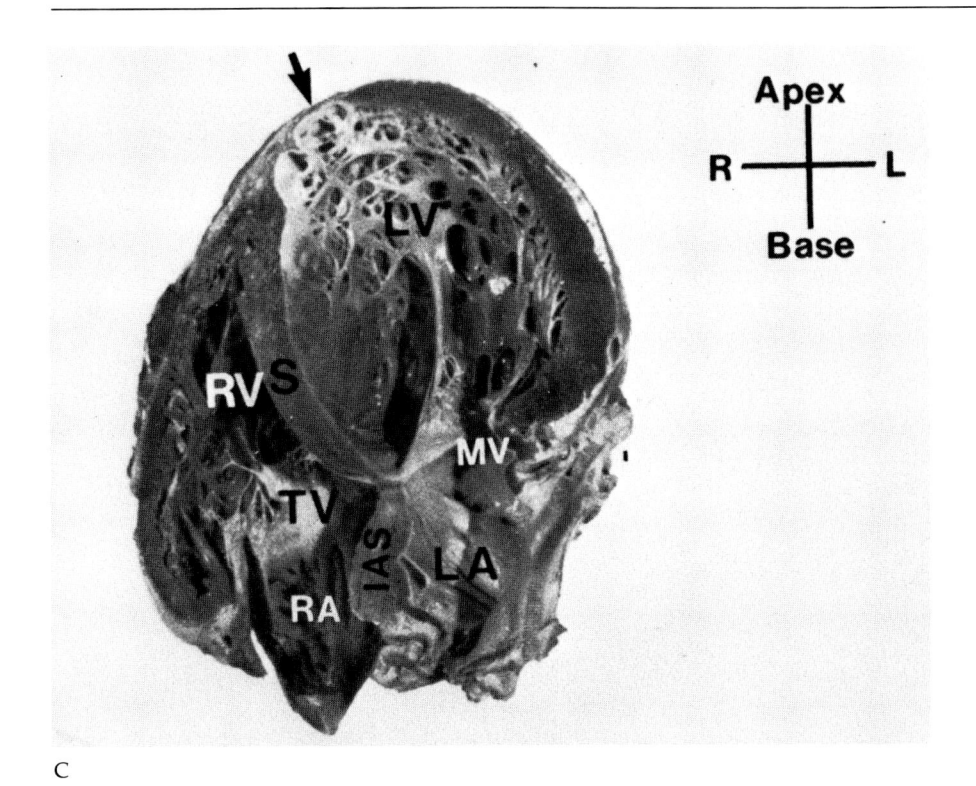

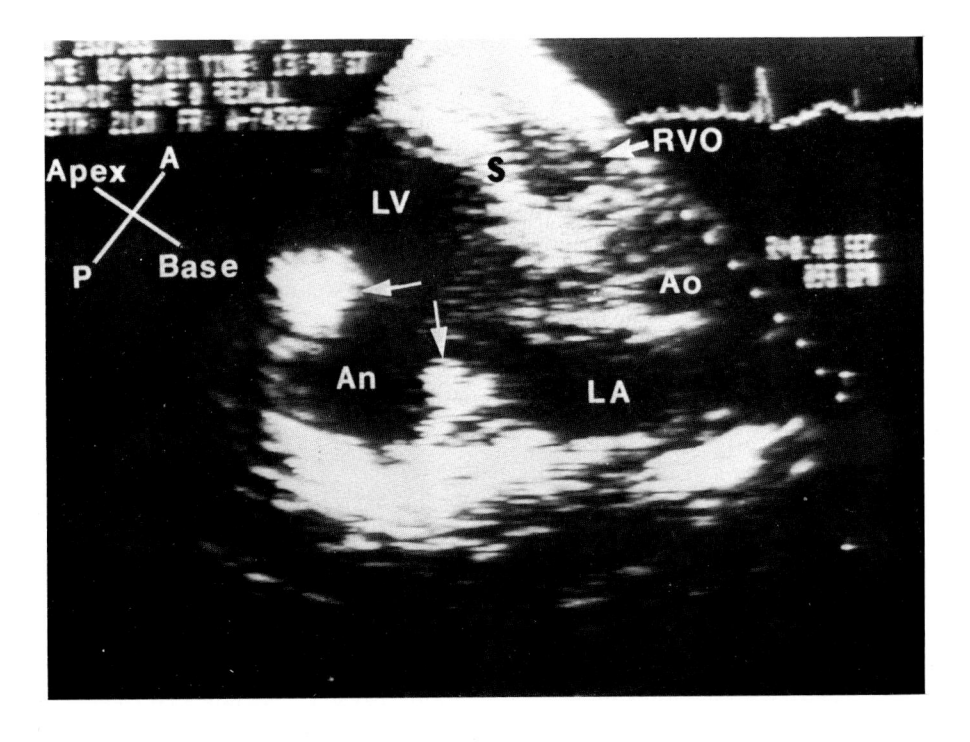

Fig. 6-11. Parasternal long axis view showing an aneurysm (An) of the posterior basilar segment of the left ventricle. Other views demonstrated some involvement of the posterolateral wall but the posterior septum was spared. The opening or neck (arrows) of the aneurysm measured 3 cm in diameter excluding a false or pseudoaneurysm, which had been the angiographic diagnosis prior to the 2-D echo study. At surgery the A–P depth of the aneurysm was greater than the echo appearance because the posterior wall was covered with 2 to 3 cm of mural thrombus.

192   6. Coronary artery disease

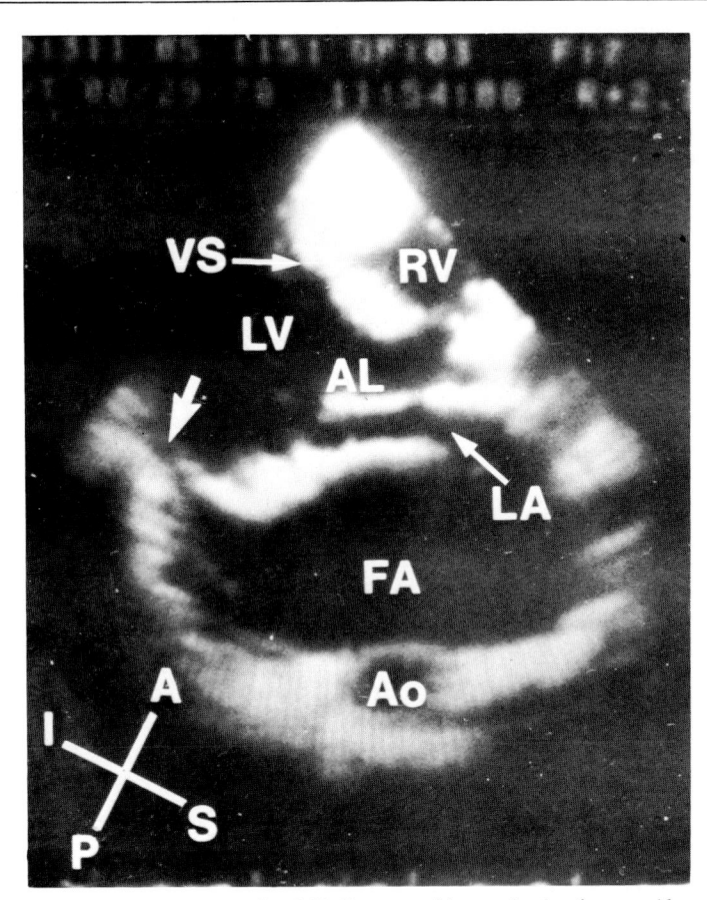

Fig. 6-12. Parasternal long axis view from a middle-age man who suffered an acute posterior myocardial infarction five days before this 2-D echo examination was performed. The white arrow within the left ventricle is pointing to the rupture site within a concave, aneurysmal area of the posterior wall, the site of the recent infarction. This rupture site communicates with the large false aneurysm (FA), which is posterior to and compressing the left atrium and entire heart anterior. The right ventricle was compressed against the anterior chest wall. The FA measured approximately 7 cm in A–P dimension, slightly larger than the short axis dimension of the left ventricle. The very narrow neck of the aneurysm identifies it as a false aneurysm. VS = interventricular septum; Ao = descending aorta.

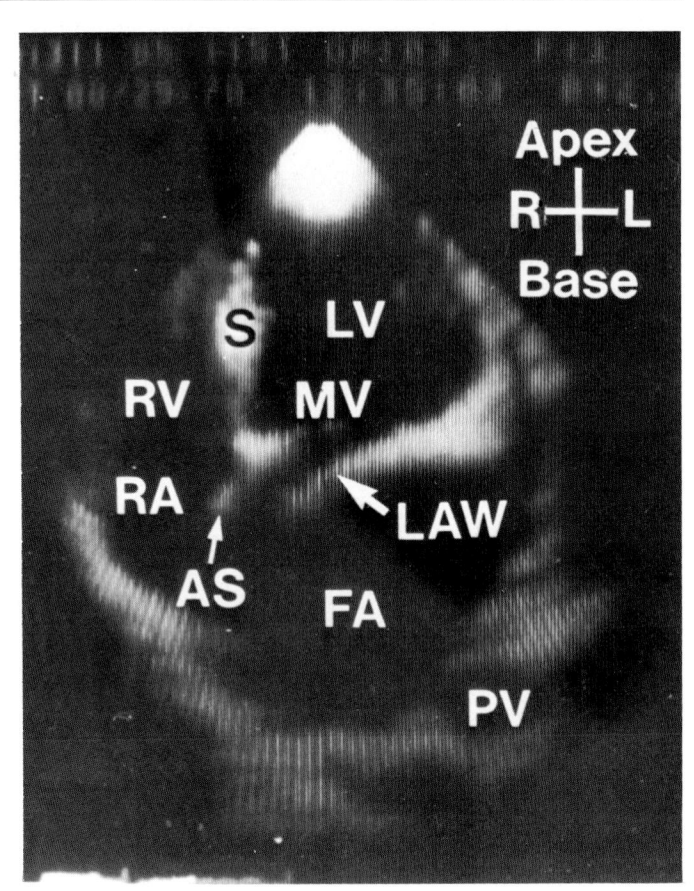

Fig. 6-13. Apical 4-chamber view of same patient as in Fig. 6-12 showing displacement of left atrial wall (LAW) and interatrial septum (AS) by the large false aneurysm (FA). It is difficult to determine right ventricular size in this view; however, it was markedly compressed in an A–P dimension with no evidence of pericardial effusion surrounding either right ventricle or right atrium. The pulmonary vein (PV) was dilated owing to compression from the massive false aneurysm.

aneurysm include (1) sharp discontinuity of the endocardial image at the site of the pseudoaneurysm communication with the left ventricular cavity; (2) a saccular or global contour of the false aneurysmal chamber; (3) the presence of a narrow orifice compared with the diameter of the pseudoaneurysm; and (4) occasional displacement of other cardiac chambers or compression of the right ventricle (Fig. 6-13).

LEFT VENTRICULAR THROMBUS. A mural thrombus represents an important, potentially dangerous complication of acute myocardial infarction. Left ventricular thrombi have been detected in 20 to 60 percent of patients at autopsy following transmural infarction [137, 138]. In the presence of left ventricular aneurysm the incidence of mural thrombi is reported between 44 and 78 percent as documented at autopsy or cardiac surgery [139–141].

Although many embolic events may be clinically silent, particularly those in the spleen or kidneys [142], systemic emboli caused or contributed to death in 12 to 33 percent of autopsy patients with myocardial infarction or left ventricular aneurysm [140, 143]. Clinically diagnosed systemic emboli occurred in 2 to 12 percent of patients following acute myocardial infarction [142–145].

Two-dimensional echocardiography is a sensitive method for identifying left ventricular thrombi and is probably superior to left ventricular angiography in diagnosing small clots [146–152]. Reeder and colleagues [152] reported two-dimensional echocardiographic and clinical features of 60 patients with left ventricular thrombi and observed superior predictive accuracy of two-dimensional echocardiography (79%) versus biplane angiography (57%) in detecting left ventricular thrombus. In another study Reeder and associates [153] reported that in 100 consecutive patients with left ventricular aneurysm operated on at the Mayo Clinic preoperative angiography correctly identified thrombus with a sensitivity of only 31 percent and a predictive accuracy of only 54 percent.

There is a high incidence of congestive heart failure in patients with associated left ventricular thrombi [138]. Reeder and coworkers [152] reported that physical examination, chest x-ray, and electrocardiography were not sensitive to or predictive of the presence of thrombus. The thrombi visualized in their study were rarely mobile and were typically found in the apex. Furthermore, these authors noted that the incidence of large thrombi was higher in patients with congestive cardiomyopathy than in patients with coronary artery disease and believed it to be related to more serious generalized reduction of left ventricular function in that group. There are currently no proven diagnostic techniques that reliably predict risk of embolization from intracardiac thrombi.

Drobac and colleagues [147] studied four different types of clots in cadaveric left ventricles, including fibrin, whole blood, platelet, and organized thrombus, and observed that two-dimensional echocardiography was able to detect all clots regardless of composition and could visualize clots as small as 2 mm in diameter.

Although the echocardiographic features of a left ventricular thrombus may be characteristic, there are instances in which these features are not specific or the quality of the images is suboptimal; hence the examination is not diagnostic (Fig. 6-14). Asinger and associates [150] have recommended using a grading scale to indicate index of suspicion for left ventricular thrombus: Class 0 = thrombus definitely not present, technically good examination; Class 1 = definite left ventricular echo mass but probably not thrombus, examination technically not good enough to classify as 0 (probably represents cardiac structure other than thrombus); Class 2 =

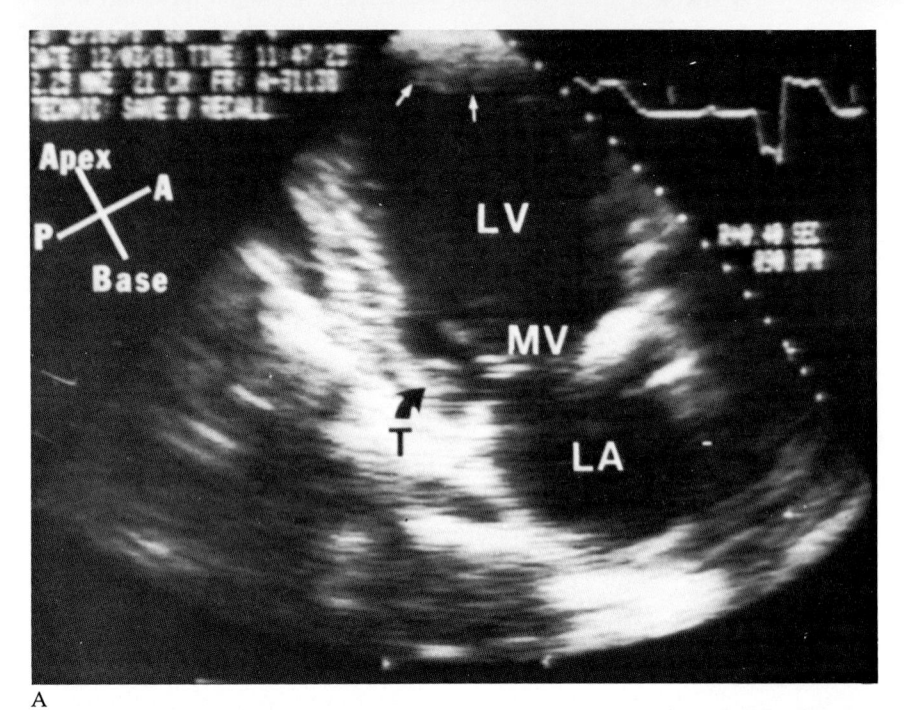

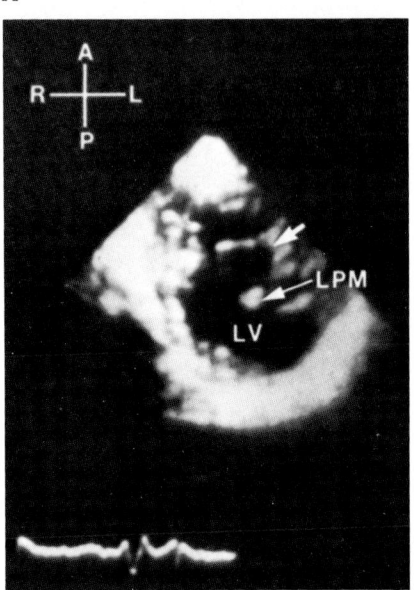

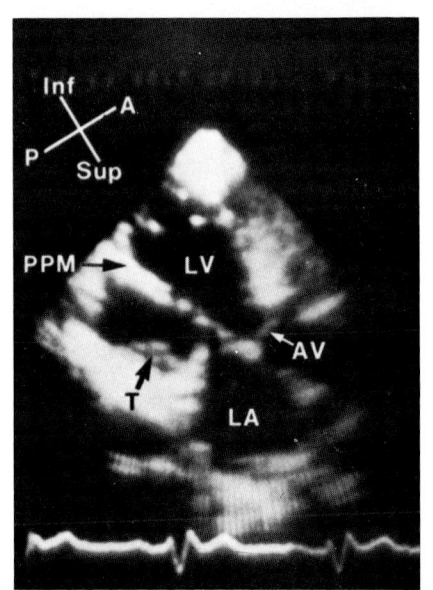

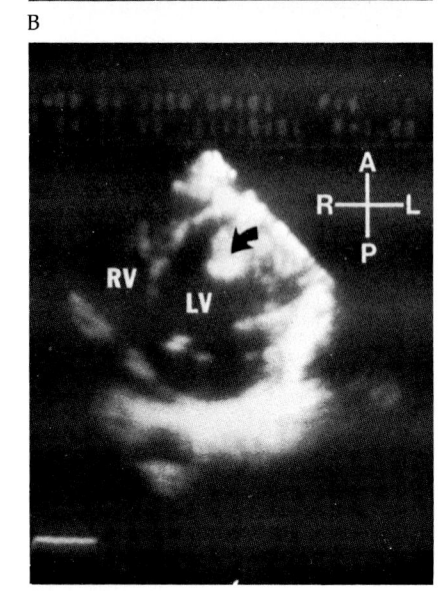

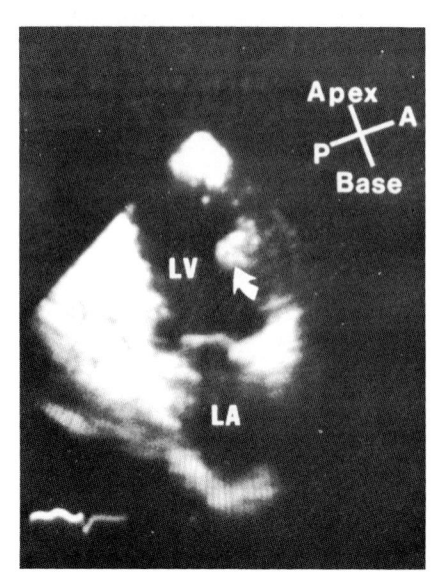

Fig. 6-14A. Apical long axis view in a patient with previous anterior and posterior myocardial infarctions showing a small but distinct mass extending from the endocardial surface of the akinetic posterior-basilar wall indicative of a thrombus (T). The anteroapical region of the left ventricle reveals some apparent increased reflectances (white arrows); however, the apex is not sufficiently outlined to distinguish whether these echo targets are generated by a thrombus or by reflectances from an oblique plane through a scarred apical wall. B. Low left sternal border parasternal short axis (left panel) and long axis (right panel) views in a patient with severe coronary artery disease and previous myocardial infarctions. The left panel shows the anterolateral papillary muscle (LPM) and some additional strong reflectances (arrow) within an obvious infarct zone, but it is not certain whether thrombus is present; the recordings are suggestive but not diagnostic. The right panel shows a prominent, scarred posteromedial papillary muscle (PPM) and a distinct mass visible in several views that represents a thrombus (T) adherent to the infarcted posterior-basilar wall. C. Low sternal border parasternal short axis view (left panel) and an apical long axis view (right panel) of the same patient demonstrating a large thrombus (arrows) attached to an akinetic anterolateral wall. Any target suggestive of mass or thrombus should be reproducible in two tomographic planes 90° to each other to confirm whether the target is an actual mass.

definite abnormality of uncertain nature; Class 3 = findings highly suspicious for thrombus, examination technically not adequate to classify as diagnostic; Class 4 = findings characteristic of thrombus, technically good or adequate examination.

Wall thickness should be carefully assessed, particularly in the setting of left ventricular aneurysm; since the walls of a discrete aneurysm are usually thin, the finding of normal wall thickness in an aneurysmal segment should raise the suspicion of mural thrombus [146]. Another difficulty in identifying thrombus relates to the width of the ultrasonic beam, which may cause the image from an adjacent structure or within the myocardium to be reflected as if it were within the left ventricular cavity. These spurious echoes are commonly encountered when extensive scarring from previous infarction(s) or calcification in the myocardium or coronary arteries is present. These dense echoes can simulate the margins of a thrombus. In order to distinguish these echoes as artifacts it is very important to obtain multiple apical views to confirm apical contour and anatomy. Individual thrombi may have heterogeneous areas of echo density that occasionally give the appearance of a layered pattern. When a layered pattern is observed the most echo-dense portion of the left ventricular thrombus is usually along the intracavitary margin [150]. Furthermore, variations noted in serial observations of patients with abnormal reflectances suggesting mass have been helpful in identifying the mass as thrombus versus artifact [150, 154]. In our experience the presence of thrombus in the left ventricle is always associated with wall motion abnormalities. The features of left ventricular thrombus which can be observed with multiple two-dimensional echocardiographic views are as follows (Fig. 6-15): (1) associated wall motion abnormality; (2) left ventricular apex the most common location; (3) distinct thrombus margin that disrupts the continuity of the endocardial echo; (4) apparent increase in the thickness of the left ventricular wall caused by the thrombus; (5) occasional free motion of the intracavitary thrombus; (6) thrombus acoustically distinct from the underlying left ventricular wall. Variations may be noted on serial echocardiographic examinations.

Serial follow-up examinations in the postoperative period following excision of the aneurysm and removal of the thrombus are helpful (Fig. 6-16).

False positive diagnosis of a left ventricular thrombus may occur from incomplete or faulty imaging technique or from incorrect identification of other structures within the left ventricular apex. The apical views are by far the most useful in diagnosing left ventricular thrombi. Since the apex is only a few centimeters from the source of ultrasound in the apical views, near-field artifact must be minimized. Spurious intracavitary echoes caused by structures outside the main axis of the ultrasonic beam may also cause interpretive difficulty [155]. This problem can usually be eliminated by obtaining multiple tomographic views of the area in question.

Although recognition of papillary muscles is not difficult, if they are involved in zones of infarction with resultant scarring and fibrosis they may become very prominent in appearance, and it may be difficult to distinguish whether mural thrombus extends from the aneurysm to include a portion of one or both papillary muscles (Fig. 6-17). Imaging from the apex with posterior angulation of the transducer causes the walls to appear thicker and, if scarring exists in the left ventricular apex from previous infarction, the combination of these bright targets together with a tangential view through the wall and papillary muscle may simulate a mass protruding into the left ventricular cavity and be confused with a left ventricular thrombus.

196   6. Coronary artery disease

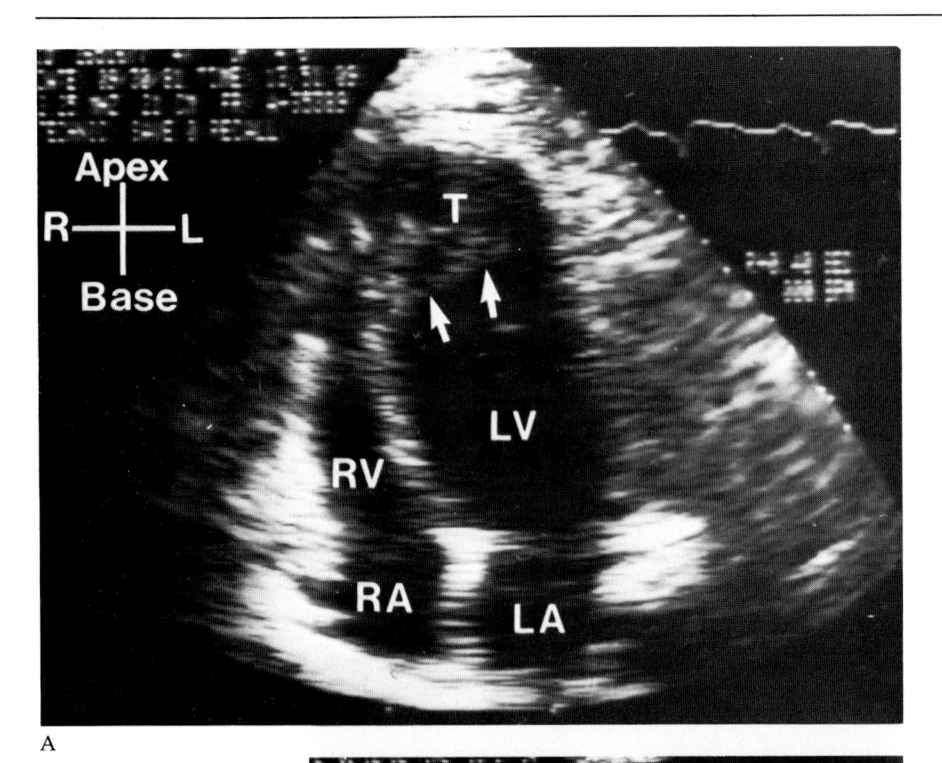

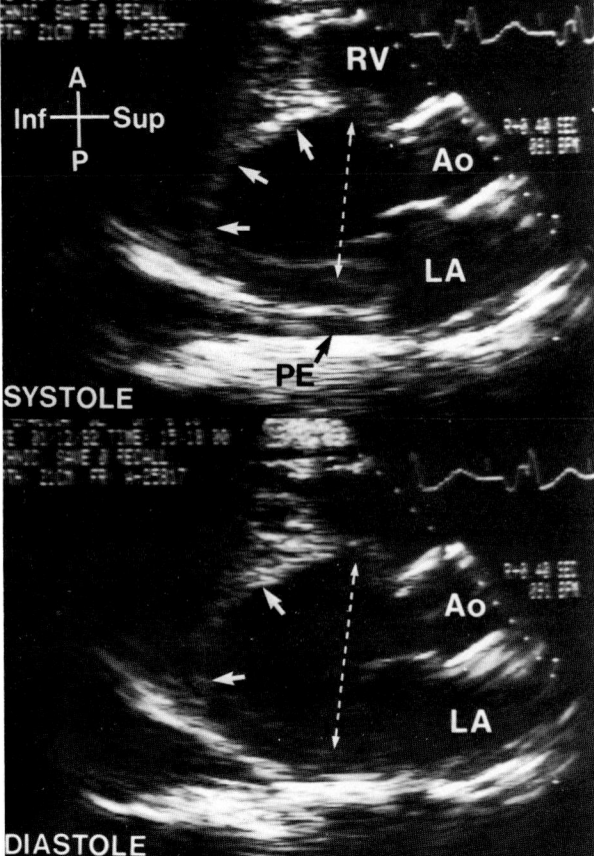

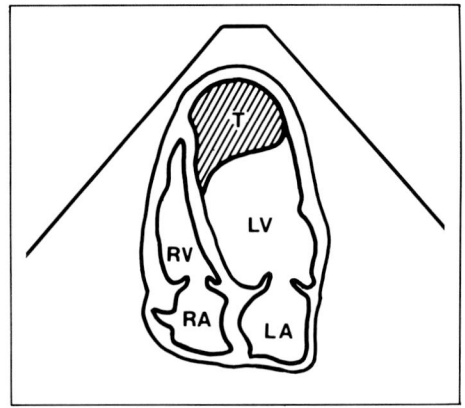

Fig. 6-15A. Apical 4-chamber view from a patient with a recent anterior-apical infarction and a large apical thrombus (T). B. Diagrammatic representation of A showing apical thrombus. C. Parasternal long axis views in systole (upper panel) and diastole (lower panel) of a patient with a huge apical thrombus extending up the anterior septum within 27 mm of the aortic valve. The end-diastolic diameter at the base measures 74 mm (dashed line of lower panel); that dimension is 60 mm at end systole (upper panel). The white arrows in both panels identify the superior margin of the thrombus; the apex is not visualized in these views. A pericardial effusion (PE) is present. D. Apical 4-chamber views during systole (upper panel) and diastole (lower panel) of the same patient as in C showing the large apical thrombus and a distinct enclosed area (white arrows) within the distal region of the thrombus that appears to be a liquified area. No significant change in the systolic and diastolic dimensions (dashed white lines) are noted in this tomographic plane through the base of the left ventricle. Although more than half the LV cavity is filled with thrombus, the superior margin of the thrombus adjacent to posterior septum is 50 mm from the aortic annulus compared to 27 mm of thrombus overlying the anterior septum (compare with C). Pericardial effusion is observed along the lateral wall of the left ventricle. E. Apical 4-chamber views of same patient as in C and D showing an irregular layer which is more echo-dense (arrows) than the thrombus in the upper panel. In real-time the dyskinetic motion of the apex was very conspicuous. An acoustically distinct narrow layer between thrombus and lateral wall of the LV (small white arrows) is present in the lower panel and suggests that the thrombus may have been loosely attached to the thin, scarred LV wall at that point. Another dense target involving the pericardium of the lateral LV wall (open arrows) noted in the lower panel may represent a site of inflammatory reaction secondary to Dressler's syndrome or a mass of unknown etiology.

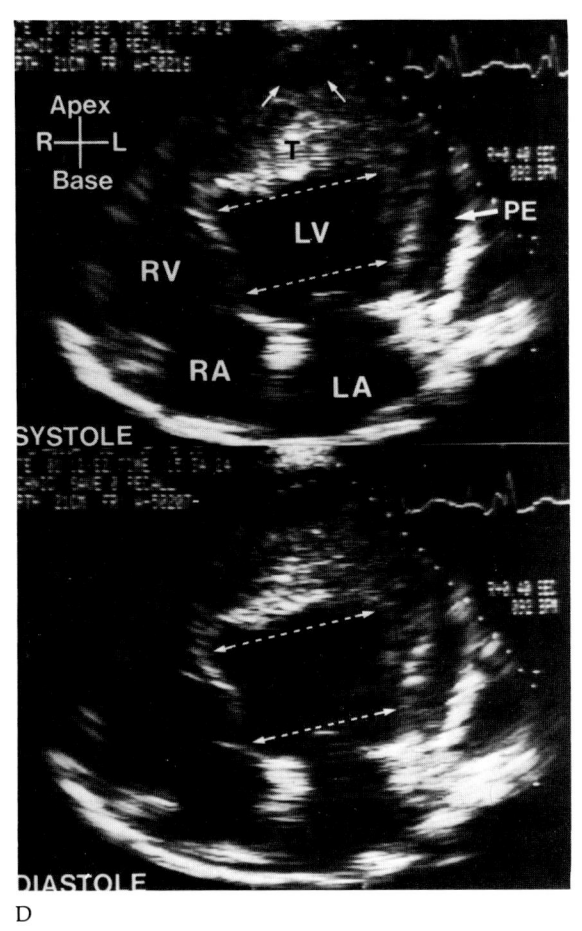

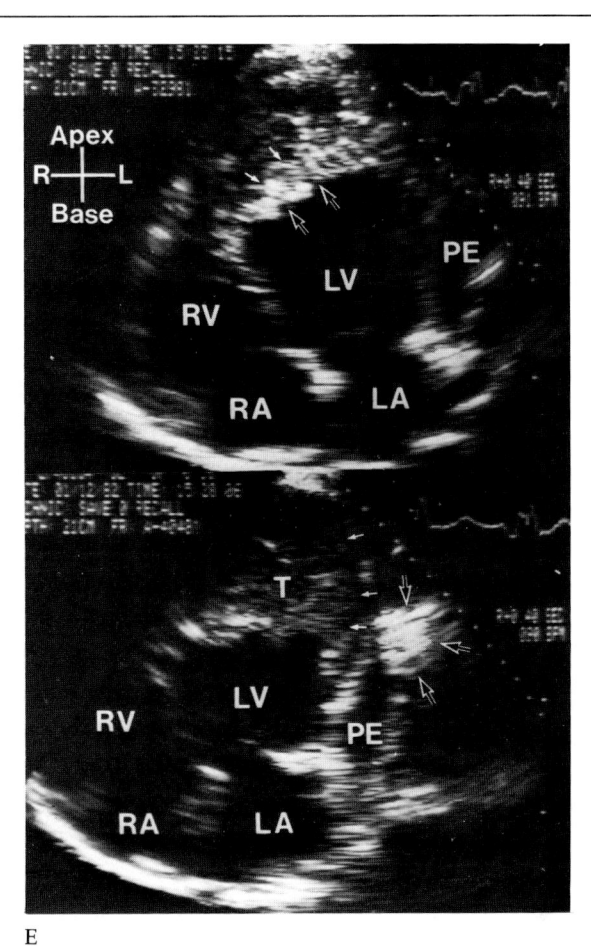

D

E

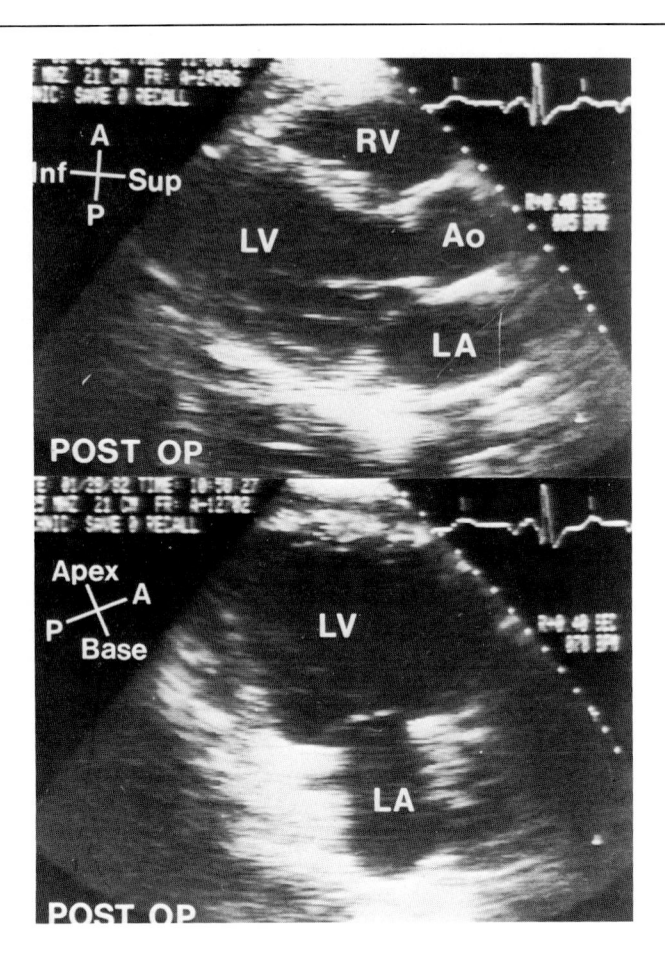

Fig. 6-16. Parasternal long axis and apical long axis views recorded 17 days later in same patient as in Fig. 6-15C–E following surgical removal of the thrombus and portion of the apical aneurysm. The long axis dimension of the left ventricle measured 117 mm preoperatively compared to 80 mm postoperatively (lower panel). The apex appears very blunted because of LV dilatation and the true apex has been excised. The anteroapical wall (lower panel) appears thickened and probably represents some recurrent thrombus overlying the suture site. Function of the LV is improved and the patient did well in the postoperative period. Notice that the inferosuperior dimension of the left atrium is 20 mm longer than the anteroposterior dimension and probably represents slight LA enlargement.

Heavy trabeculations in the apex, particularly in patients who have left ventricular hypertrophy, may present further confusion because of prominent targets; however, in the absence of any associated wall motion abnormality this should not be a diagnostic problem.

A fresh thrombus with an irregular surface is easily distinguished from the adjacent endocardium; however, when the thrombus becomes endothelialized the surface is smooth and may not be distinct from the adjacent endocardium, particularly since the surrounding endocardium is usually fibrotic and produces prominent echo reflectances (Fig. 6-18).

Ectopic chordae or muscle bridging is very commonly seen and is recognized by a thin, discrete reflectance extending from one wall to another. These thin structures resemble chordae tendineae and are attached at each end to either muscle trabeculations or papillary muscles but are not attached to the mitral valve (Fig. 6-19). These structures have a characteristic appearance on 2-D echo and should never be confused with a mass, thrombus, or abnormality. They may be observed to move or "buckle" as the cavity of the left ventricle becomes smaller with systole (Fig. 6-20). When these structures are recorded by M-mode echo they resemble a band or membrane and if located near the base of the left ventricle the flow turbulence of rapid filling during early diastole may cause a fluttering motion (Fig. 6-21).

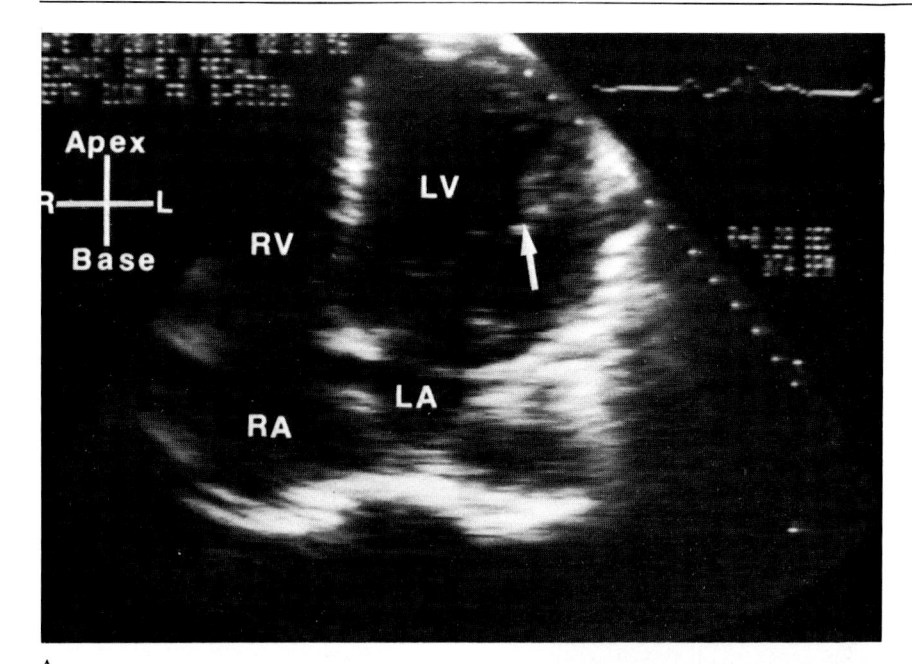

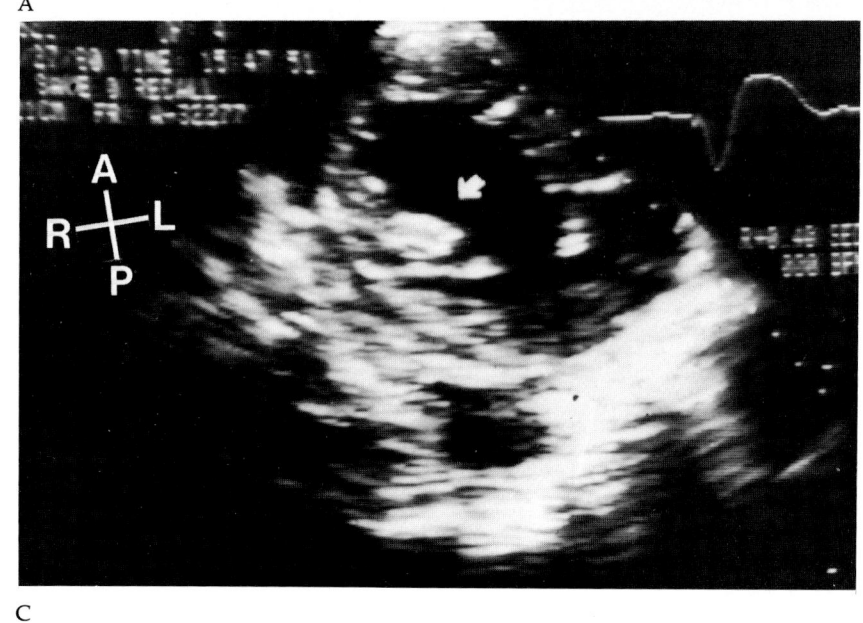

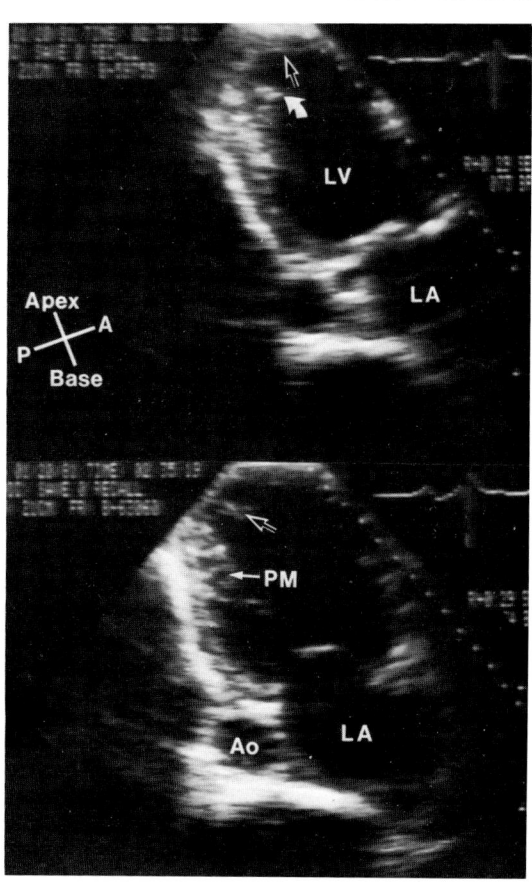

Fig. 6-17A. Apical 4-chamber view showing prominent anterolateral papillary muscle (arrow) within the infarct zone of the left ventricle. B. Apical long axis views showing prominent bulge in the distal (apical) aspect of the posteromedial papillary muscle (solid arrow, upper panel). The open arrow (upper panel) points to an area in the LV apex suggestive of additional thrombus. The apical long axis view in the same patient in the lower panel shows a normal-appearing papillary muscle with a linear target in the apex (open arrow), which is probably caused by a scarred trabeculation and does not appear to be a thrombus. The ventricle is enlarged and functions poorly. C. Oblique apical short axis view showing a prominent target (arrow), which is a normal papillary muscle. The left ventricular walls appear thick because of the tangential angle of the tomographic image.

200   6. Coronary artery disease

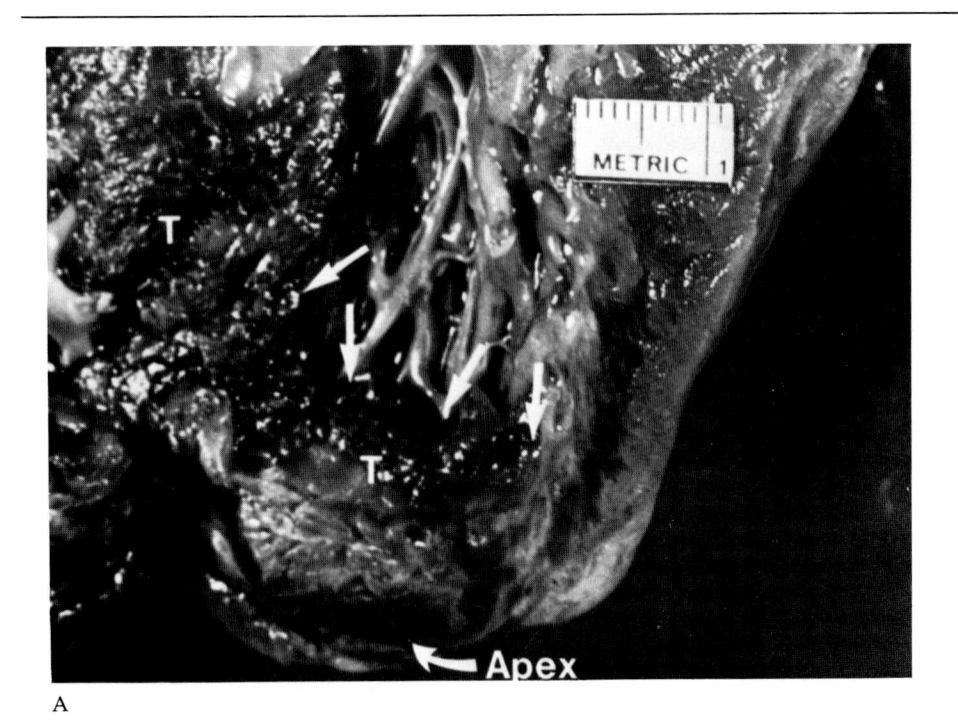

Fig. 6-18A. Large thrombus (T) secondary to an apical infarction in postmortem specimen showing irregular margins of thrombus overlying endocardium (arrows). B. Anatomic short axis section at level of chordae tendineae showing mural thrombus (MT), which is endothelialized and firmly adherent to the underlying scarred posterior wall and posterior portion of the interventricular septum. The arrows identify the margins of the thrombus. AW = anterior wall; LW = lateral wall. C. Anatomic short axis section looking into the apex, which is completely infarcted, showing thin scar but no muscle in the posterior wall (PW). The black arrow shows the margin of scar and myocardium. Because of the aneurysm and extensive scarring with superimposed mural thrombus (T), the relationship of the anterolateral (ALPM) and posteromedial (PMPM) papillary muscles is distorted and unusually distant from the interventricular septum. D. Anatomic short axis section showing left ventricular apex and large apical-lateral aneurysm filled with thrombus. The right ventricle is anterior, and a portion of the posteromedial papillary muscle (PPM) is present.

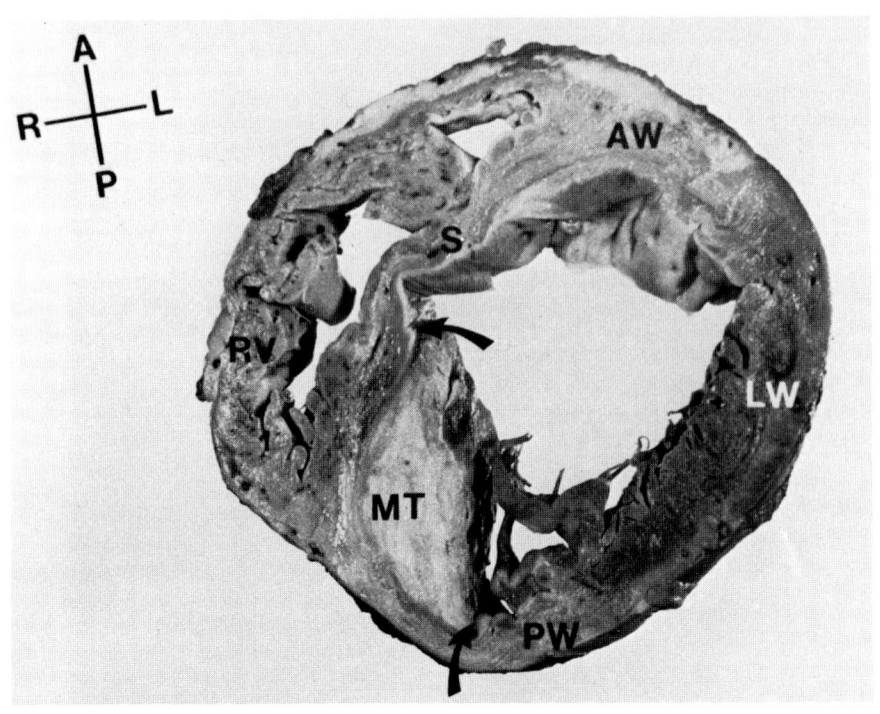

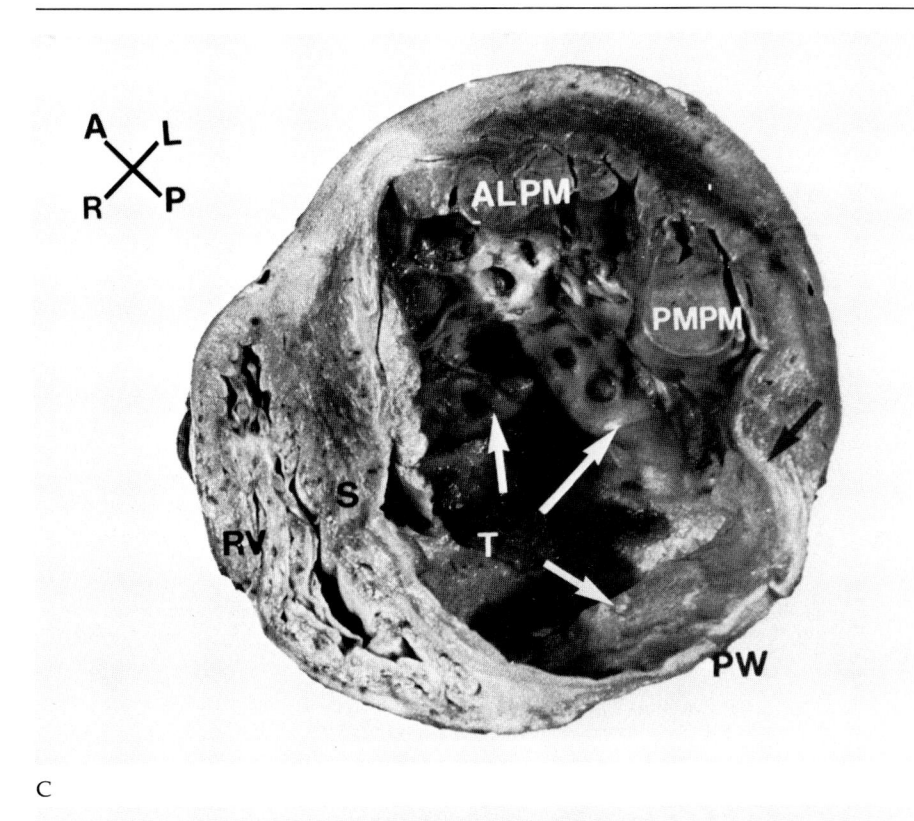

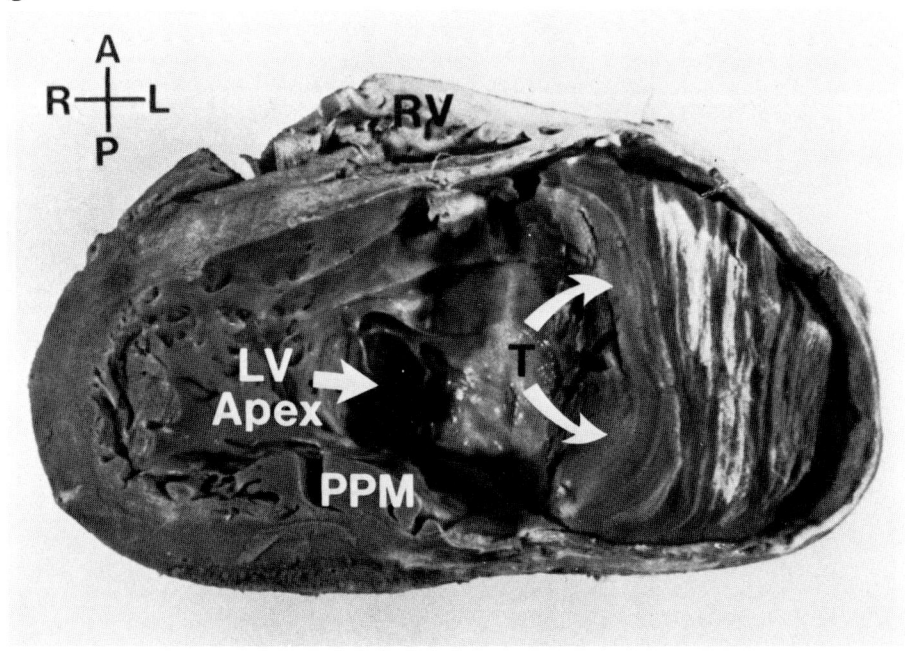

C

D

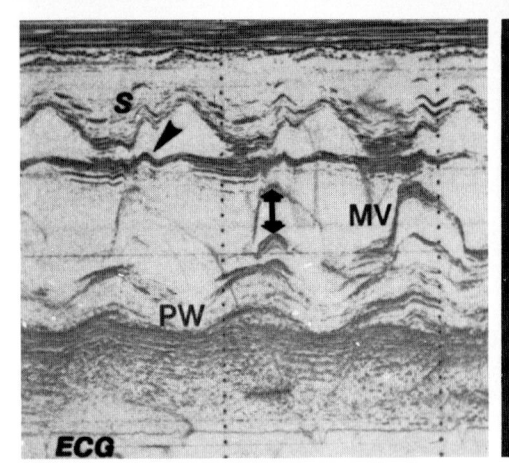

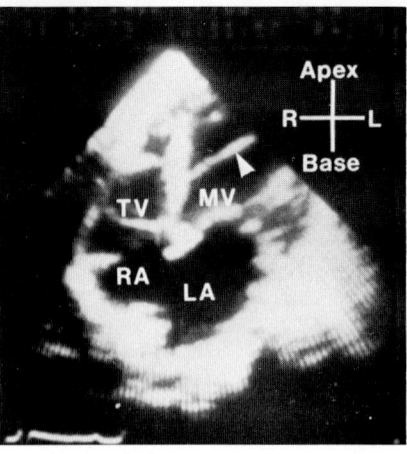

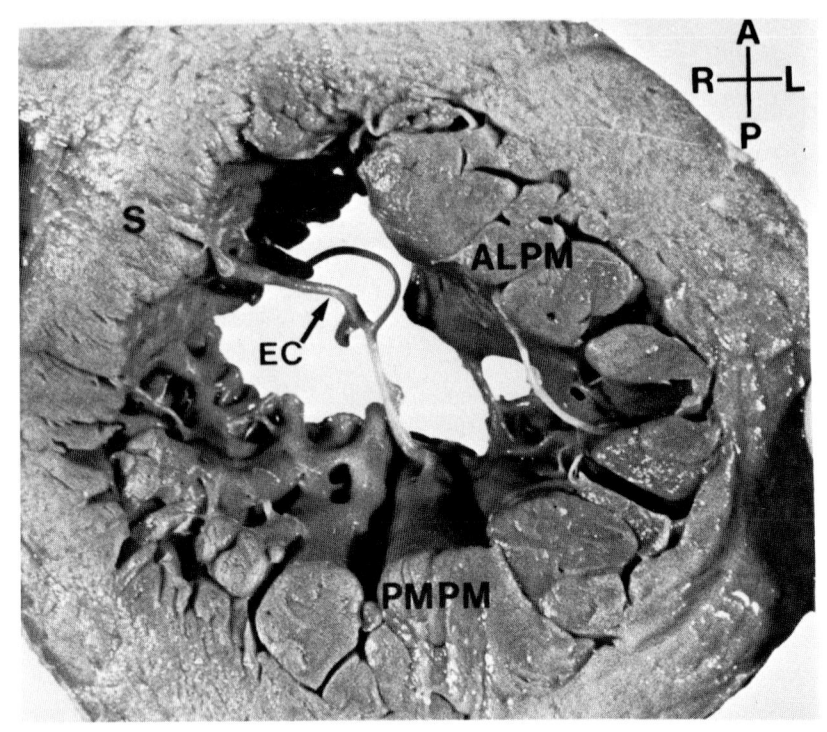

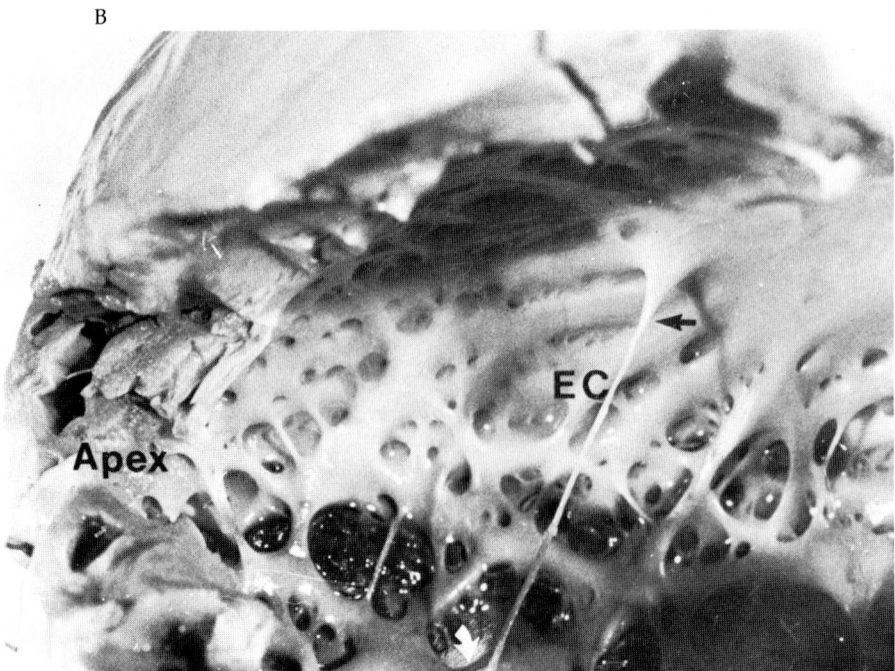

Fig. 6-19A. M-mode recording (left panel) *shows abnormal mitral valve with motion changes typical of mitral stenosis and a horizontal, membranelike structure (arrow) near the left side of the interventricular septum. The apical 4-chamber view* (right panel) *from the same patient shows the same reflectance (arrow) extending from the septum to the lateral wall of the left ventricle; it is caused by an ectopic chordae. Left atrial enlargement is present due to mitral stenosis. B. Short axis anatomic section showing an ectopic chordae (EC) extending from the interventricular septum to the opposite wall near the posteromedial papillary muscle (PMPM). C. Close-up view looking into the left ventricular cavity showing an ectopic chordae (EC) extending from the anterior wall (black arrow) to the posterior wall (white arrow). The LV apex is to the left and the base of the heart is to the right. ALPM = anterolateral papillary muscle; PW = posterior wall.*

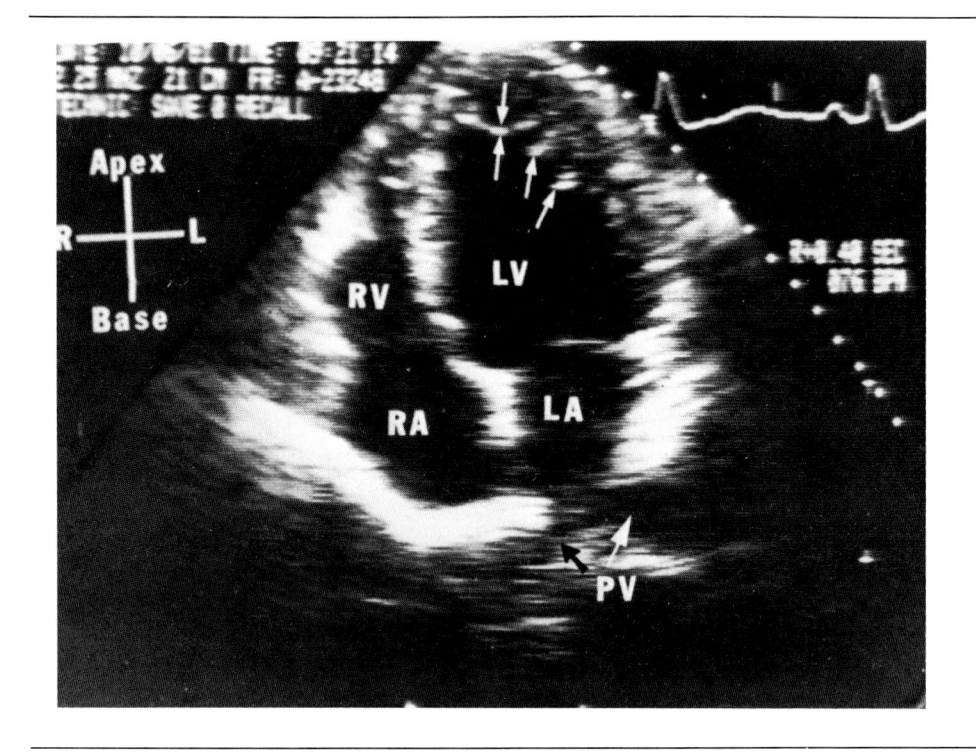

Fig. 6-20. Apical 4-chamber view of a normal subject showing an ectopic chordae "buckling" with systole (arrows). The other two white arrows point to reflectances from normal muscle trabeculations of the apical-lateral wall of the left ventricle. PV = pulmonary veins.

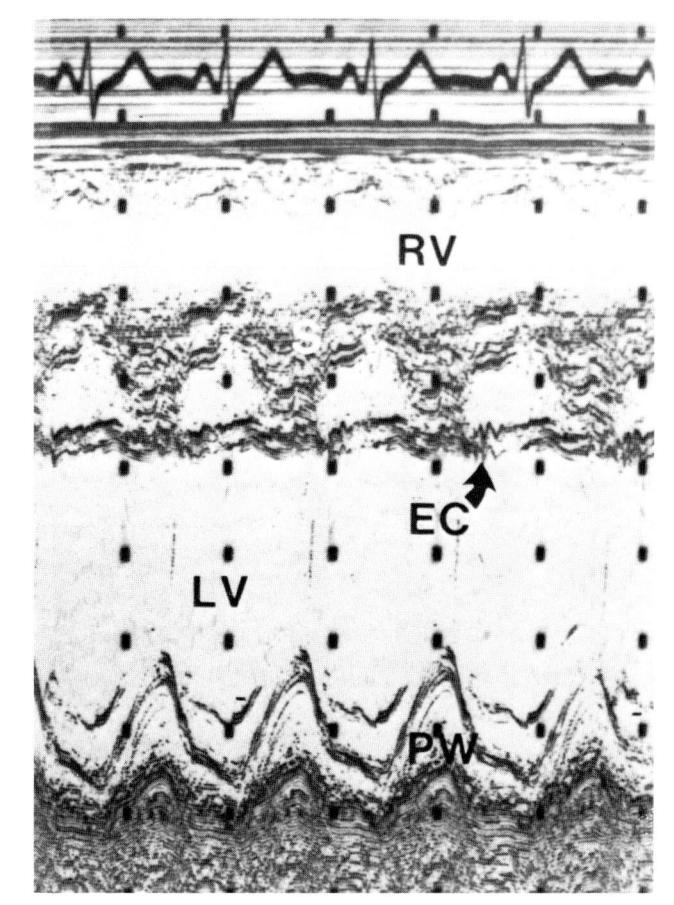

Fig. 6-21. M-mode recording in a normal adult with ectopic chordae (EC) showing brief fluttering. PW = posterior wall.

204 6. Coronary artery disease

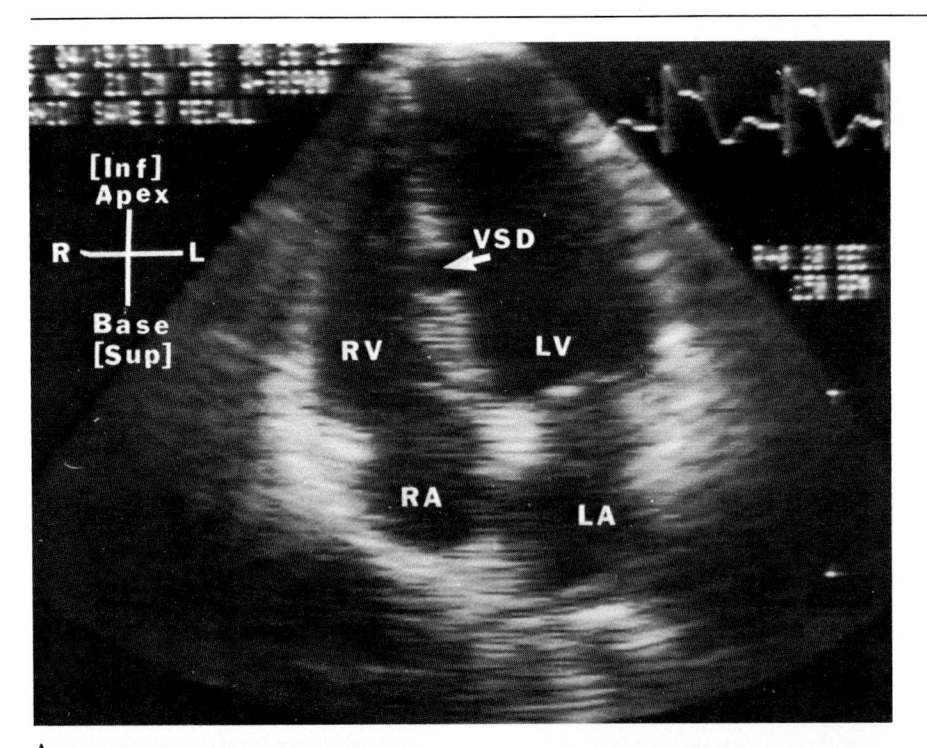

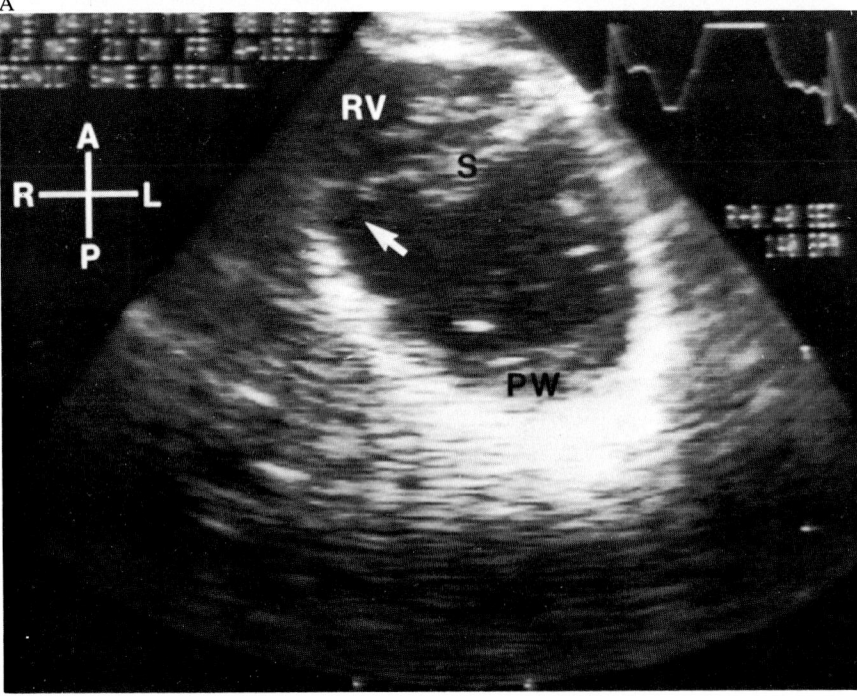

Fig. 6-22A. Apical 4-chamber view showing a ventricular septal defect secondary to rupture from an extensive posteromedial myocardial infarction. Rupture occurred earlier than usual, approximately 10 to 12 hours after onset of chest pain. B. Parasternal short axis view of same patient as in A showing the rupture site (arrow) of the posterior portion of the interventricular septum. C. Anatomic short axis section through a thin posterior wall (black arrow) and rupture site (white arrow) of the posterior interventricular septum; scarring of the septum above the rupture site from the myocardial infarction can be seen. A calcified thrombus (open arrow) is adherent to the scarred posterior wall. D. Anatomic short axis section from a patient who died as a result of rupture of the posterior septum (arrow). The posterior infarction was acute and the patient died before any significant thinning of the posterior wall (PW) had time to occur. E. Anatomic short axis section from a patient who died after acute infarction rupture of the midseptum (open arrow) together with rupture of the anterior free wall of the right ventricle (solid arrow). Right ventricular infarction causing rupture of the anterior wall is very unusual. Considerable epicardial fat (EF) can be seen surrounding the right ventricle and posterior wall of the left ventricle. AL = anterolateral wall; LW = lateral wall.

205

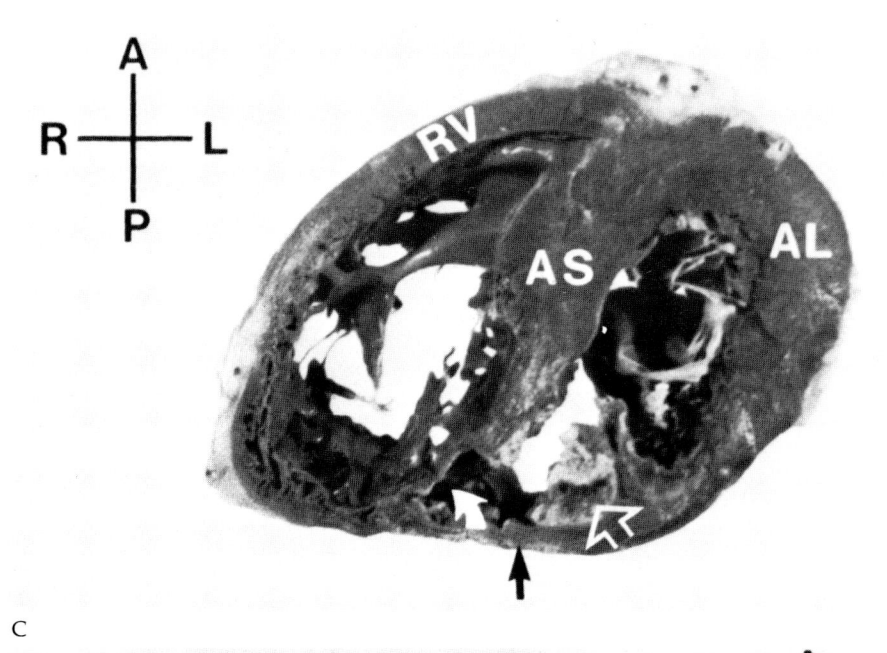

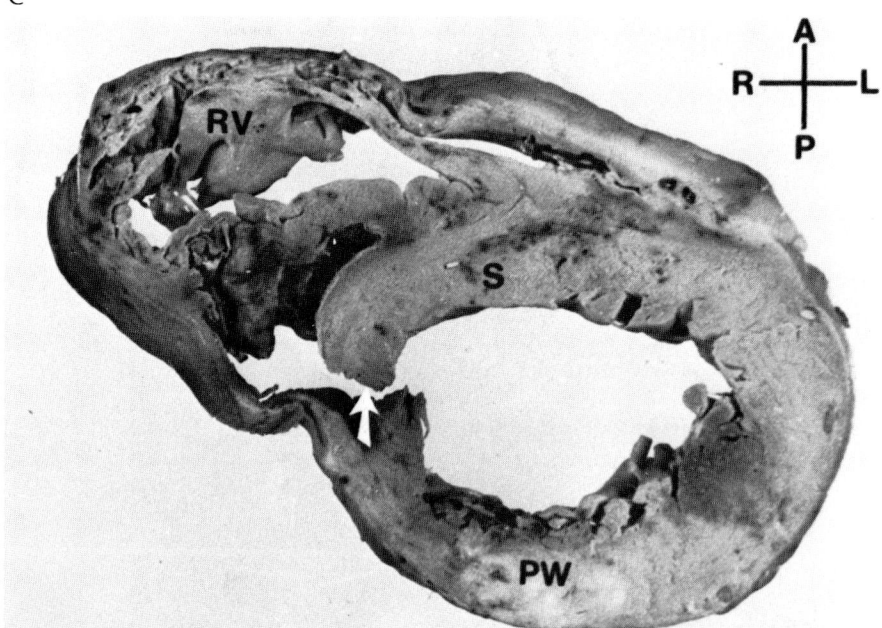

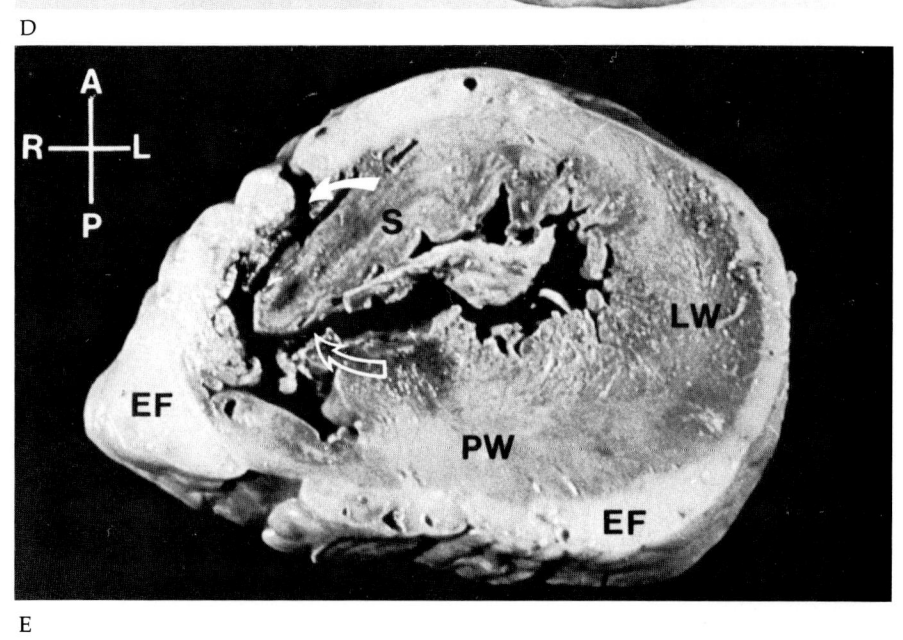

C

D

E

VENTRICULAR SEPTAL RUPTURE. Although rupture of the ventricular septum occurs quite infrequently it is a very severe complication of acute myocardial infarction. Twenty-five percent of the patients die within 24 hours and 65 percent within two weeks following ventricular septal perforation [156]. Clinically the differential diagnosis of ruptured ventricular septum and acute mitral valve regurgitation caused by a flail leaflet may be difficult, and in past years cardiac catheterization was considered essential to confirm the diagnosis [157].

Rupture of the interventricular septum is estimated to complicate from 1 to 3 percent of acute myocardial infarctions and produces approximately 5 percent of peri-infarction deaths [158]. It occurs most frequently during the first week following myocardial infarction [156]. In a study of 41 patients with postinfarction ventricular septal rupture Radford and colleagues [159] reported the presence of cardiogenic shock that developed after septal rupture in 55 percent of that group. They found that shock was unrelated to the site of infarction, extent of coronary artery disease, left ventricular ejection fraction, or pulmonary-to-systemic flow ratio, which suggested that shock was produced largely by right ventricular impairment. These investigators found the myocardial infarction to be anterior in 22 patients and inferior in 19. The onset of ventricular septal rupture occurred within 24 hours in 12 patients, between 2 and 4 days in 13 patients, between 5 and 7 days in five patients, between 8 and 10 days in four patients, between 11 and 14 days in three patients, and in the remaining two patients it occurred between 15 and 20 days following the acute infarction.

Hypertension before or after myocardial infarction has been postulated to be important in the pathogenesis of ventricular septal rupture [160, 161]. This relationship between hypertension and ventricular septal rupture did not exist, however, in the study by Radford and associates [159].

The diagnosis of ventricular septal rupture by means of bedside right heart catheterization and sequential oximetry has been commonly practiced for the past several years [162]. M-mode echocardiography may show some nonspecific findings suggesting ventricular septal rupture; however, it is usually not definitive, and two-dimensional imaging technique is much more reliable for demonstrating the rupture site [163–165]. Left-to-right shunting may also be detected by radionuclide techniques [166, 167], and the diagnosis can also be made by Doppler echocardiographic methods [168].

In patients with ventricular septal rupture in association with inferior wall myocardial infarction, necropsy findings of Radford and associates [159] suggest that more right ventricular free wall was infarcted in those in whom shock had developed than in those in whom it had not. Right ventricular aneurysm formation or right ventricular dysfunction following acute infarction may contribute to the inability of the infarcted right ventricle to sustain pulmonary blood flow necessary to maintain adequate systemic output.

In our experience ventricular septal rupture has been found more commonly in the presence of inferoposterior myocardial infarction than in anterior infarctions (Fig. 6-22). The apical four-chamber and parasternal short axis views are equally important in identifying the rupture site with two-dimensional echocardiography. The subcostal four-chamber view is also valuable for additional assessment of the right ventricle which is usually infarcted together with the posterior septal infarction which has caused the rupture.

FLAIL MITRAL VALVE CAUSED BY RUPTURED PAPILLARY MUSCLE. The clinical setting of a loud systolic murmur in the presence of an acute myocardial infarction and congestive heart failure suggests the possibility of a flail mitral valve secondary to rupture of a papillary muscle. Two-dimensional echocardiography is well suited to the evaluation of such hemodynamically unstable patients to assess the integrity of the mitral valve, chordae tendineae, and papillary muscles. The presence of the flail mitral leaflet can be distinguished from profound prolapse and mitral regurgitation by the loss of leaflet coaptation in systole with either the anterior or posterior leaflet moving back into the left atrium in a flailing systolic motion.

Papillary muscle rupture is unusual and has been reported to occur as a complication in 1 percent of acute myocardial infarctions [168]. According to Sanders and associates [168], the posterior medial papillary muscle is involved 2½ times more often than the anterior lateral papillary muscle. Rupture of an entire papillary muscle is usually fatal; most patients who survive the acute event have rupture of only one or two heads of one of the papillary muscles [169]. A ruptured papillary muscle or chordae tendineae produces a flail mitral leaflet, which is easily detectable by two-dimensional echocardiography [170, 171] (Fig. 6-23). Although the exact sensitivity and specificity of echocardiographic findings differentiating a ruptured papillary muscle from ruptured chordae tendineae are unknown, the clinical implications of each are similar. Mintz and colleagues [171] reported that the length of the flail leaflet segment was longer and the tip of the segment thicker than usual in ruptured chordae tendineae, suggesting that part of the papillary muscle was attached to the leaflet. Wei and associates [172] suggested that a ruptured papillary muscle usually occurs with a small myocardial infarction and that early surgical intervention should be considered in all of these patients. An important determinant in the surgical prognosis of these patients is the extent of left ventricular scarring [173].

The acute development of irreversible papillary muscle dysfunction and severe mitral regurgitation is an unusual extreme form of papillary muscle dysfunction [174, 175]. Mittal and coworkers [176] have demonstrated in experimental studies that papillary muscle infarction does not produce significant mitral regurgitation unless both papillary muscles or left ventricular myocardium adjacent to a single infarcted papillary muscle are also involved. These experimental studies coincide with our own clinical experience. Furthermore, clinical studies by Shelburne and associates [177] suggested that severe left ventricular dysfunction must coexist in order to produce significant mitral regurgitation. However, Sanders and colleagues [178] reported that in some cases papillary muscle necrosis may lead to acute fibrosis, shortening, and retraction of one of the mitral leaflets into the body of the left ventricle, which can lead to significant valvular insufficiency. This type of resultant disruption of the normal coaptation line of the anterior and posterior leaflet closure is identifiable on two-dimensional echocardiography.

The more common forms of papillary muscle dysfunction associated with a mild to moderate degree of mitral regurgitation are commonly noted if both papillary muscles are involved with adjacent zones of wall motion abnormality from previous infarction. The 2-D echo features in such patients include left ventricular dilatation, severe left ventricular dysfunction, reduced or absent motion of the papillary muscles, and sometimes increased reflectance of one or both papillary muscles, probably owing to fibrosis and/or calcification (Fig. 6-24).

Fig. 6-23. A low sternal border parasternal long axis view showing the rupture site (open arrow) of the posterior papillary muscle with prominent reflectance caused by the tip of the papillary muscle and chordae tendineae attached to the anterior mitral leaflet. C = catheter. (From GS Mintz et al.: Two-dimensional echocardiographic identification of surgically correctable complications of acute myocardial infarction. Circulation 64:91, 1981, by permission of the American Heart Association, Inc.)

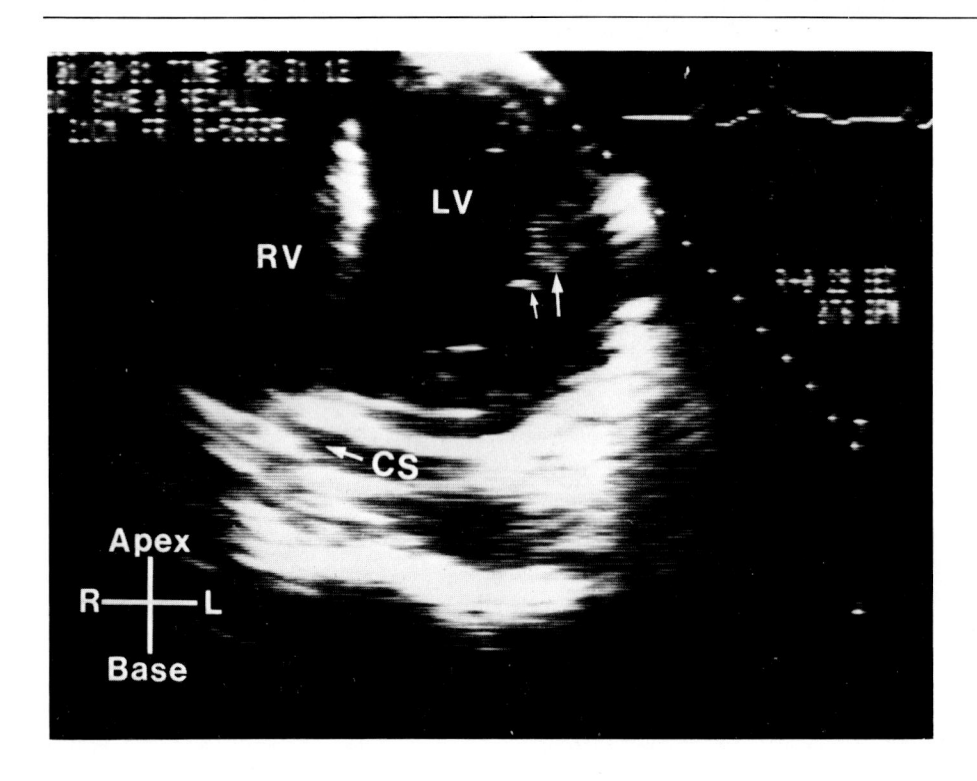

Fig. 6-24. Apical 4-chamber view with posterolateral angulation of the transducer to image the lateral papillary muscle (two arrows), which has some increased reflectances secondary to scarring from an extensive infarction.

POSTINFARCTION PERICARDITIS (DRESSLER'S SYNDROME). The echocardiogram often shows a small pericardial effusion following a transmural myocardial infarction. Most of the time this has little if any clinical significance. On rare occasions the postmyocardial infarction (Dressler's) syndrome occurs. It usually presents from two to four weeks following the infarct, but relapses of pericarditis associated with the syndrome may occur at intervals for as long as 28 months [179, 180]. The clinical features may be confused with extension or recurrence of myocardial infarction or with hemorrhagic pericardial and pleural effusions from anticoagulant therapy. Cardiac tamponade is rare (Fig. 6-25).

RIGHT VENTRICULAR INFARCTION. Right ventricular infarction often represents an interesting diagnostic and treatment challenge. Its diagnosis is based upon characteristic clinical, hemodynamic, echocardiographic, and radionuclide data [181–195]. In a review of 2000 autopsies, Wartman and Hellerstein [196] described 22 cases of right ventricular infarction out of 164 cases of myocardial infarction for a 13.8 percent prevalence.

Isner and Roberts [194] reported 33 cases of right ventricular infarction among 236 patients at necropsy and observed that infarction of the right ventricle was exclusively a complication of posterior left ventricular myocardial infarction. These authors reported that in 97 hearts with isolated anterior wall infarction there was no extension into the right ventricular wall; however, right ventricular infarction occurred in 33 of 139 patients (24%) with posterior infarction. Furthermore, these authors noted that in 65 patients with posterior infarction having transmural involvement of the septum 33 hearts (50%) demonstrated right ventricular infarction as well (Fig. 6-26).

The bedside diagnosis of right ventricular infarction has usually been based on the recognition of right ventricular enlargement associated with right ventricular dysfunction and resultant right-sided heart failure. The presence of elevated right atrial pressure equal to or greater than left ventricular filling pressure has been suggested as the characteristic hemodynamic profile of right ventricular infarction [181]. Lorell and associates [197] reported that four of 12 patients with right ventricular infarction were initially diagnosed as manifesting cardiac tamponade.

The standard 12-lead electrocardiogram is of little benefit in diagnosing right ventricular infarction; however, Candell-Riera and colleagues [191] have stressed the additional value of an electrocardiogram in diagnosing right ventricular infarction if the additional lead V4R is obtained in order to evaluate evidence of S–T segment elevation. Erhardt and associates [198] have also documented the presence of S–T segment elevation in right precordial leads as indicative of right ventricular infarction in patients with acute inferior myocardial infarction and confirmation of right ventricular involvement at necropsy examination. The S–T segment elevation in the V4R probably represents ischemic injury of the posterior basal septum since this area of contiguous myocardium is invariably damaged in patients with pathological evidence of inferior infarction with right ventricular involvement [194].

Right ventricular infarction which contributes to reduced compliance of the right ventricle and right ventricular dysfunction causes right ventricular third and fourth heart sounds, which are present in the majority of such patients [189]. The presence of a positive Kussmaul's sign, which is caused by an elevation of the right ventricular end-diastolic pressure during inspiration that is transmitted to the right atrium and hence reflected in an increased jugular venous pulse during inspiration,

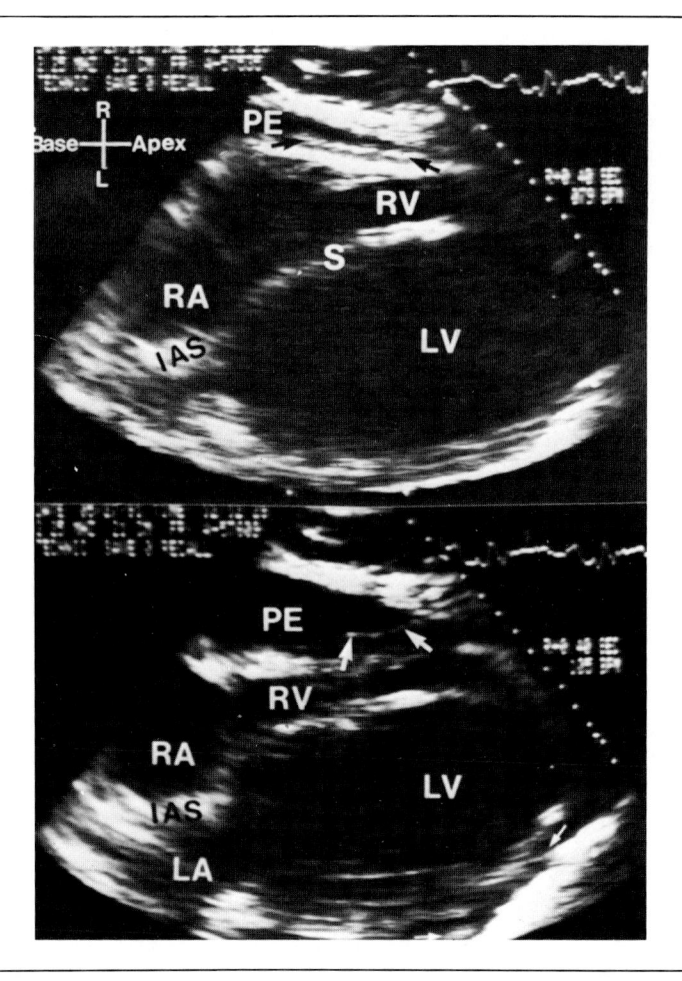

Fig. 6-25. Subcostal 4-chamber views of a patient with Dressler's syndrome and secondary pericardial effusion (PE) plus many epicardial-to-pericardial fibrinous adhesions (black arrows, upper panel) (white arrows, lower panel). The left ventricle is significantly enlarged from previous myocardial infarction. IAS = interatrial septum.

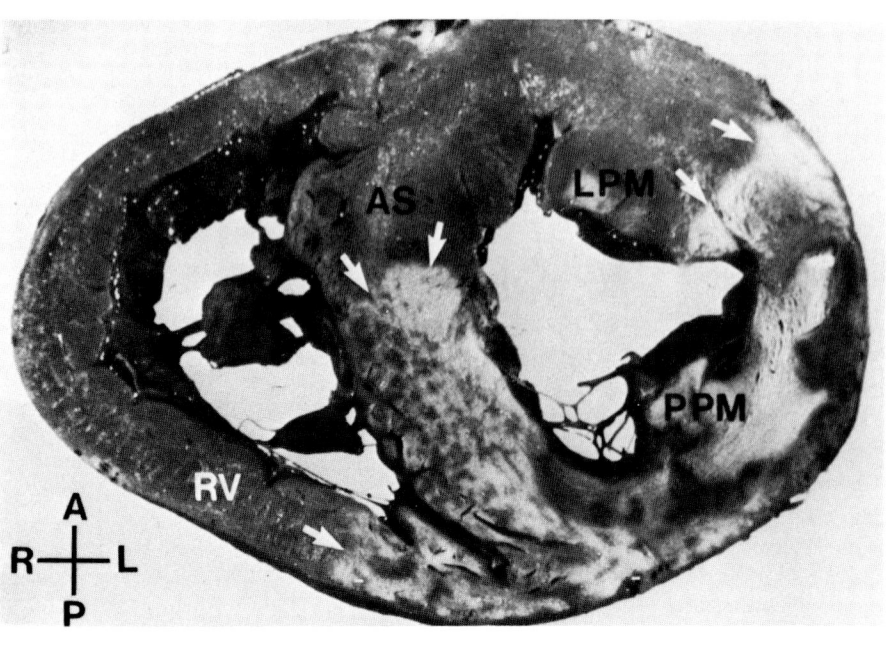

Fig. 6-26. Anatomic short axis section through the papillary muscles showing an acute posterolateral myocardial infarction. The patient died before any wall thinning occurred. The boundaries of the extensive infarction are obvious (arrows) and include the diaphragmatic (posterior) wall of the right ventricle as well as the posterior half of the interventricular septum and all of the posterior papillary muscle (PPM). LPM = anterolateral papillary muscle.

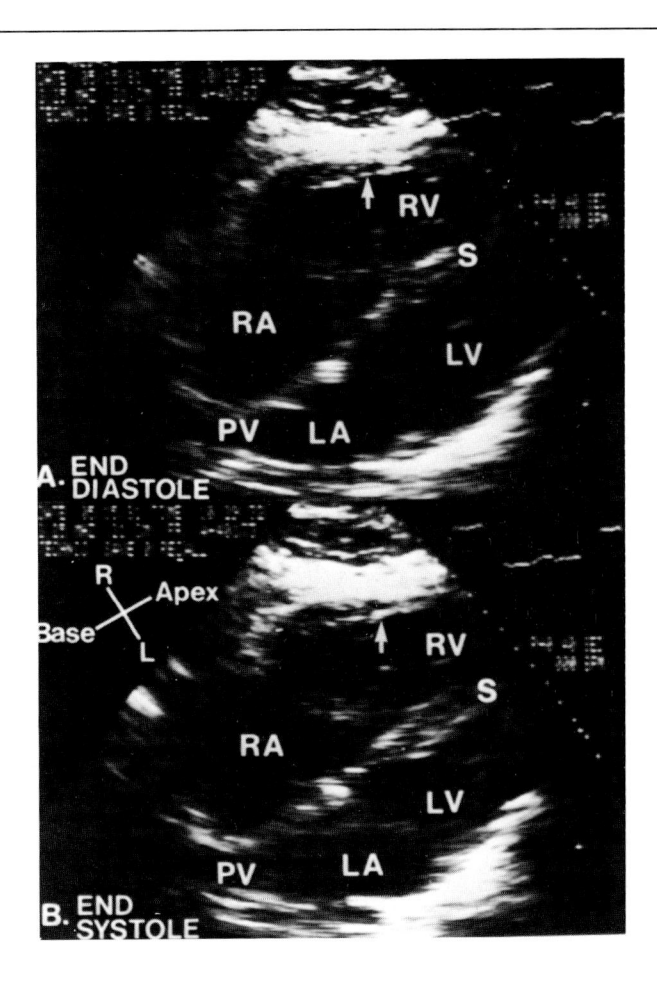

Fig. 6-27. Subcostal 4-chamber views of a patient with a right ventricular infarction manifested by enlargement of both RV and right atrium and akinesis of the free wall of the RV (white arrow, lower panel). PV = pulmonary vein.

has also been found in patients with right ventricular infarction. Lopez-Sendon and colleagues [190] reported that a severe form of noncompliance was found in 54 percent of patients with right ventricular infarction and that it may be the only hemodynamic sign leading to the suspicion of right ventricular involvement in the presence of an acute inferior myocardial infarction.

Wackers and coworkers [186] in a study of 64 patients with acute inferior myocardial infarction observed positive pyrophosphate scans involving the right ventricle in 24 patients (37.5%) and observed that patients with right ventricular infarction did not necessarily have associated right ventricular failure.

Segmental wall motion abnormalities manifested by either hypokinesis or akinesis involving the right ventricular free wall can be observed on either gated blood pool scan [185] or with two-dimensional echocardiography [192] (Fig. 6-27).

Right ventricular infarction may also be complicated by tricuspid regurgitation. If this is suspected contrast echocardiographic studies will be helpful in confirming or excluding this diagnosis. Furthermore, it is important to evaluate the dimensions and respiratory dynamics of the inferior vena cava with subcostal imaging to seek evidence of abnormalities that would suggest right ventricular dysfunction or right ventricular failure (Fig. 6-28). The free wall of the right ventricle should be carefully

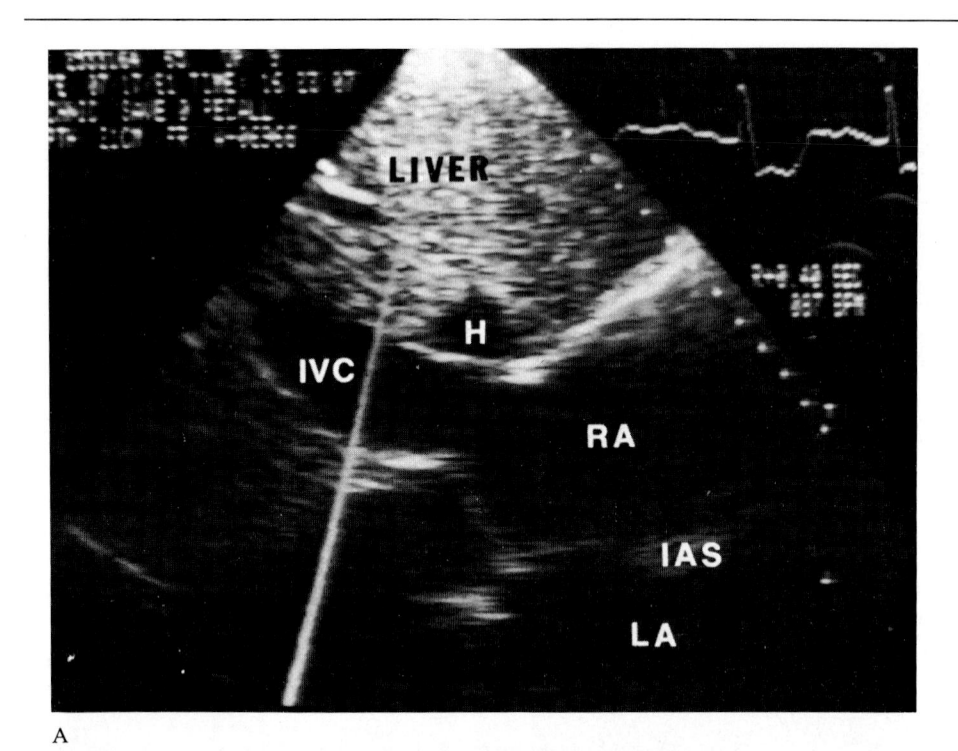

Fig. 6-28A. Subcostal view of the inferior vena cava entering the right atrium. The M-mode cursor should be positioned in a perpendicular fashion through the IVC to record diameter and affects of respiration. IVC is dilated (30 mm diameter) secondary to right ventricular infarction. B. M-mode recording of the IVC in a patient with right ventricular dysfunction secondary to RV infarction and showing the IVC at upper normal limits in diameter (19 mm); however, there is no significant decrease in diameter with inspiration (In) compared to exhalation (Ex) because of elevated right atrial pressure. H = hepatic vein; IAS = interatrial septum.

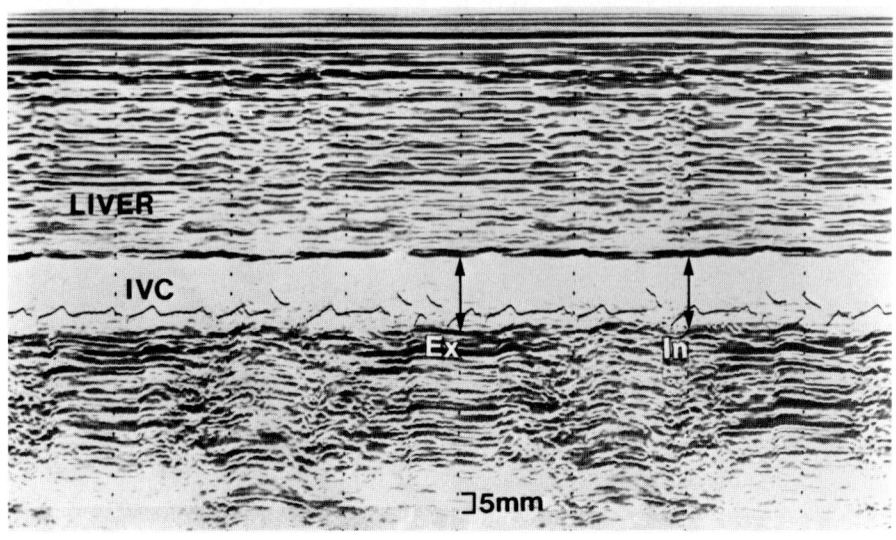

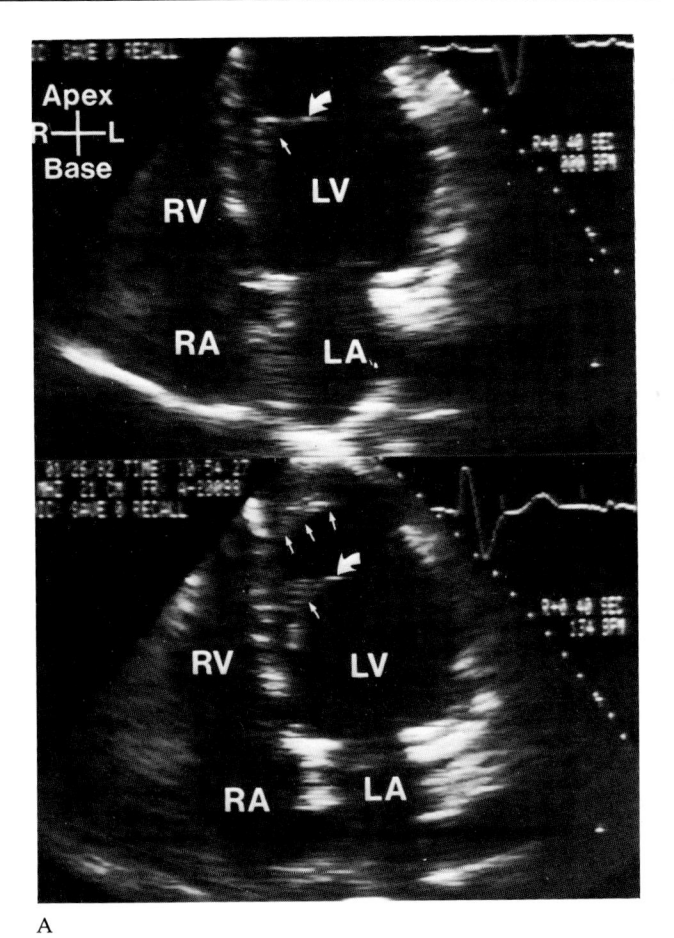

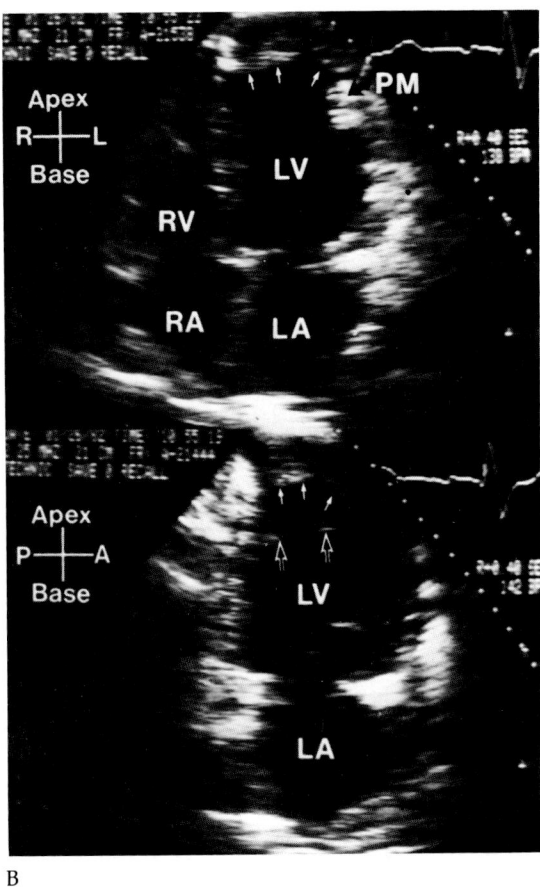

Fig. 6-29A. Apical 4-chamber views of a patient before coronary artery bypass graft surgery (upper panel) showing questionable thrombus adjacent to the infarcted midposterior septum (small arrow) and a linear reflectance from a trabeculation or ectopic chordae (large arrow). Five days after surgery (lower panel) the abnormal reflectance adjacent to the septum is unchanged; however, there is a new thrombus in the left ventricular apex (three arrows), and real-time assessment shows findings of a new apical infarction. B. Apical 4-chamber (upper panel) and apical long axis (lower panel) views of the postoperative study of the patient in A. The new apical thrombus (solid arrows) can be confirmed with the mass identifiable in both planes. The ectopic chordae (open arrows) of no clinical significance can be seen in the lower panel.

imaged from all available views, including the parasternal right ventricular inflow and outflow, parasternal short axis apical four-chamber, subcostal four-chamber, and subcostal short axis views.

Postoperative assessment of patients following coronary artery bypass graft. Echocardiography can be used for serial determinations of left ventricular function before and following coronary artery bypass graft surgery to assess the influence of surgery on left ventricular performance. Very little echocardiographic data have been published on the assessment of left ventricular function or wall motion abnormalities in such postoperative patients [199, 200]. As with changes noted following operation for cardiac valve replacement, abnormal septal motion is also frequently seen in patients following coronary artery bypass graft surgery [200].

Patients whose course is complicated by a perioperative myocardial infarction should be imaged to assess infarct size and left ventricular function and to detect aneurysm or thrombus (Fig. 6-29).

Examination of coronary arteries. Two-dimensional echocardiography is capable of delineating the proximal portions of the coronary arteries [201–206]. Parasternal short axis imaging through the aortic annulus demonstrates the origin of the left main coronary artery (Fig. 6-30). The right coronary orifice is usually more difficult to image (Fig. 6-31). Both the right and left coronary arteries are difficult to image because the vessels are constantly moving in and out of the plane of the examination.

Patients with coronary artery disease may have high-intensity echoes originating from the proximal portion of the left main coronary artery [204, 205]. If the equipment does not have good gray scale it may be difficult to distinguish high-intensity echoes from the surrounding reflectances. With low gain setting only the high-intensity echoes are seen. Rogers and associates [204] have reported a strong correlation between the findings of high-intensity echoes and calcium in the coronary artery at fluoroscopy. Another development in echocardiographic technique for examining coronary arteries has been the use of a strobe freeze and gating on diastole to better record the coronary artery [206]. This application has been shown to be helpful since the extraneous echoes recorded during systole do not obstruct and confuse the examination of the coronary artery. Aneurysms of the coronary arteries may also be detected by two-dimensional echocardiography [207] (Fig. 6-32).

In addition to parasternal short-axis imaging at the base for visualization of the coronary arteries, the left main coronary artery may also be visualized with a modification of apical four-chamber imaging [202, 203].

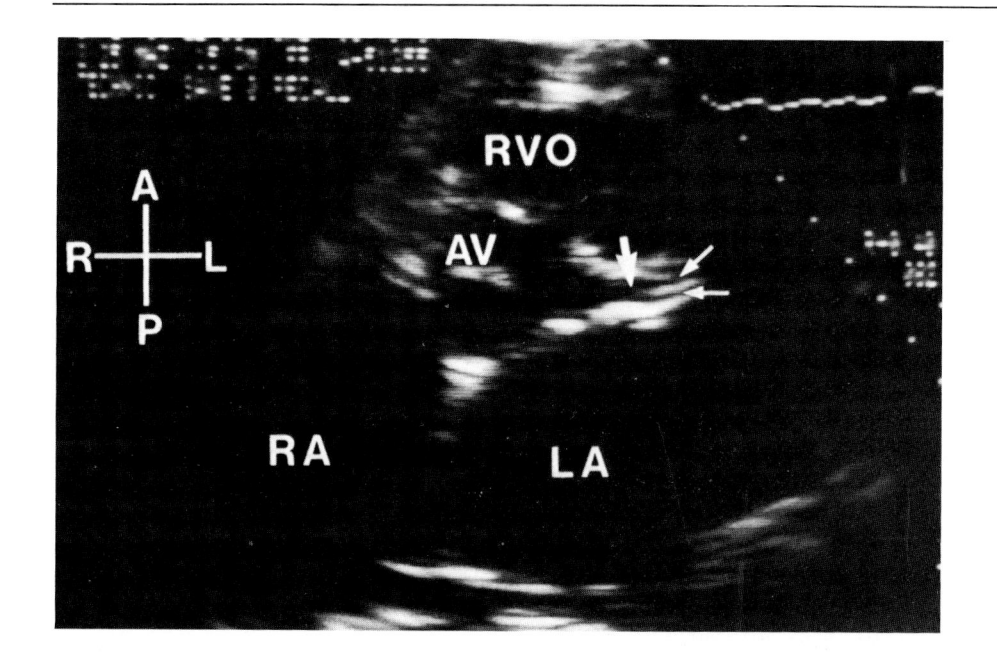

Fig. 6-30. Parasternal short axis view at the base of the orifice and short left main coronary artery (large arrow) and of the left anterior descending (small upper arrow) and the left circumflex (lower small arrow) coronary arteries.

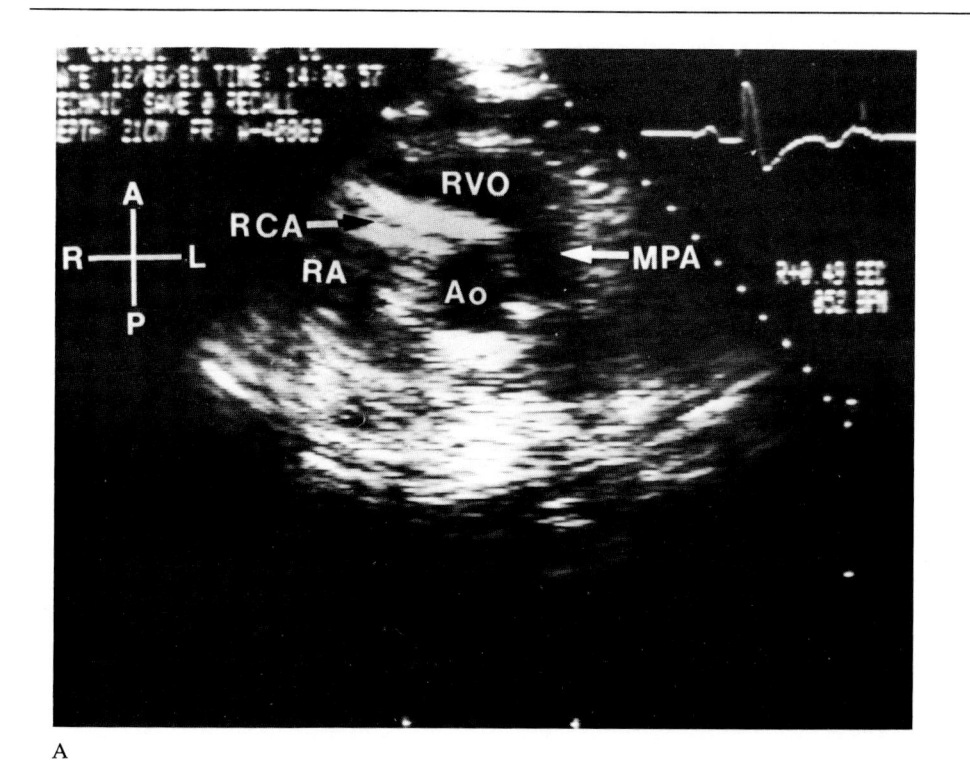

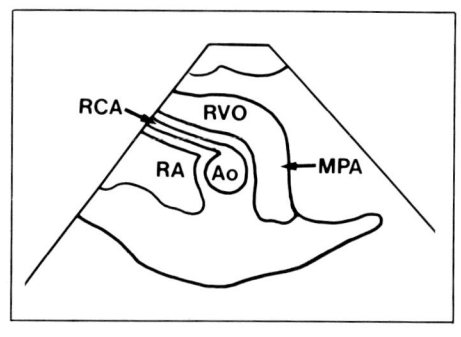

Fig. 6-31A. Parasternal short axis view at the base of the aorta with orifice and proximal portion of the right coronary artery (RCA). B. Diagram illustrating the structures in A. MPA = main pulmonary artery.

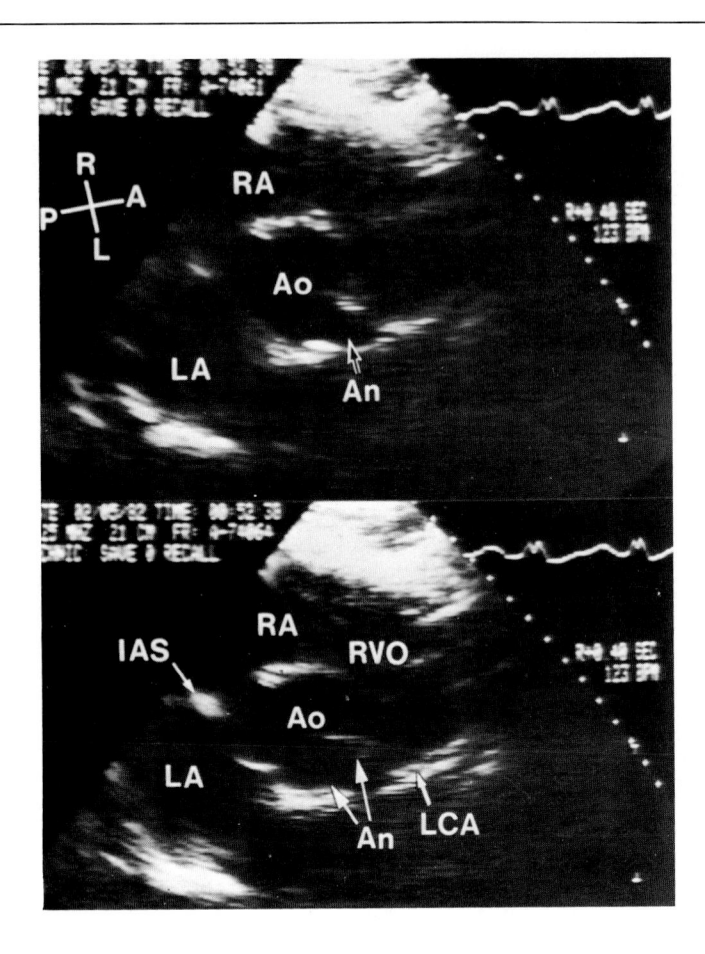

Fig. 6-32. Subcostal short axis views through the aorta and aneurysmal orifice (An) of the left main coronary artery (LCA) (both panels). IAS = interatrial septum.

References

1. Corya BC, Feigenbaum H, Rasmussen S, Black MJ: Anterior left ventricular wall echoes in coronary artery disease: Linear scanning with a single element transducer. *Am J Cardiol* 34:652, 1974
2. Sweet RL, Moraski RE, Russell RO, Rackley CE: Relationship between echocardiography, cardiac output, and abnormally contracting segments in patients with ischemic heart disease. *Circulation* 52:634, 1975
3. Teichholz LE, Kreulen TH, Herman MV, Gorlin R: Problems in echocardiographic volume determinations: Echo-angiographic correlations. *Circulation* 46(Suppl II):II-75, 1972
4. Popp RL, Alderman EL, Brown OR, Harrison DC: Sources of error in calculation of left ventricular volumes by echocardiography. *Am J Cardiol* 31:152, 1973
5. Henning H, Schelbert H, Crawford MH, Karliner JS, Ashburn W, O'Rourke RA: Left ventricular performance assessed by radionuclide angiocardiography and echocardiography in patients with previous myocardiol infarction. *Circulation* 52:1069, 1975
6. Ludbrook P, Karliner JS, London A, Peterson KL, Leopold GR, O'Rourke RA: Posterior wall velocity: An unreliable index of total left ventricular performance in patients with coronary artery disease. *Am J Cardiol* 33:475, 1974
7. Fogelman AM, Abbasi AS, Pearce ML, Kattus AA: Echocardiographic study of the abnormal motion of the posterior left ventricular wall during angina pectoris. *Circulation* 46:905, 1972
8. Belenkie I, Nutter DO, Clark DW, McCraw DB, Raizner AE: Assessment of left ventricular dimensions and function by echocardiography. *Am J Cardiol* 31:755, 1973
9. Rasmussen S, Corya BC, Feigenbaum H, Knoebel SB: Detection of myocardial scar tissue by M-mode echocardiography. *Circulation* 57:230, 1978
10. Heikkila J, Nieminen M: Echoventriculographic detection, localization, and quantification of left ventricular asynergy in acute myocardial infarction: A correlative echo- and electrocardiographic study. *Br Heart J* 37:46, 1975
11. Stack R, Kisslo J: Evaluation of the left ventricle with two dimensional echocardiography. *Am J Cardiol* 46:1117, 1980
12. Mason SJ, Weiss JL, Weisfeldt ML, Garrison JB, Fortuin NJ: Exercise echocardiography: Detection of wall motion abnormalities during ischemia. *Circulation* 59:50, 1979
13. Amon KW, Crawford MH: Upright exercise echocardiography. *JCU* 7:373, 1979
14. Sugishita Y, Koseki S: Dynamic exercise echocardiography. *Circulation* 60:743, 1979
15. Crawford MH, White DH, Amon KW: Echocardiographic evaluation of left ventricular size and performance during handgrip and supine and upright bicycle exercise. *Circulation* 59:1188, 1979
16. Mitamura H, Ogawa S, Hori S, Yamazaki H, Handa S, Nakamura Y: Two dimensional echocardiographic analysis of wall motion abnormalities during handgrip exercise in patients with coronary artery disease. *Am J Cardiol* 48:711, 1981
17. Berberich SN, Zager JRS: Hybrid exercise echocardiograph. *Angiology* 32:1, 1981
18. Zwehl W, Gueret P, Meerbaum S, Holt D, Corday E: Quantitative two dimensional echocardiography during bicycle exercise in normal subjects. *Am J Cardiol* 47:866, 1981
19. Bishop HL, Gibson RS, Stamm RB, Martin RP: Is two-dimensional echocardiography useful in the detection or exclusion of acute myocardial infarction? *Clin Res* 29:178A, 1981
20. Gibson RS, Bishop HL, Stamm RB, Beller GA, Martin RP: Predicting hemodynamic deterioration during acute myocardial infarction by early two dimensional echocardiography. *Clin Res* 29:195A, 1981
21. Pombo JF, Russell RO Jr, Rackley CE, Foster GL: Comparison of stroke volume and cardiac output determination by ultrasound and dye dilution in acute myocardial infarction. *Am J Cardiol* 27:630, 1971
22. Stack RS, Lee CC, Reddy BP, Taylor ML, Weissler AM: Left ventricular performance in coronary artery disease evaluated with systolic time intervals and echocardiography. *Am J Cardiol* 37:331, 1976
23. Lew W, Henning H, Schelbert H, Karliner JS: Assessment of mitral valve E point-septal separation as an index of left ventricular performance in patients with acute and previous myocardial infarction. *Am J Cardiol* 41:836, 1978

24. Conetta DA, Christie LG, Feldman RL, Nichols WW, Pepine CJ, Conti CR: Effects of transient regional ischemia on left ventricular diastolic function. *JCU* 8:233, 1980
25. Gueret P, Meerbaum S, Wyatt HL, Uchiyama T, Lang TW, Corday E: Two-dimensional echocardiographic quantitation of left ventricular volumes and ejection fraction. *Circulation* 62:1308, 1980
26. Visser CA, Lie KI, Kan G, Meltzer R, Durrer D: Detection and quantification of acute, isolated myocardial infarction by two dimensional echocardiography. *Am J Cardiol* 47:1020, 1981
27. Heger JJ, Weyman AE, Wann LS, Dillon JC, Feigenbaum H: Cross-sectional echocardiography in acute myocardial infarction: Detection and localization of regional left ventricular asynergy. *Circulation* 60:531, 1979
28. Meltzer RS, Woythaler JN, Buda AJ, Griffin JC, Harrison WD, Martin RP, Harrison DC, Popp RL: Two dimensional echocardiographic quantification of infarct size alteration by pharmacologic agents. *Am J Cardiol* 44:257, 1979
29. Lieberman AN, Weiss JL, Jugdutt BI, Becker LC, Bulkley BH, Garrison JG, Hutchins GM, Kallman CA, Weisfeldt ML: Two-dimensional echocardiography and infarct size: Relationship of regional wall motion and thickening to the extent of myocardial infarction in the dog. *Circulation* 63:739, 1981
30. Norris RM, Sammel NL: Predictors of late hospital death in acute myocardial infarction. *Prog Cardiovasc Dis* 23:129, 1980
31. Weiss JL, Bulkley BH, Hutchins GM, Mason SJ: Two-dimensional echocardiographic recognition of myocardial injury in man: Comparison with postmortem studies. *Circulation* 63:401, 1981
32. Morganroth J, Chen CC, David D, Sawin HS, Naito M, Parrotto C, Meixell L: Exercise cross-sectional echocardiographic diagnosis of coronary artery disease. *Am J Cardiol* 47:20, 1981
33. Hecht HS, Taylor R, Wong M, Shah PM: Comparative evaluation of segmental asynergy in remote myocardial infarction by radionuclide angiography, two-dimensional echocardiography, and contrast ventriculography. *Am Heart J* 101:740, 1981
34. Edwards WD, Tajik AJ, Seward JB: Standardized nomenclature and anatomic basis for regional tomographic analysis of the heart. *Mayo Clin Proc* 56:479, 1981
35. Maurer G, Nanda NC: Two dimensional echocardiographic evaluation of exercise-induced left and right ventricular asynergy: Correlation with thallium scanning. *Am J Cardiol* 48:720, 1981
36. Pichler M: Noninvasive assessment of segmental left ventricular wall motion: Its clinical relevance in detection of ischemia. *Clin Cardiol* 1:173, 1978
37. Kerber RE, Marcus ML, Ehrhardt J, Wilson R, Abboud FM: Correlation between echocardiographically demonstrated segmental dyskinesis and regional myocardial perfusion. *Circulation* 52:1097, 1975
38. Kerber RE, Marcus ML, Wilson R, Ehrhardt J, Abboud FM: Effects of acute coronary occlusion on the motion and perfusion of the normal and ischemic interventricular septum: An experimental echocardiographic study. *Circulation* 54:928, 1976
39. Corya BC, Phillips JF, Black MJ, Weyman AE, Rasmussen S: Prevalence of regional left ventricular dysfunction in patients with coronary artery disease. *Chest* 79:631, 1981
40. Morganroth J, Chen CC, David D, Naito M, Mardelli TJ: Echocardiographic detection of coronary artery disease: Detection of effects of ischemia on regional myocardial wall motion and visualization of left main coronary artery disease. *Am J Cardiol* 46:1178, 1980
41. Horowitz RS, Morganroth J, Parrotto C, Chen CC, Soffer J, Pauletto FJ: Immediate diagnosis of acute myocardial infarction by two-dimensional echocardiography. *Circulation* 65:323, 1982
42. Heger J, Weyman AE, Noble RJ, Dillon JC, Feigenbaum H: An analysis of the site, extent, and hemodynamic consequences of acute myocardial infarction by cross-sectional echocardiography. *Circulation* 56(Suppl III):III-152, 1977
43. Wynne J, Birnholz J, Finberg H, Alpert JS: Regional left ventricular wall motion in acute myocardial infarction as assessed by two dimensional echocardiography. *Circulation* 56 (Suppl III):III-152, 1977
44. Wyatt HL, Forrester JS, da Luz PL, Diamond GA, Chagrasulis R, Swan HJC: Functional abnormalities in nonoccluded regions of myocardium after experimental coronary occlusion. *Am J Cardiol* 37:366, 1976

45. Guth B, Savage R, White F, Hagan AD, Samtoy L, Bloor C: Detection of ischemic wall dysfunction: A comparison between M-mode echocardiography and sonomicrometry. *Am Heart J* (in press)
46. Savage RM, Guth B, White FC, Hagan AD, Bloor CM: Correlation of regional myocardial blood flow and function with myocardial infarct size during acute myocardial ischemia in the conscious pig. *Circulation* 64:699, 1981
47. Guth BD, White FC, Gallagher KP, Bloor CM: Abnormal wall thickening in myocardium adjacent to ischemic zones in conscious swine during brief coronary artery occlusion. *Fed Proc* 40:485, 1981
48. Herman MV, Gorlin R: Implications of left ventricular asynergy. *Am J Cardiol* 23:538, 1969
49. Hutchins GM, Bulkley BH, Ridolfi RL, Griffith LSC, Lohr FT, Piasio MA: Correlation of coronary arteriograms and left ventriculograms with postmortem studies. *Circulation* 56:32, 1977
50. Stinson EB, Billingham ME: Correlative study of regional left ventricular histology and contractile function. *Am J Cardiol* 39:378, 1977
51. Kerber RE, Marcus ML: Evaluation of regional myocardial function in ischemic heart disease by echocardiography. *Prog Cardiovasc Dis* 20:441, 1978
52. Dove JT, Shah PM, Schreiner BF: Effects of nitroglycerin on left ventricular wall motion in coronary artery disease. *Circulation* 49:682, 1974
53. Dumesnil JG, Laurenceau JL, Labatut A, Gagne S: Echocardiographic study of changes in regional ventricular function following nitroglycerin and surgical correlation.
54. Dodge HT, Sandler H, Ballew DW, Lord JD: The use of biplane angiocardiography for the measurement of left ventricular volume in man. *Am Heart J* 60:762, 1960
55. Dodge HT, Sandler H, Buxley WA, Hawley RR: Usefulness and limitations of radiographic methods for determining left ventricular volumes. *Am J Cardiol* 18:10, 1966
56. Falsetti HL, Marcus ML, Kerber RE, Skorton DJ: Editorial: Quantification of myocardial ischemia and infarction by left ventricular imaging. *Circulation* 63:747, 1981
57. Vatner SF: Correlation between acute reductions in myocardial blood flow and function in conscious dogs. *Circ Res* 47:201, 1980
58. Heyndrickx GR, Millard RW, McRitchie RJ, Maroko PR, Vatner SF: Regional myocardial function and electrophysiological alterations after brief coronary artery occlusion in conscious dogs. *J Clin Invest* 56:978, 1975
59. Heng MK, Lang TW, Toshimitsu T, Meerbaum S, Wyatt HL, Lee SS, Davidson R, Corday E: Quantification of myocardial ischemic damage by two dimensional echocardiography. *Circulation* 56(Suppl III):III-125, 1977
60. Weyman AE, Franklin TD, Egenes KM, Green D: Correlation between extent of abnormal regional wall motion and myocardial infarct size in chronically infarcted dogs. *Circulation* 56(Suppl III):III-72, 1977
61. Holman BL, Wynne J, Idoine J, Neill J: Disruption in the temporal sequence of regional ventricular contraction. I. Characteristics and incidence in coronary artery disease. *Circulation* 61:1075, 1980
62. Franklin T, Wiske PS, Clendenon JL, Hogan RD, Avery KS, Burke KM, Sanghvi NT, Weyman AE: Variation in cross-sectional echocardiographic radial target motion relative to a calculated mean centroid of the left ventricle. *Circulation* 62(Suppl III):III-132, 1980
63. Glover MU, Hagan AD, Cohen A, Mazzoleni A, Schvartzman M, Warren SE, Vieweg WVR: Two-dimensional echocardiography in predicting left ventricular wall motion abnormalities and left ventricular function. *South Med J* 75:313, 1982
64. Kisslo JA, Robertson D, Gilbert BW, VonRamm O, Behar VS: A comparison of real-time, two dimensional echocardiography and cineangiography in detecting left ventricular asynergy. *Circulation* 55:134, 1977
65. Wyatt HL, Meerbaum S, Heng MK, Rit J, Gueret P, Corday E: Experimental evaluation of the extent of myocardial dyssynergy and infarct size by two-dimensional echocardiography. *Circulation* 63:607, 1981
66. Eaton LW, Weiss JL, Bulkley BH, Garrison JB, Weisfeldt ML: Regional cardiac dilatation after acute myocardial infarction: Recognition by two-dimensional echocardiography. *N Engl J Med* 300:57, 1979
67. Bizarro RO: Myocardial scar: Morphologic and vectorcardiographic study. Thesis, Mayo Graduate School of Medicine, University of Minnesota, Minneapolis, 1971
68. De Sonza e Silva NA: A quantitative morphologic, vectorcardiographic and clinical study

of some malconformations of the human myocardium. Thesis, Mayo Graduate School of Medicine, University of Minnesota, Minneapolis, 1974
69. Vieweg WVR, Alpert JS, Johnson AD, Dennish GW, Nelson DP, Warren SE, Hagan AD: Distribution and severity of left ventricular wall motion abnormalities according to age and coronary arterial pattern in 500 patients with coronary artery disease and angina pectoris. *Am Heart J* 99:707, 1980
70. Bruschke AVG, Proudfit WL, Sones FM Jr: Progress study of 590 consecutive nonsurgical cases of coronary disease followed 5–9 years. I. Arteriographic correlations. *Circulation* 47:1147, 1973
71. Bruschke AVG, Proudfit WL, Sones FM Jr: Progress study of 590 consecutive nonsurgical cases of coronary disease followed 5–9 years. II. Ventriculographic and other correlations. *Circulation* 47:1154, 1973
72. Kolibash AJ, Beaver BM, Fulkerson PK, Khullar S, Leighton RF: The relationship between abnormal echocardiographic septal motion and myocardial perfusion in patients with significant obstruction of the left anterior descending artery. *Circulation* 56:780, 1977
73. Jacobs JJ, Feigenbaum H, Corya BC, Phillips JF: Detection of left ventricular asynergy by echocardiography. *Circulation* 48:263, 1973
74. DeMaria A, King JF, Bonanno JA, Lies JE, Zelis R, Vismara LA, Miller RR, Massumi RA, Amsterdam EA, Mason DT: Left anterior descending involvement in coronary disease: Detection by abnormal ventricular septal motion on echocardiogram. *Clin Res* 22:272a, 1974
75. Gordon MJ, Kerber RE: Interventricular septal motion in patients with proximal and distal left anterior descending coronary artery lesions. *Circulation* 55:338, 1977
76. Hamilton GW, Ritchie JL, Allen D, Lapin E, Murray JA: Myocardial perfusion imaging with ^{99m}Tc or ^{113m}In macroaggregated albumin: Correlation of the perfusion image with clinical, angiographic, surgical, and histological findings. *Am Heart J* 89:708, 1975
77. Widlansky S, McHenry PL, Corya BC, Phillips JF: Coronary angiographic, echocardiographic, and electrocardiographic studies on a patient with variant angina due to coronary artery spasm. *Am Heart J* 90:631, 1975
78. Dortimer AC, DeJoseph RL, Shiroff RA, Liedtke AJ, Zelis R: Distribution of coronary artery disease: Prediction by echocardiography. *Circulation* 54:724, 1976
79. Redwood DR, Henry WL, Epstein SE: Evaluation of the ability of echocardiography to measure acute alterations in left ventricular volume. *Circulation* 50:901, 1974
80. DeMaria AN, Vismara LA, Auditore K, Amsterdam EA, Zelis R, Mason DT: Effects of nitroglycerin on left ventricular cavity size and cardiac performance determined by ultrasound in man. *Am J Med* 57:754, 1974
81. Helfant RH, Pine R, Meister SG, Feldman MS, Trout RG, Banka VS: Nitroglycerin to unmask reversible asynergy: Correlation with post coronary bypass ventriculography. *Circulation* 50:108, 1974
82. McAnulty JH, Hattenhauer MT, Rosch J, Kloster FE, Rahimtoola SH: Improvement in left ventricular wall motion following nitroglycerin. *Circulation* 51:140, 1975
83. Morrison CA, Bodenheimer MM, Feldman MS, Banka VS, Helfant RH: The use of echocardiography in determination of reversible posterior wall asynergy. *Am Heart J* 94:140, 1977
84. Hardarson T, Wright KE: Effect of sublingual nitroglycerin on cardiac performance in patients with coronary artery disease and non-dyskinetic left ventricular contraction. *Br Heart J* 38:1272, 1976
85. Goldstein RE, Bennett ED, Leech GL: Effect of glyceryl trinitrate on echocardiographic left ventricular dimensions during exercise in the upright position. *Br Heart J* 42:245, 1979
86. Komer RR, Edalji A, Hood WB Jr: Effects of nitroglycerin on echocardiographic measurements of left ventricular wall thickness and regional myocardial performance during acute coronary ischemia. *Circulation* 59:926, 1979
87. Kerber RE, Martins JB, Marcus ML: Effect of acute ischemia, nitroglycerin and nitroprusside on regional myocardial thickening, stress and perfusion. Experimental echocardiographic studies. *Circulation* 60:121, 1979
88. Hillis LD, Braunwald E: Myocardial ischemia. *N Engl J Med* 296:1034, 1977
89. Kerber RE, Abboud FM, Marcus ML, Eckberg DL: Effect of inotropic agents on the localized dyskinesis of acutely ischemic myocardium. An experimental ultrasound study. *Circulation* 49:1038, 1974

90. Maroko PR, Kjekshus JK, Sobel BE, Watanabe T, Covell JW, Ross J, Braunwald E: Factors influencing infarct size following experimental coronary artery occlusions. *Circulation* 43:67, 1971
91. Maroko PR, Libby P, Ginks WR, Bloor CM, Shell WE, Sobel BE, Ross J Jr: Coronary artery reperfusion. Early effects on local myocardial function and the extent of myocardial necrosis. *J Clin Invest* 51:2710, 1970
92. Kerber RE, Abboud FM: Effect of alterations of arterial blood pressure and heart rate on segmental dyskinesis during acute myocardial ischemia and following coronary reperfusion. *Circ Res* 36:145, 1975
93. Kerber RE, Marcus ML, Ehrhardt J, Abboud FM: Effect of intraaortic balloon counterpulsation on the motion and perfusion of acute ischemic myocardium. An experimental echocardiographic study. *Circulation* 53:853, 1976
94. Parisi AF, Moynihan PF, Folland ED, Feldman CL: Assessment of Regional Wall Motion in Coronary Artery Disease by Two Dimensional Echocardiography. In CT Lancec (Ed), *Echocardiography*. The Hague, Netherlands: Martinus Nijhoff, 1979. Pp. 125, 129
95. Garrison JB, Weiss JL, Maughan WL, Tuck OM, Guier WH, Fortuin NJ: Quantifying Regional Wall Motion and Thickening in Two-dimensional Echocardiography with a Computer-aided Contouring System. In H Ostrow, K Ripley (Eds), *Proceedings of Computers in Cardiology*. Long Beach, California: IEEE, 1977. Pp. 25–35
96. Moynihan PF, Parisi AF, Feldman CL: Quantitative detection of regional left ventricular contraction abnormalities by two dimensional echocardiography. I. Analysis of methods. *Circulation* 63:752, 1981
97. Rogers WJ, Smith LR, Hood WP, Mantle JA, Rackley CE, Russell RO: Effect of filming projection and interobserver variability on angiographic biplane left ventricular volume determination. *Circulation* 59:96, 1979
98. Sullivan W, Vlodaver Z, Tuna N, Long L, Edwards JE: Correlation of electrocardiographic and pathologic findings in healed myocardial infarction. *Am J Cardiol* 42:724, 1978
99. Roberts WC, Gardin JM: Location of myocardial infarcts: A confusion of terms and definitions. *Am J Cardiol* 42:868, 1978
100. Vieweg WVR, Alpert JS, Johnson AD, Dennish GW, Nelson DP, Warren SE, Hagan AD: Electrocardiographic and left ventriculographic correlations in 245 patients with coronary artery disease. *Comput Biomed Res* 13:105, 1980
101. Kisslo JA, Ideker R, Harrison L, Scallion R, VonRamm OT, Pilkington T: Serial wall changes after acute myocardial infarction by two-dimensional echo. *Circulation* 60(Suppl II):II-151, 1979
102. Hutchins GM, Bulkley BH: Infarct expansion versus extension: Two different complications of acute myocardial infarction. *Am J Cardiol* 41:1127, 1978
103. Willerson JT: Echocardiography after acute myocardial infarction. *N Engl J Med* 300:87, 1979
104. Parisi AF, Moynihan PF, Folland ED, Strauss WE, Sharma GVRK, Sasahara AA: Echocardiography in acute and remote myocardial infarction. *Am J Cardiol* 46:1205, 1980
105. Grossman W, McLaurin LP, Moos SP, Stefadouros M, Young DT: Wall thickness and diastolic properties of the left ventricle. *Circulation* 49:129, 1974
106. Gaasch WH, Bernard SA: The effect of acute changes in coronary blood flow on left ventricular end-diastolic wall thickness: An echocardiographic study. *Circulation* 56:593, 1977
107. Sasayama S, Franklin D, Ross J Jr, Kemper WS, McKown D: Dynamic changes in left ventricular wall thickness and their use in analyzing cardiac function in the conscious dog: A study based on a modified ultrasonic technique. *Am J Cardiol* 38:870, 1976
108. Gueret P, Meerbaum S, Corday E, Uchiyama T, Wyatt HL, Broffman J: Differential effects of nitroprusside on ischemic and nonischemic myocardial segments demonstrated by computer-assisted two dimensional echocardiography. *Am J Cardiol* 48:59, 1981
109. Wyatt HL, Heng MK, Meerbaum S, Gueret P, Hestenes J, Dula E, Corday E: Cross-sectional echocardiography. II. Analysis of mathematic models for quantifying volume of the formalin-fixed left ventricle. *Circulation* 61:1119, 1980
110. Schiller NB, Acquatella H, Ports TA, Drew D, Goerke J, Ringertz H, Silverman NH, Brundage B, Botvinick EH, Boswell R, Carlsson E, Parmley WW: Left ventricular volume from paired biplane two-dimensional echocardiography. *Circulation* 60:547, 1979

111. Parisi AF, Moynihan PF, Feldman CL, Folland ED: Approaches to determination of left ventricular volume and ejection fraction by real-time two-dimensional echocardiography. *Clin Cardiol* 2:257, 1979
112. Erbel R, Schweizer P, Meyer J, Grenner H, Krebs W, Effert S: Left ventricular volume and ejection fraction determination by cross-sectional echocardiography in patients with coronary artery disease: A prospective study. *Clin Cardiol* 3:377, 1980
113. Starling MR, Crawford MH, Sorensen SG, Levi B, Richards KL, O'Rourke RA: Comparative accuracy of apical biplane cross-sectional echocardiography and gated equilibrium radionuclide angiography for estimating left ventricular size and performance. *Circulation* 63:1075, 1981
114. Quinones MA, Waggoner AD, Reduto LA, Nelson JG, Young JB, Winters WL Jr, Ribeiro LG, Miller RR: A new, simplified and accurate method for determining ejection fraction with two dimensional echocardiography. *Circulation* 64:744, 1981
115. Massie BM, Schiller NB, Ratshin RA, Parmley WW: Mitral-septal separation: New echocardiographic index of left ventricular function. *Am J Cardiol* 39:1008, 1977
116. D'Cruz IA, Lalmalani GG, Sambasivan V, Cohen HC, Glick G: The superiority of mitral E point-ventricular septum separation to other echocardiographic indicators of left ventricular performance. *Clin Cardiol* 2:140, 1979
117. Child JS, Krivokapich J, Perloff JK: Effect of left ventricular size on mitral E point to ventricular septal separation in assessment of cardiac performance. *Am Heart J* 101:797, 1981
118. Beeder C, Charuzi Y, Loh IK, Staniloff H, Swan HJC: Relationship between segmental abnormalities and global left ventricular function in coronary artery disease: Validation of a theoretical model. *Am Heart J* 102:330, 1981
119. Fujii J, Watanabe H, Kato K: Detection of the site and extent of the left ventricular asynergy in myocardial infarction by echocardiography and B-scan imaging. *Jpn Heart J* 17:630, 1976
120. Weyman AE, Peskoe SM, Williams ES, Dillon JC, Feigenbaum H: Detection of left ventricular aneurysms by cross-sectional echocardiography. *Circulation* 54:936, 1976
121. Rakowski H, Martin RP, Schapira JN, Wexler L, Silverman JF, Cipriano PR, Guthaner DF, Popp RL: Left ventricular aneurysm: Detection and determination of resectability by two-dimensional ultrasound. *Circulation* 56(Suppl III):III-153, 1977
122. Barrett MJ, Charuzi Y, Corday E: Ventricular aneurysm: Cross-sectional echocardiographic approach. *Am J Cardiol* 46:1133, 1980
123. Feigenbaum H: *Echocardiography* (3rd ed). Philadelphia: Lea & Febiger, 1981. P. 435
124. Cooperman M, Stinson EB, Griepp RB, Shumway NE: Survival and function after left ventricular aneurysmectomy. *J Thorac Cardiovasc Surg* 69:321, 1975
125. Mullen DC, Posey L, Gabriel R, Singh HM, Fleming RJ, Lepley D: Prognostic considerations in the management of left ventricular aneurysms. *Ann Thorac Surg* 23:455, 1977
126. Watson LE, Dickhaus DW, Martin RH: Left ventricular aneurysm. *Circulation* 52:868, 1975
127. Lee DC, Johnson RA, Boucher CA, Wexler LF, McEnany MT: Angiographic predictors of survival following left ventricular aneurysmectomy. *Circulation* 56(Suppl II):II-12, 1976
128. Roberts WC, Morrow AG: Pseudoaneurysm of the left ventricle. An unusual sequel of myocardial infarction and rupture of the heart. *Am J Med* 43:639, 1967
129. Van Tassel RA, Edwards JE: Rupture of heart complicating myocardial infarction. Analysis of 40 cases including nine examples of left ventricular false aneurysm. *Chest* 61:104, 1972
130. Davidson KH, Parisi AF, Harrington JJ, Barsamian EM, Fishbein MC: Pseudoaneurysm of the left ventricle: An unusual echocardiographic presentation. Review of the literature. *Ann Intern Med* 86:430, 1977
131. MacNeil DJ, Vieweg WVR, Oury JH, Folkerth TL, Hagan AD: Pseudomitral regurgitation due to false aneurysm of the left ventricle treated successfully by surgery. *Chest* 66:724, 1974
132. Higgins CB, Lipton MJ, Johnson AD, Peterson KL, Vieweg WVR: False aneurysms of the left ventricle. Identification of distinctive clinical, radiographic, and angiographic features. *Radiology* 127:21, 1978
133. Martinez-Lopez JI: Pulsatory and auscultatory phenomena in pseudoaneurysm of the heart. *Am J Cardiol* 15:422, 1965

134. Katz RJ, Simpson A, DiBianco R, Fletcher KD, Bates HR, Sauerbrunn BJL: Noninvasive diagnosis of left ventricular pseudoaneurysm. Role of two dimensional echocardiography and radionuclide gated pool imaging. *Am J Cardiol* 44:372, 1979
135. Catherwood E, Mintz GS, Kotler MN, Parry WR, Segal BL: Two-dimensional echocardiographic recognition of left ventricular pseudoaneurysm. *Circulation* 62:294, 1980
136. Glover MU, Hagan AD, Vieweg WVR, Ceretto WJ: Pseudoaneurysm of the left ventricle diagnosed by two-dimensional echocardiography: Case report. *Milit Med* 146:696, 1981
137. Yater WM, Welsh PP, Stapleton JF, Clark ML: Comparison of clinical and pathologic aspects of coronary artery disease in men of various age groups: A study of 950 autopsied cases from the Armed Forces Institute of Pathology. *Ann Intern Med* 34:352, 1951
138. Jordan RA, Miller RD, Edwards JE, Parker RL: Thromboembolism in acute and in healed myocardial infarction. I. Intracardiac mural thrombosis. *Circulation* 6:1, 1952
139. Schlichter J, Hellerstein HK, Katz LN: Aneurysm of the heart: Correlative study of one hundred and two proved cases. *Medicine* 33:43, 1954
140. Dubnow MH, Burchell HB, Titus JL: Postinfarction ventricular aneurysm: Clinicopathologic and electrocardiographic study of 80 cases. *Am Heart J* 70:753, 1965
141. Loop FD, Effler DB, Navia JA, Sheldon WC, Groves LK: Aneurysms of the left ventricle: Survival and results of a ten-year surgical experience. *Ann Surg* 178:399, 1973
142. Miller RD, Jordan RA, Parker RI, Edwards JE: Thromboembolism in acute and in healed myocardial infarction. II. Systemic and pulmonary arterial occlusion. *Circulation* 6:7, 1952
143. Hellerstein HK, Martin JW: Incidence of thromboembolic lesions accompanying myocardial infarction. *Am Heart J* 33:443, 1947
144. VA Cooperative Clinical Study Group: Anticoagulants in acute myocardial infarction. *JAMA* 225:724, 1973
145. Frishman WH, Ribner HS: Anticoagulation in myocardial infarction: Modern approach to an old problem. *Am J Cardiol* 43:1207, 1979
146. DeMaria AN, Bommer W, Neumann A, Grehl T, Weinart L, DeNardo S, Amsterdam EA, Mason DT: Left ventricular thrombi identified by cross-sectional echocardiography. *Ann Intern Med* 90:14, 1979
147. Drobac M, Rakowski H, Gilbert BW, Glynn MX, Silver MD: Two-dimensional echocardiographic recognition of mural thrombi: In-vivo and in-vitro studies. *Am J Cardiol* 45:435, 1980
148. Reeder GS, Lengyel M, Tajik AJ, Seward JB, Smith HC, Danielson GK: Mural thrombus in left ventricular aneurysm: Incidence, role of angiography, and relation between anticoagulation and embolization. *Mayo Clin Proc* 56:77, 1981
149. Stratton JR, Ritchie JL, Hamilton GW, Hammermeister KE, Harker LA: Left ventricular thrombi: In vivo detection by Indium-III platelet imaging and two dimensional echocardiography. *Am J Cardiol* 47:874, 1981
150. Asinger RW, Mikell FL, Sharma B, Hodges M: Observations on detecting left ventricular thrombus with two dimensional echocardiography: Emphasis on avoidance of false positive diagnoses. *Am J Cardiol* 47:145, 1981
151. vanWoezik HVM, Meltzer RS, van den Brand M, Essed CE, Michels RHM, Roelandt J: Superiority of echocardiography over angiocardiography in diagnosing a left ventricular thrombus. *Chest* 80:321, 1981
152. Reeder GS, Tajik AJ, Seward JB: Left ventricular mural thrombus: Two-dimensional echocardiographic diagnosis. *Mayo Clin Proc* 56:82, 1981
153. Reeder GS, Lengyel M, Tajik AJ, Smith HC, Danielson GK, Seward JB: Incidence of thrombus in left ventricular aneurysm: Sensitivity of the angiogram and relation between anticoagulation and embolization. *Am J Cardiol* 45:423, 1980
154. Asinger RW, Mikell FL, Francis G, Elsperger J, Hodges M, Sharma B: Serial evaluation for left ventricular thrombus during acute transmural myocardial infarction using two dimensional echocardiography. *Am J Cardiol* 45:483, 1980
155. Roelandt J, vanDorp WG, Bom N, Larid JD, Hugenholtz PG: Resolution problems in echocardiography: A source of interpretation errors. *Am J Cardiol* 37:256, 1976
156. Sanders RJ, Kern WH, Blount SG Jr: Perforation of the interventricular septum complicating myocardial infarction. *Am Heart J* 51:736, 1956
157. Dugall JC, Pryor R, Blount SG: Systolic murmur following myocardial infarction. *Am Heart J* 87:577, 1974
158. Hutchins GM: Rupture of the interventricular septum complicating myocardial infarc-

tion: Pathological analysis of 10 patients with clinically diagnosed perforations. *Am Heart J* 97:165, 1979
159. Radford MJ, Johnson RA, Daggett WM Jr, Fallon JT, Buckley MJ, Gold HK, Leinbach RC: Ventricular septal rupture: A review of clinical and physiologic features and an analysis of survival. *Circulation* 64:545, 1981
160. Edmondson HA, Hoxie HJ: Hypertension and cardiac rupture. *Am Heart J* 24:719, 1942
161. Roberts WC, Ronan JA Jr, Harvey WP: Rupture of the left ventricular free wall (LVFW) or ventricular septum (VS) secondary to acute myocardial infarction (AMI): An occurrence virtually limited to the first transmural AMI in a hypertensive individual. *Am J Cardiol* 35:166, 1975
162. Meister SG, Helfant RH: Rapid bedside differentiation of ruptured interventricular septum from acute mitral insufficiency. *N Engl J Med* 287:1024, 1972
163. Scanlan JG, Seward JB, Tajik AJ: Visualization of ventricular septal rupture utilizing wide-angle two-dimensional echocardiography. *Mayo Clin Proc* 54:381, 1979
164. Farcot JC, Boisante L, Rigaud M, Bardet J, Bourdarias JP: Two dimensional echocardiographic visualization of ventricular septal rupture after acute anterior myocardial infarction. *Am J Cardiol* 45:370, 1980
165. Hodsden J, Nanda NC: Dissecting aneurysm of the ventricular septum following acute myocardial infarction: Diagnosis by real time two-dimensional echocardiography. *Am Heart J* 101:671, 1981
166. Bedynek JL, Fenoglio JJ, McAllister HA: Rupture of the ventricular septum as a complication of myocardial infarction. *Am Heart J* 97:773, 1979
167. Boucher CA, Ahluwalia B, Block PC, Brownell GL, Beller GA: Inhalation imaging with oxygen-15 labeled carbon dioxide for detection and quantitation of left-to-right shunts. *Circulation* 56:632, 1977
168. Sanders RJ, Neuberger KT, Ravin A: Rupture of papillary muscles: Occurrence of rupture of the posterior muscle in posterior myocardial infarction. *Dis Chest* 31:316, 1957
169. Kremkau EL, Gilbertson PR, Bristow JD: Acquired, nonrheumatic mitral regurgitation: Clinical management with emphasis on evaluation of myocardial performance. *Prog Cardiovasc Dis* 15:403, 1973
170. Mintz GS, Kotler MN, Parry WR, Segal BL: Statistical comparison of M mode and two dimensional echocardiographic diagnosis of flail mitral leaflets. *Am J Cardiol* 45:253, 1980
171. Mintz GS, Victor MF, Kotler MN, Parry WR, Segal BL: Two-dimensional echocardiographic identification of surgically correctable complications of acute myocardial infarction. *Circulation* 64:91, 1981
172. Wei JY, Hutchins GM, Bulkley BH: Papillary muscle rupture in fatal acute myocardial infarction. A potentially treatable form of cardiogenic shock. *Ann Intern Med* 90:149, 1979
173. Fox AC, Glassman E, Isom OW: Surgically remediable complications of myocardial infarction. *Prog Cardiovasc Dis* 21:461, 1979
174. Selzer A, Katayama F: Mitral regurgitation: Clinical patterns, pathophysiology and natural history. *Medicine* 51:337, 1972
175. Cheng TO, Bashour T, Adkins PC: Acute severe mitral regurgitation from papillary muscle dysfunction in acute myocardial infarction. Successful early surgical treatment by combined mitral valve replacement and aortocoronary saphenous vein bypass graft. *Circulation* 46:491, 1972
176. Mittal AK, Lanston M Jr, Cohn KE, Selzer A, Kerth WJ: Combined papillary muscle and left ventricular wall dysfunction as a cause of mitral regurgitation: An experimental study. *Circulation* 44:174, 1971
177. Shelburne JC, Rubinstein D, Gorlin R: A reappraisal of papillary muscle dysfunction. Correlative clinical and angiographic study. *Am J Med* 46:862, 1969
178. Sanders CA, Armstrong PW, Willerson JT, Dinsmore RE: Etiology and differential diagnosis of acute mitral regurgitation. *Prog Cardiovasc Dis* 14:129, 1971
179. Dressler W: The post-myocardial infarction syndrome: A report of 44 cases. *Arch Intern Med* 103:28, 1959
180. Dressler W, Leavitt SS: Pericarditis after acute myocardial infarction. *JAMA* 173:129, 1960
181. Cohn JN, Guiha NH, Broder MI, Limas CJ: Right ventricular infarction: Clinical and hemodynamic features. *Am J Cardiol* 33:209, 1974
182. Rackley CE, Russell RO: Right ventricular function in acute myocardial infarction. *Am J Cardiol* 33:927, 1974

183. Rotman M, Ratliff NB, Hawley J: Right ventricular infarction: A hemodynamic diagnosis. *Br Heart J* 36:941, 1974
184. Rigo P, Murray M, Taylor DR, Weisfeldt ML, Kelly DT, Strauss HW, Pitt B: Right ventricular dysfunction detected by gated scintiphotography in patients with acute inferior myocardial infarction. *Circulation* 52:268, 1975
185. Sharpe DN, Botvinick EH, Shames DM, Schiller NB, Massie BM, Chatterjee K, Parmley WW: The noninvasive diagnosis of right ventricular infarction. *Circulation* 57:483, 1978
186. Wackers FJT, Lie KI, Sokole EB, Res J, van der Schoot JB, Durrer D: Prevalence of right ventricular involvement in inferior wall infarction assessed with myocardial imaging with thallium-201 and technetium-99m pyrophosphate. *Am J Cardiol* 42:358, 1978
187. Cohn JN: Right ventricular infarction revisited. *Am J Cardiol* 43:666, 1979
188. Coma-Canella I, Lopez-Sendon J: Ventricular compliance in ischemic right ventricular dysfunction. *Am J Cardiol* 45:555, 1980
189. Cintron GB, Hernandez E, Linares E, Aranda JM: Bedside recognition, incidence and clinical course of right ventricular infarction. *Am J Cardiol* 47:224, 1981
190. Lopez-Sendon J, Coma-Canella I, Gamallo C: Sensitivity and specificity of hemodynamic criteria in the diagnosis of acute right ventricular infarction. *Circulation* 64:515, 1981
191. Candell-Riera J, Figueras J, Valle V, Alvarez A, Gutierrez L, Cortadellas J, Cinca J, Salas A, Rius J: Right ventricular infarction: Relationships between ST segment elevation in V_{4R} and hemodynamic, scintigraphic, and echocardiographic findings in patients with acute inferior myocardial infarction. *Am Heart J* 101:281, 1981
192. D'Arcy BJ, Gondi B, Nanda NC, Gatewood RP, Biddle T: Real time two-dimensional echocardiography in right ventricular infarction. *Am J Cardiol* 45:436, 1980
193. Rackley CE, Russell RO Jr, Mantle JA, Rogers WJ, Papapietro SE, Schwartz KM: Right ventricular infarction and function. *Am Heart J* 101:215, 1981
194. Isner JM, Roberts WC: Right ventricular infarction complicating left ventricular infarction secondary to coronary heart disease. *Am J Cardiol* 42:885, 1978
195. Strauss HD, Sobel BE, Roberts R: The influence of occult right ventricular infarction on enzymatically estimated infarct size, hemodynamics, and prognosis. *Circulation* 62:503, 1980
196. Wartman WB, Hellerstein HK: The incidence of heart disease in 2000 consecutive autopsies. *Ann Intern Med* 28:41, 1948
197. Lorell B, Leinbach RC, Pohost GM, Gold HK, Dinsmore RE, Hutter AM Jr, Pastore JO, Desanctis RW: Right ventricular infarction: Clinical diagnosis and differentiation from cardiac tamponade and pericardial constriction. *Am J Cardiol* 43:465, 1979
198. Erhardt LR, Sjogren A, Wahlberg I: Single right-sided precordial lead in the diagnosis of right ventricular involvement in inferior myocardial infarction. *Am Heart J* 91:571, 1976
199. Kisslo J, Wolfson S, Ross A, Pasternak R, Hammond G, Cohen LS: Ultrasound assessment of left ventricular function following aortocoronary saphenous vein bypass grafting. *Circulation* 47(Suppl III):III-156, 1973
200. Righetti A, Crawford MH, O'Rourke RA, Schelbert H, Daily PO, Ross J Jr: Interventricular septal motion and left ventricular function after coronary bypass surgery: Evaluation with echocardiography and radionuclide angiography. *Am J Cardiol* 39:372, 1977
201. Weyman AE, Feigenbaum H, Dillon JC, Johnston KW, Eggleton RC: Noninvasive visualization of the left main coronary artery by cross-sectional echocardiography. *Circulation* 54:169, 1976
202. Ogawa S, Chen CC, Hubbard FE, Pauletto FJ, Mardelli TJ, Morganroth J, Dreifus LS, Akaishi M, Nakamura Y: A new approach to visualize the left main coronary artery using apical cross-sectional echocardiography. *Am J Cardiol* 45:301, 1980
203. Chen CC, Morganroth J, Ogawa S, Mardelli TJ: Detecting left main coronary artery disease by apical, cross-sectional echocardiography. *Circulation* 62:288, 1980
204. Rogers EW, Feigenbaum H, Weyman AE, Godley RW, Vakili ST: Evaluation of left coronary artery anatomy in vitro by cross-sectional echocardiography. *Circulation* 62:782, 1980
205. Friedman MJ, Sahn DJ, Goldman S, Eisner DR, Gittinger NC, Lederman FL, Puckette CM, Tiemann JJ: High frequency, high resolution cross-sectional echo for evaluation of left main coronary artery disease: Is resolution alone enough? *Circulation* 60(Suppl II):II-153, 1979

206. Rink LD, Feigenbaum H, Marshall JE, Godley RW, Doty D, Dillon JC, Weyman AE: Improved echocardiographic technique for examining the left main coronary artery. *Am J Cardiol* 45:435, 1980
207. Yoshikawa J, Yanagihara K, Owaki T, Kato H, Takagi Y, Okumachi F, Fukaya T, Tomito Y, Baba K: Cross-sectional echocardiographic diagnosis of coronary artery aneurysms in patients with the mucocutaneous lymph node syndrome. *Circulation* 59:133, 1979

Left ventricular function 7

One of the most valuable clinical applications of two-dimensional echocardiography is the noninvasive assessment of left ventricular performance. The left ventricular function indices comprise global and regional (segmental) parameters. The determinants of left ventricular function include: (1) left ventricular volume or preload, (2) systemic resistance or afterload, (3) left ventricular mass, and (4) contractility.

Left ventricular cavity size, wall thickness, and mass. An extensive number of studies have been performed with M-mode echocardiography to determine normal criteria for left ventricular chamber size, wall thickness, and mass in infants, children, and adults [1–12]. Although these measurements are potentially accurate, several investigators have examined sources of variability and possible error that fall into three categories: technical [10, 13, 14], interpretive [5, 14–16], and physiologic [6, 8, 9, 17].

Wong and colleagues [10] used an inclinometer to measure the effect of transducer angulation on the reproducibility of left ventricular internal dimensions. They found that if other recording variables were controlled, there was a 20-degree tolerance for transducer angulation in reproducing left ventricular internal dimensions in smaller ventricles; however, a 20-degree difference in recordings of large hearts resulted in poorer reproducibility. These investigators observed that changing body position does not introduce variability in the measurement of left ventricular dimensions, provided that the spatial orientation between the heart and transducer remains constant. Varying reports suggest that body position can become a variable if the alignment of the transducer with the target shifts [14, 18, 19].

A common clinical problem encountered in patients who are technically difficult to image is the necessity of placing the transducer in a low left sternal border interspace, which routinely causes the echo beam to intersect the interventricular septum and left ventricular cavity obliquely, producing a falsely thick septum and falsely increased internal dimensions. For that reason the quality control of M-mode measurements can be improved with simultaneous imaging with two-dimensional echo [20] (Fig. 7-1).

Bett and Dryburgh [9] recommend using five or more consecutive cycles to provide representative values for left ventricular dimensions. They also reported that the derived indices of function from one or two cardiac cycles are often not representative.

DeMaria and associates [17] examined the changes in left ventricular dimensions produced by changes in heart rate in normal subjects. These investigators found that by using right atrial pacing to vary heart rate from 70 to 150 beats/min that a linear regression of a 2.7 percent decrease in left ventricular dimensions occurred for every increase of 10 beats/min in heart rate.

It is well established that inspiration causes an increase in right ventricular volume and a decrease in left ventricular volume. Ruskin and colleagues [21] noted a 10 percent average inspiratory decrease in stroke volume in a group of 11 normal subjects undergoing cardiac catheterization. Brenner and Waugh [6], in a study of 30 normal subjects 5 to 47 years of age, found a mean inspiratory decrease of 2.9 ± 0.4 mm in diastolic dimension; however, the mean decrease in systolic dimension

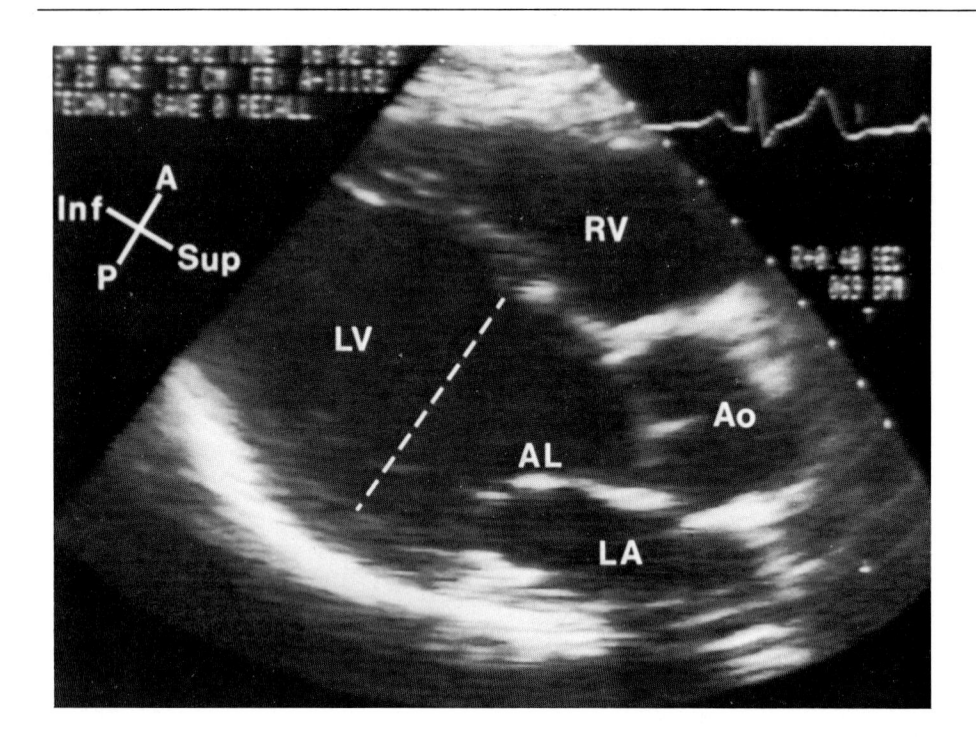

Fig. 7-1. Parasternal long axis view from a low left sternal border transducer position demonstrating an upturned ventricular septum, which prevents an M-mode echo beam from intersecting the septum in a perpendicular manner. Left ventricular internal dimension would be recorded in an oblique anterior-inferior to posterior-superior direction. The only way to obtain a true short axis dimension is from an end-diastolic 2-D video image (dashed line).

was only 0.7 ± 0.4 mm, which was not statistically significant. This inspiratory decrease in left ventricular size is caused by a physiologic shifting of the ventricular septum; however, in the absence of simultaneous 2-D echo imaging, an artifact component due to respiratory shifting of heart position cannot be excluded.

Although the American Society of Echocardiography has recommended that end-diastolic dimensions be measured at the onset of the QRS complex, Friedman and associates [11] found that the measurement did not differ at the peak of the R wave or at the onset of the QRS complex. They did find that the end-diastolic dimension measured as the largest diameter was significantly larger. These investigators reported that the end-systolic dimension measured at the nadir of septal motion did not differ from that measured from sonomicrometer crystal signals; however, when measured at the most anterior ascent of posterior wall motion or as the smallest dimension, it was significantly smaller than end-systolic dimension measured from sonomicrometer crystal signals (Fig. 7-2).

Increasing age correlates with increased aortic root diameter, left ventricular wall thickness, and left atrial size; aging does not affect left ventricular cavity dimensions or global function indices [8, 22].

The determination of left ventricular muscle mass is the accepted standard for identifying the presence or absence of left ventricular hypertrophy. The biplane angiographic method of Rackley and colleagues [23] and Kennedy and coworkers [24] is accurate by comparison with autopsy but has limited use because of its technical complexity and invasive methodology. An accurate echocardiographic method for determination of left ventricular mass with postmortem anatomic validation has been reported [7, 12]. Devereux and Reichek [12] found the best method for determination of left ventricular mass (LVM) combined cube function geometry

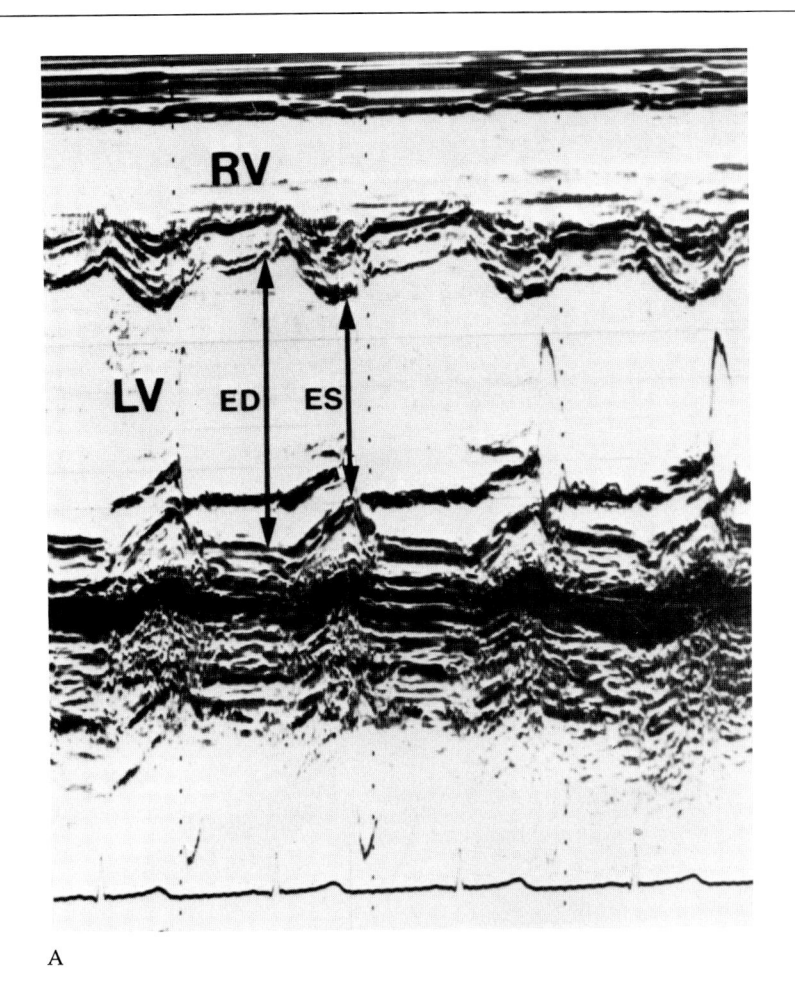

Fig. 7-2A. M-mode recording of the left ventricle in a normal adult subject demonstrating end-diastolic and end-systolic dimensions. The calibration dots are 5 mm apart. B. Parasternal short axis view with M-mode cursor properly positioned through the center of the left ventricle at end systole at the level of the chordae tendineae (C). The M-mode cursor is intersecting the septum and posterior wall in a perpendicular manner; the endocardium and epicardium of the posterior wall are identified by the white and black arrows, respectively. The white arrow in the right ventricle points to a trabeculation that makes the septum appear thicker at that point and can contribute to variations in septal thickness on M-mode recordings.

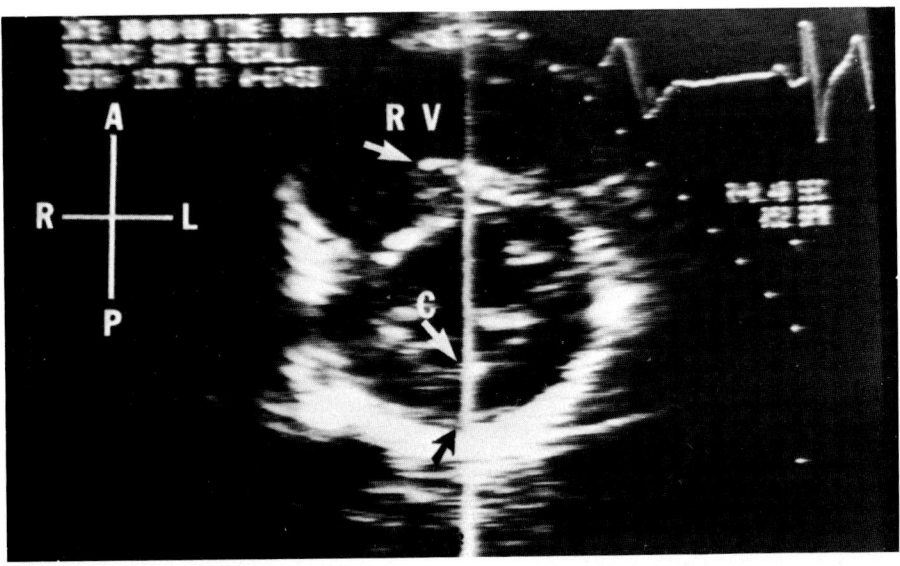

with a modified convention for determination of left ventricular internal dimensions (LVID), posterior wall thickness (PWT), and interventricular septal thickness (IVST), which excluded the thickness of endocardial echo lines from wall thicknesses and included the thickness of left septal and posterior wall endocardial echo line in LVID (Penn Convention):

$$\text{Anatomic LVM} = 1.04\,[(LVID + PWT + IVST)^3 - (LVID)^3] - 13.6\text{ gm} \quad (1)$$

By this method, the echocardiographic correlation with postmortem weight was excellent ($r = 0.96$, SD = 29 gm) in 34 patients with a wide range of anatomic left ventricular mass (101–505 gm). It should be emphasized, however, that none of these subjects had massive myocardial infarction, ventricular aneurysm, severe right ventricular volume overload, or hypertrophic cardiomyopathy.

Because of asymmetrical or segmental hypertrophy, localized thinning from myocardial infarctions, or altered geometry of the cavity due to an aneurysm, determination of left ventricular mass is limited with one-dimensional M-mode echocardiography. For these same reasons two-dimensional echo is superior for quantitative assessment of left ventricular volume and mass. Validation studies of 2-D echocardiography in several laboratories have demonstrated the accuracy of in vitro canine left ventricular volume and mass in symmetric and asymmetric ventricles [25], in vivo canine left ventricular volume and mass (26–28), in vitro human left ventricular cast volume [29], and in vitro anatomic validation of left ventricular volume and mass in postmortem human hearts [30]. Helak and Reichek [30] concluded that 2-D echo can provide reliable estimates of left ventricular volume and mass using the short axis Simpson's rule or area-length methods and appropriate regression corrections.

Aerobic training of college-age men [31] and athletes involved in isotonic exercise [32] develops an increase in end-diastolic volume and mass; however, left ventricular wall thickness remains normal. Athletes involved in isometric exercise, such as wrestling and shot putting, have normal left ventricular end-diastolic volumes but increased wall thickness and mass [32]. Other investigators, in comparing sedentary controls with endurance-trained athletes during supine bicycle exercise, have observed a mean increase in end-diastolic volume to 124 percent of that at rest in the controls in contrast to no change during exercise in the athletes [33]. Although trained and untrained healthy subjects had similar increases in the left ventricular ejection fraction during exercise, different mechanisms were used to achieve these increases. The investigators observed that untrained subjects had increased end-diastolic volumes, whereas trained subjects had decreased end-systolic volumes. Accordingly, they postulated that the ability of athletes to exercise without increasing preload may be an effect of training and might have important implications in reducing myocardial oxygen demand during exercise.

DeMaria and colleagues [34] and Ikaheimo and associates [35] have reported that endurance runners develop increased left ventricular dimensions and mass as well as systolic function parameters. Ikaheimo and associates [35] noted that endurance running causes left ventricular dilatation equal to that of sprinter training but greater wall hypertrophy, and it also produces left atrial dilatation, possibly because of decreased left ventricular compliance.

Left ventricular wall stress. The noninvasive determination of left ventricular wall stress has been validated [36, 37]. The force per unit area, or stress, acting along the circumference of the left ventricle at its minor axis is directly dependent on intracavitary pressure and radius of curvature and inversely dependent on wall thickness [38]. Conditions leading to either chronic pressure or volume overload result in an increase in stress and, thus, a decrease in left ventricular performance unless compensatory hypertrophy develops. Noninvasive indices of circumferential wall stress were developed from systolic arterial pressure and echocardiographic left ventricular diameter and thickness (average of septum and posterior wall), applying the basic formula [36]:

$$\text{Stress} = \frac{\text{pressure} \times \text{radius}}{\text{wall thickness}} \qquad (2)$$

Gould and colleagues [39], in an angiographic study of 122 patients with various forms of heart disease, analyzed wall dynamics and directional components of left ventricular contraction. They calculated three components of work or power: meridional (longitudinal), equatorial (circumferential), and radial (wall thickening). To compute these components, stresses and velocities in each of the three directions were determined. Meridional stress and equatorial stress were computed as defined by Sandler and Dodge [40]. Stress in the radial direction is directly related to the pressure within the wall against which myocardial fibers thicken. The radial stress is equal to midwall myocardial tissue pressure, previously shown to be approximately equal to intraventricular pressure [41, 42]; radial stress therefore equals left ventricular pressure. Gould and associates [39] found the percent contribution of directional components to total work or power developed by a midwall equatorial element of myocardium to be: longitudinal, 14 percent in normal and diseased ventricles; circumferential, 45 percent in normal, increasing to 55 percent in dilated ventricles; wall thickening, 40 percent in normal, decreasing to 31 percent in dilated ventricles. The rate and amount of ventricular wall thickening correlated closely with both ejection fraction and velocity of circumferential shortening.

Quinones and associates [36] calculated three indices of stress at end diastole (WSed), end systole (WSes), and mean as follows:

$$(\text{WSed}) \text{ Wall stress index I} = \frac{\text{systolic arterial pressure} \times \text{radius}}{\text{end-diastolic wall thickness}} \qquad (3)$$

$$(\text{WSes}) \text{ Wall stress index II} = \frac{\text{systolic arterial pressure} \times \text{radius}}{\text{end-systolic wall thickness}} \qquad (4)$$

$$(\text{mean stress}) \text{ Wall stress index III} = \frac{\text{systolic arterial pressure} \times \text{mean radius}}{\text{mean wall thickness}} \qquad (5)$$

where mean radius and mean wall thickness represent the average of end-diastolic and end-systolic measurements. These investigators reported that peak circumferential wall stress can be accurately estimated noninvasively in a variety of cardiac conditions. The assumption of a stress constant allows assessment of severity of aortic stenosis but only when the pressure stimulus has been chronically sustained and left ventricular cavity size and function remain normal [36, 43].

Reichek and colleagues [37] developed a noninvasive method for estimating end-systolic left ventricular meridional wall stress based upon M-mode echocardiographic end-systolic diameter and posterior wall thickness, and cuff systolic arterial pressure. End-systolic meridional wall stress is a quantitative index of true myocardial afterload that can be plotted against left ventricular end-systolic diameter to give an index of contractility independent of loading conditions [37]. These investigators observed that cuff systolic pressure correlated well with end-systolic left ventricular micromanometer pressure ($r = 0.89$) and noninvasive end-systolic stress correlated extremely well with invasive stress ($r = 0.97$).

Left ventricular oxygen consumption per mass unit (M$\dot{V}$O$_2$) is significantly correlated with the systolic force per unit cross-sectional area of the left ventricular wall, that is, to left ventricular systolic wall stress [44]. The relations between left ventricular mass, mass-to-volume ratio, systolic wall stress, and myocardial oxygen consumption were analyzed in 187 patients with chronic heart disease. Strauer [44] described three types of left ventricular hypertrophy in chronic hypertrophic heart disease: (1) appropriate hypertrophy with peak systolic stress normal even at extreme pressure load because of an appropriate increase in mass-to-volume ratio parallel with pressure load; (2) low-stress hypertrophy (inappropriate excess hypertrophy) associated with a marked increase in left ventricular mass out of proportion to volume; (3) high-stress hypertrophy (inappropriate low hypertrophy), which is characterized by excess ventricular dilatation out of proportion to ventricular mass development. This investigator concludes that peak systolic wall stress represents one of the major determinants of myocardial oxygen consumption and of ventricular performance.

Left ventricular volumes and performance. Although M-mode echocardiography has been useful for determining left ventricular volumes and function in children and adults [45–47], other studies have challenged the reliability of M-mode methods, particularly in the presence of coronary artery disease [48–50, 54]. Numerous experimental [50–53] and clinical [54–58] studies have documented the reliability of two-dimensional echocardiography for the quantitation of left ventricular volumes. Various methods have been employed; however, the biplane area-length and Simpson's rule methods have generally proved more accurate for determining volumes and ejection fraction [54–57]. Other methods utilizing mechanical cross-sectional echocardiography have been less reliable for measuring left ventricular end-diastolic volume [59]. Two-dimensional echocardiographic techniques tend to underestimate the left ventricular end-diastolic volume [54, 57].

Schiller and colleagues [54] used the parasternal short axis and apical long axis views as the two planes to obtain paired tomographic images of the left ventricle. Other investigators have preferred using apical long axis and apical four-chamber views for biplane volume determinations [56, 57] (Fig. 7-3).

Mercier and associates [58] evaluated eight algorithms utilizing five geometric models to determine left ventricular volumes and ejection fraction in 25 children with congenital heart disease (Fig. 7-4). These investigators found the degree of correlation with biplane cineangiography varied with the algorithm used. They reported that four algorithms estimated left ventricular volumes with equal accuracy (Simpson's rule assuming the ventricle to be a truncated cone, Simpson's rule assuming the ventricle to be a truncated ellipse, hemisphere cylinder, and ellipsoid biplane). All methods employed in this study underestimated end-diastolic volume, end-systolic volume, and ejection fraction. The degree of underestimation depended upon the algorithm used; the method that provided the best ejection fraction data was the ellipsoid biplane model using the short axis plane at the

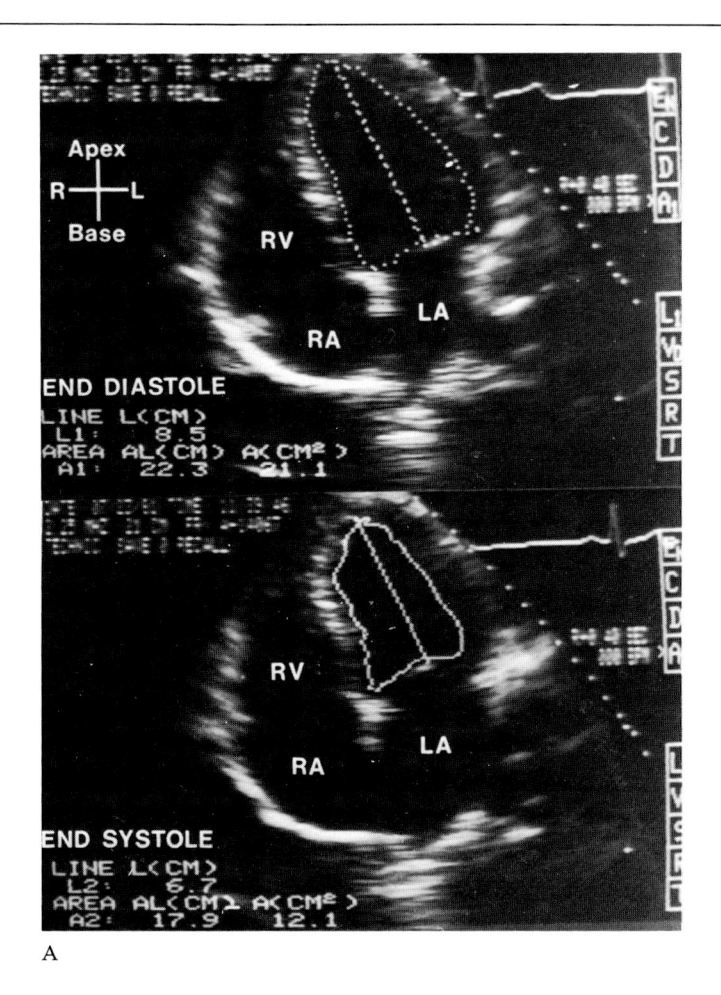

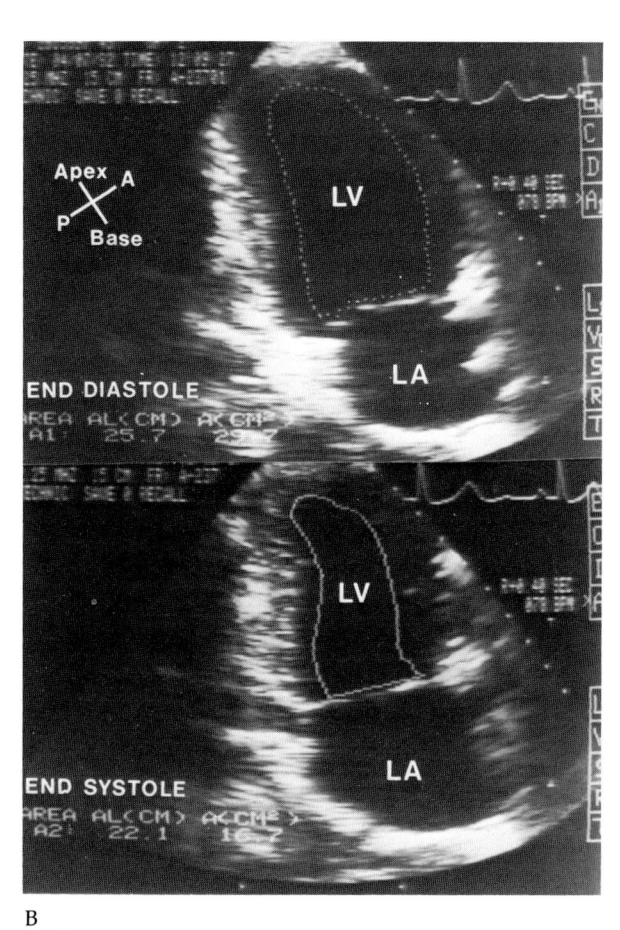

Fig. 7-3A. Apical 4-chamber views in a normal subject at end diastole (upper panel) and end systole (lower panel) demonstrating technique of planimetry of these areas. B. Apical long axis views at end diastole (upper panel) and end systole (lower panel) in a normal adult subject.

234   7. Left ventricular function

Algorithm	Formula	Geometric model
Simpson's rule I	$V = \dfrac{L}{4}\left[Am + \dfrac{Am + Ap_1}{2} + \dfrac{Ap_1 + Ap_2}{2} + 1/3\, Ap_2\right]$	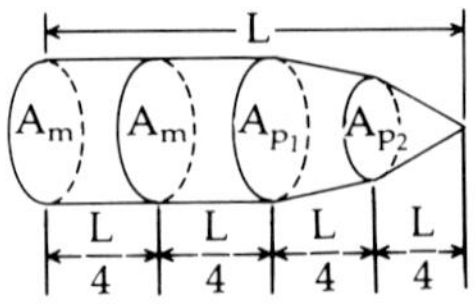
Simpson's rule II	$V = (Amv + Ap_1)\dfrac{L}{3} + \dfrac{Ap_2}{2}\dfrac{L}{3} + \dfrac{\pi}{6}\left(\dfrac{L}{3}\right)^3$	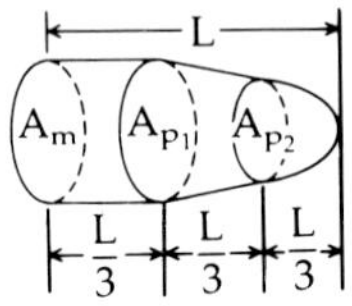
Hemisphere cylinder (MV)	$V = 5/6\, AL\,(MV)$	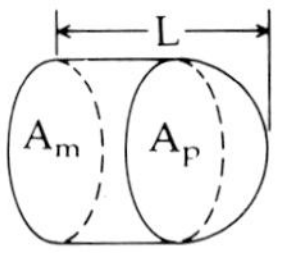
Hemisphere cylinder (PM)	$V = 5/6\, AL\,(PM)$	
Ellipsoid single plane Four-chamber view	$V = 0.85\, A^2/L$	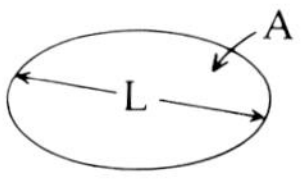
Ellipsoid single plane Two-chamber view	$V = 0.85\, A^2/L$	
Ellipsoid biplane (MV) Area-length	$V = \pi/6\, L\, D_1\, D_2(MV)$	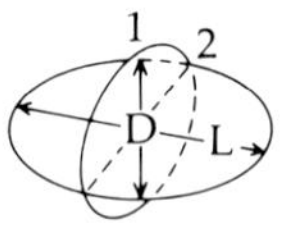
Ellipsoid biplane (PM) Area-length	$V = \pi/6\, L\, D_1\, D_2(PM)$	

Fig. 7-4. Algorithms for determination of left ventricular volumes and ejection fraction. Am = area of short axis at mitral valve level; Ap_1 = area of short axis at high papillary muscle level; Ap_2 = area of short axis at low papillary muscle level; D_1 = minor axis diameter right-left; D_2 = minor axis diameter anteroposterior; L = longest length from the apical 4-chamber view; V = volume. (From JC Mercier et al, Two-dimensional echocardiographic assessment of left ventricular volumes and ejection fraction in children. Circulation 65:962, 1982 by permission of the American Heart Association, Inc.)

papillary muscle level and apical four-chamber view. Since echocardiography underestimated end-diastolic and end-systolic volumes to the same degree, ejection fraction correlated well with cineangiographic data.

Three-dimensional computer reconstructions for spatial visualization and volume calculation of cardiac chambers have been reported [60–62]; however, there has not yet been any significant clinical application.

Peterson and coauthors [63] compared isovolumic indices (derived from developed pressure [DP] including V max, dp/dt/DP) with some ejection phase indices (mean velocity of circumferential fiber shortening [$\overline{Vcf}$] and mean normalized systolic ejection rate). They observed that, in patients with diffuse myocardial involvement, isovolumic indices are not reliable for detecting depressed myocardial function and the ejection phase indices are preferable for assessing myocardial function in the basal state.

The sensitive portion of the normal left ventricular function curve lies below the normal supine filling pressure, and peak performance is achieved near a filling pressure considered to be normal at rest [64]. In the upright position, with a reduced left ventricular filling pressure, cardiac output is sensitive to volume changes. Filling pressure can easily be altered by relatively minor changes in heart rate and other influences. The ventricular function curve in the failing or noncompliant ventricle differs from the normal in that the failing ventricle reaches its peak performance at a much higher filling pressure [64].

The left ventricular global function indices can be divided into volume-dependent and non-volume-dependent measurements. The volume-dependent indices include ejection fraction and stroke volume. M-mode echo methods to determine volumes and ejection fraction are not sufficiently accurate for routine clinical purposes; accordingly, echocardiographic volumes and ejection fraction determinations should be derived from biplane 2-D echo methods previously discussed. The clinically important non-volume-dependent parameters include the circumferential indices (percent fractional shortening and circumferential fiber shortening rate [Vcf], E point septal separation [EPSS], and the wall motion index) [65–73].

From the time Cooper and colleagues [65] reported echocardiographic determination of mean Vcf to be a valid method for distinguishing normal from abnormal left ventricular performance, it has been a valuable index of contractile state. Many investigators have been advocates of mean Vcf as a valuable index of left ventricular performance in infants and children [67, 74] as well as in adults [65, 72]. By adding the element of time to the measurement of change in left ventricular dimensions, Vcf reportedly offers better separation of normal from abnormal patients than ejection fraction alone [65, 66]. Mean Vcf is calculated from the following formula:

$$\overline{Vcf} = \frac{EDD - ESD}{EDD \times LVET} = circ/sec \qquad (6)$$

where EDD = end-diastolic dimension, ESD = end-systolic dimension, LVET = left ventricular ejection time, and the resultant value is expressed in circumferences per second. Since LVET is directly related to age and inversely related to heart rate, infants and children with a faster heart rate have a shorter ejection time and thus a higher value for mean Vcf [67].

DeMaria and associates [75], in a study of 25 normal subjects during atrial pacing, evaluated left ventricular performance at heart rates from 50 to 150 beats/min and observed the mean Vcf to be 1.0 circ/sec at a heart rate of 50 beats/min and up to 1.7 circ/sec at 150 beats/min. These investigators reported no change in blood pressure or percent fractional shortening during pacing. They also reported that left ventricular end-diastolic and end-systolic dimensions decreased with increasing heart rate from a group mean of 48 mm and 30 mm respectively, at a rate of 70/min to 30 mm and 23 mm at a rate of 150/min.

Nixon and associates [72], in a study of 12 healthy young men subjected to head-down tilt at 5 degrees and during progressive lower body negative pressure to −40 mm Hg, noted the mean Vcf to be an index of contractility which is independent of preload, whereas stroke volume and ejection fraction are significantly altered by changes in preload. These authors found that during head-down tilt end-diastolic volume increased 23 percent, stroke volume increased 35 percent, and ejection fraction increased 10 percent; during lower body negative pressure, end-diastolic volume decreased 28 percent, end-systolic volume decreased 21 percent, and stroke volume decreased 33 percent.

The left ventricular end-diastolic dimension and its percentage change with systole (percent fractional shortening [%FS]) has been reported to be as sensitive as Vcf in detecting depressed left ventricular function [76, 77]. This short axis dimensional change measured at the level of the chordae tendineae is calculated in the same manner as the mean Vcf except that ejection time is not taken into consideration:

$$\%FS = \frac{EDD - ESD}{EDD} \times 100 \qquad (7)$$

The %FS can be measured easily and quickly and clinically represents a very useful quantitative left ventricular function index; in contrast to Vcf, it is not dependent on accurate measurement of ejection time. The %FS is potentially inaccurate whenever paradoxical septal motion is present or in the presence of segmental wall motion abnormalities, particularly if the measured systolic dimensional changes are not representative of the rest of the ventricle.

The mitral E point-septal separation (EPSS) has proved to be a very useful indicator of left ventricular performance [69–71]. As recommended by D'Cruz and coworkers [71], we routinely measure the mitral-septal separation at the instant of inscription of the E point (Fig. 7-5). All three of these studies have demonstrated good sensitivity and specificity of EPSS for left ventricular function; in fact, Lew and associates [70] and D'Cruz and colleagues [71] found EPSS superior to other echocardiographic indicators of left ventricular function. All of these studies have demonstrated a good linear relationship of EPSS and either angiographic or radionuclide ejection fractions; however, EPSS correlates poorly with left ventricular size. Accordingly, increased EPSS is not due simply to a dilated left ventricle. Practical advantages of EPSS are: easy recording of anterior mitral leaflet and the left border of the ventricular septum in nearly all patients; lack of dependence on or influence by segmental wall motion abnormalities or left ventricular size; and lack of dependence on mathematical formulas or geometric assumptions. It has been suggested that EPSS is determined by the interplay of multiple factors; however, the precise mechanism of increased EPSS has never been explained. Two-dimensional echo can be employed to improve the specificity of EPSS in a small number of patients who have an increased EPSS (false positive) caused by a low transducer position with resultant upturned septum (Fig. 7-6).

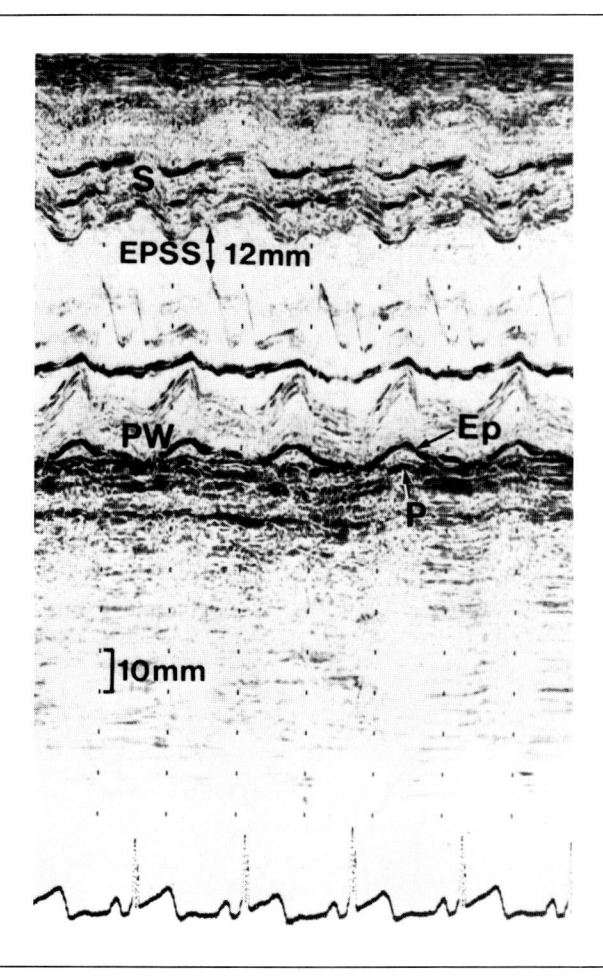

Fig. 7-5. M-mode recording of a patient with normal end-diastolic dimension as well as normal motion of the septum and posterior wall demonstrating an increased E point-septal separation (EPSS) (12 mm), which indicates reduced left ventricular function (ejection fraction). P = pericardium.

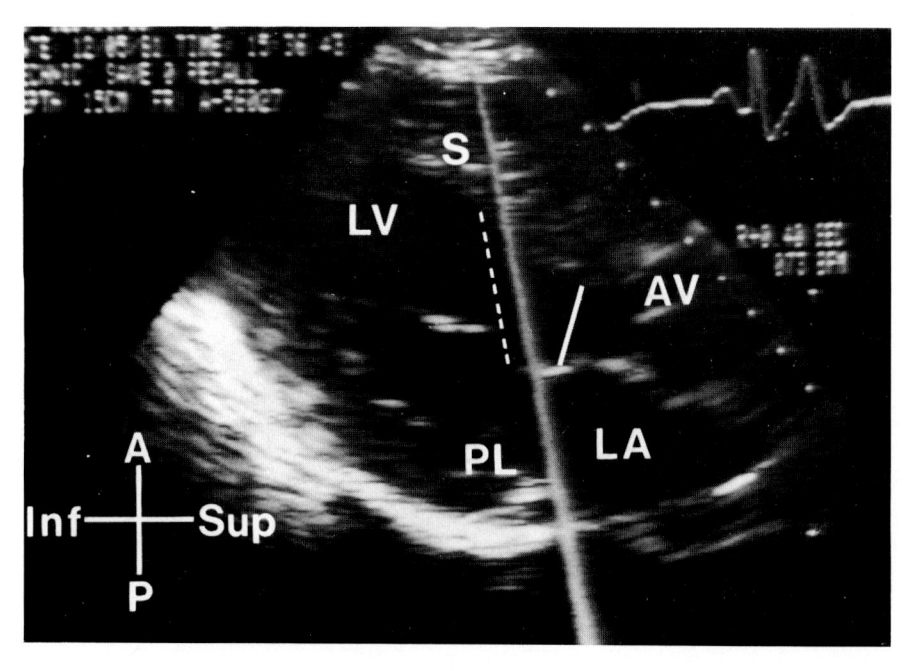

Fig. 7-6. Parasternal long axis view from a low left sternal border transducer position with M-mode demonstrating how a false positive E point-septal separation (EPSS) could occur because the beam intersects the septum at a more distal location and, due to the oblique angle through the left ventricle, cause an increased EPSS (dashed line). When the correct (shortest) distance (solid line) to the septum is measured from the 2-D echo image, it is normal. Distances in this photograph are even greater because the anterior leaflet is farther from the septum at mid diastole.

Echocardiographic and Doppler estimates of cardiac output. Accurate measurement of volume flow using a pulsed Doppler flowmeter requires determination of the angle of the Doppler beam with respect to the vector representing flow velocity, the cross-sectional area of the vessel, and the flow profile at the cross section being investigated [78–80]. By combining a pulsed Doppler flowmeter with a phased-array sector scanner, an image of a vessel is produced with a cursor line, corresponding to the path of the Doppler sound beam superimposed on it.

Magnin and colleagues [80] evaluated a pulsed Doppler–phased-array (DPA) system in vitro and in patients undergoing cardiac catheterization and found DPA estimates of cardiac output compared favorably with Fick estimates in 11 patients ($r = 0.83$). The range cursor was positioned within the ascending aorta just above the aortic valve leaflets at the point that had the greatest analog-net-flow (ANF) output to ensure that it was centered in the vessel. Angles from 40 to 68 degrees were used. These investigators emphasized that, although these preliminary results were encouraging, several limitations of the DPA combined approach were apparent: (1) potential for error in angle measurement, that is, angle errors have a more detrimental effect on the flow estimate as angles approach 90 degrees than for smaller angles; (2) potential for error in measuring the diameter of the vessel (cardiac output has a squared dependence on this variable) and the possibility that the vessel is not a perfect cylinder; (3) potential for nonuniform flow profile at the sample site or nonlinearities within the pulsed Doppler unit; and (4) variations in cardiac output with transducer location which are presumably caused by errors associated with angle, attenuation of the ANF signal caused by tissue absorption, and acoustic noise caused by rib reflections.

Steingart and colleagues [81] have demonstrated experimentally that pulsed Doppler echocardiography is an excellent measurement of stroke volume changes.

Darsee and associates [82] described the technique and clinical value of noninvasive continuous wave Doppler measurements for monitoring changes in cardiac output in patients with acute myocardial infarction. The basic Doppler equation, $v = \Delta fc/2f_o \cos\theta$, indicates that flow velocity can be calculated from the observed Doppler shifts with an accuracy of ± 10 percent if the beam is within 25 degrees of the direction of flow because of the small variation of $\cos\theta$ when θ is near 0: c = sound velocity; f = the Doppler shift (Hz); f_o = the center frequency (Hz); θ = the angle between the beam vector and velocity; and v = flow velocity. For the measurement of volume flow ($\dot{Q}$), the Doppler equation must be multiplied by the cross-sectional area (A) of the vessel:

$$\dot{Q} = \frac{(A)(\Delta fc)}{(2f_o \cos\theta)} \tag{8}$$

The mean frequency shift (Δf) in this case is the average over the total vessel lumen; and θ is the average angle over the total lumen [82]. Although this study clearly demonstrated the clinical value of this procedure for the initial evaluation and frequent monitoring of patients who are hemodynamically unstable, the Doppler signals were noisy at heart rates exceeding 150/min and produced less satisfactory results.

Methods for estimating cardiac output and stroke volume using the mitral valve and aortic root echo have been reported [83–85]. Corya and colleagues [85] developed a method for calculating aortic valve stroke volume (AVSV) using the M-

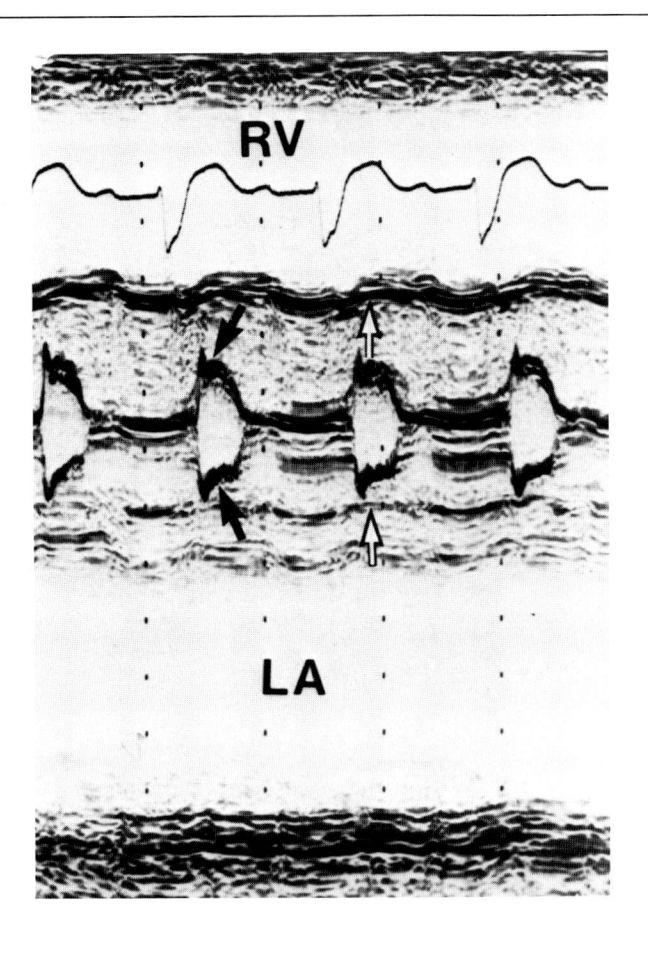

Fig. 7-7. M-mode recording in a patient with poor cardiac output and left atrial enlargement. The reduced stroke volume is indicated by the reduced aortic leaflet opening (solid arrows) *and by the decreased systolic amplitude of the aortic root* (open arrows).

mode echo recordings of initial and late aortic cusp separation (AVO), ejection time (ET), and amplitude of posterior aortic root motion during ejection (AA):

$$AVSV = (\text{average AVO [cm]} \times ET [sec]) \times 100 + AA \text{ (mm)} \tag{9}$$

These investigators found an excellent linear correlation between this method and the Fick or thermodilution method for stroke volume ($r = 0.96$) and for cardiac output ($r = 0.92$).

The findings of Pratt and colleagues [86] indicate that the aortic root motion is an index of stroke volume and they further demonstrated that root motion is acutely sensitive to variations in stroke volume. These investigators, in a study of 24 normal subjects, reported that the systolic amplitude of the anterior aortic wall at rest was 11.2 ± 0.5 mm and the posterior wall was 9.5 ± 0.3 mm; during the strain phase of the Valsalva maneuver, anterior wall amplitude decreased to 8.2 ± 0.4 mm and the posterior wall to 7.3 ± 0.5 mm; following inhalation of amyl nitrite the amplitude of the anterior wall increased to 13.5 ± 0.8 mm and the posterior wall to 11.9 ± 0.6 mm. In addition to the reduced motion of the aortic root in patients with poor stroke volume, the reduced flow through the mitral valve also produces a characteristic appearance in patients with poor cardiac output (Figs. 7-7 and 7-8).

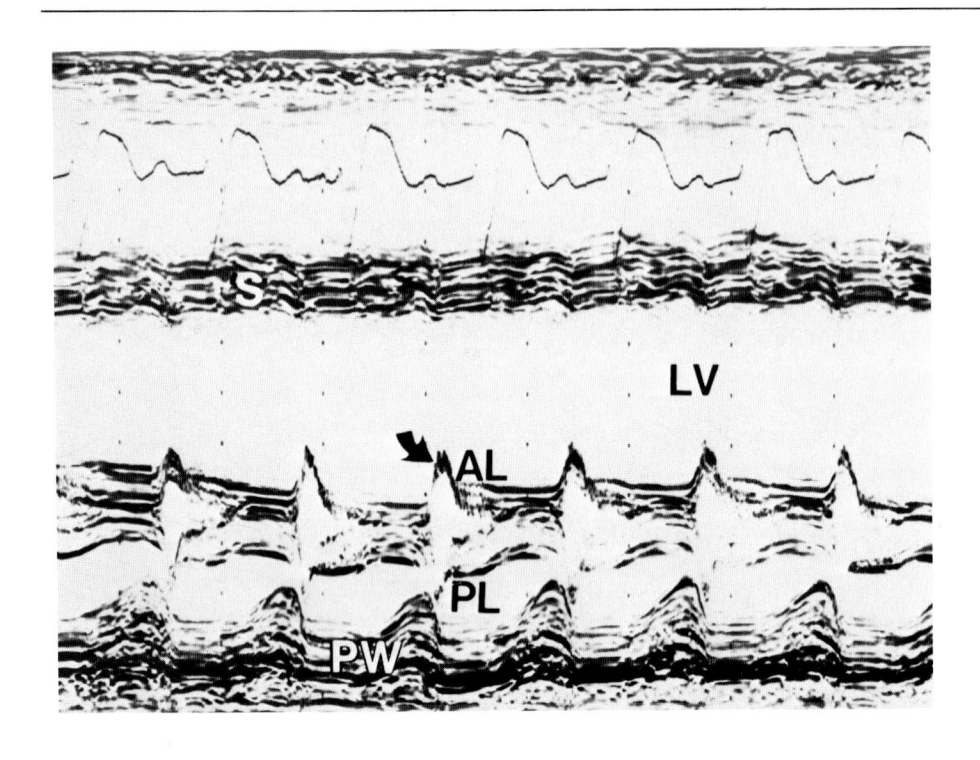

Fig. 7-8. *M-mode recording from a patient with poor left ventricular function and reduced cardiac output demonstrating the characteristic appearance of the mitral valve with low flow in such patients. Besides the reduced separation of the anterior and posterior mitral leaflets during diastole, the increased EPSS also indicates a reduced ejection fraction. The opening of the AL (arrow) does not occur until after the P wave in this patient with first-degree AV block.*

Influence of cardiovascular drugs and exercise on left ventricular function. Echocardiography is well suited for evaluating acute alterations or serial changes of cardiovascular drugs on left ventricular dimensions and performance [18, 87–96].

Redwood and colleagues [87] found that sublingual nitroglycerin reduced both end-diastolic and end-systolic dimensions, whereas phenylephrine increased end-diastolic dimensions but did not alter end-systolic dimensions. They observed that mean Vcf was not altered significantly by phenylephrine but was increased by nitroglycerin (from 1.3 ± 0.1 to 1.7 ± 0.1 circ/sec). Hirshleifer and associates [89] emphasized that when echocardiographic measurements are used for serial assessment of left ventricular performance, the heart rate and blood pressure at which studies are obtained are very important. Hardarson and associates [91], in an acute study of 11 patients with previous myocardial infarctions, found that both oral isosorbide dinitrate (20 mg) and nitroglycerin ointment (12.5 to 40 mg) produced a significant decrease in systolic blood pressure, end-diastolic dimension, end-systolic dimension, and left ventricular wall stress but no change in heart rate during 4 hours of study. The triple product of heart rate, systolic blood pressure, and left ventricular ejection time decreased by 21 percent after administration of isosorbide dinitrate and 19 percent after administration of nitroglycerin ointment. Wei and Reid [96] have demonstrated the existence of a close relationship between plasma nitroglycerin levels and variables that reflect the known responses to this drug.

Frishman and coworkers [88] reported that the echocardiographic assessment of left ventricular function was more valuable than determinations of propranolol blood levels in managing patients with angina pectoris and provided a guide to optimal adjustment of dosage. In a study of 19 patients with severe but stable angina pectoris, these investigators found that with propranolol, 80 mg daily, total work performance increased by 128 percent, whereas with 160 mg daily, total work performance decreased but remained higher than at control levels. They reported exercise tolerance was maximally improved with doses of 80 to 160 mg daily and higher dose levels caused deterioration of left ventricular function and exercise work decreased.

Crawford and colleagues [90] have demonstrated the utility of echocardiography for studying the effects of oral maintenance digoxin therapy on left ventricular performance. In ten normal subjects they found that digoxin increased ejection fraction (74 ± 2 to 79 ± 1%) and fractional shortening increased from 37 ± 2 to 41 ± 1 percent.

Chaignon and coinvestigators [97] used echocardiography to monitor the acute effects of hemodialysis on left ventricular performance. Hemodialysis for 5 hours led to no change in either ejection fraction or percent fractional shortening whereas the mean Vcf and mean systolic ejection rate were both significantly increased (1.17 ± 0.2 to 1.38 ± 0.28 circ/sec and 2.38 ± 0.27 to 2.80 ± 0.40 end-diastolic volume/sec respectively).

Left ventricular diastolic filling and compliance. The term ventricular compliance refers to the distensibility of the relaxed ventricle, defined in terms of its diastolic pressure-volume relationship. Although it is well known that left ventricular failure causes elevated diastolic filling pressures, other conditions without depressed systolic function such as hypertrophic cardiomyopathy, left ventricular hypertrophy, or constrictive pericarditis may have marked elevations of end-diastolic pressures and normal end-diastolic volumes.

The expression dv/dp, representing the change in ventricular volume per unit change in diastolic filling pressure, is considered an index of distensibility of the entire ventricle. The reciprocal of this expression (dp/dv) has been used as an index of stiffness or elasticity of the ventricle [98]. The diastolic pressure-volume curve is not linear, and the compliance of the ventricle falls as the filling pressure rises. A structurally normal ventricle then may exhibit the same low compliance as a scarred or hypertrophied ventricle if its filling pressure is elevated sufficiently.

Experimental studies of Hood and associates [99] demonstrated that elevated filling pressures of the left ventricle following acute myocardial infarction may not signify ventricular failure; and the observed fall in compliance 3 to 5 days after coronary ligation may represent a mechanism for improving ventricular function during recovery from acute myocardial infarction. The role played by altered compliance of the left ventricle is essential to the clinical distinction between myocardial failure and congestive failure [98].

Mann and colleagues [100] demonstrated relaxation abnormalities during angina pectoris induced by atrial pacing.

Myocardial relaxation is an energy-dependent process that consumes high-energy phosphate, and calcium released from the troponin is sequestered in the sarcoplasmic reticulum during this period [101].

The quantitative assessment of left ventricular diastolic thickness in patients with coronary artery disease and chronic valve disease correlates well with the presence or absence of left ventricular hypertrophy [102, 103]. The findings of Hess and associates [104] suggest that diastolic myocardial stiffness in myocardial hypertrophy is related more to the interstitial than to the muscular tissue.

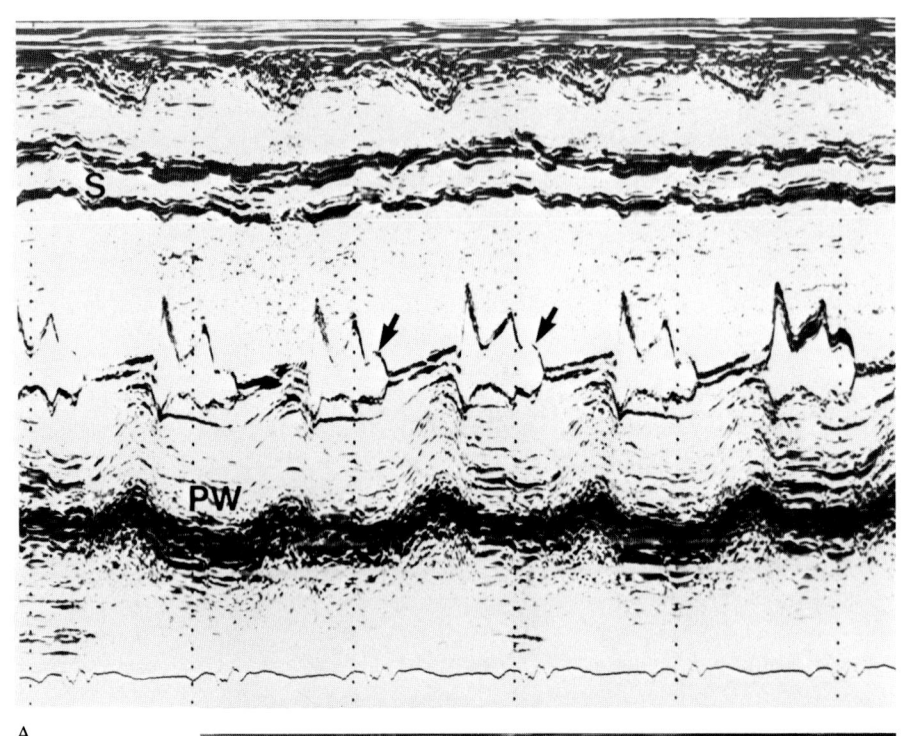

Fig. 7-9A. M-mode recording in a patient with left ventricular enlargement (calibration dots 5 mm apart), poor left ventricular function, akinetic septum, and very large "B" notch (arrows) with prolongation of the A–C interval, which is indicative of an elevated end-diastolic pressure. B. M-mode recording in a patient with borderline enlargement of the left ventricle (calibration dots 10 mm apart), abnormal LV function, and prominent "B" notch (arrows) with prolongation of the A–C interval, which in this case is not indicative of elevated end-diastolic pressure but is caused by first-degree AV block, which can be seen in the accompanying ECG.

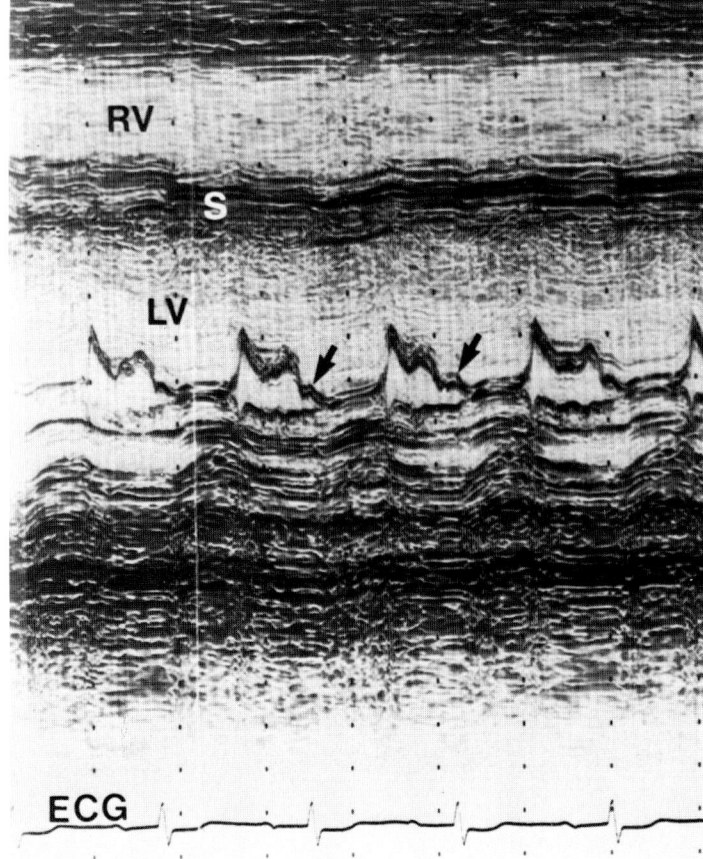

M-mode echocardiography is particularly well suited for evaluating early diastolic filling (mitral valve E–F slope) [105, 106], left atrial emptying index [107], left ventricular end-diastolic pressure (abnormal PR–AC interval) [108, 109], and delay in opening of the mitral valve following aortic valve closure (see discussion in Chapter 6) (Fig. 7-9). Quinones and coworkers [105] found that in every instance in which mitral valve slope was less than 60 mm/sec, in the absence of mitral valve obstruction, an abnormality of the left ventricular pressure-volume relation was present. These investigators also observed that mitral valve slope correlated well with the pressure-volume relation ($r = 0.72$, $p < 0.001$) and with the end-diastolic distensibility index ($r = 0.59$, $p < 0.001$), but poorly when compared with end-diastolic compliance or left ventricular end-diastolic pressure.

DeMaria and colleagues [106] measured transmitral flow of 52 ± 25 ml during the initial third of diastole in normal subjects representing 48 ± 10 percent of total flow; flow was diminished in patients with coronary artery disease and hypertrophic cardiomyopathy to 23 ± 16 ml ($25 \pm 24\%$) and 24 ± 20 ml ($20 \pm 11\%$), respectively. They found the E–F slope could not be related to compliance in individual patients; however, those with an E–F slope of less than 75 mm/sec nearly always had diminished compliance.

Rapid filling of the left ventricle is reduced in hypertension, even before electrocardiographic or systolic function abnormalities are detectable [20, 107]. The atrial emptying index appears to be an early indicator of abnormalities of left ventricular diastolic compliance in uncomplicated hypertension [107] (see discussion and Fig. 6-1C in Chap. 6).

In studies of subjects in the resting state, a PR–AC interval greater than 0.06 second has been associated with a left ventricular end-diastolic pressure of less than 20 mm Hg; and a PR–AC interval of 0.06 second or less is predictive of an end-diastolic pressure of 20 mm Hg or greater [108, 110]. Lewis and colleagues [109], in a study of 22 patients undergoing cardiac catheterization, infused dextran and administered nitroglycerin to alter left ventricular end-diastolic pressure to determine the predictive value of the PR–AC interval for the end-diastolic pressure during acute hemodynamic manipulations and found a poor correlation ($r = -0.33$, $p < 0.01$).

Interdependence of the right and left ventricles. The functional integration of the right ventricle, lungs, and left ventricle is fostered by their anatomic arrangement and mechanical interaction. The mobile interventricular septum and pericardium promote the interaction between the ventricles, while intrathoracic or pleural pressure surrounds the entire unit and creates a second interaction between the ventricles as well as between the heart and lungs [111].

Five potential mechanisms have been suggested to explain the nonlinear relationship between pressure and volume in the diastolic left ventricle [112]: (1) changes in the heart's geometry, (2) changes in the myocardium's passive mechanical properties, (3) engorgement of the coronary circulation, (4) incomplete relaxation from the previous systole, and (5) interaction between the two ventricles. The pericardium restricts expansion of the entire heart and increases the extent to which one ventricle can affect the other. Glantz and associates [113], in an experimental dog study, evaluated the relationship between left and right ventricular diastolic pressures with the pericardium closed and open. With the pericardium closed, right ventricular pressure was a more powerful predictor of left ventricular pressure than were left ventricular dimensions. In addition, the left ventricle appeared much more compliant with the pericardium open.

Diastolic bulging of the interventricular septum toward the left ventricle is commonly seen in patients with severe pulmonary hypertension with or without associated right ventricular volume overload [114]. Brinker and colleagues [115] used the Müller maneuver (forced inspiration against a closed airway) to increase right ventricular volume loading and observed secondary flattening of the septum which persisted during systole. These authors postulated that changed septal shape may be an important mechanism of, and evidence for, ventricular interdependence in normal man.

Both experimental and clinical studies have demonstrated that high levels of positive expiratory pressure (PEEP) produce elevation of left atrial pressure, reduced stroke work, and decreased cardiac output [116–120]. Left atrial pressure increases when measured relative to pleural pressure during PEEP. Scharf and coworkers [118], in anesthetized, mechanically ventilated dogs, observed that pericardial pressure did not rise more during PEEP than did pleural pressure, which indicated a true increase in transmural left atrial pressure. Jardin and associates [120] studied ten patients with adult respiratory distress syndrome with a stepwise increase in PEEP from 0 to 30 cm H_2O to evaluate the effect on left ventricular output. They reported that increasing PEEP was associated with progressive declines in cardiac output, mean blood pressure, left ventricular dimensions, and with equalization of right and left ventricular filling pressures. The radius of septal curvature decreased at both end diastole and end systole secondary to a leftward shift of the interventricular septum. These investigators noted that at the highest PEEP blood volume expansion did not restore cardiac output, although left ventricular filling pressures had returned to baseline values. Because of this interdependence of the right and left ventricles and the problem with interpreting pulmonary wedge pressures in such patients receiving PEEP, it is important to obtain additional anatomic and functional information about the left ventricle with two-dimensional echocardiography.

References

1. Hagan AD, Deely WF, Sahn D, Friedman WF: Echocardiographic criteria for normal newborn infants. *Circulation* 48:1221, 1973
2. Henry WL, Ware J, Gardin JM, Hepner SI, McKay J, Weiner M: Echocardiographic measurements in normal subjects: Growth-related changes that occur between infancy and early adulthood. *Circulation* 57:278, 1978
3. Goldberg SJ, Allen HD, Sahn DJ: *Pediatric and Adolescent Echocardiography.* Chicago: Year Book, 1975
4. Bahler AS, Teichholz LE, Gorlin R, Herman MV: Correlations of electrocardiography and echocardiography in determination of left ventricular wall thickness: Study of apparently normal subjects. *Am J Cardiol* 39:189, 1977
5. Monoson PA, O'Rourke RA, Crawford MH, White DH: Measurements of left ventricular wall thickness and systolic thickening by M-mode echocardiography: Interobserver and intrapatient variability. *JCU* 6:252, 1978
6. Brenner JI, Waugh RA: Effect of phasic respiration on left ventricular dimension and performance in a normal population: An echocardiographic study. *Circulation* 57:122, 1978
7. Reichek N, Devereux RB: Left ventricular hypertrophy: Relationship of anatomic, echocardiographic and electrocardiographic findings. *Circulation* 63:1391, 1981

8. Gerstenblith G, Frederiksen J, Yin FCP, Fortuin NJ, Lakatta EG, Weisfeldt ML: Echocardiographic assessment of a normal adult aging population. *Circulation* 56:273, 1977
9. Bett JHN, Dryburgh LG: Beat-to-beat variation in echocardiographic measurements of left ventricular dimensions and function. *JCU* 9:119, 1981
10. Wong M, Shah PM, Taylor RD: Reproducibility of left ventricular internal dimensions with M-mode echocardiography: Effects of heart size, body position and transducer angulation. *Am J Cardiol* 47:1068, 1981
11. Friedman MJ, Roeske WR, Sahn DJ, Larson D, Goldberg SJ: Accuracy of M-mode echocardiographic measurements of the left ventricle. *Am J Cardiol* 49:716, 1982
12. Devereux RB, Reichek N: Echocardiographic determination of left ventricular mass in man: Anatomic validation of the method. *Circulation* 55:613, 1977
13. Popp RL, Filly K, Brown OR, Harrison DC: Effect of transducer placement on echocardiographic measurement of left ventricular dimensions. *Am J Cardiol* 35:537, 1975
14. Felner JM, Blumenstein BA, Schlant RC, Carter AD, Alimurung BN, Johnson MJ, Sherman SW, Klicpera MW, Kutner MH, Drucker LW: Sources of variability in echocardiographic measurements. *Am J Cardiol* 45:995, 1980
15. Valdez RS, Motta JA, London E, Martin RP, Haskell WL, Farquhar JW, Popp RL, Horlick L: Evaluation of the echocardiogram as an epidemiologic tool in an asymptomatic population. *Circulation* 60:921, 1979
16. Vignola PA, Bloch A, Kaplan AD, Walker HR, Chlotellis PN, Myers GS: Interobserver variability in echocardiography. *JCU* 5:238, 1977
17. DeMaria AN, Neumann A, Schubart PJ, Lee G, Mason DT: Systematic correlation of cardiac chamber size and ventricular performance determined with echocardiography and alterations in heart rate in normal persons. *Am J Cardiol* 43:1, 1979
18. Martin MA, Fieller NRJ: Echocardiography in cardiovascular drug assessment. *Br Heart J* 41:536, 1979
19. Katz R, Karliner JS, Resnik R: Effects of a natural volume overload state (pregnancy) on left ventricular performance in normal human subjects. *Circulation* 58:434, 1978
20. Cohen A, Hagan AD, Watkins J, Mitas J, Schvartzman M, Mazzoleni A, Cohen IM, Warren SE, Vieweg WVR: Clinical correlates of hypertensive patients with left ventricular hypertrophy diagnosed with echocardiography. *Am J Cardiol* 47:335, 1981
21. Ruskin J, Bache RF, Rembert JC, Greenfield JC: Pressure flow studies in man: Effect of respiration on left ventricular stroke volume. *Circulation* 48:79, 1973
22. Henry WL, Gardin JM, Ware JH: Echocardiographic measurements in normal subjects from infancy to old age. *Circulation* 62:1054, 1980
23. Rackley CE, Dodge HT, Coble YD, Hay RE: A method for determining left ventricular mass in man. *Circulation* 29:666, 1964
24. Kennedy JW, Reichenbach DD, Baxley WA, Dodge HT: Left ventricular mass: A comparison of angiocardiographic measurements with autopsy weight. *Am J Cardiol* 19:221, 1967
25. Wyatt HL, Heng MK, Meerbaum S, Hestenes J, Davidson R, Corday E: Quantitation of volumes in asymmetric left ventricles by 2-D echocardiography. *Circulation* 57(Suppl II):II-188, 1978
26. Gueret P, Wyatt HL, Meerbaum S, Corday E: A practical two-dimensional echocardiographic model to assess volume in the ischemic left ventricle. *Am J Cardiol* 45:471, 1980
27. Wyatt HL, Heng MK, Meerbaum S, Hestenes JD, Cobo JM, Davidson RM, Corday E: Cross-sectional echocardiography. I. Analysis of mathematic models for quantifying mass of the left ventricle in dogs. *Circulation* 60:1104, 1979
28. Schiller NB, Skioldebrand C, Schiller E, Mavroudis C, Silverman N, Rahimtoola S, Lipton M: In vivo assessment of left ventricular mass by two-dimensional echocardiography. *Circulation* 59(Suppl II):II-18, 1979
29. Bommer W, Chun T, Kwan OL, Neumann A, Mason DT, DeMaria AN: Biplane apex echocardiography versus biplane cineangiography in the assessment of left ventricular volume and function: Validation by direct methods. *Am J Cardiol* 45:471, 1980
30. Helak JW, Reichek N: Quantitation of human left ventricular mass and volume by two-dimensional echocardiography: In vitro anatomic validation. *Circulation* 63:1398, 1981
31. Adams TD, Yanowitz FG, Fisher AG, Ridges JD, Lovell K, Pryor TA: Noninvasive evaluation of exercise training in college-age men. *Circulation* 64:958, 1981
32. Morganroth J, Maron BJ, Henry WL, Epstein SE: Comparative left ventricular dimensions in trained athletes. *Ann Intern Med* 82:521, 1975

33. Bar-Shlomo B-Z, Druck MN, Morch JE, Jablonsky G, Hilton JD, Feiglin DHI, McLaughlin PR: Left ventricular function in trained and untrained healthy subjects. *Circulation* 65:484, 1982
34. DeMaria AN, Neumann A, Lee G, Fowler W, Mason DT: Alterations in ventricular mass and performance induced by exercise training in man evaluated by echocardiography. *Circulation* 57:237, 1978
35. Ikaheimo MJ, Palatsi IJ, Takkunen JT: Noninvasive evaluation of the athletic heart: Sprinters versus endurance runners. *Am J Cardiol* 44:24, 1979
36. Quinones MA, Mokotoff DM, Nouri S, Winters WL Jr, Miller RR: Noninvasive quantification of left ventricular wall stress: Validation of method and application to assessment of chronic pressure overload. *Am J Cardiol* 45:782, 1980
37. Reichek N, Wilson J, Sutton MSJ, Plappert TA, Goldberg S, Hirshfeld JW: Noninvasive determination of left ventricular end-systolic stress: Validation of the method and initial application. *Circulation* 65:99, 1982
38. Hood WP Jr, Rackley CE, Rolett EL: Wall stress in the normal and hypertrophied human left ventricle. *Am J Cardiol* 22:550, 1968
39. Gould KL, Kennedy JW, Frimer M, Pollack GH, Dodge HT: Analysis of wall dynamics and directional components of left ventricular contraction in man. *Am J Cardiol* 38:322, 1976
40. Sandler H, Dodge HT: Left ventricular tension and stress in man. *Circ Res* 13:91, 1963
41. Armour JA, Randall WC: Canine left ventricular intramyocardial pressures. *Am J Physiol* 220:1833, 1971
42. Kirk ES, Honig CR: An experimental and theoretical analysis of myocardial tissue pressure. *Am J Physiol* 207:361, 1964
43. Hagan AD, DiSessa TG, Samtoy L, Friedman WF, Vieweg WVR: Reliability of echocardiography in diagnosing and quantitating valvular aortic stenosis. *Cardiovasc Med* 5:391, 1980
44. Strauer BE: Myocardial oxygen consumption in chronic heart disease: Role of wall stress, hypertrophy and coronary reserve. *Am J Cardiol* 44:730, 1979
45. Pombo JF, Troy BL, Russell RO Jr: Left ventricular volumes and ejection fraction by echocardiography. *Circulation* 43:480, 1971
46. Meyer RA, Stockert J, Kaplan S: Echographic determination of left ventricular volumes in pediatric patients. *Circulation* 51:297, 1975
47. Bennett DH, Rowlands DJ: Test of reliability of echocardiographic estimation of left ventricular dimensions and volumes. *Br Heart J* 38:1133, 1976
48. Linhart JW, Mintz GS, Segal BL, Kawai N, Kotler MN: Left ventricular volume measurement by echocardiography: Fact or fiction? *Am J Cardiol* 36:114, 1975
49. Teichholz LE, Kreulen T, Herman MV, Gorlin R: Problems in echocardiographic volume determinations: Echocardiographic-angiographic correlations in the presence or absence of asynergy. *Am J Cardiol* 37:7, 1976
50. Schapira JN, Kohn MS, Beaver WL, Popp RL: In vitro quantitation of canine left ventricular volume by phased-array sector scan. *Cardiology* 67:1, 1981
51. Eaton LW, Maughan WL, Shoukas AA, Weiss JL: Accurate volume determination in the isolated ejecting canine left ventricle by two-dimensional echocardiography. *Circulation* 60:320, 1979
52. Gueret P, Meerbaum S, Zwehl W, Wyatt HL, Davidson RM, Uchiyama T, Corday E: Two-dimensional echocardiographic assessment of left ventricular stroke volume: Experimental correlation with thermodilution and cineangiography in normal and ischemic states. *Cathet Cardiovasc Diagn* 7:247, 1981
53. Wyatt HL, Heng MK, Meerbaum S, Gueret P, Hestenes J, Dula E, Corday E: Cross-sectional echocardiography. II. Analysis of mathematic models for quantifying volume of the formalin-fixed left ventricle. *Circulation* 61:1119, 1980
54. Schiller NB, Acquatella H, Ports TA, Drew D, Goerke J, Ringertz H, Silverman NH, Brundage B, Botvinick EH, Boswell R, Carlsson E, Parmley WW: Left ventricular volume from paired biplane two-dimensional echocardiography. *Circulation* 60:547, 1979
55. Erbel R, Schweizer P, Meyer J, Grenner H, Krebs W, Effert S: Left ventricular volume and ejection fraction determination by cross-sectional echocardiography in patients with coronary artery disease: A prospective study. *Clin Cardiol* 3:377, 1980

56. Silverman NH, Ports TA, Snider AR, Schiller NB, Carlsson E, Heilbron DC: Determination of left ventricular volume in children: Echocardiographic and angiographic comparisons. *Circulation* 62:548, 1980
57. Starling MR, Crawford MH, Sorensen SG, Levi B, Richards KL, O'Rourke RA: Comparative accuracy of apical biplane cross-sectional echocardiography and gated equilibrium radionuclide angiography for estimating left ventricular size and performance. *Circulation* 63:1075, 1981
58. Mercier JC, DiSessa TG, Jarmakani JM, Nakanishi T, Hiraishi S, Isabel-Jones J, Friedman WF: Two-dimensional echocardiographic assessment of left ventricular volumes and ejection fraction in children. *Circulation* 65:962, 1982
59. Carr KW, Engler RL, Forsythe JR, Johnson AD, Gosink B: Measurement of left ventricular ejection fraction by mechanical cross-sectional echocardiography. *Circulation* 59:1196, 1979
60. Heintzen PH, Moldenhauer K, Lange PE: Three-dimensional computerized contraction pattern analysis. *Eur J Cardiol* 1:229, 1974
61. Heintzen PH, Brennecke P, Bursch JH: Automated video-angiographic image analysis. *Computer* 8:54, 1975
62. Matsumoto M, Inoue M, Tamura S, Tanaka K, Abe H: Three-dimensional echocardiography for spatial visualization and volume calculation of cardiac structures. *JCU* 9:157, 1981
63. Peterson KL, Skloven D, Ludbrook P, Uther JB, Ross J Jr: Comparison of isovolumic and ejection phase indices of myocardial performance in man. *Circulation* 49:1088, 1074
64. Parker JO, Case RB: Normal left ventricular function. *Circulation* 60:4, 1979
65. Cooper RH, O'Rourke RA, Karliner JS, Peterson KL, Leopold GR: Comparison of ultrasound and cineangiographic measurements of the mean rate of circumferential fiber shortening in man. *Circulation* 46:914, 1972
66. Quinones MA, Gaasch WH, Alexander JK: Echocardiographic assessment of left ventricular function: With special reference to normalized velocities. *Circulation* 50:42, 1974
67. Gutgesell HP, Paquet M, Duff DF, McNamara DG: Evaluation of left ventricular size and function by echocardiography: Results in normal children. *Circulation* 56:457, 1977
68. Wilson JR, Reichek N: Echocardiographic indices of left ventricular function. *Chest* 76:441, 1979
69. Massie BM, Schiller NB, Ratshin RA, Parmley WW: Mitral-septal separation: New echocardiographic index of left ventricular function. *Am J Cardiol* 39:1008, 1977
70. Lew W, Henning H, Schelbert H, Karliner JS: Assessment of mitral valve E point-septal separation as an index of left ventricular performance in patients with acute and previous myocardial infarction. *Am J Cardiol* 41:836, 1978
71. D'Cruz IA, Lalmalani GG, Sambasivan V, Cohen HC, Glick G: The superiority of mitral E point-ventricular septum separation to other echocardiographic indicators of left ventricular performance. *Clin Cardiol* 2:140, 1979
72. Nixon JV, Murray RG, Leonard PD, Mitchell JH, Blomqvist CG: Effect of large variations in preload on left ventricular performance characteristics in normal subjects. *Circulation* 65:698, 1982
73. Glover MU, Hagan AD, Cohen A, Mazzoleni A, Schvartzman M, Warren SE, Vieweg WVR: Two-dimensional echocardiography in predicting left ventricular wall motion abnormalities and left ventricular function. *South Med J* 75:313, 1982
74. Sahn DJ, Deely WJ, Hagan AD, Friedman WF: Echocardiographic assessment of left ventricular performance in normal newborns. *Circulation* 49:232, 1974
75. DeMaria AN, Neumann A, Schubart PJ, Lee G, Mason DT: Systematic correlation of cardiac chamber size and ventricular performance determined with echocardiography and alterations in heart rate in normal persons. *Am J Cardiol* 43:1, 1979
76. Sahn DJ, Vaucher Y, Williams DE, Allen HD, Goldberg SJ, Friedman WF: Echocardiographic detection of large left to right shunts and cardiomyopathies in infants and children. *Am J Cardiol* 38:73, 1976
77. Rosenblatt A, Clark R, Burgess J, Cohn K: Echocardiographic assessment of the level of cardiac compensation in valvular heart disease. *Circulation* 54:509, 1976
78. Baker DW, Johnson SL, Strandness DE: Prospects for quantitations of transcutaneous pulsed Doppler techniques in cardiology and peripheral vascular disease. In RS Reneman (Ed), *Cardiovascular Applications of Ultrasound*. Amsterdam: North-Holland, 1974, Chapter 8

79. Griffith JM, Henry WL: An ultrasound system for combined cardiac imaging and Doppler blood flow measurement in man. *Circulation* 57:925, 1978
80. Magnin PA, Stewart JA, Myers S, VonRamm O, Kisslo JA: Combined Doppler and phased-array echocardiographic estimation of cardiac output. *Circulation* 63:388, 1981
81. Steingart RM, Meller J, Barovick J, Patterson R, Herman MV, Teichholz LE: Pulsed Doppler echocardiographic measurement of beat-to-beat changes in stroke volume in dogs. *Circulation* 62:542, 1980
82. Darsee JR, Walter PF, Nutter DO: Transcutaneous doppler method of measuring cardiac output. II. Noninvasive measurement by transcutaneous doppler aortic blood velocity integration and M-mode echocardiography. *Am J Cardiol* 46:613, 1980
83. Lalani AV, Lee SJK: Echocardiographic measurement of cardiac output using the mitral valve and aortic root echo. *Circulation* 54:738, 1976
84. Rasmussen S, Corya BC, Feigenbaum H, Black MJ, Lovelace DE, Phillips JF, Noble RJ, Knoebel SB: Stroke volume calculated from the mitral valve echogram in patients with and without ventricular dyssynergy. *Circulation* 58:125, 1978
85. Corya BC, Rasmussen S, Phillips JF, Black MJ: Forward stroke volume calculated from aortic valve echograms in normal subjects and patients with mitral regurgitation secondary to left ventricular dysfunction. *Am J Cardiol* 47:1215, 1981
86. Pratt RC, Parisi AF, Harrington JJ, Sasahara AA: The influence of left ventricular stroke volume on aortic root motion: An echocardiographic study. *Circulation* 53:947, 1976
87. Redwood DR, Henry WL, Epstein SE: Evaluation of the ability of echocardiography to measure acute alterations in left ventricular volume. *Circulation* 50:901, 1974
88. Frishman W, Smithen C, Befler B, Kligfield P, Killip T: Noninvasive assessment of clinical response to oral propranolol therapy. *Am J Cardiol* 35:635, 1975
89. Hirshleifer J, Crawford M, O'Rourke RA, Karliner JS: Influence of acute alterations in heart rate and systemic arterial pressure on echocardiographic measures of left ventricular performance in normal human subjects. *Circulation* 52:835, 1975
90. Crawford MH, Karliner JS, O'Rourke RA: Favorable effects of oral maintenance digoxin therapy on left ventricular performance in normal subjects: Echocardiographic study. *Am J Cardiol* 38:843, 1976
91. Hardarson T, Henning H, O'Rourke RA: Prolonged salutary effects of isosorbide dinitrate and nitroglycerin ointment on regional left ventricular function. *Am J Cardiol* 40:90, 1977
92. Hirota Y, Suwa M, Hori K, Takatsu T: Dynamic echoventriculography: Noninvasive assessment of effects of nitroglycerin, phenylephrine, isoproterenol, and propranolol on the human cardiovascular system. *Jpn Heart J* 19:719, 1978
93. Gomes JAC, Carambas CR, Moran HE, Dhatt MS, Calon AH, Caracta AR, Damato AN: The effect of isosorbide dinitrate on left ventricular size, wall stress and left ventricular function in chronic refractory heart failure: An echocardiographic study. *Am J Med* 65:794, 1978
94. Goldstein RE, Bennett ED, Leech GL: Effect of glyceryl trinitrate on echocardiographic left ventricular dimensions during exercise in the upright position. *Br Heart J* 42:245, 1979
95. Ryan WF, Karliner JS: Effects of tocainide on left ventricular performance at rest and during acute alterations in heart rate and systemic arterial pressure: An echocardiographic study. *Br Heart J* 41:175, 1979
96. Wei JY, Reid PR: Relation of time course of plasma nitroglycerin levels to echocardiographic, arterial pressure and heart rate changes after sublingual administration of nitroglycerin. *Am J Cardiol* 48:778, 1981
97. Chaignon M, Chen W-T, Tarazi RC, Nakamoto S, Salcedo E: Acute effects of hemodialysis on echographic-determined cardiac performance: Improved contractility resulting from serum increased calcium with reduced potassium despite hypovolemic-reduced cardiac output. *Am Heart J* 103:374, 1982
98. Levine HJ: Compliance of the left ventricle. *Circulation* 46:423, 1972
99. Hood WB Jr, Bianco JA, Kumar R, Whiting RB: Experimental myocardial infarction. IV. Reduction of left ventricular compliance in the healing phase. *J Clin Invest* 49:1316, 1970
100. Mann T, Goldberg S, Mudge GH Jr, Grossman W: Factors contributing to altered left ventricular diastolic properties during angina pectoris. *Circulation* 59:14, 1979
101. Schwartz A, Sordahl LA, Entman ML, Allen JC, Reddy YS, Goldstein MA, Luchi RJ, Wyborny LE: Abnormal biochemistry in myocardial failure. *Am J Cardiol* 32:407, 1973

102. Grossman W, Stefadouros MA, McLaurin LP, Rolett EL, Young DT: Quantitative assessment of left ventricular diastolic stiffness in man. *Circulation* 47:567, 1973
103. Grossman W, McLaurin LP, Stefadouros MA: Left ventricular stiffness associated with chronic pressure and volume overloads in man. *Circ Res* 35:793, 1974
104. Hess OM, Schneider J, Koch R, Bamert C, Grimm J, Krayenbuehl HP: Diastolic function and myocardial structure in patients with myocardial hypertrophy: Special reference to normalized viscoelastic data. *Circulation* 63:360, 1981
105. Quinones MA, Gaasch WH, Waisser E, Alexander JK: Reduction in the rate of diastolic descent of the mitral valve echogram in patients with altered left ventricular diastolic pressure-volume relations. *Circulation* 49:246, 1974
106. DeMaria AN, Miller RR, Amsterdam EA, Markson W, Mason DT: Mitral valve early diastolic closing velocity in the echocardiogram: Relation to sequential diastolic flow and ventricular compliance. *Am J Cardiol* 37:693, 1976
107. Dreslinski GR, Frohlich ED, Dunn FG, Messerli FH, Suarez DH, Reisin E: Echocardiographic diastolic ventricular abnormality in hypertensive heart disease: Atrial emptying index. *Am J Cardiol* 47:1087, 1981
108. Konecke LL, Feigenbaum H, Chang S, Corya BC, Fisher JC: Abnormal mitral valve motion in patients with elevated left ventricular diastolic pressure. *Circulation* 47:989, 1973
109. Lewis JR, Parker JO, Burggraf GW: Mitral valve motion and changes in left ventricular end-diastolic pressure: A correlative study of the PR–AC interval. *Am J Cardiol* 42:383, 1978
110. Corya BC, Rasmussen S, Knoebel SB, Feigenbaum H, Black MJ: Echocardiography in acute myocardial infarction. *Am J Cardiol* 36:1, 1975
111. Weber KT, Janicki JS, Shroff S, Fishman AP: Contractile mechanics and interaction of the right and left ventricles. *Am J Cardiol* 47:686, 1981
112. Glantz SA, Parmley WW: Factors which affect the diastolic pressure-volume curve. *Circ Res* 42:171, 1978
113. Glantz SA, Misbach GA, Moores WY, Mathey DG, Lekven J, Stowe DF, Parmley WW, Tyberg JV: The pericardium substantially affects the left ventricular diastolic pressure-volume relationship in the dog. *Circ Res* 42:433, 1978
114. Tanaka H, Tei C, Nakao S, Tahara M, Sakurai S, Kashima T, Kanehisa T: Diastolic bulging of the interventricular septum toward the left ventricle: An echocardiographic manifestation of negative interventricular pressure gradient between left and right ventricles during diastole. *Circulation* 62:558, 1980
115. Brinker JA, Weiss JL, Lappe DL, Rabson JL, Summer WR, Permutt S, Weisfeldt ML: Leftward septal displacement during right ventricular loading in man. *Circulation* 61:626, 1980
116. Lozman J, Powers SR, Older T, Dutton RE, Roy RJ, English M, Marco D, Eckert C: Correlation of pulmonary wedge and left atrial pressures. *Arch Surg* 109:270, 1974
117. Robotham JL, Lixfeld W, Holland L, MacGregor D, Bromberger-Barnea B, Permutt S, Rabson JL: The effects of positive end-expiratory pressure on right and left ventricular performance. *Am Rev Respir Dis* 121:677, 1980
118. Scharf SM, Brown R, Saunders N, Green LH, Ingram RH Jr: Changes in canine left ventricular size and configuration with positive end-expiratory pressure. *Circ Res* 44:672, 1979
119. Manny J, Patten MT, Liebman PR, Hechtman HB: The association of lung distention, PEEP and biventricular failure. *Ann Surg* 187:151, 1978
120. Jardin F, Farcot J-C, Boisante L, Curien N, Margairaz A, Bourdarias J-P: Influence of positive end-expiratory pressure on left ventricular performance. *N Engl J Med* 304:387, 1981

Diseases of the right heart

M-mode echocardiography has had very limited clinical value in the evaluation of right-sided cardiac chambers, valves, and function. Because the right atrium and pulmonary artery are largely inaccessible and the right ventricle is an irregular geometric shape, M-mode echo has been inadequate for evaluation of right heart structures. For that reason, imaging information about these structures provided by two-dimensional echocardiography represents an important clinical contribution.

Single-dimensional M-mode studies have identified right ventricular enlargement in some patients [1, 2]. In addition to dimension measurements, considerable importance has been attached to the presence of paradoxical septal motion as an indicator of right ventricular volume overload [3–5]. If both endocardial and epicardial surfaces are properly recorded, M-mode echo is fairly reliable for determining wall thickness of the right ventricle [6–9]. However, because of technical difficulties in obtaining satisfactory recordings as well as other variables, such as transducer position and angulation, patient position, and phase of respiration, the overall clinical value of M-mode echocardiography for evaluating the right ventricle has remained quite limited.

Normal criteria for dimensions of right heart structures. Since two-dimensional echocardiography provides comprehensive imaging of all three dimensions from different transducer positions, evaluation of the size of all cardiac chambers is more reliable with 2-D imaging [10–15].

Bommer and associates [14] studied rubber casts fashioned from the right atrium and right ventricle of human necropsy hearts to confirm that the echocardiographic dimensions obtainable from these chambers by two-dimensional echo correlated with actual volume, and that accurate measurements of these dimensions could be determined by ultrasound. Their findings, as well as our own unpublished data, confirm that the apical four-chamber view is the single most important 2-D echo view for evaluating the size of both right ventricle and right atrium. Our findings agree with those of Bommer and colleagues [14] regarding the normal range of right atrial and right ventricular dimensions. The right ventricular long axis dimension, measured from the apical four-chamber view, does not reliably distinguish normal from abnormal. The maximum short axis dimension of the right ventricle obtained from the apical four-chamber view ranged from 22 mm to 44 mm in the two study groups (25 normal hearts in the Bommer group and 98 normal hearts in our group). The body surface area of these normal adults ranged from 1.2 to 2.25 m^2. The end-diastolic planimetered areas of the right ventricle were similar in the two normal groups (10 to 27 cm^2 for the Bommer group) compared to those in our group, which ranged from 12 to 29 cm^2. We found the ratio of equal to or less than 0.9 of the end-diastolic area of the right ventricle to left ventricle measured in the apical four-chamber view to be the most sensitive indicator in distinguishing a normal from a dilated right ventricle. This area ratio is only valid for use when the left ventricular size is verified as normal.

Our data for normal right atrial dimensions and area also compare very closely with those of Bommer and colleagues [14]. They found the upper normal limit of right atrial short axis (right-to-left dimension in the apical four-chamber view) to be 45 mm while the maximum normal long axis dimension (inferosuperior) in the

Table 8-1. Normal criteria for adult right heart structures

Structure	Mean	Two standard deviations	Number of patients
RV area	21.3 cm^2	10.6	112
RV area index	11.5 cm^2/m^2	5.0	112
RV/LV area ratio	0.7	0.2	109
RV short axis dimension	35.8 mm	10.6	77
RV/LV short axis dimension ratio	0.8	0.2	113
RV wall thickness	4.0 mm	2.0	36
RA area	13.8 cm^2	5.6	112
RA area index	7.5 cm^2/m^2	2.6	112
RA/LA area ratio	1.0	0.2	108
RA inf/sup dimension	43.8 mm	12.2	115
PA diameter	22.1 mm	7.0	74
Ao diameter	23.5 mm	7.6	76
PA/Ao ratio	1.0	0.2	73
IVC diameter	18.0 mm	9.8	38

Note: Body surface area = 1.3–2.2 m^2.

same view was 50 mm; we found the maximum inferosuperior dimension in 98 normal subjects to be 54 mm. The planimetered area of the right atrium in their normal group ranged from 10 to 21 cm^2 compared to our normal subjects whose right atrial area ranged from 9 to 19 cm^2. When the areas of the left atrium and right atrium were compared in this normal group, the ratio of the right atrial to left atrial area ranged from 0.75 to 1.17; this ratio was not influenced by age or body surface area.

When we compared the diameter of the ascending aorta to that of the main pulmonary artery in 70 normal subjects, we found the mean to be 1.0. An aorta-to-pulmonary artery ratio less than 0.84 was indicative of a dilated pulmonary artery. This measurement was nearly as reliable as either right atrial or right ventricular measurements in identifying patients with a right ventricular volume overload.

Right ventricular volumes can be reliably determined from either angiographic or two-dimensional echocardiographic methods [16–18]. Hiraishi and associates [18] observed good correlation between right ventricular volumes derived from planimetry of the areas in the apical four-chamber view corrected by three different equations when compared to volumes derived from biplane cineangiography.

The normal criteria for dimensions and areas of the right heart chambers and vessels derived from 134 normal subjects in our laboratory are shown in Table 8-1.

Imaging techniques of right heart structures. In discussing the imaging techniques of right heart structures, transducer positions from the four major locations—left parasternal (precordial) area, apex, subcostal region, and suprasternal notch—are considered. The structures that are identified as right heart structures for the purpose of this discussion include the following: right ventricle, right atrium, tricuspid valve, pulmonic valve, main pulmonary artery, right and left pulmonary arteries, interatrial septum, inferior vena cava, and superior vena cava.

Imaging techniques of these structures will be reviewed in the same sequence that we normally employ in the laboratory; obviously this sequence can be in different order as long as comprehensive imaging is obtained. All of these planes are demonstrated in Chapter 1.

Parasternal long axis imaging views a portion of the right ventricular outflow tract, but no quantitative measurements are attempted in this limited view. From this position the transducer is rotated slightly counterclockwise and aimed toward the tricuspid valve with orientation of the sector fan in the right ventricular inflow tract and right atrium. This sector plane provides good visualization of the anteroposterior dimension of the right ventricular inflow tract together with a large segment of the anterior free wall of the right ventricle. In addition, this plane provides excellent visualization of the right atrium as well as of the anterior and septal leaflets of the tricuspid valve.

Clockwise rotation of the transducer from the same parasternal position coupled with lateral-superior angulation demonstrates the right ventricular outflow tract and pulmonic valve. The plane of the sector fan is oriented in the supracristal region of the ventricular septum and visualizes the subpulmonic region and portion of the pulmonary artery. The anterior mitral leaflet is imaged; however, the sector plane is lateral to the aortic annulus, so that the aortic valve is not visualized in this view.

Both inflow and outflow views of the right ventricle provide excellent opportunities to obtain M-mode recordings of the tricuspid and pulmonic valves, respectively.

The parasternal short axis view at the level of the base is an essential view for demonstration of the normal relationship of the great arteries by simultaneously visualizing the tricuspid valve, right ventricular outflow tract, and pulmonic valve. Medial angulation from this position enables visualization of variable amounts of the tricuspid valve, right ventricular inflow tract, and right atrium. Lateral angulation from the same transducer position to bring the lateral wall of the main pulmonary artery into the middle of the sector, and orientation of the fan in the plane of the pulmonary artery usually affords visualization of the proximal portion of the right and left pulmonary arteries. This maneuver also provides good visualization of the pulmonic valve. Because of the lateral angulation the tricuspid valve and right atrium are no longer present in the plane when the pulmonary arteries are optimally visualized. This view through the base in the plane of the pulmonary artery may require locating the transducer in more lateral and/or inferior precordial interspace positions. Parasternal short axis views through the basal and middle thirds of the left ventricle provide additional views of the right ventricle that may be of value for measuring anterior and posterior wall thickness as well as another short axis dimension of the right ventricle.

The single most valuable view of the right ventricle and right atrium is the apical four-chamber plane. This view is preferred for obtaining long and short axis dimension measurements of both chambers as well as planimetered area and volume determinations. It requires transducer positioning, rotation, and angulation to maximize the size of both right ventricle and right atrium; both chambers are not always optimally visualized in the same tomographic plane. We do not measure the long axis dimension of the right ventricle since it is a poor measurement for distinguishing normal from abnormal [14]. The maximum short axis dimension of the normal right ventricle in the apical four-chamber view varies from 37 to 45 mm depending upon the body surface area. The primum portion of the interatrial septum near the endocardial cushion is well visualized in this view; however, there is frequently echo dropout in the mid to superior portion because of the parallel angle of the ultrasound beam.

The subcostal views are very important for evaluating the diaphragmatic free wall of the right ventricle, the right atrium, the interatrial septum, and the inferior vena cava. Positioning the right ventricular wall perpendicular to the M-mode cursor while in the four-chamber plane enables accurate recording of diastolic and systolic wall thickness. With medial angulation and by locating the atria centrally with sector, both atria and interatrial septum are imaged very well. From this view an M-mode recording can be obtained from the interatrial septum, and the entire length of the septum can be scanned for evidence of an atrial septal defect. Rightward angulation and slight counterclockwise rotation to image the inferior vena cava-right atrial junction affords another valuable subcostal view. It is also important to record the IVC in short axis as well as long axis to assess true diameter and observe the effects of respiration. A dilated IVC and/or loss of normal collapse with inspiration usually means elevated right atrial pressures. In addition to the patient's respiration and state of hydration, positional changes can influence the venous return and diameter of the inferior vena cava. An M-mode recording positioned perpendicularly through the inferior vena cava just distal to the junction of the hepatic vein near the IVC-RA junction is the best method for measuring IVC size. Investigative data are incomplete regarding the effect of various physiologic maneuvers on IVC size. The upper limits of normal for IVC diameter in adults are approximately 20 to 25 mm. A fourth subcostal view for evaluating right heart structures is the short axis of the left ventricle which includes the right ventricular outflow tract, pulmonic valve, and a small portion of the pulmonary artery.

Finally, the superior vena cava and right pulmonary artery are both imaged in the suprasternal short axis view of the ascending aorta.

Right ventricular function and pulmonary hypertension.

Right ventricular ejection time (RVET) is normally longer than left ventricular ejection time (LVET) [19]. Right ventricular preejection period (RPEP) is shorter than left ventricular preejection period (LPEP). Hirshfeld and colleagues [19], in a group of normal children aged 3 to 14 years, reported average ratios of LVET to RVET to be 0.80 and LPEP to RPEP to be 1.25. The RPEP/RVET ratio is of some limited value in predicting pulmonary arterial pressure or resistance [20]. Mills and associates [20] observed that right ventricular isovolumic contraction time increased as pulmonary arterial pressure increased; this interval is unreliable for accurately predicting the pulmonary artery pressure in adults. However, an echo-determined isovolumic contraction time of less than 25 msec suggests a normal pulmonary arterial pressure.

Other studies [21–23] have reported that an RPEP/RVET ratio of less than 0.30 could be used to predict a pulmonary arterial end-diastolic pressure less than 30 mm Hg. However, intermediate and higher ratios could not be used to quantitate reliably changes in pulmonary artery pressure. Determination of right ventricular systolic time intervals in adults by traditional M-mode echocardiography is difficult because closure of the pulmonic valve is frequently not seen. Complete recording of pulmonic valve motion is considerably easier with a movable cursor and simultaneous two-dimensional imaging from different transducer positions.

Wroblewski and colleagues [24] found that contractile performance of the right ventricle in mitral stenosis remains normal with moderate pressure overload when there is no clinical evidence of right ventricular failure.

Olivari and associates [25], in a study of pulmonary and systemic hemodynamics in hypertensive subjects with left ventricular hypertrophy, noted a functional interdependence of the two ventricles. These investigators noted that systemic hypertension is associated with elevation of pulmonary arterial pressure and of pulmonary arteriolar resistance, which is not necessarily a consequence of impairment in left ventricular function. Atkins and coworkers [26] suggested that a sustained elevation of left ventricular end-diastolic pressure had significant importance in determining pulmonary vascular resistance in hypertension. They found a high degree of correlation between pulmonary vascular resistance and wedge pressures greater than 20 mm Hg. Taylor and associates [27] have documented in animals a functional interdependence of the right and left ventricles.

Some investigators [28, 29] have reported the presence of poor right ventricular compliance manifested by a pressure wave form in the right ventricle and right atrium similar to that observed in constrictive pericarditis and restrictive cardiomyopathy. Coma-Canella and Lopez-Sendon [28] diagnosed ischemic right ventricular dysfunction in 54 patients with acute myocardial infarction who had a right atrial pressure disproportionately increased in relation to the pulmonary capillary pressure. The right atrial pressure curve was M- or W-shaped in 40 of these patients (74%), termed a noncompliant pattern. Kussmaul's sign was found in the patients whose respiration was recorded. This pattern of poor right ventricular compliance was severe in 30 cases (Y descent > X descent) and slight in 10 cases (Y descent = X descent). These investigators believe that the severe noncompliant pattern indicates a poor prognosis as a result of a more severe degree of right ventricular stiffness.

Marmor and colleagues [30] found that patients with anterior infarction had persistent regional and global impairment of left ventricular function but only transient impairment of the right ventricle, whereas inferior infarction was associated with severe, persistent regional and global dysfunction of the right ventricle.

Starling and associates [31] reported the presence of a B notch or hump in the resting tricuspid valve echogram when the right ventricular end-diastolic pressure was 9 mm Hg or greater. They observed that in nine patients with right heart failure the PR–AC interval was 21 ± 16 msec in contrast to 68 ± 18 msec in normal controls.

Echocardiography can differentiate posterior myocardial infarction from right ventricular hypertrophy or normal subjects who display an anterior loop on vectorcardiography [32]. Two-dimensional echocardiography, in contrast to both electrocardiography and vectorcardiography, more effectively separates these three conditions by direct analysis of chamber dimensions, wall thickness, and segmental wall motion.

M-mode echocardiographic patterns of pulmonic valve motion caused by pulmonary hypertension have been well known for several years [33–35] (Fig. 8-1). Abnormal echo patterns of the pulmonic valve, including an absent "A" dip, decreased or negative diastolic slope, prolonged preejection period, and mid-systolic semiclosure, have been found useful in assessment of pulmonary hypertension.

Tahara and coworkers [36] reported that pulmonic valve motion during systole may be instantaneously determined by pulmonary artery flow change and the

256   8. Diseases of the right heart

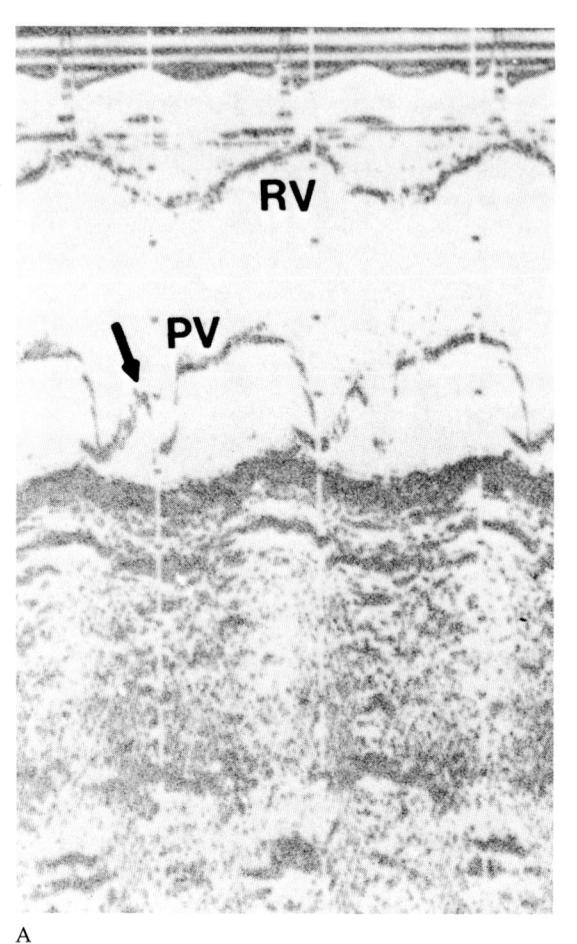

Fig. 8-1A. *M-mode recording of the pulmonic valve (PV) in a patient with pulmonary hypertension showing mid-systolic closure notch (arrow), which is fairly specific for the diagnosis of pulmonary hypertension. A portion of the right ventricular outflow tract is present anterior to the pulmonic valve leaflet. B. M-mode recording of the pulmonic valve in a patient with pulmonary hypertension and severe right ventricular dysfunction demonstrating prolongation of the preejection period (PEP) and shortening of the ejection time (ET). Although the diastolic slope is flat and there is no "A" dip in either patient, neither of these findings is as specific as mid-systolic closure for the diagnosis of pulmonary hypertension.*

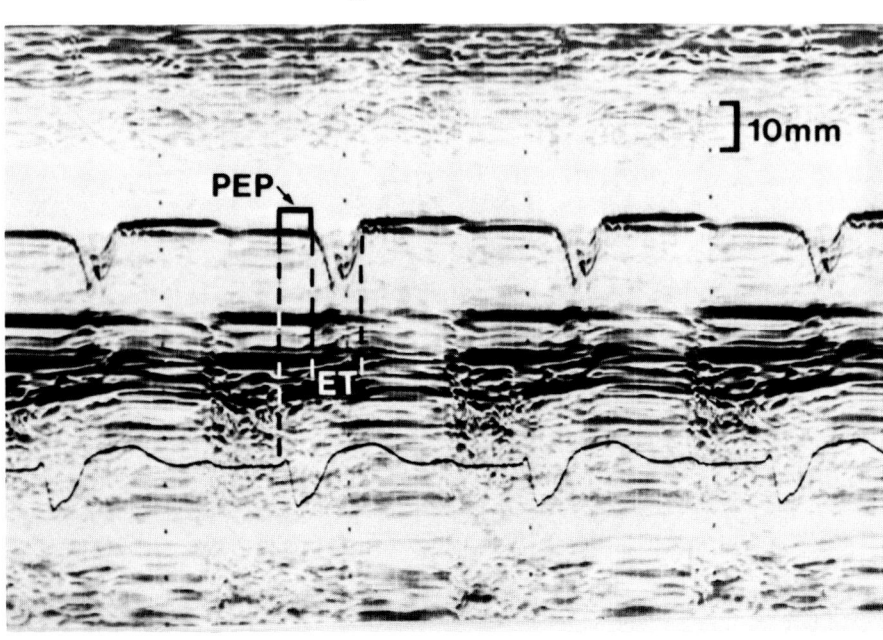

pulmonary artery–right ventricular pressure gradient during the cardiac cycle in experimental pulmonary hypertension. Mid-systolic notching of the pulmonic valve occurs more commonly in advanced degrees of pulmonary hypertension and is specific, but not sensitive, for that condition [37]. Acquatella and colleagues [37] found no significant correlation between hemodynamic measurements and the echographic pulmonary valve "A" wave amplitude, diastolic E point slope, or the systolic opening velocity. Changes in hemodynamic measurements observed in serial observations were not associated with predictable changes in configuration of the pulmonic valve echogram.

Right ventricular volume overload. One of the useful clinical findings in patients with right ventricular volume overload is the presence of abnormal motion of the interventricular septum, which is easily diagnosed with M-mode echocardiography [4, 5, 38–42]. This abnormal systolic motion consists of an anterior-rightward movement in contrast to the normal posterior-leftward direction. Segmental thickening of the septum is normal. Sometimes the anterior or paradoxical systolic motion is minimal or absent in the presence of a right ventricular volume overload. Several years ago we demonstrated that most patients who had an atrial septal defect and a left-to-right shunt greater than 2:1 exhibited paradoxical septal motion; however, patients with small shunts (less than 2:1) frequently have normal septal motion [5].

Pearlman and associates [42] reported that paradoxical systolic septal motion is not a diagnostic marker for right ventricular volume overload, but merely reflects right ventricular dilatation of any cause. These investigators noted a linear relation between the end-diastolic intracardiac position of the ventricular septum and the direction and magnitude of systolic septal motion in (1) 43 patients with an atrial septal defect ($r = 0.80$); (2) 14 patients with other causes of right ventricular volume overload ($r = 0.82$); (3) 19 patients with left ventricular volume overload ($r = 0.74$); (4) 10 patients with right ventricular pressure overload ($r = 0.93$); (5) 10 patients with left ventricular pressure overload ($r = 0.80$); (6) 28 normal subjects ($r = 0.82$). They concluded that, in the presence of normal ventricular activation and contraction, the direction and magnitude of septal motion during systole is determined by the intracardiac position of the septum at end diastole.

Other conditions which cause paradoxical motion of the ventricular septum include cardiac surgery (particularly prosthetic valve replacement), left bundle branch block [43], absence of the pericardium [44], and type B Wolff-Parkinson-White syndrome [45].

Weyman and associates [46] suggested that paradoxical septal motion in patients with right ventricular volume overload occurs as a result of a change in the diastolic shape of the left ventricle. This change in shape varies from flattening of the septum and left ventricle during diastole to total reversal of normal direction of septal curvature so that the septum becomes concave toward the right ventricle and convex toward the left ventricle. During systole the left ventricle and septum return to their normal, relatively circular configuration. This change in left ventricular shape from diastole to systole results in net motion of the ventricular septum toward the right ventricle (paradoxically).

Septal flattening can also be visualized well in the parasternal long axis view (Fig. 8-2). In addition to the narrowed anteroposterior diameter of the left ventricle

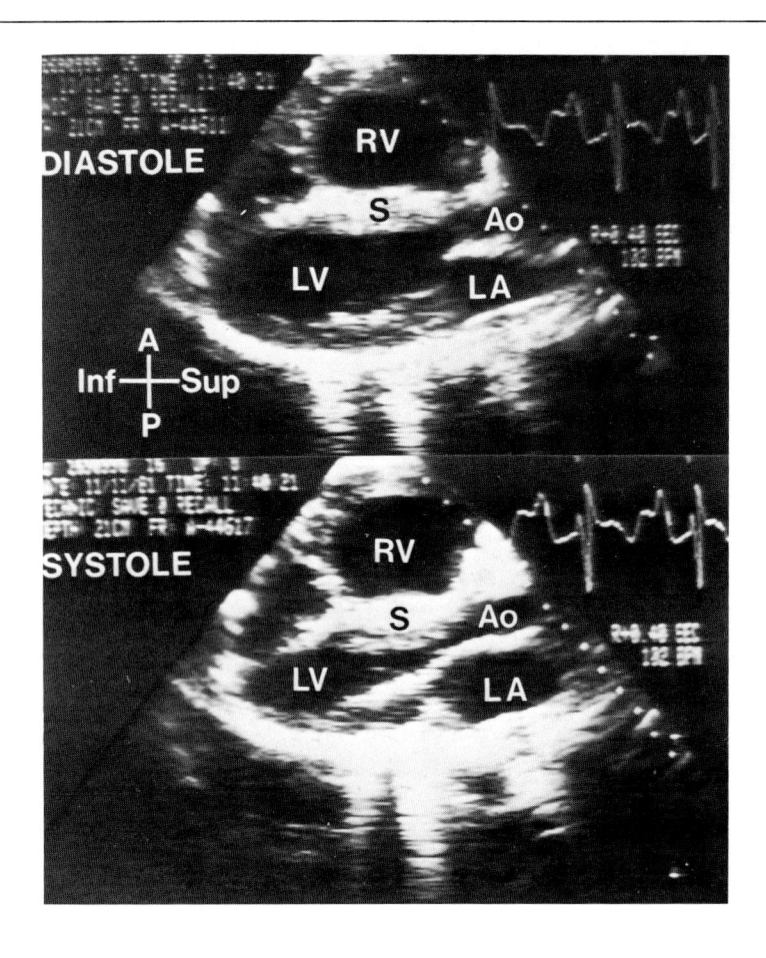

Fig. 8-2. Parasternal long axis views in diastole (upper panel) and systole (lower panel) showing marked enlargement of the right ventricle with secondary flattening of the interventricular septum and narrowed left ventricular outflow tract during systole. The septum is thickened because of pulmonary hypertension. The left ventricle appears small and the LV apex is imaged in the parasternal window.

caused by the flattened septum, the left ventricle may also be displaced leftward and the apex imaged from the parasternal long axis position.

The parasternal right ventricular inflow view provides an excellent opportunity to image the anterior free wall of the right ventricle, the anteroposterior dimension of the inflow tract, the anterior and septal leaflets of the tricuspid valve, and the right atrium (Fig. 8-3).

The parasternal right ventricular outflow view shows the wall thickness and outflow diameter of the right ventricle. Epicardial fat is commonly seen on the surface of the right ventricle and care must be taken not to confuse the reflectances from the fat with those caused by the right ventricular myocardium (Fig. 8-4). Localized sites of reflectances on the right ventricular epicardial surface which do not thicken during systole help distinguish the fat deposits from the myocardium.

Parasternal short axis imaging through the left ventricle demonstrates several abnormal features in the presence of right ventricular dilatation. In addition to the flattened septum and altered geometric shape of the left ventricle during systole and diastole, the free wall of the right ventricle also extends farther leftward than normal (Fig. 8-5A). As the right atrium and right ventricle dilate, the tricuspid annulus is shifted leftward and inferiorly, which enables simultaneous visualization of tricuspid and mitral valves in the parasternal short axis plane at the level of the mitral valve. On those occasions when the right heart chambers are

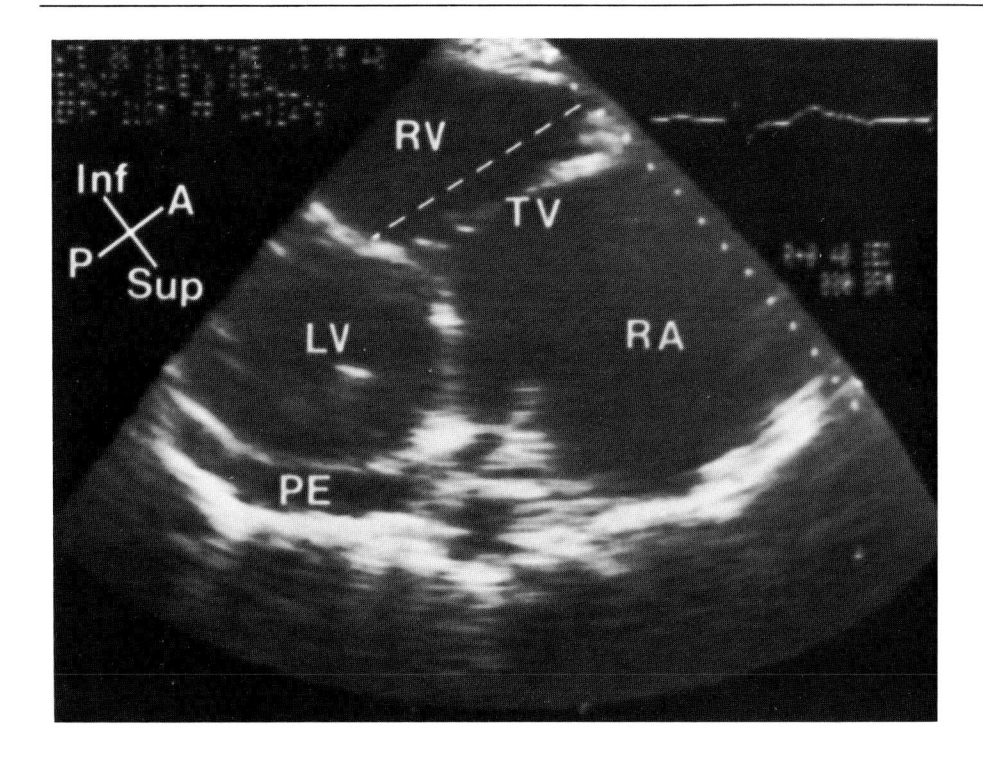

Fig. 8-3. Parasternal right ventricular inflow view showing enlarged anteroposterior (AP) dimension (70 mm) of the RV and dilated right atrium with inferosuperior dimension of 90 mm in a patient with a large right ventricular volume overload. Calibration dots are 1 cm apart.

significantly enlarged it is often possible to image all three leaflets of the tricuspid valve simultaneously (Fig. 8-5B). Under normal circumstances the echocardiographer is able to image only two of the three leaflets from any single tomographic plane. It is apparent from either parasternal long or short axis imaging positions that, depending upon beam angulation of the M-mode cursor, it is possible to record a wide range of right ventricular dimensions. Accordingly, short axis dimensions of the right ventricle as measured from parasternal windows (particularly from an M-mode machine) may be unreliable for evaluation of right ventricular size. Although the parasternal right ventricular inflow and outflow views are valuable in assessing those particular portions of right ventricular anatomy, the best single tomographic plane for determining right ventricular size, area, or volume is the apical four-chamber view.

When the transducer is positioned directly overlying the left ventricular apex and angled toward the patient's right shoulder with the patient in a steep left lateral decubitus position, all four chambers and both atrioventricular valves can be imaged. It is often necessary to slide the transducer slightly medially, that is, closer to the right ventricular apex, to image all of the free wall of the right ventricle during systole and diastole (Fig. 8-6A, B). From this position it is possible to measure both long and short axis dimensions as well as the planimetered area of the right ventricle (Fig. 8-6C, D). Since it has been shown that the long axis dimension is an unreliable measurement in distinguishing normal from abnormal chambers, we do not make that determination. When right ventricular dilatation is present, the left ventricular apex is nearly always deleted from view in this imaging plane. With right ventricular hypertrophy the prominent trabeculations, papillary muscles, and moderator band are easily imaged and usually become very conspicuous with 2-D

260   8. Diseases of the right heart

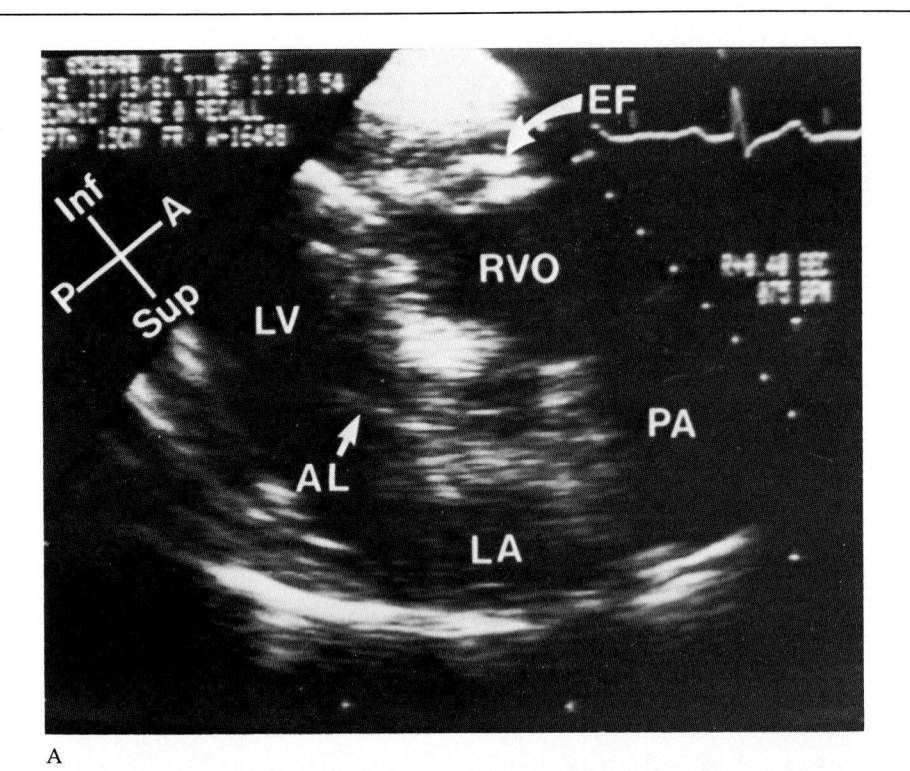

Fig. 8-4A. Parasternal right ventricular outflow view showing an extra reflectance separated by a thin, linear echo-free space from underlying RV anterior wall; during real-time it does not demonstrate systolic thickening and is typical for epicardial fat (EF). B. Parasternal RVO view in a patient with right ventricular volume overload demonstrating an enlarged RVO dimension (50 mm) and pulmonic valve (PV), and oblique portion of the main pulmonary artery; however, the anterolateral wall of the PA is not adequately imaged in this photograph. A small portion of the left ventricular outflow above the anterior mitral leaflet and below the interventricular septum is routinely imaged in this plane.

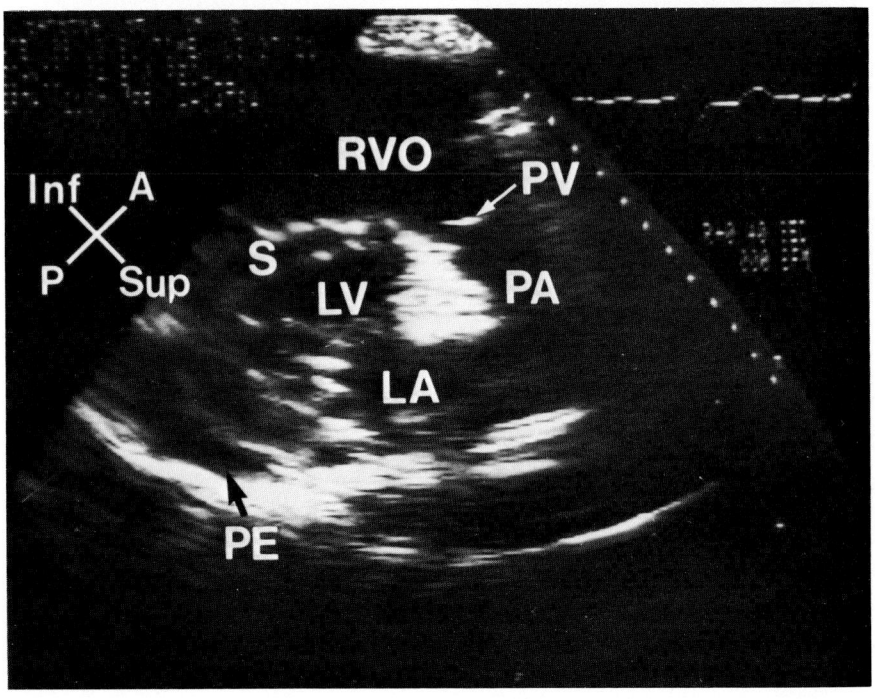

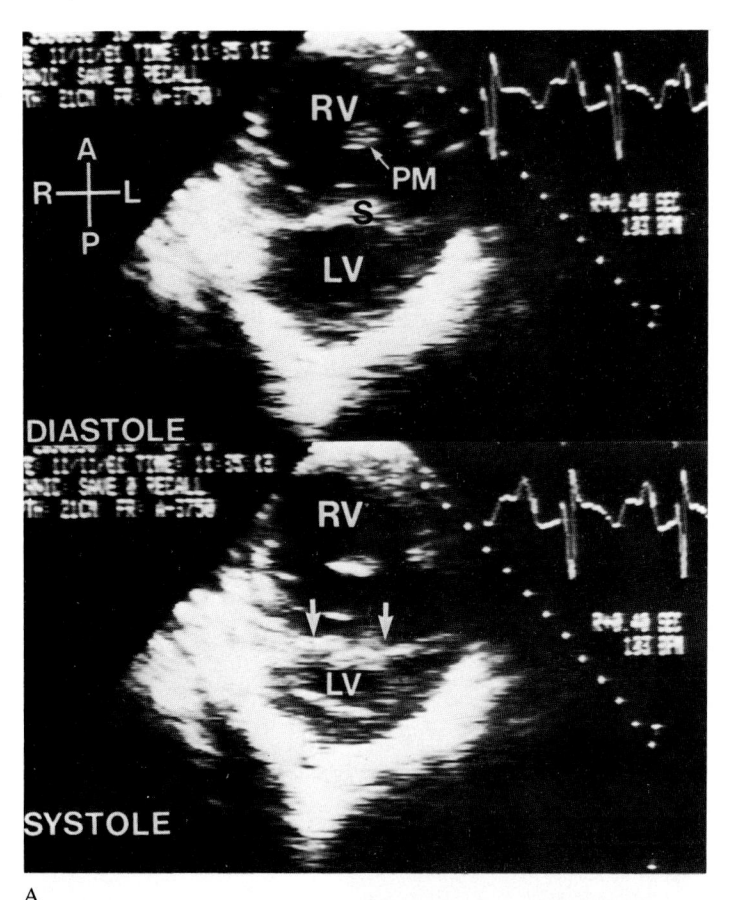

Fig. 8-5A. Parasternal short axis views during diastole (upper panel) and systole (lower panel) demonstrating marked right ventricular enlargement and flattening of the interventricular septum during systole (arrows, lower panel). The left ventricular cavity is small and has a distorted, flattened shape during systole. B. Parasternal short axis view through the left ventricle and orifice of the tricuspid valve demonstrating all three tricuspid leaflets (SL = septal; PL = posterior; AL = anterior) in the presence of marked dilatation of the right ventricle. The RV extends farther leftward than the LV but the lateral wall is not included within this sector plane. Calibration dots are 1 cm apart.

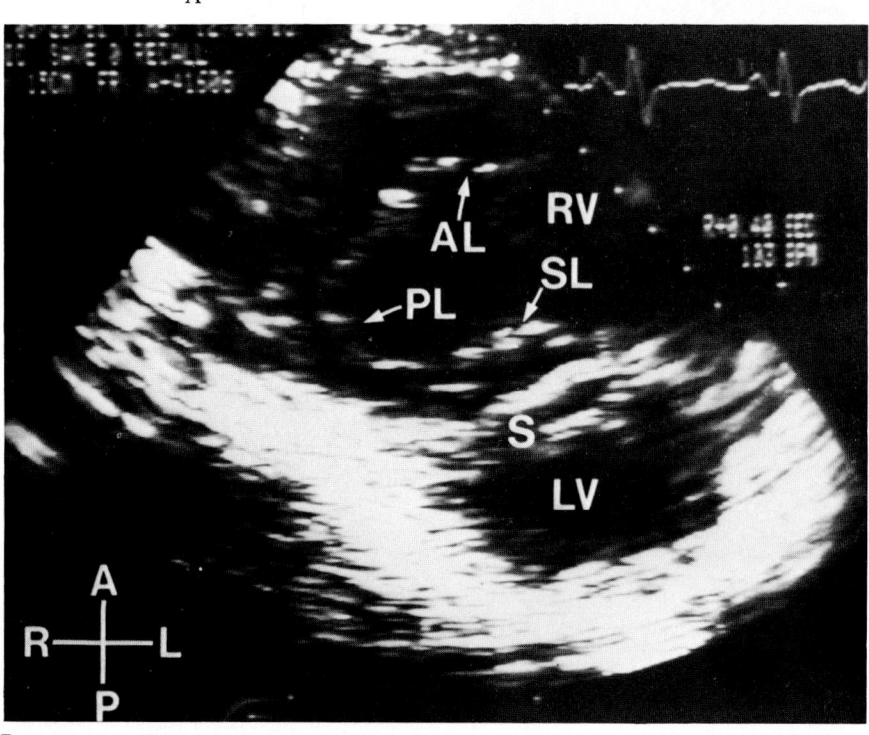

262   8. Diseases of the right heart

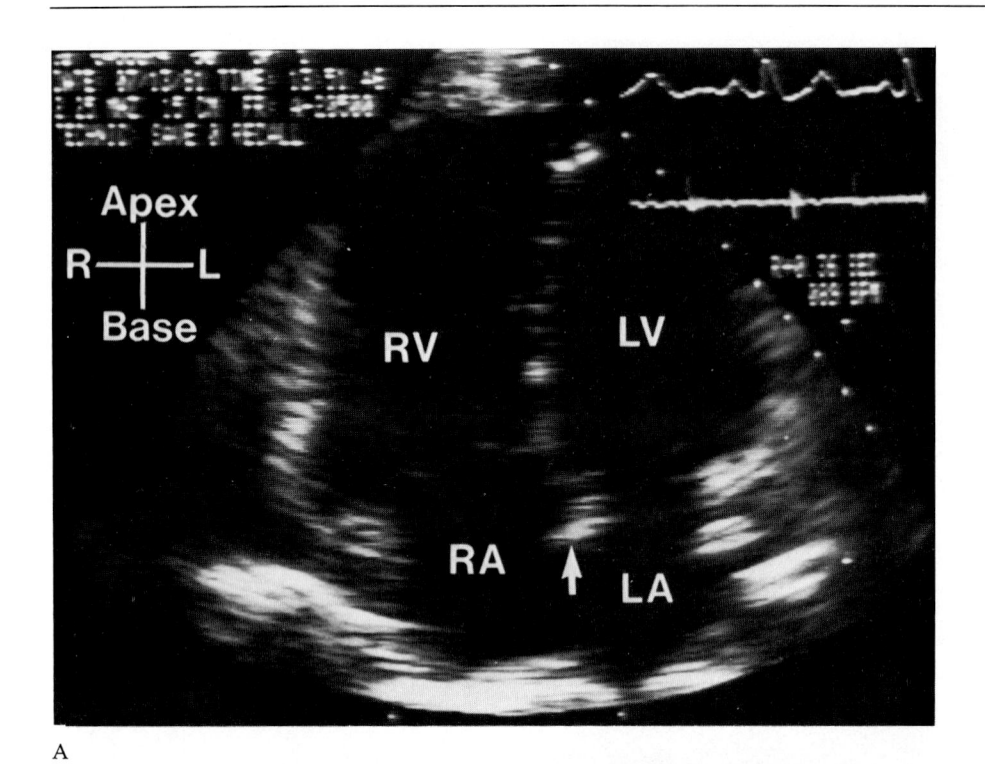

Fig. 8-6A. Apical 4-chamber view with the transducer positioned over the right ventricular apex in a patient with a large RV due to atrial septal defect; note the bright echo of atrial septum (arrow), which has been designated "T artifact" and suggests an actual ASD rather than normal echo dropout. This end-diastolic view shows the RV to be larger than the left ventricle. B. Apical 4-chamber view in same patient at end systole demonstrating right atrial enlargement and the flattened area (arrow) where in the absence of an atrial septal defect (sinus venosus or secundum types) a reflectance would normally be seen from the atrial septum. C. Apical 4-chamber view of a normal subject demonstrating technique of measuring maximum short axis dimension of both right ventricle and left ventricle at end diastole. D. Apical 4-chamber view of a normal adult subject demonstrating the technique of planimetering the end-diastolic area of the right ventricle. This is more reliable than any dimension measurement for distinguishing normal from abnormal cavity size.

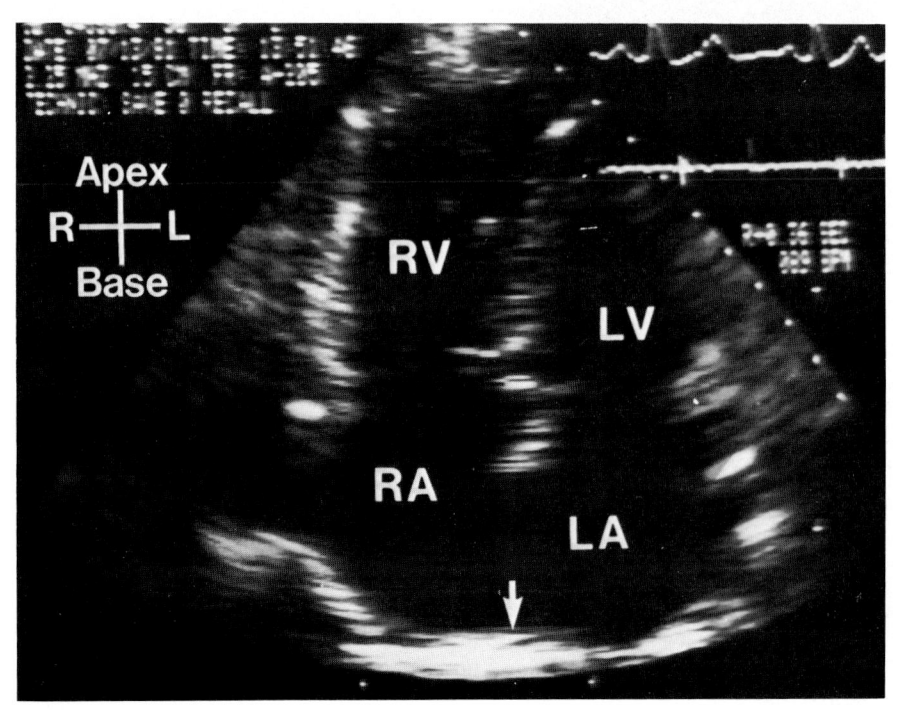

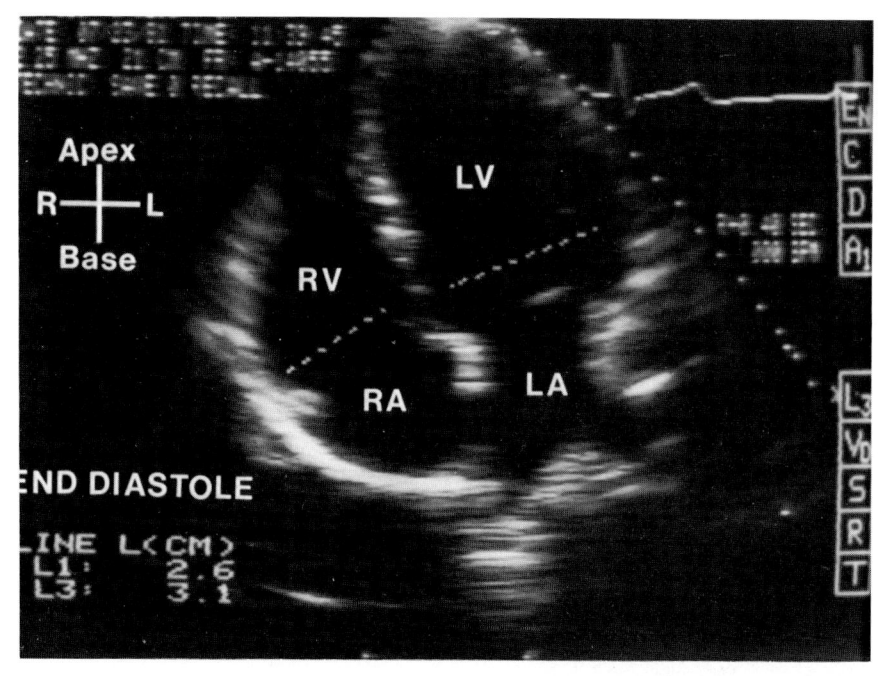

263

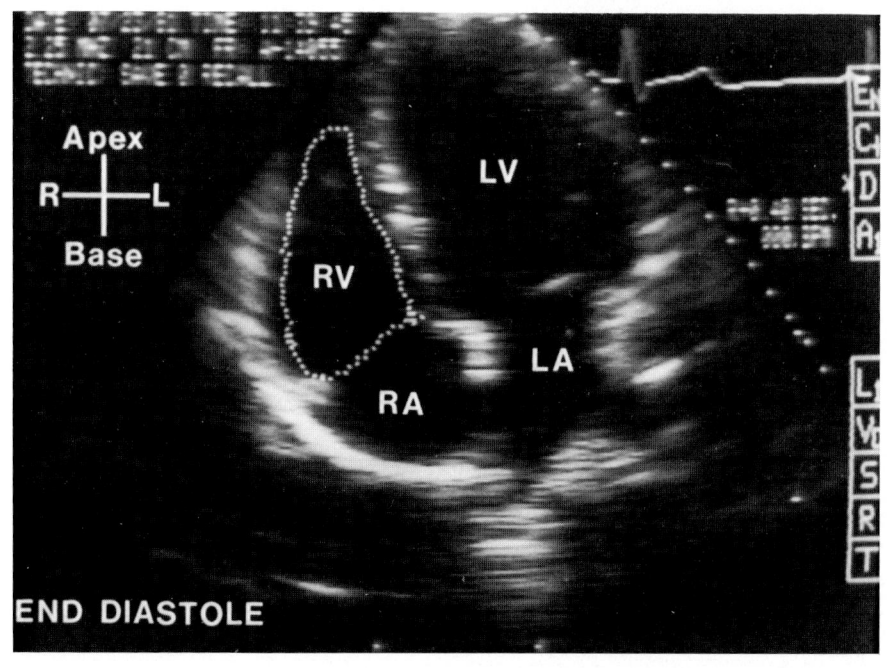

C

END DIASTOLE

L1: 2.6
L3: 3.1

D

END DIASTOLE

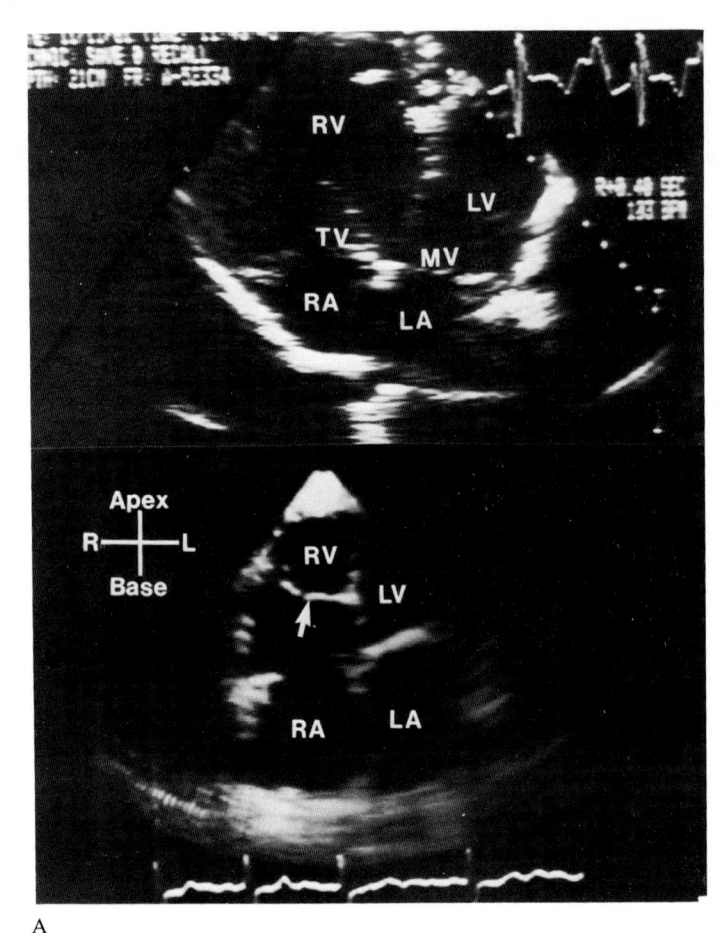

Fig. 8-7A. Apical 4-chamber view showing a patient with a huge right ventricle caused by an atrial septal defect (upper panel) *and an elderly woman with severe rheumatic mitral disease, pulmonary hypertension, enlarged left atrium, right atrium, and right ventricle; a prominent reflectance due to a hypertrophied moderator band* (arrow, lower panel) *is commonly seen in patients with right ventricular hypertrophy. The apex of the left ventricle is not visible in either of these apical 4-chamber planes. B. Anatomic section of apical 4-chamber plane in a patient who died with severe right ventricular hypertrophy. The RV free wall trabeculations and papillary muscle are very hypertrophied. The true apex of the left ventricle is not present in this tomographic plane. IAS = interatrial septum.*

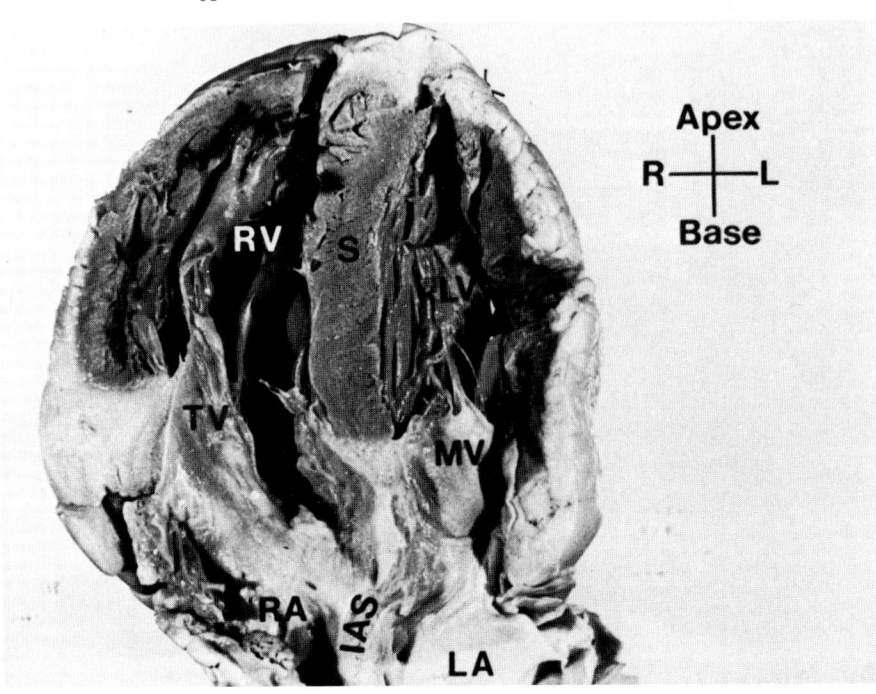

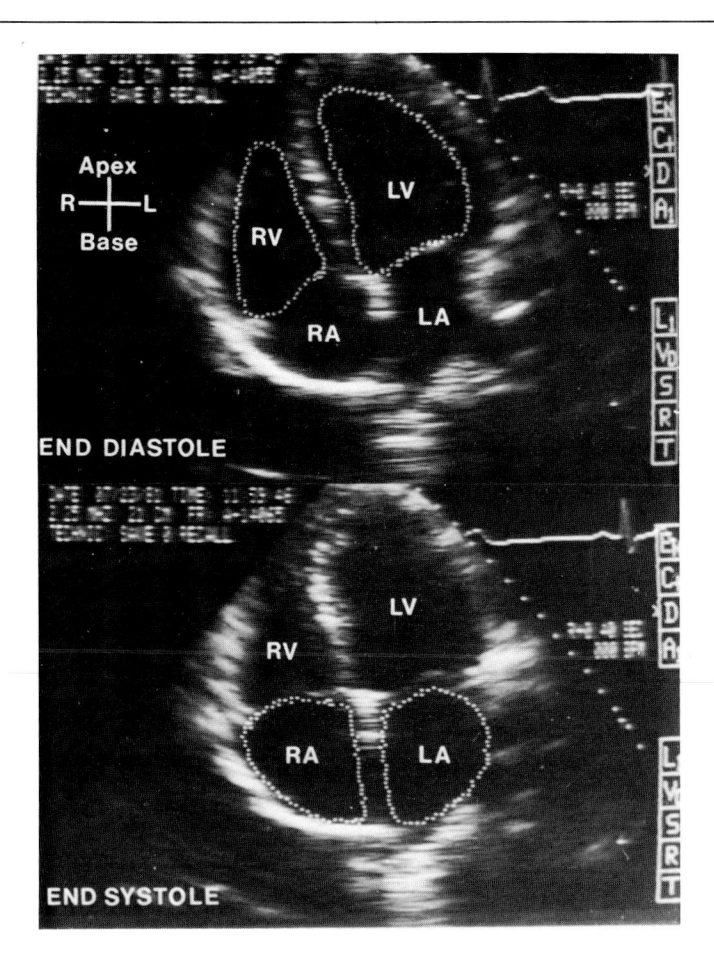

Fig. 8-8. Apical 4-chamber views of a normal adult subject to demonstrate technique of planimetry of both right ventricle and left ventricle at end diastole (upper panel) and of right atrium and left atrium at end systole (lower panel). Notice that the RA and LA are equal in area and have slightly longer apex (inferior) to base (superior) dimension than the short axis or right-to-left dimension.

echo (Fig. 8-7). The single best measurement of the right ventricle is the end-diastolic planimetered area from the apical four-chamber view. This area correlates well with right ventricular volume determined from biplane cineangiography [47].

The apical four-chamber view is also the single best view for evaluating the size of the right atrium. In this view the right atrium normally appears the same size as the left atrium and the areas of the two chambers are equal. Usually the long axis (inferosuperior dimension) is slightly greater than the short axis (right–left dimension). The two most valuable measurements of the right atrium for distinguishing normal from abnormal are the inferosuperior dimension and the planimetered area. The single best measurement for distinguishing normal from abnormal of either right ventricle or right atrium is the planimetered area in the apical four-chamber view. Because of the parallel beam angle, the mid to superior portions of the interatrial septum are often not well visualized because of echo dropout in the apical four-chamber view. However, when the atrial wall is particularly flat where the interatrial septum should be present, there is usually the presence of an atrial septal defect (either sinus venosus or secundum types) (Fig. 8-6B); this observation should be made if the right atrium or right ventricle is enlarged. Definitive diagnosis of an atrial septal defect using contrast echocardiography is discussed in Chapter 13.

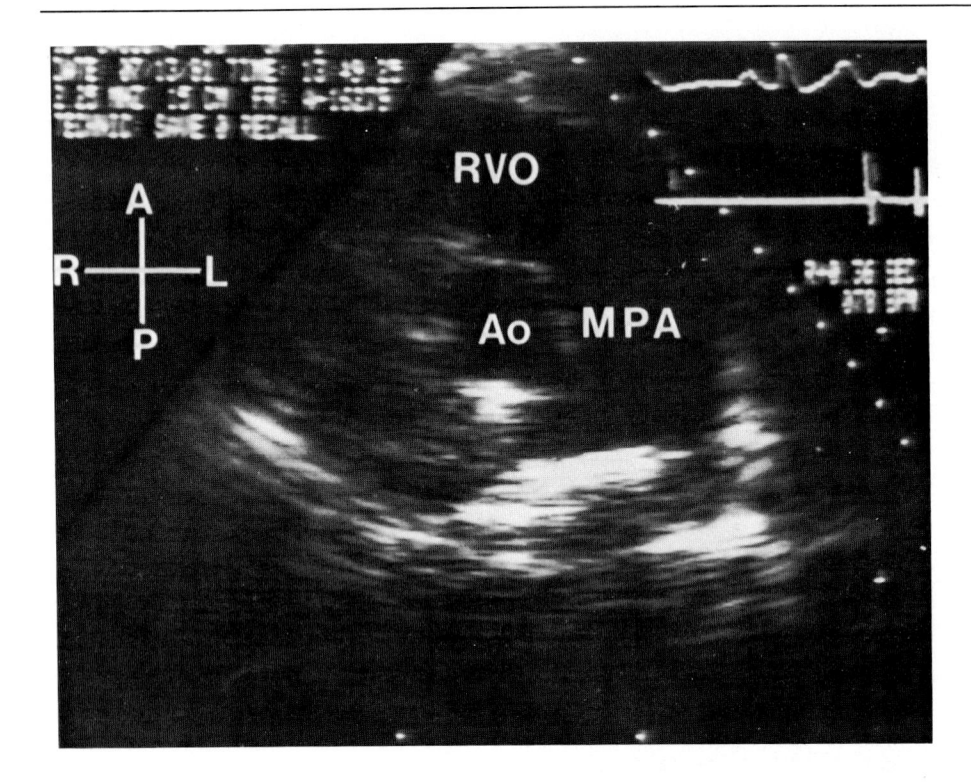

Fig. 8-9. Parasternal short axis view at the base with lateral angulation toward the enlarged pulmonary artery in a patient with right ventricular volume overload. The ratio of the MPA diameter (30 mm) to the aortic diameter (22 mm) is abnormal at 1.36 (upper limit of normal is approximately 1.2).

If there is sufficient clinical information and adequate imaging of the left atrium and left ventricle further confirms normal left heart anatomy, then area determinations of the chambers in the apical four-chamber view to derive RV to LV and RA to LA ratios are one of the most sensitive methods of identifying subtle enlargement of either right ventricle or right atrium. End-diastolic planimetry of both right ventricle and left ventricle in an apical four-chamber view is performed in a manner so as to maximize the cavity size of both ventricles (Fig. 8-8). Planimetry of the atria is also performed when the chambers are the largest, which occurs at the end of ventricular systole just before the opening of the atrioventricular valves. The chamber sizes are correlated with body surface area; however, the ratios of the right heart structure to the corresponding left heart structure are not related to body surface area.

The diameter of the main pulmonary artery is increased in the presence of right ventricular volume overload (Fig. 8-9). The extent of that increase appears to be directly related to the magnitude of the left-to-right shunt. Of course an enlarged pulmonary artery is not specific for a right ventricular volume overload, since pulmonary hypertension in the absence of increased volume in the right heart also produces significant dilatation of the pulmonary artery.

Subcostal imaging is particularly valuable in the overall anatomic and functional assessment of the right heart structures. The subcostal four-chamber view is one of the best tomographic planes for measuring the free wall thickness of the right ventricle (Fig. 8-10).

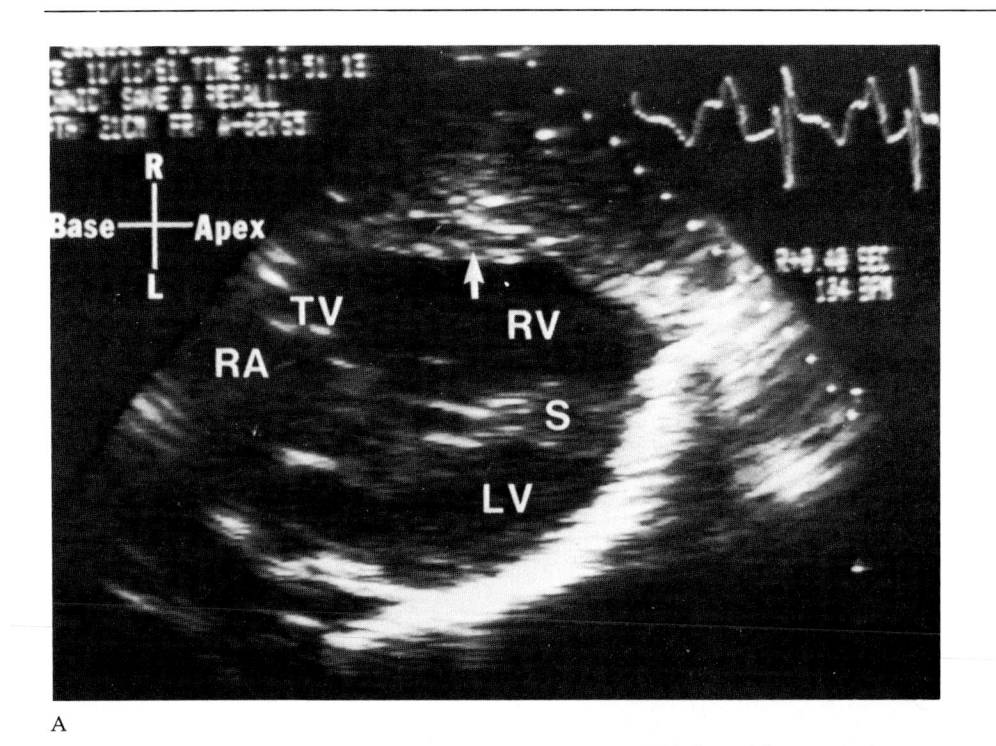

Fig. 8-10A. Subcostal 4-chamber view of a patient with enlargement of the right ventricle and demonstrating a good view of RV wall thickness (arrow). This 4-chamber plane is superior to the apical 4-chamber plane for measuring free wall thickness of the RV but inferior for measuring RV cavity size. B. Subcostal 4-chamber view of a normal adult subject to demonstrate the technique of positioning the M-mode cursor perpendicularly through the RV free wall with the benefit of simultaneous 2-D imaging; in this way, the M-mode records can be used to reliably measure RV wall thickness. AS = interatrial septum.

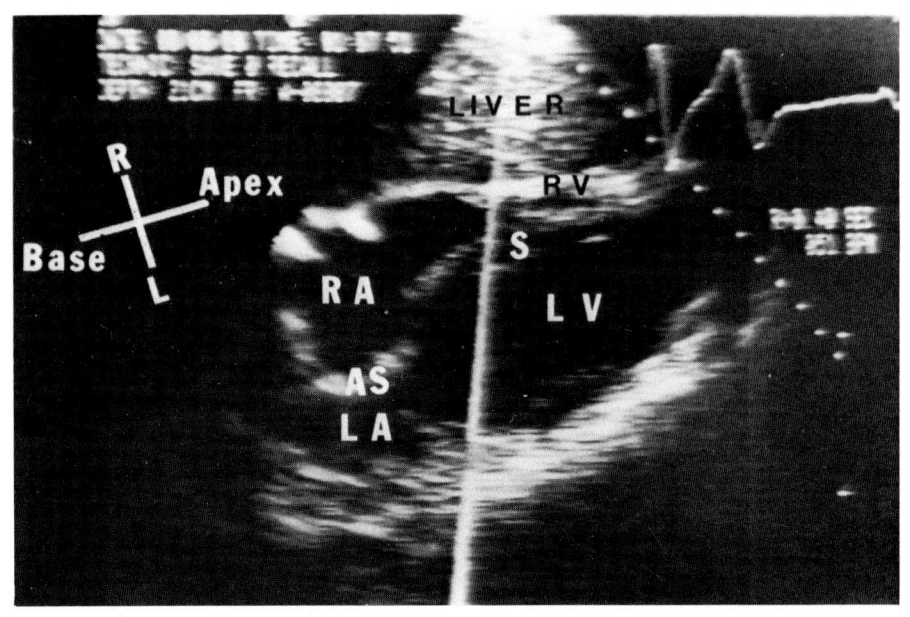

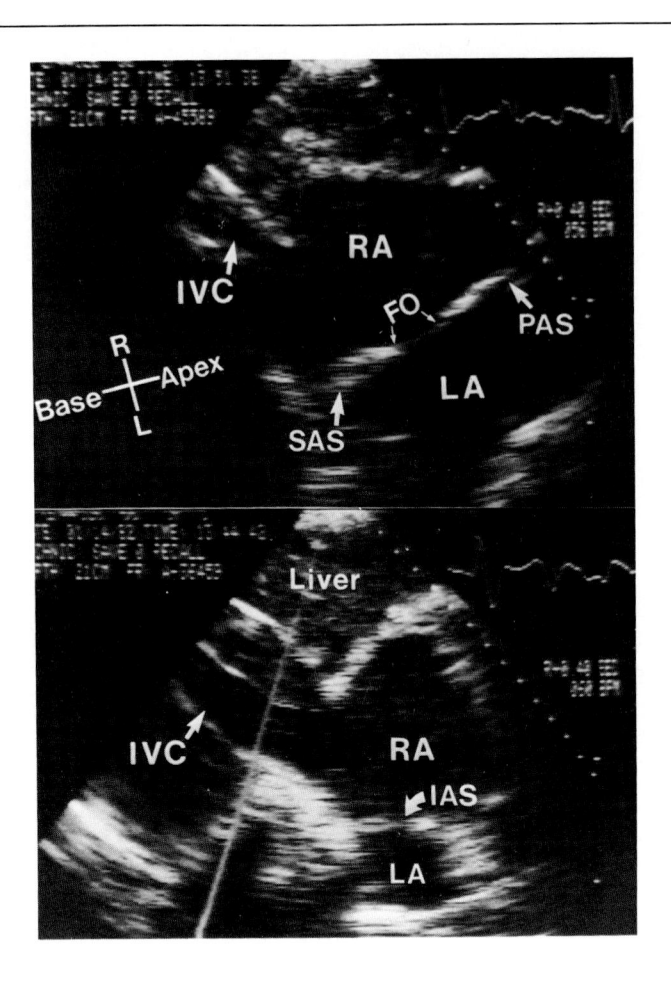

Fig. 8-11. Subcostal views of both atria and interatrial septum (IAS) (upper panel) and the IVC entering the right atrium (lower panel). When the sector beam is directed in the proper perpendicular fashion through the IAS, the primum (PAS) and secundum (SAS) portions of the atrial septum can be seen and a thinner, central portion of the IAS which is the fossa ovalis (FO) (upper panel). With slight counterclockwise rotation and rightward angulation of the sector the IVC-RA junction can be viewed (lower panel) with a small portion of the IAS and left atrium. The M-mode cursor is directed through the IVC.

Interatrial septum, inferior vena cava, and superior vena cava. Although the primum portion of the interatrial septum is optimally visualized in the apical four-chamber plane, the remainder of the septum is best imaged in the subcostal position with the sector beam directed in a perpendicular fashion toward the interatrial septum. Thinning of the interatrial septum in the region of the fossa ovalis can usually be seen (Fig. 8-11). The inferior vena cava is usually not seen or is only partially imaged when the atrial septum is being visualized. Simultaneous recording of the M-mode cursor through the atrial septum provides thickness and motion information that can be timed with the electrocardiogram and may be clinically useful (Fig. 8-12A, B). The motion of the interatrial septum may be quite exaggerated at times, change with respiratory dynamics, and have altered motion due to arrhythmias (Fig. 8-12C, D).

In normal subjects the interatrial septum is slightly convex toward the right atrium at end systole and slightly convex toward the left atrium at end diastole [48]. During acute mitral regurgitation the systolic bulge toward the right atrium may be accentuated, and the motion of the interatrial septum may be markedly decreased as a result of pulmonary hypertension [49].

Aneurysms of the interatrial septum are uncommon but have been observed at angiography as a filling defect in the right or left atrium that can be mistaken for a tumor mass [50]. If the aneurysm is sufficiently large it may protrude into either the mitral or tricuspid orifice, resulting in obstruction simulating atrioventricular valve stenosis [51]. Since some of these aneurysms may have fenestrations with associated left-to-right shunting, patients should also be evaluated for evidence of an atrial septal defect. Such patients are theoretically at increased risk of catheter entanglement in the fenestrated aneurysm at the time of cardiac catheterization.

A few cases of atrial septal aneurysm have been reported with the use of two-dimensional echocardiography [52, 53]. One of these patients was found to have a loud mid-systolic click at the lower left sternal border simulating mitral valve prolapse on physical examination [53]. Bulging of this aneurysm into the right atrium was associated with the production of the systolic click; the intensity of the click increased with inspiration and decreased slightly with the Valsalva maneuver. We have observed an atrial septal aneurysm in a few patients. The extent of motion may be quite significant when observed in real-time (Fig. 8-13).

The inferior vena cava represents an index of right atrial pressure and right ventricular function. Subcostal imaging of the inferior vena cava should include both long and short axis views during normal and held respiration. Simultaneous M-mode recordings should be obtained while the IVC is being imaged with 2-D echo to ensure that correct dimensions are recorded. Normal subjects have a small presystolic "A" wave (less than 125% of the end-diastolic IVC dimension), a small systolic V wave (less than 140% of the end-diastolic IVC dimension), and a 50 percent inspiratory decrease in IVC dimension [54] (Fig. 8-14). Mintz and coinvestigators [54] found an "A" wave greater than or equal to 125 percent of end-diastolic IVC dimension in 71 percent of patients with sinus rhythm and an elevated right ventricular end-diastolic pressure of 10 mm Hg or greater. These investigators also found a V wave greater than or equal to 140 percent of end-diastolic IVC dimension in 75 percent of patients with severe tricuspid insufficiency. Minimal or no inspiratory collapse of the IVC dimension is seen in patients with significant right ventricular dysfunction, constrictive pericarditis, or pericardial tamponade (Fig. 8-15A–C). Cannon "A" waves may be confused with V waves in the presence of ventricular bigeminy (Fig. 8-15D).

The superior vena cava can be imaged from the suprasternal notch position (see Chap. 1). Although qualitative evaluation of the superior vena cava can usually be made from this tomographic plane, it is more difficult to image and normal echocardiographic criteria have not yet been published. Furthermore it is not possible to obtain M-mode recordings of the superior vena cava since the structure lies superiorly-inferiorly in a parallel direction to the echo beam from the suprasternal notch.

Pulmonic valve and tricuspid valve. Considerable attention has been paid in past years to the diastolic wave form of the pulmonic valve echocardiogram to make diagnoses of pulmonary hypertension and pulmonic stenosis [55–57]. Acquatella and colleagues [37] have shown the lack of correlation between echocardiographic pulmonic valve motion and pulmonary artery pressure. Green and Popp [58] demonstrated that the pulmonic valve "A" wave does not represent independent valvular displacement, but rather reflects motion of the entire cardiac base. They also reported that variations in "A" wave morphology may result, at

270   8. Diseases of the right heart

A

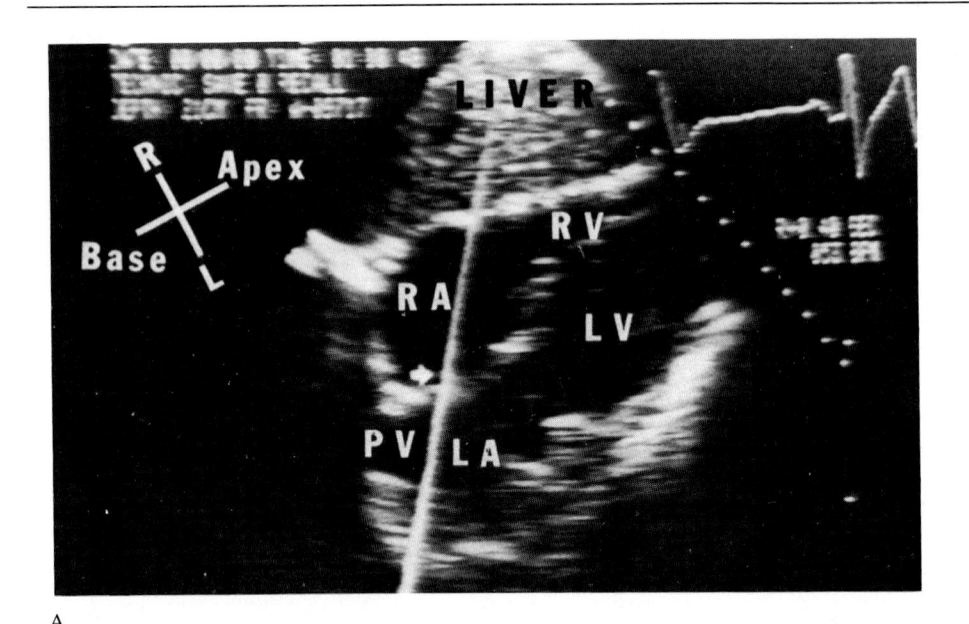

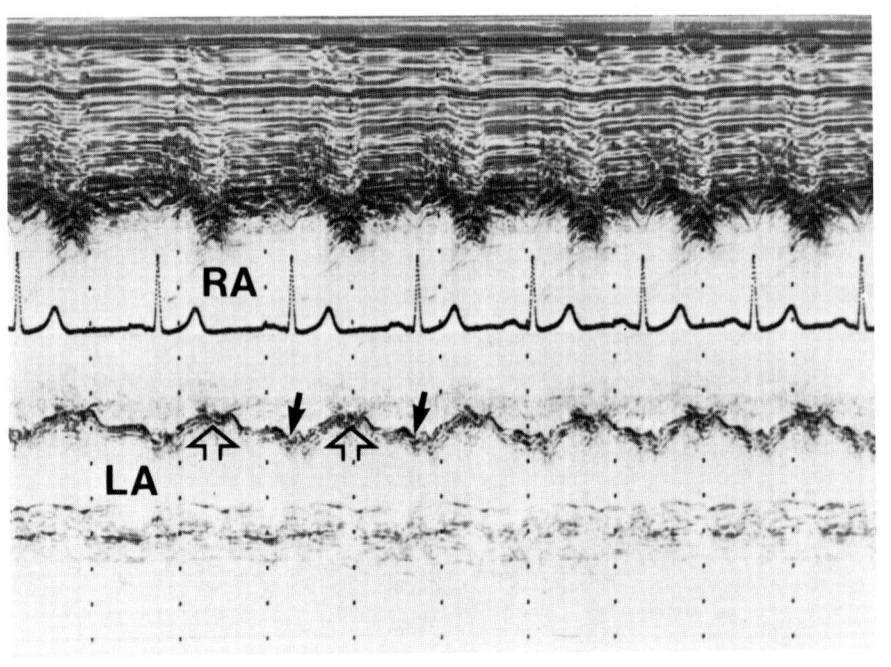

B

Figure 8-12A. Subcostal 4-chamber view demonstrating the M-mode cursor through the interatrial septum (arrow). B. M-mode recording of right atrium, interatrial septum, and left atrium obtained from subcostal position in a normal adult demonstrating normal motion of the interatrial septum; it moves toward the RA during ventricular systole (open arrows) and then toward the LA following atrial contraction (solid arrows). The calibration dots are 1 cm apart. C. M-mode recording of RA, interatrial septum, and LA obtained from the subcostal position in a patient with mitral regurgitation and accentuated V wave motion of the IAS toward the RA during ventricular systole. A = "A" wave. Calibration dots are 5 mm apart. D. M-mode recording of RA, IAS, and LA obtained from the subcostal position in a patient with atrial flutter demonstrating flutter waves on ECG (solid arrows) and flutter waves of the IAS (open arrows). The effects of respiration can also be seen with the RA becoming smaller with exhalation (Ex) and larger with inspiration (In). PV = pulmonic vein.

271

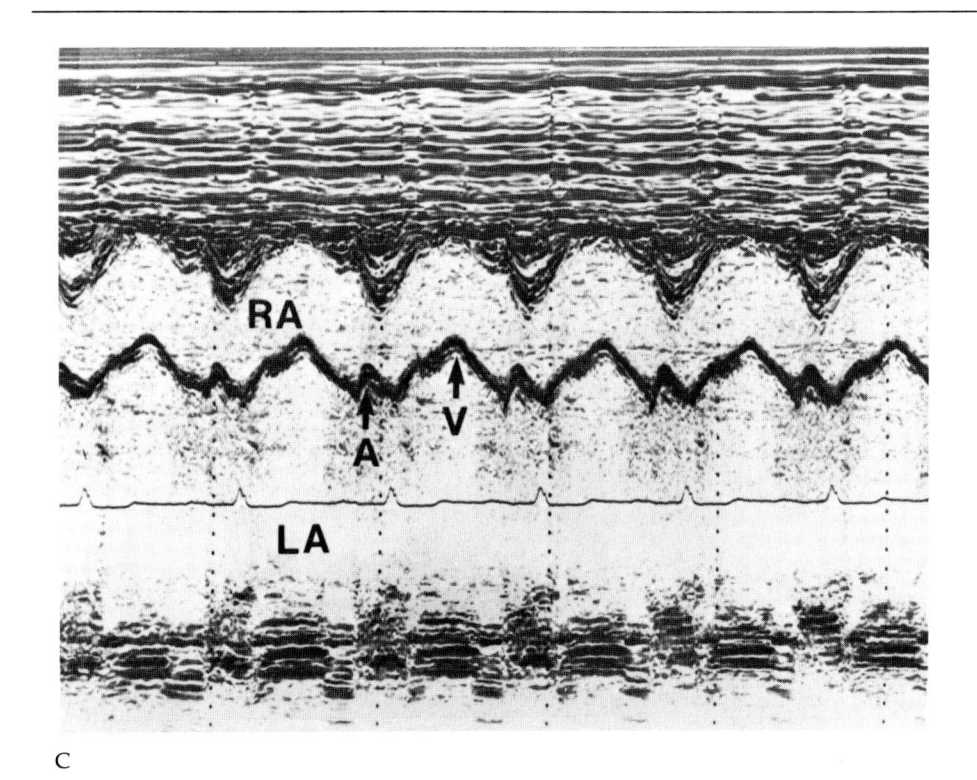

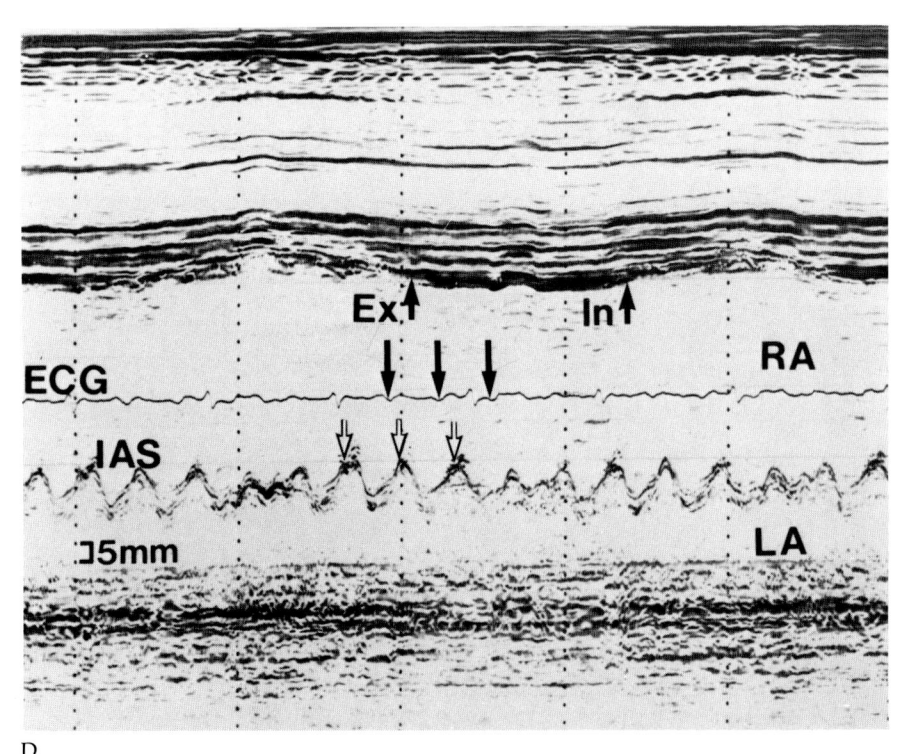

C

D

272   8. Diseases of the right heart

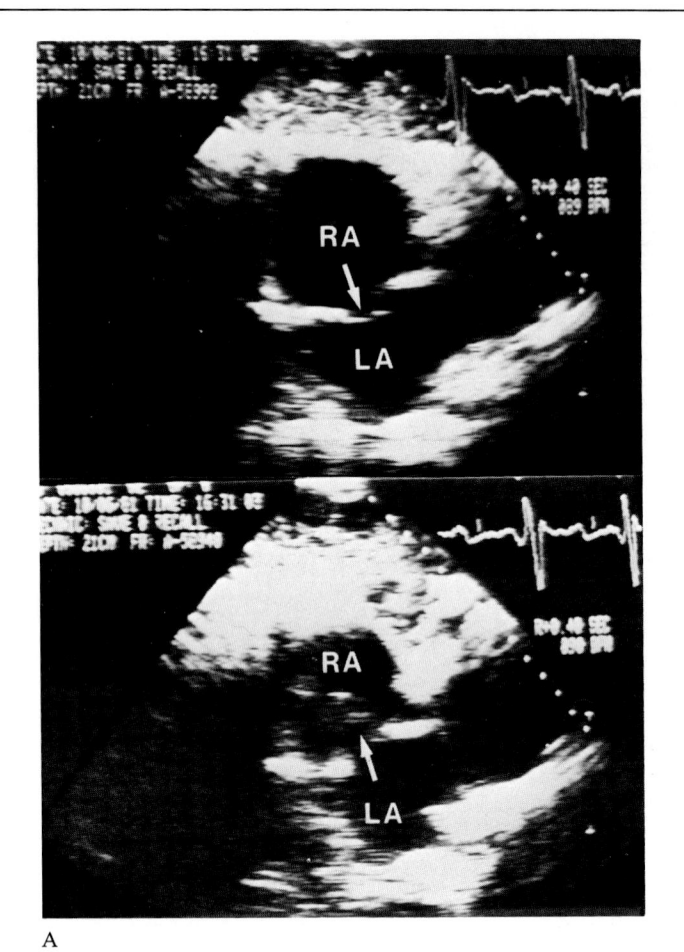

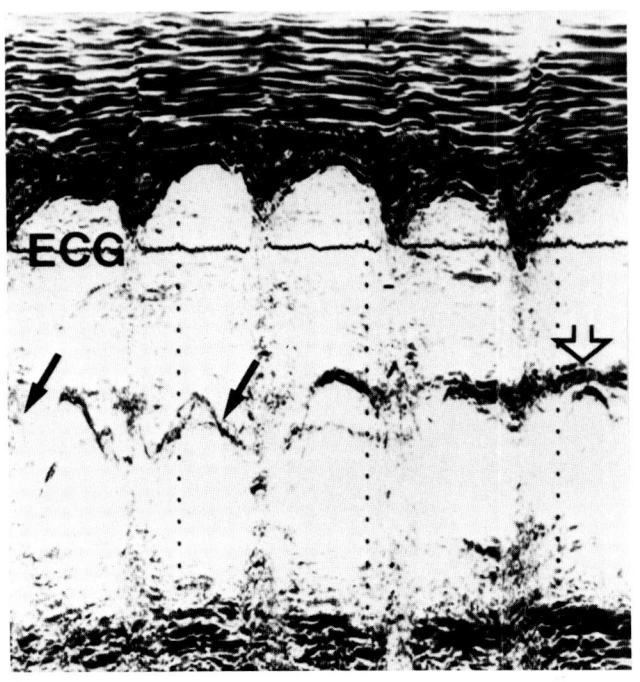

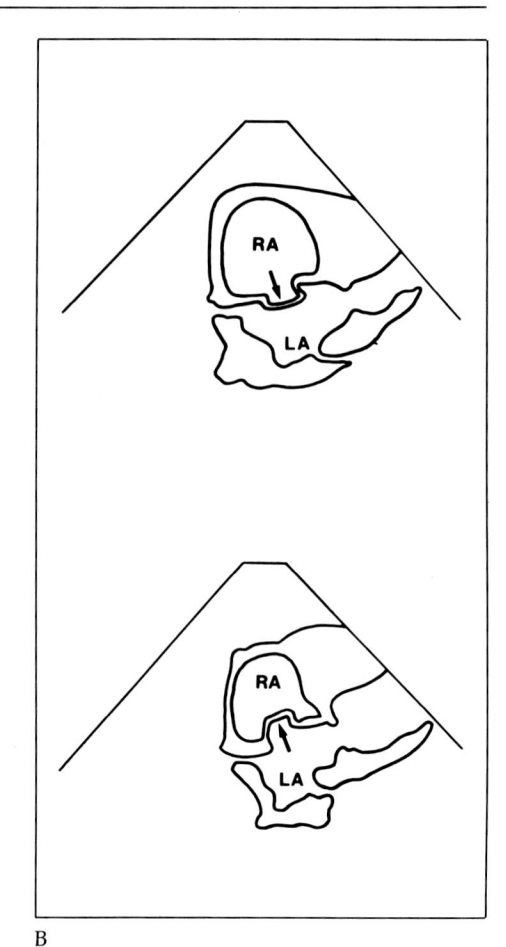

Fig. 8-13A. Subcostal view of right atrium, interatrial septum, and left atrium demonstrating an aneurysm of the fossa ovalis which moves into the LA (arrow, upper panel) during diastole and *into the RA (arrow, lower panel) during systole. B. Diagram of structures shown in A. C. M-mode recording of the same patient showing exaggerated motion and thin wall of the fossa ovalis aneurysm (two solid arrows) and normal motion and thickness of adjacent interatrial septum (IAS) (open arrow). Right atrium is above and left atrium below the IAS. The calibration dots are 5 mm apart.*

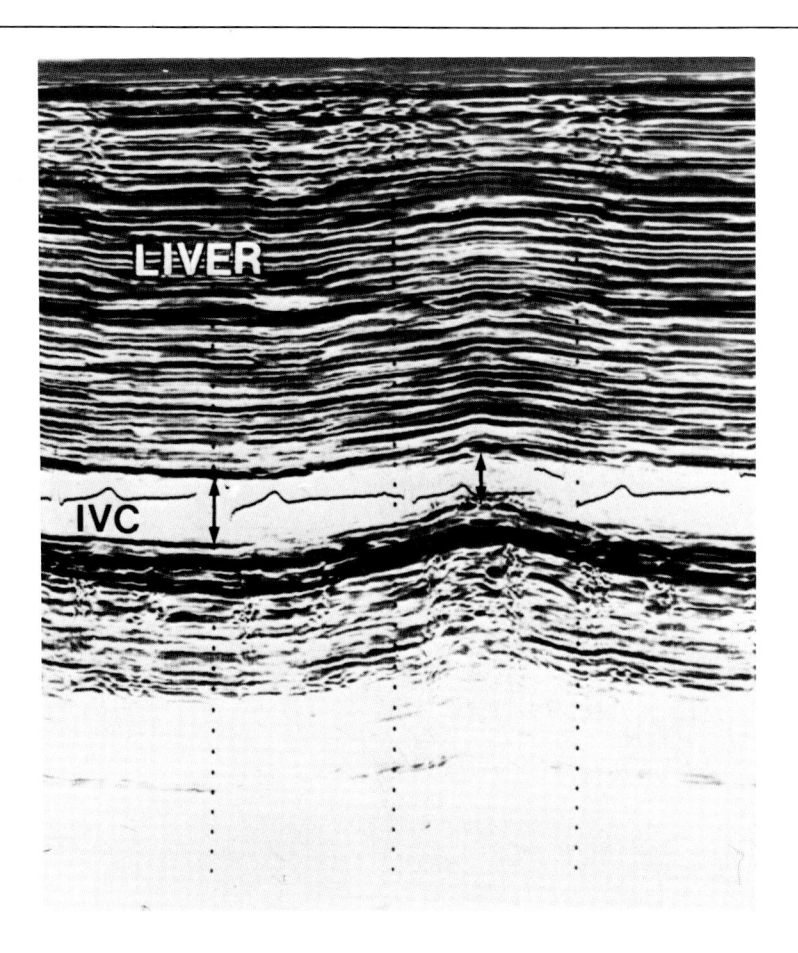

Fig. 8-14. M-mode recording from subcostal position showing normal diameter of the IVC (17 mm), which collapses normally with inspiration to 10 mm. The calibration dots are 5 mm apart.

274   8. Diseases of the right heart

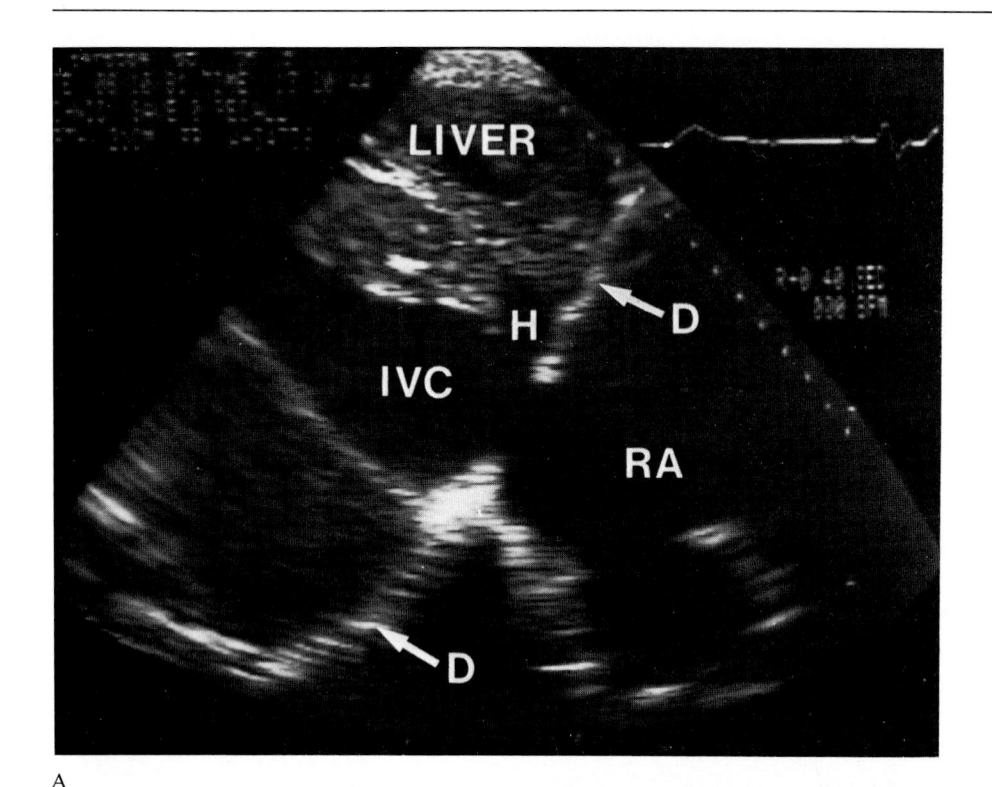

Fig. 8-15A. Subcostal view of IVC entering the right atrium and liver separated from the heart by the diaphragm (D). The patient had severe right ventricular dysfunction with secondary enlargement of the IVC caused by high right atrial pressures. The calibration dots to the right of the sector are 1 cm apart. B. Subcostal view of IVC entering the RA in a young adult suffering acute pericardial tamponade following chest contusion in an automobile accident. The IVC was within normal limits (diameter = 22 to 23 mm); however, there was no inspiratory collapse consistent with high right atrial pressures. C. M-mode recording of the IVC in a patient with elevated right atrial pressures and tricuspid regurgitation. The diameter of the IVC is 22 mm, increases to 25 mm during V waves (arrows), and does not reveal inspiratory collapse with normal respiration. D. M-mode recording of the IVC in a patient with normal right atrial pressures and normal IVC diameter (12 mm). Cannon waves (arrows) (IVC diameter = 23 mm) are caused by right atrial contraction against a closed tricuspid valve.

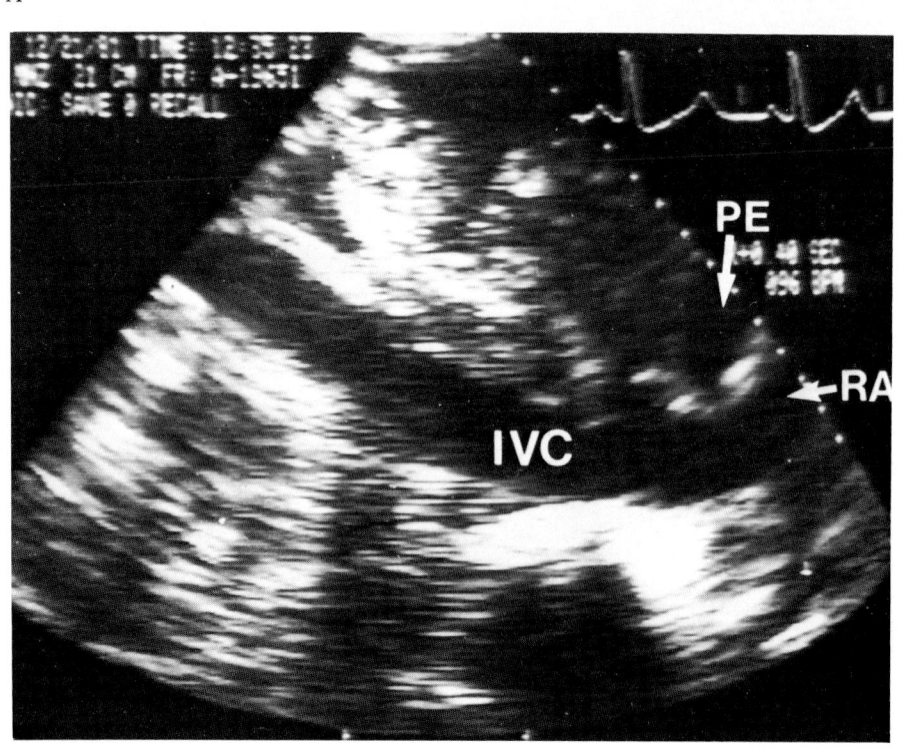

275

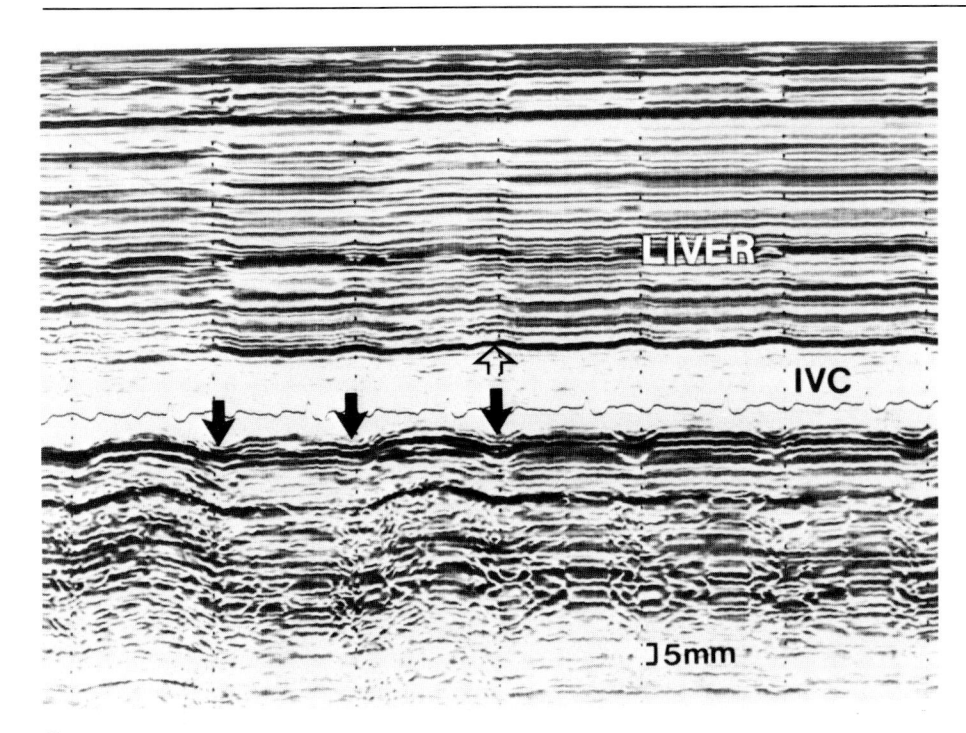

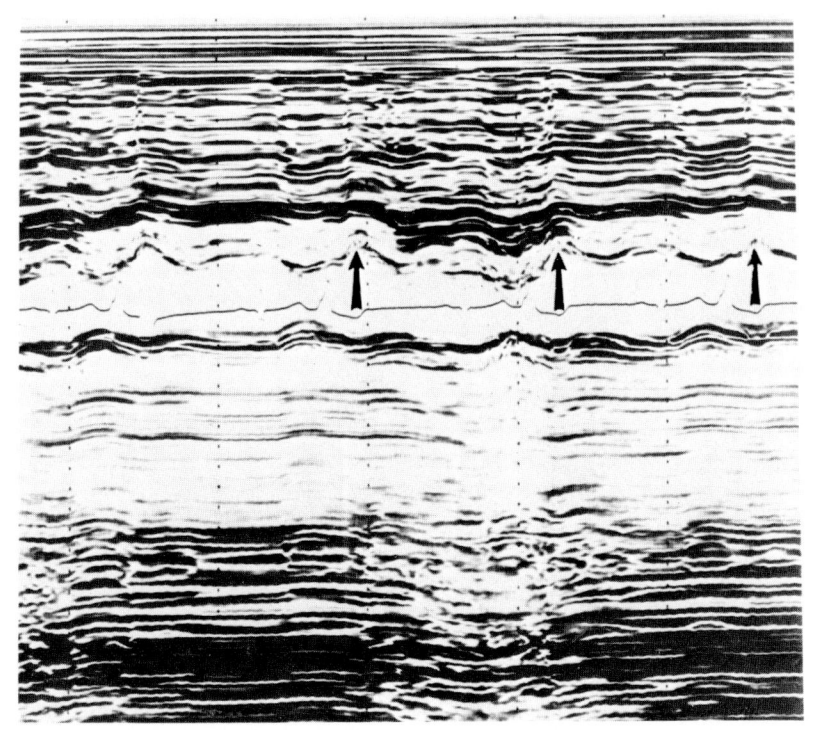

LIVER

IVC

] 5mm

C

D

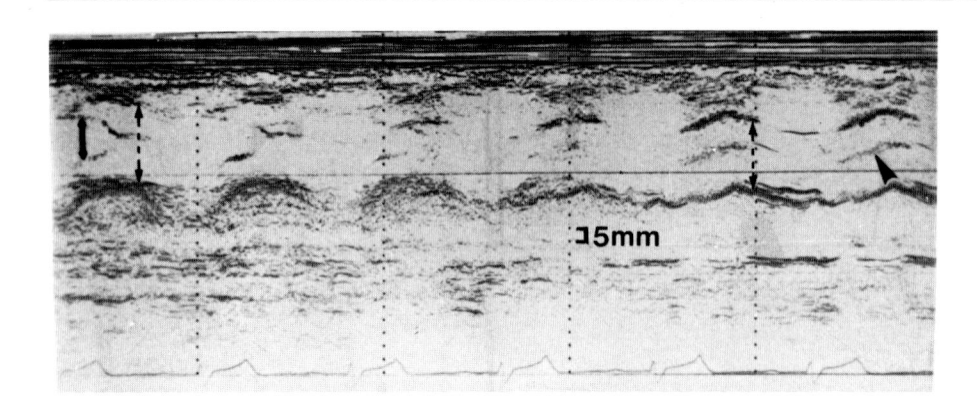

Fig. 8-16. M-mode recording of both semilunar valves during continuous sweeping from the normal aortic valve (left side of figure) to the smaller pulmonary artery and stenotic pulmonary valve showing systolic fluttering (arrow at right margin of figure) *in an adult with corrected transposition and pulmonary stenosis.*

least in part, from the effects of altered ventricular geometry and compliance on left atrial emptying. Significant variations in the depth of the "A" waves may occur with normal respiration. Extreme respiratory variation in the depth of the "A" wave has been demonstrated in a patient with constrictive pericarditis [59]. These authors suggest that during inspiration a small increase in right ventricular volume can produce a disproportionate increase in right ventricular diastolic pressure, which may be further increased by atrial contraction, producing a deep pulmonic "A" wave during inspiration.

Two-dimensional echocardiography is significantly better than M-mode echo for making the diagnosis of pulmonary stenosis. Weyman and associates [60] observed systolic doming and failure of the leaflets to move fully open and lie parallel to the margins of the pulmonary artery. Multiple transducer positions from parasternal and subcostal windows provide excellent opportunities to visualize the pulmonic valve and subpulmonic region. Simultaneous M-mode recordings may reveal additional abnormalities of increased thickness, reduced motion, or fluttering of the leaflets (Fig. 8-16).

Diastolic fluttering of the pulmonic valve may be caused by a patent ductus arteriosus. Fisher and colleagues [61] made this observation in 15 of 39 (38%) children with confirmed diagnosis of patent ductus arteriosus. This fluttering disappeared after ligation of the ductus.

Vegetations of the pulmonic valve are discussed in Chapter 5.

The anatomy of the tricuspid valve and its supporting structures differs from that of the mitral valve. The mitral valve is supported by chordae tendineae, all of which insert into the two papillary muscles. Traditionally the right ventricle is expected to have three papillary muscles (posterior, anterior, and septal); however, they are not always as well defined as their counterparts in the left ventricle, and sometimes only two are found. Furthermore, all the chordae tendineae from the three tricuspid leaflets do not insert into the papillary muscles. Many of the chordae insert directly into the endocardial surface of the interventricular septum or into the coarse trabeculations of the free wall of the right ventricle (Fig. 8-17).

The tricuspid valve is imaged quite easily from several different tomographic planes. The right ventricular inflow view is one of the best planes for evaluation of evidence of tricuspid stenosis (Fig. 8-18A). Thickened leaflets and restricted diastolic opening are the most conspicuous abnormalities. Careful attention must be

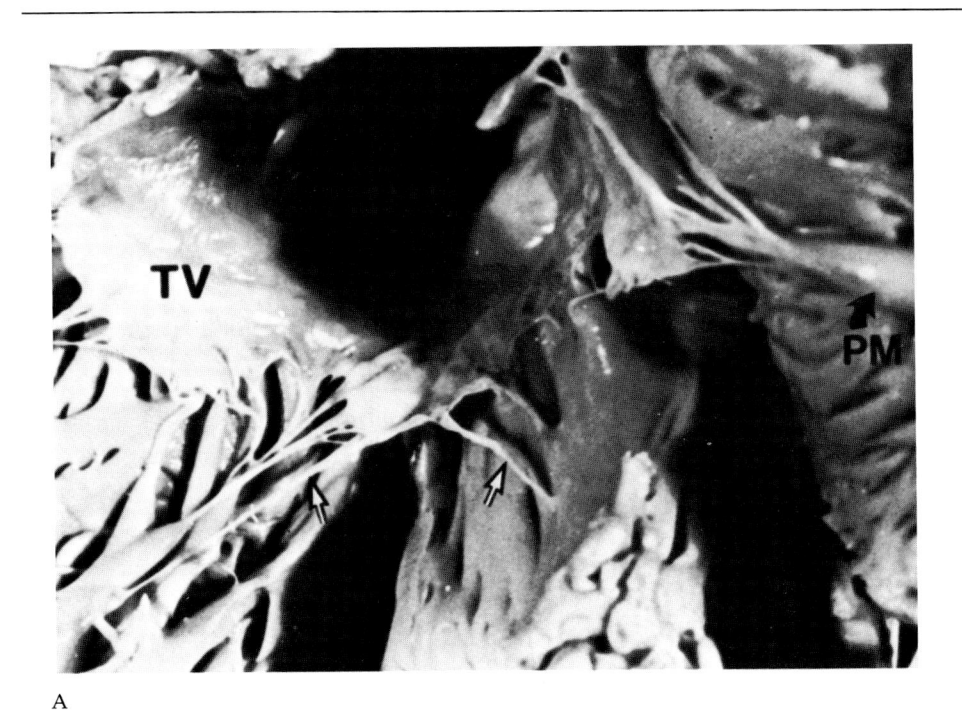

Fig. 8-17A. Close-up anatomic view of tricuspid valve showing chordae tendineae inserting into the right ventricular wall (open arrows) and other chordae inserting into a papillary muscle. B. Anatomic view of TV with chordae tendineae inserting directly into the right side of the interventricular septum (two black arrows).

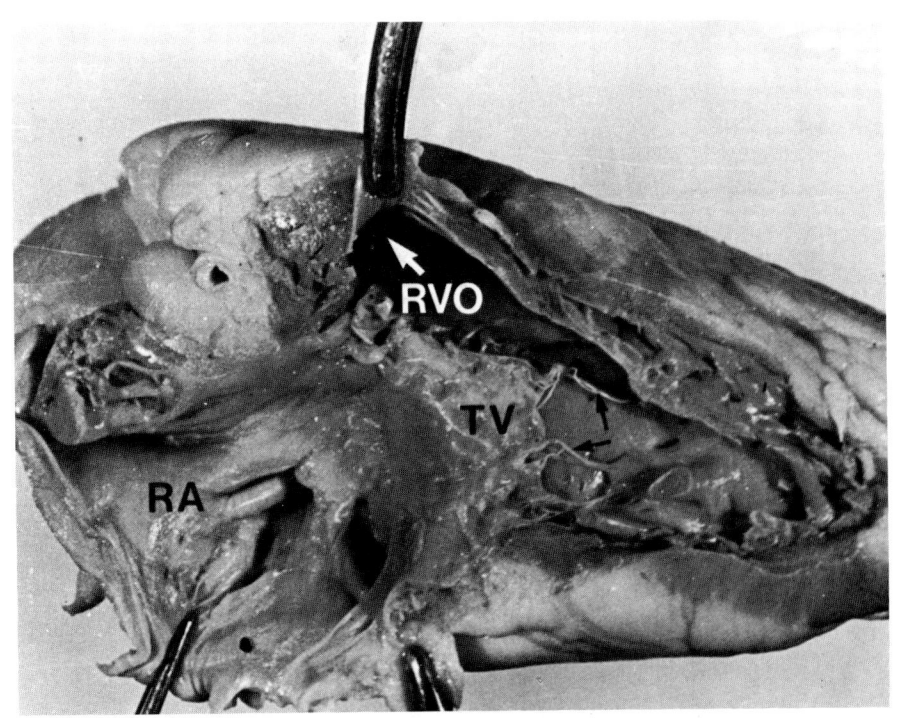

278 8. Diseases of the right heart

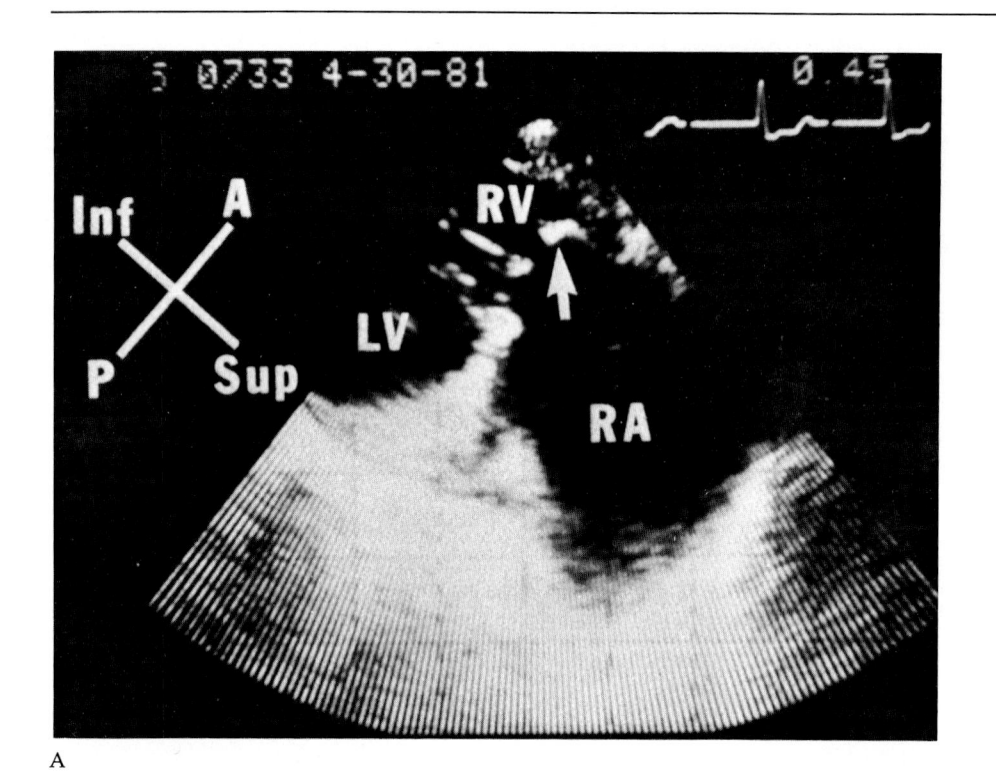

Fig. 8-18A. Parasternal right ventricular inflow view of a patient with tricuspid stenosis demonstrating increased thickness of the tip of the anterior tricuspid leaflet (arrow), restricted opening of both anterior and septal leaflets, doming contour of anterior tricuspid leaflet, and right atrial enlargement. B. M-mode recordings of the tricuspid valve in the same patient on two different occasions a few days apart. The left panel shows reduced excursion and apparent increased thickness (open arrows) of the TV because the beam was directed too close to the tricuspid annulus, producing pseudo tricuspid stenosis. In the right panel, although the heart rate is faster, the tricuspid valve demonstrates normal thickness and motion (arrows) because the M-mode cursor was directed through the leaflet tips. C. M-mode recording of TV demonstrating actual tricuspid stenosis (arrows) with properly directed M-mode cursor and showing very large right atrium.

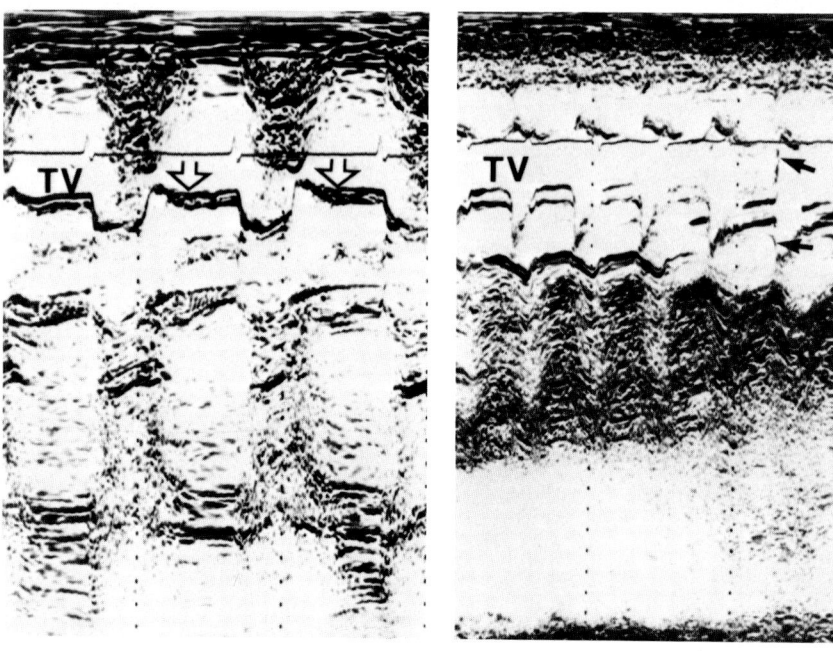

C

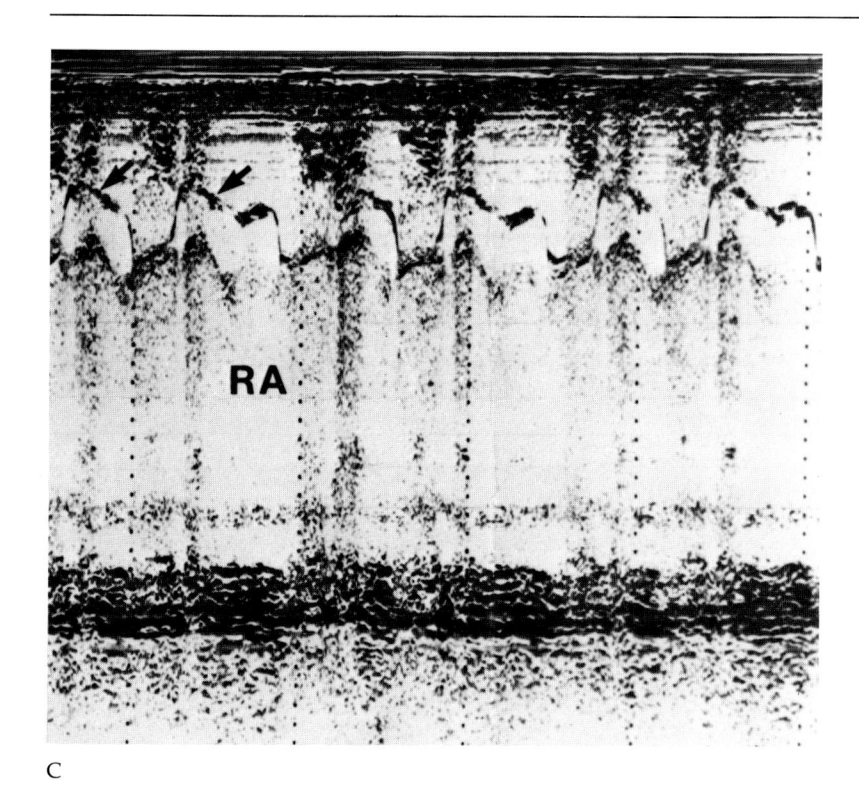

given to imaging leaflet motion from more than one plane; the right ventricular inflow and apical four-chamber are the best. Failure to direct the beam through the leaflet tips and imaging too close to the tricuspid annulus may simulate tricuspid stenosis with either 2-D imaging or M-mode recordings (Fig. 8-18B, C).

The utilization of right ventricular inflow and apical four-chamber views has been recommended for evaluation of the tricuspid valve for evidence of prolapse [62, 63] (Fig. 8-19). Werner and associates [64] found that 21 percent of patients with mitral valve prolapse had concomitant tricuspid valve prolapse; Mardelli and associates [63] and Ogawa and colleagues [65] reported an incidence of 48 percent and 40 percent, respectively. Chen and coworkers [62] found that patients with tricuspid valve prolapse had a 40 percent prevalence rate of tricuspid regurgitation.

Echocardiographic findings of increased thickness and reduced motion of the tricuspid valve have been reported in carcinoid heart disease [66, 67] (Fig. 8-20).

The diagnosis of tricuspid regurgitation by cineangiography may be inconclusive because of valvular incompetence induced by the catheter as it crosses the tricuspid valve. The most sensitive method and currently the diagnostic procedure of choice for diagnosing tricuspid insufficiency is contrast echocardiography to record systolic reflux into the inferior vena cava [62, 68–70]. Subcostal imaging of the IVC and right atrium with the M-mode cursor directed through the IVC to record systolic reflux during held respiration is the technique to follow (Fig. 8-21). (This procedure will be discussed in greater detail in Chapter 13.) Atrial fibrillation or premature ventricular contractions may cause false positive reflux into the IVC.

280   8. Diseases of the right heart

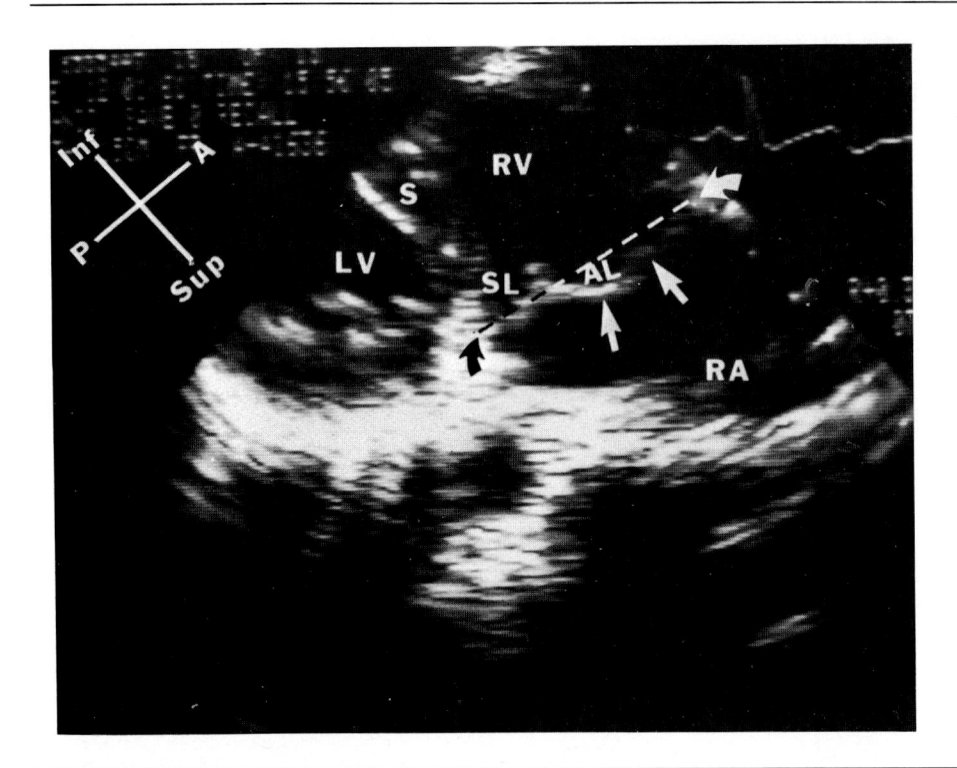

Fig. 8-19. Parasternal right ventricular inflow demonstrating prolapse (straight white arrows) of the anterior tricuspid leaflet (AL) and probably prolapse of the septal leaflet; the dashed line shows the tricuspid annulus (curved white and black arrows).

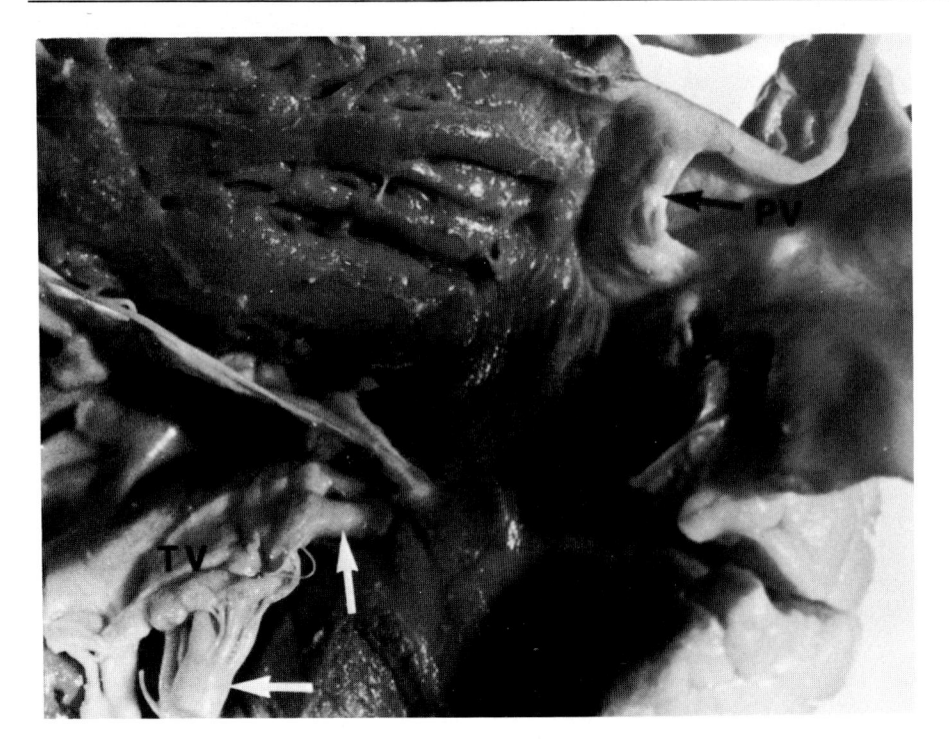

Fig. 8-20. Anatomic view of marked increased thickening of pulmonic valve (PV), tricuspid valve, and chordae tendineae (white arrows) in a patient who died of carcinoid heart disease.

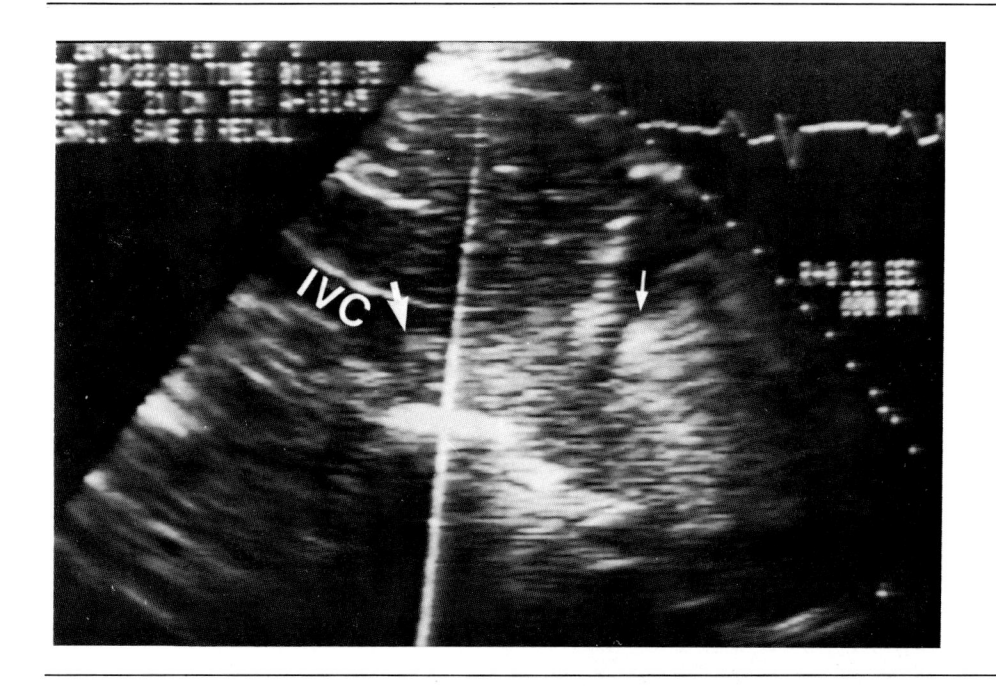

Fig. 8-21. Subcostal view of contrast echocardiogram with M-mode cursor through the IVC demonstrating systolic reflux from right atrium into the IVC (large arrow) *and right atrial wall* (small arrow) *apart from adjacent small pericardial space and diaphragm.*

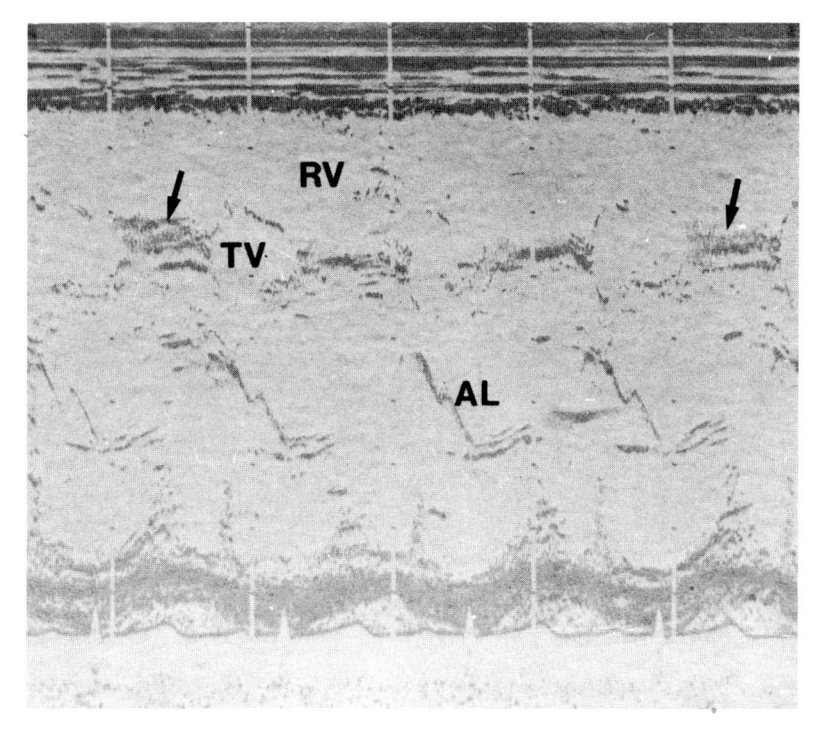

Fig. 8-22. M-mode recording in a patient with a large ventricular septal defect, right ventricular enlargement, and high frequency systolic fluttering of the tricuspid valve (arrows).

282   8. Diseases of the right heart

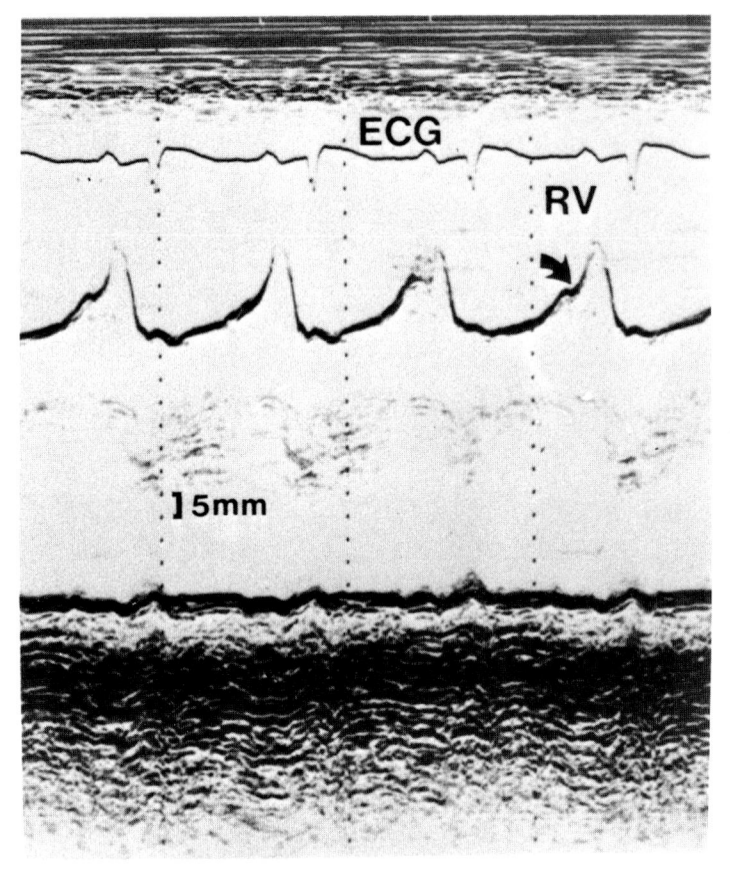

Fig. 8-23A. *M-mode recording of tricuspid valve in a patient with right ventricular failure, enlargement of both right ventricle and right atrium, and marked slowing and delay in the diastolic opening of the tricuspid valve (arrow). B. M-mode recording of a patient with right ventricular failure showing an enlarged RV and delayed opening of the tricuspid valve following atrial contraction (arrow). The left ventricular cavity and flow through the mitral valve diminishes during inspiration (In) and increases during exhalation (Ex).*

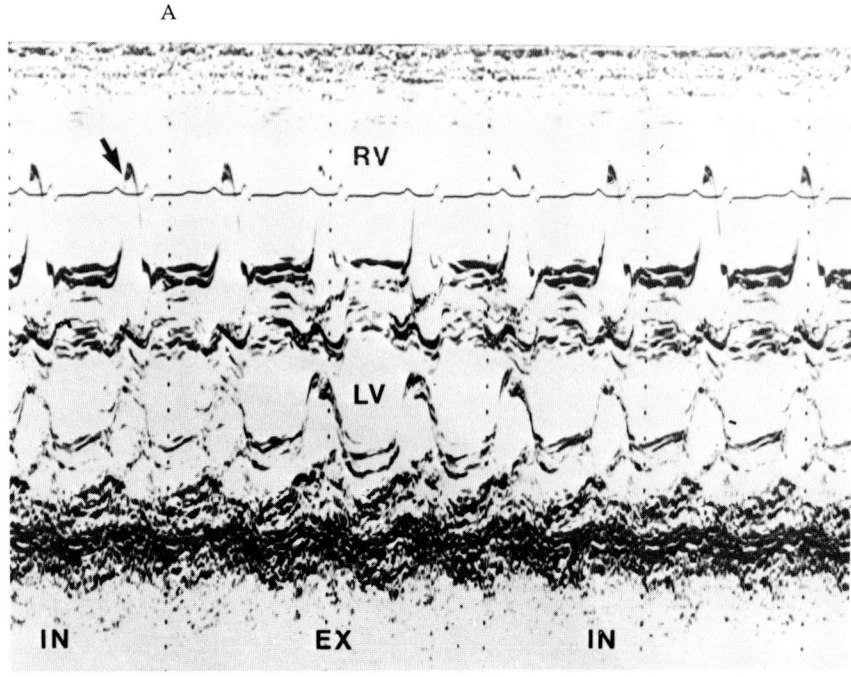

Elevated right atrial pressures in the presence of sinus rhythm may produce diastolic reflux following atrial contraction.

On rare occasions systolic fluttering of the tricuspid valve may be caused by the jet from a ventricular septal defect (Fig. 8-22).

The tricuspid valve may also demonstrate secondary motion abnormalities as a result of right ventricular dysfunction (Fig. 8-23).

References

1. Pearlman AS, Chester CE, Henry WL, Morganroth J, Itscoitz SB, Epstein SE: Determinants of ventricular septal motion: Influence of relative right and left ventricular size. *Circulation* 53:83, 1976
2. Popp RL, Wolfe SB, Hirata T, Feigenbaum H: Estimation of right and left ventricular size by ultrasound. *Am J Cardiol* 24:523, 1969
3. Meyer RH, Schwartz DC, Benzing G, Kaplan S: Ventricular septum in right ventricular volume overload. *Am J Cardiol* 30:349, 1972
4. Kerber RE, Dippel WF, Abboud FM: Abnormal motion of the interventricular septum in right ventricular volume overload: Experimental and clinical echocardiographic studies. *Circulation* 48:86, 1973
5. Hagan AD, Francis GS, Sahn D, Karliner J, Friedman WF, O'Rourke RA: Ultrasound evaluation of systolic anterior septal motion in patients with and without right ventricular volume overload. *Circulation* 50:248, 1974
6. Hagan AD, Deely WJ, Sahn DJ, Friedman WF: Echocardiographic criteria for the normal newborn infant. *Circulation* 48:1221, 1973
7. Matsukubo H, Matsuura T, Endo N, Asayama J, Watanabe T, Furukawa K, Kunishige H, Katsume H, Ijichi H: Echocardiographic measurement of right ventricular wall thickness: A new application of subxyphoid echocardiography. *Circulation* 56:278, 1977
8. Prakash R: Determination of right ventricular wall thickness in systole and diastole: Echocardiographic and necropsy correlation in 32 patients. *Br Heart J* 40:1257, 1978
9. Prakash R: Echocardiographic diagnosis of right ventricular hypertrophy: Correlation with ECG and necropsy findings in 248 patients. *Cath Cardiovasc Diag* 7:179, 1981
10. Kisslo J, VonRamm OT, Thurstone FL: Cardiac imaging using a phased-array ultrasound system: Clinical technique and application. *Circulation* 53:1262, 1976
11. Silverman NH, Schiller NB: Apex echocardiography: A two-dimensional technique for evaluation of congenital heart disease. *Circulation* 57:503, 1978
12. Tajik AJ, Hagler DJ, Mair DD, Lie JT: Two-dimensional real-time ultrasonic imaging of the heart and great vessels—technique, image orientation, structure identification, and validation. *Mayo Clin Proc* 53:271, 1978
13. Starling M, Sorensen S, Crawford M, Amon W, O'Rourke RA: Cross-sectional echocardiographic assessment of right ventricular size and performance in obstructive pulmonary disease patients. *Circulation* 60(Suppl II):II-202, 1979
14. Bommer W, Weinert L, Neumann A, Neef J, Mason DT, De Maria A: Determination of right atrial and right ventricular size by two-dimensional echocardiography. *Circulation* 60:91, 1979
15. Di Sessa TG, Kirkman JH, Ti CC, Hagan AD, Kirkpatrick SE, Friedman WF: Evaluation of cardiac chamber size and left ventricular function in children using two-dimensional apex echocardiography. *Am J Cardiol* 45:468, 1980
16. Graham TP Jr, Jarmakani JM, Atwood GF, Canent RV Jr: Right ventricular volume determinations in children: Normal valves and observations with volume or pressure overload. *Circulation* 47:144, 1973
17. Horn V, Mullins CB, Saffer SI, Jones DC, Freeborn WA, Knapp RS, Nixon JV: A comparison of mathematical models for estimating right ventricular volumes in animals and man. *Clin Cardiol* 2:341, 1979
18. Hiraishi S, Di Sessa TG, Jarmakani JM, Nakanishi T, Isabel-Jones J, Friedman WF: Two-dimensional echocardiographic assessment of right ventricular volume in children with congenital heart disease. *Am J Cardiol* 50:1368, 1982
19. Hirschfeld S, Meyer R, Schwartz DC, Korfhagen J, Kaplan S: Measurement of right and left ventricular systolic time intervals by echocardiography. *Circulation* 51:304, 1975

20. Mills P, Amara I, McLaurin LP, Craige E: Noninvasive assessment of pulmonary hypertension from right ventricular isovolumic contraction time. *Am J Cardiol* 46:272, 1980
21. Hirschfeld S, Meyer R, Schwartz DC, Korfhagen J, Kaplan S: The echocardiographic assessment of pulmonary artery pressure and pulmonary resistance. *Circulation* 52:642, 1975
22. Riggs T, Hirschfeld S, Borkat G, Knoke J, Liebman J: Assessment of the pulmonary vascular bed by echocardiographic right ventricular systolic time intervals. *Circulation* 57:939, 1978
23. Johnson GL, Mayer RA, Korfhagen J, Schwartz DC, Kaplan S: Echocardiographic assessment of pulmonary arterial pressure in children with complete right bundle branch block. *Am J Cardiol* 41:1264, 1978
24. Wroblewski E, James F, Spann JF, Bove AA: Right ventricular performance in mitral stenosis. *Am J Cardiol* 47:51, 1981
25. Olivari MT, Fiorentini C, Polese A, Guazzi MD: Pulmonary hemodynamics and right ventricular function in hypertension. *Circulation* 57:1185, 1978
26. Atkins JM, Mitchell HC, Pettinger WA: Increased pulmonary vascular resistance with systemic hypertension: Effect of Minoxidil and other antihypertensive agents. *Am J Cardiol* 39:802, 1977
27. Taylor RR, Covell JW, Sonnenblick EH, Ross J Jr: Dependence of ventricular distensibility on filling of the opposite ventricle. *Am J Physiol* 213:711, 1967
28. Coma-Canella I, Lopez-Sendon J: Ventricular compliance in ischemic right ventricular dysfunction. *Am J Cardiol* 45:555, 1980
29. Jensen DP, Goolsby JP, Oliva PB: Hemodynamic pattern resembling pericardial constriction after acute inferior myocardial infarction with right ventricular infarction. *Am J Cardiol* 42:858, 1978
30. Marmor A, Geltman EM, Biello DR, Sobel BE, Siegel BA, Roberts R: Functional response of the right ventricle to myocardial infarction: Dependence on the site of left ventricular infarction. *Circulation* 64:1005, 1981
31. Starling MR, Crawford MH, Walsh RA, O'Rourke RA: Value of the tricuspid valve echogram for estimating right ventricular end-diastolic pressure during vasodilator therapy. *Am J Cardiol* 45:966, 1980
32. Kramer NE, Chawla KK, Patel R, Khan M, Mayer T, Towne WD: Differentiation of posterior myocardial infarction from right ventricular hypertrophy and normal anterior loop by echocardiography. *Circulation* 58:1057, 1978
33. Weyman AE, Dillon JC, Feigenbaum H, Chang S: Echocardiographic patterns of pulmonic valve motion with pulmonary hypertension. *Circulation* 50:905, 1974
34. Goodman DJ, Harrison DC, Popp RL: Echocardiographic features of primary pulmonary hypertension. *Am J Cardiol* 33:438, 1974
35. Pocoski DJ, Shah PM: Physiologic correlates of echocardiographic pulmonary valve motion in diastole. *Circulation* 58:1064, 1978
36. Tahara M, Tanaka H, Nakao S, Yoshimura H, Sakurai S, Tei C, Kashima T: Hemodynamic determinants of pulmonary valve motion during systole in experimental pulmonary hypertension. *Circulation* 64:1249, 1981
37. Acquatella H, Schiller NB, Sharpe DN, Chatterjee K: Lack of correlation between echocardiographic pulmonary valve morphology and simultaneous pulmonary arterial pressure. *Am J Cardiol* 43:946, 1979
38. Diamond MA, Dillon JC, Haine CL, Chang S, Feigenbaum H: Echocardiographic features of atrial septal defect. *Circulation* 43:129, 1971
39. Tajik AJ, Gau GT, Ritter DG, Schattenberg TT: Echocardiographic pattern of right ventricular diastolic volume overload in children. *Circulation* 46:36, 1972
40. Kerber RE, Dippel WF, Abboud FM: Abnormal motion of the interventricular septum in right ventricular volume overload: Experimental and clinical echocardiographic studies. *Circulation* 48:86, 1973
41. Assad-Morell J, Tajik AJ, Giuliani ER: Echocardiographic analysis of the ventricular septum. *Prog Cardiovasc Dis* 17:219, 1974
42. Pearlman AS, Clark CE, Henry WL, Morganroth J, Itscoitz SB, Epstein SE: Determinants of ventricular septal motion: Influence of right and left ventricular size. *Circulation* 54:83, 1976

43. Abbasi AS, Eber LM, MacAlpin RN, Kattus AA: Paradoxical motion of interventricular septum in left bundle branch block. *Circulation* 49:423, 1974
44. Payvandi MN, Kerber RE: Echocardiography in congenital and acquired absence of the pericardium: An echocardiographic mimic of right ventricular volume overload. *Circulation* 53:86, 1972
45. Francis G, Theroux P, Hagan AD, Johnson A, O'Rourke R: Echocardiographic study of interventricular septal motion in Wolff-Parkinson-White Syndrome. *Circulation* 54:174, 1976
46. Weyman AE, Wann S, Feigenbaum H, Dillon JC: Mechanism of abnormal septal motion in patients with right ventricular volume overload: A cross-sectional echocardiographic study. *Circulation* 54:179, 1976
47. Fontana G, Kirkman JH, DiSessa TG, Hagan AD, Hiriashi S, Isabel-Jones J, Friedman WF: Evaluation of right ventricular and right atrial size in children with atrial septal defect using two-dimensional apex echocardiography. *JCU* 10:385, 1982
48. Tei C, Tanaka H, Kashima T, Yoshimura H, Minagoe S, Kanehisa T: Real-time cross-sectional echocardiographic evaluation of the interatrial septum by right atrium-interatrial septum-left atrium direction of ultrasound beam. *Circulation* 60:539, 1979
49. Tei C, Tanaka H, Kashima T, Nakao S, Tahara M, Kanehisa T: Echocardiographic analysis of interatrial septal motion. *Am J Cardiol* 44:472, 1979
50. Thompson JI, Phillips LA, Melmon KL: Pseudotumor of the right atrium: Report of a case and review of its etiology. *Ann Intern Med* 64:665, 1966
51. Lev M: *Autopsy Diagnosis of Congenitally Malformed Hearts*. Springfield, Ill: Thomas, 1953. Pp. 22–23
52. Gondi B, Nanda NC: Two-dimensional echocardiographic features of atrial septal aneurysms. *Circulation* 63:452, 1981
53. Alexander MD, Bloom KR, Hart P, D'Silva F, Murgo JP: Atrial septal aneurysm: A cause for midsystolic click. Report of a case and review of the literature. *Circulation* 63:1186, 1981
54. Mintz GS, Kotler MN, Parry WR, Iskandrian AS, Kane SA: Real-time inferior vena caval ultrasonography: Normal and abnormal findings and its use in assessing right-heart function. *Circulation* 64:1018, 1981
55. Nanda NC, Gramiak R, Robinson TI, Shah PM: Echocardiographic evaluation of pulmonary hypertension. *Circulation* 50:575, 1974
56. Weyman AE, Dillon JC, Feigenbaum H, Chang S: Echocardiographic patterns of pulmonic valve motion with pulmonary hypertension. *Circulation* 50:905, 1974
57. Weyman AE, Dillon JC, Feigenbaum H, Chang S: Echocardiographic patterns of pulmonary valve motion in valvular pulmonary stenosis. *Am J Cardiol* 34:644, 1974
58. Green SE, Popp RL: The relationship of pulmonary valve motion to the motion of surrounding cardiac structures: A two-dimensional and dual M-mode echocardiographic study. *Circulation* 64:107, 1981
59. Doi YL, Sugiura T, Spodick DH: Motion of pulmonic valve and constrictive pericarditis. *Chest* 80:513, 1981
60. Weyman AE, Hurwitz RA, Girod DA, Dillon JC, Feigenbaum H, Green D: Cross-sectional echocardiographic visualization of the stenotic pulmonary valve. *Circulation* 56:769, 1977
61. Fisher EA, Sepehri B, Barron S, Hastreiter AR: Echocardiographic diastolic flutter of the pulmonary valve in isolated patent ductus arteriosus. *Chest* 81:74, 1982
62. Chen CC, Morganroth J, Mardelli TJ, Naito M: Tricuspid regurgitation in tricuspid valve prolapse demonstrated with contrast cross-sectional echocardiography. *Am J Cardiol* 46:983, 1980
63. Mardelli TJ, Morganroth J, Chen CC, Naito M, Vergel J: Tricuspid valve prolapse diagnosed by cross-sectional echocardiography. *Chest* 79:201, 1981
64. Werner JA, Schiller NB, Prasquier R: Occurrence and significance of echocardiographically demonstrated tricuspid valve prolapse. *Am Heart J* 96:180, 1978
65. Ogawa S, Hayashi J, Sasaki H, Tani M, Akaishi M, Mitamura H, Sano M, Hoshino T, Handa S, Nakamura Y: Evaluation of combined valvular prolapse syndrome by two-dimensional echocardiography. *Circulation* 65:174, 1982
66. Okada RD, Ewy GA, Copeland JG: Echocardiography and surgery in tricuspid and pulmonary valve stenosis due to carcinoid syndrome. *Cardiovasc Med* 4:871, 1979
67. Baker BJ, McNee VD, Scovil JA, Bass KM, Watson JW, Bissett JK: Tricuspid insufficiency in carcinoid heart disease: An echocardiographic description. *Am Heart J* 101:107, 1981

68. Lieppe W, Behar VS, Scallion R, Kisslo JA: Detection of tricuspid regurgitation with two-dimensional echocardiography and peripheral vein injection. *Circulation* 57:128, 1978
69. Reeves WC, Leaman DM, Buonocore E, Babb JD, Dash H, Schwiter EJ, Ciotola TJ, Hallahan W: Detection of tricuspid regurgitation and estimation of central venous pressure by two-dimensional contrast echocardiography of the right superior hepatic vein. *Am Heart J* 102:374, 1981
70. Meltzer RS, vanHoogenhuyze D, Serruys PW, Hallebos MMP, Hugenholtz PG, Roelandt J: Diagnosis of tricuspid regurgitation by contrast echocardiography. *Circulation* 63:1093, 1981

Cardiomyopathies 9

Hypertrophic cardiomyopathy. It has been more than two decades since Teare [1] originally reported the first description of a heart disease characterized by asymmetric hypertrophy of the heart and nondilated ventricular cavities. His observations were made on postmortem studies of eight patients, seven of whom died suddenly. During the next 20 years subsequent investigations have led to significant evolution of concepts concerning the clinical and pathophysiologic spectrum of this disease to which at least 58 different names have been attached in the process [2].

For many years following Teare's initial report, the majority of terms used to describe hypertrophic cardiomyopathy emphasized left ventricular outflow obstruction, a finding that was thought to be highly characteristic of this disease. Accordingly, the terms *idiopathic hypertrophic subaortic stenosis* (IHSS) [3, 4], *hypertrophic obstructive cardiomyopathy* [5–7], and *muscular subaortic stenosis* [8] became widely used.

The first application of M-mode echocardiography by Moreya and colleagues [9] in patients with hypertrophic cardiomyopathy noted the abnormal diastolic pattern of the anterior mitral leaflet and its relationship to the ventricular septum; the first recognition of abnormal systolic anterior motion (SAM) of the mitral valve by echocardiography was reported by Shah and associates [10]. The widespread application of M-mode echocardiography in the early 1970s further documented the hypertrophic nature of this disease and showed that a hypertrophied ventricular septum measuring at least 1.3 times the thickness of the posterior wall was invariably present [11–17]. It was also reported that in the majority of patients about half of the first-degree relatives of patients with hypertrophic cardiomyopathy also showed an abnormal septal-to-free wall thickness ratio [18, 19].

Although Henry and associates [12] introduced the term *asymmetric septal hypertrophy* and its acronym *ASH* to describe the disease hypertrophic cardiomyopathy, it soon became evident that disproportionate septal thickening was not pathognomonic of hypertrophic cardiomyopathy.

PATHOPHYSIOLOGY. The occurrence of an abnormal forward movement of the anterior mitral leaflet during systole in hypertrophic obstructive cardiomyopathy was first suspected by Bjork in 1964 [20], and later was angiographically documented by Dinsmore and associates [21]. Simon and coworkers [22] also observed that the mitral valve abnormality involved the posterior leaflet and postulated that the abnormal systolic motion of the mitral valve resulted from abnormal traction on the chordae tendineae secondary to maldirection of the hypertrophied papillary muscles. These investigators suggested that the abnormal systolic position of the mitral leaflets together with the asymmetric septal hypertrophy played an important part in the production of the intraventricular pressure gradient. These findings were supported by the echocardiographic findings of Shah and colleagues [10] who suggested that the abnormal anterior displacement of the mitral leaflets toward the ventricular septum during systole was responsible not only for the left ventricular outflow tract obstruction but also for the mitral valve regurgitation that is commonly seen in this disease. These observations and interpretations were supported by Popp and Harrison [23] as well as by Pridie and Oakley [24].

Echocardiographic evidence of narrowing of the left ventricular outflow tract in hypertrophic cardiomyopathy was first presented by Gramiak and associates [25]. These investigators also reported abnormal aortic valve motion with the aortic cusps moving toward a closed position in mid systole and then reopening in late systole, which they suggested was secondary to obstruction of the left ventricular outflow tract.

Although left ventricular outflow tract obstruction in hypertrophic cardiomyopathy has received considerable attention in the literature, left ventricular inflow tract obstruction may also occur. The inflow tract obstructive component has been attributed to impaired left ventricular filling secondary to reduced cavity size and to loss of ventricular wall compliance associated with the extreme hypertrophy [26–28]. Feizi and Emanuel [29] believed that the mechanical left ventricular inflow tract obstruction was due to incomplete valve opening secondary to severe ventricular septal hypertrophy. These investigators also reported that two of five patients who had left ventricular inflow tract obstruction suffered acute hemiparesis from embolic origin and suggested that such patients may be at greater risk for embolization; this finding may assist in the selection of patients to be recommended for septal myotomy-myectomy. Patients with hypertrophic cardiomyopathy who have left ventricular inflow tract obstruction may have mid-diastolic murmurs that simulate mitral stenosis.

Patients with hypertrophic cardiomyopathy classically demonstrate three hallmarks of the disease: asymmetric septal hypertrophy, septal disorganization of cells, and systolic anterior motion of the mitral valve apparatus [30]. Although none of these findings is pathognomonic of hypertrophic cardiomyopathy, each one is uncommonly found in patients with other forms of cardiac disorders. Disproportionate septal thickening has been found to occur in about 10 percent of older children and adults with various acquired and congenital heart diseases [30–33]. In these patients it usually appears to be secondary to the underlying hemodynamic state, whereas disproportionate septal thickening is a common finding in the developing embryonic and fetal heart (prevalence rate approximately 25%), in normal neonates, and in infants with congenital heart disease [30–34].

Although cell disorganization in the ventricular septum may occur with other cardiac malformations, extensive disorganization is present in approximately 90 percent of patients with hypertrophic cardiomyopathy and in approximately 5 percent of patients with other forms of cardiac disease [30]. In an analysis of 1664 patients Maron and Epstein [30] reported that the specificity of asymmetric septal hypertrophy, marked septal disorganization, and systolic anterior motion of the mitral valve was 90 percent, 93 percent, and 97 percent, respectively.

The etiology of cardiac muscle cell disorganization is not definitely known. Maron and Epstein [30] have suggested that extensive cell disorganization may be a primary derangement of septal architecture, that is, a morphologic manifestation of the underlying genetic defect known to be present in a large proportion of patients with hypertrophic cardiomyopathy. Other investigators believe that septal disorganization results secondarily from unique mechanical stresses to which the left ventricle in hypertrophic cardiomyopathy is exposed. Bulkley and associates [35] have proposed that septal disorganization in hypertrophic cardiomyopathy is due to a prolonged period of isometric contraction during mid and late ventricular systole. Although some investigators have questioned the usefulness of septal disorganization as a diagnostic marker of hypertrophic cardiomyopathy [36, 37],

Maron and Roberts [38] have emphasized the importance of a quantitative histologic method that permits a more critical assessment of the relative area of septal myocardium occupied by disorganized cells. These investigators further emphasize that the disordered septal architecture specifically pertains to malalignment between cardiac muscle cells and not to the disarray of myofibrils and myofilaments that have been described in normally arranged muscle cells in human beings and animals with a variety of normal or diseased cardiac states [39–41]; the disorganization appears to be a relatively nonspecific morphologic alteration.

In patients with hypertrophic cardiomyopathy left ventricular outflow tract narrowing and obstruction are produced by apposition of the anterior mitral leaflet tip together with the chordae tendineae against the hypertrophied ventricular septum during mid systole [14, 21, 22, 42–45]. Systolic anterior motion of the mitral valve apparatus has also been used to estimate the severity of left ventricular outflow tract obstruction in hypertrophic cardiomyopathy [43, 46]. The magnitude and duration of systolic anterior motion has been shown to correlate well with the magnitude of the intraventricular gradient measured at cardiac catheterization under basal conditions and with provocative maneuvers [43]. This predictive relationship between systolic anterior motion of the mitral valve and outflow obstruction has been disputed by others [16, 29, 47]. Systolic anterior motion of the mitral valve apparatus has also been shown to occur in a variety of other diseases and hemodynamic states. These conditions, as well as the phenomenon "pseudo SAM," will be discussed later in this chapter. Systolic anterior motion of the mitral valve, together with hemodynamically proven left ventricular outflow obstruction, has also been described in patients without evidence of ventricular hypertrophy on echocardiographic examination [48, 49], as well as in patients with concentric hypertrophy of the left ventricle [16, 50–52]. Some of the patients with concentric hypertrophy have evidence of genetic transmission of asymmetric septal hypertrophy; therefore their condition appears to represent a variant of hypertrophic cardiomyopathy [50]. Others have no evidence of genetic transmission and must be regarded as having an idiopathic form of left ventricular hypertrophy.

Distinguishing secondary disproportionate septal thickening from primary hypertrophic cardiomyopathy may present a diagnostic dilemma. The various clinical conditions that cause secondary disproportionate septal thickening will be discussed later in the chapter. Some investigators have reported that in the vast majority of patients hypertrophic cardiomyopathy is genetically transmitted as an autosomal dominant trait with a high degree of penetrance [18, 19]. Accordingly, the absence of asymmetric septal hypertrophy in five or more first-degree adult relatives of a patient with an abnormal septal-to-free wall ratio with acquired or congenital heart disease strongly suggests that the septal thickening present is not a manifestation of genetically transmitted disease. Conversely, the presence of an abnormal septal/free wall ratio in one or more relatives suggests the presence of a primary cardiomyopathy in the case being evaluated.

In a study of 151 normal hearts at various stages of development (embryo, fetus, and young infant), Maron and associates [53] reported that a septal-to-free wall ratio of 1.3 or greater was present in more than 90 percent of embryos and young fetuses. They found disproportionate septal thickening in 65 percent of older fetuses and in 25 pecent of live born infants without congenital heart disease; of the latter, the number of affected infants decreased to 12 percent after two weeks of age. This decrease in septal-to-free wall ratio appears to occur because the ventricular septum, which is markedly thicker than the left ventricular free wall in the earliest stages of development, increases in thickness at a slower rate than the left ventricular free wall during subsequent cardiac growth.

Hypertrophic cardiomyopathy may become clinically apparent during early infancy with congestive heart failure and cardiomegaly and may lead to infant death [54]. The clinical and hemodynamic spectrum of hypertrophic cardiomyopathy in childhood is broad. Deterioration in the clinical condition or sudden death has been relatively common in children with overt signs of cardiac disease [55]. Maron and coauthors followed 35 children from one to 16 years (average 7.4 years) and observed the following: 14 (40%) improved or remained stable, 10 (29%) deteriorated clinically, and 11 (31%) died suddenly (4% mortality per year). They noted that neither symptomatology, electrocardiographic abnormalities, heart size, left ventricular ejection or upstroke time, magnitude of outflow gradient, or left ventricular end-diastolic pressure proved to be predictive of sudden death.

ECHOCARDIOGRAPHIC SUBCLASSIFICATION OF HYPERTROPHIC CARDIOMYOPATHY. Gilbert and associates [56] reported that a noninvasive classification of patients with hypertrophic cardiomyopathy into hemodynamic subgroups of obstruction at rest, latent obstruction, and no obstruction can be made by assessing the degree of systolic anterior motion, the presence of aortic valve mid-systolic notching, and left atrial size. These authors noted that mitral leaflet contact with the ventricular septum exceeding 30 percent of echocardiographic systole occurred in all 27 patients with obstruction at rest but in no patient with latent or no obstruction. They also observed mid-systolic notching of the aortic valve in all patients with obstruction at rest but in only 3 of 17 patients with latent obstruction and in no patients without obstruction. The third most useful differentiating feature, namely left atrial enlargement, occurred in 25 of 27 in the group with obstruction at rest but in only 4 of 28 in the group with latent obstruction and in 2 of 15 in the group without obstruction.

Some patients with hypertrophic cardiomyopathy may have hypertrophy present in unusual locations of the left ventricular wall. With the use of wide-angle two-dimensional echocardiography, Maron and colleagues [57] reported segmental hypertrophy involving regions of the left ventricle through which the M-mode ultrasound beam does not pass, the posterior ventricular septum (seven patients), anterior or anterolateral free wall (seven patients), and ventricular septum near the apex (two patients). No echocardiographic or hemodynamic evidence of left ventricular outflow tract obstruction was present in any of these patients.

MECHANISM OF LEFT VENTRICULAR OUTFLOW OBSTRUCTION. Angiographic and echocardiographic observations have suggested that the left ventricular outflow obstruction in patients with hypertrophic cardiomyopathy was caused by systolic apposition of the anterior mitral leaflet and the asymmetrically hypertrophied ventricular septum [10, 21–23, 43, 46]. Using both M-mode and two-dimensional echocardiography, Henry and associates [58] studied 100 patients with hypertrophic cardiomyopathy and 22 normal subjects to determine the mitral valve position at the onset of systole from the ventricular septum and the distance from the mitral valve to the posterior left ventricular wall. They found that none of the normal subjects and only 3 of 51 patients with nonobstructive hypertrophic cardiomyopathy had a septal–mitral valve distance of less than 20 mm compared with

23 of 35 (66%) patients with obstructive hypertrophic cardiomyopathy. These authors did not find that shortening of the papillary muscles along their long axis caused any right angle bending of the mitral valve leaflet tip as viewed with two-dimensional echocardiography. Therefore they postulated that the mitral leaflets were either sucked forward by a Venturi effect or pushed forward from behind by the stream of blood being ejected. The degree to which these hemodynamic forces exceed the resistance of the valve apparatus should determine the extent of the systolic anterior motion and hence the degree of obstruction. Accordingly, they proposed that left ventricular outflow obstruction occurred in patients with hypertrophic cardiomyopathy as a result of the interaction of two factors: narrowing of the left ventricular outflow tract at the onset of systole, and hydrodynamic forces generated by contraction of the left ventricle.

Some investigators have described the systolic anterior motion as movement caused by chordal buckling without involvement of the body of the leaflet in some patients with hypertrophic cardiomyopathy [59].

Utilizing two-dimensional echocardiography in the apical four-chamber and apical long axis views, Shah and colleagues [60] described abnormal mitral valve coaptation in patients with hypertrophic obstructive cardiomyopathy. They observed that the posterior leaflet coapted with a midportion of the anterior leaflet thus leaving a distal "residual" anterior leaflet in the left ventricle during systole. A sharp angulation of this distal leaflet in mid systole toward the interventricular septum is thought to represent the systolic anterior motion. The Bernoulli effect may well play an active role in angulating the residual distal anterior mitral leaflet along with its chordal attachments into the outflow space. Shah and associates postulate that the left ventricular outflow obstruction in these patients occurs as a result of the sequence of abnormal coaptation, "residual" distal leaflet, rapid early ejection through narrow outflow space, and sharp angulation of the distal anterior mitral leaflet. The precise mechanism for valve coaptation abnormalities observed in the study remains to be elucidated. The authors suggest the following possibilities: (1) elongation of the anterior mitral leaflet; (2) elongation of the posterior mitral leaflet; (3) anterior displacement of the posterior mitral annulus so that the posterior leaflet plays a larger role in mitral orifice closure; and (4) greater than normal reduction in the size of the mitral annulus in early systole.

Three theories have been invoked recurrently in the literature to explain the mechanism of systolic anterior motion: (1) vigorous contraction of the posterior basilar left ventricular wall, forcing the anterior and posterior mitral leaflets into a nearly emptied left ventricular outflow tract; (2) hypertrophy of the superior interventricular septum leading to a malalignment of the papillary muscles so that during systole the hypertrophied septum acts as a fulcrum on the taut chordae to pull the mitral valve apparatus forward to meet the downward contracting septum; and (3) the Venturi effect, in which the mitral valve leaflet is forced forward into the low pressure caused by the high velocity flow of blood through the narrowed left ventricular outflow tract. Martin and colleagues [61], employing wide-angle two-dimensional echocardiographic imaging, consistently observed in long axis views that the systolic anterior movement primarily involved the area of attachment of the free edge of the mitral valve to the chordae tendineae thus involving both leaflet tip and chordal structures. These authors noted that both papillary muscles appeared to be equally displaced anteriorly in short axis views and found no evidence of papillary malorientation-traction abnormalities; they favor the theory that the Venturi effect resulting from the high velocity of flow through a narrowed left ventricular outflow tract is primarily operative in producing the systolic anterior motion.

REGIONAL MYOCARDIAL FUNCTION. Hypertrophic cardiomyopathy is characteristically associated with increased myocardial contractility, small left ventricular cavity size, and increased ejection fraction. Other global function ejection phase indices such as mean circumferential fiber shortening rate (mean Vcf) and percent fractional shortening (%FS) are also usually increased above normal. Cohen and associates [62] found that the mean Vcf of patients with hypertrophic cardiomyopathy averaged 1.62 circ/second while the normal subjects in their study averaged 1.24 circ/second. The mean Vcf as determined by echocardiography has been shown to be a reliable quantitative index of global left ventricular function [63, 64].

The interventricular septum in hypertrophic cardiomyopathy does not thicken normally during systolic contraction. Cohen and colleagues [62] observed the normal septums to thicken by 76 percent whereas thickening averaged only 22 percent in patients with hypertrophic cardiomyopathy. These findings, which were also confirmed by Tajik and Guilani [14] as well as by Rossen and coworkers [65], demonstrated that individual contributions of septal and posterior wall contraction to overall ventricular function in hypertrophic cardiomyopathy patients are not comparable. The velocity of septal contraction in such patients is also depressed. Systolic thickening of the posterior wall averages 75 percent in the hypertrophic cardiomyopathy ventricles and 85 percent in normal hearts [62]. Thus anatomic, histologic, and functional evidence supports the concept that hypertrophic cardiomyopathy is an asymmetric entity. The abnormal septum moves as expected in a myopathic ventricle while the remainder of left ventricular myocardium appears to compensate by contracting vigorously with the overall result being a hyperdynamic, hypercontractile ventricle.

Henry and colleagues [15] studied the distribution of wall thickening of the septum and left ventricular posterior free wall in patients with hypertrophic cardiomyopathy with varying degrees of outflow obstruction. In addition, the configuration and thickness of the ventricular septum and left ventricular free wall were evaluated in necropsy specimens from 23 patients with obstructive and nonobstructive hypertrophic cardiomyopathy. Maximum thickness of the ventricular septum in 13 hearts with obstructive ASH ranged from 20 to 45 mm (mean 29.8), and maximum left ventricular free wall thickness ranged from 17 to 32 mm (mean 20.5). No significant difference was noted in any heart between the free wall thickness directly behind the posterior mitral leaflet and maximum posterior wall thickness elsewhere. In the same study, maximum thickness of the ventricular septum in ten hearts with nonobstructive ASH was found to range from 17 to 40 mm (mean 25.4), and maximum thickness of the left ventricular free wall ranged from 13 to 26 mm (mean 17.7). In contrast to the obstructive group, however, the thickness of the posterior basilar free wall as measured directly behind the posterior leaflet was significantly less, ranging from 6 to 14 mm (mean 9.3), than the posterior wall thickness elsewhere.

Henry and associates [15] and Maron and colleagues [66] proposed the hypothesis that left ventricular posterior wall thickening in patients with obstructive ASH is a consequence of left ventricular outflow obstruction while thickening in patients with nonobstructive ASH is due to the underlying myocardial abnormality. These investigators noted that the portion of the left ventricular free wall directly behind the posterior mitral leaflet was thickened in patients with resting obstruction, and tended to be less so in patients with only provocable gradients, and finally differed only slightly from normal in patients without obstruction. They also observed that the posterior basilar wall thickness in patients whose left ventricular outflow obstruction had been abolished several years previously by operation was significantly less than that measured preoperatively in a similar group of patients with obstruction operated upon within the past year, suggesting that the thickening present in patients with obstructive ASH may be at least partially reversed by operative abolition of the obstruction. It should be noted, however, that the latter hypothesis is only tentative because the authors have not performed sufficient serial follow-up evaluations of patients following surgery to document the presence of such regression of hypertrophy in that segment of the ventricle. Furthermore, these authors found the configuration of the left ventricular posterior wall in hearts with obstructive ASH examined at necropsy to be indistinguishable from that seen in valvular aortic stenosis. The microscopic data revealed that hypertrophied, bizarrely shaped, and abnormally arranged cells were abundantly present in the ventricular septum but not in the left ventricular posterior wall. The myocardial cells in the posterior wall were hypertrophied and morphologically identical to those found in patients with valvular aortic stenosis. The investigators concluded that anatomic, echocardiographic, and microscopic evidence were all consistent with the concept that left ventricular free wall thickening in obstructive ASH is a consequence of left ventricular outflow obstruction.

When Henry and colleagues [15] and Maron and associates [66] examined the left ventricular posterior wall of patients with nonobstructive ASH, a different mechanism was suggested that leads to wall thickening in these patients. Necropsy examination of hearts from patients with nonobstructive hypertrophic cardiomyopathy, revealed that the portion of the left ventricular free wall directly behind the posterior mitral leaflet was normal in thickness; however, major portions of the remainder of the left ventricular free wall were thickened. Furthermore, the microscopic morphology of the left ventricular free wall in the nonobstructive hypertrophic cardiomyopathy was distinctly different from that observed in the obstructive form, in that the hypertrophied, bizarrely shaped, and abnormally arranged cells not only were present in the septum but were also extensively distributed in the free wall. There was no secondary cause to explain this additional abnormal process such as systemic hypertension; thus these investigators concluded from the gross anatomic and microscopic evidence that the left ventricular free wall thickening in nonobstructive hypertrophic cardiomyopathy was due to the underlying myocardial abnormality. In symptomatic patients with nonobstructive ASH the data suggest that the left ventricle, including the free wall, is extensively involved with a primary myocardial abnormality. It would be logical to conclude from these data that regional function would also be disturbed in such patients with nonobstructive ASH; however, the authors did not investigate this hypothesis in their studies.

Shah and associates [67] studied 35 patients with asymmetric hypertrophy of the left ventricle diagnosed by two-dimensional echocardiography for regional distribution of hypertrophy and wall motion. The study group consisted of 19 patients with evidence of resting obstruction and 16 without. The distribution of asymmetric left ventricular hypertrophy was similar in both groups: upper septum in 13, midseptum in 16, upper anterolateral wall in 5, midanterolateral wall in 4, lower septum and anterolateral wall in 4 patients each, and posterior inferior wall in 2 patients. They also noted that more than one segment was involved in 17 patients. Hyperkinesis of the anterolateral or posteroinferior walls was significantly more prevalent in the obstructive group (79%) compared to the nonobstructive group (38%). In addition, the obstructive group demonstrated evidence of increased ejection fraction. Radionuclide angiography in the obstructive group showed ejection fraction to be 85 percent compared to 76 percent for the nonobstructive group, maximum ejection velocities (volume/second) was 6.36 compared to 5.09, respectively, and average ejection velocities were 3.05 compared to 2.41, respectively.

CATENOID SHAPE OF THE INTERVENTRICULAR SEPTUM. Hutchins and Bulkley [68] studied eight autopsied hearts from patients with hypertrophic cardiomyopathy for curvature and thickness of free walls and septum, and suggested that the interventricular septa resembled catenoids. They suggested for that reason that this unique configuration of the septum in hypertrophic cardiomyopathy is distinctive and may be the primary event leading to development of the condition. Every point on a catenoid has net 0 curvature. The radii of curvature of mutually perpendicular planes at a point are equal and opposite; this property of 0 curvature determines, as shown by the Laplace relation, that tension within the catenoid exerts no pressure. The investigators postulated that the mechanics of net 0 curvature of the septum would produce hypertrophic obstructive cardiomyopathy. They found that in all eight hearts with hypertrophic cardiomyopathy the septum was concave to the left in the transverse plane but convex to the left in the apex-to-base plane. Such a catenoid configuration of the septum was not observed in any of the other 80 hearts they examined. They further postulated that this distinctive shape of the septum would account for isometric contraction, since adjacent fiber tracts with oppositive curvatures would develop maximum tension but would not have motion (Fig. 9-1). They further speculated that the fiber disarray and local hypertrophy would result from such isometric contraction. These authors also suggested that, since ventricular configuration is acquired early in cardiogenesis, hypertrophic cardiomyopathy might therefore result from a genetic or embryonic determination of a catenoid septum.

CLINICAL FEATURES. Symptoms of hypertrophic cardiomyopathy characteristically consist of one or more of the following: chest pain, dyspnea on exertion, fatigue, orthopnea, paroxysmal nocturnal dyspnea, palpitations, lightheadedness, or syncope. The cause of symptoms in patients with hypertrophic cardiomyopathy is largely unexplained. St. John Sutton and associates [69] found no clear correlation between the incidence of symptoms and hemodynamic data, namely, left ventricular end-diastolic pressure and left ventricular outflow gradients. These investigators noted that systolic function was consistently normal or above normal even in the presence of severe diastolic abnormalities. On the basis of wide variation in diastolic function in patients with hypertrophic cardiomyopathy, the authors separated the patients into three groups on the basis of left ventricular peak filling rate: group 1 had rapid left ventricular filling rates, group 2 had normal filling rates, and group 3 had slow filling rates. Because of the severe septal hypertrophy and hypokinesia, peak left ventricular filling rate was noted to be predominantly determined by the rate of free wall thinning. These investigators noted that angina and

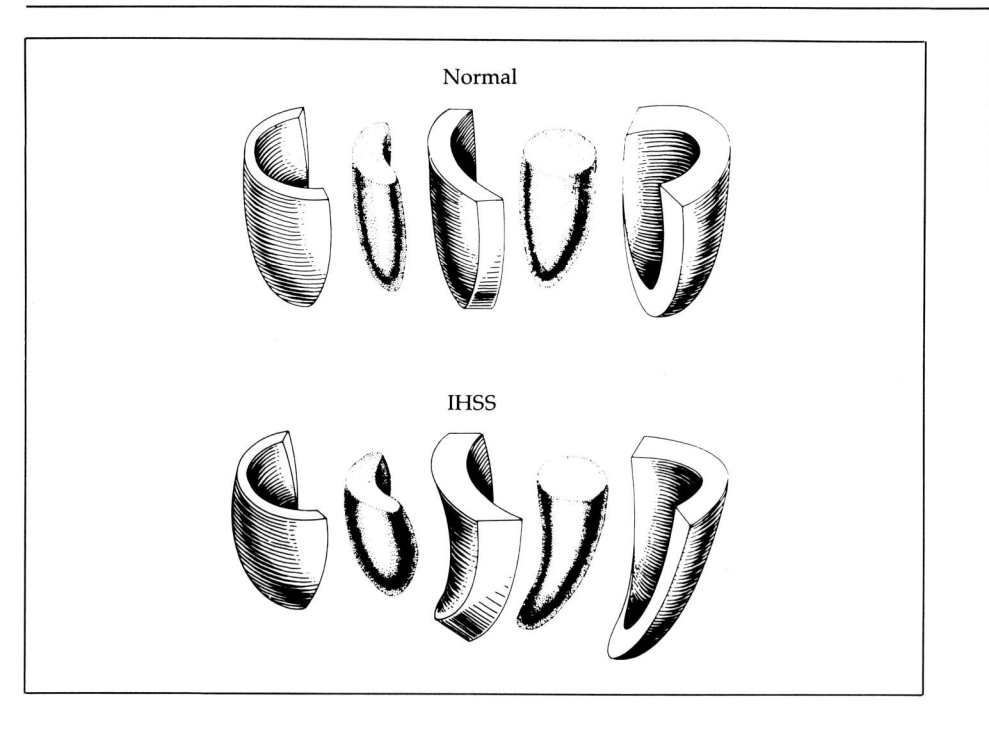

Fig. 9-1. Diagram of configurations of catenoid septum and left ventricular free wall and cavity in normal and IHSS hearts. (From GM Hutchins, BH Bulkley, Catenoid shape of the interventricular septum. Circulation 58:392, 1978, by permission of the American Heart Association, Inc.)

atrial fibrillation were most frequent in group 3 while dyspnea was most common in group 1. There were 29 patients with hypertrophic cardiomyopathy in the study group, 7 of whom were women and 22 were men; age range was 16 to 69 years with a median age of 45 years. Twenty-three of the patients were taking propranolol with similar dose ranges in the three groups. There was no correlation between the dose of propranolol and the incidence of angina, syncope, or dyspnea, and no relation between the doses of propranolol and systolic or diastolic ventricular dynamics. The authors postulated that the higher incidence of angina in the group with slow filling was possibly due to a combination of two factors: (1) significantly decreased normalized peak rate of posterior wall thinning in this group which could cause a slower release of systolic wall tension, thereby shortening the time available for diastolic coronary blood flow; and development of incoordinate septal contraction and relaxation, which was most severe in group 3, and also could have contributed to a reduction of intramyocardial blood flow. Paroxysmal atrial fibrillation was observed to occur in patients only in groups 2 and 3. It was also noted that atrial size in the three groups increased with reduction of peak filling rates; the increased left atrial size, which caused a propensity for atrial fibrillation to develop, therefore represents increased resistance to left ventricular filling resulting from impaired wall dynamics which was most severe in group 3. Other investigators have reported that atrial fibrillation tends to occur late in the natural history of hypertrophic cardiomyopathy and its development may be regarded as an index of advanced left ventricular disease [70, 71].

In hypertrophic cardiomyopathy the septum makes little contribution to either ejection or filling, and peak filling rates and periods reflect the properties and dynamics of the free wall upon which both filling and ejection depend. St. John Sutton and others [69] suggest in their study that rapid filling occurs in patients in whom the histopathologic process remains predominantly confined to the septum and involves the free wall only minimally, thus allowing compensatory increase in systolic thickening and rapid rates of change of the posterior wall thickness during systole and diastole. These authors propose that as the myopathic process progressively involves the free wall this compensatory mechanism is limited by reduction in posterior wall dynamics with earlier and disproportionately greater effect on diastolic function. The result is a decrease in peak filling rate, prolongation of the filling and isovolumic relaxation periods, and finally, development of asynchrony between septal and posterior wall contraction. Although it is not fully understood, they suggested that the asynchrony between the septum and posterior wall may possibly reflect the prolonged rate of repolarization observed electrophysiologically [72] to occur differentially in the septum and the posterior wall. Accordingly, the natural history of this disease may be determined by the degree of pathological change involving the free ventricular wall; as this change increases it imposes progressive mechanical restraint on wall dynamics and cavity function.

Early in the course of hypertrophic cardiomyopathy, before the patient develops any abnormal symptoms, there may be no abnormal physical findings. One of the earliest abnormal physical findings may be the development of an abnormal fourth heart sound and by the time symptoms develop this is very commonly present. However, a third heart sound would not be expected to be present until much later in the course of the disease or when the patient develops congestive heart failure. A systolic ejection murmur is commonly found and is usually located along the left sternal border or at the apex or both. Depending upon whether or not there is associated mitral regurgitation the systolic murmur may have some holosystolic characteristics and be more prominent at the apex if mitral regurgitation is present.

The prevalence of abnormal electrocardiograms in patients with hypertrophic cardiomyopathy has been reported to be from 10 percent [73] to 18 percent [74] to nearly 100 percent [4, 75]. In a study of 144 patients with hypertrophic cardiomyopathy Savage and colleagues [76] found normal electrocardiograms in fewer than 7 percent of each subgroup of patients (those with or without either symptoms or obstruction to left ventricular outflow), with the exception of those who were both asymptomatic and had no left ventricular outflow obstruction; normal electrocardiograms were obtained in 27 percent of these patients. They found that repolarization abnormalities and left ventricular hypertrophy were the most common abnormalities, occurring in 81 and 62 percent respectively of the total population. Other common electrocardiographic abnormalities in patients with hypertrophic cardiomyopathy include left atrial enlargement, left axis deviation, and prominent Q waves.

Goodwin and colleagues [77] have suggested that electrocardiographic findings of combined right atrial enlargement and left ventricular hypertrophy are suggestive of hypertrophic cardiomyopathy since it is so rare in valvular aortic stenosis, which is often included in the differential diagnosis of this disease. Prominent septal Q waves in young patients are another helpful diagnostic electrocardiographic finding that suggests the presence of hypertrophic cardiomyopathy. Neither Halpern and colleagues [75] nor Savage and coworkers [76] could demonstrate a significant relationship between the presence or absence of prominent septal Q waves and the relative thickening of the ventricular septum compared with the free wall.

Maron and associates [78] reported that premature cardiac death occurs frequently in certain families with hypertrophic cardiomyopathy. These investigators studied a total of 69 first-degree relatives in eight families with 41 having evidence of hypertrophic cardiomyopathy. A total of 31 (75%) died of their heart disease and 18 were less than 25 years of age at the time of death. They further reported that death was sudden and unexpected in 23 of the 31 patients and in 15 of these 23 patients sudden death was the initial manifestation of cardiac disease. Although this study by Maron and associates does not establish the prevalence with which "malignant" hypertrophic cardiomyopathy occurs, such families appear to be uncommon.

IMAGING TECHNIQUES EMPLOYING COMBINED M-MODE AND TWO-DIMENSIONAL ECHOCARDIOGRAPHY. Multiple two-dimensional views are necessary for comprehensive imaging and adequate clinical assessment of patients with hypertrophic cardiomyopathy. Two views, the parasternal long axis and parasternal short axis views (Figs. 9-2, 9-3), are mandatory, since without them even technically adequate imaging will not provide sufficient clinical information.

The parasternal long axis view is particularly important because of the opportunity it affords to view the profile of the ventricular septum and left ventricular outflow tract together with the mitral valve and chordae tendineae (Fig. 9-4). In this view it is possible to measure the diameter of the left ventricular outflow tract and determine whether any systolic movement of the mitral-chordal structures is occurring. It is also important to obtain simultaneous imaging with the M-mode cursor sweeping through the structures from the level of the chordae superiorly to the aortic valve in order to further look for evidence of SAM or mid-systolic notching of the aortic valve. Maintaining directional control during two-dimensional imaging affords the opportunity to ensure that the M-mode record is being taken precisely in the location and from that part of the structure that best portrays the anatomy or motion to be evaluated. The parasternal short axis view is equally important because it provides the opportunity to determine whether segmental hypertrophy exists in other areas of the left ventricle, such as the posterior septum, anterolateral free wall, and posterolateral free wall (Fig. 9-5A). Multiple parasternal short axis views from the atrioventricular groove to the level of the papillary muscles will permit good visualization of these other areas. Furthermore, the ventricular septum can be evaluated from its anterior to posterior extent to determine how diffuse or localized the septal hypertrophy is. The parasternal short axis position is often superior to the parasternal long axis for obtaining M-mode recording of the ventricular septum and posterior wall because of its ability to ensure that the cursor intersects the septum and posterior wall in a perpendicular fashion (Fig. 9-5B). If the patient is technically very difficult to image and adequate parasternal windows cannot be obtained, the apical views become even more important. The traditional apical long axis view results in the plane of the sector passing through the anterolateral and posteromedial walls of the ventricle (Fig. 9-6). Therefore, in order to identify the anterior septum from the apical long axis position, the transducer must be rotated more in a counterclockwise direction; this orientation causes the sector to pass through the anterior portion of the septum, thus making the tomographic plane essentially identical to the parasternal long axis view except that the transducer has been positioned over the apex instead of along the left sternal border

298   9. Cardiomyopathies

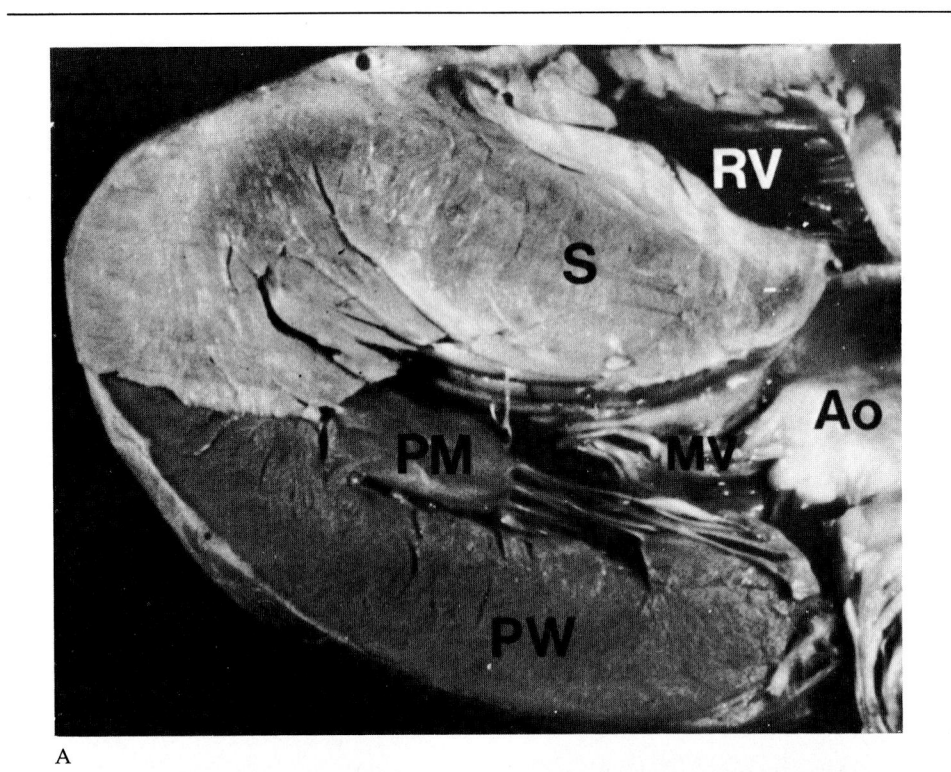

Fig. 9-2A. Anatomic view of parasternal long axis plane in a patient who died of severe hypertrophic cardiomyopathy demonstrating marked increase in thickness of the interventricular septum as well as hypertrophy of the posterior medial papillary muscle and posterior wall. The left ventricular cavity and outflow tract are small. B. Parasternal long axis view in a patient with hypertrophic cardiomyopathy demonstrating marked disproportionate thickening of the septum, which measures approximately 28 mm at end diastole (bracket). The left ventricular outflow tract is only borderline narrowed (20 mm diameter).

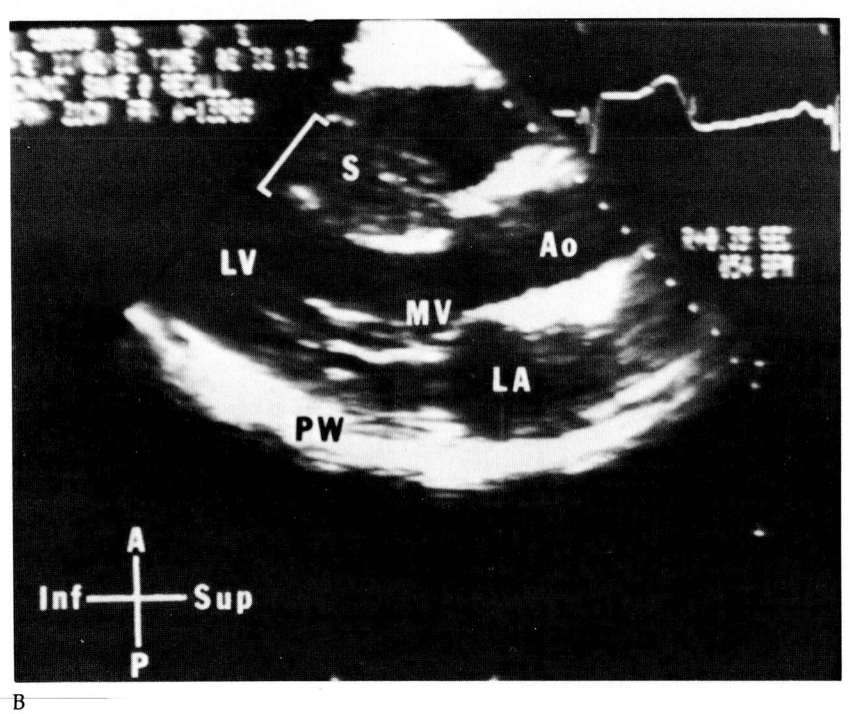

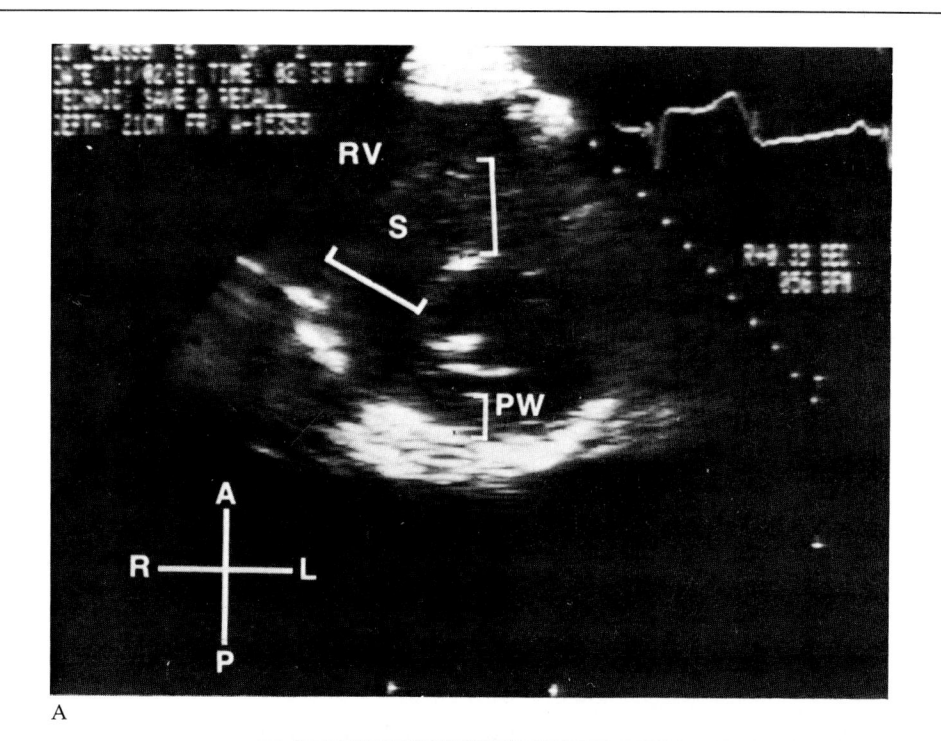

Fig. 9-3A. Parasternal short axis view from same patient as in Fig. 9-2B demonstrating that septal hypertrophy diffusely involves both anterior and posterior components as well as the anterolateral free wall of the left ventricle. The posterior wall demonstrates mild hypertrophy with end-diastolic thickness approximately 14 mm. B. M-mode recording obtained from parasternal short axis imaging in another patient with hypertrophic nonobstructive cardiomyopathy demonstrating not only a disproportionately thick septum (21–22 mm) but also poor systolic thickening of the septum. The posterior wall is mildly hypertrophic (15 mm diastolic thickness) and very hyperkinetic, but there is no systolic anterior motion of the mitral valve. First degree AV block is present on the ECG.

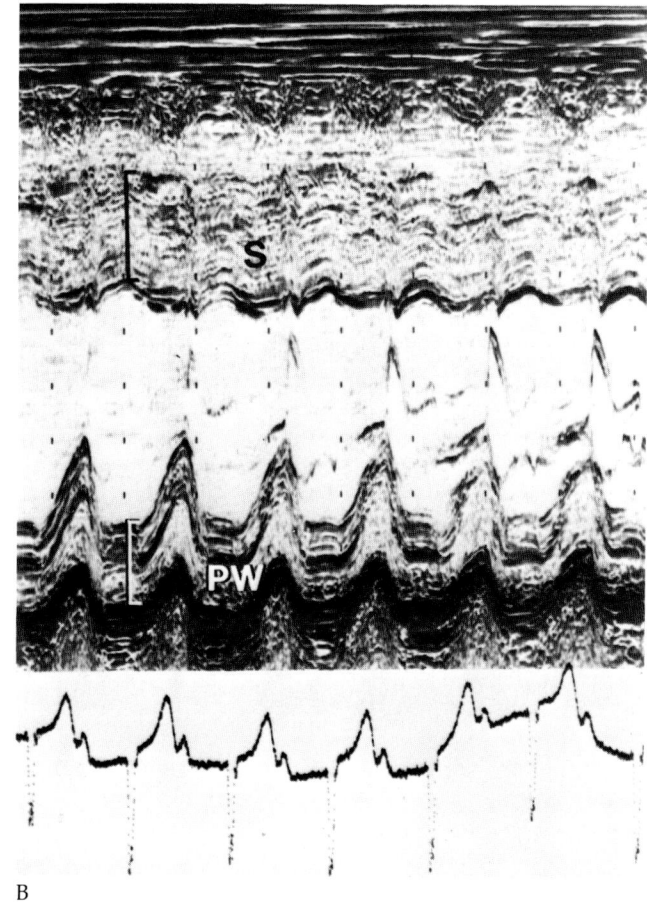

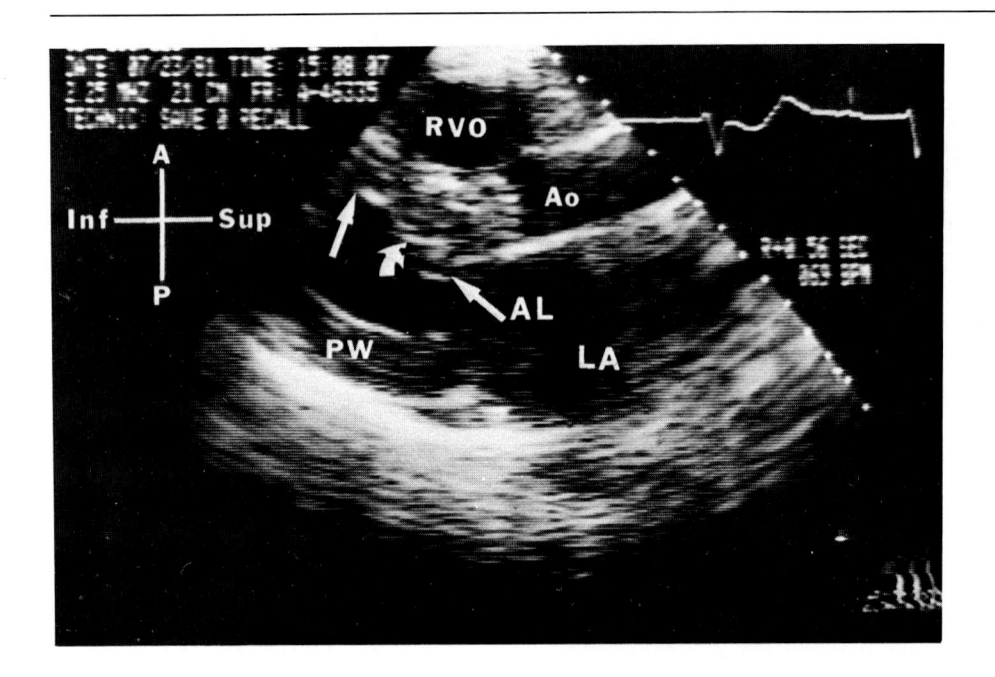

Fig. 9-4. Parasternal long axis view in a patient with hypertrophic cardiomyopathy demonstrating more severe localized hypertrophy of the anterior basal septum (curved arrow); the septal hypertrophy is less extensive in the midportion (straight arrow) as well as the distal and posterior portions observed in other views. PW = posterior wall.

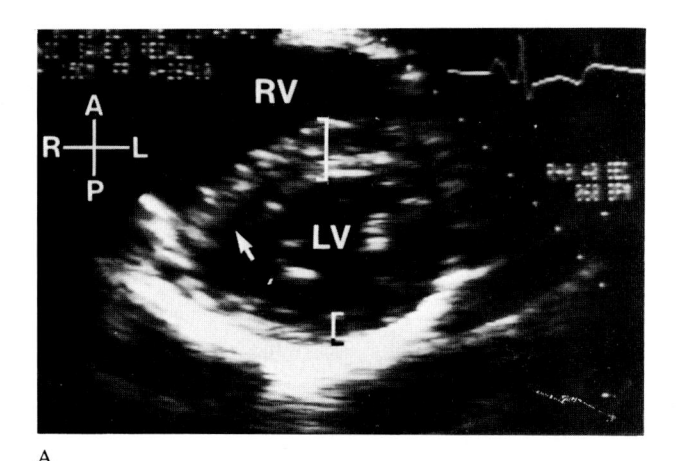

Fig. 9-5A. Parasternal short axis view from an adult patient with hypertrophic nonobstructive cardiomyopathy demonstrating an abnormally thick septum except for a small posterior segment (arrow) where the septal thickness is normal and the same as the posterior and lateral walls (10 mm). Calibration dots are 1 cm apart. B. M-mode recording obtained from the parasternal short axis view in a patient with hypertrophic nonobstructive cardiomyopathy demonstrating asymmetric septal hypertrophy (15 mm) and normal posterior wall (PW) thickness (9 mm) and S:PW ratio of 1.67. Systolic thickening of S is reduced (28%) vs. normal PW (67%). Calibration dots are 5 mm apart.

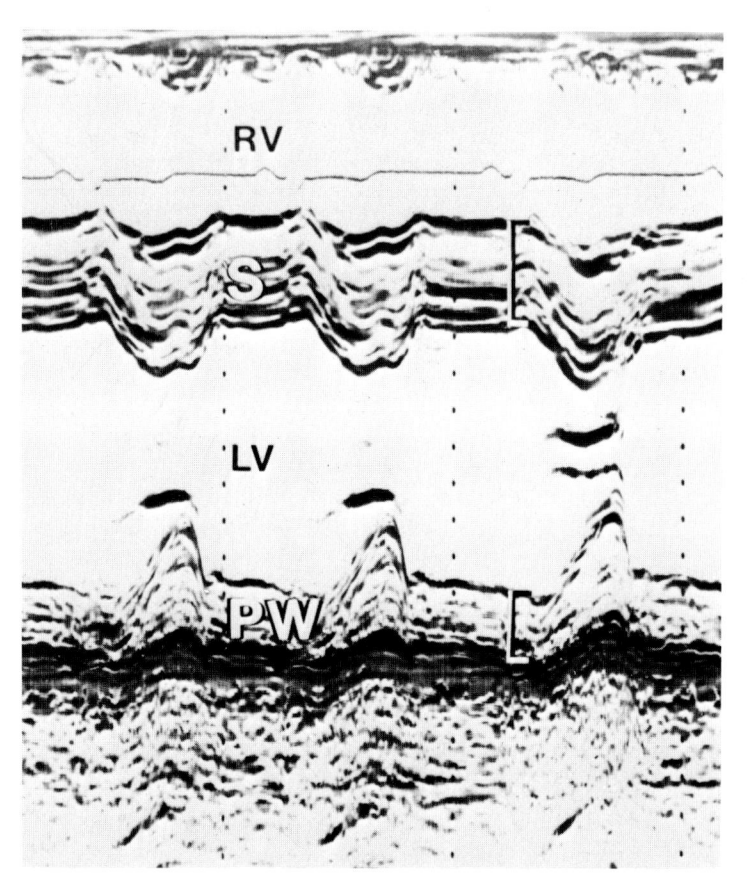

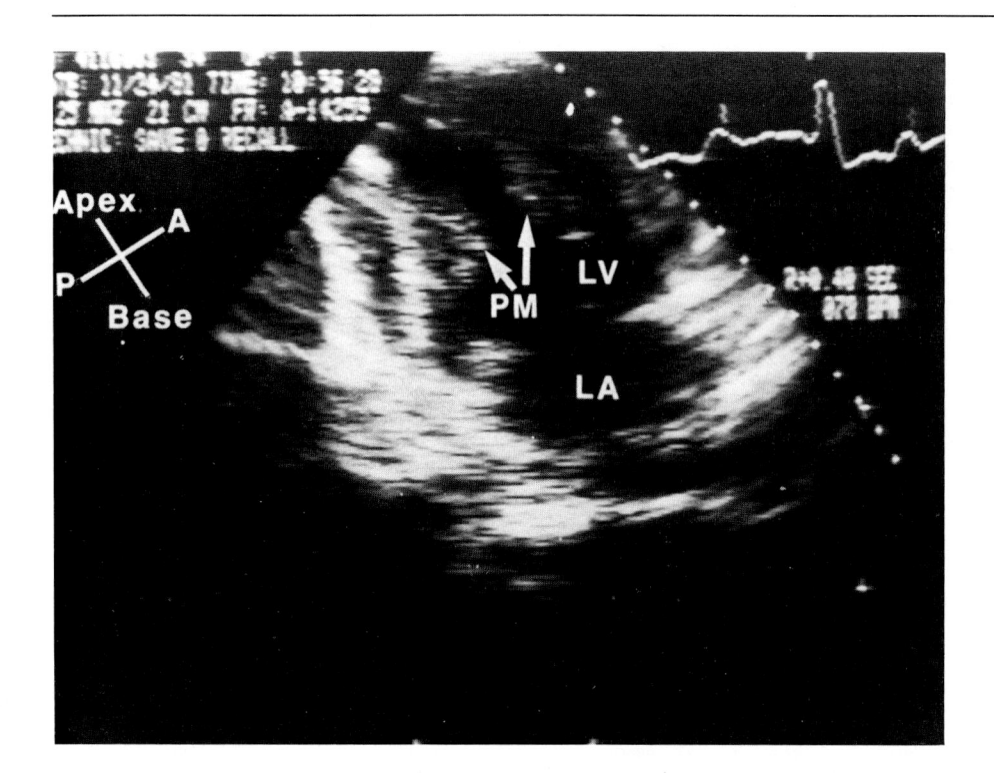

Fig. 9-6. Apical long axis view in a patient with left ventricular hypertrophy, small cavity left ventricle, and significant hypertrophy of both papillary muscles, resulting in simultaneous imaging of both in this plane. Calibration dots are 1 cm apart.

(Fig. 9-7). Multiple views through the apical four-chamber view will provide a good opportunity for visualizing the posterior portion of the ventricular septum as well as the lateral and posterolateral portions of the left ventricle (Fig. 9-8A). Anterior angulation from this position enables imaging through the anterior portion of the septum and the aortic valve (Fig. 9-8B). If parasternal imaging has failed to obtain good-quality recordings of the aortic valve with M-mode, it may be possible to record the motion of a single cusp from either the apical long axis or apical four-chamber position. Although the classic mid-systolic closure motion on the M-mode record has reasonably good specificity for patients with resting outflow obstruction, it should not be confused with other types of nonspecific notching motion or the movement of the early systolic closure caused by membranous subvalvular stenosis (Fig. 9-9).

It must be remembered that there are some inherent limitations of two-dimensional echo equipment because of reduced resolution in the margins of the sector; this limitation may lead to error in obtaining precise measurements of the lateral wall thickness in comparison to those of the septum and posterior wall, which are directly under the beam in a more central portion of the sector when imaging in the parasternal short axis position. The echocardiographer can minimize these sources of error in measuring the free wall thickness near the lateral boundary of the sector by merely positioning the lateral free wall closer to the center of the field of view where lateral resolution is best. It may take several short axis images with variable positioning of the ventricle toward the center of the sector to optimize measurement opportunities both medially and laterally of the ventricle. Obviously

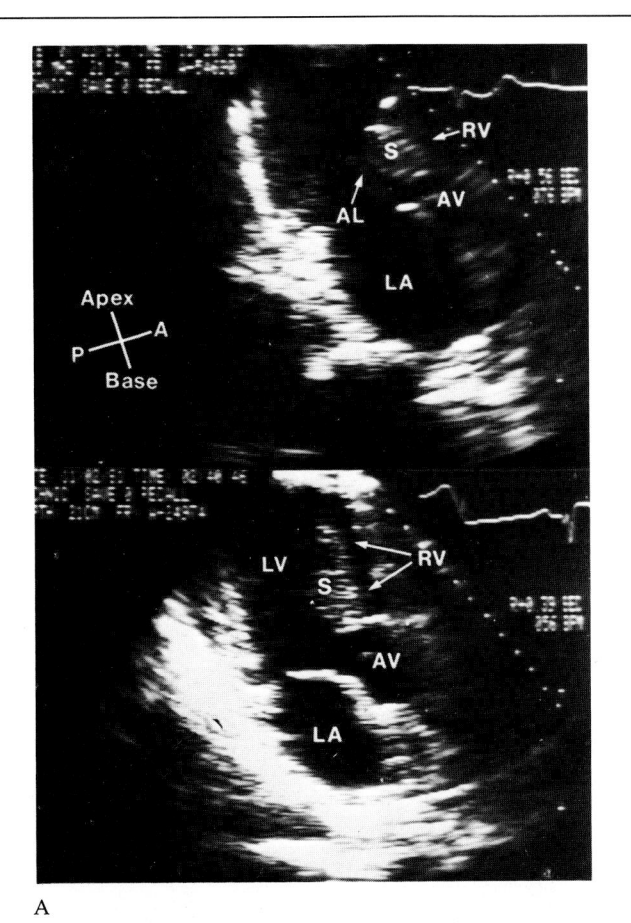

Fig. 9-7A. Apical long axis views with aorta during diastole (upper panel) and systole (lower panel) in a patient with hypertrophic nonobstructive cardiomyopathy. A small portion of the right ventricle can be seen. The septum is thick and the left atrium mildly enlarged. No systolic anterior motion of mitral valve or chordae tendineae can be seen during systole (lower panel). B. Apical long axis with aorta and left ventricular apex deleted from view in a patient with a thick septum; however, owing to the oblique plane of this view the septal thickness appears greater than it actually is, and the LV outflow tract also appears falsely narrow. The mitral valve, chordae, and papillary muscle are normal. The proximal ascending aorta measures approximately 40 mm in diameter in this view; other views showed it to be even larger, with aneurysmal enlargement of 45 mm diameter. Calibration dots are 1 cm apart.

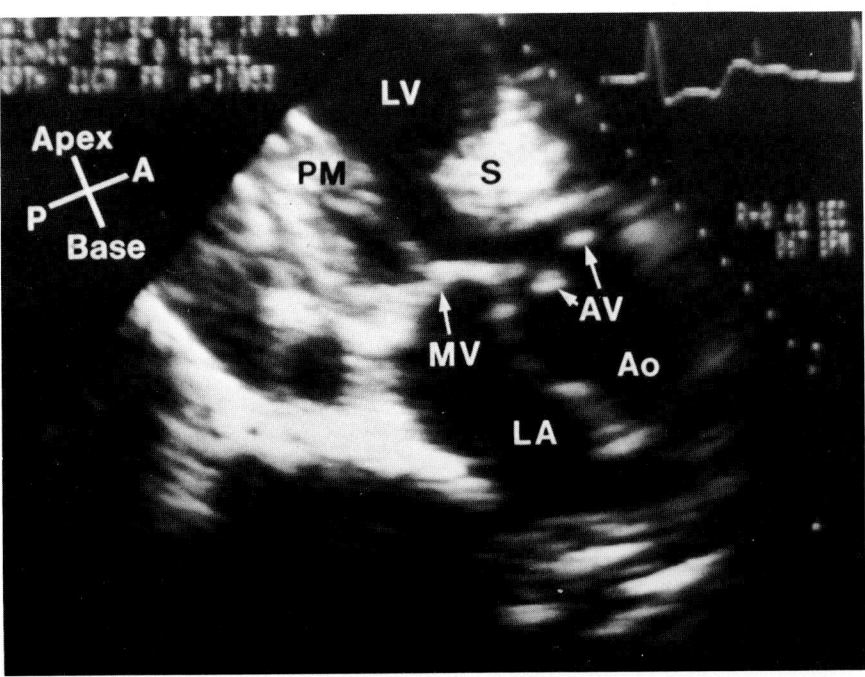

assessment of the extent of left ventricular segmental hypertrophy depends greatly upon the reliable definition of the endocardial and epicardial surfaces.

Studies have shown that some patients with hypertrophic cardiomyopathy may have significant hypertrophy present in unusual locations of the left ventricular wall [57, 79, 80]. Although left ventricular hypertrophy is "asymmetric" in most patients with hypertrophic cardiomyopathy, it is usually not confined to the ventricular septum and often involves the anterolateral free wall, but it rarely involves the posterior portion of the free wall [79]. Wide-angle two-dimensional echocardiography is capable of detecting myocardial hypertrophy that involves a variety of patterns. Maron and colleagues [79], in a study of 125 patients, identified four patterns of distribution of left ventricular hypertrophy: type I hypertrophy was confined to the anterior portion of the ventricular septum in 12 of 25 patients (10%); type II hypertrophy involved both anterior and posterior portions of the ventricular septum in 25 of 125 patients (20%); type III hypertrophy involved substantial portions of both the ventricular septum and the left ventricular free wall in 65 of 125 patients (52%); type IV hypertrophy involved portions of the septum not accessible to the M-mode beam or the anterolateral free wall in 23 of 125 patients (18%). The anterior basal portion of the ventricular septum and the posterior free wall had normal thickness in 22 of these 23 patients. In this latter group all patients appeared normal by M-mode echocardiography.

Employing two-dimensional echocardiography together with M-mode measurements taken from two-dimensional systems will improve quality control of M-mode measurements and help to eliminate many of the problems that have been long recognized in obtaining ultrasonic estimates of ventricular septal thickness from M-mode machines [81].

A number of studies have been performed comparing echocardiographic features with angiographic and hemodynamic findings in patients with hypertrophic cardiomyopathy [52, 82, 83]. Chahine and associates [82] reported that six of eight (75%) patients with angiographic evidence of outflow obstruction had echocardiographic findings of mid-systolic closure of the aortic valve. These investigators reported that although the incidence of mid-systolic closure of the aortic valve in hypertrophic cardiomyopathy is relatively low (40%), this finding appears to be a moderately sensitive sign of left ventricular outflow obstruction and is a more specific predictor of outflow obstruction than asymmetric septal hypertrophy and systolic anterior motion of the mitral valve.

Doppler ultrasound has been shown to demonstrate a characteristically abnormal aortic velocity profile in patients with obstructive forms of hypertrophic cardiomyopathy [84–86] characterized by a rapid early systolic velocity followed by an abrupt decrease in flow velocity in mid-systole with a slower late systolic velocity.

The aortic root M-mode echocardiogram has been shown to be abnormal in patients with hypertrophic cardiomyopathy manifested by a flatter slope in early diastole caused by a slower than normal rate of atrial emptying during early diastole together with a steeper slope at the end of diastole caused by forceful atrial contraction [87] (Fig. 9-10). Investigators also noted a steep initial anterior motion of the aortic root during early systole corresponding to rapid ventricular ejection followed by a relatively flat segment resulting from a decrease in the aortic flow caused by the obstruction of the left ventricular outflow tract. These echocardiographic features correspond to the abnormal flow measurements determined by Hsu [88], who observed that 80 to 85 percent of stroke volume is ejected during the

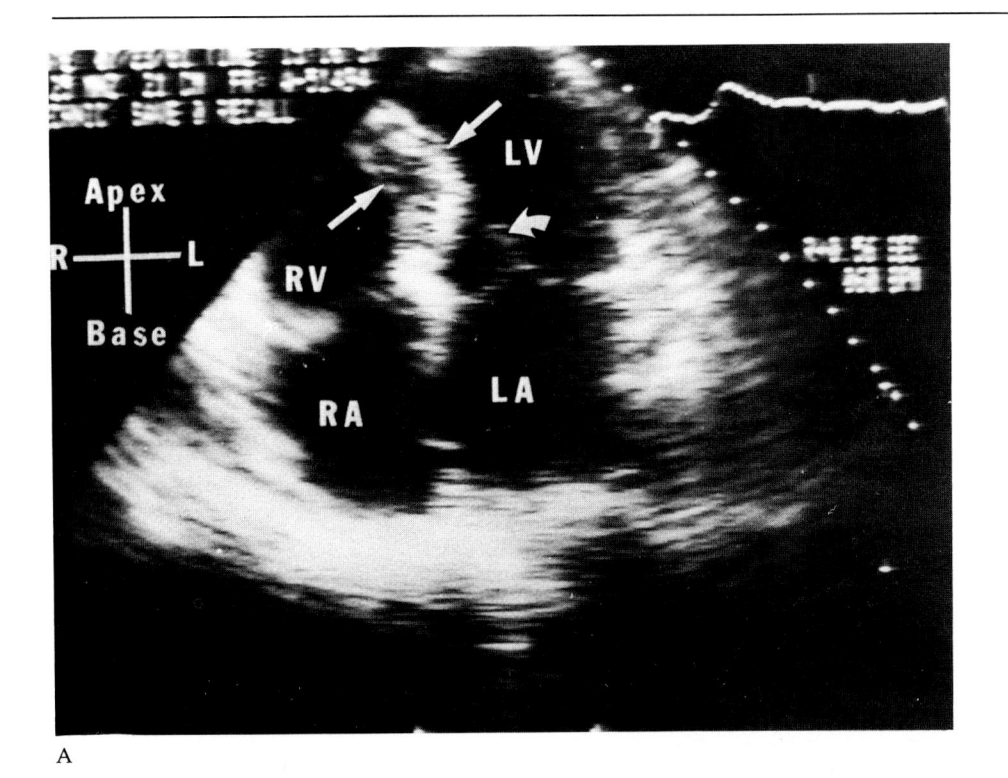

Fig. 9-8A. Apical 4-chamber view in a patient with hypertrophic obstructive cardiomyopathy demonstrating diffuse increased thickness of the ventricular septum (straight arrows) plus systolic anterior motion (SAM) of the tips of the mitral valve (curved arrow); since the chordae and papillary muscle are not seen in this view and in the absence of an anteroposterior dimension, this view is often suboptimal for demonstrating SAM. This is also a good view for evaluating left atrial size; LA enlargement is usually present in those patients with obstruction. Calibration dots are 1 cm apart. B. Apical 4-chamber with aortic valve view in a different patient with hypertrophic obstructive cardiomyopathy demonstrating tips of mitral valve (arrow) in the left ventricular outflow tract near the septum. The distal (apical) portion of the septum appears thinner. When the aortic valve is imaged in the apical 4-chamber view, the anterior septum is viewed primarily rather than the posterior portion, which is imaged in the standard 4-chamber plane.

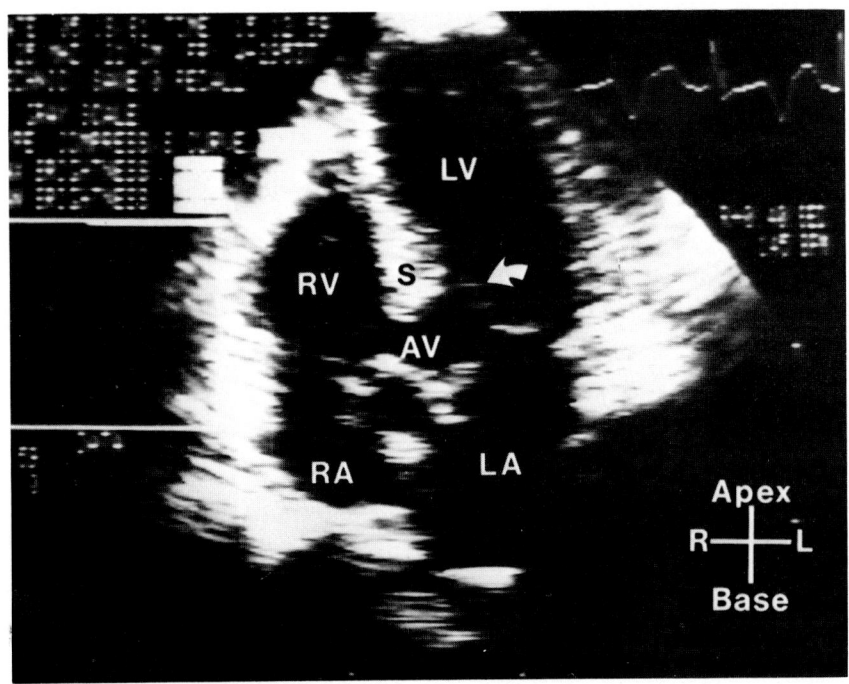

306   9. Cardiomyopathies

Fig. 9-9A. M-mode recording in a patient with hypertrophic obstructive cardiomyopathy demonstrating mid-systolic closure (arrows) followed by reopening of the aortic valve. B. M-mode recording in an elderly patient with left ventricular hypertrophy of unknown etiology but no findings to suggest hypertrophic cardiomyopathy demonstrates nonspecific coarse fluttering (arrows) of the aortic valve. Dotted line and bracket show aortic valve closure and delay in left atrial emptying. C. M-mode recording of aortic valve in a patient with membranous subaortic stenosis producing early systolic closure (black arrows) of the aortic valve. Typically the AV does not reopen in this type of subvalvular obstruction and can usually be distinguished from the mid-systolic closure and reopening of the hypertrophic cardiomyopathy patients. The open arrow (right panel) demonstrates some variation in this patient and late systolic reopening is observed.

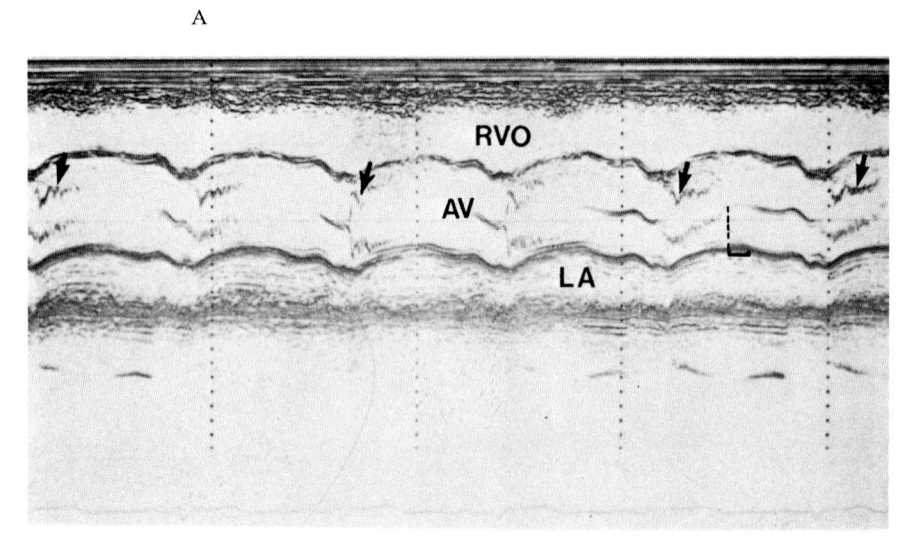

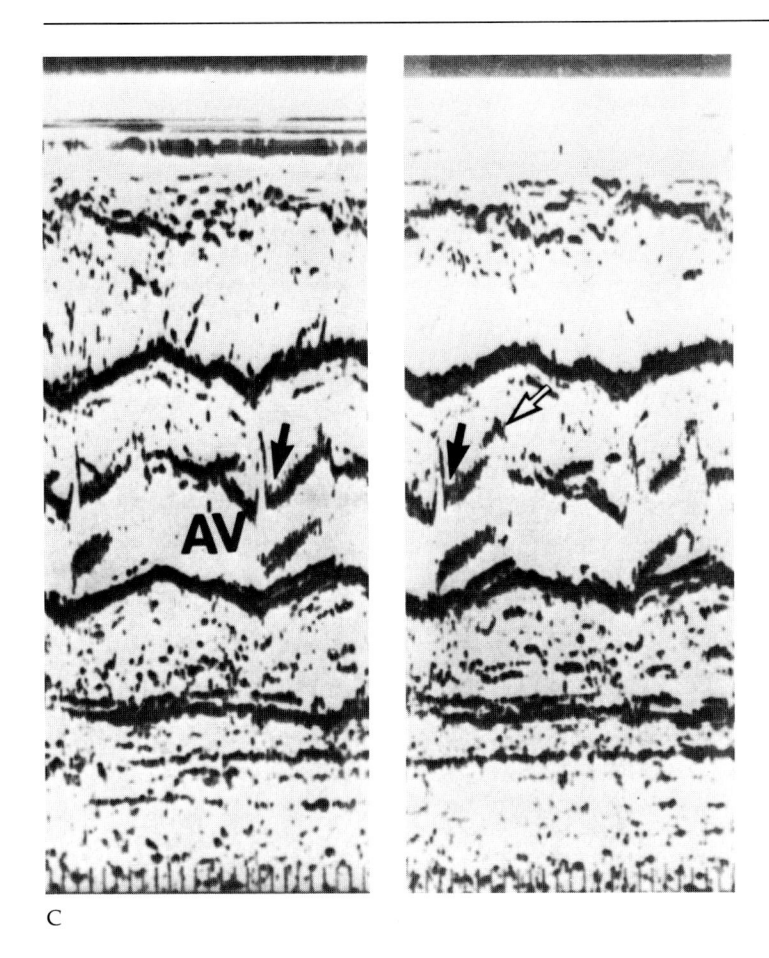

C

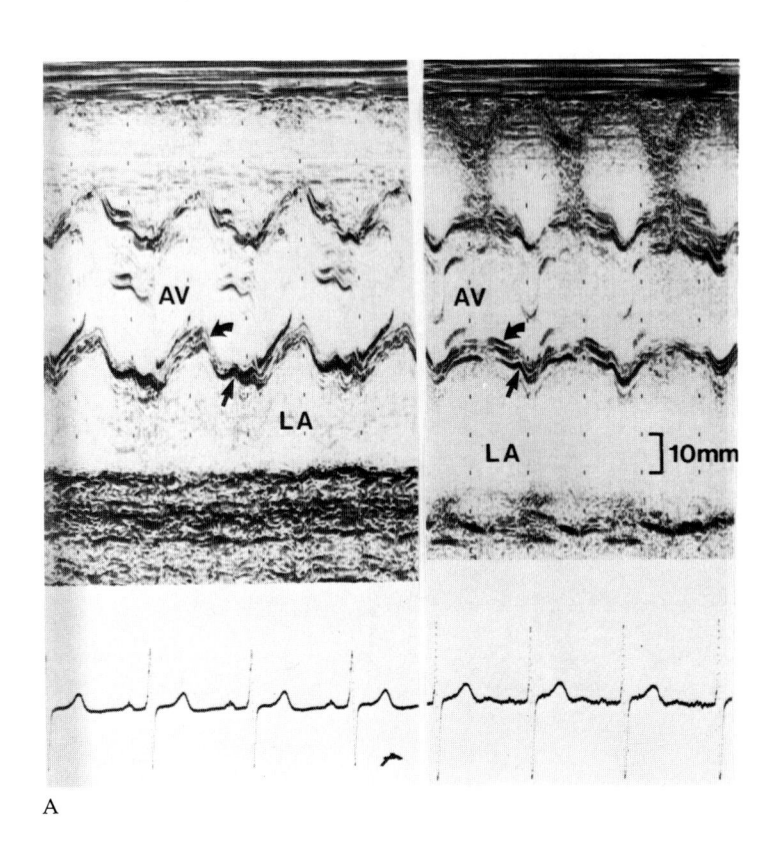

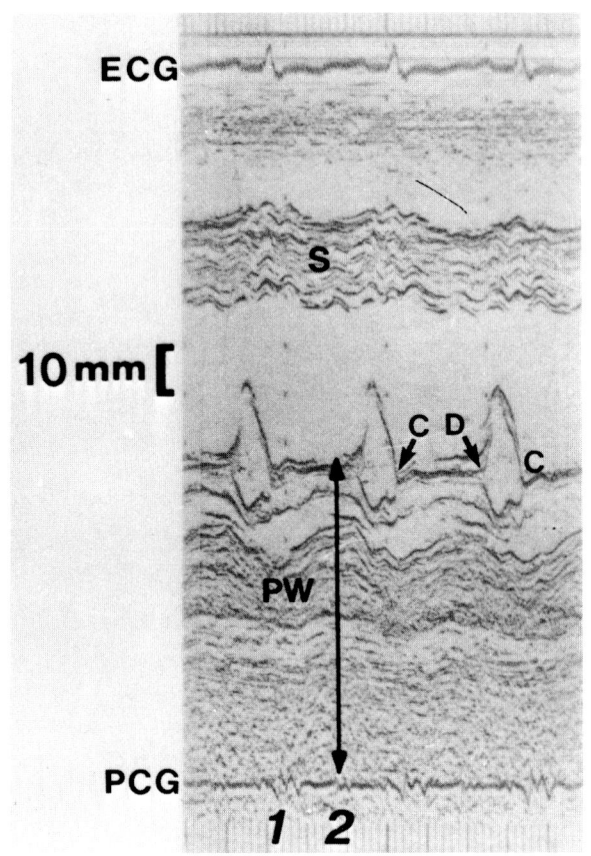

Fig. 9-10A. M-mode recordings of aortic valve and left atrium from a normal adult (left panel) and a hypertrophic cardiomyopathy patient (right panel). The steep slope of the posterior aortic root (curved arrow, left panel) shows normal left atrial emptying and only a small reduction in LA size with atrial contraction (straight arrow, left panel). In contrast, the recording in the right panel demonstrates very slow LA emptying (upper, curved arrow) owing to poor compliance and slow filling of the left ventricle with most of the decrease in LA size occurring with atrial contraction (lower, straight arrow). B. M-mode recording in a hypertensive patient with concentric hypertrophy of the left ventricle demonstrating a marked delay in the mitral valve opening following the second heart sound. Part of the slowed left atrial emptying observed in A (right panel) is often caused by the delay in the opening of the mitral valve, a finding frequently observed in hypertrophic cardiomyopathy as well as in patients with left ventricular hypertrophy and poor compliance from other etiologies. The duration of the C–D interval is longer than the D–C interval in such patients. PCG = phonocardiogram.

first half of systole and flow in the latter half of systole is markedly attenuated in patients with hypertrophic obstructive cardiomyopathy. The reduction of early diastolic slope of the posterior wall of the aortic root has also been reported in patients with systemic hypertension [89]; this results from a reduced rate of ventricular filling caused by decreased left ventricular compliance. Since Strunk and colleagues [90] observed a good correlation between the posterior aortic wall movement and change in left atrial volume, the findings of Chandraratna and coworkers [87] suggest that a greater amount of left ventricular filling occurred in the patients with hypertrophic cardiomyopathy during atrial contraction than during the early phase of diastole. This underscores the importance of atrial contraction to ventricular filling in patients with hypertrophic cardiomyopathy and shows why serious clinical deterioration usually occurs if atrial fibrillation develops.

Yamaguchi and associates [91] have reported a study of 30 patients with an unusual form of nonobstructive hypertrophic cardiomyopathy manifested by marked concentric hypertrophy in the apex but with a different septal shape and contraction pattern from those seen in obstructive types. The echocardiographic features of apical hypertrophic cardiomyopathy have been reported by these same investigators [92]. Although this type of hypertrophy appears to be fairly common in Japan it has been reported only rarely in the United States. Yamaguchi and colleagues [91] noted that the average thickness in these patients (24.8 ± 6.6 mm) was significantly greater than in normal subjects (9.4 ± 3.1 mm) or in patients with obstructive hypertrophic cardiomyopathy (14.7 ± 5.0 mm). Obstruction of the outflow tract does not occur because the upper half of the septum remains essentially normal during systole and does not bulge into the left ventricle, nor is there any systolic anterior motion of the mitral valve apparatus (Fig. 9-11). The electrocardiogram in these patients showed a characteristic giant negative T wave (> 10 mm) associated with high QRS voltage in the precordial leads despite the absence of hypertension or coronary artery disease; also the prominent septal Q waves commonly seen in IHSS are not present.

CONDITIONS MIMICKING HYPERTROPHIC CARDIOMYOPATHY. Numerous clinical conditions have been reported that may mimic hypertrophic cardiomyopathy either because of disproportionate septal thickening greater than 1.3 of the posterior wall thickness or because of systolic anterior motion of the mitral valve apparatus, which occurs in various conditions and has commonly been referred to as "pseudo-SAM" [31, 33, 34, 93–105].

Nongenetically transmitted disproportionate septal thickening is relatively common in infants with congenital heart disease [31, 34], and some investigators have recommended that the only practical and reliable way a distinction can be made between genetically transmitted asymmetric septal hypertrophy and nongenetically transmitted disproportionate septal thickening is to examine the first-degree relatives for ASH by echocardiography [31, 106]. The overall prevalence of disproportionate septal thickening in one study involving echocardiography and necropsy measurements among patients with congenital heart disease was 10 percent (30 of 304 patients) [31]. The investigators found the prevalence of disproportionate septal thickening to be greater than 20 percent in patients with pulmonic valvular stenosis or primary pulmonary hypertension and relatively low (< 15%) in patients with Eisenmenger's syndrome, isolated aortic or mitral valve disease, or combined aortic and mitral valve disease. In another study by Maron and associates

310   9. Cardiomyopathies

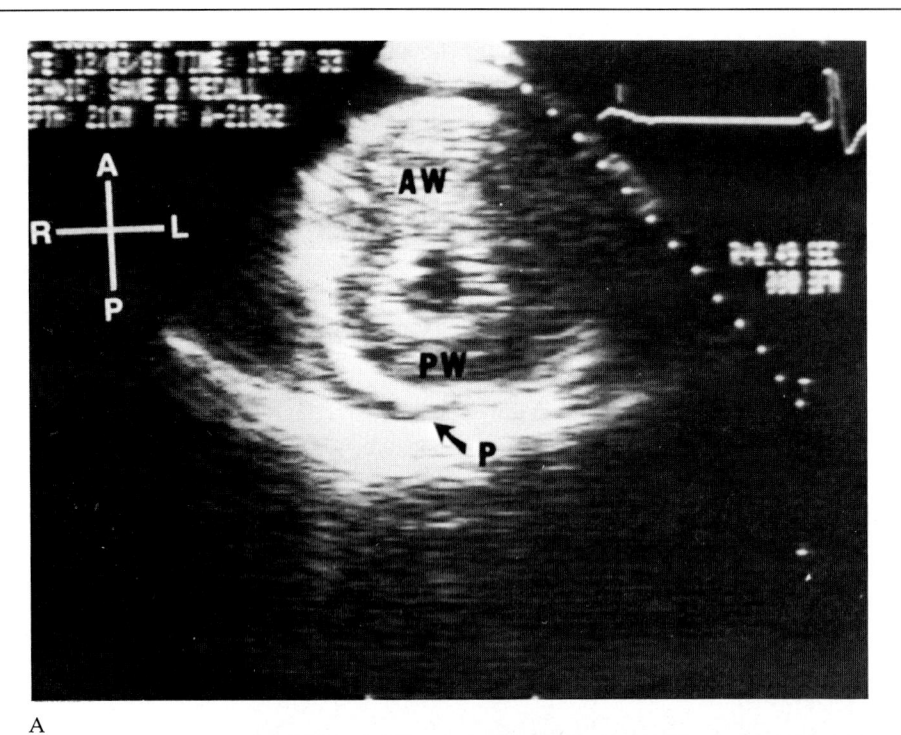

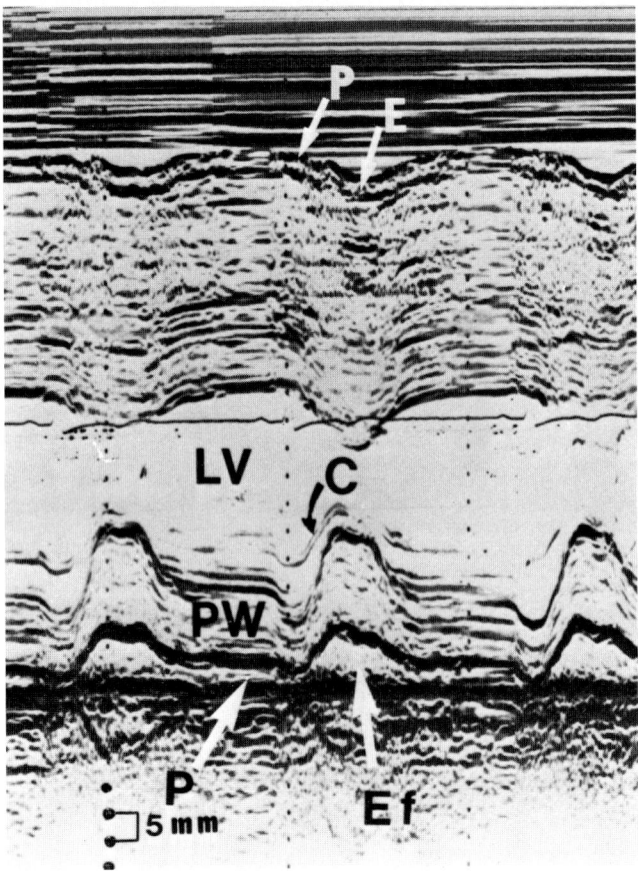

Fig. 9-11A. Parasternal short axis view in the middle third of the left ventricle; the right ventricle and septum are not identified in this view. The pericardium (P) is separated from the posterior wall by a small pericardial effusion. The cavity of the left ventricle is very small and the anterior wall (AW) is extremely thick. B. M-mode recording from same view shown in A demonstrating that anterior wall thickness and left ventricular cavity dimension at end diastole are the same (40 mm). The posterior wall is only slightly increased (12–13 mm). A small pericardial effusion (Ef) is present. C. Apical 4-chamber view in same patient demonstrating enormous apical hypertrophy with completely normal mitral valve and chordae tendineae (C) at end systole and only minimal increase in wall thickness at the base but massive hypertrophy of the apical half of the left ventricle with very small cavity. D. Apical long axis view at end diastole showing marked hypertrophy of the anterolateral wall near the apex, small pericardial effusion, and small segment of the ascending aorta. An area of the anterolateral wall of the left ventricle is brightly reflective (illustrated in E). E. Diagram of D illustrating the segment of the anterolateral wall, which is brightly reflective. F. Apical long axis view at end systole in same patient showing cavity obliteration in the apex of the left ventricle; however, there is no systolic anterior motion of the mitral valve or chordae and a wide open outflow tract. E = epicardium; PM = lateral papillary muscle.

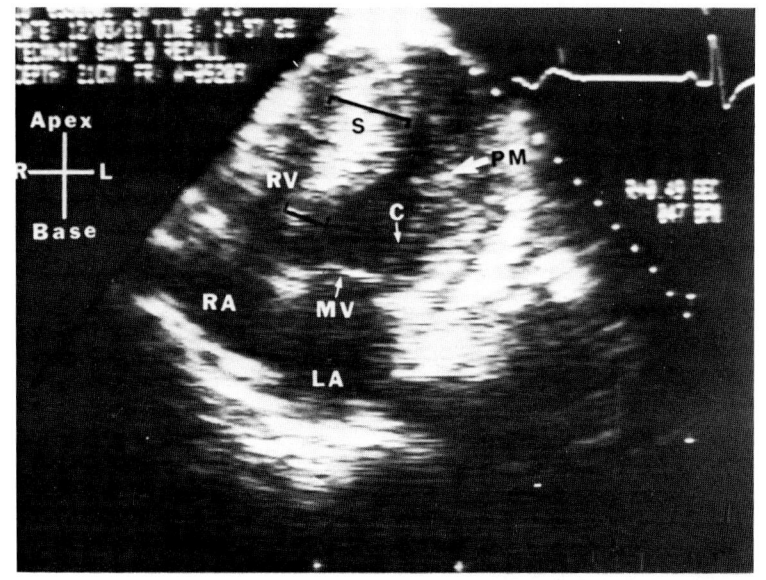

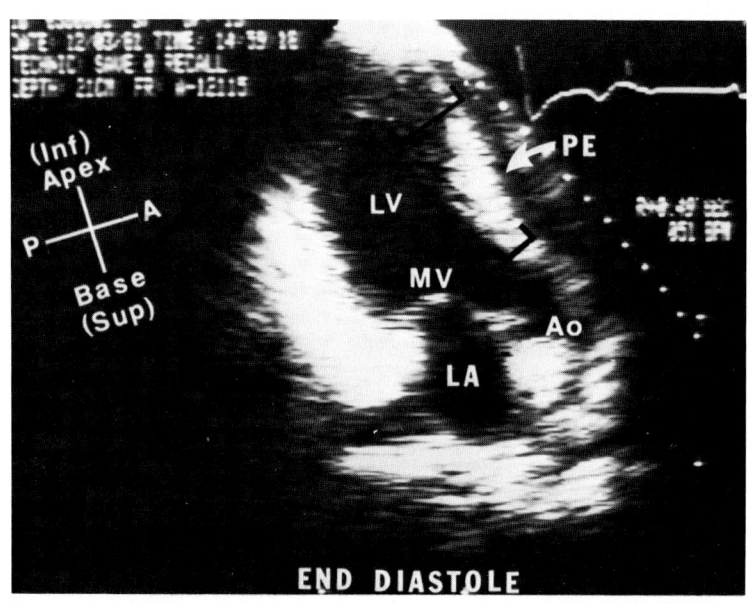

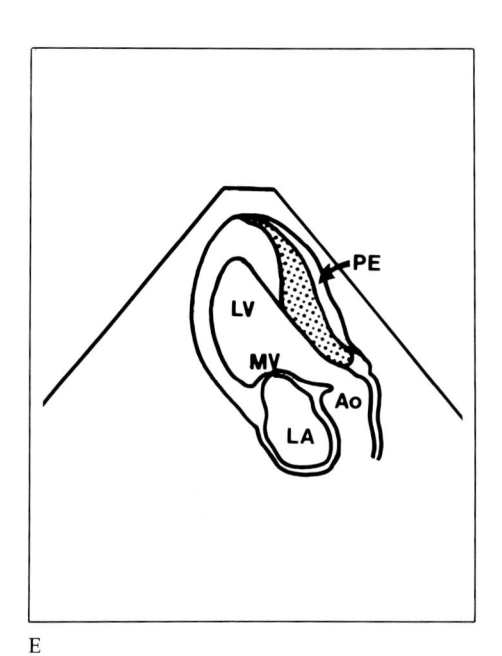

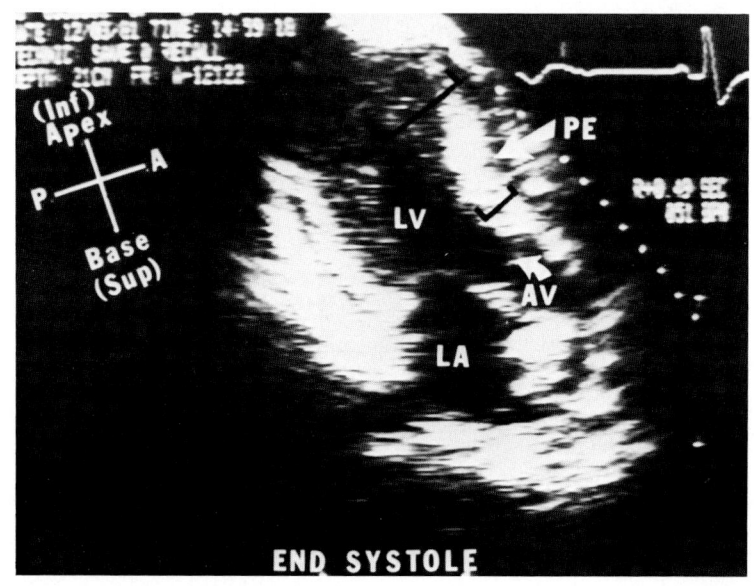

C

D

END DIASTOLE

E

F

END SYSTOLE

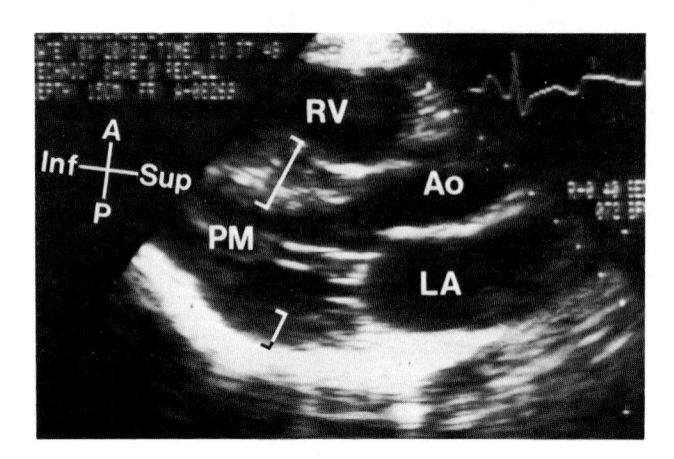

Fig. 9-12. Parasternal long axis view showing an adult hypertensive patient with disproportionate septal thickening and minimal increased thickness of the posterior wall with an S:PW ratio of 1.67. The posteromedial papillary muscle is hypertrophied.

[34], the hearts of 31 of 125 infants with congenital cardiac malformations were found to have abnormal septal-to-free wall ratio greater than 1.3 at necropsy. In this study the age of the patients ranged from 1 day to 2½ years at death and 92 were under 2 months of age with 76 male and 49 female patients. The congenital malformations found to have disproportionate septal thickening included the following: pulmonic valve atresia in 3, complete d-transposition of the great vessels with ventricular septal defect in 1, aortic valve atresia with hypoplastic left ventricle in 2, coarctation of the aorta in 2, truncus arteriosus in 4, total anomalous pulmonary venous return in 4, aortic valve stenosis with normal-sized left ventricle in 1, Ebstein's malformation in 1, double-outlet right ventricle in 1, valvular pulmonic stenosis with intact septum in 4, tetralogy of Fallot in 1, ventricular septal defect plus pulmonic stenosis in 3, cor triatriatum in 1, and congenital mitral valve stenosis plus ventricular septal defect in 1.

Ten Cate and colleagues [106] reported that asymmetric septal hypertrophy could be considered the anatomic marker for hypertrophic cardiomyopathy only when in addition there were decreased systolic septal thickening (<25%) and a characteristically abnormal left ventricular shape that could be identified with two-dimensional echocardiography. These investigators found an incidence of 8 percent in the general population of 100 patients with various forms of cardiac disease having a ventricular septal-to-posterior free wall ratio greater than 1.3. They noted that in the so-called borderline cases with echocardiographic signs of an abnormal ventricular septal-to-posterior wall ratio, a definitive clinical diagnosis of hypertrophic cardiomyopathy could be made only after echocardiographic screening of family members for the presence of asymmetric septal hypertrophy.

Systemic hypertension is one of the most common causes of disproportionate septal thickening encountered among adult patients referred to an echocardiography laboratory (Fig. 9-12). The actual incidence of disproportionate septal thickening among hypertensive patients is probably around 15 percent [107]. Some studies have reported a low incidence from 4 to 10 percent [108–110], although other studies have reported a much higher incidence (30–47%) in hypertensive patients [111–113]. One explanation for such a wide range (4–47%) is measurement error, because all determinations with one exception [107] were obtained from M-mode recordings without additional benefit of two-dimensional imaging in order to

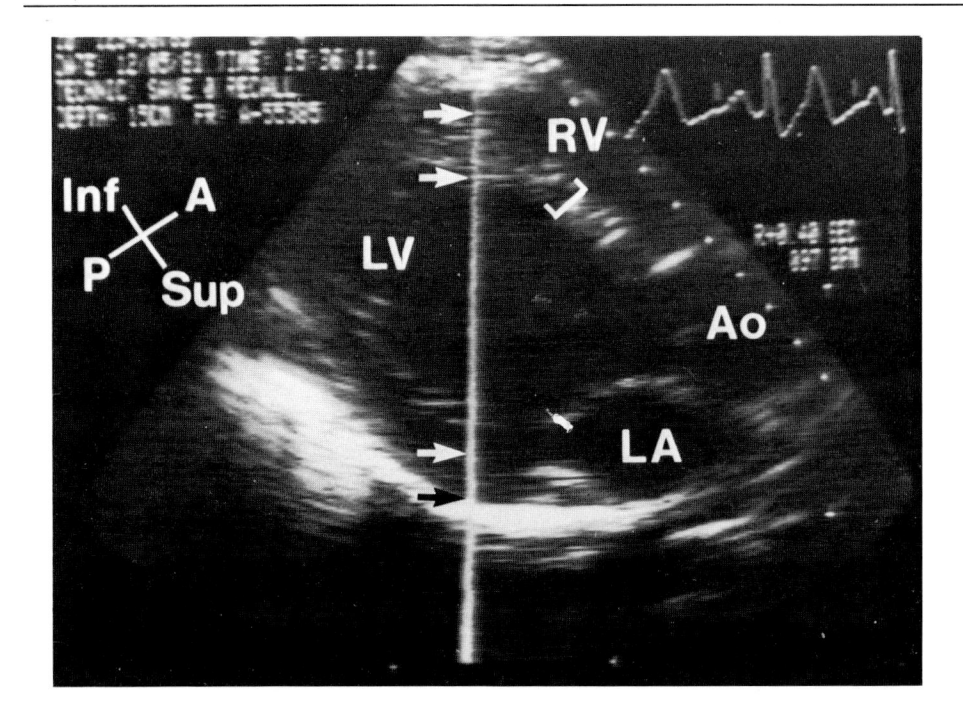

Fig. 9-13. Parasternal long axis view from a low left sternal border transducer position demonstrating the oblique angle of the M-mode beam intersecting the septum (white arrows) *producing false increased thickness compared to posterior left ventricular wall (white and black arrows). Bracket shows the true thickness of the septum.*

ensure accuracy of septal thickness measurements. A common error in measurement of ventricular septal thickness with only M-mode echocardiography is to direct the beam at a tangent or oblique angle through the septum; this happens most commonly when the transducer is positioned low along the left sternal border with the result that the beam is directed slightly superiorly, usually causing the septum to be recorded as thicker than it actually is (Fig. 9-13). On the other hand, if echo dropout occurs as a result of improper machine setting or beam angulation through the septum, the full thickness may not be properly recorded and the anatomic thickness may be underestimated. This type of underestimation or overestimation of septal thickness can be essentially eliminated with technically adequate imaging utilizing two-dimensional echocardiography.

In addition to systemic hypertension another very common cause of disproportionate septal thickening in the absence of hypertrophic cardiomyopathy is coronary artery disease [33, 97, 98]. The incidence of disproportionate septal thickening in patients with coronary artery disease has been reported to be between 11 and 52 percent [33, 97]. There are two reasons why this abnormal septal-to-posterior wall ratio is commonly encountered in patients with coronary artery disease, segmental hypertrophy of the septum existing in the presence of normal posterior wall thickness, and infarction of the posterior wall causing thinning producing an abnormal ratio even in the presence of normal septal thickness. Even in the absence of two-dimensional imaging, the M-mode echocardiographer can easily differentiate coronary artery disease from hypertrophic cardiomyopathy by observing the absolute systolic thickening of the left ventricular posterior free wall, relative wall motions during systole, and increased thickening and motion of the ventricular septum compared to the left ventricular posterior wall during systole in patients with inferior myocardial infarctions.

Both cardiac sarcoma and lymphoma have been reported to produce disproportionate septal thickening with resultant mimicking of hypertrophic cardiomyopathy [101, 102]. Primary cardiac involvement with tumor in both of these case reports was demonstrated at autopsy to have preferential infiltration of the ventricular septum, thus creating the asymmetric thickening of the septum and abnormal septal-to-posterior wall ratio. One of these patients [102] had a murmur and clinical findings strongly suggesting hypertrophic cardiomyopathy manifested by worsening of heart failure symptoms, intensification of the systolic murmur by digitalis and diuretics, and lessening of both by propranolol. Before the patient's death a diagnosis of lymphoma was never suspected clinically, and at autopsy the neoplasm was found to be limited to the heart. The case report of the cardiac sarcoma [101] was also unique in that the patient's disease had clinical features simulating coronary artery disease. At autopsy the tumor was found to be compressing a segment of left anterior descending coronary artery, which explained the clinical symptomatology since there was no evidence of any significant coronary atherosclerosis.

Further controversy has existed regarding the septal-to-posterior wall thickness ratio as to what represents an abnormal ratio, 1.3 or 1.5 [113]. It has been shown that the ventricular septal-to-left ventricular posterior wall ratio of 1.3 or greater is commonly found in healthy weight lifters [99]. However, Menapace and colleagues [99] found that the ratio of the ventricular septum to the left ventricular systolic dimension was not significantly different in the weight lifters compared to normal subjects (0.41 versus 0.31). In contrast those investigators found that this ratio was 0.60 in patients with asymmetric septal hypertrophy and 0.78 in patients with IHSS.

Systolic anterior motion (SAM) has been reported in numerous conditions other than hypertrophic cardiomyopathy: mitral valve prolapse [93], left ventricular aneurysm [114], normal subjects [49], hypercontractile state [51, 104], aortic regurgitation [115], concentric left ventricular hypertrophy [50], Pompe's disease [94], Friedreich's ataxia [116], infants of diabetic mothers [117], d-transposition [118], abnormal left ventricular ejection dynamics [96], hypovolemia [119], mitral valve vegetations [56], aortic disc prosthesis [56], and chordal SAM [93, 121] (Fig. 9-14A). The phenomenon of "pseudo-SAM" is also well recognized and has been caused by such things as hyperdynamic motion of the posterior left ventricular wall [93], atrial septal defect [103], aortic root [56], and pericardial effusion [120] (Fig. 9-14B).

Mintz and colleagues [96], in a study of seven patients, reported individuals without asymmetric septal hypertrophy having hemodynamic findings typical of obstructive hypertrophic cardiomyopathy. In addition to noting the vigorous posterior left ventricular wall motion in these patients, they observed increased left ventricular ejection fraction and ejection rate as well as narrowed left ventricular outflow tract and small left ventricular volume. For these reasons the investigators suggested that the unifying link among the various causes of this dynamic left ventricular outflow obstruction may not necessarily be asymmetric septal hypertrophy but rather abnormal ventricular ejection dynamics.

Wei and associates [105] have noted the lack of predictive value of M-mode echocardiography in correctly identifying hypertrophic cardiomyopathy in an unselected population. These investigators performed nine autopsy examinations of hearts in which M-mode echocardiographic diagnosis of IHSS had been made. The patients had ranged in age from 1 month to 74 years and six were women. Seven

315

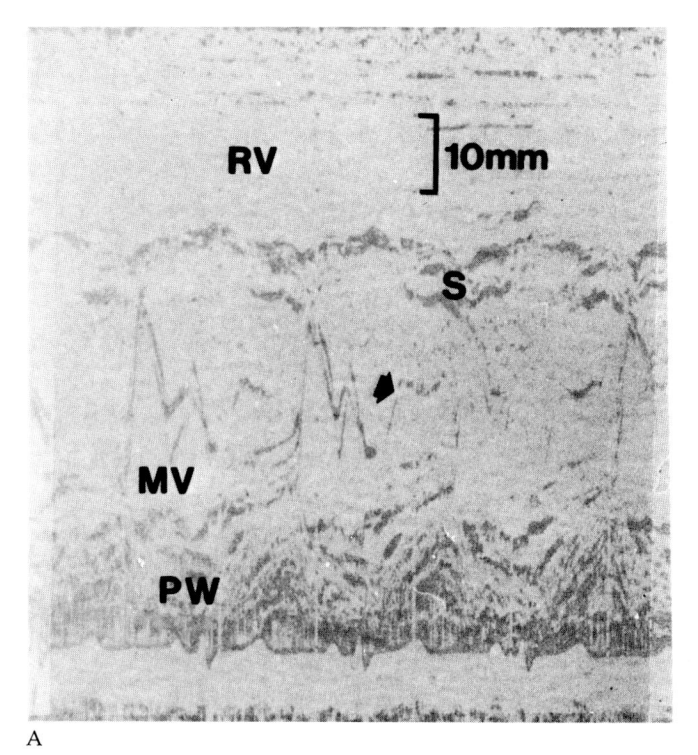

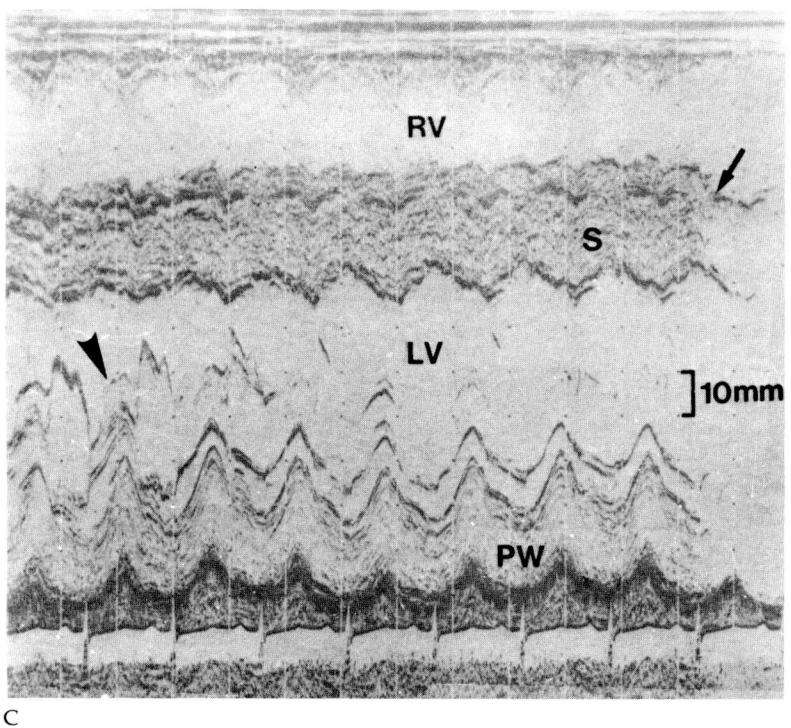

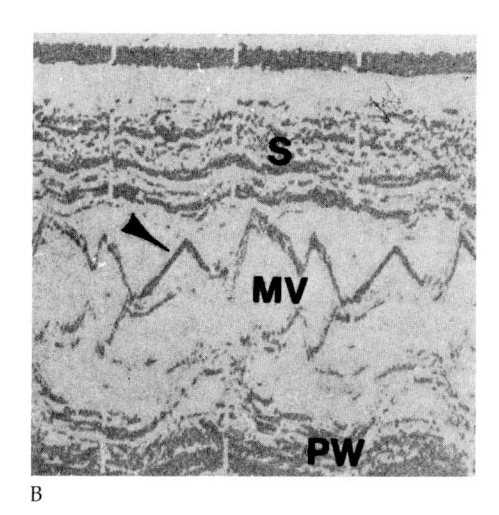

Fig. 9-14. M-mode recordings from two different subjects demonstrating (A) a normal individual with "chordal SAM" (arrow) vs. (B) a patient with hypertrophic cardiomyopathy and true SAM (arrow). "Chordal SAM," found in normal subjects as well as in individuals with mitral valve prolapse, is characterized by an abrupt anterior motion of chordae at onset of systole followed by a short plateau and then disappearance of the echo; with 2-D imaging it is confirmed that the motion is entirely from chordae tendineae and no anterior motion of the mitral valve occurs during systole. C. M-mode recording in a patient with concentric hypertrophy of the left ventricle due to hypertension and false or "pseudo" SAM (arrow). PW = posterior wall.

had been diagnosed as having systolic anterior motion of the mitral valve, eight asymmetric septal hypertrophy, three mid-systolic aortic valve closure, and all nine had had a systolic murmur at the apex together with an abnormal electrocardiogram. However, at autopsy only two hearts actually had asymetic septal hypertrophy and myocardial fiber disarray, while the other seven had no evidence of hypertrophic cardiomyopathy on either gross examination or on light microscopy. Of the seven hearts in which the clinical diagnosis and echocardiographic findings had been falsely positive for hypertrophic cardiomyopathy the following conditions were found: two had concentric left ventricular hypertrophy, one had coronary artery disease, one had cardiac amyloidosis, and three had no cardiac disease.

It is important to note that, although no studies have been reported yet to define the predictive value of two-dimensional echocardiography for correctly diagnosing hypertrophic cardiomyopathy, most of the obvious errors in measuring septal thickness and identifying systolic anterior motion of the total mitral valve apparatus can be avoided with two-dimensional imaging.

Rakowski and colleagues [122] have reported the value of employing two-dimensional echocardiography in attempting to make the crucial distinction between obstructive and nonobstructive systolic anterior motion. They observed in a study involving 84 patients with asymmetric septal hypertrophy that there was no evidence of obstruction in 16 of these patients as identified by absence of any prolonged SAM septal contact (> 30% of systole) and, if SAM was noted, it was observed on two-dimensional imaging involving only the leaflet tip and/or the chordae tendineae without significant change after amyl nitrite inhalation. ASH was absent in 16 of 100 (16%) in whom SAM was observed on both M-mode and two-dimensional echocardiography. One of these patients demonstrated a hyperkinetic heart and obstruction after amyl nitrite provocation with the development of prolonged SAM septal contact involving the body of the mitral leaflet.

THE ROLE OF PHARMACOLOGIC AND MANEUVER INTERVENTIONS IN PATIENTS WITH HYPERTROPHIC CARDIOMYOPATHY. The evaluation of dynamic left ventricular outflow tract obstruction using noninvasive techniques must be done with care using a variety of methods. Two of the most valuable maneuvers, which have been employed both at the bedside and in the echocardiography laboratory for clinical diagnosis, have been amyl nitrite inhalation and the Valsalva maneuver [123–125]. Amyl nitrite causes peripheral vasodilatation and transient pooling of blood in the extremities with resultant temporary reduction of venous return to the right heart; this reduced volume of blood in the left ventricle results in aggravation of outflow obstruction or it may induce a temporary gradient in patients with latent obstruction. The Valsalva maneuver also results in decreased venous return to the heart and causes reduction in volume with a similar physiologic effect.

The effect of post extrasystolic potentiation of myocardial contractility on left ventricular outflow tract obstruction is one of the well recognized physiologic characteristics of hypertrophic cardiomyopathy. Brockenbrough and colleagues [126] were the first to describe a decrease in the arterial pulse pressure of the post extrasystolic beat despite an increased intraventricular pressure. When present this sign is specific and has been correlated with the echocardiographic findings of obstruction [127, 128]. This post premature ventricular contraction response can be identified by M-mode echo with the development of mid-systolic closure of the aortic valve and SAM of the mitral valve in beats following premature systoles (Fig.

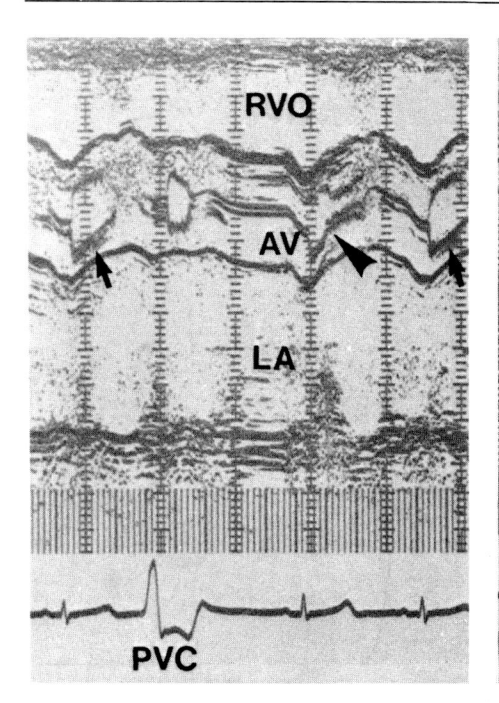

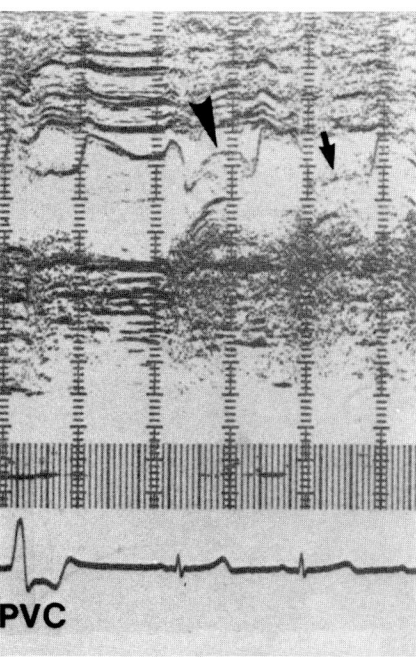

Fig. 9-15. M-mode recording in a patient with hypertrophic cardiomyopathy and provocable obstruction demonstrating mid-systolic closure of the aortic valve (left panel) *in the post-PVC beat and no mid-systolic notching motion on any of the other beats. Spontaneous PVCs also provoked systolic anterior motion (SAM) of the mitral valve in the post-PVC beat but no SAM was present on any other beats* (right panel).

9-15). White and Zimmerman [127] used the post extrasystolic beat phenomena in a slightly different fashion; they reported that prolongation of ejection time of the post extrasystolic beat by more than 20 msec was more sensitive than change in pulse pressure as an indicator of hypertrophic subaortic stenosis. Angoff and associates [129] emphasized the value of employing an external mechanical cardiac stimulator during echocardiographic and phonocardiographic assessment of patients with IHSS. They demonstrated that this technique is easily performed and clinically useful in evaluating the dynamic left ventricular outflow tract obstruction and correlates very well with cardiac catheterization findings in patients with IHSS.

Joye and associates [130] have reported that nitroprusside infusion provides improved accuracy and safety compared to amyl nitrite inhalation in the diagnosis and assessment of outflow tract obstruction in patients with IHSS. They found that controlled intravenous infusion of nitroprusside was more valuable than amyl nitrite in evaluation of hypertrophic cardiomyopathy in nine patients. No significant hypotension occurred nor was there any significant increase in heart rate or left ventricular end-diastolic pressure with appropriate titration of intravenous nitroprusside. In three patients these authors noted that amyl nitrite did not increase left ventricular outflow tract gradient, whereas nitroprusside raised the left ventricular outflow tract gradient more than 55 mm without adverse effects.

A study by de la Calzada and coworkers [131] showed that in 17 patients with hypertrophic obstructive cardiomyopathy, the intravenous injection of propranolol (5 mg) produced shortening of the isovolumic relaxation time and increases in both the diastolic closure rate of the mitral valve and the left ventricular systolic and diastolic diameters, indicating improvement in distensibility and rate of left ventricular filling.

ECHOCARDIOGRAPHIC ASSESSMENT OF MEDICAL AND SURGICAL THERAPY IN PATIENTS WITH HYPERTROPHIC CARDIOMYOPATHY. Echocardiography is a valuable noninvasive tool for long-term follow-up of patients with hypertrophic cardiomyopathy as well as for the preoperative and postoperative assessment of such patients. Frank and colleagues [132] reported favorable results in 22 patients with hypertrophic obstructive cardiomyopathy followed for 2 to 8 years on "complete" beta-blocking doses of propranolol (average dose 462 mg per day). Additional measures were required in some patients to provide adequate control of arrhythmias.

Hanrath and associates [133] reported that abnormal prolongation of the isovolumic relaxation period in patients with hypertrophic cardiomyopathy can be shortened by intravenous administration of verapamil, which improves left ventricular relaxation and filling and may improve left ventricular function.

The mid-systolic closure of the aortic valve in patients with hypertrophic subaortic stenosis has been shown to correlate with preoperative and postoperative hemodynamics [134]. Other studies have demonstrated the value of M-mode and two-dimensional echocardiography in evaluating the effects of septal myectomy in patients with IHSS [135–137]. Bolton and coworkers [135] have shown that the markedly abnormal systolic anterior motion of the mitral valve apparatus present in all patients preoperatively was diminished or absent following operation. Schapira and colleagues [137] showed that by defining the geometry of the septal myectomy with two-dimensional echocardiography that M-mode studies could be more reliably interpreted. In all patients who had pre- and postoperative 2-D echocardiographic studies the postoperative region of septal thinning could be easily appreciated. One important advantage of wide-angle two-dimensional imaging is that the entire septum can be viewed from an apical to base orientation as well as anterior to posterior portions of the septum throughout. The group in this study also demonstrated postoperative changes in the left ventricular outflow tract configuration and size, mitral valve systolic anterior motion, mitral E–F slope, and left ventricular percent fractional shortening from both M-mode and two-dimensional echocardiography (Fig. 9-16).

Maron and associates [138] reported long-term postoperative results in 124 patients who underwent septal myotomy-myectomy for IHSS in the period from 1960 to 1975. Their study showed that the large majority of patients reported distinct symptomatic improvement and nearly all manifested marked reduction in left ventricular outflow gradients at rest; however, the operative mortality was 8 percent; 12 percent of the patients had persistent, or subsequently developed, recurrent severe functional limitation. Late cardiac death continued to occur despite abolition of the gradient and the annual mortality following operation was 1.8 percent. Of the 11 late postoperative cardiac deaths these authors reported six to be sudden and five due to progressive congestive heart failure.

In a 19-year postsurgical survivorship study in hypertrophic obstructive cardiomyopathy patients, Beahrs and associates [139] reported that 9 (25%) postoperative deaths had occurred with sudden death in 4, intractable heart failure with atrial fibrillation in 4, and 1 noncardiac death. Of the 27 surviving patients, 12 do not take cardiac medications and 15 are taking propranolol or digitalis or both. Three patients have required permanent pacemakers and 5 other patients are in atrial fibrillation. Therefore the investigators continue to recommend surgery in such patients when clinically indicated on the basis of their study showing that 75 per-

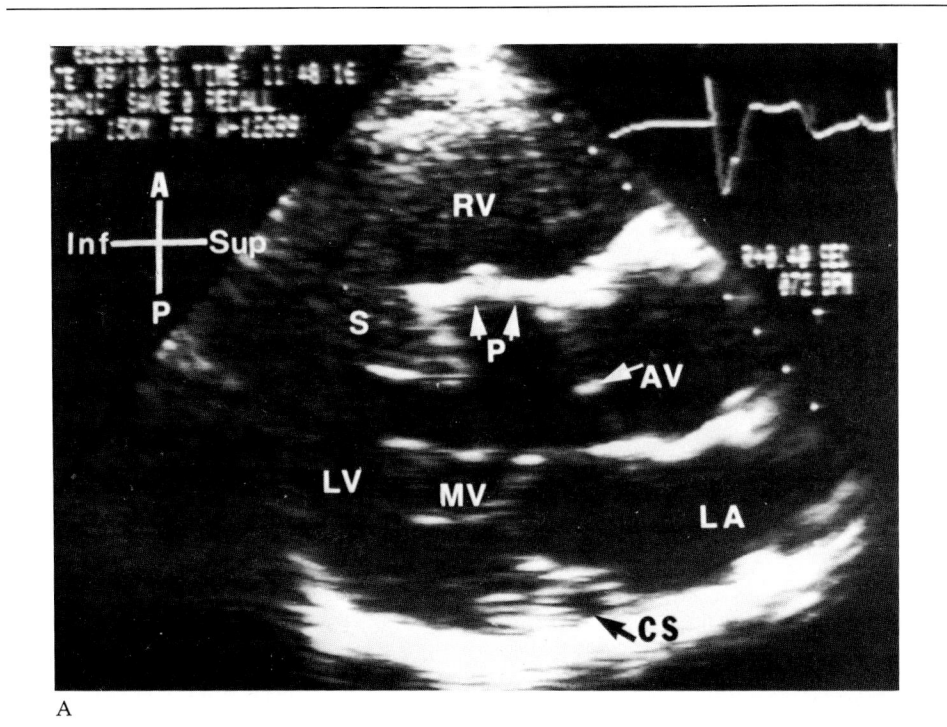

Fig. 9-16A. Parasternal long axis view from a patient after myectomy complicated by iatrogenic ventricular septal defect which was closed by a patch (P). The thick septum inferior to the site of resection can be seen but no SAM of the mitral valve or chordae is present. B. Parasternal short axis view in same patient demonstrating that the residual thick septum is very localized (open arrow). The posterior septum (solid arrow) is normal thickness; the site of the myectomy (M) is easily imaged. The patient has no lateral wall involvement in the hypertrophic process.

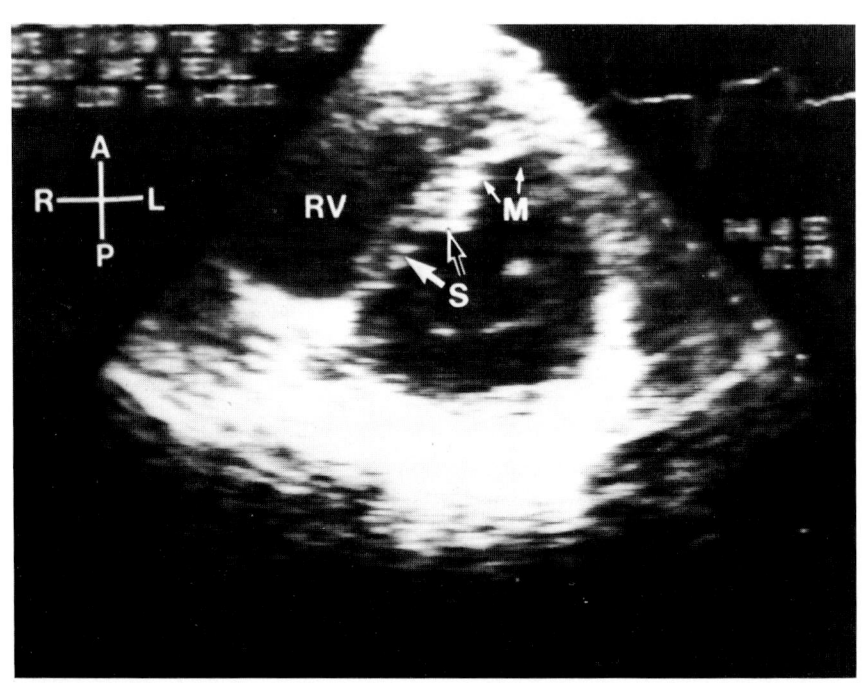

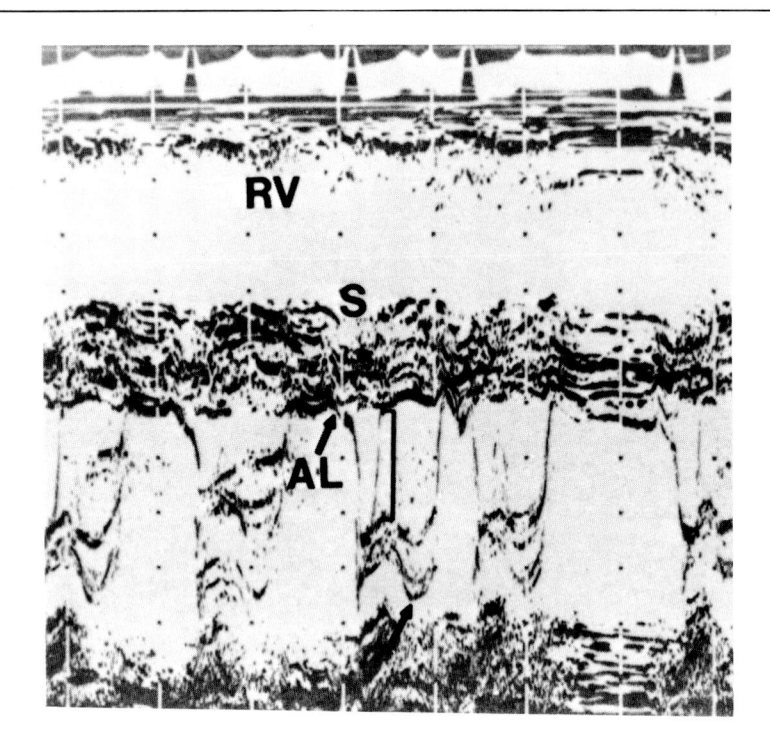

Fig. 9-17. M-mode recording in a patient with hypertrophic nonobstructive cardiomyopathy demonstrating classic late systolic prolapse of the mitral valve (arrow). The bracket identifies marked anterior motion at onset of systole, which (with 2-D echo) was caused by "chordal SAM" but there is no evidence of any actual obstruction in the LV outflow tract from either mitral valve or chordae.

cent of their patients undergoing surgery are alive with good-to-excellent alleviation of their symptoms for as long as 19 years; 22 patients were followed for more than 10 years.

Hypertrophic cardiomyopathy in association with other cardiac disorders. Hypertrophic cardiomyopathy has been reported to coexist with a number of other cardiac disorders, including coronary artery disease, hypertension, aortic valve regurgitation, discrete subvalvular aortic stenosis, aortic stenosis, mitral regurgitation, mitral valve prolapse (Fig. 9-17), and subpulmonic stenosis [29, 140–146]. It is obvious that conditions such as hypertension or obstructive lesions in the left ventricular outflow tract, aortic stenosis, or any supravalvular obstruction such as coarctation may cause a variable degree of left ventricular hypertrophy. These same conditions may also have some degree of disproportionate septal thickening; when they coexist with hypertrophic cardiomyopathy it is difficult or impossible to distinguish the extent of the left ventricular hypertrophy that can be attributed to each disease process. Assessment of the early closing movement of the aortic valve leaflets can be helpful in distinguishing discrete membranous subaortic stenosis from idiopathic hypertrophic subaortic stenosis [141].

The recognition of diastolic mitral regurgitation in some patients with hypertrophic cardiomyopathy may have clinical importance. If the timing is not appreciated it may be mistaken for systolic mitral regurgitation, and the severity of concomitant systolic mitral regurgitation may be overestimated because of partial filling of the atrium during diastole [144]. Since the end-diastolic volume may be reduced by the diastolic mitral regurgitation, this reduction in volume may aggravate the outflow pressure gradient in some patients with hypertrophic cardiomyopathy [147].

Right-sided hypertrophic subpulmonic stenosis has been reported in patients with hypertrophic obstructive cardiomyopathy; however, its pathophysiology has not been well characterized. Brik and colleagues [146] reported a case in which SAM of the anterior tricuspid leaflet was found in a patient with right-sided outflow obstruction together with left-sided outflow obstruction because of hypertrophic cardiomyopathy.

Hypertension and miscellaneous forms of hypertrophic cardiomyopathies. The echocardiographic differentiation of hypertensive heart disease and hypertrophic cardiomyopathy may be a problem [107, 108, 113, 148, 149]. Doi and associates [148] did not find SAM of the mitral valve or mid-systolic closure of the aortic valve in patients with hypertensive heart disease. The hypertrophic response to a chronic increase in systemic arterial pressure does not by itself result in depression of the basal inotropic state of the left ventricle [150]. Meerson [151] reported that the immediate response to a hypertrophy-inducing stimulus imposed on a normally functioning heart was one of physiologic hyperfunction associated with an increase in myocardial protein synthesis. Even before the hypertrophic process causes an increase in left ventricular mass, myocardial function is enhanced in order to overcome its increased pressure workload. This enhancement of left ventricular performance may be observed in patients with aortic stenosis as well as in hypertensive patients [152].

Echocardiography is not only the most sensitive noninvasive means of identifying increased left ventricular mass in hypertensive patients but also the most reliable method of identifying early evidence of decreased left ventricular function before clinical manifestations of left ventricular failure [107–109, 153, 154]. Two-dimensional echocardiography is more reliable than M-mode recordings for estimating left ventricular weight [153], and when M-mode measurements are obtained they can be derived more reliably from a 2-D echo system that allows simultaneous 2-D imaging to ensure better quality control of the M-mode records [107].

Safar and colleagues [110] reported that asymmetric septal hypertrophy was more commonly encountered in borderline hypertension in comparison to those patients with sustained hypertension in whom symmetric cardiac hypertrophy was more commonly encountered.

We have found no relationship between the incidence of asymmetric septal hypertrophy and the level of blood pressure or the duration of hypertension [107]. In our study of 73 hypertensive patients 89 percent of those with normal left ventricular mass were taking two or more antihypertensive drugs, whereas only 59 percent of those with evidence of left ventricular hypertrophy were taking two or more drugs, suggesting that control of hypertension regardless of the number of medications is more important in preventing the development of left ventricular hypertrophy than the duration of the disease. No dilatation of the left ventricular cavity was found in any of the patients with left ventricular hypertrophy or decreased left ventricular performance. Of 37 patients with left ventricular hypertrophy documented by echocardiography, only 19 percent showed evidence of left ventricular hypertrophy by electrocardiogram. A finding of left ventricular hypertrophy by echocardiography is a clinically useful predictive index that suggests there will be target organ disease elsewhere.

Strauer [155], in a study of ventricular function and coronary hemodynamics in hypertensive heart disease patients, reported that left ventricular function was impaired only when regional contraction abnormalities or ventricular dilatation or both occurred and was inversely related to both cardiac size and systolic wall stress. He concluded that the extent of left ventricular hypertrophy, a result of mass-to-volume ratio and stress, is a major determinant of left ventricular performance and of myocardial oxygen consumption. He described two types of left ventricular hypertrophy in patients with hypertensive heart disease: low-stress hypertrophy, with an increased mass-to-volume ratio, normal left ventricular function, and normal or reduced myocardial oxygen consumption; and high-stress hypertrophy, with normal or low mass-to-volume ratio, impaired left ventricular function, and increased myocardial consumption.

Guazzi and associates [156] reported a similar functional pattern of the right and left ventricles in hypertensive patients; this parallel functional pattern of both ventricles suggested a functional interdependence of the two sides that cannot be interpreted in terms of afterload but is probably best explained by changes in the contractile state of the entire heart. Olivari and associates [157] observed that systemic hypertension was associated with mild increases in pulmonary artery pressure and pulmonary arterial resistance that were not apparently the consequences of impaired left ventricular function.

In a study of 234 asymptomatic patients with mild to moderate systemic hypertension Savage and colleagues [109] found increased left ventricular mass in 51 percent by echocardiography; however, only 5 percent had increased left ventricular internal dimensions. These investigators found probable or definite left ventricular hypertrophy by electrocardiogram in only 6 of 108 (6%) hypertensive patients who had increased left ventricular mass by echocardiography. Furthermore, they found left ventricular enlargement by chest x-ray in only 6 of 81 (7%) hypertensive patients who had left ventricular enlargement or increased left ventricular mass or both by echocardiography.

It is obvious that the early detection of cardiac abnormalities in hypertensive patients can be more reliably determined by M-mode and two-dimensional echocardiography than any other diagnostic method, and that both 12-lead electrocardiograms and chest x-rays are quite insensitive for recognition of these abnormalities. In addition, approximately two-thirds of patients with echocardiographic evidence of left ventricular hypertrophy will have other manifestations of target organ disease such as hypertensive retinopathy or elevated serum creatinine levels.

Cardiomyopathy of hypothyroidism. Patients suffering from hypothyroidism commonly demonstrate a clinical picture of fatigue, lethargy, mental slowness, and cold intolerance. Less commonly, symptoms suggesting cardiac dysfunction such as exertional dyspnea, dizziness, syncope and anginalike chest pain may be prominent [158]. Santos and associates [159] reported 19 patients with untreated hypothyroidism of whom 17 had features of hypertrophic cardiomyopathy manifested by disproportionate thickening of the septum, reduced systolic thickening of the septum, reduced amplitude of septal excursion, reduced left ventricular outflow tract dimension, and systolic anterior motion of the mitral valve. In ten patients who returned to euthyroid state following therapy these abnormalities disappeared. The presence of pericardial effusion has been commonly observed in patients with hypothyroidism and effusions observed in seven of ten patients before treatment completely disappeared after normalization of thyroid function, which was consistent with findings reported in other studies [160, 161]. Low cardiac output and reduced left ventricular stroke volume have been demonstrated in patients with myxedema. These cardiovascular manifestations have been ascribed to diminished peripheral metabolic demands or to depression of myocardial contractility [162–164].

Although left ventricular hypertrophy has been demonstrated, most of the autopsy studies have showed the chambers to be dilated with little hypertrophy and no asymmetric septal hypertrophy or outflow tract obstruction [165–168]. However, gross anatomic examination at autopsy of three hearts demonstrated left ventricular hypertrophy with marked thickening of the interventricular septum [169], which supported the echocardiographic features reported by Santos and colleagues [159].

Cardiac abnormalities in scleroderma. No clinical symptoms are characteristic of scleroderma heart disease. Interpretations of cardiovascular symptoms may be complicated by abnormalities of pulmonary function and systemic hypertension secondary to involvement of the lung and kidney [170, 171]. In a study of 24 patients with scleroderma and related disorders, Gottdiener and associates [172] reported one or more of the following cardiac abnormalities: increased left ventricular wall thickness (57%), decreased left ventricular compliance (42%), left atrial enlargement (52%), pericardial effusion (21%), and increased left ventricular end-diastolic dimension (13%); however, normal left ventricular systolic performance was noted in all patients. These investigators found right ventricular enlargement by M-mode echocardiography in ten of 24 patients; only five of these had increased left ventricular wall thickness. In the same study, of six patients with progressive systemic sclerosis and right ventricular enlargement, three had pulmonary insufficiency causing severe hypoxia. At autopsy chronic adhesive pericarditis has been the most frequent cardiac finding while myocardial fibrosis has been noted less frequently and may be either focal or diffuse [173–175].

Congestive cardiomyopathy. Congestive cardiomyopathy is a disease of varied etiology that may primarily or secondarily affect left ventricular performance with resultant left ventricular dilatation and clinical manifestations of heart failure. The basic disorder in congestive cardiomyopathy appears to be a generalized disease of the myocardium with impaired contractile function, cardiac dilatation, and no significant change in left ventricular wall thickness. The echocardiographic features in these patients show diffuse involvement with dilatation of the left ventricle, normal left ventricular wall thickness, and reduced posterior wall thickening as well as reduced or absent systolic thickening of the ventricular septum [93, 176–179]. The echocardiographic features of congestive cardiomyopathy are remarkably constant regardless of the underlying etiology.

Ghafour and Gutgesell [180] reported the value of performing serial echocardiograms in evaluating left ventricular size and function in children with congestive cardiomyopathy.

One of the complications of chronic alcoholism is the development of a dilated congestive cardiomyopathy. The hemodynamic features of the disease reflect depression of myocardial contractile function and ventricular dilatation with reduced left ventricular ejection fraction and increased diastolic pressure in both ventricles. Left ventricular angiography has demonstrated an increase in left ventricular wall thickness and overall myocardial mass [181]. Mathews and colleagues [182] reported in 22 asymptomatic chronic alcoholics that 15 (68%) demonstrated significant increases in at least one of the following echocardiographic variables: left ventricular mass, left ventricular dimensions, septal and left ventricular wall thickness, and left atrial dimension. These authors showed that echocardiographic abnormalities in asymptomatic chronic alcoholics did not correlate with the presence or absence of auscultatory abnormalities on physical examination and appeared to reflect an earlier stage in the spectrum of alcoholic disease before the development of dilated cardiomyopathy. These investigators found no significant difference in left ventricular wall thickness in the symptomatic group of alcoholics compared to the normal controls; in contrast, in the asymptomatic chronic alcoholic subjects, the mean ventricular septal thickness was 10 percent above normal, a statistically significant difference. In a similar fashion this asymptomatic group demonstrated an 11 percent mean increase in thickness of the left ventricular posterior wall. Eight of 11 symptomatic patients in this study had mild to moderate regurgitation; however, the presence of mitral regurgitation was not necessary for left ventricular dilatation and decompensation to be seen. Mathews and associates [182] speculate that two models might explain the response in the left ventricle to the toxic effects of alcohol: the first model postulates that every asymptomatic subject goes through an initial stage in which there is mild left ventricular dilatation associated with an increase in left ventricular wall thickness that is proportionately greater than the increase in internal dimension, resulting in an increased thickness-to-radius ratio. At this time the left ventricular function is normal. Subsequently, with continued alcohol consumption, left ventricular dilatation progresses but wall thickening does not keep pace, yielding a thickness-to-radius ratio that is slightly decreased. Left ventricular wall stress at this stage is presumably normal or nearly normal, and systolic function is beginning to be impaired. Finally, with left ventricular failure, the enlargement of the left ventricle is markedly increased but the left ventricular thickness-to-radius ratio is decreased which results in a marked increase in left ventricular wall stress. In the second model, there are two distinct subgroups of asymptomatic subjects whose hearts respond differently to the toxic effects of alcohol. One group exhibits a mild left ventricular dilatation with a proportionately greater increase in wall thickness associated with an increased thickness-to-radius ratio, which results in a normal or reduced wall stress with resultant normal or increased percent fractional shortening. These patients may have a stable clinical course and may be relatively resistant to the toxic effects of alcohol on the heart. A second group, destined to have left ventricular decompensation with continued alcohol consumption, responds with a moderately increased left ventricular dimension and a proportionately smaller increase in wall thickness, which results in a normal or slightly decreased left ventricular thickness-to-radius ratio with the percent fractional shortening in the lower range of normal.

Other causes of congestive cardiomyopathy besides alcohol include postpartum cardiomyopathy, idiopathic cardiomyopathy, myocarditis, rheumatic heart disease, coronary artery disease, and Chagas' disease [93, 179, 180, 183–185].

M-mode echocardiography is usually adequate for the diagnosis of congestive cardiomyopathy (Fig. 9-18). Certain features such as abnormal motion of the mitral valve, aortic valve, or aorta are usually better appreciated on M-mode recording than with two-dimensional imaging. A small pericardial effusion is also very commonly found. The markedly dilated left ventricular cavity is obvious with very little change in the cavity size with systole.

Two-dimensional echocardiography provides complementary information to M-mode imaging by viewing the entire ventricle and observing the diffuse involvement of the entire chamber. Typically the only significant segmental thickening observed is in the region of the base near the mitral annulus with the entire septum, with the rest of the ventricle and the apex appearing akinetic. As a result of the marked dilatation of the left ventricle, mitral valve coaptation is realigned, resulting in closer anterior and posterior leaflet coaptation with the anterior and posterior annulus than the coaptation at a lesser angle on the ventricular side that would normally be the case (Fig. 9-19). Imaging in the apical four-chamber and the apical long axis view can provide valuable diagnostic information because some patients with congestive cardiomyopathy may have mural thrombi in the apex (Fig. 9-20). The apical four-chamber view is also valuable for demonstrating four-chamber cardiomegaly, which is present in many patients.

Benjamin and associates [186] have reported that the spectrum of hypertrophy that occurs in dilated congestive cardiomyopathy may have implications for clinical evaluation, pathophysiology, and prognosis. In their study of 30 autopsied hearts, 15 were from short-term survivors with the average duration of symptoms before death being six months; the other 15 were from long-term survivors in whom the average duration of symptoms was six years. Clinical findings consisted of the following: recent viral illness in 8, recent pregnancy in 2, alcohol abuse in 14, chest pain in 12, and diabetes mellitus in 5. The causes of death were: congestive heart failure in 10, pulmonary emboli in 8, ventricular arrhythmias in 8, sudden death in 2, and cerebrovascular accident in 2. The investigators calculated a left ventricular hypertrophy-dilatation index (average left ventricular wall thickness/maximal left ventricular cavity diameter) for the short-term and long-term survivors. They observed the hypertrophy-dilatation index to be 0.48 ± 0.19 for the normal control subjects, 0.38 ± 0.07 for patients with volume overload, 0.21 ± 0.07 for the long-term cardiomyopathy survivors, and 0.17 ± 0.07 for short-term cardiomyopathy patients. They observed that when patients were divided into those with a left ventricular diameter greater than 6 cm and those with a left ventricular diameter less than 6 cm there was no difference in the survival. An index of equal to or greater than 0.18 was more frequent in long-term survivors than in short-term survivors of congestive cardiomyopathy. No long-term survivors had an index of less than 0.14. The investigators postulated that patients with higher hypertrophy-dilatation indices are likely to tolerate cavity dilatation better, to have less wall stress, and thus decreased oxygen demand. Accordingly, in patients with idiopathic dilated congestive cardiomyopathy, cardiac function, survival, and response to therapy may be predicted by the extent of hypertrophy.

Cardiac catheterization studies have also shown that in patients with congestive cardiomyopathy, thick left ventricular walls and a large myocardial mass carry

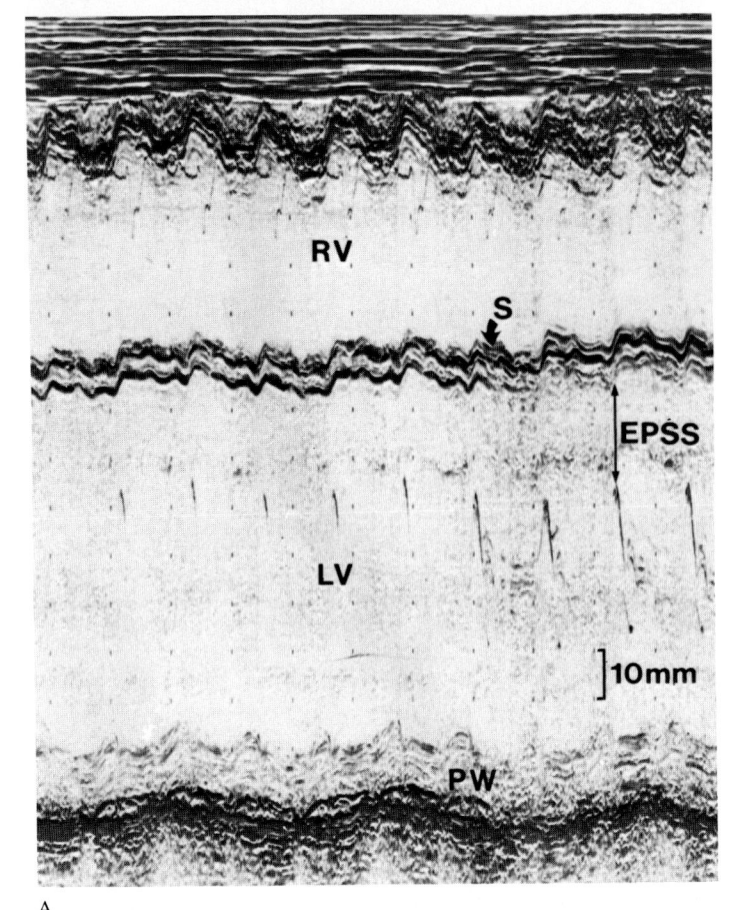

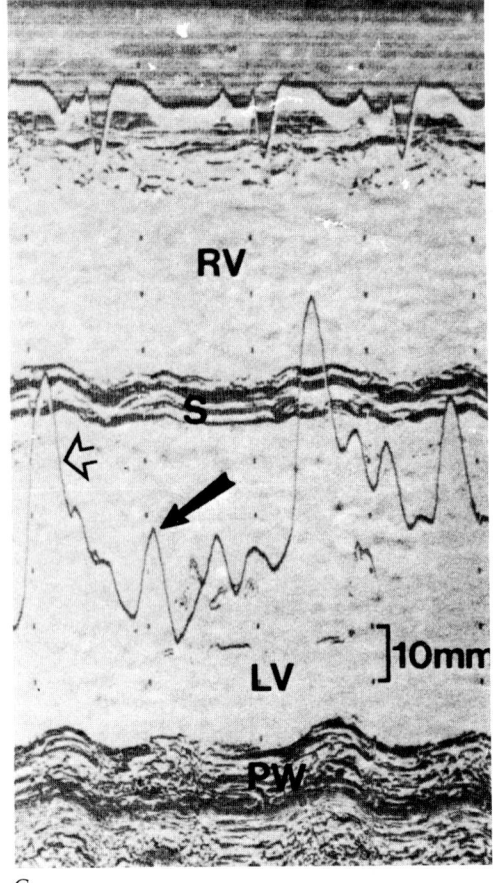

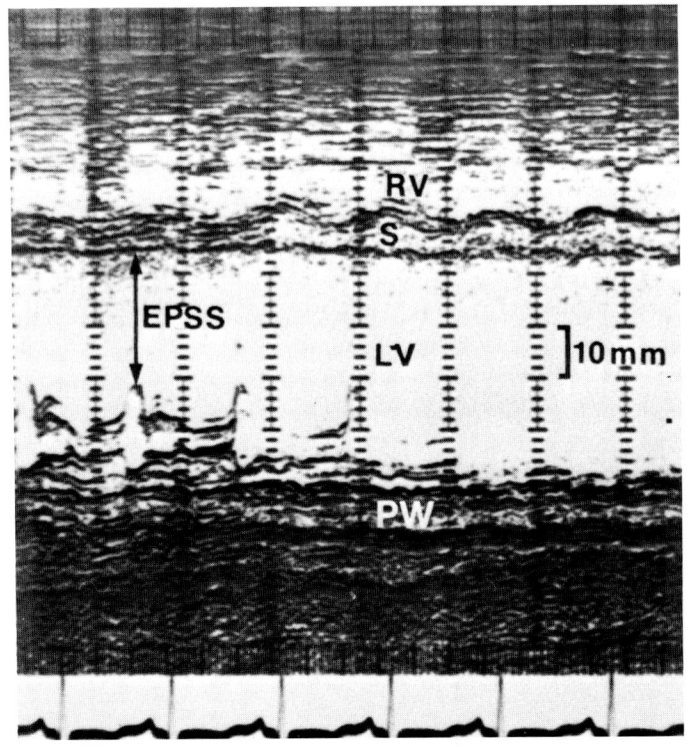

Fig. 9-18A. M-mode recording of the right ventricle and left ventricle in a patient with congestive cardiomyopathy demonstrating diffusely poor wall motion of both septum and posterior wall (PW), dilated LV, and abnormal E-point septal separation (EPSS) owing to poor global function. B. M-mode recording from a young woman with postpartum cardiomyopathy demonstrating an EPSS of 26 mm consistent with a markedly reduced ejection fraction; both septum and posterior wall appear essentially akinetic in this view; however, left ventricular size is still normal. C. M-mode recording in a patient with congestive cardiomyopathy demonstrating mild left ventricular dilatation (EDD = 58 mm), akinetic and mildly paradoxical septum, and severe hypokinesis of the posterior wall and very poor global function of the LV. Simultaneous carotid artery pulse recording (open arrow) shows pulsus alternans (solid arrow).

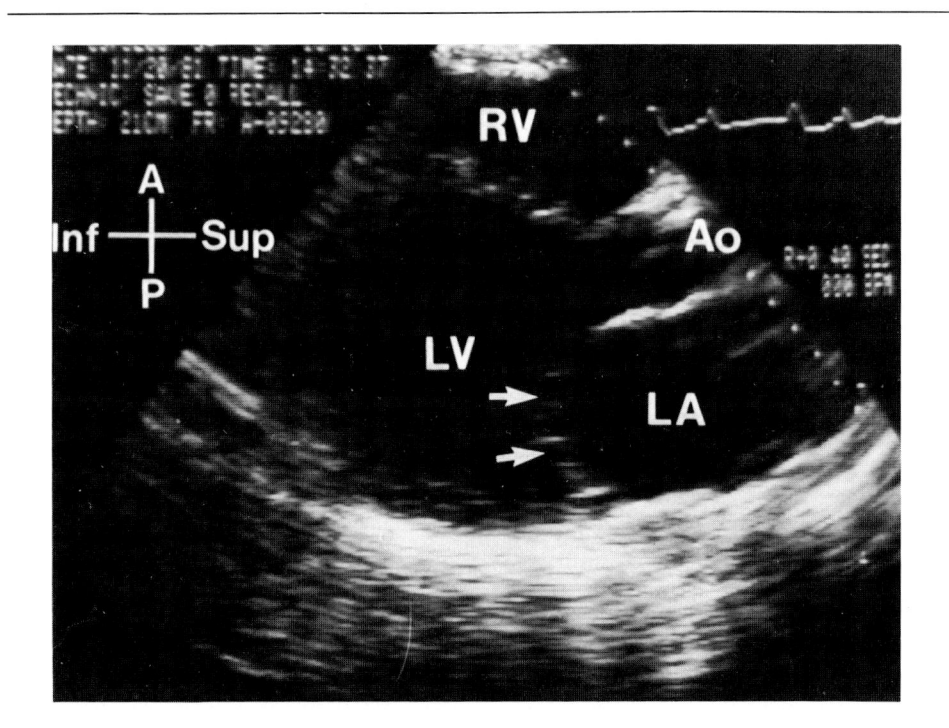

Fig. 9-19. Parasternal long axis view of a dilated left ventricle, normal LV wall thickness, and straightened alignment of mitral valve (arrows) during systole, typical features of a congestive cardiomyopathy. Left atrial enlargement is present.

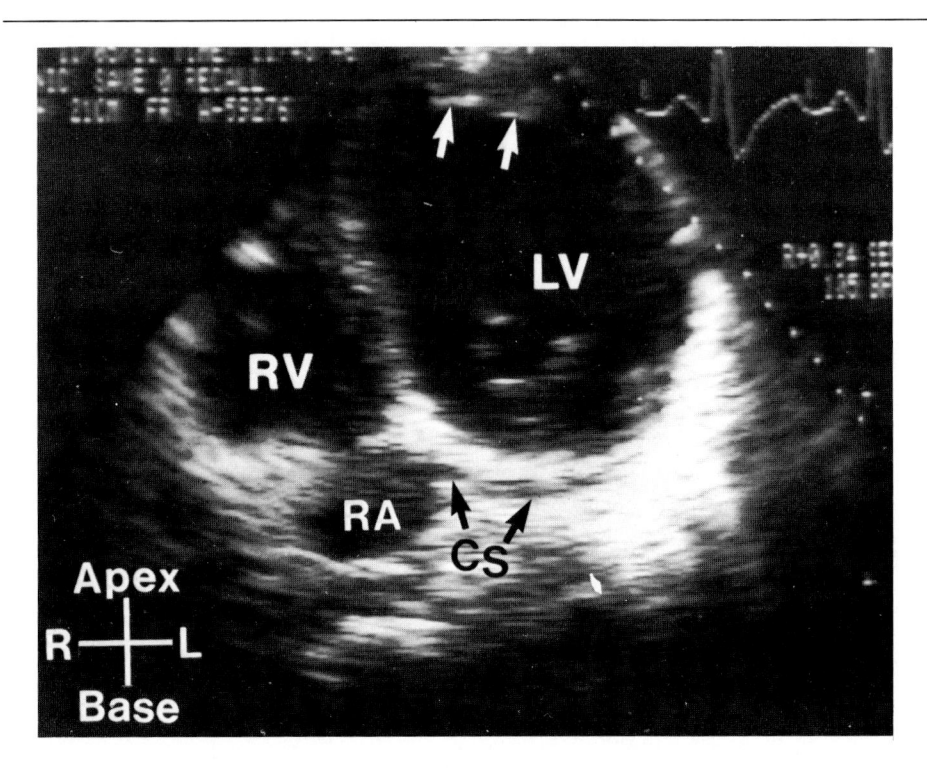

Fig. 9-20. Apical 4-chamber view with slight posterior angulation of the transducer in a patient with a dilated congestive cardiomyopathy and mural thrombus (white arrows) in the left ventricular apex.

a more favorable prognosis [187, 188]. Benjamin and colleagues [186] found no difference in the left ventricular volume or left ventricular dimensions in the short-term and long-term survivors whereas left ventricular wall thickness averaged 1 cm in the short-term survivors compared to 1.3 cm in the long-term survivors; the heart weight averaged 540 gm in the short-term survivors compared to 759 gm in the long-term survivors.

Restrictive or infiltrative cardiomyopathy. Restrictive cardiomyopathy is a form of myocardial disease that may simulate constrictive pericarditis. Restrictive cardiomyopathy may be idiopathic or it may be secondary to disease processes such as amyloidosis or hemochromatosis. In this disease an abnormal infiltrate and/or fibrosis of the myocardium or endocardium restricts the cardiac size, limits ventricular filling, and alters diastolic compliance.

In addition to amyloidosis and hemochromatosis, other etiologies include sarcoidosis, Loeffler's eosinophilic endomyocardial disease, and endomyocardial fibrosis [189]. Except for hemochromatosis the other conditions have no known specific therapy and are associated with progressive deterioration and poor prognosis.

In the United States restrictive cardiomyopathy is rare; however, in Africa where it is a common cause of death, an important cause of restrictive cardiomyopathy is endomyocardial fibrosis [190].

The hemodynamic pattern of restrictive cardiomyopathy is characterized by an elevated filling pressure in the ventricles associated with normal or nearly normal systolic function. Ventricular pressure declines significantly at the onset of diastole and then rises abruptly and rapidly in early diastole, producing a dip-and-plateau filling pattern in the ventricular diastolic pressure tracing that is manifested in the atrial pressure tracing as a prominent Y descent followed by a rapid rise and plateau. This rapid rise and abrupt plateau give rise to the "square root," in which both right and left ventricular diastolic pressures may be superimposable on or within 3 to 4 mm of one another when simultaneously recorded. The hemodynamic findings may closely simulate constrictive pericarditis [191, 192].

Benotti and colleagues [193] reported a study of nine patients with restrictive hemodynamic features who had symptoms of left and/or right ventricular failure, chest pain in the absence of any significant coronary artery disease, and/or symptoms from atrial arrhythmias. They found echocardiographic evidence of various degrees of left ventricular wall thickening but no significant pericardial effusion, pericardial thickening, or calcification. The common pathophysiologic feature for this syndrome appears to be a reduced ventricular compliance; however, the etiology in many cases remains unclear. It appears that when restrictive cardiomyopathy is associated with a specific infiltrative or fibrotic process it carries a worse prognosis [189, 194].

Borer and associates [195] evaluated 19 patients with one of various systemic infiltrative diseases: 4 with systemic amyloidosis, 10 with idiopathic hypereosinophilia, and 5 with iron overload. Among these 19 patients 10 had no clinical evidence of cardiac disease, but all 19 subjects had echocardiographic abnormalities. The left ventricle was symmetrically thickened and left ventricular mass was increased in all, the left ventricular internal dimension was slightly increased (>52 mm) in 5 patients, and evidence of reduced compliance was present in 5 patients. Ejection fraction was normal in 18 of the 19 patients.

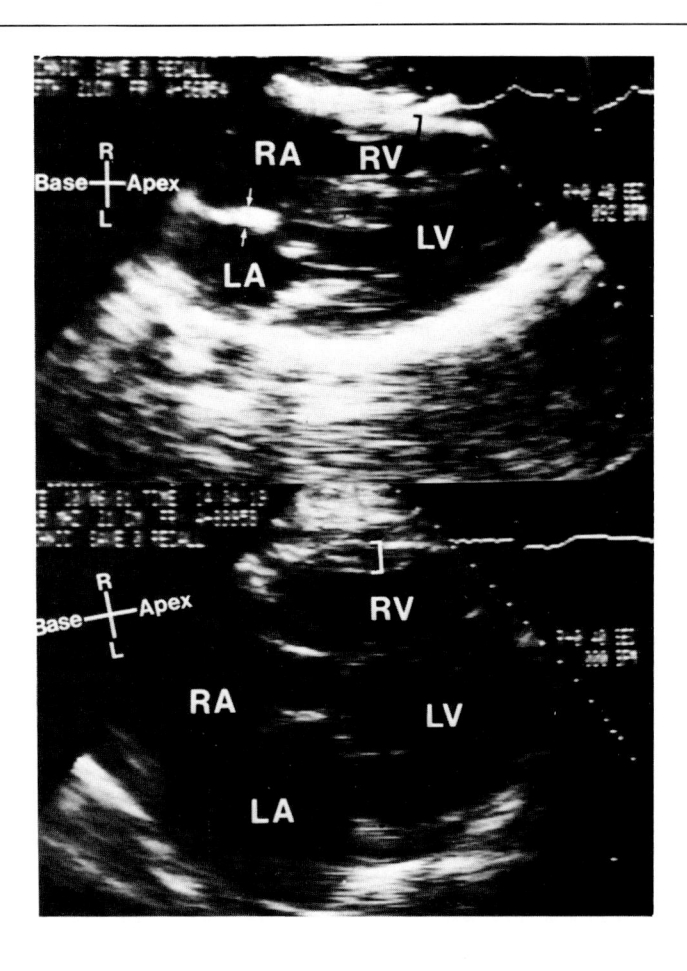

Fig. 9-21. Subcostal 4-chamber views from two patients with confirmed amyloid heart disease (upper panel) and possible amyloid heart disease (lower panel). Significant findings in upper panel include concentric hypertrophy of the left ventricle, poor LV function; increased thickness of right ventricular free wall (bracket), and bright reflectance and increased thickness of interatrial septum (arrows). Patient in lower panel suffers from right- and left-sided heart failure, has only mild LV hypertrophy with diffuse hypokinesis, enlargement of both right atrium and left atrium, and marked increase in the thickness of the RV free wall.

Tyberg and associates [196] showed a significantly different profile of diastolic left ventricular filling volume and rate curves during the first half of diastole in patients with restrictive cardiomyopathy and those with constrictive pericarditis. Analysis of the left ventricular filling rate during the first half of diastole revealed significant differences in patients with restrictive amyloid cardiomyopathy or constrictive pericarditis, and normal subjects: those with restrictive amyloid cardiomyopathy had 45 percent, those with constrictive pericarditis had 85 percent, and normal subjects had 65 percent of left ventricular filling completed during the first 50 percent of diastole.

Siqueira-Filho and associates [197] studied 28 patients with cardiac amyloidosis by echocardiography, all of whom had heart failure and biopsy-proven amyloidosis. The echocardiographic features in this study included the following: (1) normal left ventricular dimension in all; (2) thickened ventricular septum (88%), left ventricular posterior wall (77%), and right ventricular anterior wall (79%); (3) decreased systolic thickening of the ventricular septum (96%) and of the left ventricular posterior wall (65%) and reduced left ventricular global function in 62%; (4) left atrial enlargement (50%); and (5) pericardial effusion (58%). The investigators found that two-dimensional echocardiography provided the following additional information: thickened papillary muscles (5 of 13); thickened valves (4 of 13); improved evaluation of thickened right ventricular wall; and a characteristic granular sparkling appearance of the thickened cardiac walls, presumably secondary to the amyloid deposit, could be appreciated in 12 of 13 patients. The investigators believe that in an older patient with unexplained congestive heart failure, two-dimensional echocardiographic findings of thickened right and left ventricular myocardium, normal left ventricular cavity dimension, and a diffuse hyper-refractive granular sparkling appearance are virtually diagnostic of amyloid heart disease. Child and associates [198] further emphasized the importance of recognizing the increased right ventricular wall thickness as a diagnostic marker of amyloid infiltrative cardiomyopathy (Fig. 9-21). Another characteristic finding which has been recognized by two-dimensional echocardiography in these patients is hypertrophy of the interatrial septum, which is best detected by subcostal imaging [199].

Endomyocardial fibrosis. Patients with endomyocardial fibrosis may have a primary congestive cardiomyopathy or a restrictive form of cardiomyopathy with abnormal filling characteristics [194, 200]. Hess and colleagues [200] demonstrated abnormal thickening of the anterior right ventricular wall as well as dense echoes from the posterior left ventricular endocardial wall. Following surgical removal of the fibrous tissue, the right ventricular wall thickness was markedly reduced, and the size of the right ventricular cavity was increased. Also, the left ventricular cavity was increased in size postoperatively following the removal of some of the fibrous tissue on the surface of the left ventricular endocardium.

The distribution of fibrous tissue in this condition is not necessarily uniform throughout the heart; Eterovic and coworkers [201] reported successful surgical removal of an obliterative restrictive form of endomyocardial fibrosis in the apex of the left ventricle.

Acquatella and associates [202] reported that some patients with chronic Chagas' heart disease had echocardiographic features indistinguishable from those of a congestive cardiomyopathy; however, in the majority, a characteristic apical abnormality was observed with involvement of the posteroinferior left ventricular wall and relative sparing of the interventricular septum. These investigators observed that two-dimensional echocardiography was valuable for detecting early changes of the left ventricular apex in asymptomatic patients. Although Chagas' heart disease does not occur in the United States, it is a significant public health problem in South America, where it is estimated that more than 10 million people are afflicted [202].

Puigbo and colleagues [203] found the most characteristic 2-D echocardiographic finding in endomyocardial fibrosis to be obliteration of the right and/or left ventricular apices by echogenic material that behaved as a specular reflector near its endocardial border. In their study of seven patients they observed the noninvolved basal ventricular cavity to be significantly reduced in size, and most of the noninvolved ventricular walls and septum were hyperdynamic.

References

1. Teare RD: Asymmetrical hypertrophy of the heart in young adults. *Br Heart J* 20:1, 1958
2. Maron BJ, Epstein SE: Hypertrophic cardiomyopathy: A discussion of nomenclature. *Am J Cardiol* 43:1242, 1979
3. Braunwald E, Morrow AG, Cornell WP, Aygen MM, Hilbish TF: Idiopathic hypertrophic subaortic stenosis: Clinical, hemodynamic and angiographic manifestations. *Am J Med* 29:924, 1960
4. Braunwald E, Lambrew CT, Rockoff SF, Ross J Jr, Morrow AG: Idiopathic hypertrophic subaortic stenosis. I. A description of the disease based upon an analysis of 64 patients. *Circulation* 30(Suppl IV):IV-3, 1964
5. Cohen J, Effat H, Goodwin JF, Oakley CM, Steiner RE: Hypertrophic obstructive cardiomyopathy. *Br Heart J* 26:16, 1964
6. Goodwin JF: Congestive and hypertrophic cardiomyopathies: A decade of study. *Lancet* 1:731, 1970
7. Goodwin JF, Oakley CM: The cardiomyopathies. *Br Heart J* 34:545, 1972
8. Wigle ED, Heimbecker RO, Gunton RW: Idiopathic ventricular septal hypertrophy causing muscular subaortic stenosis. *Circulation* 26:325, 1962
9. Moreyra E, Klein JJ, Shimada H, Segal BL: Idiopathic hypertrophic subaortic stenosis diagnosed by reflected ultrasound. *Am J Cardiol* 23:32, 1969
10. Shah PM, Gramiak R, Kramer DH: Ultrasound localization of left ventricular outflow obstruction in hypertrophic obstructive cardiomyopathy. *Circulation* 40:3, 1969
11. Abbasi AS, MacAlpin RN, Eber LM, Pearce ML: Echocardiographic diagnosis of idiopathic hypertrophic cardiomyopathy without outflow obstruction. *Circulation* 46:897, 1972
12. Henry WL, Clark CE, Epstein SE: Asymmetric septal hypertrophy: Echocardiographic identification of the pathognomonic anatomic abnormality of IHSS. *Circulation* 47:225, 1973
13. Henry WL, Clark CE, Epstein SE: Asymmetric septal hypertrophy (ASH): The unifying link in the IHSS disease spectrum. Observations regarding its pathogenesis, pathophysiology, and course. *Circulation* 47:827, 1973
14. Tajik AJ, Giuliani ER: Echocardiographic observations in idiopathic hypertrophic subaortic stenosis. *Mayo Clin Proc* 49:89, 1974
15. Henry WL, Clark CE, Roberts WC, Morrow AG, Epstein SE: Differences in distribution of myocardial abnormalities in patients with obstructive and nonobstructive asymmetric septal hypertrophy (ASH): Echocardiographic and gross anatomic findings. *Circulation* 50:447, 1974
16. Rossen RM, Goodman DJ, Ingham RE, Popp RL: Echocardiographic criteria in the diagnosis of idiopathic hypertrophic subaortic stenosis. *Circulation* 50:747, 1974
17. Abbasi AS, MacAlpin RN, Eber LM, Pearce ML: Left ventricular hypertrophy diagnosed by echocardiography. *N Engl J Med* 289:118, 1973
18. Clark CE, Henry WL, Epstein SE: Familial prevalence and genetic transmission of idiopathic hypertrophic subaortic stenosis. *N Engl J Med* 289:709, 1973
19. van Dorp WG, ten Cate FJ, Vletter WB, Dohmen H, Roelandt J: Familial prevalence of asymmetric septal hypertrophy. *Eur J Cardiol* 4:349, 1976
20. Bjork VO: Discussion on RJ Linden's Related Physiology of Cardiac Contraction. In GEW Wolstenholme and M O'Connor (eds), *Cardiomyopathies* (Ciba Symposium). London: Churchill, 1970
21. Dinsmore RE, Sanders CA, Harthorne JW: Mitral regurgitation in idiopathic hypertrophic subaortic stenosis. *N Engl J Med* 275:1225, 1966
22. Simon AL, Ross J Jr, Gault JH: Angiographic anatomy of the left ventricle and mitral valve in idiopathic subaortic stenosis. *Circulation* 36:852, 1967
23. Popp RL, Harrison DC: Ultrasound in the diagnosis and evaluation of therapy of idiopathic hypertrophic subaortic stenosis. *Circulation* 40:905, 1969
24. Pridie RB, Oakley CM: Mechanism of mitral regurgitation in hypertrophic obstructive cardiomyopathy. *Br Heart J* 32:203, 1970
25. Gramiak R, Shah PM, Kramer DH: Ultrasound cardiography: Contrast studies in anatomy and function. *Radiology* 92:939, 1969

26. Hansen PF, Davidsen AG, Fabricius J: Subvalvular aortic stenosis of muscular type. *Acta Med Scand* 171:743, 1962
27. Goodwin JF: Cardiac function in primary myocardial disorders. Part I. *Br Med J* 1:1527, 1964
28. Wigle ED: Muscular Subaortic Stenosis: The Clinical Syndrome, with Additional Evidence of Ventricular Septal Hypertrophy. In GEW Wolstenholme and M O'Connor (eds), *Cardiomyopathies* (Ciba Symposium). London: Churchill, 1970
29. Feizi O, Emanuel R: Echocardiographic spectrum of hypertrophic cardiomyopathy. *Br Heart J* 37:1286, 1975
30. Maron BJ, Epstein SE: Hypertrophic cardiomyopathy. Recent observations regarding the specificity of three hallmarks of the disease: Asymmetric septal hypertrophy, septal disorganization and systolic anterior motion of the anterior mitral leaflet. *Am J Cardiol* 45:141, 1980
31. Maron BJ, Clark CE, Henry WL, Fukuda T, Edwards JE, Mathews EC, Redwood DR, Epstein SE: Prevalence and characteristics of disproportionate ventricular septal thickening in patients with acquired or congenital heart diseases: Echocardiographic and morphologic findings. *Circulation* 55:489, 1977
32. Maron BJ, Edwards JE, Epstein SE: Disproportionate ventricular septal thickening in patients with systemic hypertension. *Chest* 73:466, 1978
33. Maron BJ, Savage DD, Clark CE, Henry WL, Vlodaver Z, Edwards JE, Epstein SE: Prevalence and characteristics of disproportionate ventricular septal thickening in patients with coronary artery disease. *Circulation* 57:250, 1978
34. Maron BJ, Edwards JE, Moller JH, Epstein SE: Prevalence and characteristics of disproportionate ventricular septal thickening in infants with congenital heart disease. *Circulation* 59:126, 1979
35. Bulkley BH, Weisfeldt ML, Hutchins GM: Isometric cardiac contraction: A possible cause of the disorganized myocardial pattern of idiopathic hypertrophic subaortic stenosis. *N Engl J Med* 296:135, 1977
36. Bulkley BH, Weisfeldt ML, Hutchins GM: Asymmetric septal hypertrophy and myocardial fiber disarray: Features of normal, developing and malformed hearts. *Circulation* 56:292, 1977
37. van der Bel-Kahn J: Muscle fiber disarray in common heart diseases. *Am J Cardiol* 40:355, 1977
38. Maron BJ, Roberts WC: Quantitative analysis of cardiac muscle cell disorganization in the ventricular septum of patients with hypertrophic cardiomyopathy. *Circulation* 59:689, 1979
39. Ferrans VJ, Morrow AG, Roberts WC: Myocardial ultrastructure in idiopathic hypertrophic subaortic stenosis: A study of operatively excised left ventricular outflow tract muscle in 14 patients. *Circulation* 45:769, 1972
40. Adomian GE, Beazell JW, Furmanski M, Tan KS, Laks MM: The production of myofibrillar disarray in hearts of normal dogs produced by chronic electronic pacing. *Circulation* 56(Suppl III)III-205, 1977
41. Knieriem HJ: Electron-Microscopic Findings in Congestive Cardiomyopathy. In M Kaltenbach, F Loogen, EGJ Olsen (eds), *Cardiomyopathy and Myocardial Biopsy*. Berlin: Springer, 1978, p 71
42. Adelman AG, McLoughlin MJ, Marquis Y, Auger P, Wigle ED: Left ventricular cineangiographic observations in muscular subaortic stenosis. *Am J Cardiol* 24:689, 1969
43. Henry WL, Clark CE, Glancy DL, Epstein SE: Echocardiographic measurement of the left ventricular outflow gradient in idiopathic hypertrophic subaortic stenosis. *N Engl J Med* 288:989, 1973
44. King JF, DeMaria AN, Reis RL, Bolton MR, Dunn MI, Mason DT: Echocardiographic assessment of idiopathic hypertrophic subaortic stenosis. *Chest* 64:723, 1973
45. Criley JM, Lennon PA, Abbasi AS, Blaufuss AH: Hypertrophic Cardiomyopathy. In HJ Levine (ed), *Clinical Cardiovascular Physiology*. New York: Grune & Stratton, 1976. P 771
46. Shah PM, Gramiak R, Adelman AG, Wigle ED: Role of echocardiography in diagnostic and hemodynamic assessment of hypertrophic subaortic stenosis. *Circulation* 44:891, 1971
47. King JF, DeMaria AN, Miller RR, Hilliard GK, Zelis, R, Mason DT: Markedly abnormal mitral valve motion without simultaneous intraventricular pressure gradient due to un-

even mitral septal contact in idiopathic hypertrophic subaortic stenosis. *Am J Cardiol* 34:360, 1974
48. Mintz GS, Kotler MN, Segal BL, Parry WR: Systolic anterior motion of the mitral valve in the absence of asymmetric septal hypertrophy. *Circulation* 57:256, 1978
49. Boughner DR, Rakowski H, Wigle D: Mitral valve systolic anterior motion in the absence of hypertrophic cardiomyopathy. *Circulation* 57:256, 1978
50. Maron BJ, Gottdiener JS, Roberts WC, Henry WL, Savage DD, Epstein SE: Left ventricular outflow tract obstruction due to systolic anterior motion of the anterior mitral leaflet in patients with concentric left ventricular hypertrophy. *Circulation* 57:527, 1978
51. Come PC, Bulkley BH, Goodman ZD, Hutchins GM, Pitt B, Fortuin NJ: Hypercontractile cardiac states simulating hypertrophic cardiomyopathy. *Circulation* 55:901, 1977
52. Chahine RA, Raizner AE, Ishimori T, Montero AC: Echocardiographic, haemodynamic and angiographic correlations in hypertrophic cardiomyopathy. *Br Heart J* 39:945, 1977
53. Maron BJ, Verter J: Disproportionate ventricular septal thickening in the developing normal human heart. *Circulation* 57:520, 1978
54. Maron BJ, Edwards JE, Henry WL, Clark CE, Bingle GJ, Epstein SE: Asymmetric septal hypertrophy (ASH) in infancy. *Circulation* 50:809, 1974
55. Maron BJ, Henry WL, Clark CE, Redwood DR, Roberts WC, Epstein SE: Asymmetric septal hypertrophy in childhood. *Circulation* 53:9, 1976
56. Gilbert BW, Pollick C, Adelman AG, Wigle ED: Hypertrophic cardiomyopathy: Subclassification by M-mode echocardiography. *Am J Cardiol* 45:861, 1980
57. Maron BJ, Gottdiener JS, Bonow RO, Epstein SE: Hypertrophic cardiomyopathy with unusual locations of left ventricular hypertrophy undetectable by M-mode echocardiography: Identification by wide-angle two-dimensional echocardiography. *Circulation* 63:409, 1981
58. Henry WL, Clark CE, Griffith JM, Epstein SE: Mechanism of left ventricular outflow obstruction in patients with obstructive asymmetric septal hypertrophy (idiopathic hypertrophic subaortic stenosis). *Am J Cardiol* 35:337, 1975
59. Rakowski H, Gilbert BW, Drobac M, Pollick C, Boughner D, Wigle ED: Obstructive versus nonobstructive SAM: A crucial distinction. *Am J Cardiol* 45:491, 1980
60. Shah PM, Taylor RD, Wong M: Abnormal mitral valve coaptation in hypertrophic obstructive cardiomyopathy: A proposed role in systolic anterior motion of mitral valve. *Am J Cardiol* 48:258, 1981
61. Martin RP, Rakowski H, French J, Popp RL: Idiopathic hypertrophic subaortic stenosis viewed by wide-angle, phased-array echocardiography. *Circulation* 59:1206, 1979
62. Cohen MV, Cooperman LB, Rosenblum R: Regional myocardial function in idiopathic hypertrophic subaortic stenosis: An echocardiographic study. *Circulation* 52:842, 1975
63. Quinones MA, Gaasch WH, Alexander JK: Echocardiographic assessment of left ventricular function: With special reference to normalized velocities. *Circulation* 50:42, 1974
64. Cooper RH, O'Rourke RA, Karliner JS, Peterson KL, Leopold GR: Comparison of ultrasound and cineangiographic measurements of the mean rate of circumferential fiber shortening in man. *Circulation* 46:914, 1972
65. Rossen RM, Goodman DJ, Ingham RE, Popp RL: Ventricular systolic thickening and excursion in idiopathic hypertrophic subaortic stenosis. *N Engl J Med* 291:1317, 1974
66. Maron BJ, Ferrans VJ, Henry WL, Clark CE, Redwood DR, Roberts WC, Morrow AG, Epstein SE: Differences in distribution of myocardial abnormalities in patients with obstructive and nonobstructive asymmetric septal hypertrophy (ASH): Light and electron microscopic findings. *Circulation* 50:436, 1974
67. Shah PM, Taylor RD, Hecht HS, Wong M: Asymmetric left ventricular hypertrophy—a study of anatomy and function by cross-sectional echocardiography and radionuclide angiography. *Am J Cardiol* 45:491, 1980
68. Hutchins GM, Bulkley BH: Catenoid shape of the interventricular septum: Possible cause of idiopathic hypertrophic subaortic stenosis. *Circulation* 58:392, 1978
69. St. John Sutton MG, Tajik AJ, Gibson DG, Brown DJ, Seward JB, Giuliani ER: Echocardiographic assessment of left ventricular filling and septal and posterior wall dynamics in idiopathic hypertrophic subaortic stenosis. *Circulation* 57:512, 1978
70. Hardarson T, de la Calzada CS, Curiel R, Goodwin JF: Prognosis and mortality of hypertrophic obstructive cardiomyopathy. *Lancet* 2:1462, 1973
71. Swan DA, Bell B, Oakley CM, Goodwin J: Analysis of symptomatic course and prognosis and treatment of hypertrophic obstructive cardiomyopathy. *Br Heart J* 33:671, 1971

72. Coltart DJ: The electrophysiological and contractile responses of hypertrophic cardiomyopathic myocardium. *Postgrad Med J* 48:763, 1972
73. Criley JM, Lennon PA, Abbasi AS, Blaufuss AH: Hypertrophic Cardiomyopathy. In HJ Levine (ed), *Clinical Cardiovascular Physiology*. New York: Grune & Stratton, 1976. P 795
74. Joye J, DeMaria AN, Neumann A, Miller RR, Vismara LA, Mason DT: Electrocardiographic abnormalities in hypertrophic cardiomyopathy: Relation to cardiac hypertrophy and intraventricular obstruction. *Circulation* 54(Suppl II):II-209, 1976
75. Halpern SW, Mandel WJ, Allen HN, Kraus R, Charuzi Y: Disparity between echocardiographic and electrocardiographic findings in asymmetric septal hypertrophy. *Clin Res* 25:89A, 1977
76. Savage DD, Seides SF, Clark CE, Henry WL, Maron BJ, Robinson FC, Epstein SE: Electrocardiographic findings in patients with obstructive and nonobstructive hypertrophic cardiomyopathy. *Circulation* 58:402, 1978
77. Goodwin JF, Hollman A, Cleland WP, Teare D: Obstructive cardiomyopathy simulating aortic stenosis. *Br Heart J* 22:403, 1960
78. Maron BJ, Lipson LC, Roberts WC, Savage DD, Epstein SE: "Malignant" hypertrophic cardiomyopathy: Identification of a subgroup of families with unusually frequent premature death. *Am J Cardiol* 41:1133, 1978
79. Maron BJ, Gottdiener JS, Epstein SE: Patterns and significance of distribution of left ventricular hypertrophy in hypertrophic cardiomyopathy: A wide angle, two dimensional echocardiographic study of 125 patients. *Am J Cardiol* 48:418, 1981
80. DeMaria A, Bommer W, Lee G, Mason DT: Value and limitations of two dimensional echocardiography in assessment of cardiomyopathy. *Am J Cardiol* 46:1224, 1980
81. Allen JW, Kim SJ, Edmiston WA, VenKataraman K: Problems in ultrasonic estimates of septal thickness. *Am J Cardiol* 42:89, 1978
82. Chahine RA, Raizner AE, Nelson J, Winters WL Jr, Miller RR, Luchi RJ: Mid systolic closure of aortic valve in hypertrophic cardiomyopathy: Echocardiographic and angiographic correlation. *Am J Cardiol* 43:17, 1979
83. Doi YL, McKenna WJ, Gehrke J, Oakley CM, Goodwin JF: M mode echocardiography in hypertrophic cardiomyopathy: Diagnostic criteria and prediction of obstruction. *Am J Cardiol* 45:6, 1980
84. Hernandez RR, Greenfield JC, McCall BW: Pressure-flow studies in hypertrophic subaortic stenosis. *J Clin Invest* 43:401, 1964
85. Joyner CR, Harrison FS, Gruber JW: Diagnosis of hypertrophic subaortic stenosis with a Doppler velocity flow detector. *Ann Intern Med* 74:692, 1971
86. Boughner DR, Schuld RL, Persaud JA: Hypertrophic obstructive cardiomyopathy: Assessment by echocardiographic and Doppler ultrasound techniques. *Br Heart J* 37:917, 1975
87. Chandraratna PAN, Chu W, Schechter E, Langevin E: Hemodynamic correlates of echocardiographic aortic root motion: Observations on normal subjects and patients with idiopathic hypertrophic subaortic stenosis. *Chest* 74:183, 1978
88. Hsu HP: *Fourier Analysis*. New York: Simon and Schuster, 1970
89. Djalaly A, Schiller NB, Poehlmann HW, Arnold S, Gertz EW: Diastolic aortic root motion in left ventricular hypertrophy. *Chest* 79:442, 1981
90. Strunk BL, Fitzgerald JW, Lipton M, Popp RL, Barry WH: The posterior aortic wall echocardiogram: Its relationship to left atrial volume change. *Circulation* 54:744, 1976
91. Yamaguchi H, Ishimura T, Nishiyama S, Nagasaki F, Nakanishi S, Takatsu F, Nishijo T, Umeda T, Machii K: Hypertrophic nonobstructive cardiomyopathy with giant negative T waves (apical hypertrophy): Ventriculographic and echocardiographic features in 30 patients. *Am J Cardiol* 44:401, 1979
92. Nishiyama S, Yamaguchi H, Ishimura T, Nagasaki F, Takatsu F, Umeda T, Machi K: Echocardiographic features of apical hypertrophic cardiomyopathy. *J Cardiography* 8:177, 1978
93. Hagan AD: Evaluation of Hypertrophic and Congestive Cardiomyopathies by M-mode and Two-dimensional Echocardiography. In DT Mason (ed), *Advances in Heart Diseases* (Vol. 3). New York: Grune & Stratton, 1980. Pp 673–695
94. Rees A, Elbl F, Minhas K, Solinger R: Echocardiographic evidence of outflow tract obstruction in Pompe's Disease (glycogen storage disease of the heart). *Am J Cardiol* 37:1103, 1976

95. Cooperberg P, Hazell S, Ashmore PG: Parachute accessory anterior mitral valve leaflet causing left ventricular outflow tract obstruction: Report of a case with emphasis on the echocardiographic findings. *Circulation* 53:908, 1976
96. Mintz GS, Kotler MN, Segal BL, Parry WR: Systolic anterior motion of the mitral valve in the absence of asymmetric septal hypertrophy. *Circulation* 57:256, 1978
97. Henning H, O'Rourke RA, Crawford MH, Righetti A, Karliner JS: Inferior myocardial infarction as a cause of asymmetric septal hypertrophy: An echocardiographic study. *Am J Cardiol* 41:817, 1978
98. Stern A, Kessler KM, Hammer WJ, Kreulen TH, Spann JF: Septal-free wall disproportion in inferior infarction: The echocardiographic differentiation from hypertrophic cardiomyopathy. *Circulation* 58:700, 1978
99. Menapace FJ, Hammer WJ, Kessler KK, Ritzer T, Bove AA, Warner HH, Spann JF: Echocardiographic measurements of left ventricular wall thickness in weight lifters: A problem with the definition of ASH. *Am J Cardiol* 39:276, 1977
100. Goodman DJ, Rossen RM, Popp RL: Echocardiographic pseudo idiopathic hypertrophic subaortic stenosis. *Chest* 66:573, 1974
101. Isner JM, Falcone MW, Virmani R, Roberts WC: Cardiac sarcoma causing "ASH" and simulating coronary heart disease. *Am J Med* 66:1025, 1979
102. Cabin HS, Costello RM, Vasudevan G, Maron BJ, Roberts WC: Cardiac lymphoma mimicking hypertrophic cardiomyopathy. *Am Heart J* 102:466, 1981
103. Tajik AJ, Gau GT, Schattenberg TT: Echocardiographic "pseudo-IHSS" pattern in atrial septal defect. *Chest* 62:324, 1972
104. Erdin RA, Abdulla AM, Stefadouros MA: Hypercontractile cardiac state mimicking hypertrophic subaortic stenosis. *Cathet Cardiovasc Diagn* 7:71, 1981
105. Wei JY, Weiss JL, Bulkley BH: The heterogeneity of hypertrophic cardiomyopathy: An autopsy and one dimensional echocardiographic study. *Am J Cardiol* 45:24, 1980
106. ten Cate FJ, Hugenholtz PG, van Dorp WG, Roelandt J: Prevalence of diagnostic abnormalities in patients with genetically transmitted asymmetric septal hypertrophy. *Am J Cardiol* 43:731, 1979
107. Cohen A, Hagan AD, Watkins J, Mitas J, Schvartzman M, Mazzoleni A, Cohen IM, Warren SE, Vieweg WVR: Clinical correlates in hypertensive patients with left ventricular hypertrophy diagnosed with echocardiography. *Am J Cardiol* 47:335, 1981
108. Dunn FG, Chandraratna P, deCarvalho JG, Basta LL, Frohlich ED: Pathophysiologic assessment of hypertensive heart disease with echocardiography. *Am J Cardiol* 39:789, 1977
109. Savage DD, Drayer JIM, Henry WL, Mathews EC Jr, Ware JH, Gardin JM, Cohen ER, Epstein SE, Laragh JH: Echocardiographic assessment of cardiac anatomy and function in hypertensive subjects. *Circulation* 59:623, 1979
110. Safar ME, Lehner JP, Vincent MI, Plainfosse MT, Simon ACH: Echocardiographic dimensions in borderline and sustained hypertension. *Am J Cardiol* 44:930, 1979
111. Toshima H, Koga Y, Yoshioka H, Ayiyoshi T, Kimura N: Echocardiographic classification of hypertensive heart disease: A correlative study with clinical features. *Jpn Heart J* 16:377, 1975
112. Criley JM, Blaufuss AH, Abbasi AS: Nonobstructive IHSS. *Circulation* 52:963, 1975
113. Kansal S, Roitman D, Sheffield LT: Interventricular septal thickness and left ventricular hypertrophy: An echocardiographic study. *Circulation* 60:1058, 1979
114. Greenwald J, Yap JF, Franklin M, Lichtman AM: Echocardiographic mitral systolic motion in left ventricular aneurysm. *Br Heart J* 37:684, 1975
115. Feigenbaum H: *Echocardiography* (3rd ed). Philadelphia: Lea & Febiger, 1981. P 462
116. Gattiker HF, Davignon A, Bozio A, Batlle-Diaz J, Geoffroy G, Lemieux B, Barbeau A: Echocardiographic findings in Friedreich's ataxia. *Can J Neurol Sci* 3:329, 1976
117. Way GL, Ruttenberg HD, Eshaghpour E, Nora JJ, Wolfe RR: Hypertrophic obstructive cardiomyopathy in infants of diabetic mothers. *Circulation* 54(Suppl II):II-105, 1976
118. Nanda NC, Gramiak R, Manning JA, Lipchik EO: Echocardiographic features of subpulmonic obstruction in dextrotransposition of the great vessels. *Circulation* 51:515, 1975
119. Bulkley BH, Fortuin NJ: Systolic anterior motion of the mitral valve without asymmetric septal hypertrophy. *Chest* 69:694, 1976
120. Hearne MJ, Sherber HS, deLeon AD: Asymmetric septal hypertrophy in acromegaly—an echocardiographic study. *Circulation* 52(Suppl II):II-35, 1975

121. Gardin JM, Stephanides LM, Kordecki S, Talano JV: Systolic anterior motion in the absence of asymmetrical septal hypertrophy: A buckling phenomenon of the chordae tendineae. *Circulation* 58(Suppl II):II-121, 1978
122. Rakowski H, Gilbert BW, Drobac M, Pollick C, Boughner D, Wigle ED: Obstructive versus non-obstructive SAM: A crucial distinction. *Am J Cardiol* 45:491, 1980
123. Marcus FI, Westura EE, Summa J: The hemodynamic effect of the Valsalva maneuver in muscular stenosis. *Am Heart J* 67:324, 1964
124. Braunwald E, Oldham HN, Ross J, Linhart JW, Mason DT, Fort L: The circulatory response of patients with idiopathic hypertrophic subaortic stenosis to nitroglycerin and to the Valsalva maneuver. *Circulation* 29:422, 1964
125. Cohn KE, Flamm MD, Hancock EW: Amyl nitrite inhalation as a screening test for hypertrophic subaortic stenosis. *Am J Cardiol* 21:681, 1968
126. Brockenbrough EC, Braunwald E, Morrow AG: A hemodynamic technic for the detection of hypertrophic subaortic stenosis. *Circulation* 23:189, 1961
127. White CW, Zimmerman TJ: Prolonged left ventricular ejection time in the postpremature beat: A sensitive sign of idiopathic hypertrophic subaortic stenosis. *Circulation* 52:306, 1975
128. Reich F, Cabizuca SV, Benchimol A, Desser KB, Sheasby C: Diagnostic postextrasystolic carotid pulse wave change in idiopathic hypertrophic subaortic stenosis: Echocardiographic correlation. *Chest* 69:775, 1976
129. Angoff GH, Wistran D, Sloss LJ, Markis JE, Come PC, Zoll PM, Cohn PF: Value of a noninvasively induced ventricular extrasystole during echocardiographic and phonocardiographic assessment of patients with idiopathic hypertrophic subaortic stenosis. *Am J Cardiol* 42:919, 1978
130. Joye JA, Lee G, Warren D, DeMaria AN, Mason DT: Advantages of nitroprusside infusion in diagnosis and assessment of outflow obstruction in idiopathic hypertrophic subaortic stenosis: Improved accuracy and safety than amyl nitrite inhalation. *Am J Cardiol* 45:492, 1980
131. de la Calzada CS, Ziady GM, Hardarson T, Curiel R, Goodwin JF: Effect of acute administration of propranolol on ventricular function in hypertrophic obstructive cardiomyopathy measured by non-invasive techniques. *Br Heart J* 38:798, 1976
132. Frank MJ, Abdulla AM, Canedo MI, Saylors RE: Long-term medical management of hypertrophic obstructive cardiomyopathy. *Am J Cardiol* 42:993, 1978
133. Hanrath P, Mathey D, Kremer P, Sonntag F, Bleifeld W: Effect of Verapamil on left ventricular relaxation and filling in hypertrophic cardiomyopathy. *Am J Cardiol* 45:393, 1980
134. Krajcer Z, Orzan F, Pechacek LW, Garcia E, Leachman RD: Early systolic closure of the aortic valve in patients with hypertrophic subaortic stenosis and discrete subaortic stenosis: Correlation with preoperative and postoperative hemodynamics. *Am J Cardiol* 41:823, 1978
135. Bolton MR Jr, King JF, Polumbo RA, Mason D, Pugh DM, Reis RL, Dunn MI: The effects of operation on the echocardiographic features of idiopathic hypertrophic subaortic stenosis. *Circulation* 50:897, 1974
136. Schapira JN, Martin RP, Stemple DR, Rakowski H, Stinson EB, Popp RL: Assessment of septal myectomy in hypertrophic subaortic stenosis by single- and two-dimensional echocardiography. *Am J Cardiol* 41:371, 1978
137. Schapira JN, Stemple DR, Martin RP, Rakowski H, Stinson EB, Popp RL: Single and two-dimensional echocardiographic visualization of the effects of septal myectomy in idiopathic hypertrophic subaortic stenosis. *Circulation* 58:850, 1978
138. Maron BJ, Merrill WH, Freier PA, Epstein SE, Morrow AG: Long-term prognosis and symptomatic status of patients after operation for IHSS. *Am J Cardiol* 41:420, 1978
139. Beahrs MM, Tajik AJ, Seward JB, Giuliani ER, McGoon DC: Hypertrophic obstructive cardiomyopathy—19 year postsurgical survivorship. *Am J Cardiol* 45:489, 1980
140. Hamby RI, Roberts GS, Meron JM: Hypertension and hypertrophic subaortic stenosis. *Am J Med* 51:474, 1971
141. Hagaman JF, Wolfe C, Craige E: Early aortic valve closure in combined idiopathic hypertrophic subaortic stenosis and discrete subaortic stenosis. *Am J Cardiol* 45:1083, 1980
142. Chung KJ, Manning JA, Gramiak R: Echocardiography in coexisting hypertrophic subaortic stenosis and fixed left ventricular outflow obstruction. *Circulation* 49:673, 1974

143. Nanda NC, Gramiak R, Shah PM, Stewart S, DeWeese JA: Echocardiography in the diagnosis of idiopathic hypertrophic subaortic stenosis co-existing with aortic valve disease. *Circulation* 50:752, 1974
144. Wigle ED, Adelman AG, Auger P, Marquis Y: Mitral regurgitation in muscular subaortic stenosis. *Am J Cardiol* 24:698, 1969
145. Chandraratna PAN, Tolentino AO, Mutucumarana W, Gomez AL: Echocardiographic observations on the association between mitral valve prolapse and asymmetric septal hypertrophy. *Circulation* 55:622, 1977
146. Brik H, Meller J, Bahler AS, Herman MV, Teichholz LE: Systolic anterior motion of the tricuspid valve in idiopathic hypertrophic subaortic stenosis. *JCU* 6:121, 1978
147. Ross J Jr, Braunwald E, Gault JH, Mason DT, Morrow AG: The mechanism of the intraventricular pressure gradient in idiopathic hypertrophic subaortic stenosis. *Circulation* 34:558, 1966
148. Doi YL, Deanfield JE, McKenna WJ, Dargie HJ, Oakley CM, Goodwin JF: Echocardiographic differentiation of hypertensive heart disease and hypertrophic cardiomyopathy. *Br Heart J* 44:395, 1980
149. Alday LE, Wagner HR, Vlad P: Severe systemic hypertension and muscular subaortic stenosis. *Am Heart J* 83:395, 1972
150. Karliner JS, Williams D, Gorwit J, Crawford MH, O'Rourke RA: Left ventricular performance in patients with left ventricular hypertrophy caused by systemic arterial hypertension. *Br Heart J* 39:1239, 1977
151. Meerson FZ: *The Myocardium in Hyperfunction, Hypertrophy and Heart Failure.* Monograph 26. New York: American Heart Association, 1969. Pp 6–8
152. Hagan AD, DiSessa TG, Samtoy L, Friedman WF, Vieweg WVR: Reliability of echocardiography in diagnosing and quantitating valvular aortic stenosis. *J Cardiovasc Med* 5:391, 1980
153. Salcedo EE, Gockowski K, Tarazi RC: Left ventricular mass and wall thickness in hypertension: Comparison of M-mode and two-dimensional echocardiography in two experimental models. *Am J Cardiol* 44:936, 1979
154. Schlant RC, Felner JM, Heymsfield SB, Gilbert CA, Shulman NB, Tuttle EP Jr, Blumenstein BA: Echocardiographic studies of left ventricular anatomy and function in essential hypertension. *Cardiovasc Med* 2:477, 1977
155. Strauer BE: Ventricular function and coronary hemodynamics in hypertensive heart disease. *Am J Cardiol* 44:999, 1979
156. Guazzi M, Fiorentini C, Olivari MT, Polese A: Cardiac load and function in hypertension: Ultrasonic and hemodynamic study. *Am J Cardiol* 44:1007, 1979
157. Olivari MT, Fiorentini C, Polese A, Guazzi MD: Pulmonary hemodynamics and right ventricular function in hypertension. *Circulation* 57:1185, 1978
158. Watanakunakorn C, Hodges RE, Evans TC: Myxedema: A study of 400 cases. *Arch Intern Med* 116:183, 1965
159. Santos AD, Miller RP, Mathew PK, Wallace WA, Cave WT Jr, Hinojosa L: Echocardiographic characterization of the reversible cardiomyopathy of hypothyroidism. *Am J Med* 68:675, 1980
160. Kerber RE, Sherman B: Echocardiographic evaluation of pericardial effusion in myxedema. Incidence and biochemical and clinical correlations. *Circulation* 52:823, 1975
161. Crowley WF, Ridgway EC, Bough EW, Francis GS, Daniels GH, Kourides IA, Myers GS, Maloof F: Noninvasive evaluation of cardiac function in hypothyroidism. *N Engl J Med* 296:1, 1977
162. Graettinger JS, Muenster JJ, Checchia CS, Grissom RL, Campbell JA: A correlation of clinical and hemodynamic studies in patients with hypothyroidism. *J Clin Invest* 37:502, 1958
163. Buccino RA, Spann JF Jr, Pool PE, Sonnenblick EH, Braunwald E: Influence of the thyroid state on the intrinsic contractile properties and energy stores of the myocardium. *J Clin Invest* 46:1669, 1967
164. Amidi M, Leon DF, deGroot WJ, Krotez FW, Leonard JJ: Effect of the thyroid state on myocardial contractility and ventricular ejection in man. *Circulation* 38:229, 1968
165. La Due JS: Myxedema heart: A pathological and therapeutic study. *Ann Intern Med* 18:332, 1943

166. Douglass RC, Jacobson SD: Pathological changes in adult myxedema: Survey of 10 necropsies. *J Clin Endocrinol Metab* 17:1354, 1957
167. Batsakis JG: Degenerative Lesions of the Heart. In IE Gould (ed), *Pathology of the Heart and Blood Vessels*. Springfield, Ill: Thomas, 1968. P 498
168. Bloor CM: *Cardiac Pathology*. Philadelphia: Lippincott, 1978. P 135
169. Miller RP, Santos AD, Roth-Moyo L: Hypothyroid heart disease: A reversible/obstructive cardiomyopathy (Abstract). The Endocrine Society Program and Abstracts, 61st Annual Meeting, Anaheim, California, 1979. P 140
170. Oram S, Stokes W: The heart in scleroderma. *Br Heart J* 23:243, 1961
171. Sackner MA, Heinz ER, Steinberg AJ: The heart in scleroderma. *Am J Cardiol* 17:542, 1966
172. Gottdiener JS, Moutsopoulos HM, Decker JL: Echocardiographic identification of cardiac abnormality in scleroderma and related disorders. *Am J Med* 66:391, 1979
173. McWhorter JE, Leroy EC: Pericardial disease in scleroderma (systemic sclerosis). *Am J Med* 57:566, 1974
174. D'Angelo WA, Fries JF, Masi AT, Shulman LE: Pathologic observations in systemic sclerosis (scleroderma). *Am J Med* 46:428, 1969
175. Ridolfi RL, Bulkley BH, Hutchins GM: The cardiac conduction system in progressive systemic sclerosis: Clinical and pathologic features of 35 patients. *Am J Med* 61:361, 1976
176. Levisman JA: Echocardiographic diagnosis of mitral regurgitation in congestive cardiomyopathy. *Am Heart J* 93:33, 1977
177. Abbasi AS, Chahine RA, MacAlpin RN, Kattus AA: Ultrasound in the diagnosis of primary congestive cardiomyopathy. *Chest* 63:937, 1973
178. Corya BC, Feigenbaum H, Rasmussen S, Black MJ: Echocardiographic features of congestive cardiomyopathy compared with normal subjects and patients with coronary artery disease. *Circulation* 49:1153, 1974
179. Millward DK, McLaurin LP, Craige E: Echocardiographic studies of the mitral valve in patients with congestive cardiomyopathy and mitral regurgitation. *Am Heart J* 85:413, 1973
180. Ghafour AS, Gutgesell HP: Echocardiographic evaluation of left ventricular function in children with congestive cardiomyopathy. *Am J Cardiol* 44:1332, 1979
181. Peterson KL, Karliner JS, Ross J: Profile in Congestive and Hypertrophic Cardiomyopathies. In W Grossman (ed), *Cardiac Catheterization and Angiography*. Philadelphia: Lea & Febiger, 1974. P 296
182. Mathews EC Jr, Gardin JM, Henry WL, Del Negro AA, Fletcher RD, Snow JA, Epstein SE: Echocardiographic abnormalities in chronic alcoholics with and without overt congestive heart failure. *Am J Cardiol* 47:570, 1981
183. Fujino T, Ito M, Kanaya S, Imanishi J, Fujino M, Yamada K, Hamanaka Y, Kinoshita R, Oya I, Mashiba H: Echocardiographic comparison of acute myocarditis with congestive cardiomyopathy. *J Cardiogr* 7:39, 1977
184. Raftery EB, Banks DC: Occlusive disease of the coronary arteries presenting as primary congestive cardiomyopathy. *Lancet* 2:1147, 1969
185. Acquatella H, Schiller NB, Puigbo JJ, Giordano H, Suarez JA, Casal H, Arreaza N, Valecillos R, Hirschhaut E: M-mode and two-dimensional echocardiography in chronic Chagas' heart disease: A clinical and pathologic study. *Circulation* 62:787, 1980
186. Benjamin IJ, Schuster EH, Bulkley BH: Cardiac hypertrophy in idiopathic dilated congestive cardiomyopathy: A clinicopathologic study. *Circulation* 64:442, 1981
187. Feild BJ, Baxley WA, Russell RO Jr, Hood WP, Holt JH, Dowling JT, Rackley CE: Left ventricular function and hypertrophy in cardiomyopathy with depressed ejection fraction. *Circulation* 47:1022, 1973
188. Hatle L, Orjavik O, Storstein O: Chronic myocardial disease. I. Clinical picture related to long-term prognosis. II. Hemodynamic findings related to long-term prognosis. *Acta Med Scand* 199:399, 1976
189. Hurst JW, Logue RB, Schlant RC, Wenger NK: Obliterative and Restrictive Cardiomyopathies. In JW Hurst (ed), *The Heart* (4th ed). New York: McGraw-Hill, 1978. Pp 1580–1590
190. Shabetai R: Restrictive cardiomyopathy. *Practical Cardiol* 4:146, 1978
191. Hetzel PS, Wood EH, Burchell HP: Pressure pulses in the right side of the heart in a case

of amyloid heart disease and in a case of idiopathic heart failure simulating constrictive pericarditis. *Mayo Clin Proc* 28:107, 1953

192. Meaney E, Shabetai R, Bhargava V, Shearer M, Weidner C, Mangiardi LM, Smalling R, Peterson K: Cardiac amyloidosis, constrictive pericarditis and restrictive cardiomyopathy. *Am J Cardiol* 38:547, 1976
193. Benotti JR, Grossman W, Cohn PF: Clinical profile of restrictive cardiomyopathy. *Circulation* 61:1206, 1980
194. Chew CY, Ziady GM, Raphael MJ, Nellen M, Oakley CM: Primary restrictive cardiomyopathy: Non-typical endomyocardial fibrosis and hypereosinophilic heart disease. *Br Heart J* 39:399, 1977
195. Borer JS, Henry WL, Epstein SE: Echocardiographic observations in patients with systemic infiltrative disease involving the heart. *Am J Cardiol* 39:184, 1977
196. Tyberg TI, Goodyer AN, Hurst VW, Alexander J, Langou RA: Left ventricular filling in differentiating restrictive amyloid cardiomyopathy and constrictive pericarditis. *Am J Cardiol* 47:791, 1981
197. Siqueira-Filho AG, Cunha CLP, Tajik AJ, Seward JB, Schattenberg TT, Giuliani ER: M-mode and two-dimensional echocardiographic features in cardiac amyloidosis. *Circulation* 63:188, 1981
198. Child JS, Krivokapich J, Abbasi AS: Increased right ventricular wall thickness on echocardiography in amyloid infiltrative cardiomyopathy. *Am J Cardiol* 44:1391, 1979
199. Feigenbaum H: *Echocardiography* (3rd ed). Philadelphia: Lea & Febiger, 1981. P 471
200. Hess OM, Turina M, Senning A, Goebel NH, Scholer Y, Krayenbuehl HP: Pre- and postoperative findings in patients with endomyocardial fibrosis. *Br Heart J* 40:406, 1978
201. Eterovic I, Angelini P, Leachman R, Cooley DA: Obliterative restrictive endomyocardial fibrosis: A surgical approach. *Cardiovasc Dis* 6:66, 1979
202. Acquatella H, Schiller NB, Puigbo JJ, Giordano H, Suarez JA, Casal H, Arreaza N, Valecillos R, Hirschhaut E: M-mode and two-dimensional echocardiography in chronic Chagas' heart disease: A clinical and pathologic study. *Circulation* 62:787, 1980
203. Puigbo JJ, Acquatella H, Schiller NB, Tortoledo F, Combellas I, Casal H, Giordano H, Hirschhaut E: Two-dimensional echocardiographic findings in endomyocardial fibrosis. *Circulation* 64(Suppl IV):IV-48, 1981

Pericardial diseases 10

Normal anatomy and function of the pericardium. The pericardium is a double-layered membrane consisting of the visceral pericardium (epicardium) and the parietal pericardium (pericardium). The space between the layers is filled with pericardial lymph that has been thought to lubricate the surface of the heart so that motion can occur without friction or damage to the epicardial surface [1]. The heart shifts with changing position of the individual; however, the pericardium limits the extent of this mobility of the heart within the thorax. Lymph forms on the surface of the epicardium, collects in the pericardial space, and is drained into the lymphatic system [2]. Normally the pericardial sac contains 20 to 50 ml of clear serous fluid [3].

Normal intrapericardial pressure is subatmospheric, nearly equal to intrapleural pressure, and decreases during inspiration. In general the intrapericardial pressure increases when the cardiac volume is greater and decreases when the intracardiac volume is less. A sharp decrease in intrapericardial pressure accompanies the X descent of the venous pressure at the outset of ejection. This decrease, rather than the movement of the atrioventricular valve ring, may be the cause of the X descent and of the augmented venous return to the heart that occurs during systole [4].

Role of the pericardium in diastolic properties of the ventricles. The pericardium is an important determinant of the relation between diastolic pressure and the dimensions of the left and right ventricles. When either the volume or the diastolic pressure of the right ventricle is increased, changes in the shape and dimension of the left ventricle secondary to bulging of the interventricular septum are produced [4]. These changes, in turn, alter the systolic function of the left ventricle.

Holt and colleagues [5] noted an increase in diastolic pressures of the left and right ventricles and of the right atrial pressure during acute hypervolemia and observed that pericardial pressure increased during hypervolemia. The pericardium, by influencing the effects of diastolic pressure and dimensions of one ventricle on the opposite ventricle, may facilitate hemodynamic interaction between the ventricles to balance the right and left ventricular outputs.

The diastolic left ventricular pressure-volume relation can shift upward or downward acutely to an important degree [6–14]. These shifts are significant because the transmural diastolic pressure-volume relation of either ventricle determines the distending force or preload in that it relates diastolic transmural pressure to muscle fiber length. The strength of contraction is, in turn, dependent on this length, according to the Frank-Starling mechanism. In this sense the diastolic pressure-volume relation may be considered to be a determinant of ventricular performance. Some acute upward shifts, for example, increases in left ventricular diastolic pressure at a constant left ventricular volume, have been associated with increased cardiac loading and decreased performance [9]. Thus these upward shifts have been observed under conditions in which the heart might dilate and stretch the pericardium. Conversely, downward shifts have been observed after administration of vasodilators when cardiac decompression might occur. Tyberg and associates [15] proposed that these shifts were actually due to changes in pericardial pressure, due in turn to changes in heart size and pericardial volume; that is, the change in absolute left ventricular diastolic pressure may not represent a change in transmural pressure, but only the necessary effect of a change in the pressure in the pericardial space. Since this hypothesis was proposed, changes in pericardial pressure corresponding to the demonstrated shifts in the left ventricular diastolic pressure-volume relation have been reported [8]. Refsum and associates [9] measured volume changes of the pericardium and the individual cardiac chambers by computed tomography while simultaneously measuring the pericardial pressure and intracardiac pressures. These investigators found that when cardiac volume was altered by volume load and pericardial effusion, acute shifts in the left ventricular diastolic pressure-volume relation were caused by changes in pericardial pressure, which, in turn, corresponded to changes in pericardial volume.

Spotnitz and Kaiser [6] reported that the pericardium influences left ventricular filling pressure even at small volumes.

Glantz and coworkers [7] found that when the pericardium is closed, right ventricular pressure is a more powerful predictor of left ventricular pressure than are left ventricular dimensions. They also observed that the left ventricle appeared to be much more compliant when the pericardium was opened. As a result of these experiments in dogs, these investigators reported the heart in diastole to be a composite shell of stiff pericardium and compliant muscles divided into subcompartments by a relatively compliant interventricular septum.

Furthermore, these authors found that acute right ventricular distention produced by pulmonary artery constriction elevated both right and left ventricular diastolic pressures. However, they did not find this shift in left ventricular pressure-dimension relationship on distending the right ventricle by pulmonary artery constriction after opening the pericardium. Major increases in diastolic pressure were not seen in either the right or left ventricles when the pericardium was opened because each ventricle had a much flatter diastolic pressure-volume curve than the pericardium-myocardium composite shell. Accordingly, the thin right ventricle can dilate substantially in response to increased afterload with only minimal increase in diastolic pressure.

Shirato and associates [8] reported, in a study of conscious dogs following intravenous infusion of Dextran, an increase in intrapericardial pressure from a control of 1.5 mm Hg to 8.2 mm Hg falling to 4.8 mm Hg after nitroprusside administration. They found that in acute cardiac dilatation the pericardium contributed significantly to the increased left ventricular diastolic pressure and to the fall during sodium nitroprusside infusion, and appeared responsible for shifts in the diastolic pressure-segment length relation.

Relationship of the pericardium to the pathophysiology of cardiac failure. Edema and increased systemic venous pressure observed in patients with severe left ventricular dysfunction may be partially explained by elevation of the left ventricular diastolic pressure causing pulmonary hypertension with eventual failure of the right ventricle. Right ventricular performance may also be impaired in these patients by bulging of the interventricular septum into the right ventricle (Bernheim syndrome) [16]. Reversed Bernheim physiology, bulging of the interventricular septum into the left ventricle with resulting left ventricular dysfunction, has been postulated to explain findings of left ventricular failure in patients with predominantly right ventricular disease.

Adolph [17] has speculated that the pericardium may oppose the effects of left ventricular dilatation on right ventricular function in the following manner: dilatation of the left ventricle increases intrapericardial pressure, which limits right ventricular filling and thereby reduces forward flow into the lungs, perhaps preventing pulmonary edema. The pericardium thus causes reciprocal shifts of the Frank-Starling curves of the two ventricles and so balances their outputs. The Frank-Starling mechanism and the pericardium are considered important in normal cardiovascular responses to change in body posture, and the evidence for the latter's role in compensated heart failure is strongly suggested [4].

Pericardial effusion and primary left ventricular disease. Reddy and colleagues [18] noted important hemodynamic differences in patients with pericardial effusions but no cardiac tamponade, in patients with uncomplicated cardiac tamponade, and in those with cardiac tamponade complicating severe left ventricular dysfunction. They emphasize that when left ventricular diastolic pressure is severely elevated, equalization of left and right ventricular diastolic pressures, usually a characteristic sign of cardiac tamponade, no longer occurs. Under these circumstances cardiac tamponade is defined by equilibration of intrapericardial and right ventricular diastolic (or right atrial) pressures at a high level, but below that of left ventricular diastolic pressure. Furthermore, these investigators explain the absence of pulsus paradoxus in these patients as a result of lack of inspiratory increase in right heart filling and a decrease in left heart filling with reciprocal changes in expiration. These respiratory fluctuations, combined with filling of the two ventricles against a common stiffness, are essential hemodynamic markers of ordinary cardiac tamponade and must be maintained if pulsus paradoxus is to be present. When left ventricular diastolic pressure is intrinsically elevated, filling of that chamber is determined by its compliance; therefore its diastolic pressure exceeds that of the right ventricle throughout the respiratory cycle and pulsus paradoxus cannot appear.

Localized collections of blood following cardiac surgery may compress one side of the heart; the result may be that the two ventricles fill against different pressures and pulsus paradoxus is absent. In aortic valve insufficiency a major portion of left ventricular filling is independent of respiration and pulsus paradoxus is again absent. Finally, pulsus paradoxus may be absent in extreme tamponade with severe hypotension.

DIAGNOSIS OF PERICARDIAL EFFUSION BY ECHOCARDIOGRAPHY. Since Edler in 1955 [19] first reported the use of reflected ultrasound to diagnose pericardial effusion, echocardiography has become the diagnostic method of choice for detecting the presence of pericardial fluid as well as for estimating its amount [20–23]. Horowitz and associates [20] reported that more than 15 ml was always found when a posterior echo-free space persisted throughout the cardiac cycle between a flat pericardium and the epicardium. In spite of the difficulty in visualizing the pericardial fluid anterior to the right ventricle by M-mode technique, the capability

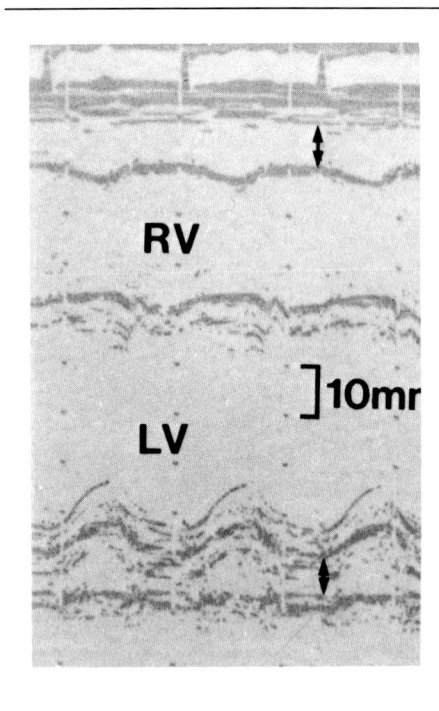

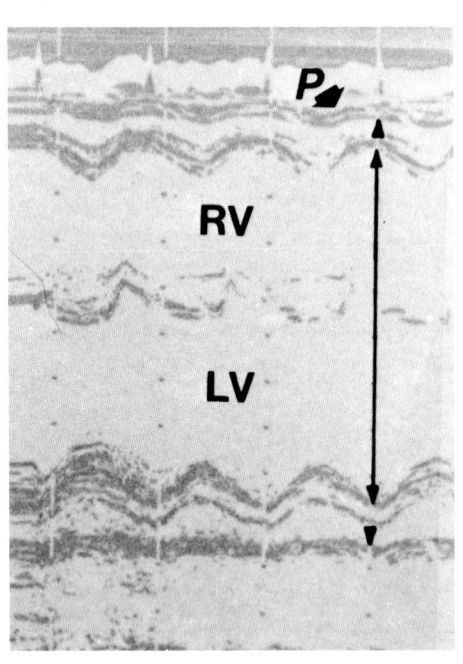

Fig. 10-1. M-mode recording in a patient with pericardial effusion. The left panel, because it demonstrates no pericardium (P) anteriorly, would overestimate the amount of fluid, whereas estimating the amount of fluid in the right panel would be more accurate because the pericardium is recorded and the pericardial-epicardial separation at end diastole can be reliably determined. Total cardiac dimension (right ventricular epicardium to left ventricular epicardium) is identified by the long arrow in right panel.

of this diagnostic method to recognize small, medium, and large effusions is good. Since the method described by Horowitz and colleagues [20] of quantitating pericardial effusions may be in error by 200 to 300 ml, it cannot be expected to provide precise estimates of the fluid content. Although echocardiography has proved more reliable than other noninvasive and invasive diagnostic procedures for recognizing pericardial fluid, criteria are currently not available for distinguishing normal pericardial fluid from an abnormal pericardial effusion. Since it is technically feasible to identify only 15 to 20 ml of pericardial fluid with echocardiography, normal amounts of fluid are frequently recognized by M-mode and 2-D echocardiography.

Riba and Morganroth [21], in a retrospective analysis of 1225 routine echocardiograms, noted a pericardial effusion in 15 percent, which was considered substantial in size in 10 percent. Sixty-one percent (68 of 111) of the latter were clinically unsuspected. Sixty percent of these patients (41 of 68) had underlying heart disease such as congestive heart failure, left ventricular hypertrophy, valvular heart disease, or asymmetric septal hypertrophy without other recognizable causes for pericardial effusion.

Since an echo-free space is often present between the chest wall and the heart, it is important to identify the pericardium in addition to the epicardial surface of the right ventricle in order to avoid overestimating intrapericardial space [24] (Fig. 10-1).

In the presence of moderate or large pericardial effusions, fluid may be seen posterior to the left atrium [24, 25] (Fig. 10-2). In addition to fluid that is superior to the atrioventricular sulcus and inferior to the junction of the pericardium and inferior pulmonary veins, fluid may also accumulate behind the left atrium in a potential space known as the oblique sinus. This sinus is closed superiorly and to

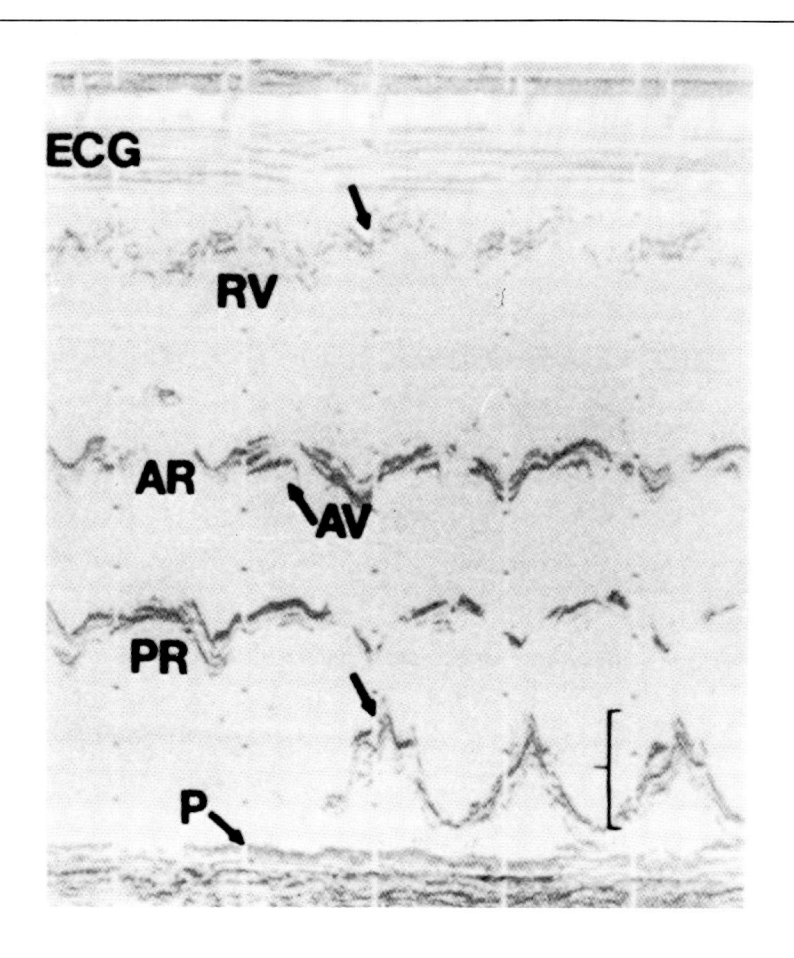

Fig. 10-2. M-mode recording in a patient with a pericardial effusion showing posterior motion (arrow) of anterior right ventricular wall during diastole and prominent anterior motion of left atrial wall with atrial contraction (arrow) with pericardial fluid between the left atrial wall posteriorly and the pericardium (P). AR = anterior root of aorta; PR = posterior root of aorta.

the right but is open inferiorly and to the left. Another potential space, the transverse sinus, exists between the posterior aortic root and the anterior wall of the left atrium and a small amount of pericardial fluid may be seen in some patients with effusions (Fig. 10-3). In most pericardial effusions this path is blocked by the tautness of the pericardium between the entrances of the left inferior pulmonary vein and the inferior vena cava and by the impression of the esophageal prominence which lies directly posterior to the oblique sinus.

Numerous conditions have been reported that mimic pericardial effusion on M-mode echocardiography [26]. These include the following normal anatomy and cardiac abnormalities: descending thoracic aorta, coronary sinus, inferior pulmonary veins, pleural effusion, coronary artery aneurysm, left atrial enlargement, mitral annulus calcification, mediastinal or pericardial cystic tumors, and pseudoaneurysm of the left ventricle. Two-dimensional echocardiography, by providing a spatial orientation of the heart, aorta, pulmonary veins, and related structures from multiple tomographic planes, sufficiently defines anatomic structures so that such conditions should not be confused with pericardial effusion.

The complementary value of 2-D echo to M-mode technique for the overall detection and evaluation of pericardial effusions has been well established [22–24, 27–30]. Lewandowski and colleagues [27], in a prospective study of 60 patients,

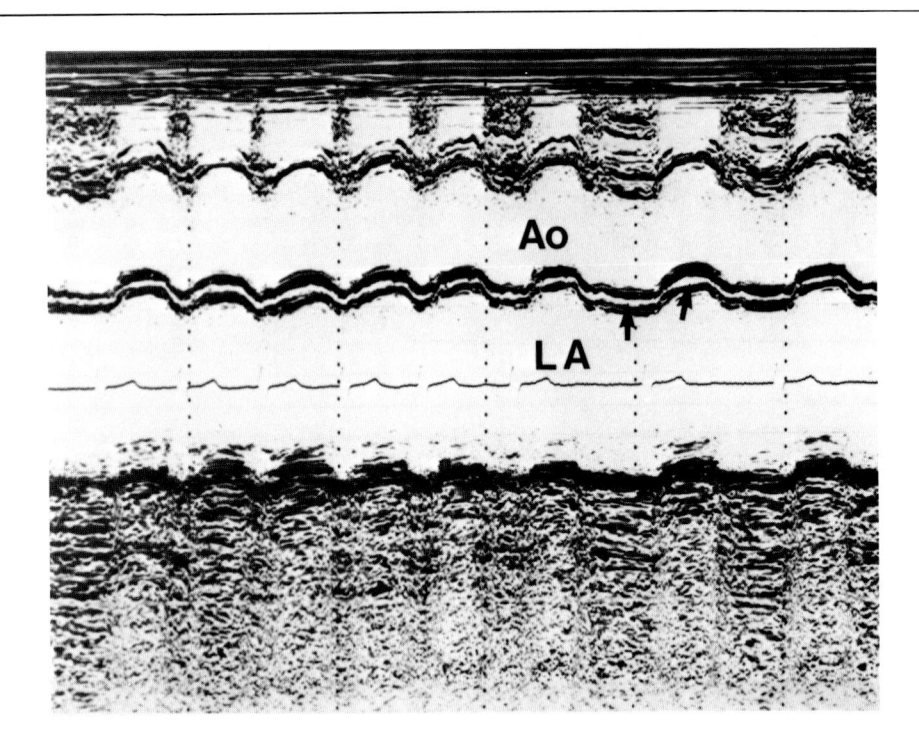

Fig. 10-3. M-mode recording of aorta and left atrium with small amount of pericardial fluid in the transverse sinus (arrows) causing a small separation between the walls of the aorta and left atrium. Calibration dots are 5 mm apart.

were able to verify with 2-D echo the relation of pericardial effusions and posterior paramediastinal pleural effusions to the descending thoracic aorta. They found that large pericardial effusions lie anterior to the descending aorta both at the level of the left atrium and the left ventricle, whereas large posterior paramediastinal pleural effusions lie posterior, lateral, or posterolateral to the descending aorta (Fig. 10-4). It may be possible to identify masses within the pleural fluid (Fig. 10-5).

Martin and associates [22] demonstrated that wide-angle phased-array echocardiography was quite effective in localizing pericardial effusions. They found that in small effusions the fluid was truly posterior at and below the atrioventricular groove. With moderate-sized effusions a more uniform distribution of the fluid was found, and with large effusions more fluid was visualized apically, posteromedially, laterally, and anteriorly. Upright redistribution of the fluid was noted by these authors with moderate to large nonloculated effusions. We have also noted considerable variation in the distribution of pericardial effusion with two-dimensional echo imaging (Fig. 10-6). The subcostal views are particularly valuable since small amounts of fluid can sometimes be seen in the pericardial space adjacent to the right ventricle or right atrium, whereas the fluid could not be identified posterior to the left ventricle. The various parasternal and apical tomographic planes with 2-D echo provide several additional views of the right ventricle, right atrium, and lateral aspect of the left ventricle that cannot be recorded with M-mode echocardiography. The characteristic motion of the right ventricle and right atrium caused by the pericardial effusion can be easily observed with 2-D echo, which further complements M-mode information.

Several studies have been conducted to evaluate echocardiographic findings in patients with impending or established cardiac tamponade [24, 29, 31–35]. Some of these studies discussed the influences of respiration on mitral valve motion in patients with large pericardial effusions; these changes have proven to be nonspecific and not indicative of cardiac tamponade. There are no specific echocardiographic findings to reliably predict the presence of tamponade. In an experimental study Martins and Kerber [34] noted that the internal diameters of both the right and left ventricles with tamponade were significantly smaller than those of controls. They also observed that the inspiratory increases of right ventricular internal dimension at end diastole and corresponding decreases in left ventricular dimensions were exaggerated during tamponade. Because of the wide range and overlap of these dimensional changes, no single expiratory value or respiratory change indicated the presence or severity of tamponade.

Schiller and Botvinick [33] found that a right ventricular end-diastolic dimension at end expiration of 7 ± 2 mm or less was strongly associated with tamponade in patients with pericardial effusions. In addition to the other nonspecific findings already discussed these authors observed that the "swinging heart" and electrical alternans, although indicative of large effusions, were not specific for tamponade (Fig. 10-7).

Subcostal imaging to evaluate the diameter of the inferior vena cava (IVC) is another important aspect of a 2-D echo examination in any patient with a pericardial effusion. In addition, it is helpful to observe the effects of respiration on the dimensions of the IVC; as the right atrial pressure increases there is reduced or absent motion with inspiration. On rare occasions we have observed an increase in diameter with inspiration (Kussmaul's sign of the IVC); this paradoxical motion of the IVC with breathing has been observed in cardiac tamponade.

As discussed earlier in this chapter, many factors play a role in the development of tamponade; the amount of fluid in the pericardial space is only one of these factors. If an effusion develops quickly, for example, following trauma, a relatively modest volume may cause tamponade (Figs. 10-6B, D; 10-8).

Pericardial thickening and constrictive pericarditis. Echocardiography has been most useful in the evaluation of patients with pericardial disease for the identification of pericardial effusion; however, the value of either M-mode or 2-D echo in identifying pericardial thickening or constrictive pericarditis has not been established with certainty. Most of the studies published to the present have been clinical ones using M-mode echocardiography [36–39].

Systolic function, measured both segmentally and globally, is normal in patients with constrictive pericarditis. Early diastolic filling of the left ventricle is normal; however, the last two-thirds of diastole has little if any additional filling. Candell-Riera and colleagues [37] studied eight patients with constrictive pericarditis and observed in seven of the eight an early diastolic motion of the interventricular septum consisting of a sudden anterior displacement followed by a brisk posterior rebound. The beginning of this abnormal movement was coincident with the pericardial knock in the phonocardiogram and its peak was coincident with the simultaneously recorded deep Y descent in the jugular venous pulse tracing.

In another study of 12 patients with constrictive pericarditis, Voelkel and associates [39] noted a "flatness" of the endocardium of the posterior left ventricular wall following the initial rapid filling period in 11 of these subjects. The net endocardial movement in these patients was less than 1 mm compared to that in

348   10. Pericardial diseases

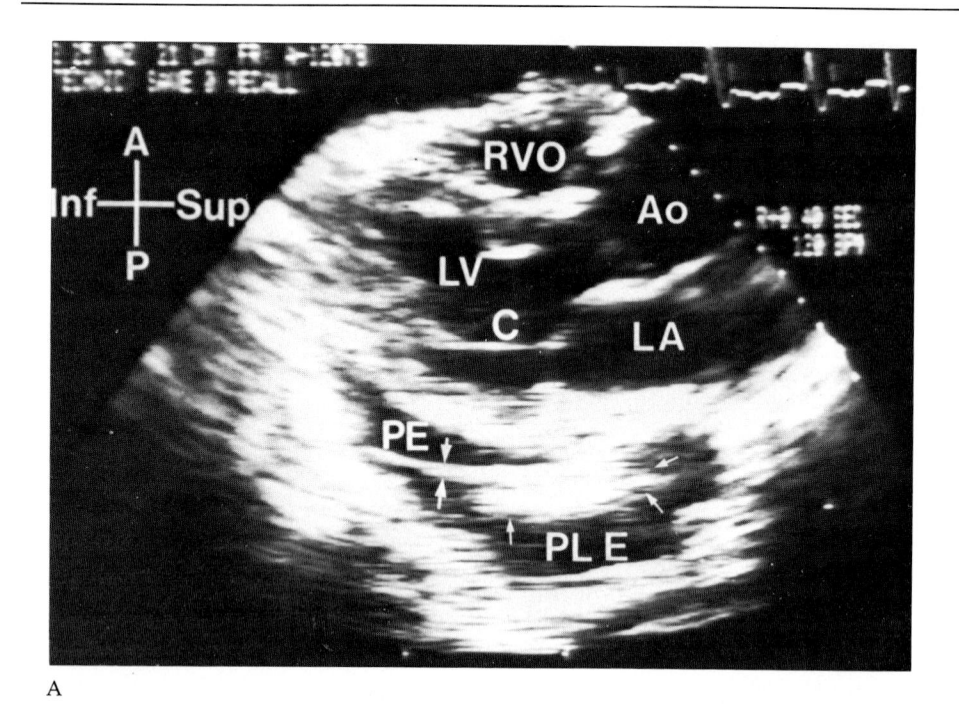

Fig. 10-4A. Parasternal long axis view demonstrating both pericardial effusion and pleural effusion (PL E) together with a prominent reflectance suggestive of a mass (arrows) adjacent to the pericardium and within the pleural fluid. B. Parasternal short axis view in same patient showing moderately large pericardial effusion (PE) and a pleural effusion. C. Parasternal long axis view in a patient with mitral stenosis and markedly thick anterior and posterior mitral leaflets. A large pleural effusion is present with several prominent linear strand-like structures (arrows) within the pleural fluid that probably represent pleural adhesions. C. = chordae tendineae.

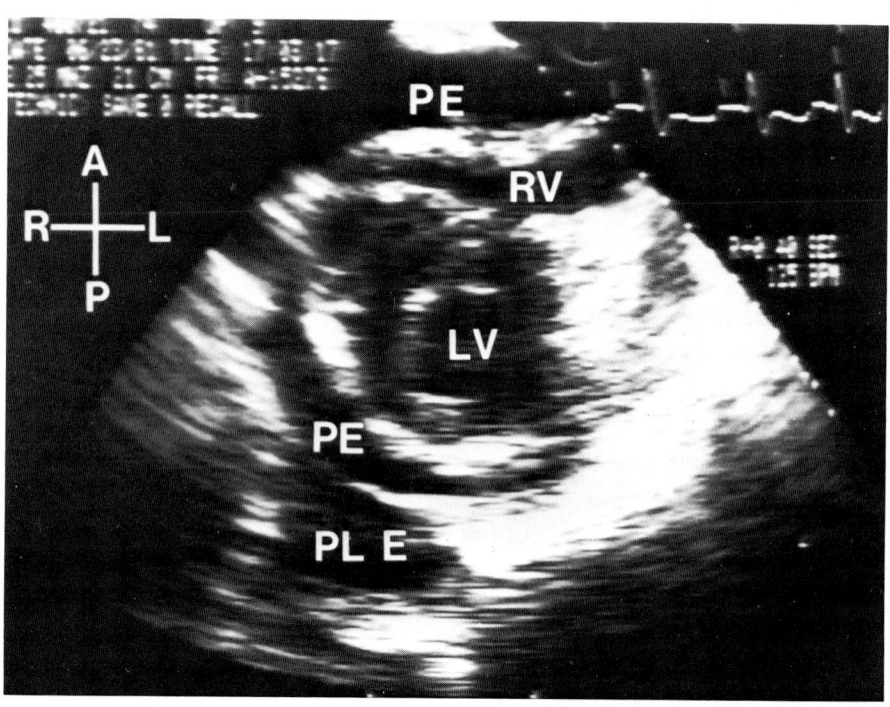

349

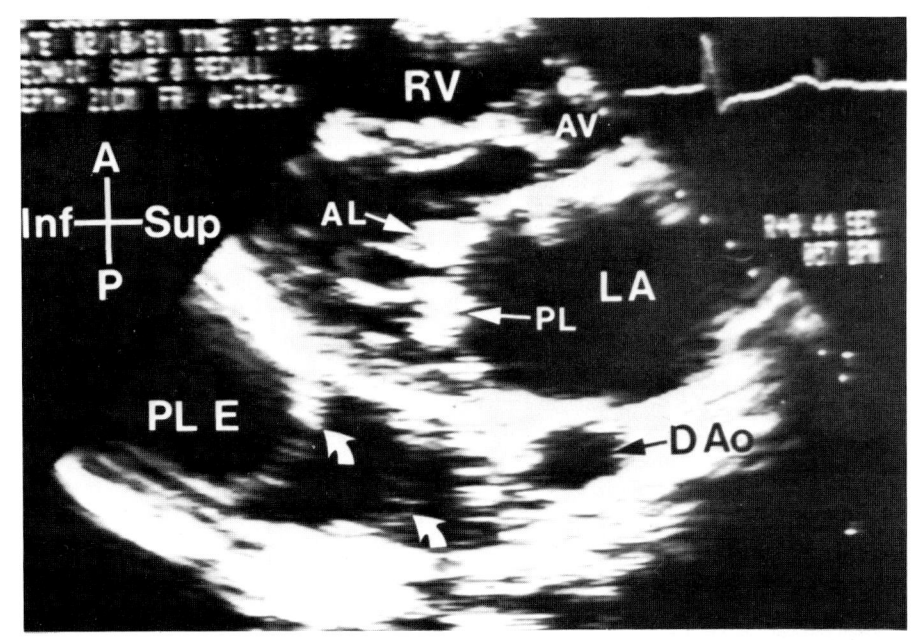

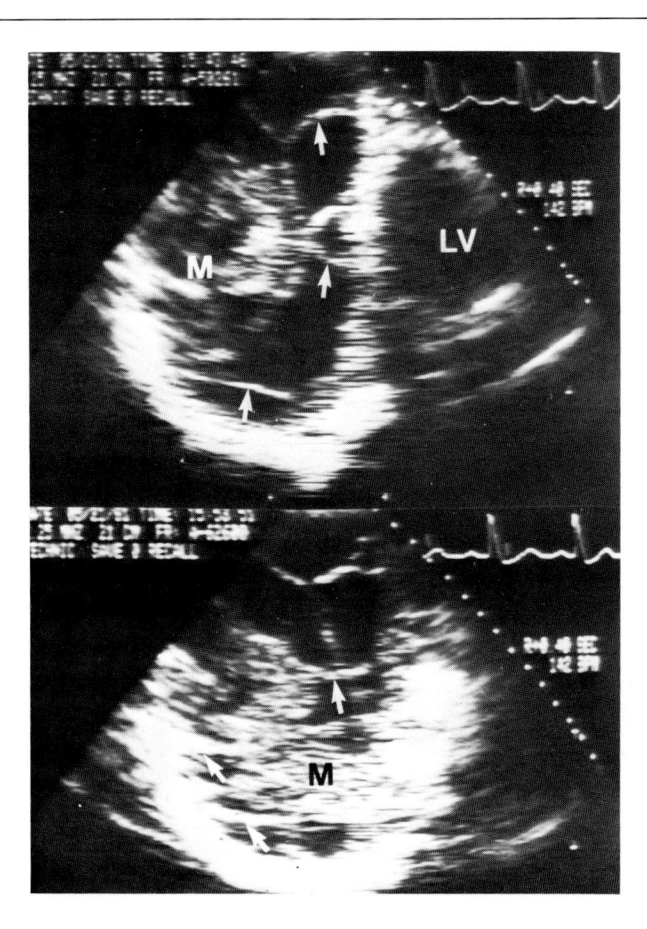

Fig. 10-5. Two views of a patient with a mass (M) or atelectasis of a lung segment with a large pleural effusion and pleural adhesions (white arrows, upper and lower panels).

350   10. Pericardial diseases

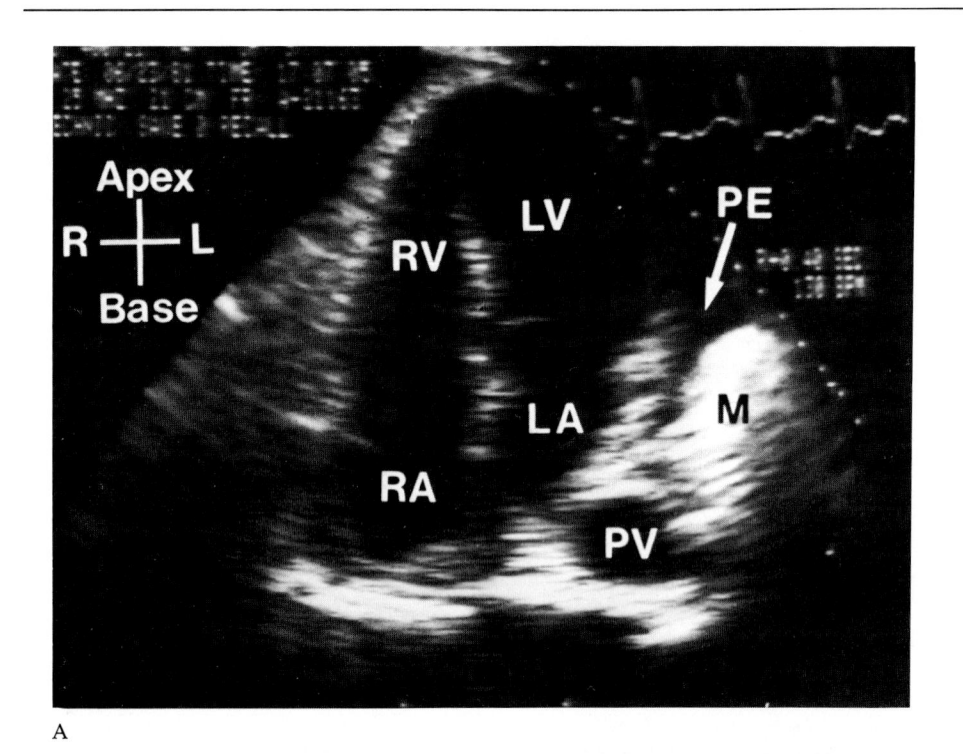

Fig. 10-6A. Apical 4-chamber view showing slight displacement of the left atrium and distended pulmonary vein (PV) because of compression from a nearby mediastinal mass (M). A localized pericardial effusion (PE) adjacent to the lateral wall of the left ventricle is present; however, no PE can be seen around the right ventricle or right atrium. B. Parasternal short axis view of the left ventricle showing a PE posteromedial to the posterior wall of the left ventricle; the PE cannot be seen lateral to the left ventricle. C. Apical 4-chamber view in a patient with a PE showing marked displacement of the right atrial wall (three arrows). D. Subcostal 4-chamber view in same patient as in B demonstrating a very large pericardial effusion around the right ventricle. No fluid is visible in either of these views adjacent to the lateral wall of the left ventricle. The pericardium (small arrows) can be seen near the diaphragm and a large thrombus can be seen attached to the epicardial surface of the RV (large arrow). Clinically the patient had pericardial tamponade.

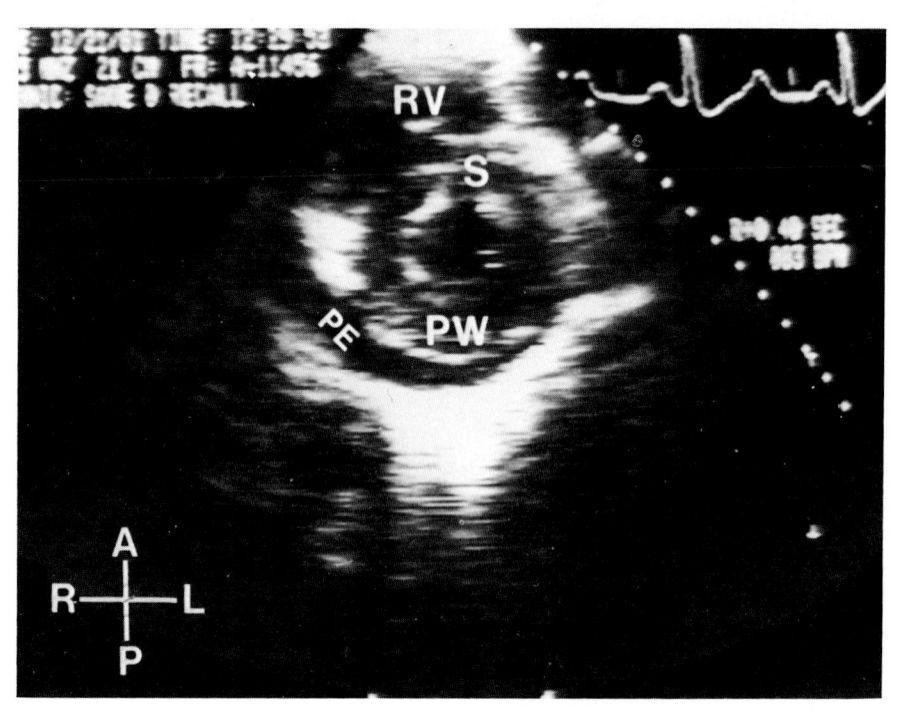

351

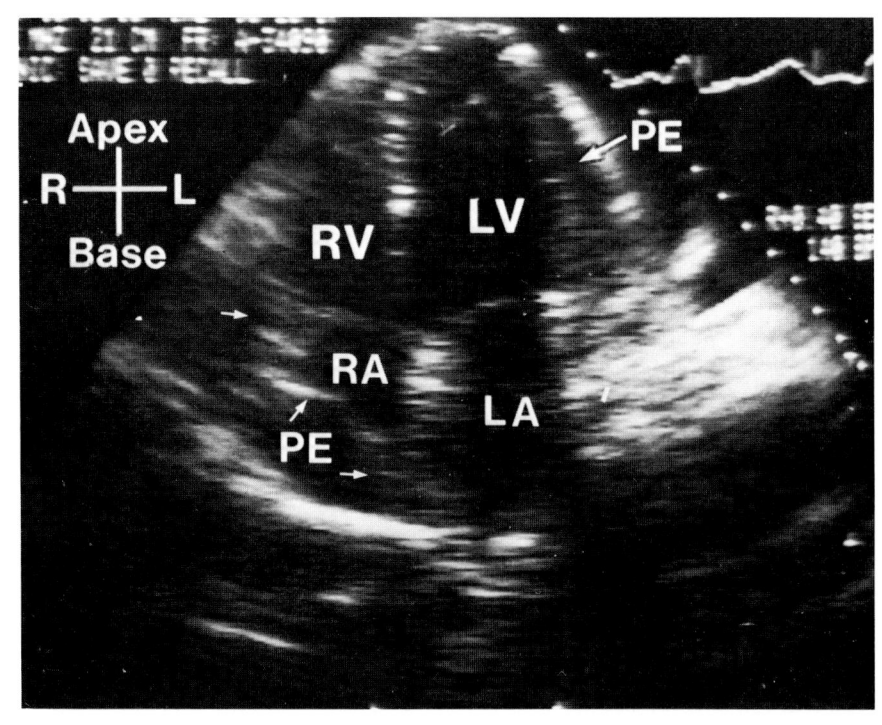

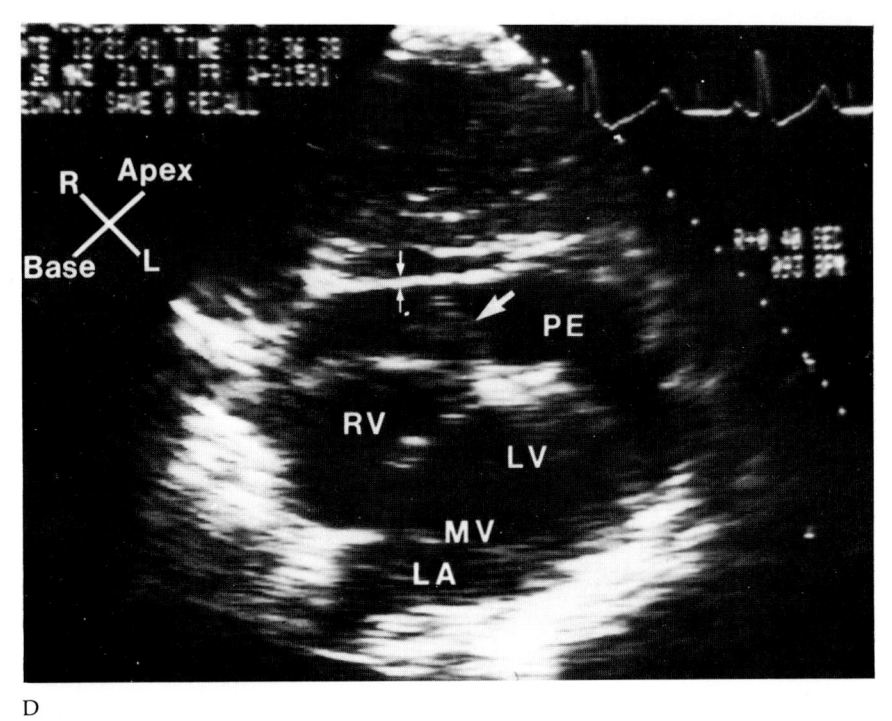

352   10. Pericardial diseases

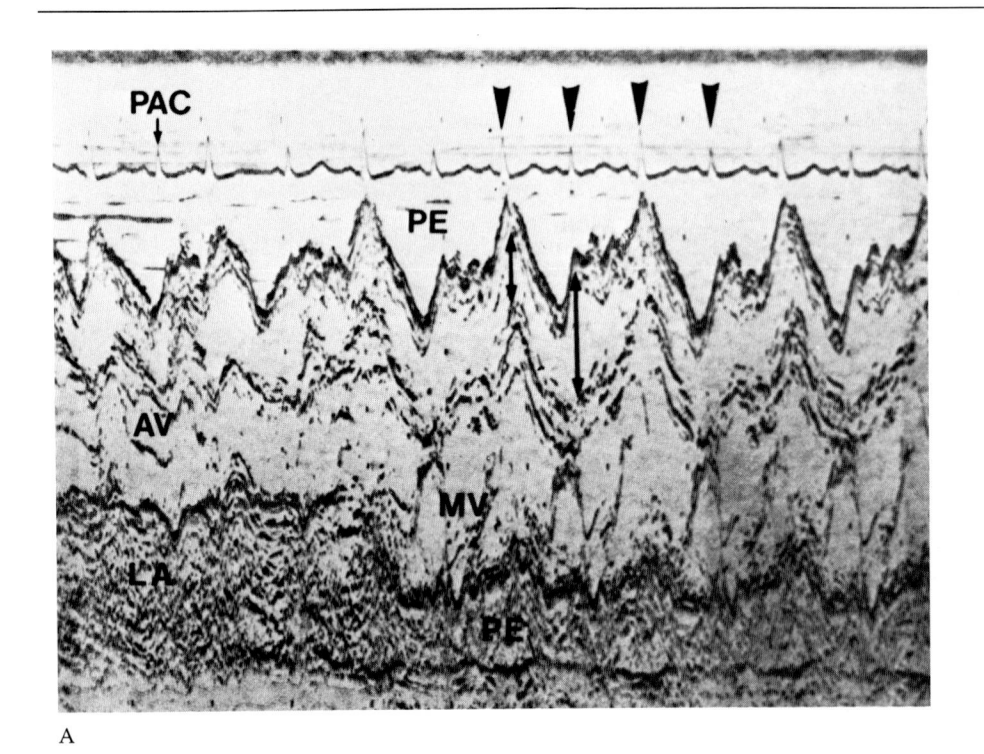

Fig. 10-7A. *M-mode recording of "swinging heart" and electrical alternans due to a large pericardial effusion; notice the changing end-diastolic dimensions of the right ventricle with alternating beats (short and long arrows). Abnormal aortic root motion and small left ventricle are also caused by the pericardial effusion. The left atrial size and posterior effusion are obscured by excessive noise on the record. B. M-mode recording of a patient in acute respiratory distress with tachypnea but no pericardial effusion demonstrating marked change in motion of the interventricular septum with respiration; upon inspiration (INSP), the right ventricle becomes larger with corresponding decrease in the size of the left ventricle. C. M-mode recording of right ventricular cavity disappearing with exhalation and increasing in dimension with inspiration primarily because of the angle of the M-mode cursor as it intersects the RV rather than because the patient is having actual RV compression from a pericardial effusion. EX = exhalation; PAC = premature atrial contraction.*

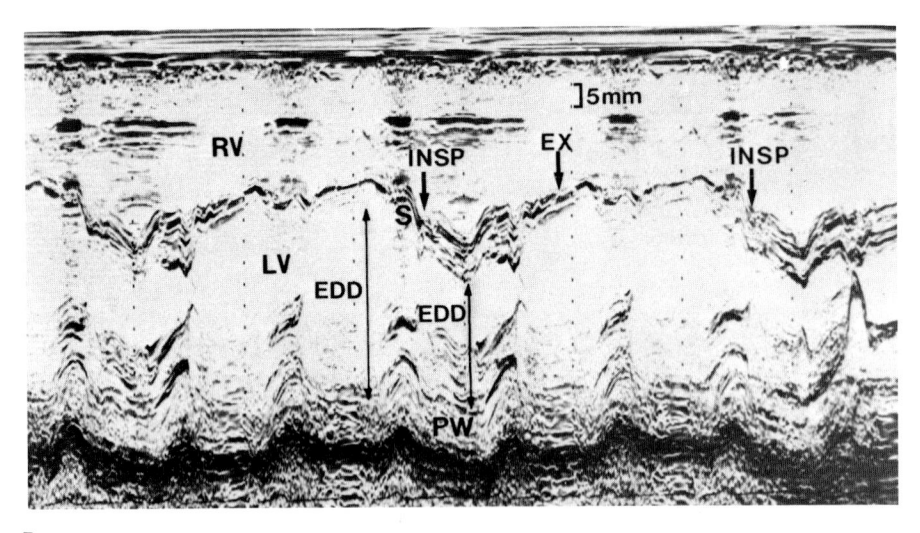

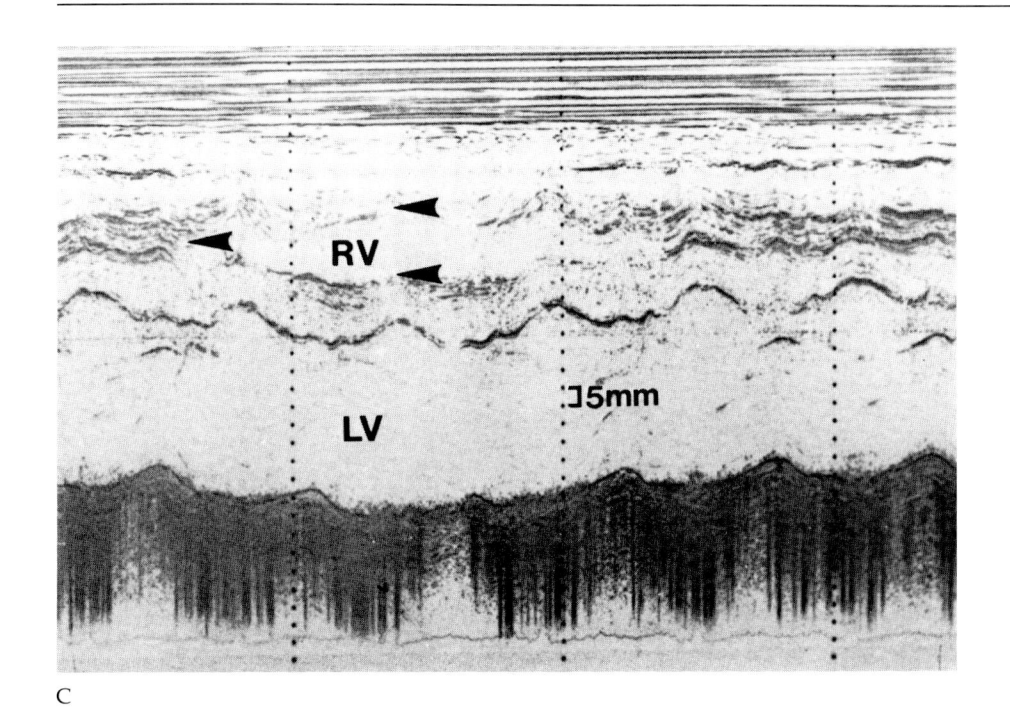

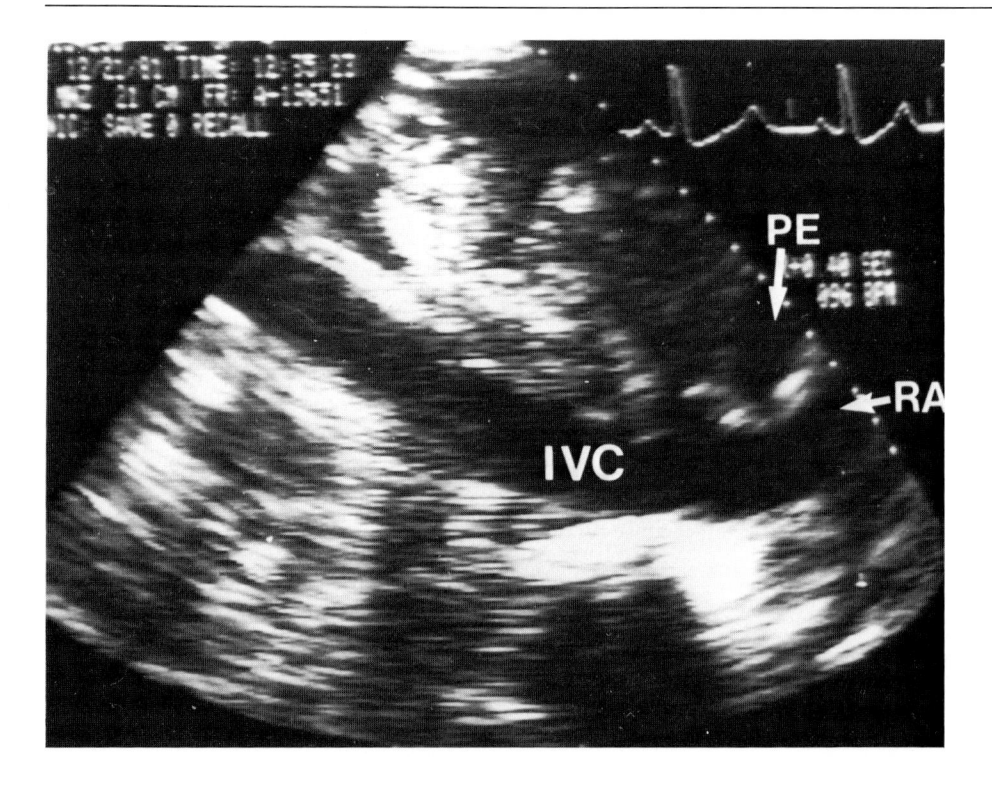

Fig. 10-8. Subcostal view of inferior vena cava, which is only minimally increased in diameter, entering the right atrium and a small portion of the pericardial effusion adjacent to the RA. This is from the same patient as in Fig. 10-6B and D.

354   10. Pericardial diseases

A

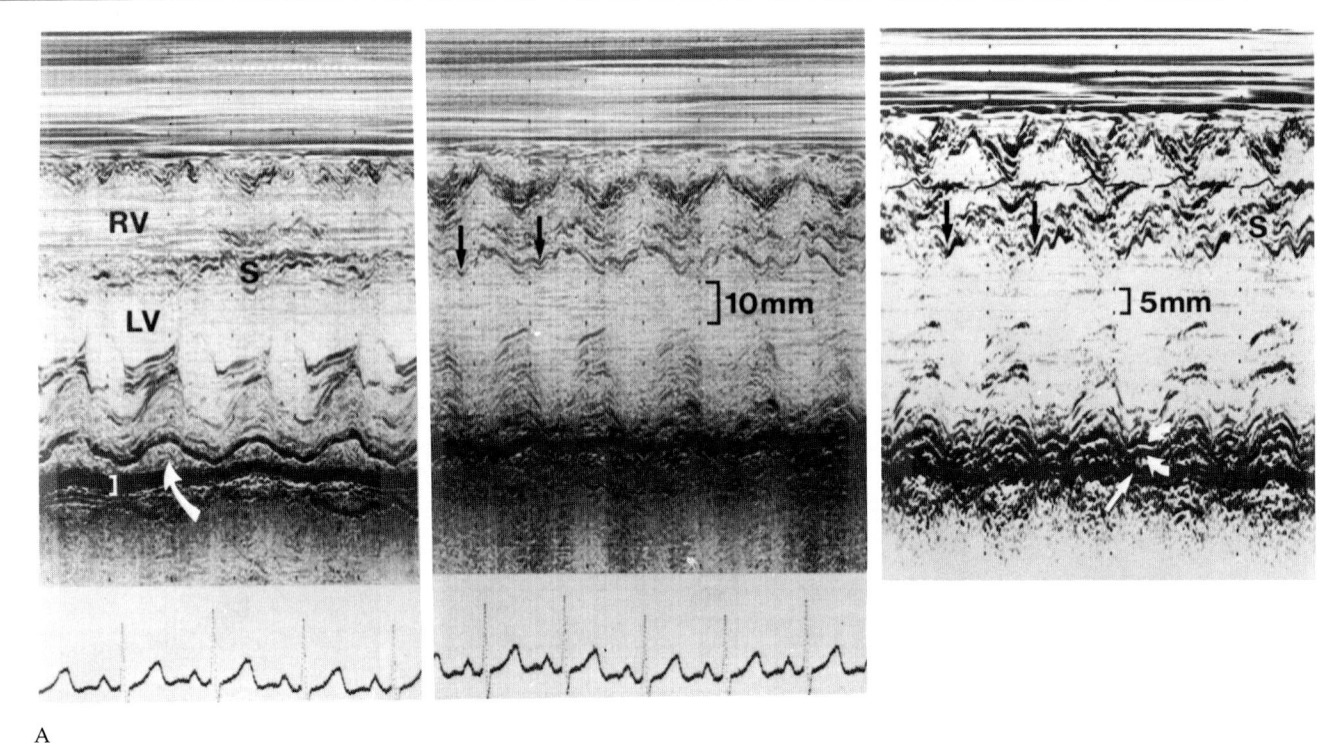

Fig. 10-9A. *M-mode recordings in two patients with constrictive pericarditis demonstrate thick pericardium* (white bracket) *and small pericardial effusion* (arrow, left panel); *posterior notches of interventricular septum in early diastole* (arrows, middle panel) *(same patient as in left panel); increased thickness of epicardium* (right panel), *particularly when associated with diastolic septal notches* (black arrows) *and/or thickened pericardium. Any or all of these findings are nonspecific and, although suggestive, are not diagnostic of constrictive pericarditis. B. M-mode recordings in a patient with documented constrictive pericarditis at autopsy demonstrating a pericardial effusion and some areas where the effusion appears large* (right panel) *with the pericardium appearing thick and irregular on the surface* (arrow, right panel). *In the left panel, the pericardium is not adequately imaged; however, the epicardial thickness is prominent* (open arrows). *The maximum posterior motion of the interventricular septum* (top arrow, left panel) *significantly precedes the peak anterior motion of the posterior wall of the left ventricle.*

355

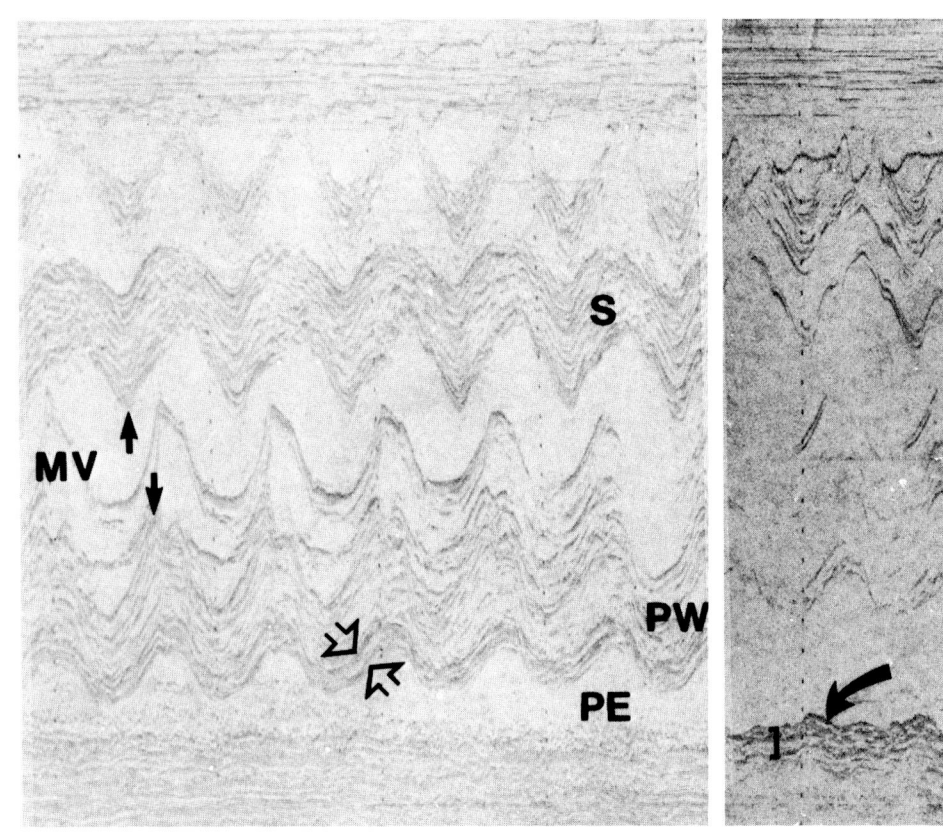

356 10. Pericardial diseases

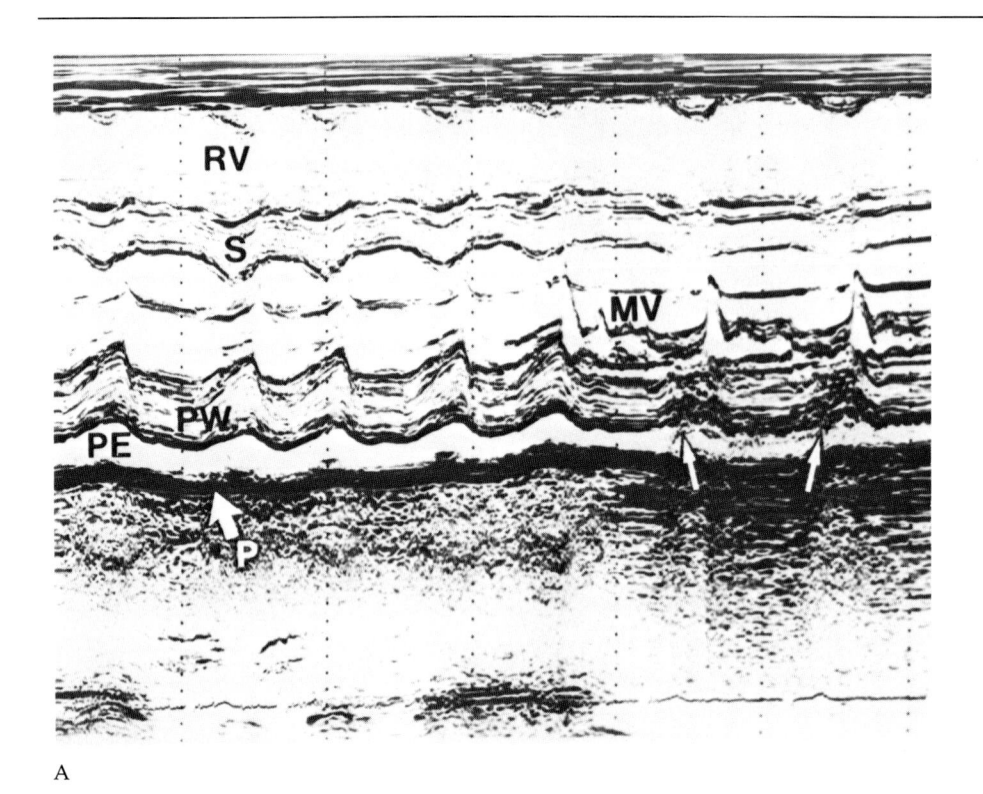

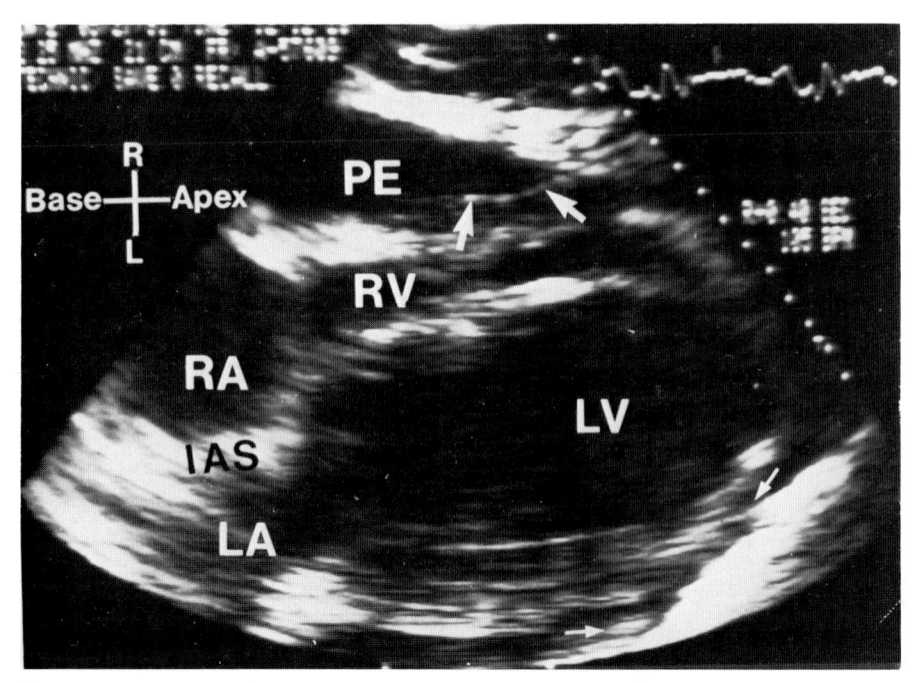

Fig. 10-10A. M-mode recording in a patient with a pericardial effusion (PE), thick pericardium (P), and adhesions with increased epicardial thickness posterior to the mitral valve (white arrows). B. Subcostal 4-chamber view showing large PE with epicardial to pericardial strands of fibrinous material or adhesions (4 white arrows around RV and LV). C. Parasternal short axis view of a patient with acute tuberculosis pericarditis showing prominent PE and thick-appearing right ventricular wall owing to shaggy epicardial inflammatory response (arrow). D. Apical long axis view from same patient as in C with left atrium deleted from view showing a very shaggy pericarditis with thick strands of inflammatory material (white arrows, upper and lower panels) extending from both the pericardium and epicardial surfaces into a large pericardial effusion. E. Apical 4-chamber view (upper panel) with leftward angulation to show pericardium and pericardial space along the lateral aspect of the left ventricle and the apical long axis view (lower panel) showing very thick pericardium and thick-appearing left ventricular wall (arrows) caused by a rapidly progressive acute pericarditis (3 weeks after D) that had developed into severe constrictive pericarditis by the time of this study. IAS = interatrial septum. (C, D, and E courtesy of Gabriel Gregoratos, M.D.)

357

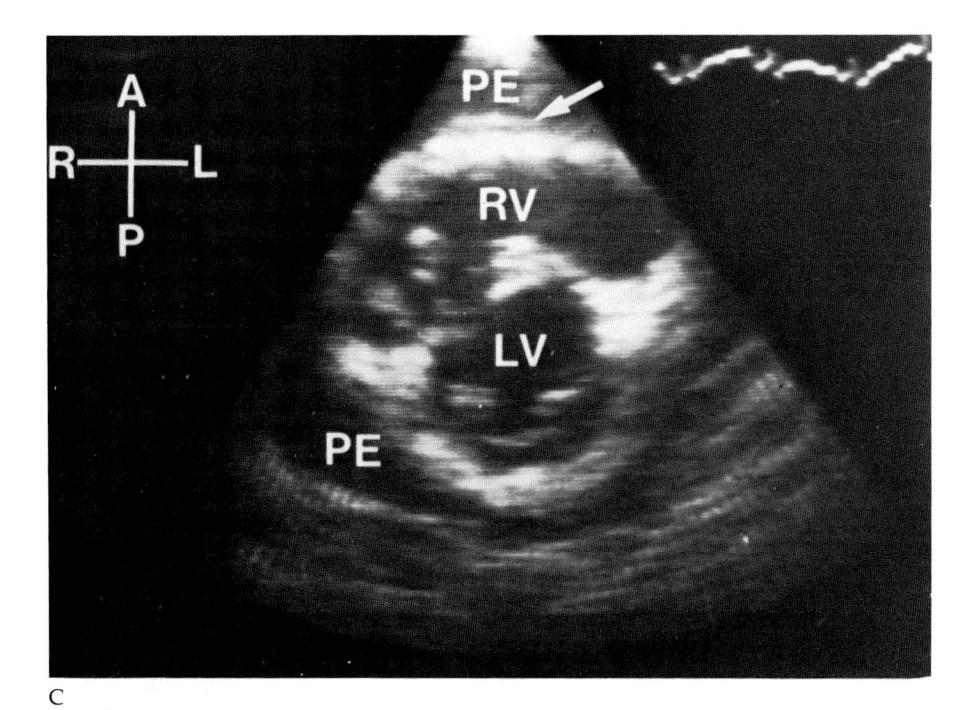

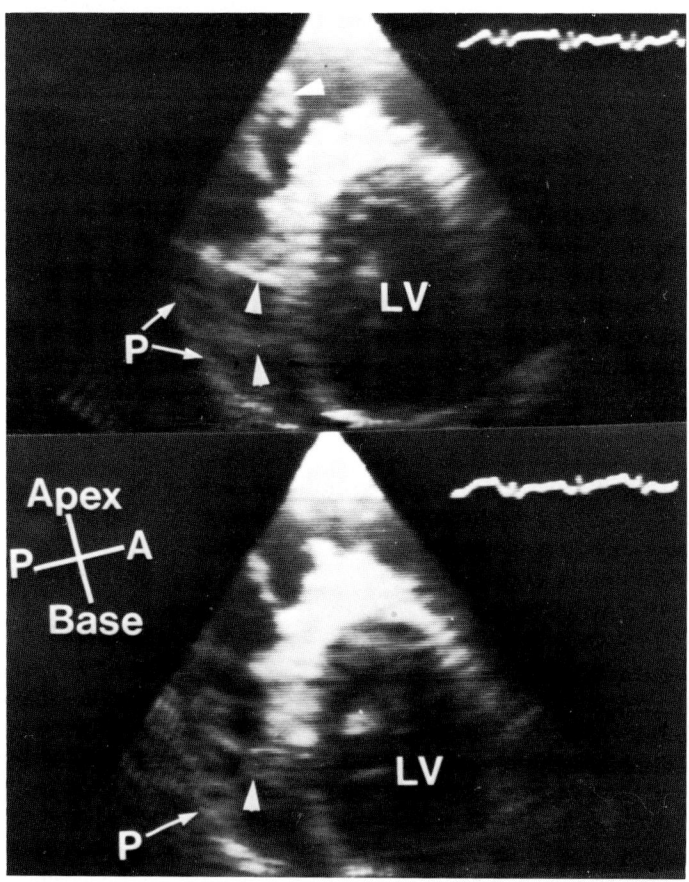

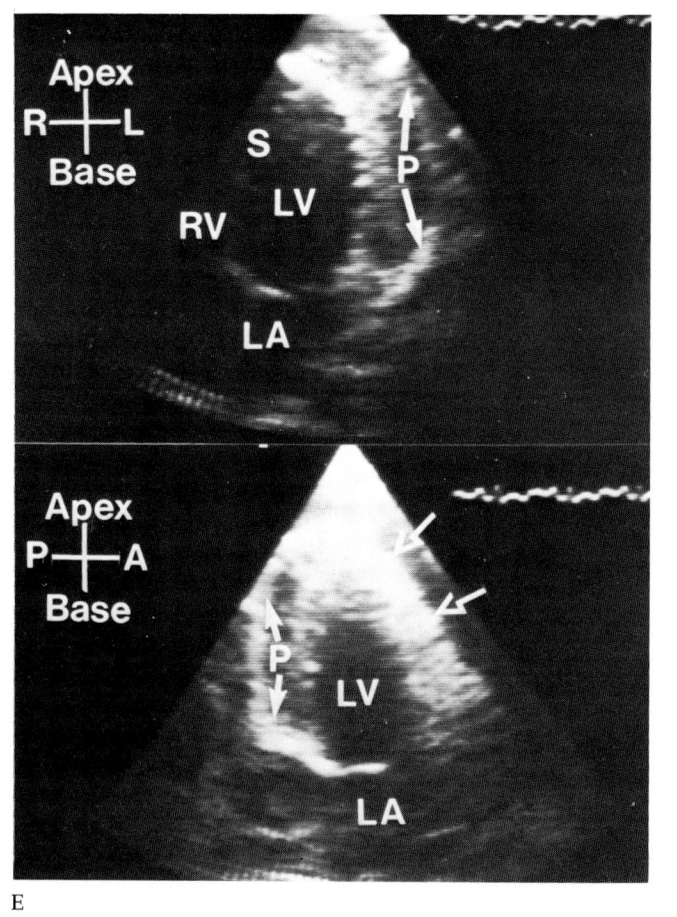

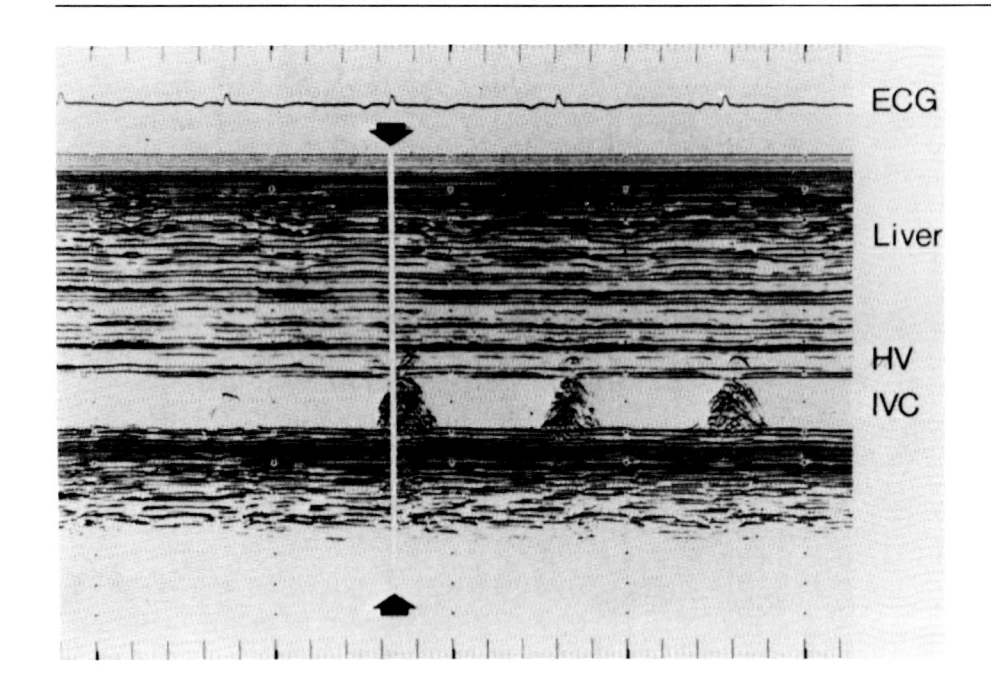

Fig. 10-11. M-mode recording in a patient with constrictive pericarditis showing diastolic reflux following atrial contraction with contrast echo examination. This is probably not specific for constrictive pericarditis but is indicative of high right atrial pressures. (From NK Wise et al, Contrast M-mode ultrasonography of the inferior vena cava. Circulation 63:1100, 1981, by permission of the American Heart Association, Inc.)

normal subjects, which moved posteriorly from 1.5 to 4 mm (mean 2.2 ± 0.8). These authors noted abnormal septal motion in only five of the 12 patients.

Schnittger and coworkers [38] described seven echocardiographic patterns consistent with pericardial adhesions or pericardial thickening. The hemodynamic diagnosis of constrictive pericardial disease was associated with the echocardiographic finding of pericardial thickening; however, there were no consistent echocardiographic patterns of pericardial thickening diagnostic of constriction.

Measurement of pericardial thickness is very much determined by the machine adjustments and imaging techniques of the echocardiographer. Simultaneous 2-D imaging can be beneficial for overall identification of the pericardium and positioning of the M-mode cursor through a certain segment; however, the actual measurements of thickness can still be determined more easily from the M-mode record (Fig. 10-9). Another distinct advantage of 2-D echo is the ability to recognize pericardial adhesions on the surface of the epicardium and extending from the epicardium to the pericardium (Fig. 10-10). Sometimes the real-time motion of the adhesions and "shaggy" appearance of a fulminant acute pericarditis are the most dramatic abnormalities noted in such a study (Fig. 10-10D, E). Another motion abnormality, which cannot be depicted in still photographs, is a diastolic "jerking" of the entire left ventricle and failure of the left ventricle to dilate together with a visual impression that total diastolic motion is restricted; when present, these findings indicate constrictive pericarditis.

In our experience one of the earlier 2-D echo findings that is recognizable in constrictive pericarditis is enlargement of the inferior vena cava, which can be viewed easily with subcostal imaging. The additional finding of diastolic reflux after atrial contraction into the inferior vena cava on contrast echo examination may prove to be beneficial in making the diagnosis of constriction (Fig. 10-11). The dilated IVC and the atrial reflux occur secondary to elevated right atrial pressure

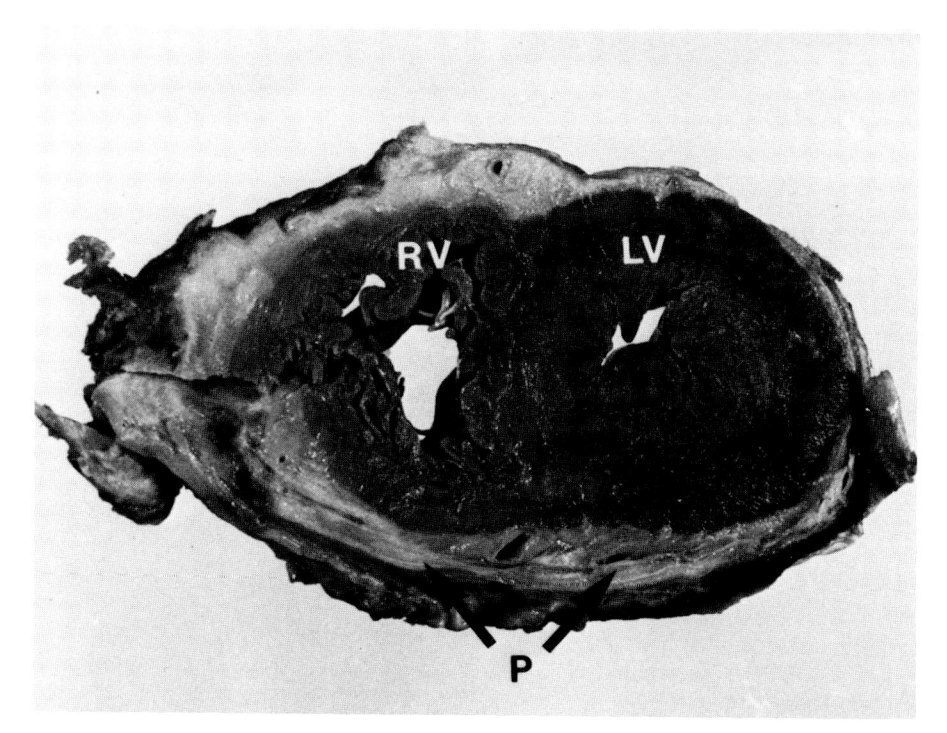

Fig. 10-12A. Anatomic short axis view in a patient who died of constrictive pericarditis demonstrating a thickened pericardium (P) firmly adherent to the right ventricle and left ventricle. B. Anatomic view of the heart with the pericardium removed showing a pericardial space and a markedly thickened (10 mm), calcified pericardium.

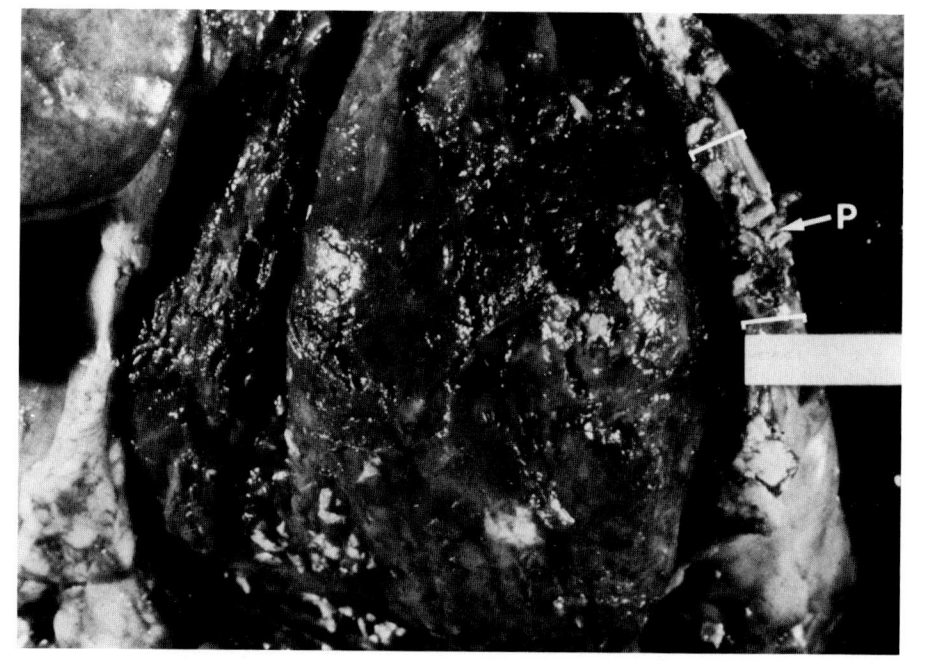

and represent nonspecific findings which may be seen in any condition causing significant elevations of right atrial pressure.

Subtle evidence of an enlarged IVC together with qualitative evidence of increased pericardial thickness in the absence of any other structural or functional abnormalities should raise the possibility of constrictive pericarditis in the overall clinical evaluation of a patient.

When a small amount of fluid separates the epicardium and pericardium, the identification of pericardial thickness is easier; however, if the two are firmly adherent, which occurs in some patients with constrictive pericarditis, measurement of pericardial thickness by echocardiography is usually difficult or impossible (Fig. 10-12).

References

1. Holt JP: The normal pericardium. *Am J Cardiol* 26:455, 1970
2. Miller AJ, Pick R, Johnson PJ: Lymphatic drainage of the heart. *Am J Cardiol* 26:463, 1971
3. Bloor CM: *Cardiac Pathology*. Philadelphia: Lippincott, 1978. P 265
4. Shabetai R: The pericardium: An essay on some recent developments. *Am J Cardiol* 42:1036, 1978
5. Holt JP, Rhode EA, Kines H: Pericardial and ventricular pressure. *Circ Res* 8:1171, 1960
6. Spotnitz HM, Kaiser GA: The effect of the pericardium on pressure-volume relations in the canine left ventricle. *J Surg Res* 11:375, 1971
7. Glantz SA, Misbach GA, Moores WY, Mathey DG, Lekven J, Stowe DF, Parmley WW, Tyberg JV: The pericardium substantially affects the left ventricular diastolic pressure-volume relationship in the dog. *Circ Res* 42:433, 1978
8. Shirato K, Shabetai R, Bhargava V, Franklin D, Ross J Jr: Alteration of the left ventricular diastolic pressure-segment length relation produced by the pericardium: Effects of cardiac distension and afterload reduction in conscious dogs. *Circulation* 57:1191, 1978
9. Refsum H, Junemann M, Lipton MJ, Skioldebrand C, Carlsson E, Tyberg JV: Ventricular diastolic pressure-volume relations and the pericardium: Effects of changes in blood volume and pericardial effusion in dogs. *Circulation* 64:997, 1981
10. Grossman W, McLaurin LP: Diastolic properties of the left ventricle. *Ann Intern Med* 84:316, 1976
11. Parmley WW, Chuck L, Chatterjee K, Klausner SC, Glantz SA, Ratshin RA: Acute changes in the diastolic pressure-volume relationship of the left ventricle. *Eur J Cardiol* 4(Suppl):105, 1976
12. Alderman EL, Glantz SA: Acute hemodynamic interventions shift the diastolic pressure-volume curve in man. *Circulation* 54:662, 1976
13. Ludbrook PA, Byrne JD, Kurnik PB, McKnight RC: Influence of reduction of preload and afterload by nitroglycerin on left ventricular diastolic pressure-volume relations and relaxation in man. *Circulation* 56:937, 1977
14. Mann T, Goldberg S, Mudge GH, Grossman W: Factors contributing to altered left ventricular diastolic properties during angina pectoris. *Circulation* 59:14, 1979
15. Tyberg JV, Misbach GA, Glantz SA, Moores WY, Parmley WW: A mechanism for shifts in the diastolic, left ventricular pressure-volume curve: The role of the pericardium. *Eur J Cardiol* 7(Suppl):163, 1978
16. East T, Bain C: Right ventricular stenosis (Bernheim's syndrome). *Br Heart J* 11:145, 1949
17. Adolph RJ: Clinical Physiology of the Circulation in Cardiac Diagnosis and Treatment. In NO Fowler (ed), *Cardiac Diagnosis and Treatment* (2nd ed). New York: Harper & Row, 1976. Pp 1–25
18. Reedy PS, Curtiss EI, O'Toole JD, Shaver JA: Cardiac tamponade: Hemodynamic observations in man. *Circulation* 58:265, 1978
19. Edler I: The diagnostic use of ultrasound in heart disease. *Acta Med Scand* 308(Suppl):32, 1955

20. Horowitz MS, Schultz CS, Stinson EB, Harrison DC, Popp RL: Sensitivity and specificity of echocardiographic diagnosis of pericardial effusion. *Circulation* 50:239, 1974
21. Riba AL, Morganroth J: Unsuspected substantial pericardial effusions detected by echocardiography. *JAMA* 236:2623, 1976
22. Martin RP, Rakowski H, French J, Popp RL: Localization of pericardial effusion with wide angle phased array echocardiography. *Am J Cardiol* 42:904, 1978
23. Schiller NB: Echocardiography in pericardial disease. *Med Clin N Am* 64:253, 1980
24. Hagan AD: Evaluation of Pericardial Diseases by M-mode and Two-dimensional Echocardiography. In DT Mason (ed), *Advances in Heart Disease* (Vol 3). New York: Grune & Stratton, 1980. Pp 699–702
25. Greene DA, Kleid JJ, Naidu S: Unusual echocardiographic manifestation of pericardial effusion. *Am J Cardiol* 39:112, 1977
26. Come PC, Riley MF, Fortuin NJ: Echocardiographic mimicry of pericardial effusion. *Am J Cardiol* 47:365, 1981
27. Lewandowski BJ, Jaffer NM, Winsberg F: Relationship between the pericardial and pleural spaces in cross-sectional imaging. *JCU* 9:271, 1981
28. Haaz WS, Mintz GS, Kotler MN, Parry WR: Two-dimensional echocardiographic recognition of the descending thoracic aorta: Value in differentiating pericardial from pleural effusions. *Am J Cardiol* 45:401, 1980
29. Matsuo H, Matsumoto M, Hamanaka Y, Ahara T, Senda S, Inoue M, Abe H: Rotational excursion of heart in massive pericardial effusion studied by phased-array echocardiography. *Br Heart J* 41:513, 1979
30. Martin RP, Bowden R, Filly K, Popp RL: Intrapericardial abnormalities in patients with pericardial effusion: Findings by two-dimensional echocardiography. *Circulation* 61:568, 1980
31. D'Cruz IA, Cohen HC, Prabhu R, Glick G: Diagnosis of cardiac tamponade by echocardiography: Changes in mitral valve motion and ventricular dimensions, with special reference to paradoxical pulse. *Circulation* 52:460, 1975
32. Settle HP, Adolph RJ, Fowler NO, Engel P, Agruss NS, Levenson NI: Echocardiographic study of cardiac tamponade. *Circulation* 56:951, 1977
33. Schiller NB, Botvinick EH: Right ventricular compression as a sign of cardiac tamponade: An analysis of echocardiographic ventricular dimensions and their clinical implications. *Circulation* 56:774, 1977
34. Martins JB, Kerber RE: Can cardiac tamponade be diagnosed by echocardiography? Experimental studies. *Circulation* 60:737, 1979
35. Shina S, Yaginuma T, Kondo K, Kawai N, Hosoda S: Echocardiographic evaluation of impending cardiac tamponade. *J Cardiogr* 9:555, 1979
36. Gibson TC, Grossman W, McLaurin LP, Moos S, Craige E: An echocardiographic study of the interventricular septum in constrictive pericarditis. *Br Heart J* 38:738, 1976
37. Candell-Riera J, Garcia Del Castillo H, Permanyer-Miralda G, Soler-Soler J: Echocardiographic features of the interventricular septum in chronic constrictive pericarditis. *Circulation* 57:1154, 1978
38. Schnittger I, Bowden RE, Abrams J, Popp RL: Echocardiography: Pericardial thickening and constrictive pericarditis. *Am J Cardiol* 42:388, 1978
39. Voelkel AG, Pietro DA, Folland ED, Fisher ML, Parisi AF: Echocardiographic features in constrictive pericarditis. *Circulation* 58:871, 1978

Cardiac tumors and masses

11

Two-dimensional echocardiography is usually the procedure of choice for detection of cardiac tumors and masses. Comprehensive two-dimensional imaging of the four chambers and valves, as well as of the immediate extracardiac spaces, affords greater sensitivity and overall reliability in the diagnosis of cardiac masses than cardiac catheterization or other noninvasive tests.

The valvular vegetation, one form of cardiac mass, is discussed in Chapter 5.

Left ventricular thrombi are discussed primarily in Chapter 6 and to a limited extent in this chapter.

Until 1950 it was believed that cardiac tumors could be recognized only at autopsy [1]. Left atrial myxoma was recognized by angiography in 1952 [2]. In 1954 the first atrial myxoma was excised using cardiopulmonary bypass [3]. With the advent of M-mode echocardiography came the first major step in the clinical recognition of cardiac tumors with a noninvasive procedure. Since the introduction of two-dimensional imaging, the reliability of echocardiography is further improved because it is possible to image all four chambers in a more comprehensive, thorough fashion.

Left atrial tumors and masses. The left atrial myxoma is the most common cardiac tumor. Bulkley and Hutchins [4] reviewed the clinical presentation and diagnosis of myxomas in 24 patients over a 50-year period. These investigators noted that the tumors occurred more frequently in women. The patients were adults ranging in age from 24 to 74 years (mean = 50 years). Twenty-two (92%) of the myxomas occurred in the left atrium and two (8%) in the right atrium. The investigators reported the clinical signs and symptoms of myxomas as follows: congestive heart failure in 13 (54%), mitral stenosis murmur in nine (38%), chest pain in seven (29%), pulmonary edema in six (25%), embolism in five (21%), stroke in four (17%), and one (4%) had a femoral artery embolus. Intracardiac myxomas may be suggested by a wide variety of signs and symptoms; Bulkley and Hutchins [4] reported that the 22 patients with left atrial myxomas had symptoms simulating mitral stenosis, collagen vascular disease, infective endocarditis, idiopathic paroxysmal atrial fibrillation, and myocarditis.

A variety of auscultatory findings accompanying left atrial myxomas have been described. The murmur often resembles either mitral stenosis, mitral regurgitation, mixed mitral valve disease, or hypertrophic cardiomyopathy. A diastolic opening snap or tumor "plop," as well as accentuation or prolongation of the first heart sound are also commonly encountered [5, 6].

Hemodynamic abnormalities include elevation of left atrial pressures, prominent c and V waves, and alterations in left atrial pressures, which vary depending upon whether the left atrial tumor is moving between the left ventricle and left atrium or remaining stationary within the left atrium throughout the entire cardiac cycle [7, 8].

Although there have been case reports in which M-mode echocardiography has been more sensitive than cardiac catheterization for identification of left atrial tumors [9, 10], cardiac catheterization was usually necessary for adequate evaluation of cardiac masses before the introduction of 2-D echocardiography [7]. Since two-dimensional echocardiography became available, it has been obvious that this noninvasive technique enables more reliable visualization of the cardiac chambers than either M-mode echo or angiography for identification of small masses [11]. Kaminsky and colleagues [12] published a case report of a 14-year-old youngster with a protracted illness characterized by tenderness and weakness of the extremities that was considered to be a collagen vascular disease; it was discovered nine months later after the development of new heart murmurs, pulmonary edema, and a stroke that the patient in fact had a left atrial myxoma [12]. Left atrial myxomas occur clinically in one of three ways [13, 14]: with constitutional effects, because of obstruction to blood flow, or by systemic embolization. Although myxomas may originate in any chamber of the heart, 75 percent arise from the left side of the interatrial septum in the region of the fossa ovalis.

Popp and Levine [15] reported a patient with long-standing symptoms of congestive heart failure and cardiac catheterization findings which had led to the erroneous diagnosis of cardiomyopathy, until a left atrial tumor was correctly diagnosed with echocardiography. Their patient was unique in that he had experienced progressively disabling symptoms for a period of 26 years. The initial stage was characterized by episodic dizziness and syncope; the second stage was manifested by symptoms of intermittent and ultimately persistent pulmonary venous hypertension; the third stage was characterized by slight improvement on digitalis and diuretic therapy for heart failure, but symptoms of right heart failure became dominant and progressive. The fourth stage consisted of severe limitations for another five years before the correct diagnosis was made.

Clinical findings in left atrial myxomas may, in unusual clinical circumstances, mimic infective endocarditis. Reports of atrial myxomas with concomitant findings of positive blood cultures and organisms in the tumor are quite rare [16, 17]. Graham and colleagues [18] reported a case of a 48-year-old woman who came to the emergency room in a delirious state with high fever and classic findings of infective endocarditis; she died within a short period of time secondary to a ruptured mycotic aneurysm and large brain abscess before the infected left atrial myxoma could be surgically removed.

Child and associates [19] have discussed the differentiation between a large mitral vegetation and a left atrial myxoma. These authors noted that a large vegetation, particularly one caused by fungus in the presence of negative blood cultures, may resemble a pedunculated left atrial myxoma. Accordingly, in certain clinical situations where a mass appears to be attached to the mitral leaflet, the differential consideration of mycotic endocarditis, marantic vegetations, valvular metastases, or thrombus should be considered along with left atrial myxoma (Figs. 11-1 to 11-3). The difficulty in distinguishing such masses is more likely to occur with M-mode echocardiography than with two-dimensional imaging (Fig. 11-4).

Atrial myxomas are usually globular in shape, but they may be slightly lobulated or villous in appearance. They are usually 4 to 8 cm in diameter, have a smooth glistening surface, and are usually pale gray in color. Myxomas are usually pedunculated and attached by fibrovascular stalks of various thicknesses and lengths. Most commonly the stalk is attached to the interatrial septum in the region of the fossa ovalis.

It may be very difficult to diagnose the etiology of a solid reflective mass within the left atrium; a thrombus may appear the same as a tumor on 2-D echo (Fig. 11-5). A large mass in a dilated left atrium in the presence of rheumatic mitral disease can be assumed to be thrombus until proved otherwise at the time of surgical removal.

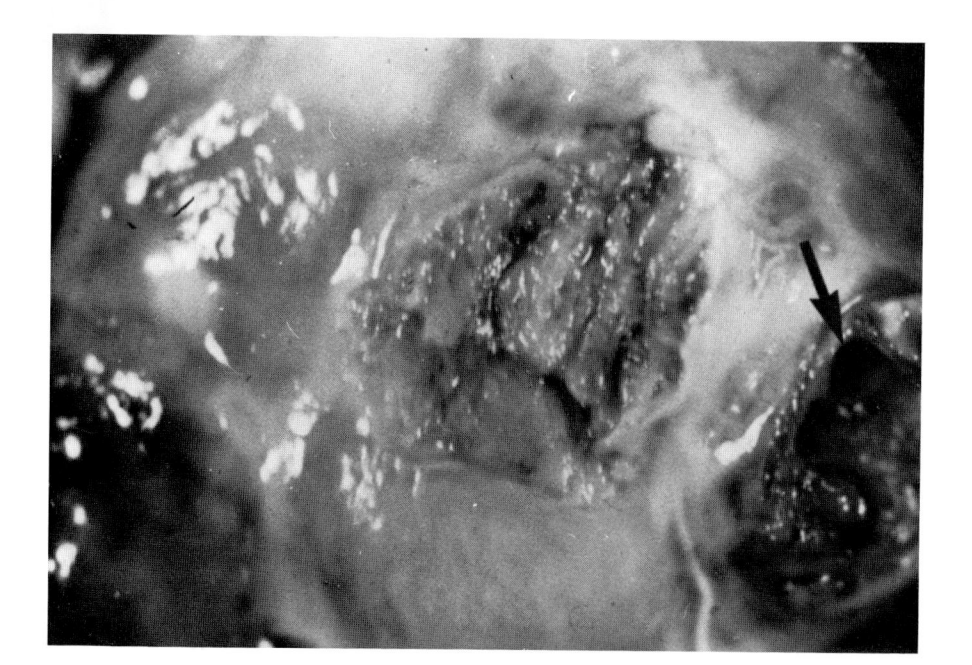

Fig. 11-1. A myxoma removed from the right atrium of a young adult male demonstrating the site of stalk attachment (arrow) and the typical appearance of a myxoma with a smooth, glistening surface. The tumor is globular in shape and measures 8 cm in diameter.

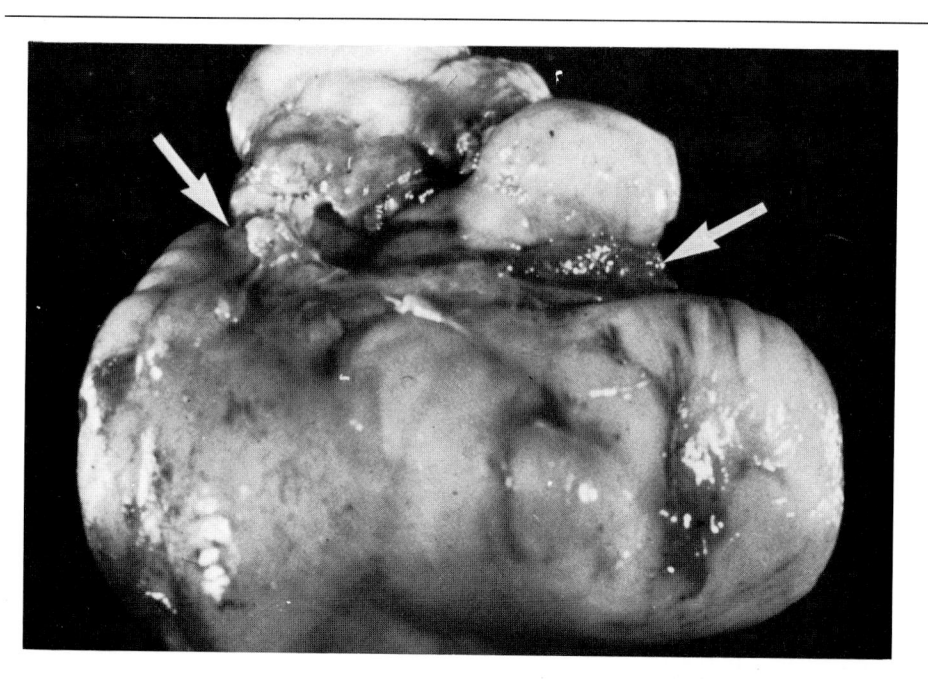

Fig. 11-2. Sarcoma removed from the left atrium of a 17-year-old male demonstrates the line of demarcation (arrows) with that portion of tumor above the arrows being within the left atrial chamber at the time of surgery and the larger portion of tumor below the arrows extrinsic to the left atrium.

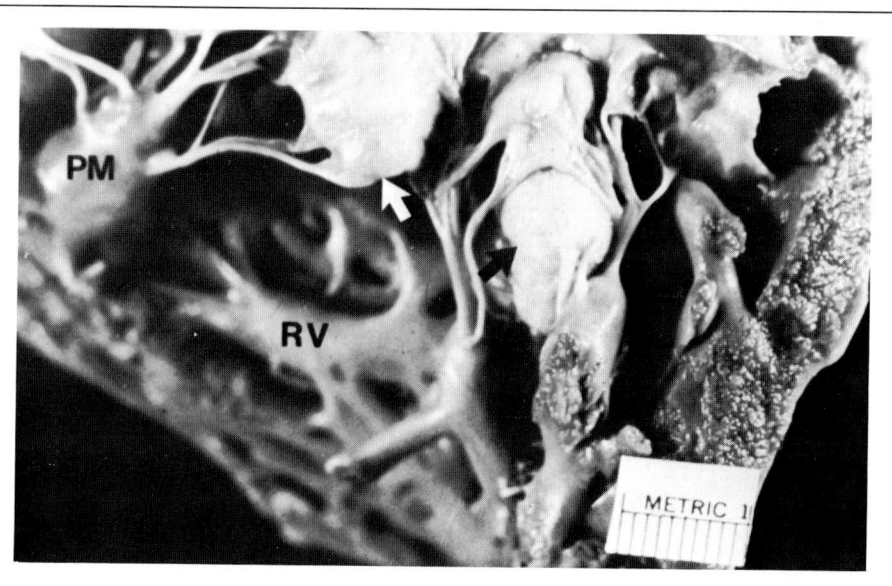

Fig. 11-3. Valvular metastases (white and black arrows) of the tricuspid valve observed at autopsy.

366   11. Cardiac tumors and masses

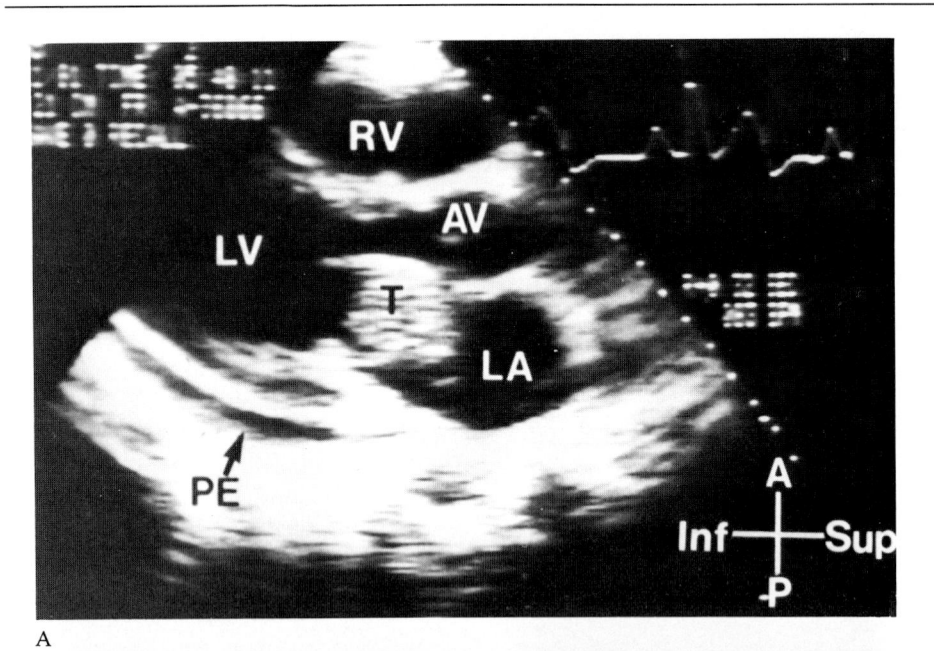

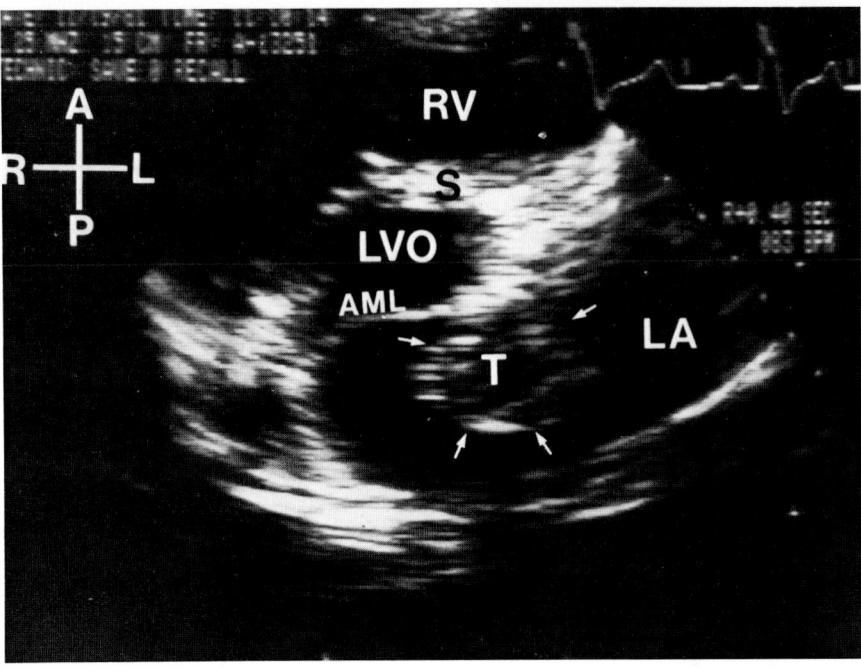

Fig. 11-4A. Parasternal long axis view showing left atrial tumor (T) passing through the mitral orifice during diastole. B. An oblique parasternal short axis view in same patient showing a large tumor mass within the left atrium. This view was obtained by angling the transducer slightly laterally (leftward) just superior to the atrioventricular sulcus and also demonstrates the anterior mitral leaflet, left ventricular outflow tract, anterosuperior portion of the ventricular septum, and right ventricle. C. Parasternal short axis view at the level of the mitral valve in same patient demonstrating the bilobed appearance of the tumor in the mitral orifice at the end of diastole immediately preceding mitral valve closure. D. Apical 4-chamber view demonstrating the tumor in the left atrium extending into the left ventricle during diastole. Three of the four pulmonary veins (PV) can be seen emptying into the LA. E. Apical long axis view of left atrial tumor extending through the mitral orifice during diastole (same patient as in D).

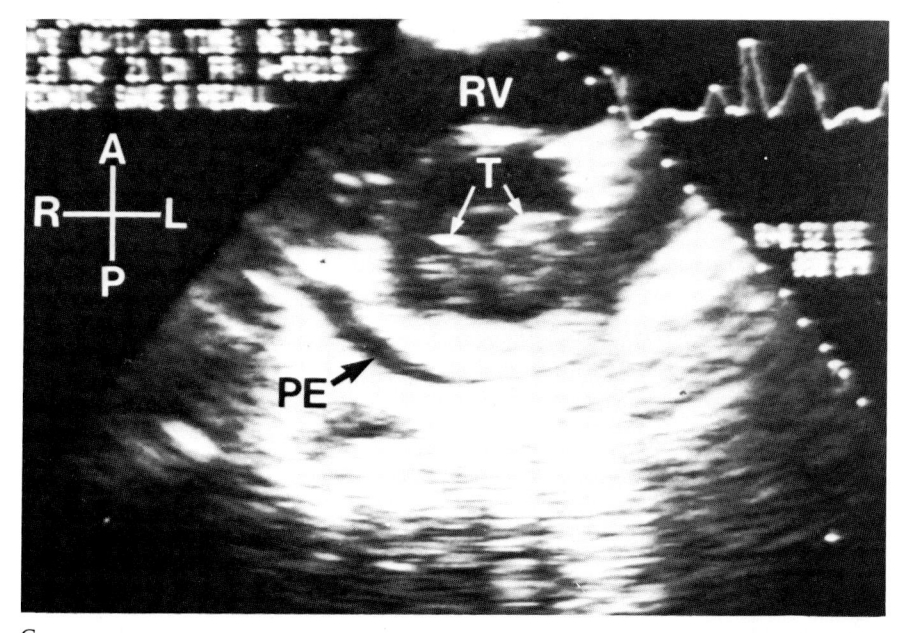

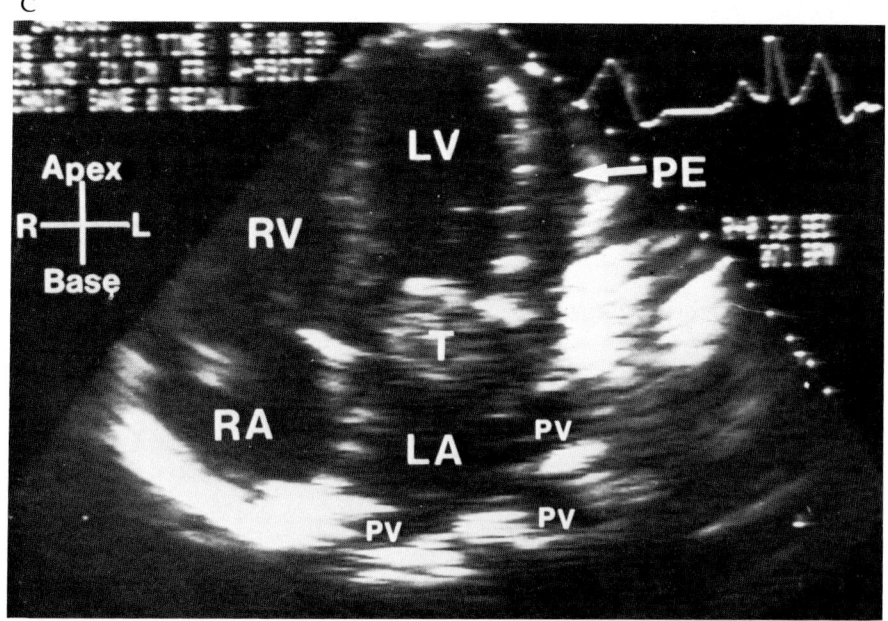

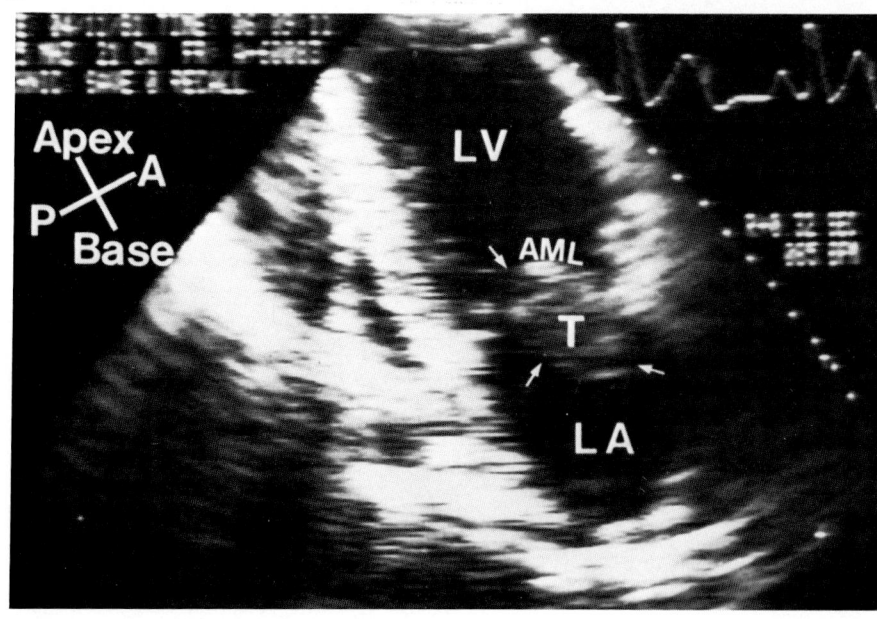

C

D

E

368 11. Cardiac tumors and masses

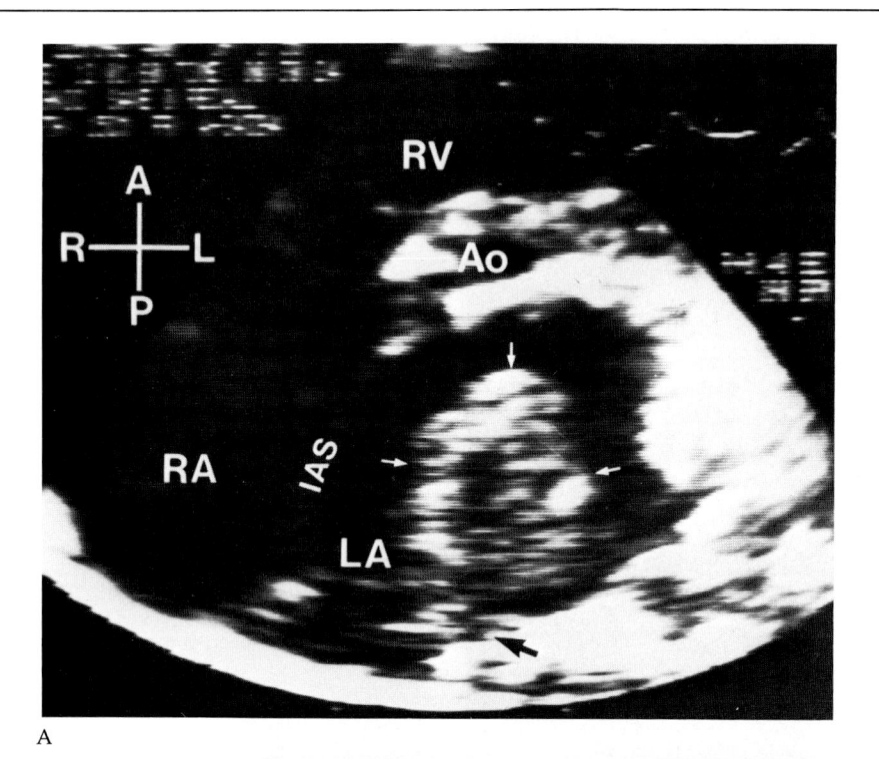

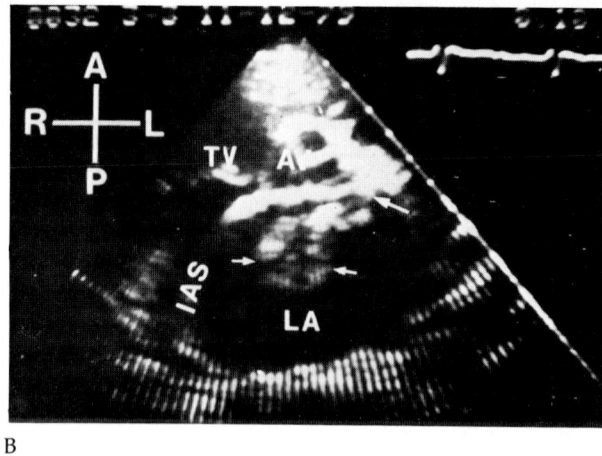

Fig. 11-5A. Parasternal short axis view at the base demonstrating a large mass (arrows) within the left atrium that measures greater than 5 cm in anteroposterior dimension and is attached to the posterior wall of the LA (black arrow). The patient has rheumatic heart disease and both RA and LA are enlarged; the large mass proved to be thrombus at surgery. B. Parasternal short axis view at the base in a patient with rheumatic mitral disease and enlarged LA containing a large pedunculated tumorlike mass (arrows) confirmed to be thrombus at surgery. C. Parasternal short axis view at the base with lateral (leftward) angulation to demonstrate pedunculated, bilobed mass (arrows) attached to the anterolateral wall of the LA and extending slightly into the left atrial appendage. The patient has mild rheumatic mitral disease, but the clinical course was complicated by a systemic embolus. M-mode recording of this mass (thrombus) was also helpful in establishing the diagnosis (see D). D. M-mode recording through the left atrial thrombus of same patient as in C demonstrating flutter motion of the mass (open arrows) owing to atrial flutter observed on electrocardiogram (solid arrows). To the right of the photograph a portion of the thrombus can be seen moving within, but not attached to, the wall of the left atrium. Calibration dots are 5 mm apart. IAS = interatrial septum.

369

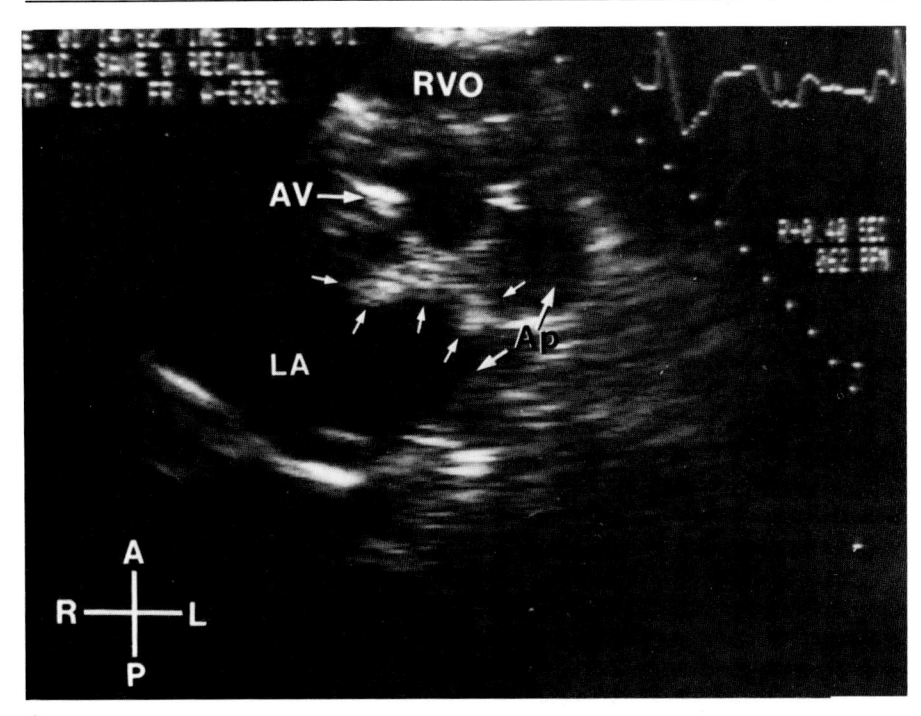

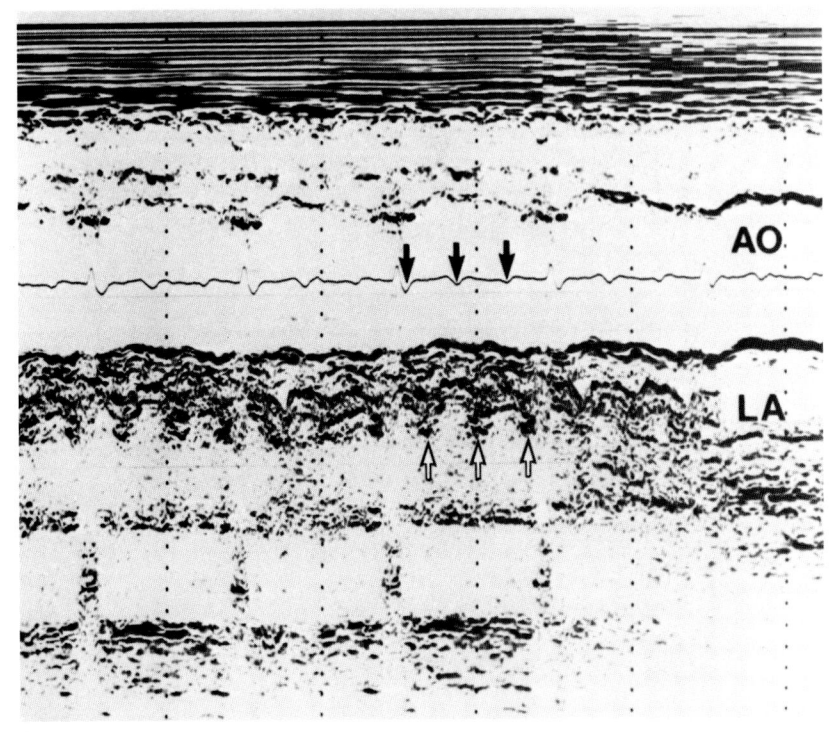

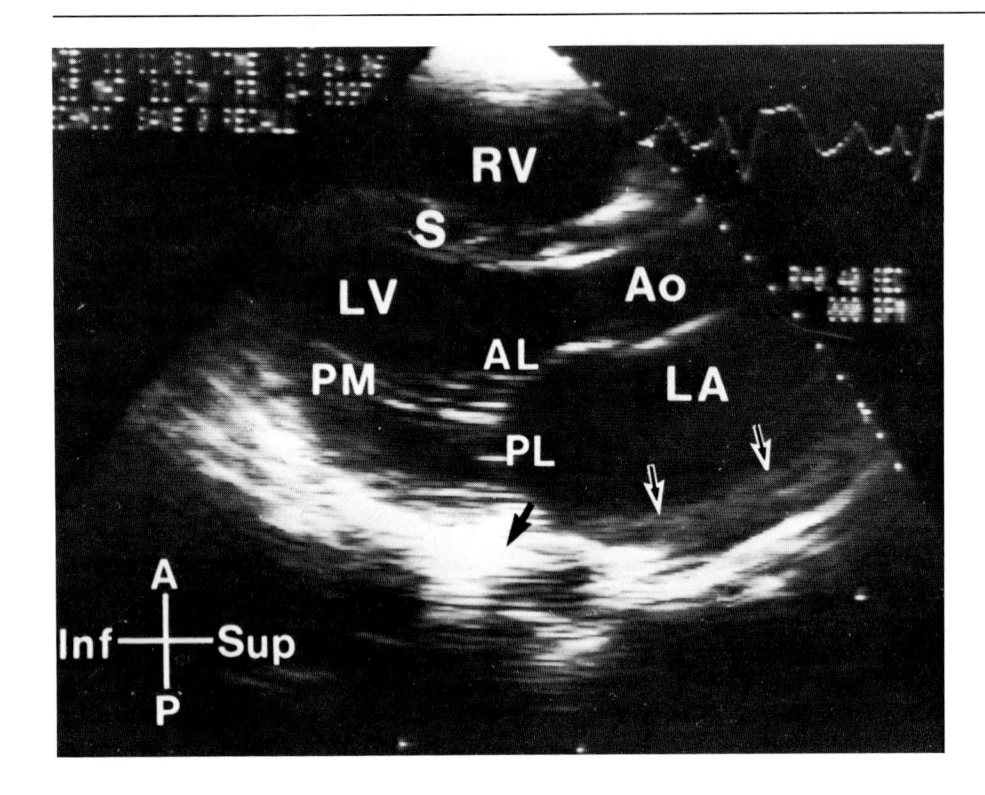

Fig. 11-6. *Parasternal long axis view of a patient demonstrating mild left atrial enlargement and a strong echo reflectance* (black arrow) *in the pericardial-atrioventricular sulcus region that produces artifact on the sector fan* (white arrows) *and can simulate a mass or structure within the left atrium.*

Particular attention must be given to imaging the left atrium in multiple views from parasternal, apical, and subcostal transducer positions in order to scan the entire chamber, including the appendage. Left atrial thrombus is very difficult to diagnose with only M-mode echo [20]. Although sensitivity and specificity data are limited with 2-D echo diagnosis of left atrial thrombi, it is clearly superior to M-mode echo for this purpose [21]. Potential limitations of 2-D echo in detecting left atrial clots do exist; flat mural thrombi closely adherent to the contour of the left atrial wall may not be adequately visualized, a shortcoming that is also well known in angiography [22]. Furthermore, it may not be possible to detect small clots within the atrial appendage, which is the most difficult anatomic region of the left atrium to image. Excessive gain control in the distal portion of the sector or artifact on the fan generated by the strong reflectances in the region of pericardium-atrioventricular sulcus may cause a pseudomass in the left atrium (Fig. 11-6).

Left ventricular tumors and masses. Primary cardiac tumors, both benign and malignant, are extremely rare, with an incidence of only 0.25 percent or less. Of the benign intracavitary tumors of the heart, myxomas are by far the most frequent. Meller and associates [23], in a review of the literature in 1977, noted the prevalence of cardiac myxomas in each chamber as follows: left atrium 75 percent, right atrium 20 percent, left ventricle 2.5 percent, and right ventricle 2.5 percent. At that time only 15 cases of left ventricular myxoma had been reported in the English and French literature with five diagnosed at autopsy and three found at surgery for clinically suspected valvular heart disease. With the availability of two-dimensional echocardiography this diagnosis can be made more easily and at less risk to the patient than with cardiac catheterization. Constitutional features, commonly present with left atrial myxomas, are usually lacking as a clinical finding with left ventricular myxomas. In a review of 16 cases of left ventricular myxoma Meller and colleagues [23] reported on a 33-year-old man who was the first patient diagnosed by echocardiography. This patient had a history of rejection from the military service, symptoms of palpitations and exertional syncope, and a systolic murmur suggestive of aortic stenosis. After the tumor was removed at surgery the heart murmur disappeared.

Whereas myxoma is the most common type of primary cardiac tumor in adults, the tumors of mesenchymal tissues predominate in infants and children [1, 24–27]. Malignant tumors constitute approximately 20 percent of the primary cardiac tumors in all age groups and they occur most commonly in adults [1, 24, 25].

Primary sarcomas of the heart are exceedingly rare. Mahar and associates [28] reported a case of a primary left atrial myxosarcoma in a 29-month-old girl in whom the diagnosis was made by two-dimensional echocardiography. However, the diagnosis was not made until after the patient suffered a stroke caused by a cerebral embolus, which resulted in her death.

The echocardiographic features of a pednunculated thrombus are essentially the same as those of a tumor mass; therefore one cannot necessarily distinguish a tumor from a polyp or thrombus (Fig. 11-7). A thrombus would be expected to occur in the presence of a myocardial infarction, left ventricular aneurysm, or congestive cardiomyopathy. Levisman and colleagues [29] reported a case of a pedunculated tumor in the left ventricle that appeared from gross morphological features to be a myxoma; however, the pathological diagnosis was pedunculated thrombus.

In addition to the nonspecific constitutional symptoms which may be caused by cardiac tumors, specific cardiac findings may include arrhythmias, pericarditis with or without effusion, systemic emboli, and left-sided inflow or outflow obstruction [30, 31]. The rhabdomyoma is the most frequent neoplasm in the pediatric age group; in 50 percent of cases this tumor occurs in association with tuberous sclerosis and is usually found in children less than 2 years of age [32, 33]. Left ventricular tumors may cause outflow obstruction with a murmur of aortic stenosis [23, 34]. Orsmond and associates [34] reported a 12-year-old girl with findings of severe aortic stenosis diagnosed by echocardiography as having a tumor involving the ventricular septum and obstructing the orifice of the aortic valve; it was difficult to distinguish histologically whether the tumor was a primary alveolar rhabdomyosarcoma or metastatic tumor from a soft tissue sarcoma that had been removed from the child's leg six years earlier. The clinical and pathological problem of distinguishing between a primary and a metastatic carcinoma is well illustrated in this case (Fig. 11-8). Approximately 40 primary rhabdomyosarcomas of the heart have been reported in the literature, and there is a tendency for these tumors, when they occur elsewhere, to metastasize to the heart [35–37].

Some investigators suggest that myxomas represent one of three possible sequences of organization of endocardial thrombi [38]. However, their site of occurrence, chiefly in the left atrium near the fossa ovalis, their lack of laminations, their complete covering by endothelium, and their containing mucopolysaccharides produced by vascular endothelial cells support the view that myxomas are neoplastic in origin [39].

372   11. Cardiac tumors and masses

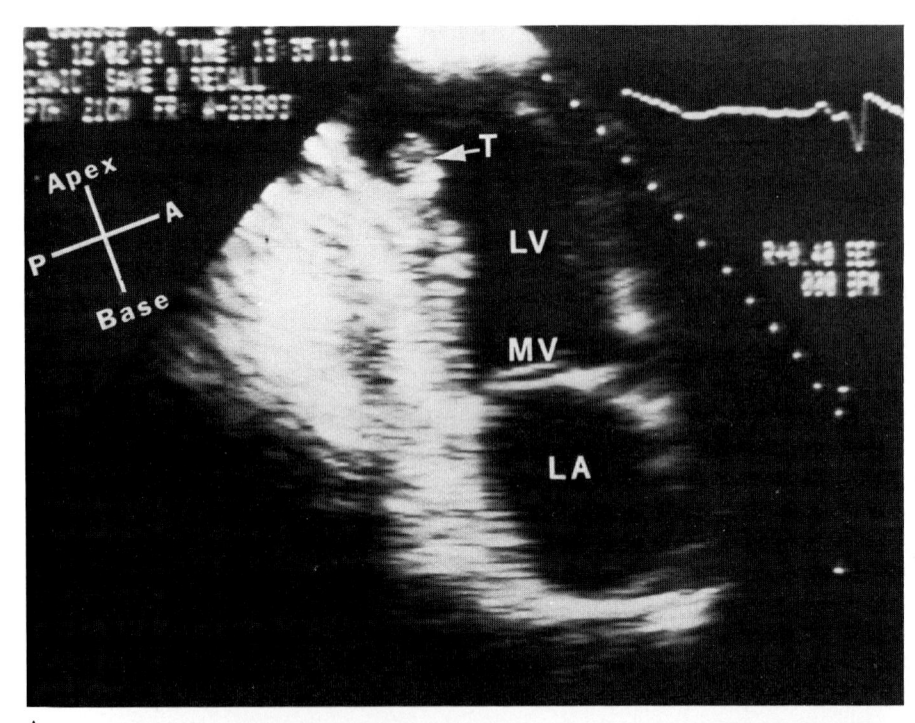

Fig. 11-7A. Apical long axis view showing pedunculated mass attached to the posterior wall of the left ventricle in the apex, the site of a previous myocardial infarction. The mass is a thrombus (T). B. Apical 4-chamber view in a 10-year-old child soon after surgery for double outlet right ventricle showing a pedunculated thrombus in the apex of the left ventricle.

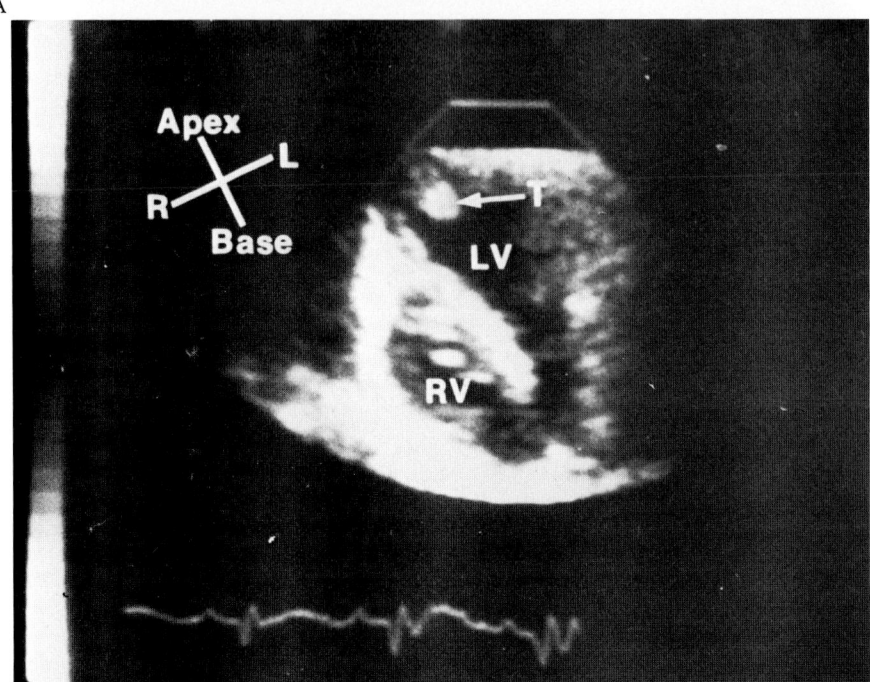

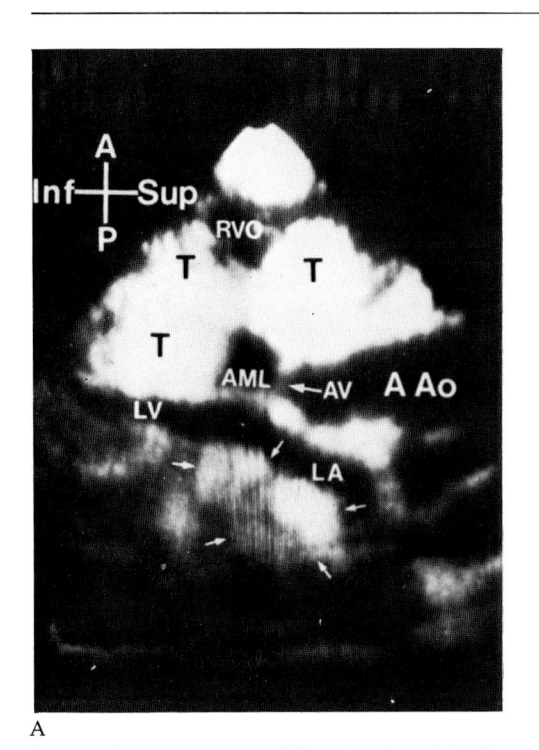

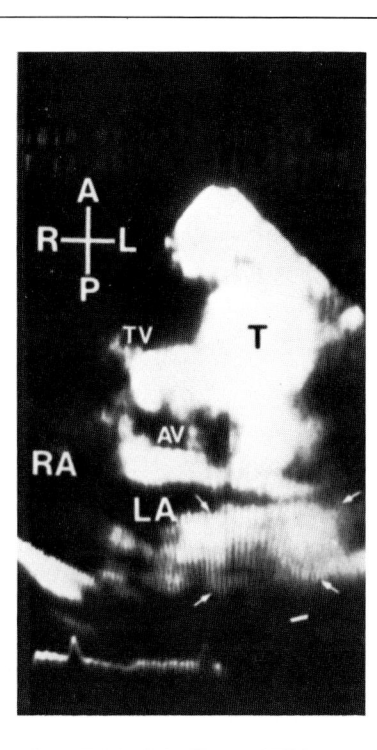

Fig. 11-8A. Parasternal long axis (left panel) *and short axis* (right panel) *views of a patient with terminal metastatic carcinoma demonstrating massive tumor (T) involvement of the right ventricular outflow tract, ventricular septum, left ventricle, and left atrium. B. M-mode recording of a calcified benign tumor (arrows) confirmed at surgery to be subendocardial in the atrioventricular sulcus.*

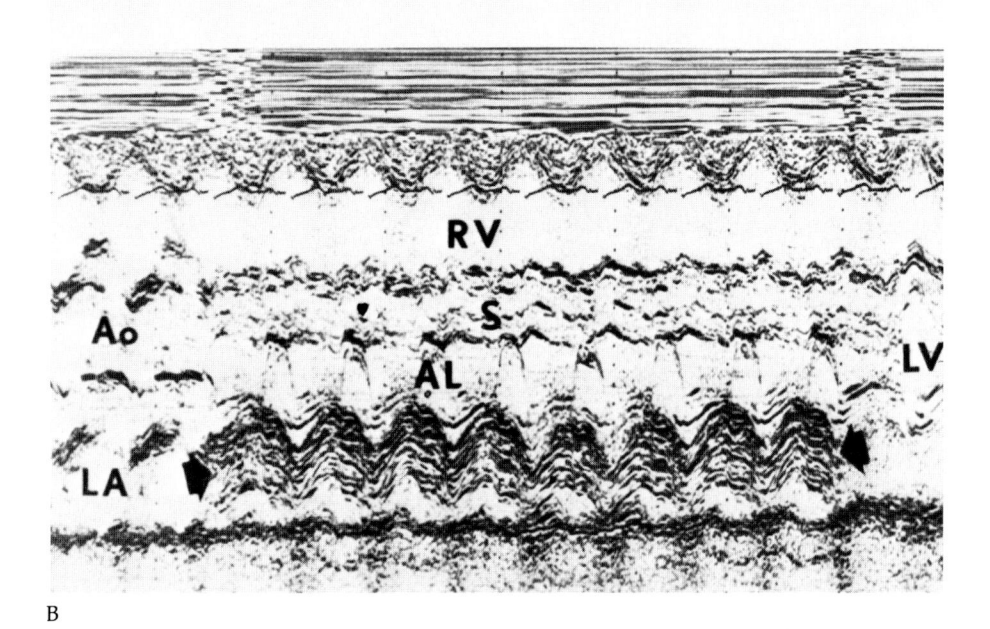

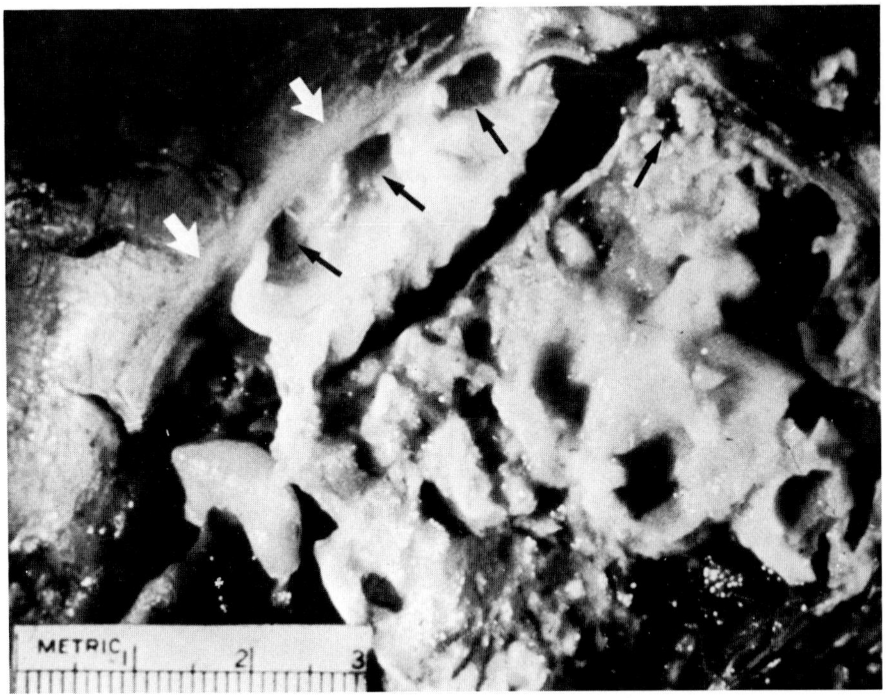

Fig. 11-9. Echinococcosis cyst of the myocardium: multiple calcified cysts (black arrows) *involving the pericardium. The dense layer at the margin of the cyst is thickened pericardium* (white arrows).

Farooki and colleagues [40] reported a case of an 8-year-old boy from the Middle East with abdominal echinococcosis who had a hydatid cyst in the ventricular septum diagnosed with echocardiography. The anatomic features of the fluid-filled hydatid cyst (Fig. 11-9) are contrasted with those of a myxoma (see Fig. 11-1).

Intramural fibrous tumors of the heart have been called a variety of names including "fibroma," "hamartoma," and "embryonic mesenchymal tumor" [39]. These tumors usually occur in children but may be seen in adults. All are located in the ventricular myocardium, usually in the interventricular septum, or less frequently in the right ventricle. Occasionally fibromas may contain calcium deposits and foci of bone formation. Despite the interdigitation of the fibroma with the myocardium, these tumors are benign (Fig. 11-10).

Tumors and cysts of heterotopic tissue may rarely occur in the heart; these include mesothelioma, epithelial cysts, teratomas, and thyroid tumors [39]. Mesotheliomas are small tumors that can form projecting nodules. Epithelial-lined cysts in the heart are quite rare. They may occur in any age group, may be located above the endocardial surface, and may contain a gelatinous material; their diameters range from 4 to 25 mm (Fig. 11-11).

Right atrial tumors, masses, and benign structures. Although right atrial myxomas are less common than the left atrial variety, tumors involving the right atrium occur more frequently than myxomas in either of the ventricular chambers. The clinical presentation of right atrial myxomas has mimicked metastatic liver disease [41], constrictive pericarditis [42], polycythemia vera [43], cyanosis and clubbing [44], pulmonary hypertension [45], tricuspid insufficiency [46], and right heart failure [47–49]. Although it is technically quite easy to image a left atrial tumor with M-mode echocardiography, it is considerably more difficult to image the right atrium or to see evidence of right atrial masses with the limitations of M-mode technique [50–52]. The echocardiographer was usually limited to imaging abnormal structures or masses during diastole behind the tricuspid valve because the right atrium was frequently not visualized. Two-dimensional echocardiography plays a very important role in the investigation of possible right atrial masses or tumors [52]. By utilizing multiple tomographic planes from different transducer positions, a structure or mass can be localized; size, shape, and motion evaluated; and site of attachment identified (Figs. 11-12 to 11-15). A minimum of five separate two-dimensional planes should be imaged for complete evaluation of the right atrium: (1) parasternal short axis at the base; (2) parasternal right ventricular inflow (RA/RV); (3) apical four-chamber; (4) subcostal biatrial-interatrial septum; and (5) inferior vena cava-right atrium.

Approximately 2 percent of normal individuals have congenital remnants of valvelike or membranous-appearing structures located within the right atrium. Congenital remnants of the sinus venosus include a weblike membrane called Chiari's network (Fig. 11-16) and valvelike structures called eustachian and thebesian valves [53–56] (Fig. 11-17). Chiari's network usually is attached to the interatrial septum and exhibits a characteristic flapping, chaotic motion. It is important to recognize the characteristic appearance, size, and location of Chiari's network because it might be confused with a vegetation or thrombus. Although there is no functional significance to Chiari's network, the multiple fenestrations may pose a theoretical hazard for entanglement of a catheter at time of cardiac catheterization. The eustachian valve is easily recognized because of its characteristic appearance and consistent location at the junction of the inferior vena cava and the right atrium. The thebesian valve is the valve to the coronary sinus.

In the embryonic development of the heart, the sinus venosus is incorporated into the wall of the right atrium. Normally the right valve of the sinus venosus forms the valve of the inferior vena cava (eustachian valve) and the valve of the coronary sinus (thebesian valve), while the left valve of the sinus venosus is incorporated into the flap tissue that seals off the fossa ovalis.

Farooki and colleagues [57] reported the echocardiographic diagnosis of right atrial extension of a Wilms' tumor in a 5-year-old girl (Fig. 11-18). A thrombus of the inferior vena cava propagating into the right atrium may also resemble a right atrial tumor [58].

A few cases of biatrial myxomas have also been reported [59–62].

Right ventricular tumors. Right ventricular tumors can be detected by echocardiography, and, here again, two-dimensional imaging is far superior compared to M-mode echo. Most tumors reported in the literature have been myxomas; however, one case of metastatic melanoma has been described [63–67]. A pedunculated myxoma may produce right ventricular outflow tract obstruction and simulate pulmonary stenosis [64, 67] (Fig. 11-19).

The antemortem diagnosis of cardiac metastases was uncommon before the advent of echocardiography. Krivokapich and associates [68] reported on two patients with metastatic carcinoma in the right ventricular cavity that was diagnosed

11. Cardiac tumors and masses

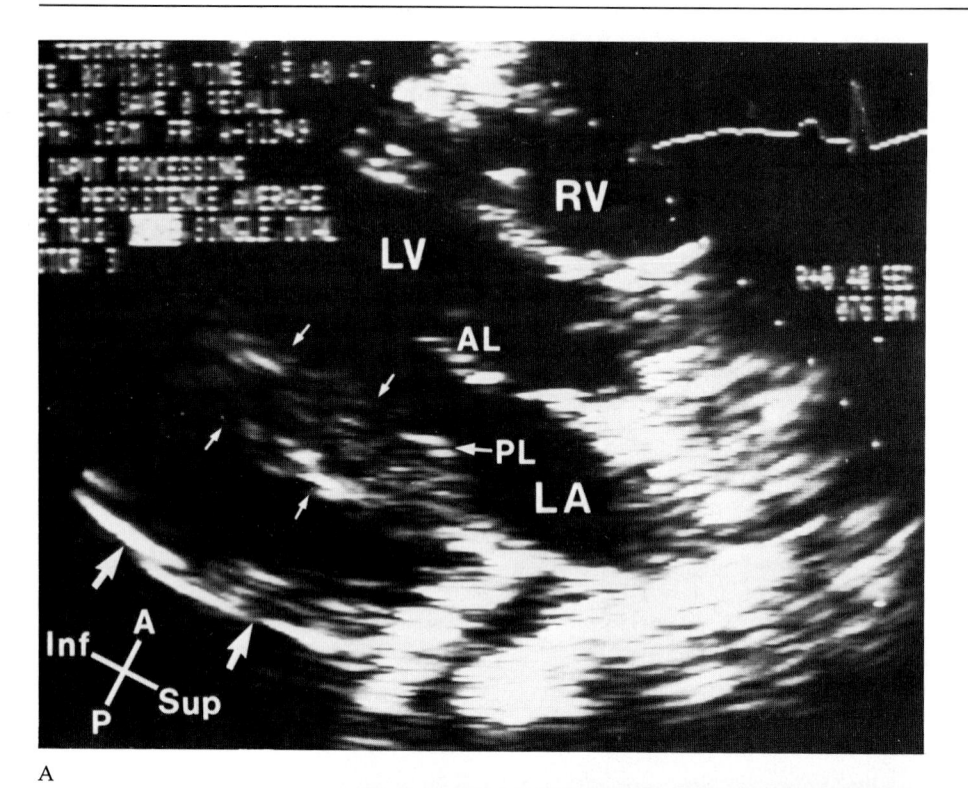

Fig. 11-10A. Parasternal long axis view of an asymptomatic young man demonstrating marked increased thickness (arrows) of the posterior basilar wall of the left ventricle with a localized fluid space posterior to the LV wall and anterior to the pericardium (two large white arrows). Some areas within this localized thickened myocardium have increased reflectance. It extends just superior to the atrioventricular sulcus and appears to involve the posterior mitral leaflet. B. Apical long axis view in same patient demonstrating the distal extent of this cystic tumor involvement of the posterior LV wall (small arrows) to the posterior medial papillary muscle (large curved arrow). The wall of this cystic tumor mass appears continuous with and cannot be distinguished from the pericardium. C. M-mode recording in same patient demonstrating the dyskinetic motion and increased thickness of the posterior left ventricular wall. It is very difficult to distinguish posterior leaflet motion (curved arrow) from the underlying myocardium, which appears to be infiltrated with tumor. Calibration dots are 5 mm apart. D. Apical 4-chamber view in same patient demonstrating the lateral involvement of the myocardium (arrows) and the adjacent fluid. The apex and septum are normal.

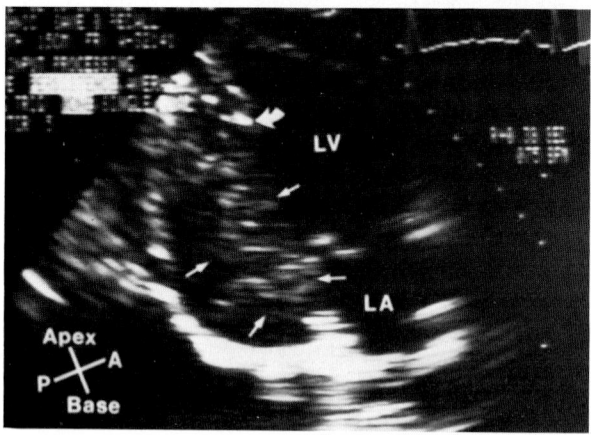

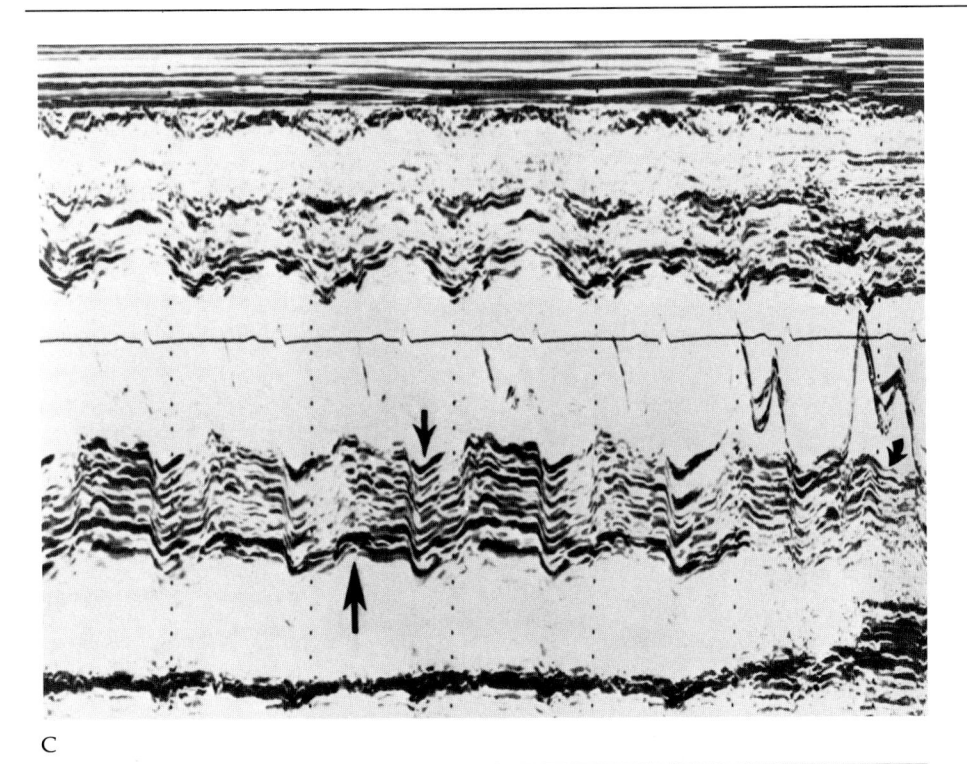

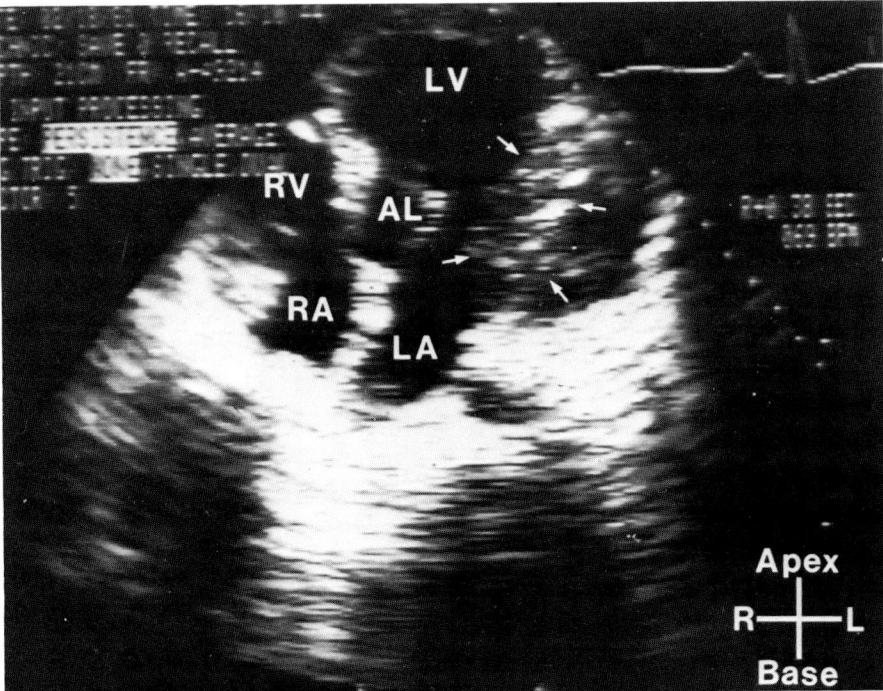

C

D

378   11. Cardiac tumors and masses

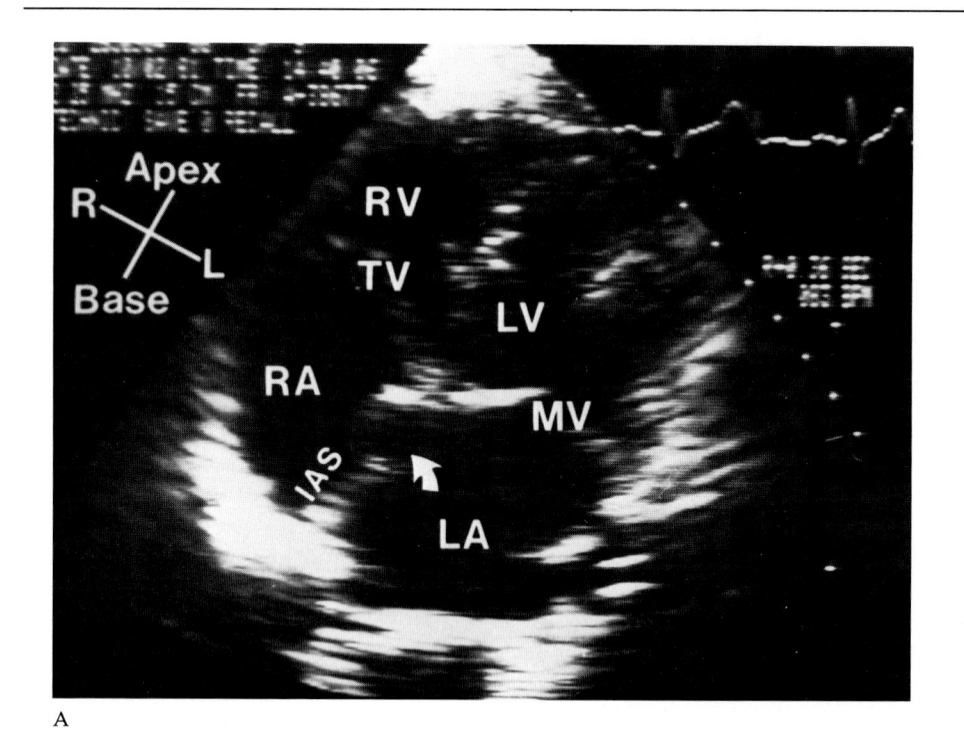

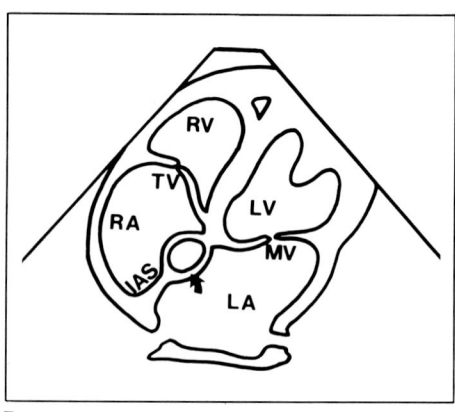

Fig. 11-11A. Apical 4-chamber view demonstrating an apparent cyst within the interatrial septum (IAS) (arrow). Internal dimensions of the cyst measure 11 mm × 10 mm. Otherwise cardiac examination was negative. B. Diagrammatic representation showing the cyst of the interatrial septum.

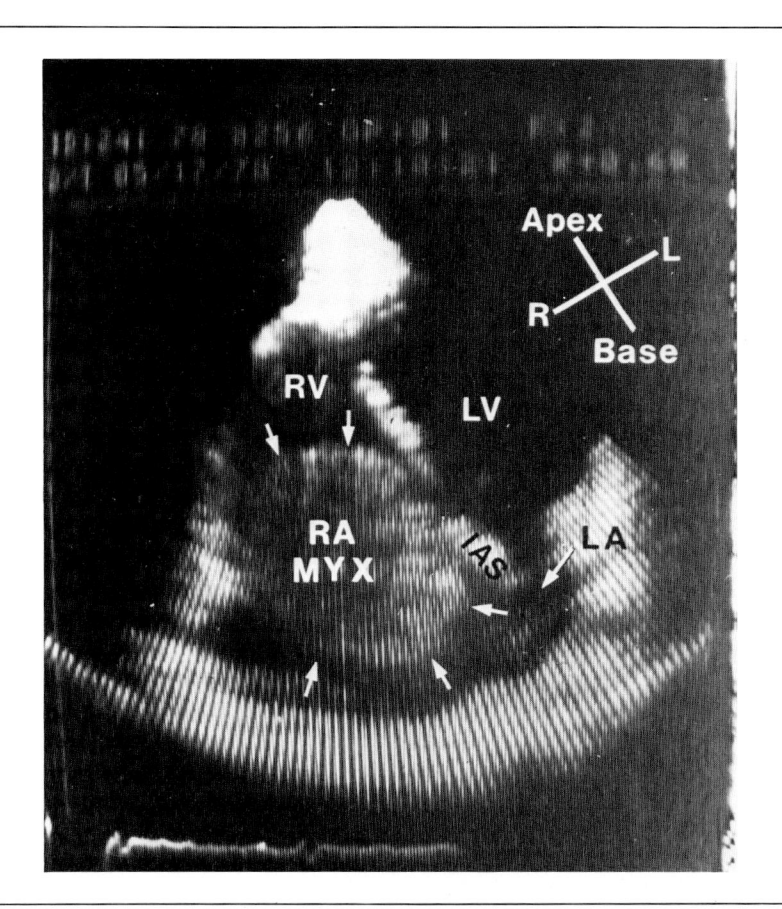

Fig. 11-12. Apical 4-chamber view obtained from a young adult male demonstrating a large (7 × 8 cm) pedunculated right atrial myxoma (RA MYX) occluding the tricuspid orifice and extending far into the right ventricle. IAS = interatrial septum.

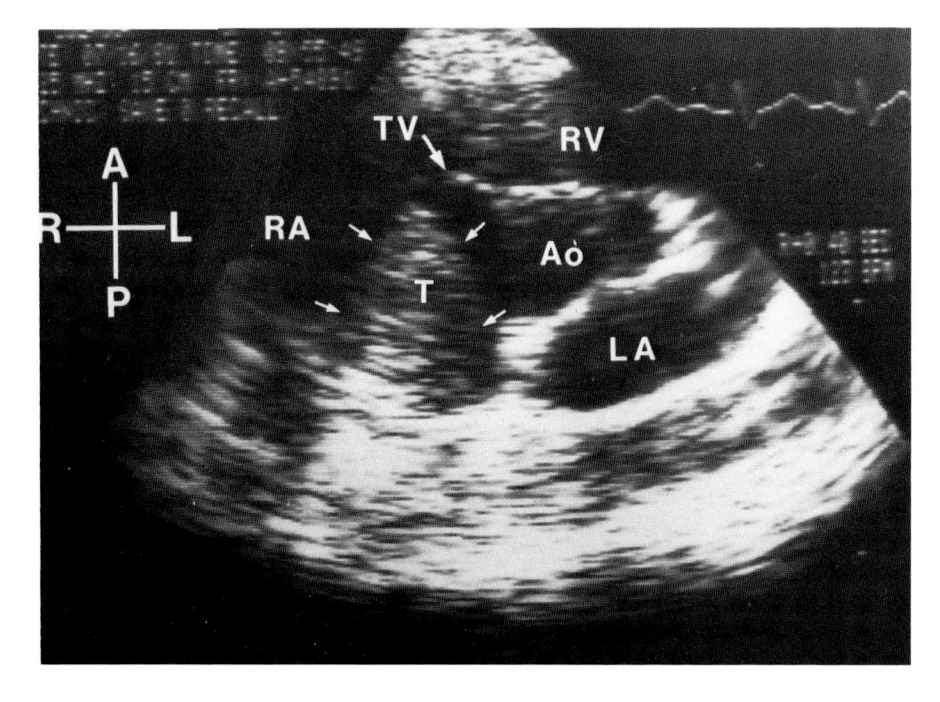

Fig. 11-13. Parasternal short axis view at the base in a patient with right ventricular failure, enlargement of the right atrium, and a huge broad-based mass (T) attached to the RA wall. The anterior end of the mass is tapered but it appeared smooth in all projections, resembling a myxoma; however, it was found to be thrombus at surgery.

380   11. Cardiac tumors and masses

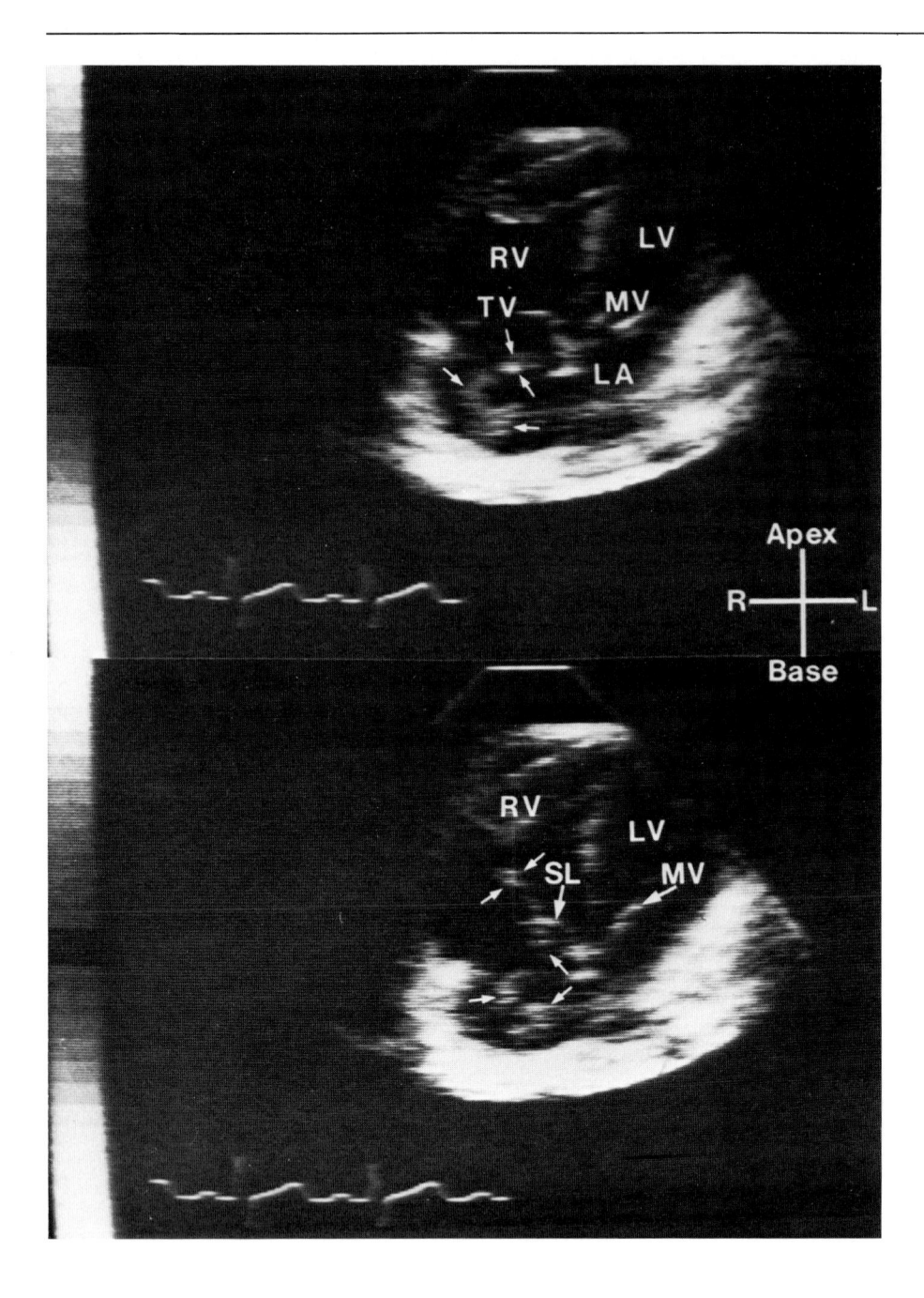

Fig. 11-14. Apical 4-chamber views obtained from a 29-year-old man demonstrating a curved, thin mass (arrows) in the right atrium during systole (upper panel). This serpentinelike mass projected far into the right ventricle (arrows, lower panel) during diastole. It was diagnosed as recent thrombus at surgery. There was no other abnormality in the right atrium where the thrombus was attached.

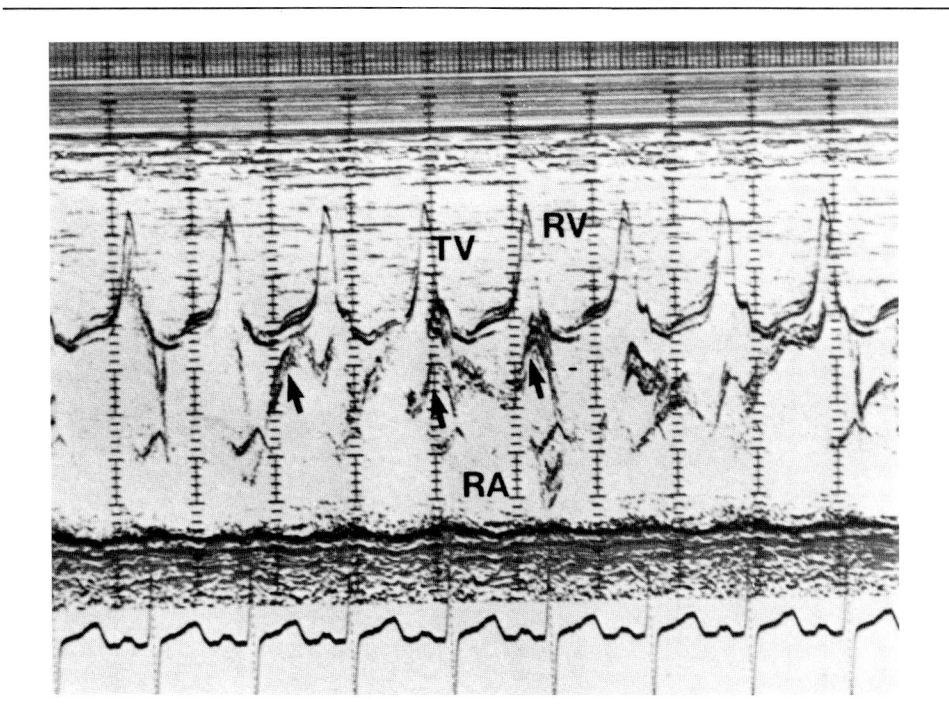

Fig. 11-15. M-mode recording from patient in Fig. 11-14 showing the thrombus (arrows) bobbing around in the right atrium.

382   11. Cardiac tumors and masses

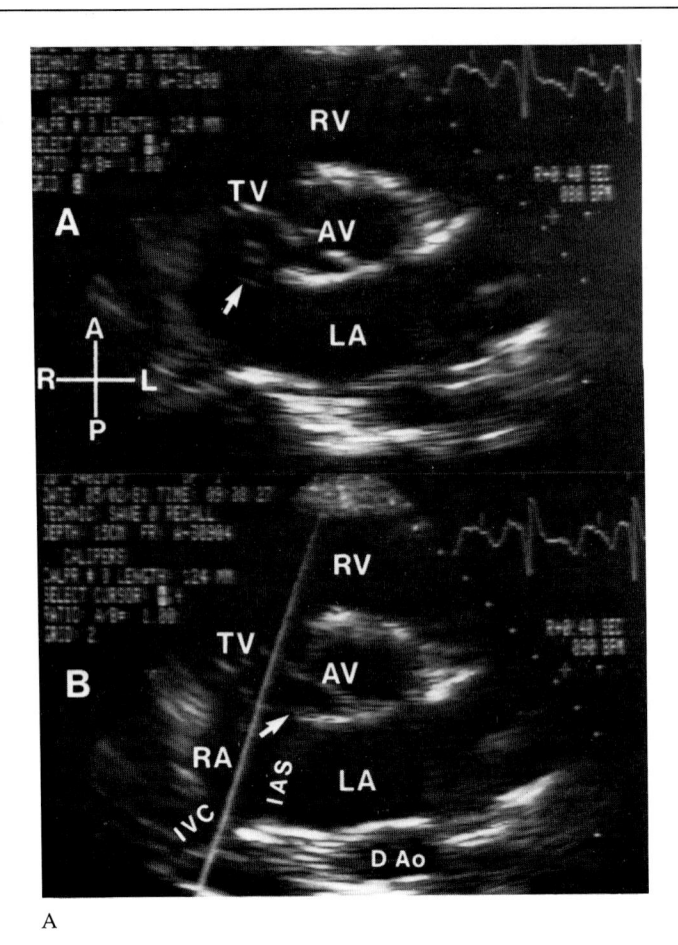

Fig. 11-16A. Parasternal short axis views at the base in the same patient demonstrating Chiari's network in the right atrium (arrow, upper panel) and its attachment to the interatrial septum (IAS) near the aortic annulus (arrow, lower panel). The motion of Chiari's network resembles a vegetation; however, it is always attached to the wall of the RA, usually the interatrial septum, and, since it is not attached to the tricuspid valve, should not be confused with a vegetation. B. Chiari's network (black arrows) showing multiple strands and fenestrations with attachments to the interatrial septum and right atrial wall. C. Close-up view of Chiari's network in different subject. It is attached to the interatrial septum and extends from a point near the coronary sinus to a more superior insertion point (black arrow). Notice the thin, weblike membrane with multiple fenestrations. The thebesian valve is overlying the opening to the coronary sinus.

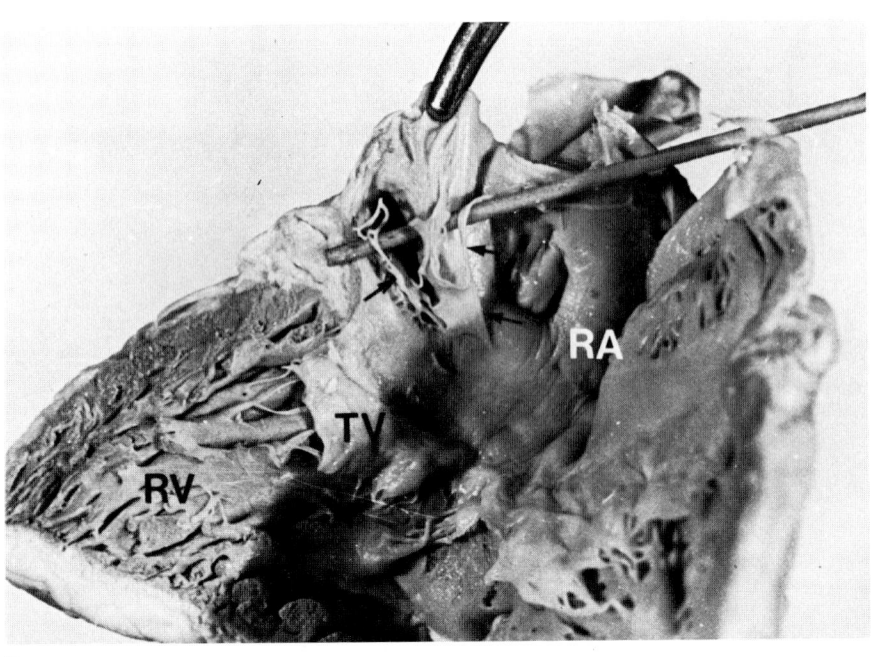

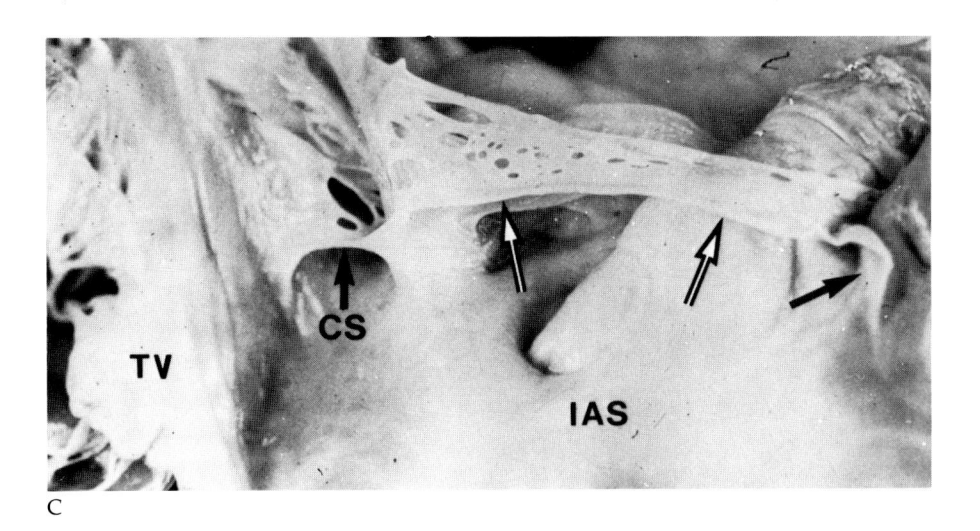

C

Fig. 11-17A. Close-up anatomic section in the subcostal 4-chamber view of a normal heart demonstrating both a thebesian valve (curved white arrow) at the opening to the coronary sinus and a eustachian valve (EV) near the junction of the right atrium and inferior vena cava. B. Subcostal view of the IVC and RA demonstrating a eustachian valve attached to the RA wall near the IVC-RA junction (single arrow, upper panel; two arrows, lower panel) in a normal adult. C. View at the low left sternal border of the right ventricular inflow tract demonstrating a eustachian valve (arrows) attached to the right atrial wall; the inferior vena cava is not visible in this view. IAS = interatrial septum.

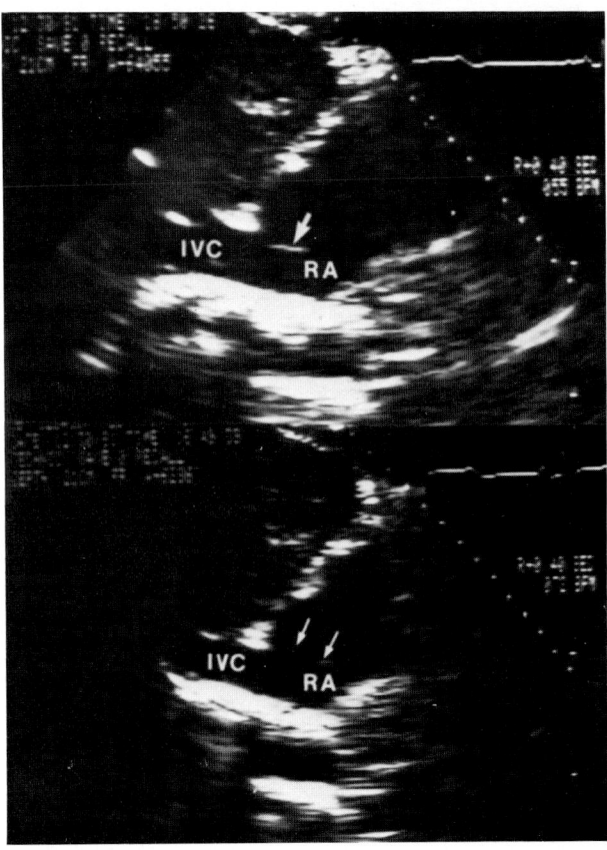

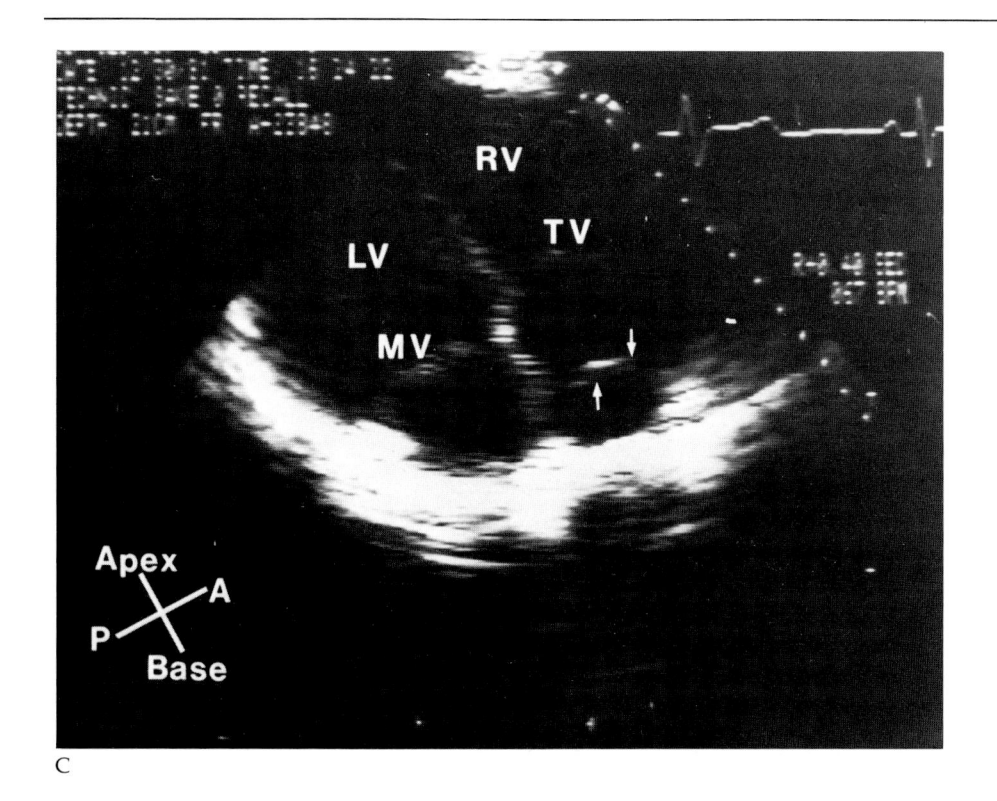

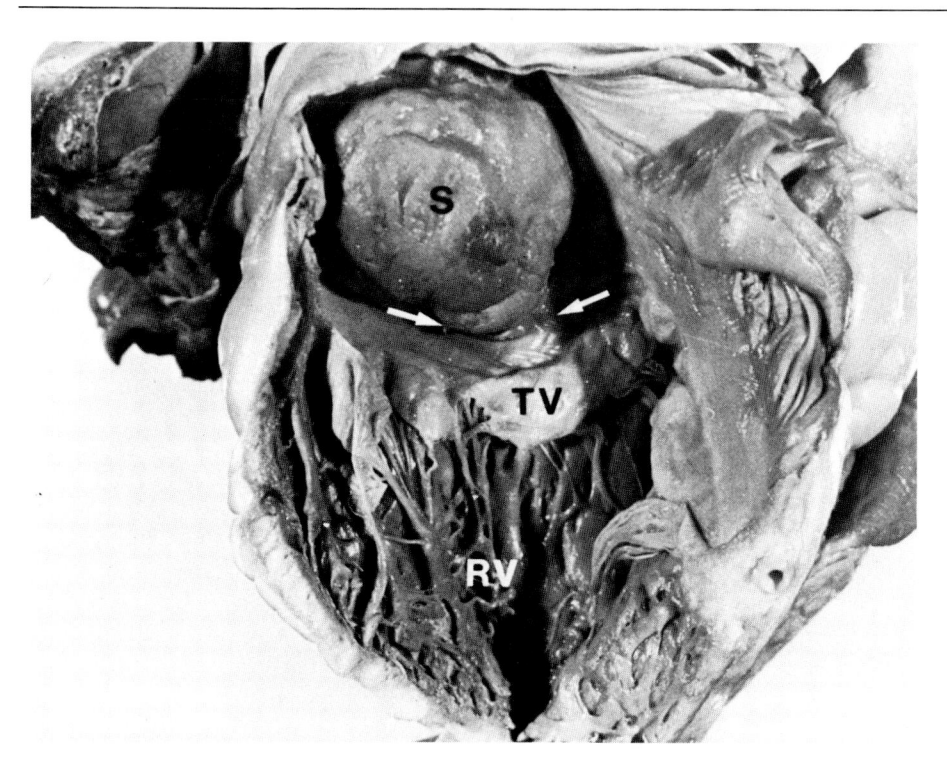

Fig. 11-18. Anatomic specimen demonstrating a large sarcoma (S) extending from the inferior vena cava (arrows) into the right atrium.

386   11. Cardiac tumors and masses

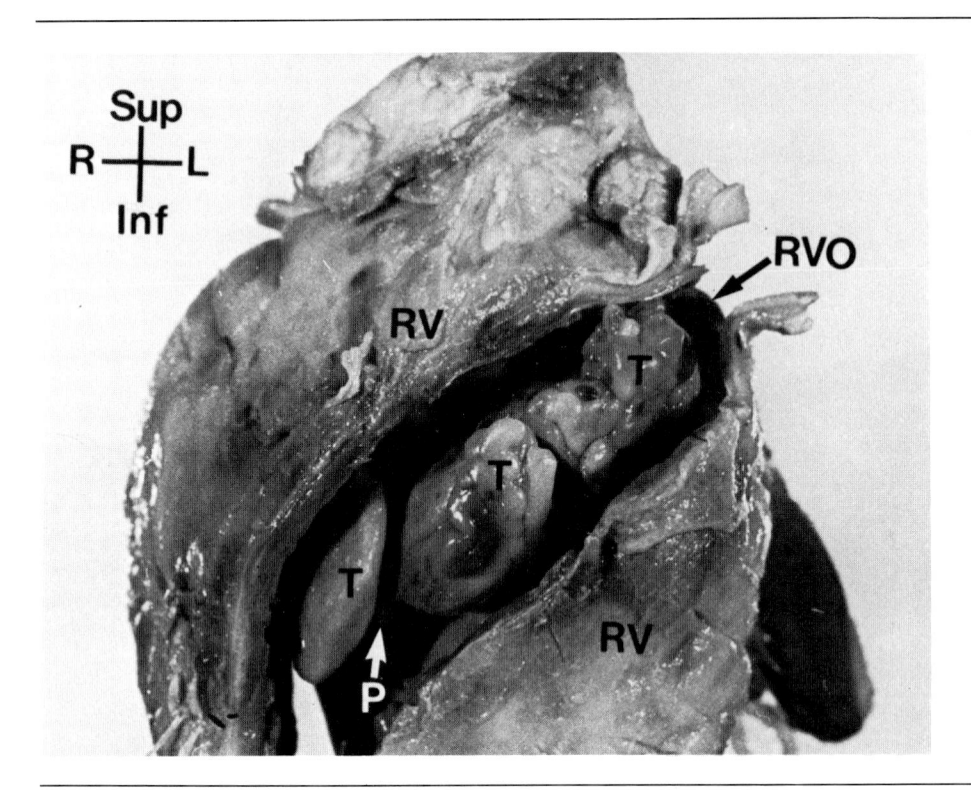

Fig. 11-19. Anatomic view of open right ventricular cavity demonstrating a large tumor (T), a small portion of a tricuspid porcine heterograft (P), and the obstructive position of the tumor in the right ventricular outflow tract.

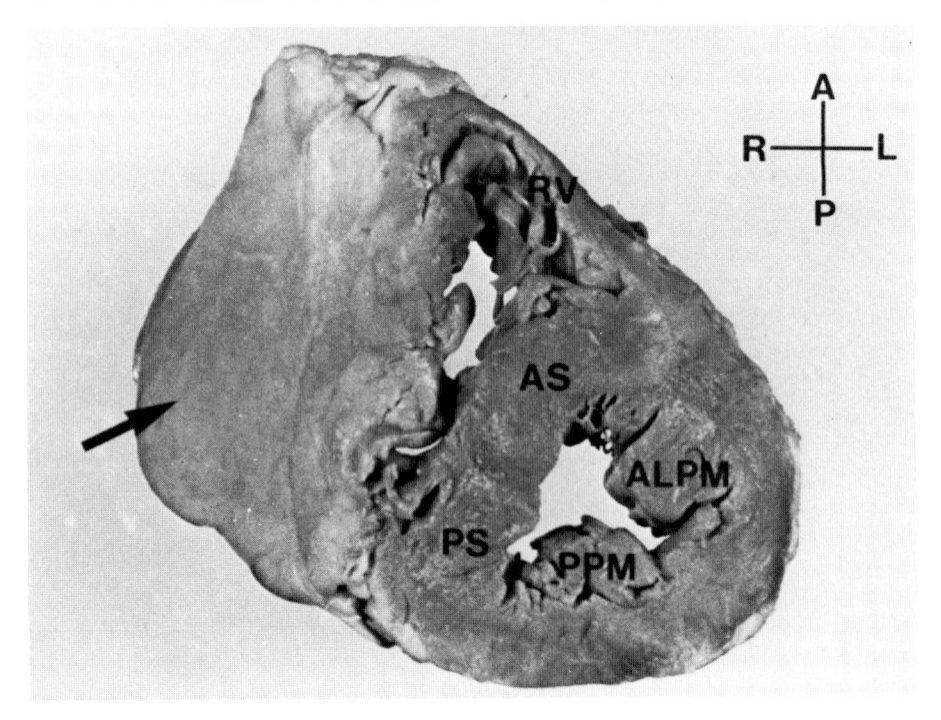

Fig. 11-20. Anatomic parasternal short axis view of Hodgkin's lymphoma (arrow) invading the free wall of the right ventricle. ALPM = anterolateral papillary muscle; AS = anterior septum; PPM = posteromedial papillary muscle; PS = posterior septum.

387

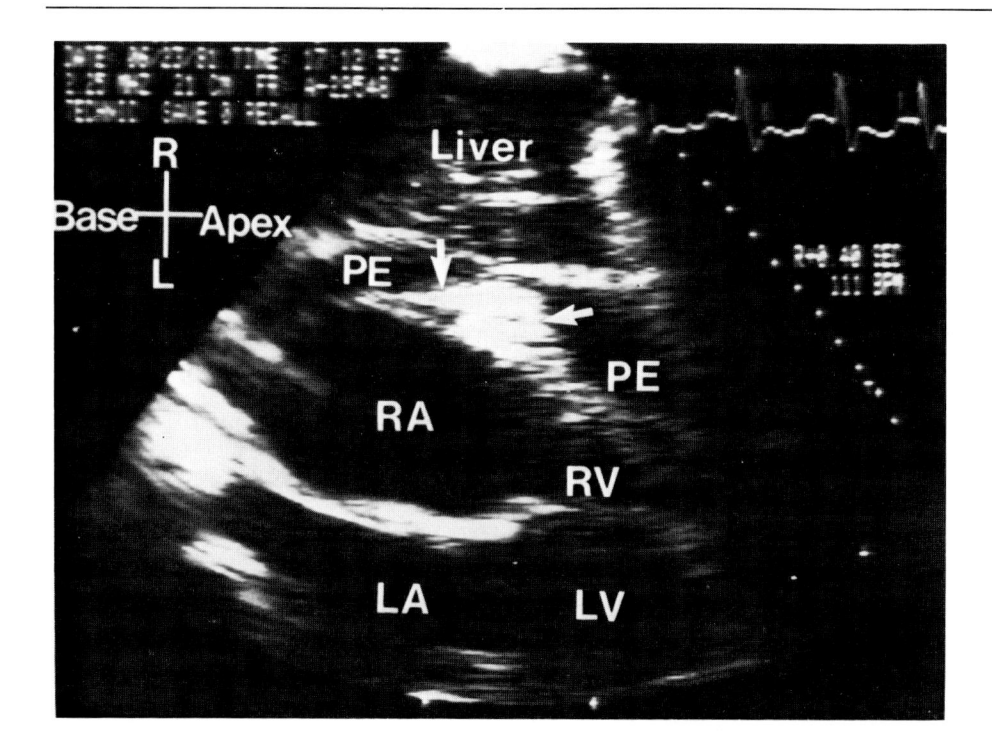

Fig. 11-21. Subcostal biatrial view in a patient with carcinoma demonstrating a pericardial effusion and metastases (arrows) on the surface of the right atrium.

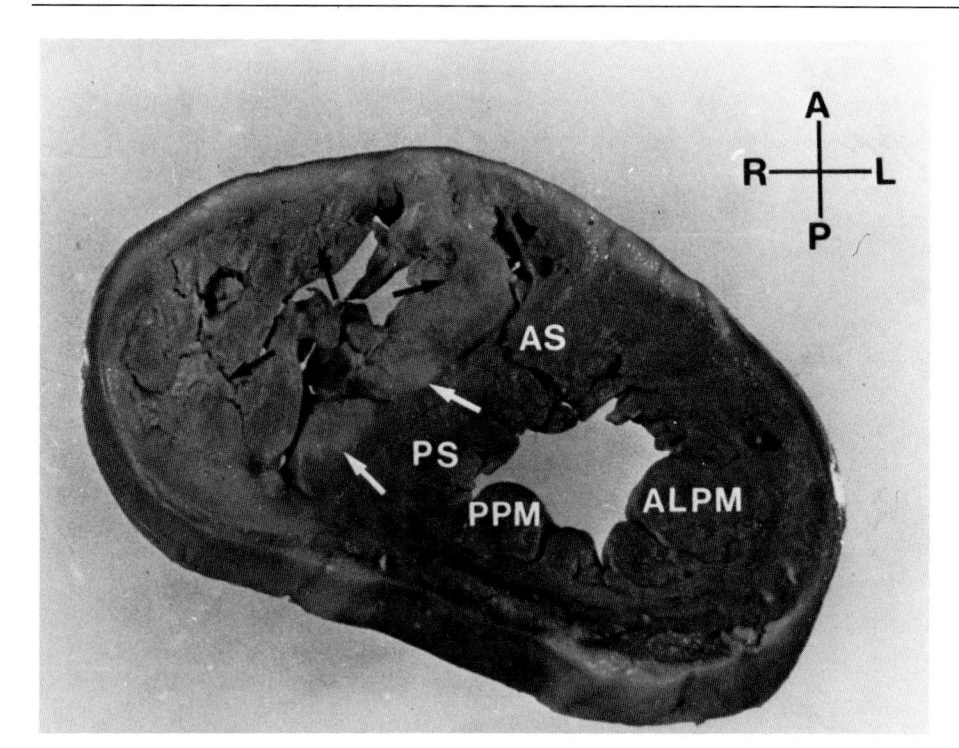

Fig. 11-22. Anatomic section in the parasternal short axis view demonstrating an extensive abscess of the right ventricle (arrows). ALPM = anterolateral papillary muscle; AS = anterior septum; PPM = posteromedial papillary muscle; PS = posterior septum.

388   11. Cardiac tumors and masses

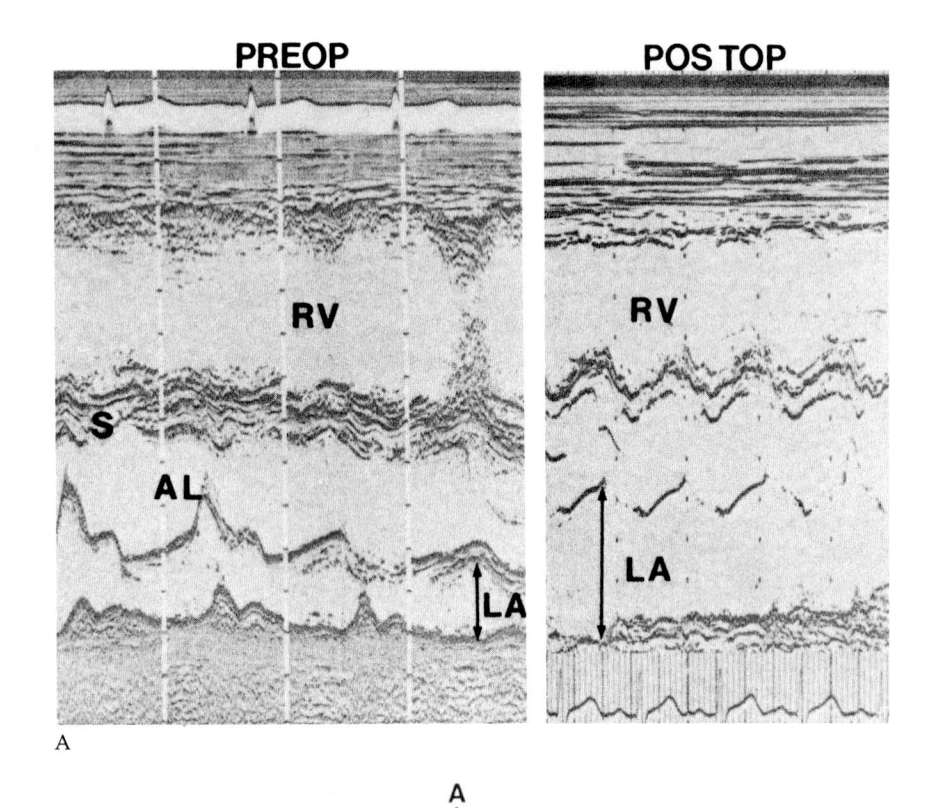

Fig. 11-23A. M-mode recordings in a patient with a mediastinal tumor displacing the heart (left panel) causing the right ventricle to be "pancaked" and to appear falsely large; there is posterior displacement of the aorta and flattening or compression of the left atrium. Following surgical removal of the tumor, the position of the heart and sizes of the cardiac chambers returned to normal (right panel). B. Parasternal short axis views in the same patient who has a cystic thymoma (CT) producing some compression of the right ventricular outflow tract. C. Subcostal 4-chamber views from a young adult with a mediastinal lymphoma demonstrating borders (arrows, both panels) of the tumor (T) and displacement of the right atrium. D. Subcostal 4-chamber (left panel) and apical 4-chamber views (right panel) of same patient with a cystic tumor (T) adjacent to the right atrium but not causing any significant displacement or compression. LPA = left pulmonary artery; RPA = right pulmonary artery.

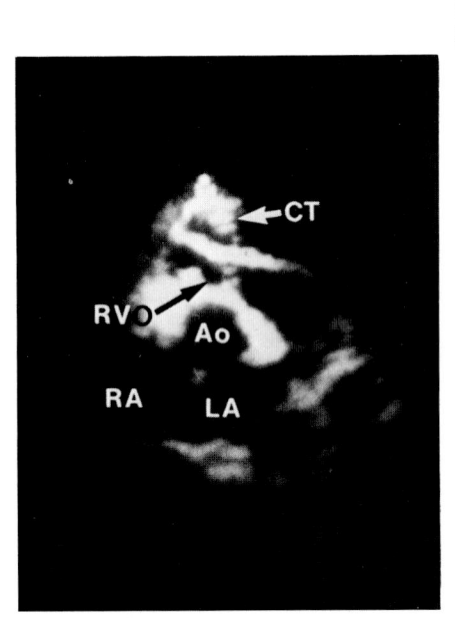

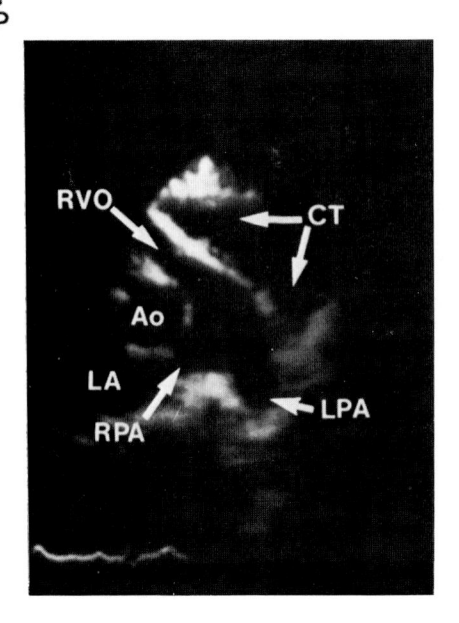

389

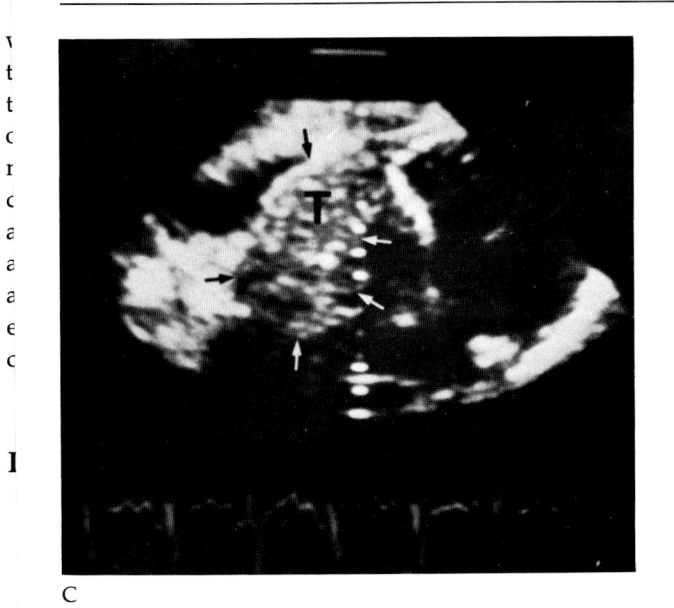

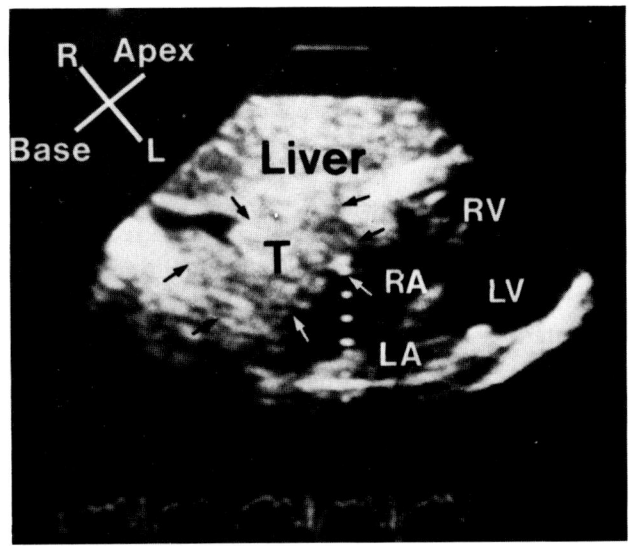

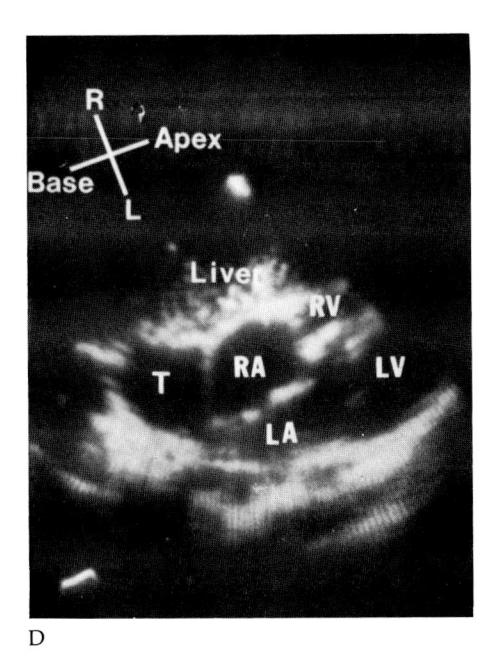

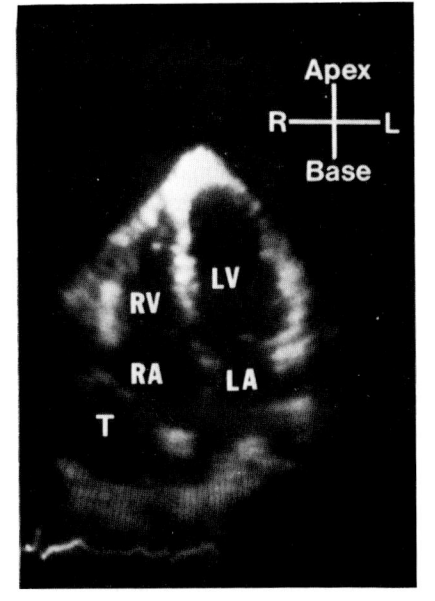

C

D

389

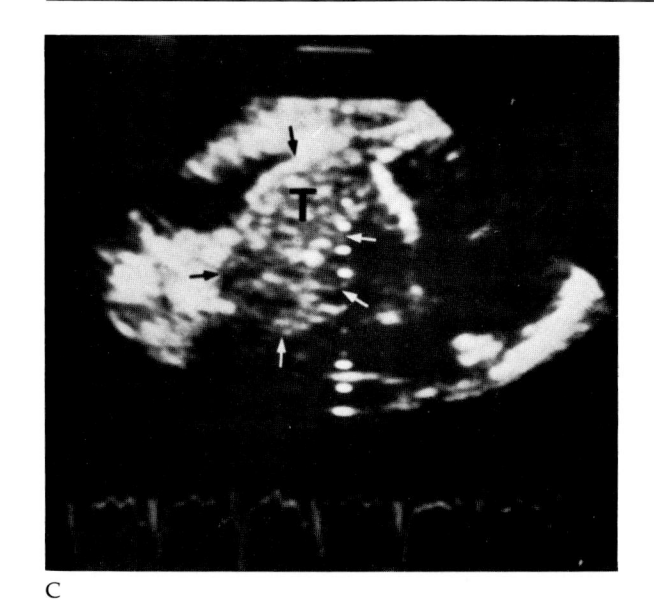

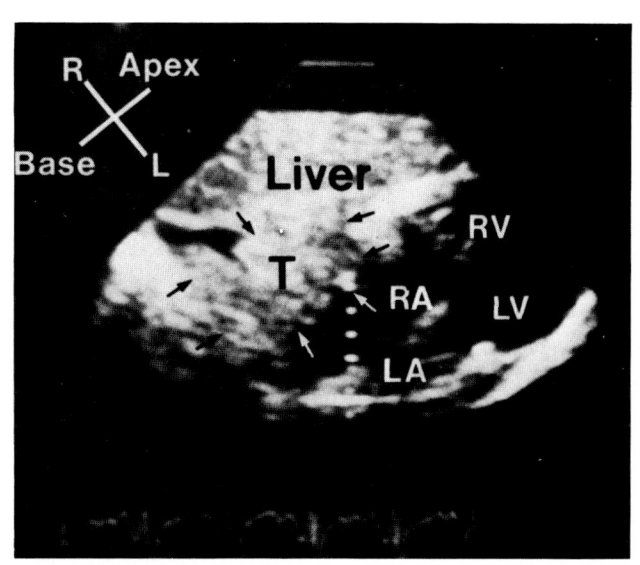

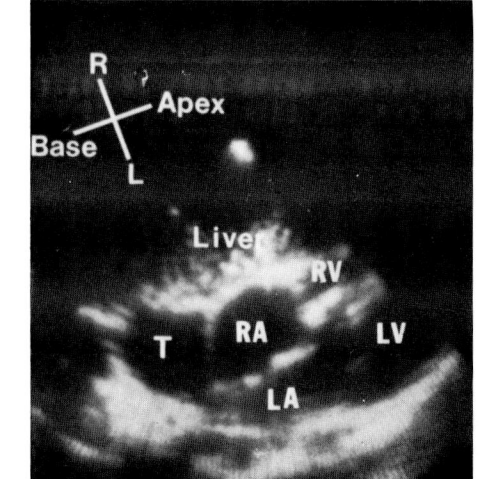

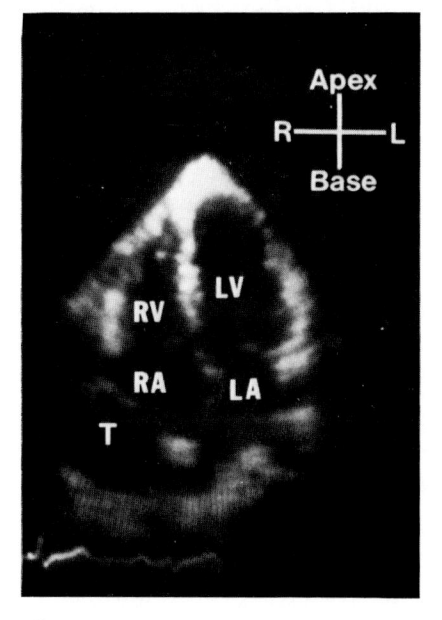

by M-mode and two-dimensional echocardiography. One of these patients, a 32-year-old woman, is of special interest since she represents the eighth reported case of metastatic carcinoma in the right ventricle causing outflow obstruction with a murmur of pulmonary stenosis and the second such reported case specifically caused by cervical carcinoma.

One should be mindful that an artifact may cause strong reflectances simulating a mass or abnormal structure within the right ventricle. Lutz and associates [69] reported a case of a pseudotumor in the right ventricular outflow tract in a 26-year-old man with congenital pulmonic valve regurgitation. In this patient a bright target was seen in the right ventricular outflow tract on two-dimensional echocardiography and was misinterpreted as a mass in the clinical presence of pulmonary regurgitation; a pulmonary artery angiogram was also misinterpreted as reflecting a mass in the right ventricular outflow tract. No mass was found at surgery; a 5 mm calcified polyplike mass was the source of the bright reflectance on the two-dimensional echocardiographic study, but no explanation could be made for the false positive interpretation of the angiogram.

Sarcomas are the most common primary malignant heart tumors and occur most frequently in the right side of the heart [70]. Sarcomas originate from the endocardium or pericardium, and rarely from the myocardium. These tumors, which include rhabdomyosarcomas, malignant vascular tumors, fibrosarcomas, fibromyxosarcomas, myxosarcomas, and lymphomas, are rapidly infiltrating and can metastasize; the prognosis is usually poor (Fig. 11-20). Metastases in rhabdomyosarcomas of the heart are usually to the lung, resulting in hemorrhagic pleural effusions. A significant percentage of these patients will have a hemopericardium. Two-dimensional echo is quite useful for detection of pericardial metastases, but the sensitivity and specificity for this abnormality have not been confirmed [71] (Fig. 11-21).

The incidence of metastases to the pericardium and heart is 0.1 to 6.4 percent in unselected autopsies, and 1.5 to 20.6 percent in autopsies with findings of malignant tumors [70]. The symptoms of metastatic cardiac tumors include progressive heart failure, acute pericarditis with a friction rub, pericardial effusion, cardiac tamponade, syncope, and vena cava obstruction. Heart metastases occur with every variety of malignant neoplasm of nearly every organ with the notable exceptions of intracranial and central nervous system tumors and parathyroid carcinoma. The tumors that tend most frequently to metastasize to the pericardium or heart are carcinoma of the lung and breast (19 to 35%), malignant melanoma (33 to 50%), malignant lymphoma (5 to 37%), and leukemia (13 to 58%) [70]. When metastases involve heart valves the tricuspid valve is most frequently affected. Metastases may reach the pericardium and myocardium via the blood stream or lymphatics, by direct extension, or by a combination of these routes.

An abscess of the right ventricle may produce an abnormal reflectance and be recognizable by 2-D echo. Septicemia or chronic conditions that predispose to development of infection may lead to a myocardial abscess (Fig. 11-22).

Extracardiac tumors. A variety of extracardiac tumors have been reported with both M-mode and two-dimensional echocardiography [72–78]. Anterior mediastinal compression may cause displacement of the cardiac structures with compression of the left atrium (Fig. 11-23A). Canedo and associates [72] described a patient with a large superior mediastinal tumor producing clinical manifestations of cardiac tamponade and obstruction of the superior vena cava in whom the solid nature of the tumor was established by echocardiography. The heart was displaced posteriorly; both left atrium and left ventricle were diminished in size; there was prominent respiratory variation in the position of the interventricular septum as well as dimensions of both ventricles, and pseudoprolapse of the mitral valve. Yoshikawa and associates [73] demonstrated that two-dimensional echocardiography is more accurate than M-mode echocardiography in the differential diagnosis of a large left atrial tumor and extracardiac tumor compressing the left atrium. Using M-mode echo we have observed mediastinal tumors displacing the heart; nearby solid or cystic masses have been observed with 2-D echo (Fig. 11-23).

References

1. Prichard RW: Tumors of the heart: Review of the subject and report of 150 cases. *Arch Pathol* 51:98, 1951
2. Goldberg HP, Glenn F, Dotter CT, Steinberg I: Myxoma of the left atrium: Diagnosis made during life with operative and postmortem findings. *Circulation* 6:762, 1952
3. Neumann HA, Cordell AR, Prichard RW: Intracardiac myxomas: Literature review and report of six cases, one successfully treated. *Am Surgeon* 32:219, 1966
4. Bulkley BH, Hutchins GM: Atrial myxomas: A fifty year review. *Am Heart J* 97:639, 1979
5. Bass NM, Sharratt GP: Left atrial myxoma diagnosed by echocardiography, with observations on tumor movement. *Br Heart J* 35:1332, 1973
6. Morgan DL, Palazola J, Reed W, Bell HH, Kindred LH, Beauchamp GD: Left heart myxomas. *Am J Cardiol* 40:611, 1977
7. Sung RJ, Ghahramani AR, Mallon SM, Richter SE, Sommer LS, Gottlieb S, Myerburg RJ: Hemodynamic features of prolapsing and nonprolapsing left atrial myxoma. *Circulation* 51:342, 1975
8. Nasser WK, Davis RH, Dillon JC, Tavel ME, Helmen CH, Feigenbaum H, Fisch C: Atrial myxoma. II. Phonocardiographic, echocardiographic, hemodynamic, and angiographic features in nine cases. *Am Heart J* 83:810, 1972
9. Popp RL, Harrison DC: Ultrasound for the diagnosis of atrial tumor. *Ann Intern Med* 71:785, 1969
10. Martinez EC, Giles TD, Burch GE: Echocardiographic diagnosis of left atrial myxoma. *Am J Cardiol* 33:281, 1974
11. Fowles RE, Miller DC, Egbert BM, Fitzgerald JW, Popp RL: Systemic embolization from a mitral valve papillary endocardial fibroma detected by two-dimensional echocardiography. *Am Heart J* 102:128, 1981
12. Kaminsky ME, Ehlers KH, Engle MA, Klein AA, Levin AR, Subramanian VA: Atrial myxoma mimicking a collagen disorder. *Chest* 75:93, 1979
13. Goodwin JF: Diagnosis of left atrial myxoma. *Lancet* 1:464, 1963
14. Peters MN, Hall RJ, Cooley DA, Leachman RD, Garcia E: The clinical syndrome of atrial myxoma. *JAMA* 230:695, 1974
15. Popp RL, Levine R: Left atrial mass simulating cardiomyopathy. *JCU* 1:96, 1973
16. Rae A: Two patients with cardiac myxoma: One presenting as bacterial endocarditis, and one as congestive cardiac failure. *Postgrad Med J* 41:644, 1965
17. Malloch CI, Abbott JA, Rapaport E: Left atrial myxoma with bacteremia. *Am J Cardiol* 25:353, 1970
18. Graham HV, vonHartitzsch B, Medina JR: Infected atrial myxoma. *Am J Cardiol* 38:658, 1976
19. Child JS, MacAlpin RN, Moyer GH, Shanley JD, Layfield LJ: Coronary ostial embolus and mitral vegetation simulating a left atrial myxoma: A case of probable cryptococcal valvulitis. *Clin Cardiol* 2:43, 1979
20. Spangler RD, Okin JT: Illustrative echocardiogram: Echocardiographic demonstration of a left atrial thrombus. *Chest* 67:716, 1975

21. Mikell FL, Asinger RW, Rourke T, Hodges M, Sharma B, Francis GS: Two-dimensional echocardiographic demonstration of left atrial thrombi in patients with prosthetic mitral valves. *Circulation* 60:1183, 1979
22. Lewis KB, Criley JM, Ross RS: Detection of left atrial thrombus by cineangiocardiography. *Am Heart J* 70:612, 1965
23. Meller J, Teichholz LE, Pichard AD, Matta R, Litwak R, Herman MV: Left ventricular myxoma: Echocardiographic diagnosis and review of the literature. *Am J Med* 63:816, 1977
24. Griffiths GC: A review of primary tumors of the heart. *Progr Cardiovasc Dis* 7:465, 1965
25. Fine G: Neoplasms of the Pericardium and Heart. In SE Gould (ed), *Pathology of the Heart* (3rd ed). Springfield, Ill: Thomas, 1968. Pp 951–883
26. Bigelow NH, Klinger S, Wright AW: Primary tumors of the heart in infancy and early childhood. *Cancer* 7:549, 1954
27. Nadas AS, Ellison RC: Cardiac tumors in infancy. *Am J Cardiol* 21:363, 1968
28. Mahar LJ, Lie JT, Groover RV, Seward JB, Puga FJ, Feldt RH: Primary cardiac myxosarcoma in a child. *Mayo Clin Proc* 54:261, 1979
29. Levisman JA, MacAlpin RN, Abbasi AS, Ellis N, Eber LM: Echocardiographic diagnosis of a mobile, pedunculated tumor in the left ventricular cavity. *Am J Cardiol* 36:957, 1975
30. Goodwin JF: The spectrum of cardiac tumors. *Am J Cardiol* 21:307, 1968
31. Harvey WP: Clinical aspects of cardiac tumors. *Am J Cardiol* 21:328, 1968
32. Harinck E, Moulaert AJ, Rohmer J, Brown AG: Cardiac rhabdomyoma in infancy. *Acta Paediatr Scand* 63:283, 1974
33. Kuehl KS, Perry LW, Chandra R, Scott LP: Left ventricular rhabdomyoma: A rare cause of subaortic stenosis in the newborn infant. *Pediatrics* 46:464, 1970
34. Orsmond GS, Knight L, Dehner LP, Nicoloff DM, Nesbitt M, Bessinger FB: Alveolar rhabdomyosarcoma involving the heart: An echocardiographic, angiographic and pathologic study. *Circulation* 54:837, 1976
35. Bale PM, Reye RDK: Rhabdomyosarcoma in childhood. *Pathology* 7:101, 1975
36. Pascuzzi CA, Parkin TW, Bruwer AJ, Edwards JE: Hypertrophic osteoarthropathy associated with primary rhabdomyosarcoma of the heart. *Mayo Clin Proc* 32:30, 1957
37. Porter GA, Berroth M, Bristow JD: Primary rhabdomyosarcoma of the heart and complete atrioventricular block: A case report and review of the literature. *Am J Med* 31:820, 1961
38. Salyer WR, Page DL, Hutchins GM: The development of cardiac myxomas and papillary endocardial lesions from mural thrombus. *Am Heart J* 89:4, 1975
39. Bloor CM: *Cardiac Pathology*. Philadelphia: Lippincott, 1978. P 396
40. Farooki ZQ, Adelman S, Green EW: Echocardiographic differentiation of a cystic and a solid tumor of the heart. *Am J Cardiol* 39:107, 1977
41. Holswade GR, Nydick I, Steinberg I: Successful removal of right atrial myxoma mistaken for liver and pericardial metastases. *J Thorac Cardiovasc Surg* 52:240, 1966
42. Emanuel RW, Lloyd WE: Right atrial myxoma mistaken for constrictive pericarditis. *Br Heart J* 24:796, 1962
43. Levinson JP, Kincaid OW: Myxoma of the right atrium associated with polycythemia: Report of successful excision. *N Engl J Med* 264:1187, 1961
44. Talley RC, Baldwin BJ, Symbas PN, Nutter DO: Right atrial myxoma: Unusual presentation with cyanosis and clubbing. *Am J Med* 48:256, 1970
45. Heath D, Mackinnon J: Pulmonary hypertension due to myxoma of the right atrium. *Am Heart J* 68:227, 1964
46. Martin CE, Hufnagel CA, deLeon AC: Calcified atrial myxoma: Diagnostic significance of the "systolic tumor sound" in a case presenting as tricuspid insufficiency. *Am Heart J* 78:245, 1969
47. Morrissey JF, Campeti FL, Mahoney EB, Yu PN: Right atrial myxoma: Report of two cases and review of the literature. *Am Heart J* 66:4, 1963
48. Miller GA, Paneth M, Gibson RV: Right atrial myxoma with right-to-left interatrial shunt and polycythemia. *Br Med J* 3:537, 1968
49. Waxler EB, Kawai N, Kasparian H: Right atrial myxoma: Echocardiographic, phonocardiographic, and hemodynamic signs. *Am Heart J* 83:251, 1972
50. Harbold NB Jr., Gau GT: Echocardiographic diagnosis of right atrial myxoma. *Mayo Clin Proc* 48:284, 1973
51. Yuste P, Asin E, Cerdan FJ, de la Fuente A: Echocardiogram in right atrial myxoma. *Chest* 69:94, 1976

52. Come PC, Kurland GS, Vine HS: Two dimensional echocardiography in differentiating right atrial and tricuspid valve mass lesions. *Am J Cardiol* 44:1207, 1979
53. Bommer WJ, Kwan OL, Mason DT, DeMaria AN: Identification of prominent eustachian valves by M-mode and two-dimensional echocardiography: Differentiation from right atrial masses. *Am J Cardiol* 45:402, 1980
54. Battle-Diaz J, Stanley P, Kratz C, Fouron J-C, Guerin R, Davignon A: Echocardiographic manifestations of persistence of the right sinus venosus valve. *Am J Cardiol* 43:850, 1979
55. Werner JA, Cheitlin MD, Gross BW, Speck SM, Ivey TD: Echocardiographic appearance of the Chiari network: Differentiation from right-heart pathology. *Circulation* 63:1104, 1981
56. Bloor CM: *Cardiac Pathology*. Philadelphia: Lippincott, 1978. P 58
57. Farooki ZQ, Henry JG, Green EW: Echocardiographic diagnosis of right atrial extension of Wilms' tumor. *Am J Cardiol* 36:363, 1975
58. Broadbent JC, Tajik AJ, Wallace RB: Thrombus of inferior vena cava presenting as right atrial tumor: Roentgenographic, phonoechocardiographic, angiographic, and surgical findings. *J Thorac Cardiovasc Surg* 72:422, 1976
59. Fitterer JD, Spicer MJ, Nelson WP: Echocardiographic demonstration of bilateral atrial myxomas. *Chest* 70:282, 1976
60. Nicholson KG, Prior AL, Normal AG, Naik DR, Kennedy A: Bilateral atrial myxomas diagnosed preoperatively and successfully removed. *Br Med J* 2:440, 1977
61. Gustafson AG, Edler IG, Dahlback OK: Bilateral atrial myxomas diagnosed by echocardiography. *Acta Med Scand* 201:391, 1977
62. Feigenbaum H: Cardiac Masses. In H Feigenbaum (ed), *Echocardiography* (3rd ed). Philadelphia: Lea & Febiger, 1981. Pp 505–527
63. Roelandt J, Bletter WB, Leuftink EW, van Dorp WG, ten Cate F, Nauta J: Ultrasonic demonstration of right ventricular myxoma. *JCU* 5:191, 1977
64. Chandraratna PAN, San Pedro S, Elkins RC, Grantham N: Echocardiographic, angiocardiographic, and surgical correlations in right ventricular myxoma simulating valvar pulmonic stenosis. *Circulation* 55:619, 1977
65. DeMaria AN, Vismara LA, Miller RR, Neumann A, Mason DT: Unusual echographic manifestations of right and left heart myxomas. *Am J Med* 59:713, 1975
66. Ports TA, Schiller NB, Strunk BL: Echocardiography of right ventricular tumors. *Circulation* 56:439, 1977
67. Jaffe CC, Kelley MJ, Taunt KA: Two-dimensional echocardiographic identification of a right ventricle tumor. *Radiology* 129:471, 1978
68. Krivokapich J, Warren SE, Child JS, Kaufman JA, Vieweg WVR, Hagan AD: M-mode and cross-sectional echocardiographic diagnosis of right ventricular cavity masses. *JCU* 9:5, 1981
69. Lutz JF, Hagan AD, Vieweg WVR, Thompson SI, Aaron BL: "Pseudo-Tumor" of the right ventricular outflow tract and congenital pulmonary valve regurgitation: A case report. *Am Heart J* 100:349, 1980
70. Bloor CM: *Cardiac Pathology*. Philadelphia: Lippincott, 1978. Pp 391–415
71. Chandraratna PAN, Aronow WS: Detection of pericardial metastases by cross-sectional echocardiography. *Circulation* 63:197, 1981
72. Canedo MI, Otken L, Stefadouros MA: Echocardiographic features of cardiac compression by a thymoma simulating cardiac tamponade and obstruction of the superior vena cava. *Br Heart J* 39:1038, 1977
73. Yoshikawa J, Sabah I, Yanagihara K, Owaki T, Kato H, Tanemoto K: Cross-sectional echocardiographic diagnosis of large left atrial tumor and extracardiac tumor compressing the left atrium. *Am J Cardiol* 42:853, 1978
74. Koch PC, Kronzon I, Winer HE, Adams P, Trubek M: Displacement of the heart by a giant mediastinal cyst. *Am J Cardiol* 40:445, 1977
75. Tingelstad JB, McWilliams NB, Thomas CE: Confirmation of a retrosternal mass by echocardiogram. *JCU* 4:129, 1976
76. Farooki ZQ, Hakimi N, Arciniegas E, Green EW: Echocardiographic features in a case of intrapericardial teratoma. *JCU* 6:108, 1978
77. Lin TK, Stech JM, Eckert WG, Lin JJ, Farha SJ, Hagan CT: Pericardial angiosarcoma simulating pericardial effusion by echocardiography. *Chest* 73:881, 1978
78. Chandraratna PAN, Littman BB, Serafini A, Whayne T, Robinson H: Echocardiographic evaluation of extracardiac masses. *Br Heart J* 40:741, 1978

Prosthetic valves

12

Clinical evaluation of a symptomatic patient with a prosthetic cardiac valve is a difficult problem. In addition to dysfunction of the prosthesis, the differential diagnosis includes ventricular dysfunction and coexistent myocardial, coronary, or other valve disease.

Several types of valve prostheses have been utilized during the past twenty years. In general there are five types of prostheses in use: caged-ball, caged-disc, tilting-disc, low-profile bileaflet, and bioprosthetic valves.

Echophonocardiography is a valuable technique for evaluating prosthetic valve malfunction, especially if early postoperative and follow-up studies are available [1–3]. Dysfunction of these valves may result from obstruction or entrapment by myocardium or thrombus formation [4, 5]. Thrombus accumulation on the prosthesis with subsequent arterial embolization, valvular incompetence resulting from dehiscence with or without exaggerated hemolysis, strut fracture, infective endocarditis, destructive changes of the disc or poppet due to wear or swelling, tissue degeneration, and fibrosis or calcification of bioprosthetic valves have all been encountered [6–25]. In order to recognize prosthetic valve dysfunction, it is important to be able to define normal motion and function characteristics of the various prostheses. Phonocardiography and echocardiography continue to play a very important clinical role in the follow-up of patients with prosthetic valves [2, 3, 7, 11, 16, 17, 25–30].

Echocardiography is also clinically useful for the assessment of left ventricular outflow width in the preoperative selection of mitral valve prosthesis [31, 32]. Nanda and colleagues [31] reported a very high postoperative mortality that was apparently related to obstruction of the left ventricular outflow tract by the caged-ball prosthesis. These investigators estimated the degree of prosthesis encroachment into the left ventricular outflow tract by comparing the length of cage and poppet expected to protrude into the outflow tract in systole with the width of the outflow tract (C point of the mitral valve to the left side of the ventricular septum). They found that the prosthesis encroachment ranged from 60 to 80 percent in the high-mortality group, whereas the group who had less than 50 percent encroachment did well clinically. Accordingly, they recommend a low-profile prosthesis when the left ventricular outflow tract width measures less than 20 mm. The problem of prosthesis-patient mismatch in valve replacement has been highlighted, with special reference to postoperative problems in patients with small valvular annuli [33]. Denbow and associates [32], in a later study of 70 patients who received mitral prostheses, found no increased surgical risk in those patients having a narrowed outflow tract (<20 mm) who received a high-profile, caged-ball prosthesis in the mitral position.

Two-dimensional echocardiography has proved clinically superior to either M-mode echocardiography or other noninvasive methods for the evaluation of porcine heterografts [19, 34–36]. Although 2-D echo offers significant advantages in imaging heterograft valves in any position, certain measurements are still more accurately derived from the M-mode recordings; therefore the clinical evaluation of these bioprostheses should include both M-mode and 2-D echo [37–39]. Homograft and fascia lata valves have been used in the past [40] (Fig. 12-1); however, the most common bioprosthetic valve in use today is the xenograft or porcine heterograft.

Discussion of normal echocardiographic criteria is subdivided according to the various types of valves. Measuring the excursion of a ball or disc in the mitral position is usually easier with an M-mode recording than with 2-D imaging. However, to record the maximum excursion of a ball valve in the aortic position with M-mode echo, the transducer would have to be placed in the right supraclavicular fossa or suprasternal notch and directed toward the aortic valve [41–43] (Fig. 12-2A). With the parasternal long axis imaging position, it is possible to view superior-inferior movement of the ball, although it is not possible to obtain M-mode recordings in the inferior-superior plane. By positioning the 2-D transducer over the left ventricular apex, directing the sector beam through the aortic valve in both apical long axis (Fig. 12-2A) and apical four-chamber views, it is also possible in some patients to direct the M-mode cursor in the inferior-superior plane through the aortic prosthesis to record disc, ball, or leaflet motion (Fig. 12-2B). Whenever any type of aortic valve prosthesis is being imaged from the parasternal long axis position, the transducer should be directed medially to exclude most of the left ventricle and thereby include as much as possible of the ascending aorta (Fig. 12-3). In addition to evaluating ball, disc, or leaflet motion of the aortic prosthesis in these views, the echocardiographer can observe any abnormal rocking motion of the prosthesis within the annulus. Much of the qualitative assessment of the aortic prosthesis is concerned with evaluating any abnormal masses attached to the sewing ring, cage, struts, stents, or leaflets (depending on the type of valve) that might suggest the presence of a thrombus or vegetation. In order to accomplish this type of comprehensive imaging additional views, including the parasternal short axis at the base, subcostal four-chamber, and subcostal short axis at tne base, should always be included (Fig. 12-4).

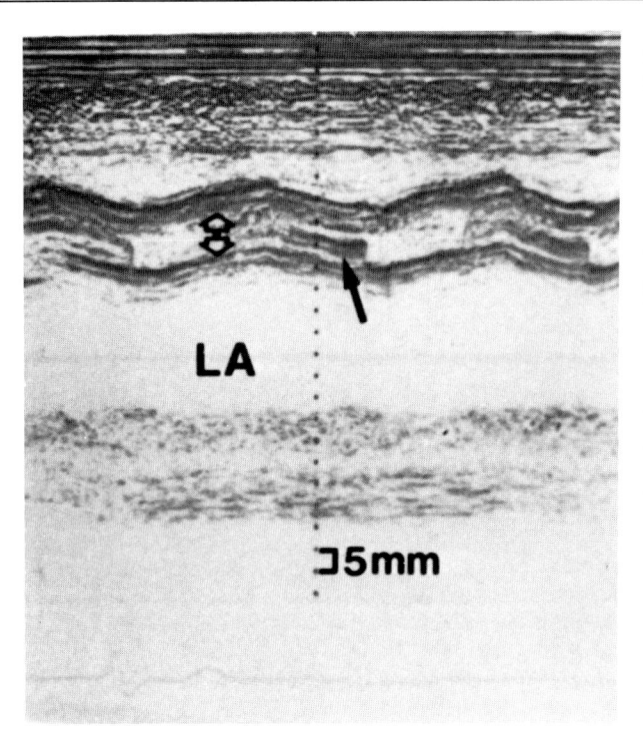

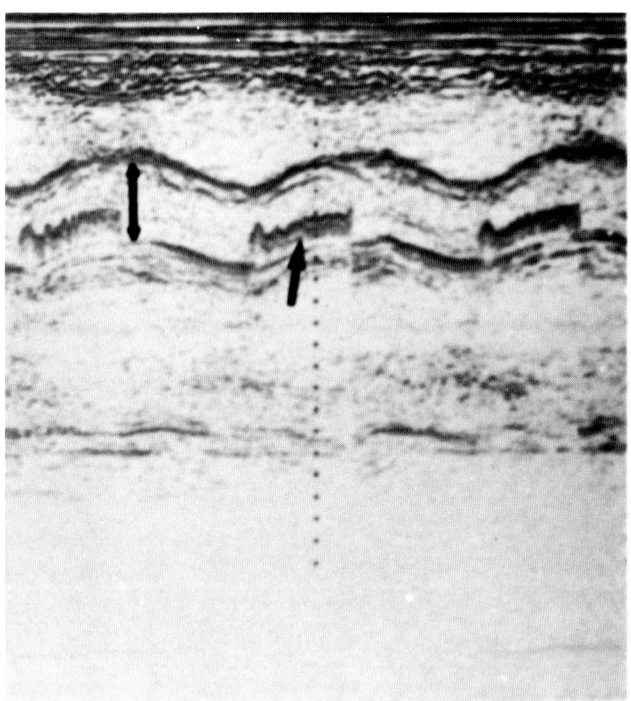

Fig. 12-1. M-mode recording through the aortic valve, aortic root, and left atrium in an adult patient who had an aortic homograft valve inserted five years earlier. The patient has recently developed severe aortic regurgitation and demonstrates thickened leaflets during diastole (left panel) and systole (right panel) (arrows). The narrow aortic annulus (11 mm diameter on the left and 17 mm in the right panel) is a result of surgery when the free fresh homograft was tailored to fit the annulus. When this valve was replaced, it was found to be calcified, but there was no vegetation or past evidence of infective endocarditis.

397

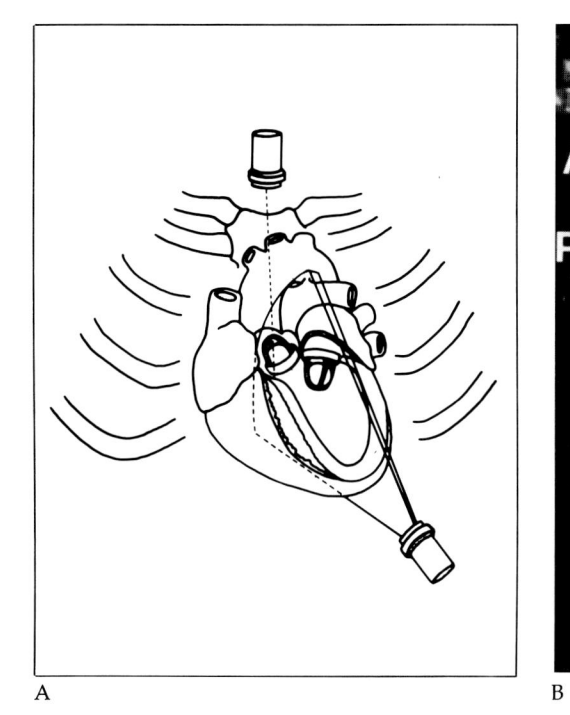

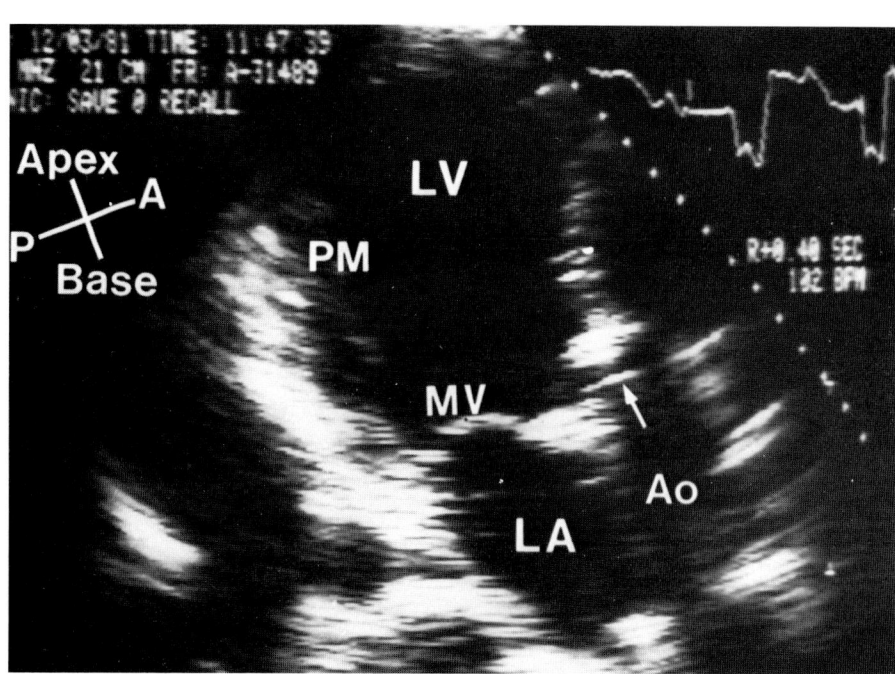

*Fig. 12-2A. Diagram illustrating M-mode transducer in suprasternal notch showing the echo beam passing through the ascending aorta and aortic prosthesis to record inferior-superior motion of the ball prosthesis. Where a 2-D echo transducer is positioned over the left ventricular apex and the sector beam directed through the aortic valve in an apical long axis view, both mitral and aortic prostheses are simultaneously imaged. B. Apical long axis view showing porcine heterograft in the aortic position with leaflet motion (**arrow**) perpendicular to the direction an M-mode cursor would have if directed through the valve.*

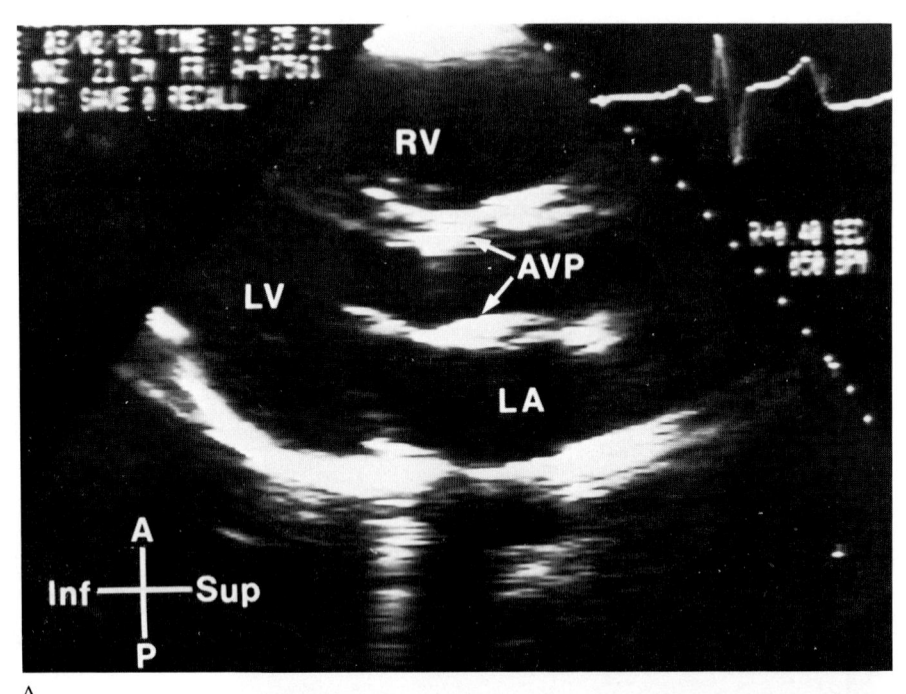

Fig. 12-3A. Parasternal long axis view with medial angulation of transducer to exclude more of the left ventricle and include more of the ascending aorta results in the aortic valve prosthesis (AVP) (porcine heterograft) being positioned centrally in sector image. B. Parasternal long axis views of a patient with normally functioning porcine heterografts in aortic and mitral positions. The stents of the aortic prosthesis (AP) are profiled best in the upper panel, whereas the profile of the stents and leaflet motion are best seen (arrow) in the lower panel.

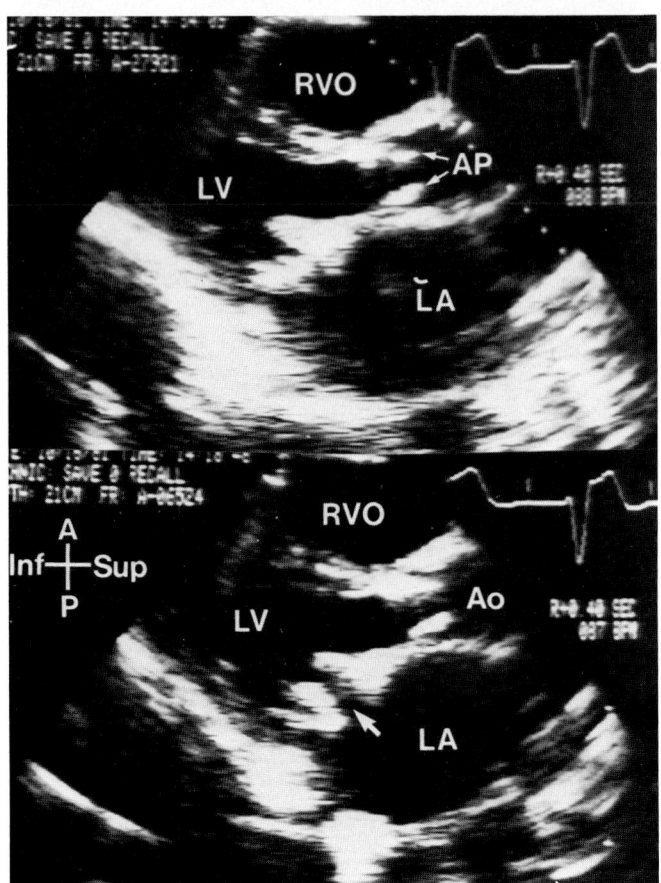

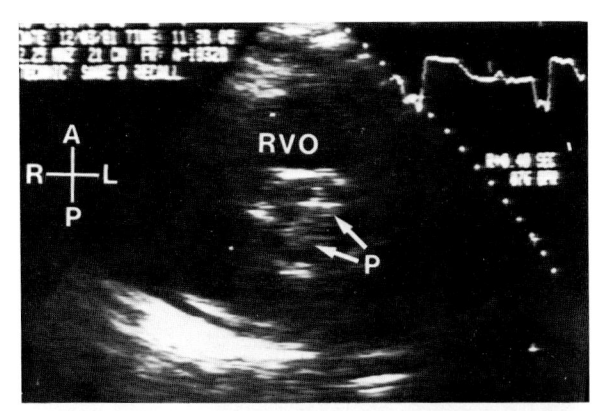

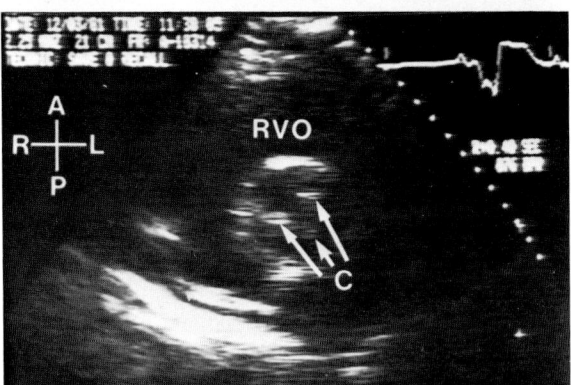

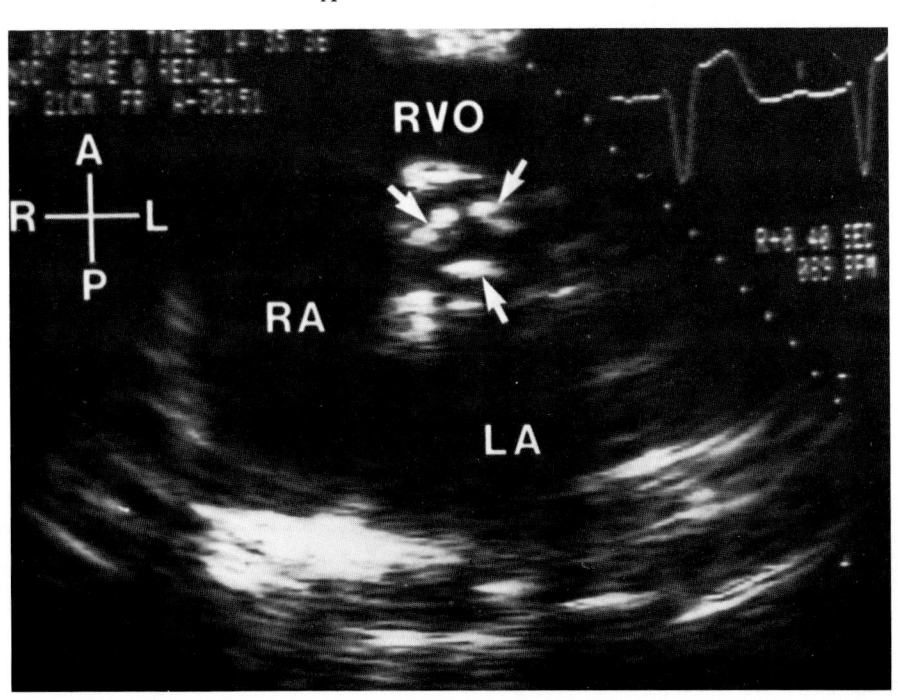

Fig. 12-4A. Parasternal short axis view at the base of ball valve aortic prosthesis in systole (upper panel) and diastole (lower panel). The ball (P) can be seen at the top of the cage (upper panel) and is absent from view (lower panel) in diastole. The three tips of the cage (C) are seen. B. Parasternal short axis view at the base showing the three stents of a porcine heterograft (arrows) in the aortic position. The leaflets are not visible in this view because the valve is closed in diastole.

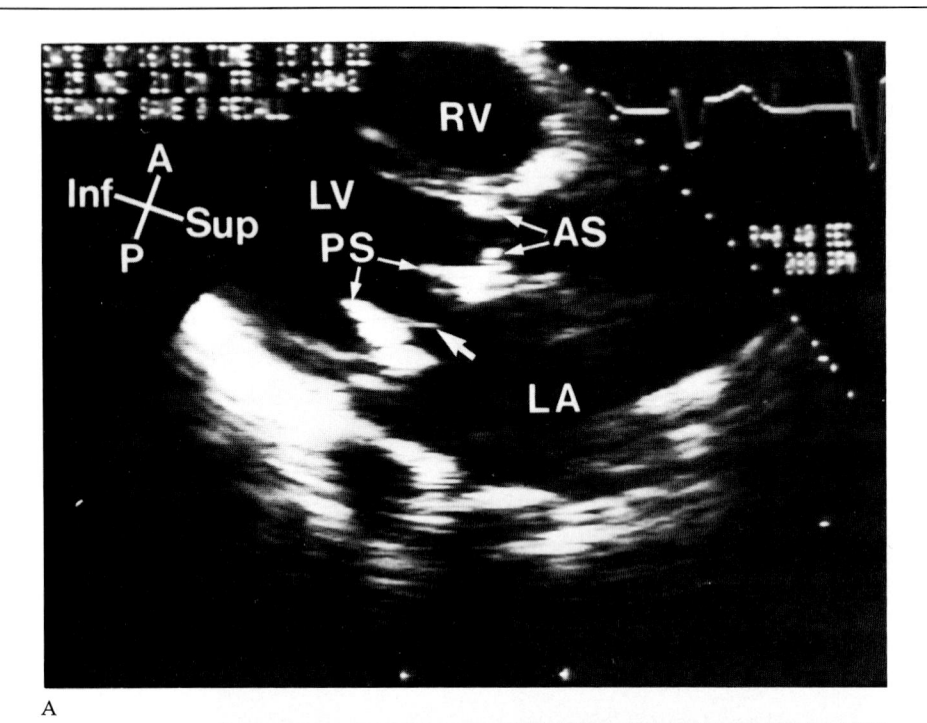

Fig. 12-5A. Parasternal long axis view demonstrating porcine heterografts in both mitral and aortic positions; only the sewing ring (AS) of the aortic prosthesis is visible; the stents of the mitral prosthesis (PS) and normal leaflet thickness (arrow) are easily visible. B. M-mode recording of porcine mitral prosthesis showing abnormal leaflets (open arrows) measuring 6–8 mm in thickness due to degenerative changes and calcification. C. M-mode recordings of normal Bjork-Shiley tilting-disc mitral prosthesis (arrows). Recordings were obtained with a movable M-mode cursor and the transducer located in the left parasternal (left panel), apical (middle panel), and subcostal (right panel) positions. R = sewing ring of heterograft valve; S = stent of heterograft valve.

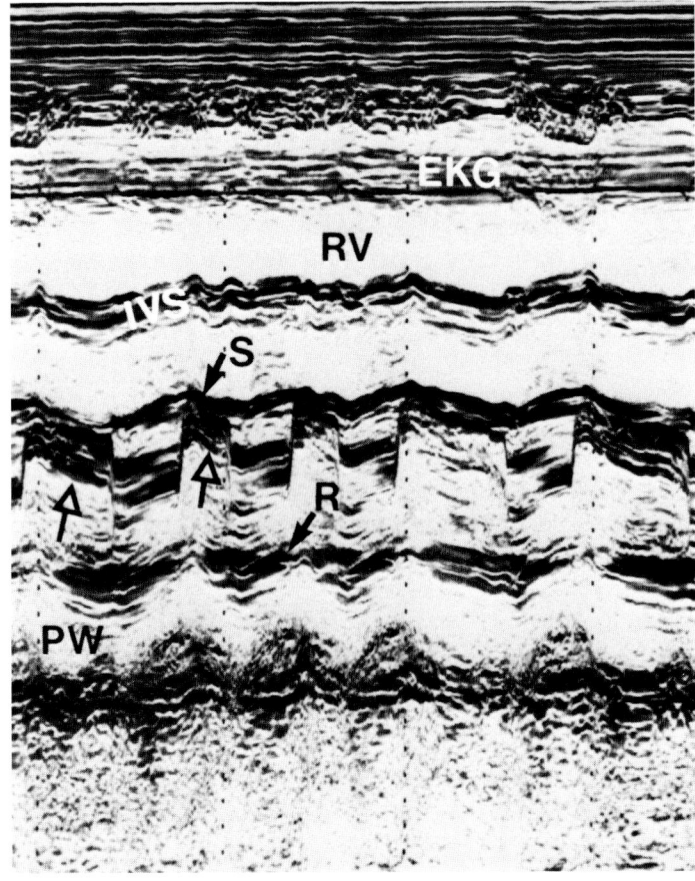

PARASTERNAL   APICAL   SUBCOSTAL

C

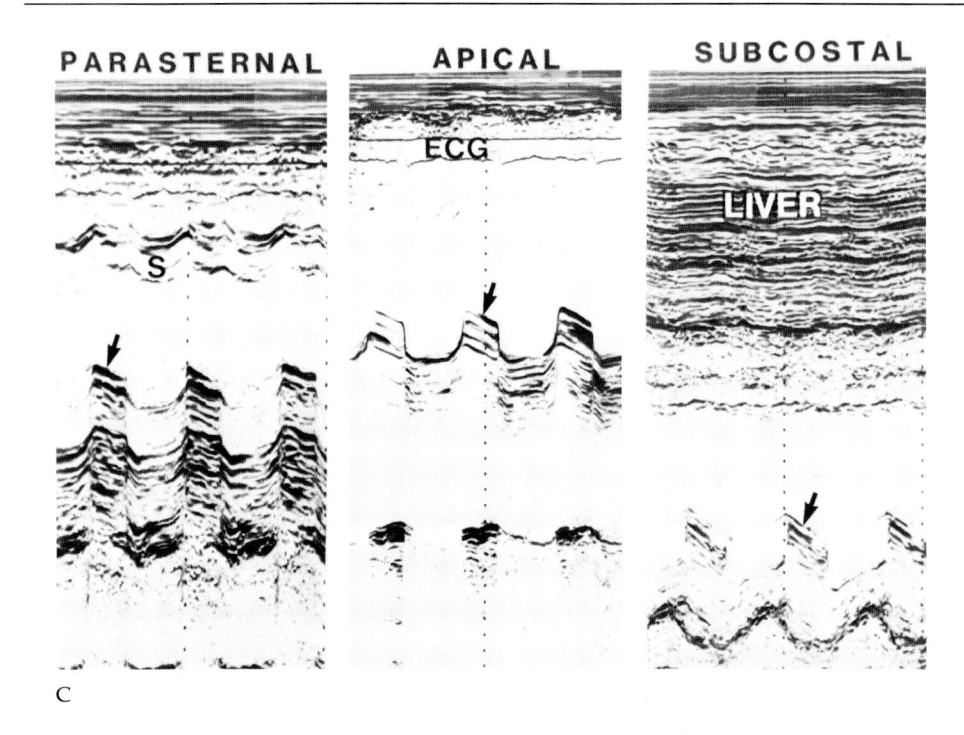

The parasternal long and short axis views of the mitral valve together with the apical long axis and four-chamber views are all important tomographic planes for evaluating any type of prosthesis in the mitral position. Overall it is easier to perform echocardiographic evaluation of mitral prostheses than of aortic prostheses. Good-quality M-mode and 2-D echo recordings can usually be obtained from porcine mitral valve prostheses (Fig. 12-5A, B). The Bjork-Shiley tilting disc presents a variety of echocardiographic M-mode patterns that depend on the exact relationship of the ultrasound beam to the tilting disc [1, 44, 45] (Fig. 12-5C). The echocardiographer should attempt to record the maximum excursion of the tilting disc.

When either a caged-ball or caged-disc mitral prosthesis is being evaluated, combining phonocardiography with echocardiography provides additional advantages of timing opening and closing sounds together with monitoring valve motion [6, 27, 46]. Some investigators have measured opening and closing velocities of mitral ball or disc prostheses [26, 28]; however, the velocities in the same patient may vary at different times because of cardiac output, heart rate, and force of ventricular contraction. These velocity measurements have very little clinical value in diagnosing malfunction of the prosthetic valve, since altered physiological conditions of the left ventricle influence ball or disc velocities in the absence of any prosthesis abnormality. The ball or disc may exhibit intermittent sticking with resultant abnormal motion on the echocardiogram that is diagnostic of malfunction of the prosthesis (Fig. 12-6). Intermittent sticking of ball prostheses was observed during the 1960s as a result of swelling from the absorption of lipids; however, this

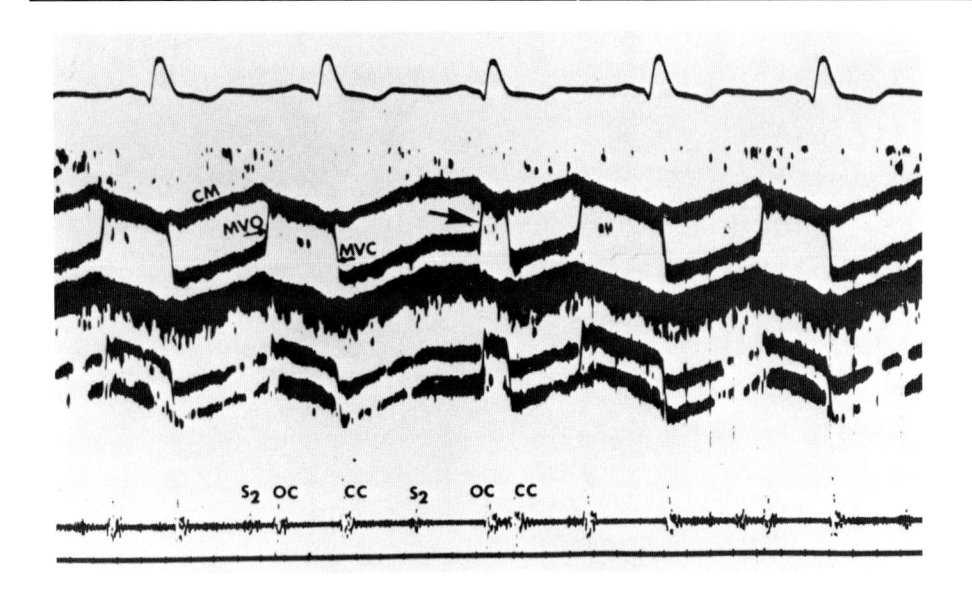

Fig. 12-6. M-mode echophonocardiogram demonstrating malfunction of mitral ball valve prosthesis with sticking of ball and delayed opening (arrow) causing delayed opening click (OC) on phono. CC = closing click; CM = cage of mitral prosthesis; MVC = mitral valve closing; S$_2$ = second heart sound. (From J Pfeifer et al, Am J Cardiol 29:95, 1972.)

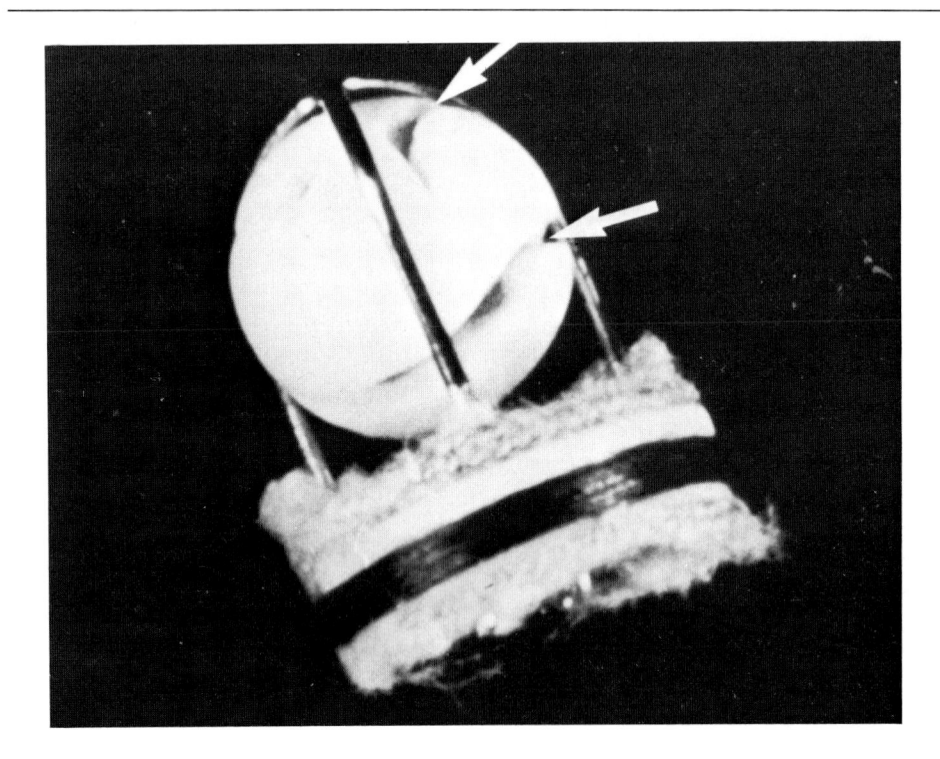

Fig. 12-7. Photograph of one of the early models of Starr-Edwards aortic prosthesis showing deep cracks (arrows) caused by swelling from lipids absorbed by the ball.

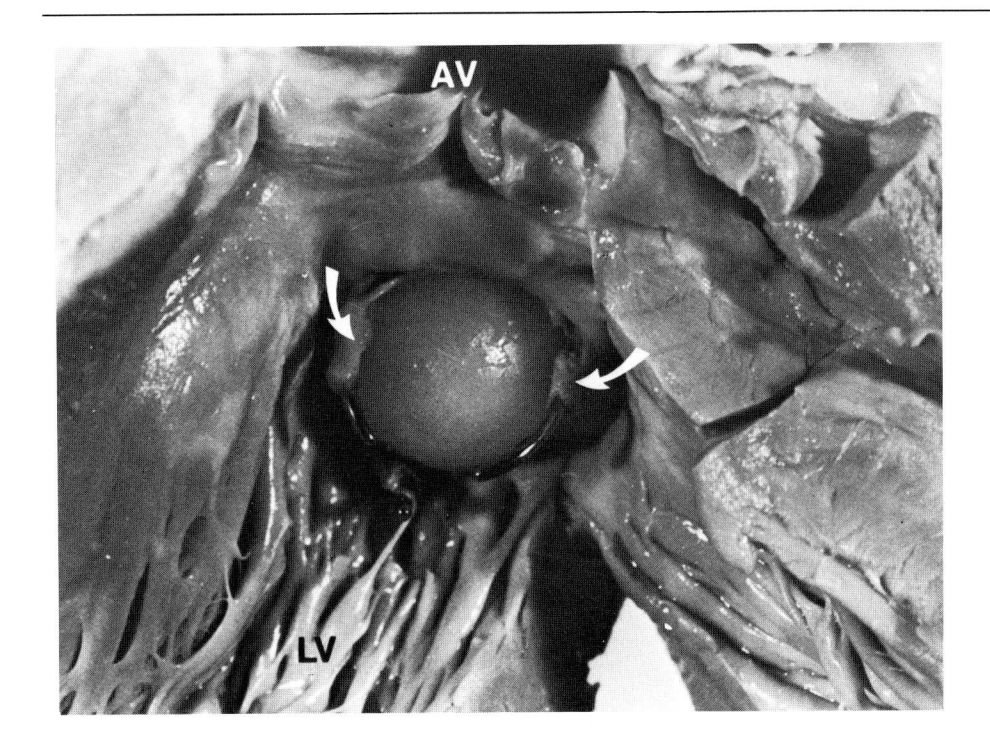

Fig. 12-8. Photograph of Cutter-Smeloff prosthesis in mitral position showing fibrin propagating along the cage (arrows), *which impinged upon poppet motion.*

has not been a clinical problem for several years (Fig. 12-7). If fibrin or thrombus propagates over the valve struts or between the cage and the ball or disc, this may also interfere with normal motion resulting in progressive mitral stenosis; if the propagation is extensive pulmonary edema or sudden death may occur (Fig. 12-8).

Any prosthetic valve with metallic components is a very strong target for reflecting sound waves. These echoes reverberate into the left atrium posteriorly when the transducer is located in the parasternal position and superiorly when the transducer is located in the apical position. Careful attention to imaging technique with selective gain reduction is required, otherwise these strong reflectances from the prosthesis can mimic a mass in the left atrium or obscure an actual abnormality in that region (Fig. 12-9). The parasternal long axis and apical four-chamber views are the two most important tomographic planes for evaluating a mitral valve prosthesis.

The interval between the aortic second sound (A_2) and the mitral valve opening (MVO) is also considered an indicator of malfunction of mitral prostheses [47]. A shortened interval has the same significance as a short A_2-opening sound interval in mitral stenosis. This interval may also be shortened in patients with poor left ventricular function as well as in patients who have a paravalvular leak around the mitral prosthesis [2]. With a long P–R interval on the electrocardiogram it is possible to see premature closure of a mitral prosthesis in the same manner in which one observes premature closure of the native mitral valve in the presence of first-degree atrioventricular block.

The St. Jude Medical (SJM) cardiac valve, a low-profile bileaflet prosthesis with central flow, was introduced in October, 1977. The two leaflets have an opening angle of 85 degrees and a closing angle of 30 to 35 degrees, depending on valve size

404 12. Prosthetic valves

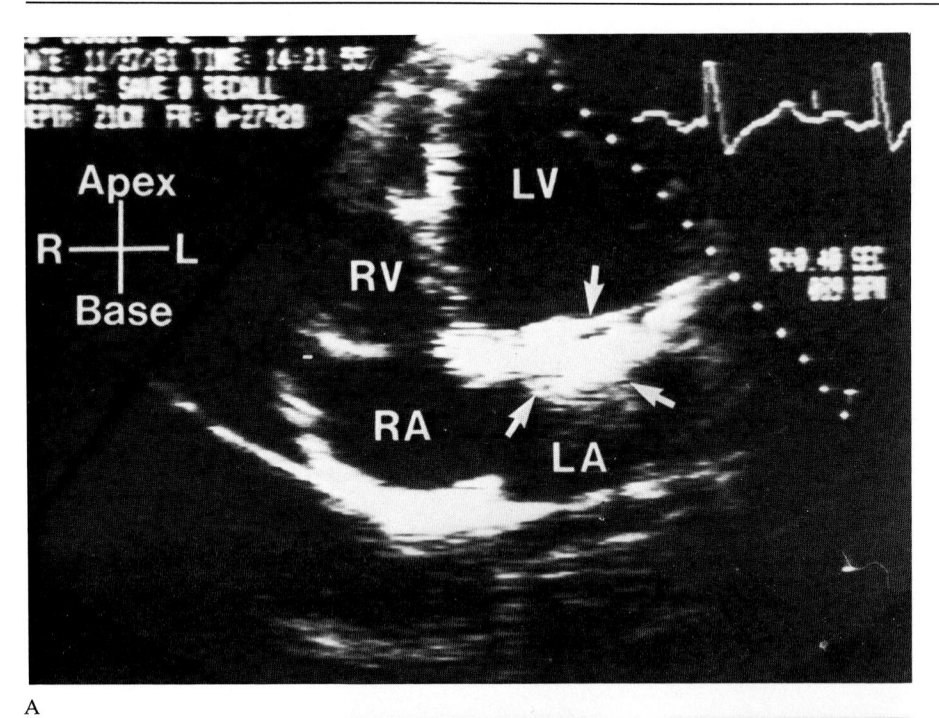

Fig. 12-9A. Apical 4-chamber view of a normally functioning caged-disc, low-profile mitral prosthesis (top arrow). Prominent reverberating reflectances (lower arrows) within the left atrium simulate a mass; real-time observation reveals this as artifact. B. Apical 4-chamber views demonstrating mid diastole (upper panel) with the poppet (P) of a mitral caged-ball prosthesis against the tip of the cage (C); the sewing ring (SR) is a strong echo producer and reverberates into the left atrium. The lower panel demonstrates the poppet in a closed position at end diastole of the same patient.

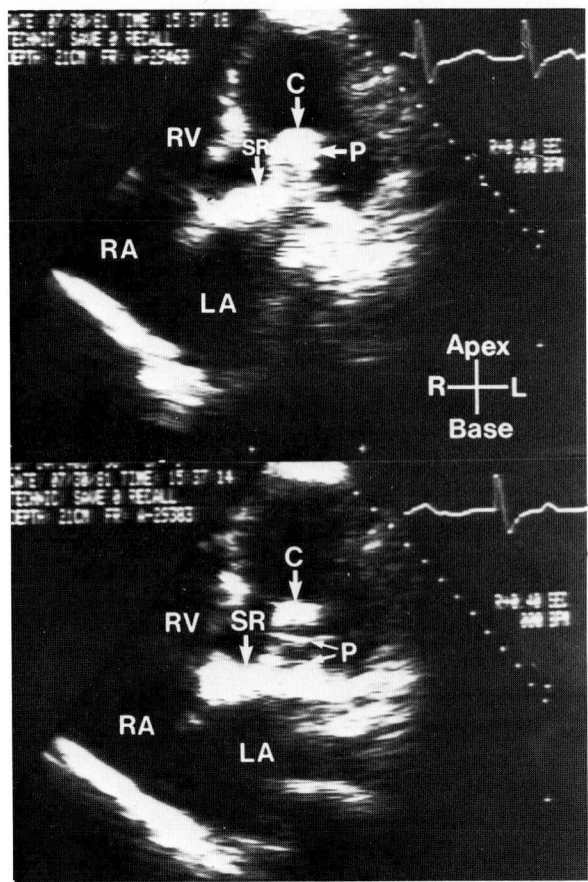

[28]. This valve is made of pyrolytic carbon, and its bileaflet design provides three orifices so that flow through the valve is entirely central. It reportedly has lower transvalvular pressure gradients for any given annulus diameter than other prostheses tested under identical conditions [48–50]. A low incidence of thromboembolic events and mild hemolysis are other advantages with this valve [50, 51]. No opening click is normally heard or recorded in any patient; however, a loud aortic or mitral closing click is normally present in all patients with either aortic or mitral SJM valves [29]. Echocardiographic evaluation of the St. Jude prosthetic valve can be facilitated if the surgeon positions the valve so that open leaflets are perpendicular to the echocardiographic plane of the long axis of the ventricle [30] (Fig. 12-10).

Ultrasound Doppler techniques can be used to determine reliably the mean diastolic gradient across mitral prosthetic valves [52–54].

The usefulness of simultaneous phonocardiography and echocardiography for the diagnosis of prosthetic valve dysfunction in patients with two prostheses has been demonstrated [55]. Using phonoechocardiography Assad-Morell and colleagues [55] were able to clearly identify the tricuspid prosthesis as the malfunctioning one, which permitted the authors to confidently recommend tricuspid prosthesis replacement without prior cardiac catheterization.

It is technically easier to obtain good-quality 2-D echo examinations in patients with porcine heterografts in the mitral position than with other types of prostheses. M-mode recordings should be obtained while imaging the mitral heterograft from the various parasternal windows. Simultaneous M-mode and 2-D imaging affords the echocardiographer the opportunity to position the cursor to record different portions of the leaflets to better evaluate both motion and thickness (Fig. 12-11). Alam and associates [22], in a study of 147 mitral and aortic porcine heterografts in 131 patients, found that leaflet thickness increased after 48 months. These authors reported that valves with thickening of 3 mm or more are at a higher risk of developing clinical evidence of valve dysfunction. Lipson and coworkers [56], in a long-term follow-up (>5 years) study of 49 patients with mitral porcine heterografts, observed a significant incidence of late valve failures requiring replacement. They also noted a high incidence of late hemodynamic deterioration even in those patients whose clinical status remained as yet unchanged.

Some investigators [18, 38] have evaluated porcine heterografts in the mitral position by measuring the motion and excursion of the anterior stent as well as the E–F slope and opening and closing velocities of the anterior leaflet. However, we have not found these specific measurements clinically useful. We primarily utilize M-mode recordings of the mitral heterograft leaflets to help evaluate leaflet thickness. This information together with the qualitative assessment of leaflet motion and stent movement from 2-D echo imaging is very important.

Schapira and colleagues [34] reported a diagnostic accuracy of 97 percent (38 of 39) with 2-D echo in evaluating porcine bioprosthetic valves compared to 67 percent accuracy (24 of 36) with M-mode echo in the same group of patients. They concluded that two-dimensional echocardiography has excellent diagnostic accuracy in assessing bioprosthetic and left ventricular function and is clearly superior to M-mode echocardiography in evaluating patients following porcine heterograft replacement in aortic and mitral positions.

A major advantage of 2-D echocardiographic imaging is its spatial orientation. By virtue of the multiple tomographic imaging planes from various precordial, apical, and subcostal transducer positions, three-dimensional anatomy of the

406 12. Prosthetic valves

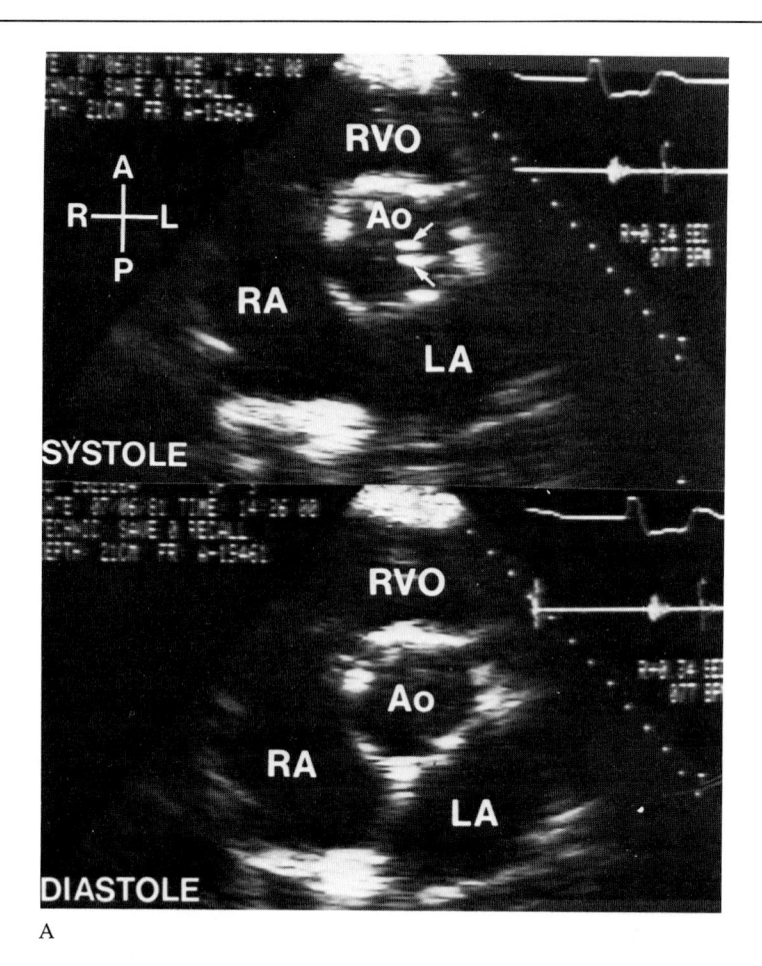

Fig. 12-10A. Parasternal short axis view at the base in a patient with a St. Jude Medical prosthesis in the aortic position during systole (upper panel) showing parallel reflectances (arrows) from the bileaflet valve and during diastole (lower panel). There is no reflectance from the closed valve. B. Parasternal long axis view in a patient with a St. Jude Medical prosthesis in the aortic position during systole showing parallel reflectances (arrows) from the normal bileaflet valve. No opening click is present from this valve; however, a prominent closing sound (S_2) is heard. A single S_2 is recorded on the accompanying phonocardiogram (PCG). C. Diagrams of St. Jude Medical prosthesis in the aortic position during systole and diastole illustrating the M-mode echo with parallel echoes during systole and no echoes from the valve during diastole. D. Diagram of the St. Jude Medical prosthesis in the mitral position showing parallel echoes during diastole and no reflectances from the valve during systole.

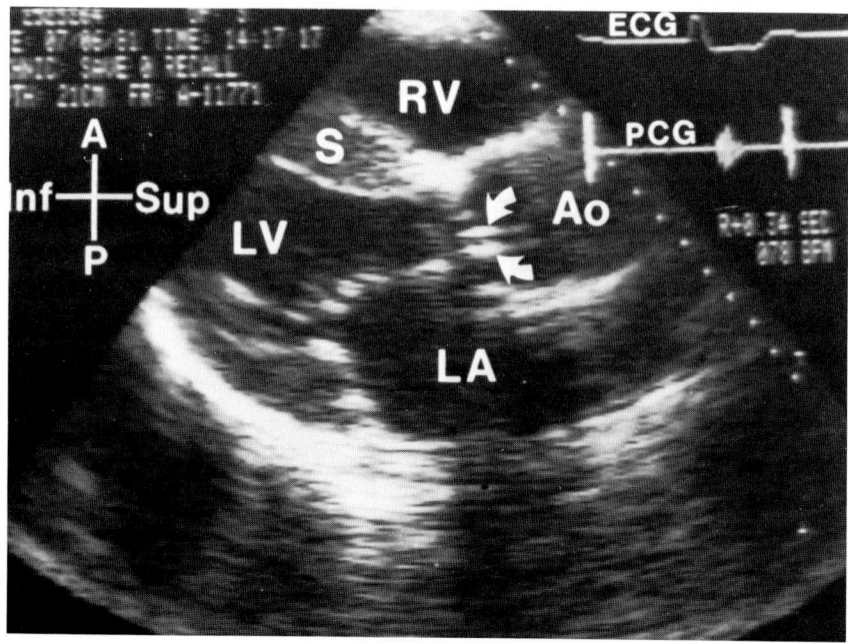

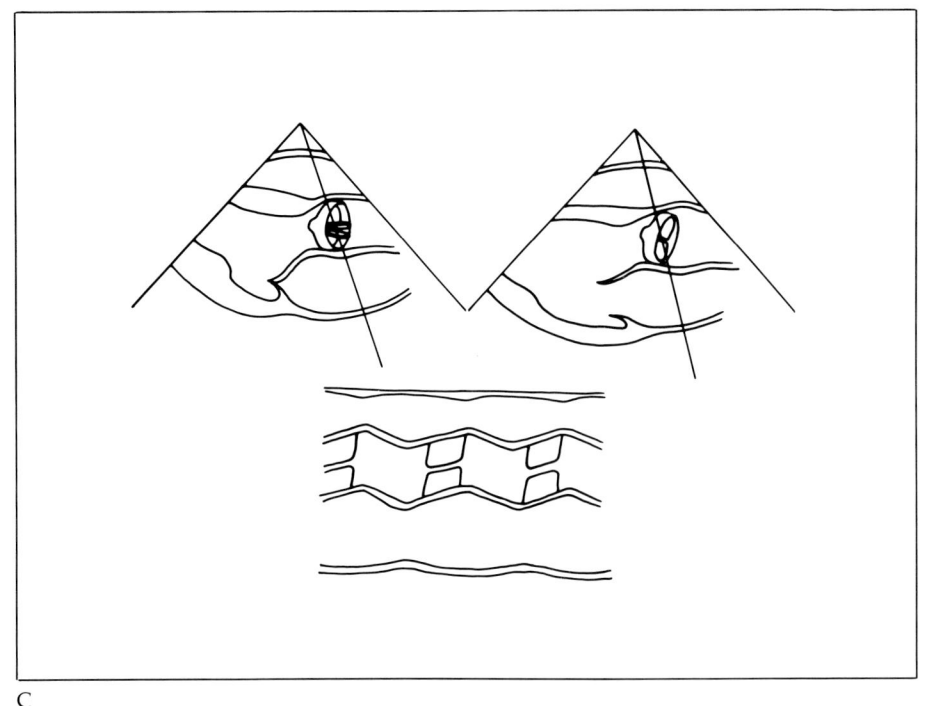

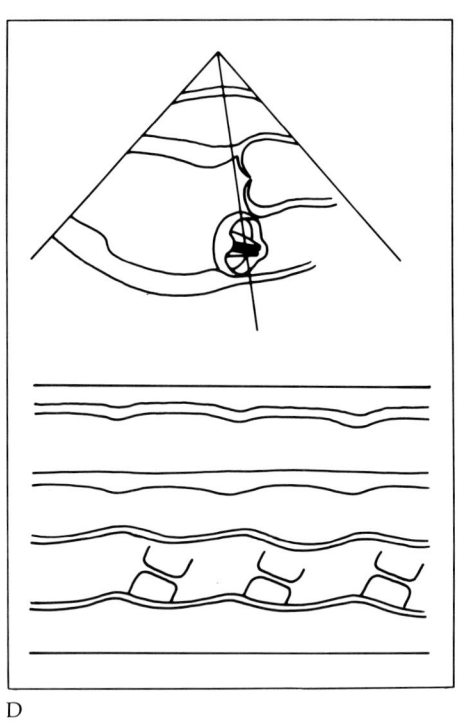

C

D

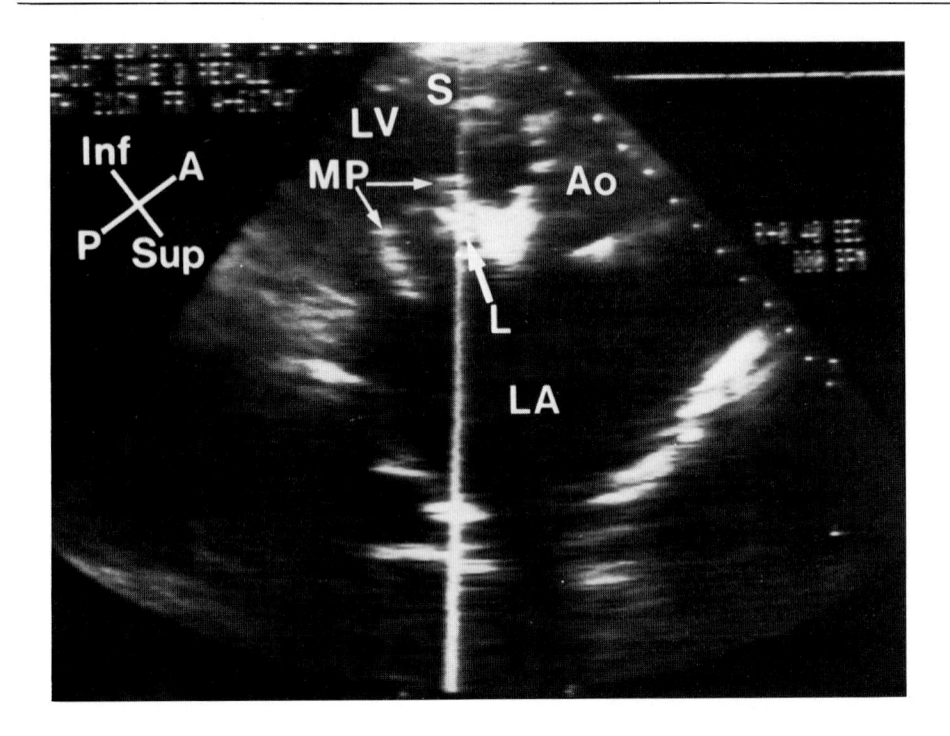

Fig. 12-11. Parasternal long axis view from low left sternal border position showing M-mode cursor through a normal mitral porcine heterograft (MP) and valve leaflet (L). Simultaneous imaging with 2-D and M-mode and positioning the cursor optimally through the leaflets enables measurement of leaflet motion and thickness.

prostheses can be appreciated (Fig. 12-12). This advantage tends to improve the chances of visualizing abnormalities of the leaflets or of detecting a small mass or abnormal echo reflective target around the sewing ring or attached to the stents. At the same time, however, the two-dimensional echocardiogram can result in a false positive or false negative diagnosis. Improperly high gain settings will lead to exaggerated reflectances, which can simulate valve masses. Although the imaging and resolution capabilities of some equipment have improved significantly since 1981, a very small mass (less than 1 or 2 mm in diameter) may still be missed by two-dimensional echocardiography. Because of equipment differences and variations of imaging techniques among clinical laboratories, the interpretation criteria and overall reliability should be established in each laboratory with whatever equipment is being used. Of course, interpretations regarding leaflet mobility and thickness, abnormal versus normal reflectances, and relative thickness of the stents and sewing ring are made primarily during real-time motion on videotape. Many of these features are difficult or impossible to portray in still-frame photographs (Fig. 12-13).

Perry and associates [35] performed measurements of stent size, orifice opening, leaflet thickness, and left atrial dimension in a two-dimensional echocardiographic assessment of mitral porcine heterografts in infants and children. In the normal bioprosthetic valves they observed leaflet thickness not exceeding 2 mm, freely moving leaflets, and normal sewing ring motion. Complications of thromboembolism, infective endocarditis, and arrhythmias are very low and occur with equal incidence in adults and children [35].

Bioprosthetic leaflet degeneration and calcification have been shown to occur more frequently and earlier in children than in adults [57, 58]. Fibrocalcific degener-

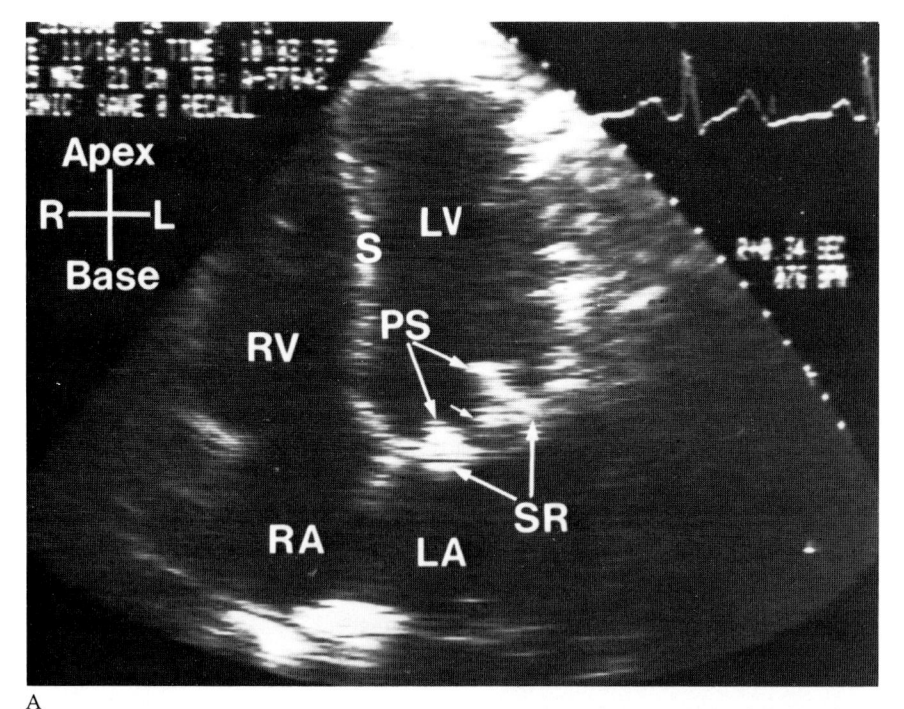

Fig. 12-12A. Apical 4-chamber view of a patient with a normally functioning mitral porcine heterograft showing the stents (PS), leaflets (small arrow), and sewing ring (SR). B. Subcostal 4-chamber view of a patient with a normal porcine mitral prosthesis (MP). IAS = interatrial septum.

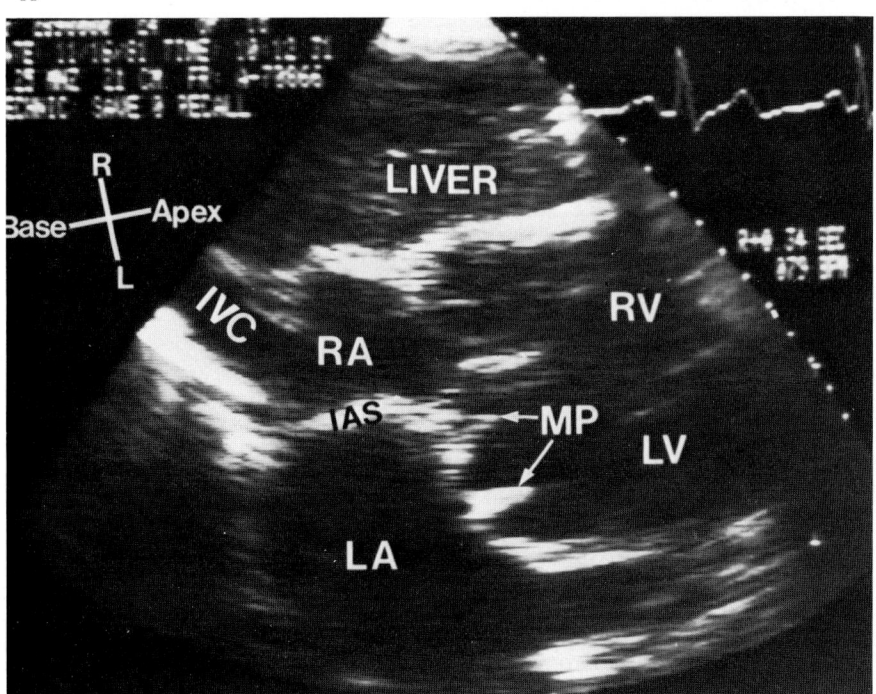

410   12. Prosthetic valves

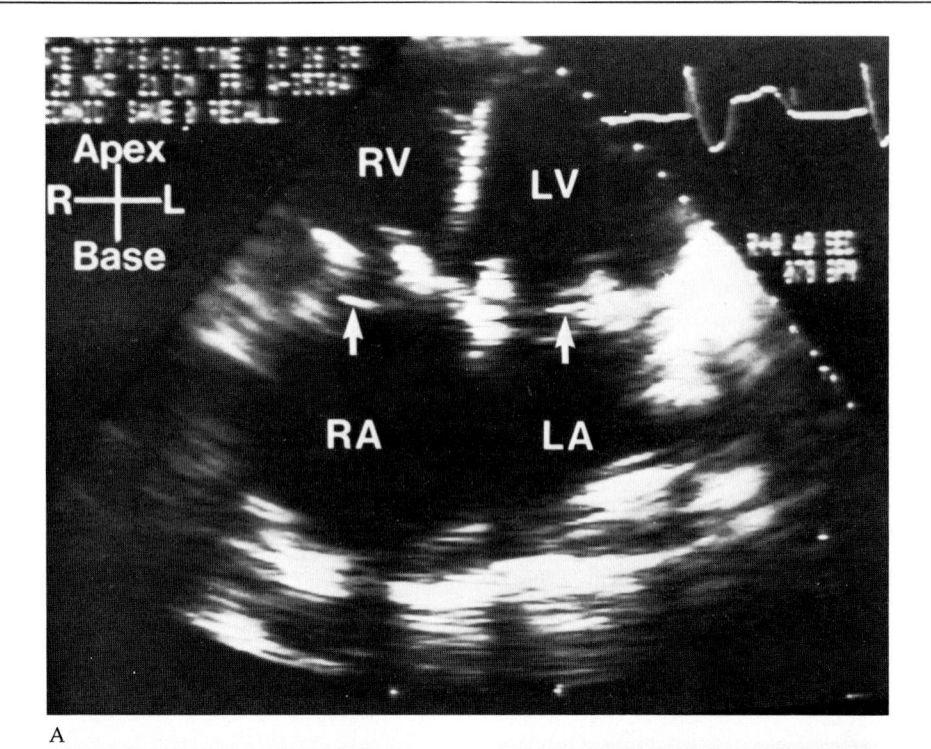

Fig. 12-13A. Apical 4-chamber view showing normal porcine heterografts in both tricuspid and mitral positions and normal leaflet thickness of both valves (arrows). Both right atrium and left atrium are enlarged. B. Apical 4-chamber view showing porcine mitral heterograft (MP) and thickened valve leaflets (L) due to calcification and secondary mitral stenosis and mitral regurgitation. Patient also has tricuspid valve porcine heterograft, which is only partially imaged in this view. C. Parasternal long axis view showing a patient with a mitral porcine heterograft who has developed infective endocarditis demonstrates a small vegetation (arrow) near the anterior stent (S) and thickened leaflet of the heterograft. Calcium is present in the aortic valve.

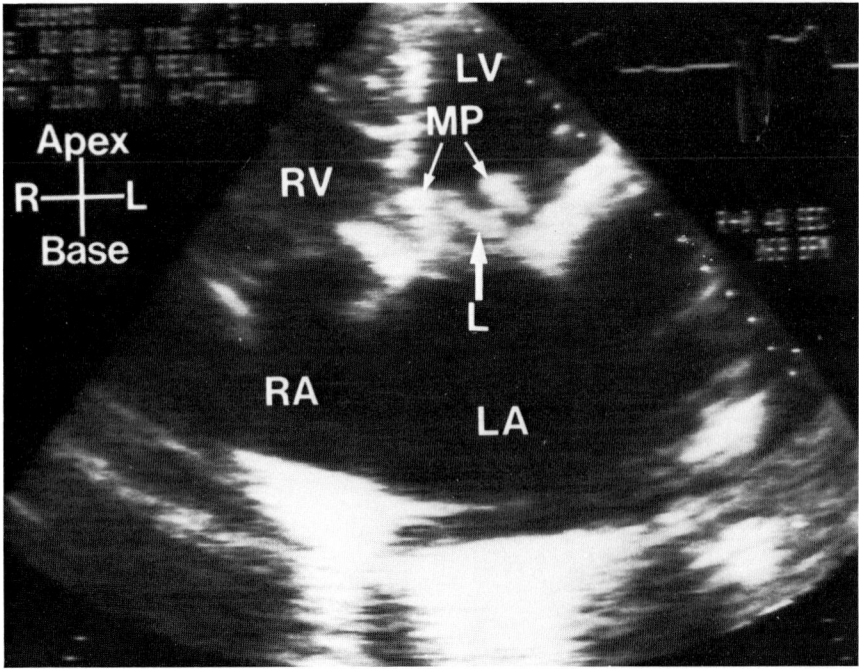

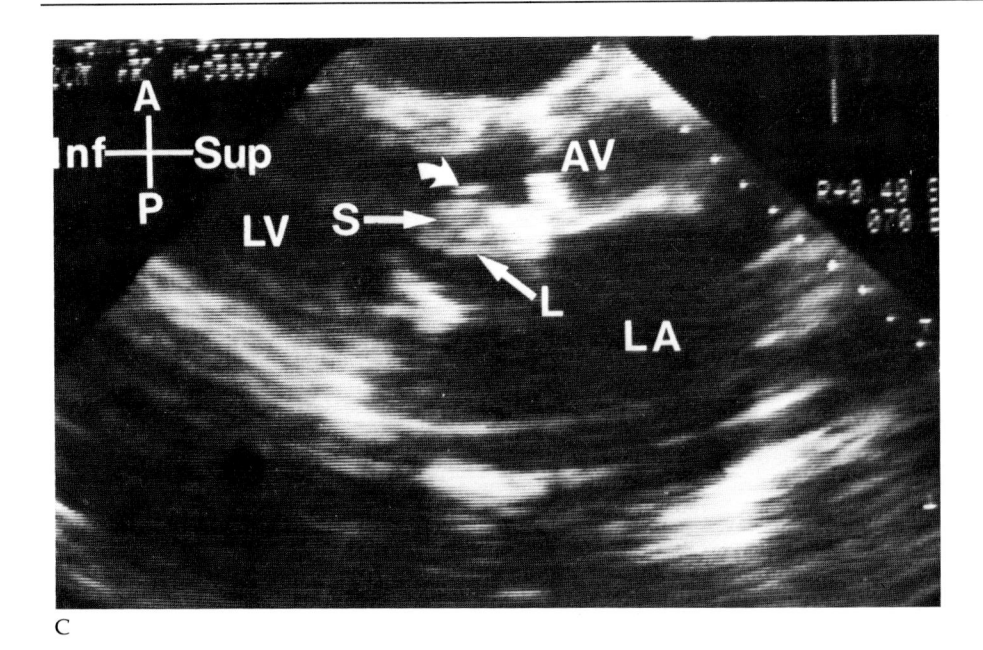

ation of mitral heterografts develops in approximately 5 percent of adult patients evaluated for up to 8 years [57–60]. In contrast, however, bioprosthetic failure (most commonly from calcification leading to stenosis) has led to repeat valve replacement in up to 38 percent of pediatric patients 30 to 56 months following implantation [57, 58, 61].

Limited information is available on the noninvasive evaluation of bioprosthetic valves in extracardiac conduits for congenital anomalies to establish continuity between the right ventricle and pulmonary artery. Canale and colleagues [62] studied 15 such patients by using 2-D echo to image the conduit diameter, valve contour, and motion as well as M-mode echo, phonocardiography, and range-gated Doppler to obtain flow information through the conduit. They were able to image the conduit and valve in all patients and could accurately determine the conduit diameter with two-dimensional echocardiography. These investigators also found thickened, stenotic heterograft leaflets in two patients and recommended serial evaluation with these noninvasive procedures to aid in planning the timing of hemodynamic follow-up studies.

In our experience the three most common clinical questions being asked which prompt referral of patients with prosthetic valves for echocardiographic evaluation are: (1) Is the prosthetic valve, left ventricle, or left atrium the source of an arterial thromboembolic complication? (2) Is there any evidence of infective endocarditis with vegetation or abscess involving the prosthesis or adjacent myocardium? and (3) Is there any evidence of or how severe is the valvular stenosis and/or regurgitation of the prosthesis? Although we cannot always answer these questions with absolute accuracy, two-dimensional echocardiographic imaging is the single most important noninvasive diagnostic procedure available which, together with the clinical information, can determine the course of treatment or decide whether cardiac catheterization is indicated.

412   12. Prosthetic valves

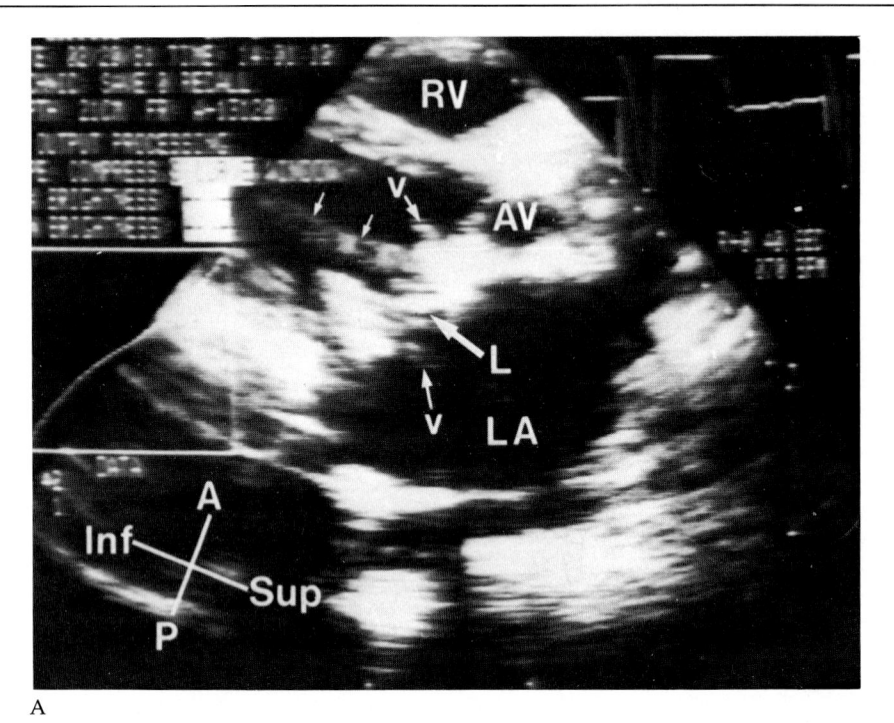

Fig. 12-14A. Parasternal long axis view of a patient with infective endocarditis of the mitral porcine heterograft demonstrating vegetations (v) on both ventricular and atrial sides of the valve. The leaflets (L) are markedly thickened. Strong reflectances from the valve produce artifact echoes on the fan projected into the left ventricular cavity (two small arrows). B. M-mode recording in the same patient of mitral porcine heterograft with thickened leaflets (white arrows) and a vegetation (black arrows) attached to one of the stents. C. Apical 4-chamber views of same patient showing thickened leaflets (arrows) of mitral porcine heterograft (MP) and vegetation (V) prolapsing into left atrium during systole (upper panel). One of the thick, infected leaflets (arrow) is more conspicuous during diastole (lower panel).

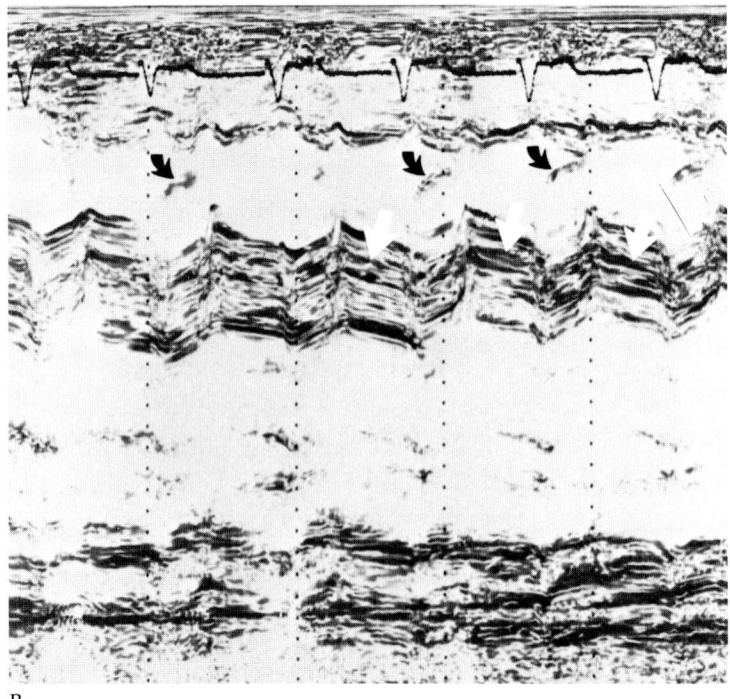

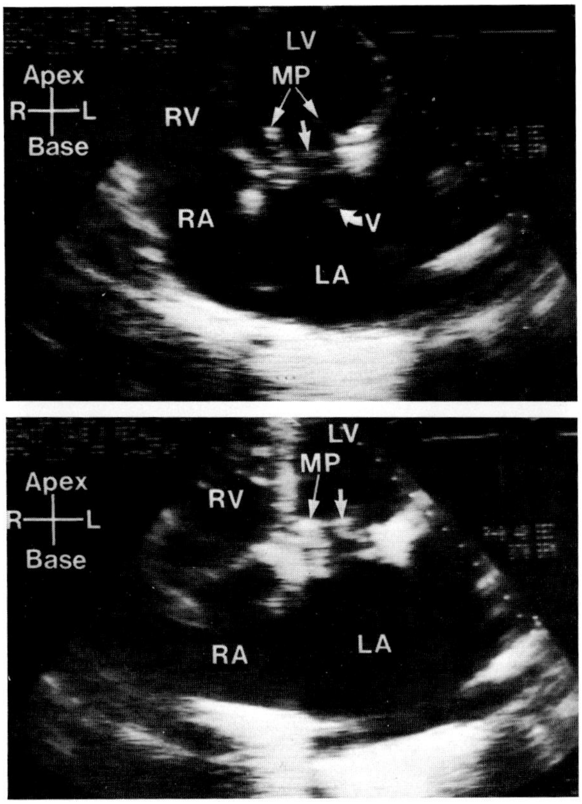

C

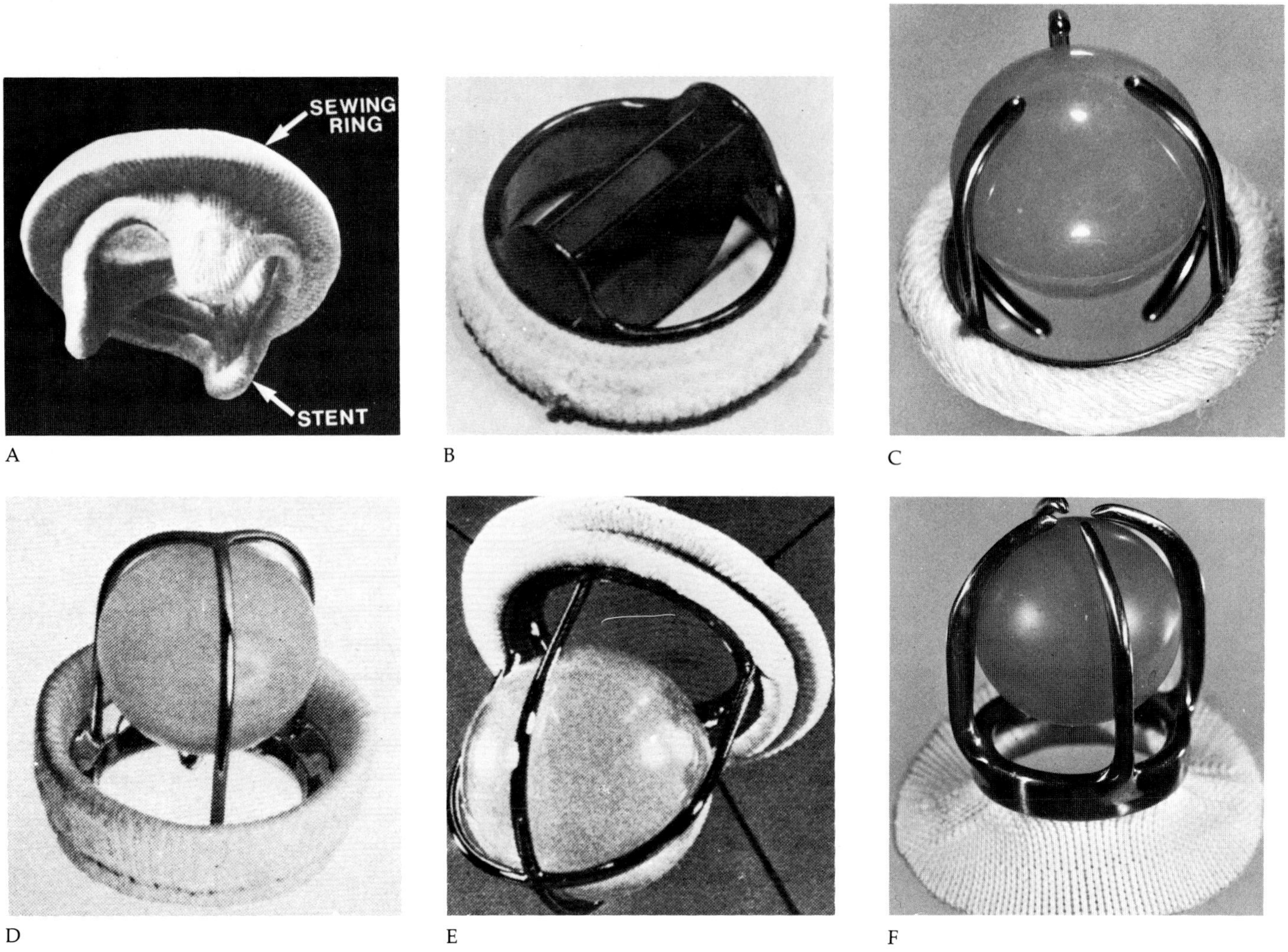

414   12. Prosthetic valves

Fig. 12-15A. Hancock porcine heterograft for mitral position. B. St. Jude Medical prosthesis. C. Smeloff-Cutter ball prosthesis. D. Starr-Edwards (model 1000, aortic position) high-profile ball prosthesis. E. Starr-Edwards (model 6120, mitral position) high-profile ball prosthesis. F. Braunwald-Cutter ball prosthesis. G. Bjork-Shiley (mitral position) low-profile tilting disc prosthesis. H. Kay-Suzuki (mitral position) low-profile disc prosthesis. I. Cooley-Cutter (mitral position) low-profile disc prosthesis. J. Beall (model 103, mitral position) low-profile disc prosthesis. K. Kay-Shiley (TGCD series, tricuspid position) disc prosthesis with two pairs of arch-like muscle guards extending from the base ring.

G

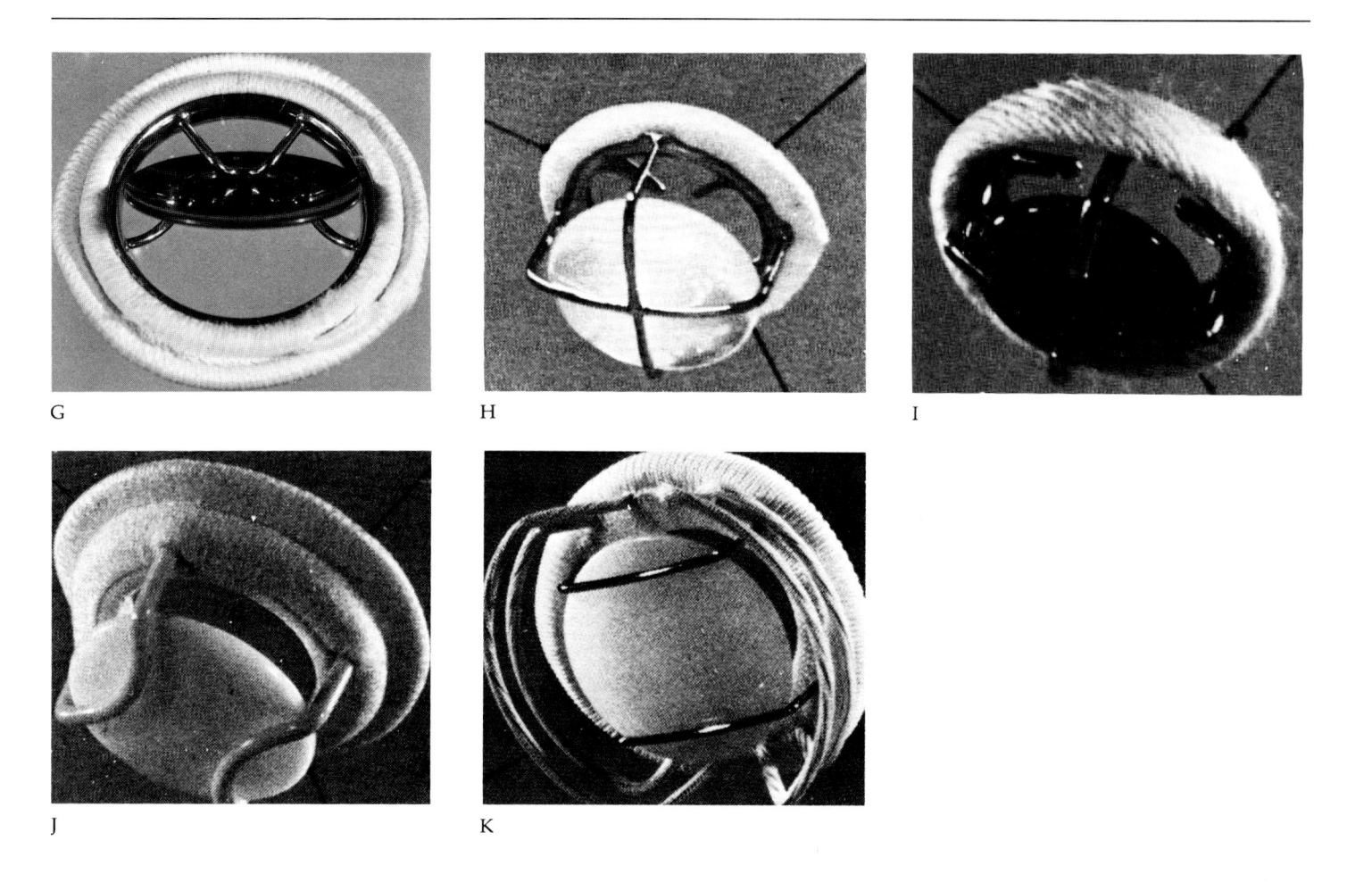

H

I

J

K

Infective endocarditis is a dreaded complication of valvular prostheses [63–65]. The incidence of early prosthetic valve infective endocarditis varies from 0 to 7.1 percent among different medical centers with an average of 1.14 percent [66]. The overall incidence (early plus late) varies from 0 to 9.2 percent among different series with an average of 2.34 percent [66]. The microbiology of the endocarditis is significantly different from that of infective endocarditis of the native valves [67]. The streptococci, the most important group of etiologic agents in infective endocarditis of natural valves, play a very minor role in early prosthetic valve infective endocarditis (7.5%), whereas these organisms are the most common cause of late endocarditis (37.1%) [66]. *Staphylococcus epidermis* is the single most important cause, accounting for 27.4 percent of the early cases and 22.9 percent of the late cases; the other important causes of early and late endocarditis respectively are: *S. aureus* 19.2 percent and 11.4 percent, gram-negative bacilli 20.5 percent and 13.6 percent, and fungi 9.6 percent and 4.3 percent [66]. In a review of 16 different studies, Watanakunakorn [66] reported a very high mortality, which has not changed significantly in recent years; mortality of early endocarditis averages 73 percent compared to the late endocarditis average of 45 percent. Surgical removal of the infected prosthesis and replacement with a new prosthesis is indicated in the following situations: fungal endocarditis, persistent infection, malfunction of the prosthetic valve, repeated major embolization, and relapse of prosthetic valve infective endocarditis [66].

Vegetations large enough to be pedunculated at their site of attachment on valvular prostheses can be quite conspicuous by their motion. Since they may be small and the motion only intermittently visible in certain views, it is obviously important that meticulous, detailed imaging be performed from many different transducer positions (Fig. 12-14).

Miller and associates [68] reported that two-dimensional echocardiography had a limited role in detecting abnormal function in prosthetic valves; 2-D echo recognized the abnormality in only 6 of 23 (26%) mechanical prostheses and in 2 of 4 (50%) heterograft valves.

Sahn and coinvestigators [69] compared two-dimensional echocardiographic findings with angiographic, hemodynamic, and surgical results in 38 patients with biologic valves in mitral and aortic positions who were undergoing reevaluation 24 to 87 months (mean 34 months) after implantation. They observed poor cusp support, gross fluttering, and prolapse behind or below the annulus which identified insufficiency in four aortic homograft valves and in three mitral homograft valves. Vegetations were easily imaged on homograft or heterograft valves; the diagnosis was confirmed in five aortic and three mitral bioprostheses. Periprosthetic abscess was identified in two patients. The investigators concluded that despite difficulties in imaging valve cusps, significant valve deterioration or infected valve prostheses were quite effectively imaged by 2-D echo.

As an aid in recognizing different types of prostheses, photographs of various models and types of prosthetic valves are included in Fig. 12-15.

References

1. Chandraratna PAN, Lopez JM, Hildner FJ, Samet P, Ben Zvi J: Diagnosis of Bjork-Shiley aortic valve dysfunction by echocardiography. *Am Heart J* 91:318, 1976
2. Brodie BR, Grossman W, McLauren L, Starek P, Craige E: Diagnosis of prosthetic mitral valve malfunction with combined echophonocardiography. *Circulation* 53:93, 1976
3. Waggoner AD, Quinones MA, Young JB, Nelson JG, Winters WL, Peterson PK, Miller RR: Echo-phonocardiographic evaluation of obstruction of prosthetic mitral valve. *Chest* 78:60, 1980
4. Ibarra-Perez C, Rodriguez-Trujillo F, Perez-Redondo H: Engagement of ventricular myocardium by struts of mitral prosthesis: Fatal complication of use of open-cage cardiac valves. *J Thorac Cardiovasc Surg* 61:403, 1971
5. Beall AC: Late results with cardiac valve replacement: Reduction of thrombo-embolic complications of mitral valve replacement. *J Cardiovasc Surg* 13:261, 1972
6. Pfeifer J, Goldschlager N, Sweatman T, Gerbode F, Selzer A: Malfunction of mitral ball valve prosthesis due to thrombus. *Am J Cardiol* 29:95, 1972
7. Miller HC, Gibson DG, Stephens JD: Role of echocardiography and phonocardiography in diagnosis of mitral paraprosthetic regurgitation with Starr-Edwards prostheses. *Br Heart J* 35:1217, 1973
8. Silver MD, Wilson GJ: The pathology of wear in the Beall model 104 heart valve prosthesis. *Circulation* 56:617, 1977
9. Nathan MJ: Strut fracture: A late complication of Beall mitral valve replacement. *Ann Thorac Surg* 16:610, 1973
10. Lee SJK, Zaragoza AJ, Callaghan JC, Couves CM, Sterns LP: Malfunction of the mitral valve prosthesis (Cutter-Smeloff): Clinical and hemodynamic observations in three cases. *Circulation* 41:479, 1970
11. Willerson JT, Kastor JA, Dinsmore RE, Mundth E, Buckley MJ, Austen WG, Sanders CA: Non-invasive assessment of prosthetic mitral paravalvular and intravalvular regurgitation. *Br Heart J* 34:561, 1972
12. Bernal-Ramirez JA, Phillips JH: Echocardiographic study of malfunction of the Bjork-Shiley prosthetic heart valve in the mitral position. *Am J Cardiol* 40:449, 1977
13. Oliva PB, Johnson ML, Pomerantz M, Levene A: Dysfunction of the Beall mitral prosthesis and its detection by cinefluoroscopy and echocardiography. *Am J Cardiol* 31:393, 1973
14. Roberts WC, Hammer WJ: Cardiac pathology after valve replacement with a tilting disc prosthesis (Bjork-Shiley type): A study of 46 necropsy patients and 49 Bjork-Shiley prostheses. *Am J Cardiol* 37:1024, 1976
15. Arnett EN, Roberts WC: Prosthetic valve endocarditis: Clinicopathologic analysis of 22 necropsy patients with comparison of observations in 74 necropsy patients with active infective endocarditis involving natural left-sided cardiac valves. *Am J Cardiol* 38:281, 1976
16. Mintz GS, Carlson EB, Kotler MN: Comparison of noninvasive techniques in evaluation of the nontissue cardiac valve prosthesis. *Am J Cardiol* 49:39, 1982
17. Wann LS, Pyhel HJ, Judson WE, Tavel ME, Feigenbaum H: Ball variance in a Harken mitral prosthesis: Echocardiographic and phonocardiographic features. *Chest* 72:785, 1977
18. Bloch WN Jr, Felner JM, Wickliffe C, Symbas PN, Schlant RC: Echocardiogram of the porcine aortic bioprosthesis in the mitral position. *Am J Cardiol* 38:293, 1976
19. Alam M, Madrazo AC, Magilligan DJ, Goldstein S: M mode and two dimensional echocardiographic features of porcine valve dysfunction. *Am J Cardiol* 43:502, 1979
20. Horowitz MS, Goodman DJ, Popp RL: Echocardiographic diagnosis of calcific stenosis of a stented aortic homograft in the mitral position. *JCU* 2:179, 1975
21. Ferrans VJ, Boyce SW, Billingham ME, Jones M, Roberts WC: Alterations in collagen of porcine valve heterografts in place from 3 to 94 months: The cause of leaflet calcific deposits and of perforations and tears. *Am J Cardiol* 45:487, 1980
22. Alam MA, Goldstein S, Lakier JB: Echocardiographic changes in the thickness of porcine valves with time. *Chest* 79:663, 1981
23. Bloch WN Jr, Felner JM, Wickliffe C, Symbas PN: Echocardiographic diagnosis of thrombus on a heterograft aortic valve in the mitral position. *Chest* 70:399, 1976
24. Copans H, Lakier JB, Kinsley RH, Colsen PR, Fritz VU, Barlow JB: Thrombosed Bjork-Shiley mitral prostheses. *Circulation* 61:169, 1980

25. Berndt TB, Goodman DJ, Popp RL: Echocardiographic and phonocardiographic confirmation of suspected cage mitral valve malfunction. *Chest* 70:221, 1976
26. Johnson ML, Holmes JH, Paton BC: Echocardiographic determination of mitral disc valve excursion. *Circulation* 47:1274, 1973
27. Estevez R, Mookherjee S, Potts J, Fulton M, Obeid AI: Phonocardiographic and echocardiographic features of Lillehei-Kaster mitral prosthesis. *JCU* 5:153, 1977
28. Amann FW, Burckhardt D, Hasse J, Gradel E: Echocardiographic features of the correctly functioning St. Jude Medical valve prosthesis. *Am Heart J* 101:45, 1981
29. DePace NL, Kotler MN, Mintz GS, Lichtenberg R, Goel IP, Segal BL: Echocardiographic and phonocardiographic assessment of the St. Jude cardiac valve prosthesis. *Chest* 80:272, 1981
30. Tri TB, Schatz RA, Watson TD, Bowen TE, Schiller NB: Echocardiographic evaluation of the St. Jude Medical prosthetic valve. *Chest* 80:278, 1981
31. Nanda NC, Gramiak R, Shah PM, DeWeese JA, Mahoney EB: Echocardiographic assessment of left ventricular outflow width in the selection of mitral valve prosthesis. *Circulation* 48:1208, 1973
32. Denbow CE, Pluth JR, Giuliani ER: The role of echocardiography in the selection of mitral valve prosthesis. *Am Heart J* 99:586, 1980
33. Rahimtoola SH: The problem of valve prosthesis-patient mismatch. *Circulation* 58:20, 1978
34. Schapira JN, Martin RP, Fowles RE, Rakowski H, Stinson EB, French JW, Shumway NE, Popp RL: Two dimensional echocardiographic assessment of patients with bioprosthetic valves. *Am J Cardiol* 43:510, 1979
35. Perry LW, Midgley FM, Galioto FM Jr, Shapiro SR, Ruckman RN, Scott LP: Two-dimensional echocardiographic evaluation of mitral bioprosthetic function in infants and children. *Am Heart J* 102:1022, 1981
36. Bommer W, Yoon D, Grehl TM, Mason DT, Neumann A, DeMaria AN: In vitro and in vivo evaluation of porcine bioprostheses by cross-sectional echocardiography. *Am J Cardiol* 41:405, 1978
37. Horowitz MS, Tecklenberg PL, Goodman DJ, Harrison DC, Popp RL: Echocardiographic evaluation of the stent mounted aortic bioprosthetic valve in the mitral position: In vitro and in vivo studies. *Circulation* 54:91, 1976
38. Harston WE Jr, Robertson RM, Friesinger GC: Echocardiographic evaluation of porcine heterograft valves in the mitral and aortic positions. *Am Heart J* 96:448, 1978
39. Yamamoto T, Tanimoto M, Ohogami T, Yasutomi N, Ando H, Iwasaki T, Yorifuji S, Shimizu Y, Horiguchi Y, Miyamoto T: Evaluation of the porcine aortic bioprosthesis by M-mode and cross-sectional echocardiography. *J Cardiogr* 7:267, 1977
40. Mary DAS, Pakrashi BC, Catchpole R, Ionescue MI: Echocardiographic studies of stented fascia lata grafts in the mitral position. *Circulation* 49:237, 1974
41. Siggers DC, Srivongse SA, Deuchar D: Analysis of dynamics of mitral Starr-Edwards valve prosthesis using reflected ultrasound. *Br Heart J* 33:401, 1971
42. Winters WL, Gimenez JL, Soloff LA: Clinical application of ultrasound in the analysis of prosthetic ball valve function. *Am J Cardiol* 19:97, 1967
43. Feigenbaum H: *Echocardiography* (3rd ed). Philadelphia: Lea & Febiger, 1981. Pp 299–300
44. Douglas JE, Williams GD: Echocardiographic evaluation of the Bjork-Shiley prosthetic valve. *Circulation* 50:52, 1974
45. Capella G, Bomba MA, Pandolfini E, Rossi P: Use of echocardiography in the study of the Bjork-Shiley disc valve prosthesis. *Boll Soc Ital Cardiol* 20:1779, 1975
46. Belenkie I, Carr M, Schlant RC, Nutter DO, Symbas PN: Malfunction of a Cutter-Smeloff mitral ball valve prosthesis: Diagnosis by phonocardiography and echocardiography. *Am Heart J* 86:399, 1973
47. Gibson TC, Starek PJ, Moos S, Craige E: Echocardiographic and phonocardiographic characteristics of the Lillehei-Kaster mitral valve prosthesis. *Circulation* 49:434, 1974
48. Emery RW, Nicoloff DM: St. Jude Medical cardiac valve prosthesis: In vitro studies. *J Thorac Cardiovasc Surg* 78:269, 1979
49. Horstkotte D, Haerten K, Herzer JA, Seipel L, Loogen F: Results after mitral valve replacement using St. Jude Medical valve in comparison to the Bjork-Shiley valve. *Circulation* 62:157, 1980
50. Chaux A, Gray RJ, Matloff JM, Feldman H, Sustaita H: An appreciation of the new St. Jude valvular prosthesis. *J Thorac Cardiovasc Surg* 81:202, 1981

51. Emery RW, Anderson RW, Lindsay WG, Jorgensen CR, Wang Y, Nicoloff DM: Clinical and hemodynamic results with the St. Jude Medical aortic valve prosthesis. *Surg Forum* 30:235, 1979
52. Holen J, Simonsen S, Froysaker T: An ultrasound Doppler technique for the noninvasive determination of the pressure gradient in the Bjork-Shiley mitral valve. *Circulation* 59:436, 1979
53. Holen J, Nitter-Hauge S: Evaluation of obstructive characteristics of mitral disc valve implants with ultrasound Doppler techniques. *Acta Med Scand* 201:429, 1977
54. Holen J, Hoie J, Semb B: Obstructive characteristics of Bjork-Shiley, Hancock, and Lillehei-Kaster prosthetic mitral valves in the immediate post-operative period. *Acta Med Scand* 204:5, 1978
55. Assad-Morell JL, Tajik AJ, Anderson MW, Tancredi RG, Wallace RB, Giuliani ER: Malfunctioning tricuspid valve prosthesis: Clinical, phonocardiographic, echocardiographic, and surgical findings. *Mayo Clin Proc* 49:443, 1974
56. Lipson LC, Kent KM, McIntosh CL, Rosing DR, Bonow RO, Condit J, Epstein SE, Morrow AG: Hemodynamic evaluation of porcine heterografts in the mitral position for more than 5 years. *Am J Cardiol* 45:486, 1980
57. Kutsche LM, Oyer P, Shumway N, Baum D: An important complication of Hancock mitral valve replacement in children. *Circulation* 60:98, 1979
58. Silver MM, Pollock J, Silver MD, Williams WG, Trusler GA: Calcification in porcine xenograft valves in children. *Am J Cardiol* 45:685, 1980
59. Cohn LH, Koster JK, Mee RBB, Collins JJ Jr: Long-term follow-up of the Hancock bioprosthetic heart valve: A 6-year review. *Circulation* 60:187, 1979
60. Cohn LH, Mudge GH, Pratter F, Collins JJ Jr: Five to eight-year follow-up of patients undergoing porcine heart valve replacement. *N Engl J Med* 304:258, 1981
61. Sanders SP, Freed MD, Norwood WI, Castaneda AR, Nadas AS: Early failure of porcine valves implanted in children. *Am J Cardiol* 45:449, 1980
62. Canale JM, Sahn DJ, Copeland JG, Goldberg SJ, Valdez-Cruz LM, Salomon N, Allen HD: Two dimensional Doppler echocardiographic/M mode echocardiographic and phonocardiographic method for study of extracardiac heterograft valve conduits in the right ventricular outflow tract position. *Am J Cardiol* 49:100, 1982
63. Killen DA, Collins HA, Koenig MG, Goodman JS: Prosthetic cardiac valves and bacterial endocarditis. *Ann Thorac Surg* 9:238, 1970
64. Amoury RA, Bowman FO Jr, Malm JR: Endocarditis associated with intracardiac prostheses. *J Thorac Cardiovasc Surg* 51:36, 1966
65. Starr A, Edwards ML, Griswold H: Mitral replacement: Late results with a ball valve prosthesis. *Prog Cardiovasc Dis* 5:298, 1962
66. Watanakunakorn C: Prosthetic valve infective endocarditis. *Prog Cardiovasc Dis* 22:181, 1979
67. Watanakunakorn C: Changing epidemiology and newer aspects of infective endocarditis. *Adv Intern Med* 22:21, 1977
68. Miller FA, Tajik AJ, Seward JB, Callahan JA, Schattenberg TT, Shub C, Giuliani ER, Pluth JR: Prosthetic valve dysfunction: Two-dimensional echocardiographic assessment. *Circulation* 64(Suppl IV):IV-315, 1981
69. Sahn DJ, Roche T, Brandt PWT, Friedman M, Valdez-Cruz LM, Allen HD, Goldberg SJ: Detection of deterioration or infection of bio-prosthetic valves in mitral and aortic positions by 2D echo. *Circulation* 64(Suppl IV):IV-315, 1981

Interventional echocardiography

A variety of diagnostic interventions to be used with M-mode and two-dimensional echocardiographic examinations have been described. These interventions can be divided into six categories: contrast echocardiography, physiologic and pharmacologic maneuvers, exercise echocardiography, echophonocardiography, esophageal echocardiography, and intraoperative echocardiography. Several of these interventions are routinely utilized in the clinical setting but others are still investigational.

Contrast echocardiography. Contrast echocardiographic techniques, initially developed by Gramiak and colleagues [1], have been used extensively for the validation of echocardiographic structure identification and the diagnosis of intracardiac shunts. If a liquid, usually normal saline or indocyanine green dye, is injected rapidly through an intravenous needle or intracardiac catheter while an ultrasound beam is traversing the chamber into which the injection is made, opacification occurs caused by the formation of microscopic bubbles. Indocyanine green dye is the preferable injectate, and a double-syringe technique is commonly employed; 1 or 2 ml of dye is manually injected through a 20 or 21 gauge needle or catheter in a peripheral arm vein, followed immediately by a vigorous manual flush of 5 to 10 ml of isotonic saline [2–5] (Fig. 13-1). Seward and colleagues [3] adjust the concentration of the green dye solution according to body weight: 5 mg/ml for patients more than 34 kg, 2.5 mg/ml for 11 to 34 kg, 1.25 mg/ml for 4.5 to 11 kg, and 0.625 mg/ml for less than 4.5 kg.

Although the concept of contrast echocardiography was introduced in the late 1960s [1], documentation of its clinical usefulness with the aid of superficial peripheral venous injections for detecting and localizing intracardiac shunts did not occur until the late 1970s [4–10]. Since the echo-producing quality of indocyanine green dye is normally lost with passage through the pulmonary capillary bed, a right-sided injection of dye should not produce echoes in the left side of the heart. For this reason any appearance of microbubbles in left heart chambers after right-sided injections indicates right-to-left shunting.

Shub and colleagues [11] were able to diagnose intrapulmonary right-to-left shunting using this technique in a patient with hereditary hemorrhagic telangiectasia and diffuse pulmonary arteriovenous fistulas. After venous injection of the green dye these authors observed the characteristic contrast flow pattern being markedly delayed before the appearance of echoes in the left ventricle.

The introduction of two-dimensional echocardiography has provided significant improvement in our ability to clinically utilize contrast techniques. Capability to record the dynamic spatial anatomy of the heart together with comprehensive imaging of the interventricular septum and interatrial septum affords a better opportunity to identify intracardiac shunts than with M-mode echo contrast techniques [5, 7, 8, 12–14]. Weyman and colleagues [5] observed negative contrast effect in nine of 11 patients who had atrial septal defects with left-to-right shunts. The phenomenon of "negative contrast effect" was produced by the non-contrast-containing blood flowing through the septum and displacing the contrast-containing blood from along the right-sided portion of the septum. In our experience, as well as that of other investigators [8, 14], the reliability of contrast 2-D echo

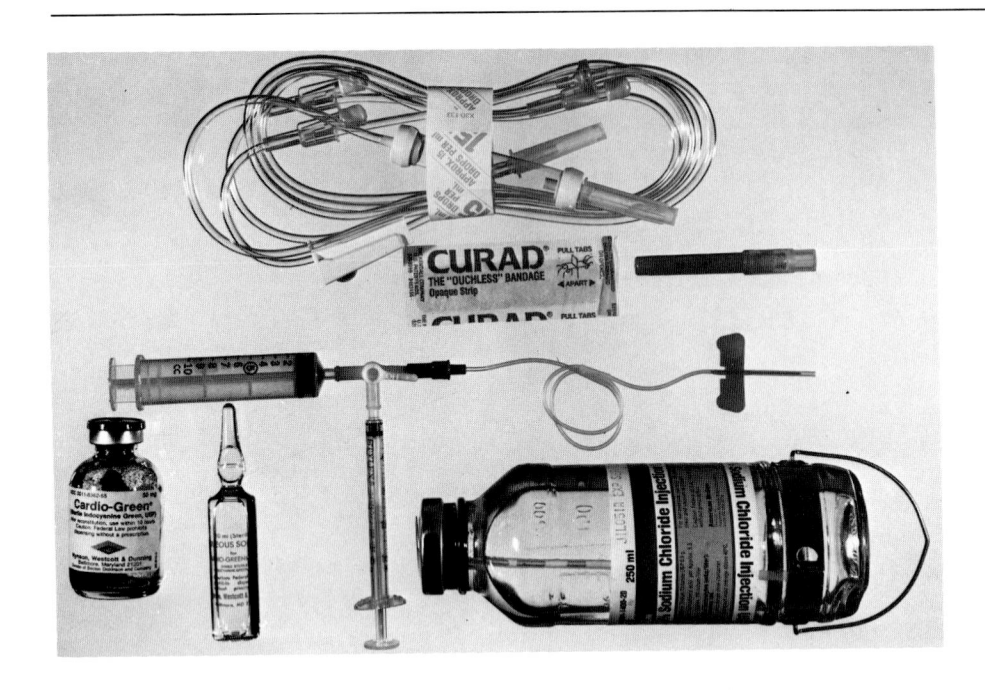

Fig. 13-1. Materials used to perform contrast echocardiography include a 20 or 21 gauge needle and minimal length of tubing connected to a three-way stopcock to permit bolus injection of 1 ml indocyanine green dye followed quickly with a bolus injection of 10 ml of normal saline.

for the detection of interatrial shunting is very good. We have found the detection of positive left atrial contrast (microbubbles moving from right atrium to left atrium) more reliable in identifying an atrial septal defect than the negative contrast effect. Gilbert and coworkers [14], in a study of 23 patients with secundum atrial septal defect, seven of whom had pulmonary hypertension, observed that all patients had either positive left atrial or negative right atrial contrast and approximately 50 percent had both. In one patient with neither positive nor negative contrast findings, anomalous pulmonary venous drainage was found at surgery. These investigators found positive left atrial contrast in all seven patients with pulmonary hypertension and interatrial shunting, but none displayed negative right atrial contrast. Shunt size cannot be predicted by positive or negative contrast alone or in combination.

Patients with predominant left-to-right atrial shunts do not always have microbubbles or microcavitations in the left atrium on a single injection. Multiple views of the atria with several bolus injections during each view may be required to prove or exclude the presence of atrial septal defect. The apical four-chamber plane is usually the best view for observing evidence of positive or negative contrast in the presence of an atrial septal defect (Fig. 13-2).

In our experience it is more difficult to identify an isolated, small ventricular septal defect (VSD) with contrast 2-D echo than to identify an atrial septal defect. Since a small VSD (less than 3 mm in diameter) may be impossible to identify, it is particularly important to image the ventricular septum in the appropriate views in an effort to show the microbubbles traversing through the defect itself. Isolated VSDs are found in three general anatomic areas: supracristal or subpulmonic, membranous or subaortic, and muscular. Imaging techniques for these zones of the ventricular septum include:

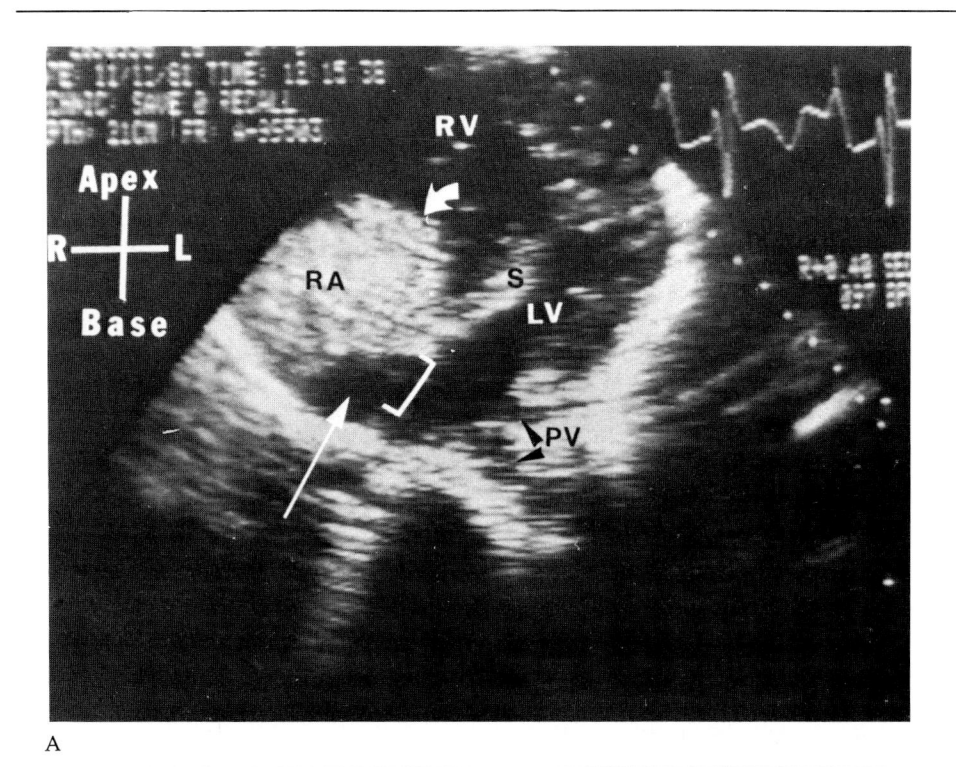

Fig. 13-2A. Apical 4-chamber view of contrast echo study showing negative contrast effect (long white arrow) *due to atrial septal defect* (bracket). *This photograph was taken during systole and shows the tricuspid valve closed* (curved arrow) *with no microbubbles in the right ventricle and no right-to-left shunting into the left atrium having yet occurred. Both RA and RV are very large; the interventricular septum is displaced leftward and posterior due to the marked RV hypertrophy. B. Apical 4-chamber view in same patient showing right-to-left shunting through a large atrial septal defect* (curved dotted arrows) *just beginning as the tricuspid valve is opening marking onset of diastole and contrast echo filling of the right ventricle. Calibration dots are 1 cm apart. PV = pulmonary veins.*

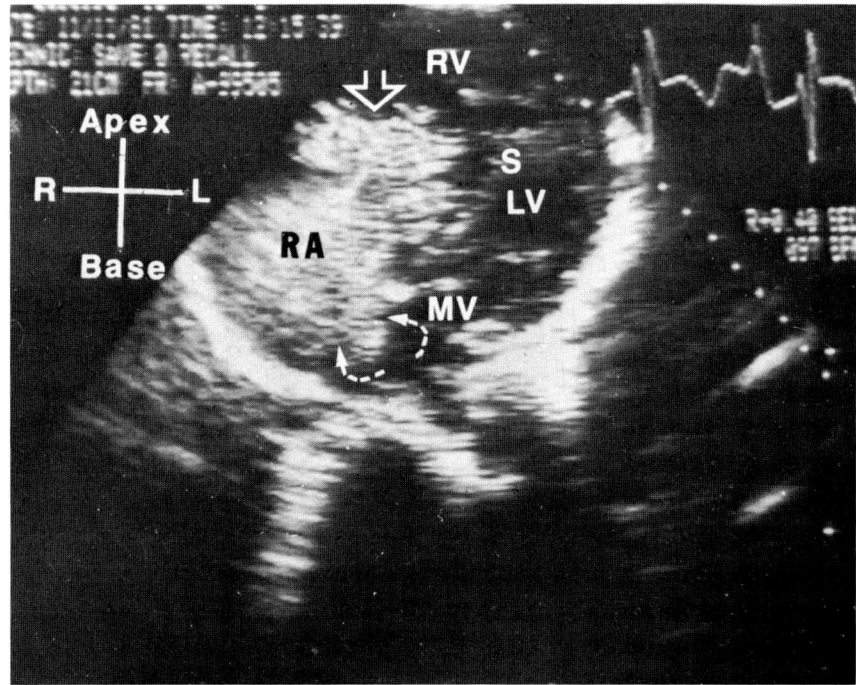

1. Subpulmonic—parasternal long axis with rotation into the right ventricular outflow view; subcostal short axis with rotation into the right ventricular outflow tract
2. Subaortic—parasternal long axis with rotation into the right ventricular inflow tract view; subcostal four-chamber showing aortic valve and tricuspid valve
3. Muscular–apical four-chamber and subcostal four-chamber views without evidence of aortic valve in either plane

Additional discussion of this topic is included in Chapter 15.

Kronik and colleagues [15] found that positive contrast echo results can be enhanced by the Valsalva maneuver in patients with atrial septal defect. These authors observed that during the Valsalva maneuver, contrast shunting was less obvious in only two patients, unchanged in three, and distinctly increased in six, including three patients in whom no diagnostic contrast shunting had been evident during quiet respiration.

When a patient performs the Valsalva maneuver the left ventricle continues to pump blood into the major arterial circulation; the venous return is significantly impeded during the strain phase by the increased intrathoracic pressure. Upon release the engorged peripheral veins rapidly empty into the right atrium while the left atrium receives little blood from the pulmonary veins. In this situation transient right-to-left shunting may occur during one or two cardiac cycles immediately following relaxation of the Valsalva effort. Although it is clear that such a Valsalva maneuver may increase the yield of positive contrast echo findings in patients with an atrial septal defect and normal pressures in the right heart, it is uncertain how many false positive contrast echo findings might occur in normal individuals who have a "probe-patent" foramen ovale. Schiller [16] has found an incidence of 17 percent positive contrast echo findings among 100 normal subjects undergoing Valsalva maneuver. He recommends that patients accomplish a 50 mm Hg straining effort before relaxation when being evaluated for potential patency of the foramen ovale. This may be a valuable technique in searching for possible paradoxical systemic embolus in the absence of clinical findings of an atrial septal defect.

Utilizing contrast echocardiography for identifying residual postoperative shunts is another valuable clinical application [17, 18]. During the early postoperative period temporary left atrial monitoring catheters can be used to inject green dye and saline to detect any residual left-to-right shunting. Valdez-Cruz and coworkers [17] found that contrast echocardiography identified the presence and level of residual shunting in 15 postoperative patients with confirmation by indicator dye dilution curves. Positive studies on the first day after surgery may represent slight temporary flow through or around the newly implanted patch or shunting across a true residual defect. Follow-up studies may be necessary for differentiation. With adequate two-dimensional echo imaging of the patch and the surrounding suture line, significant versus insignificant residual shunting can usually be identified (Fig. 13-3).

The echocardiographic detection of an enlarged coronary sinus can be helpful in the diagnosis of any congenital anomaly that causes increased coronary sinus blood flow. The most common congenital anomalies of the coronary sinus, persistent drainage from the left superior vena cava into the coronary sinus and total anomalous pulmonary venous connection to the coronary sinus, cause marked enlargement of the coronary sinus that can be detected by echocardiography [7, 19–

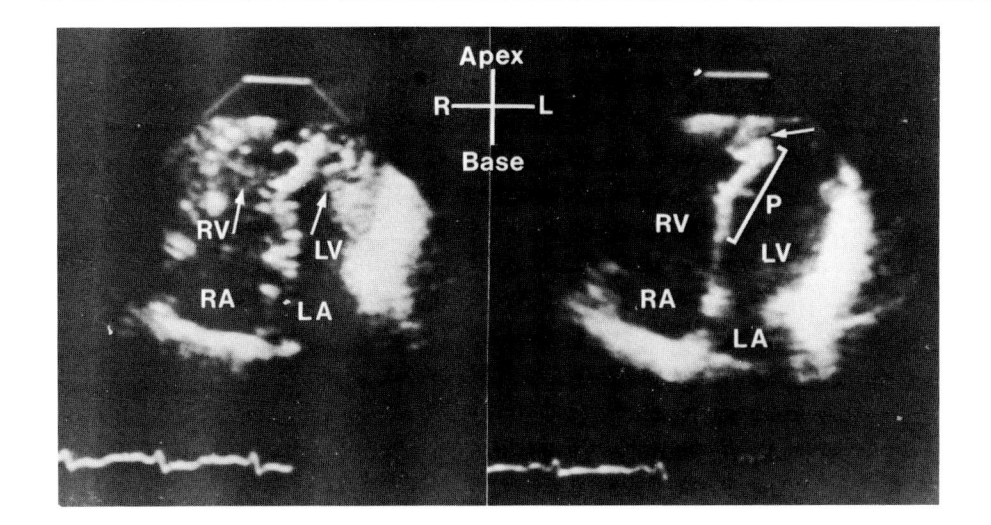

Fig. 13-3. Apical 4-chamber views of an adult male 12 hours after operative patch (P) repair of trauma-induced large ventricular septal defect. Right panel, prior to injection of saline and green dye solution through an indwelling left atrial line, shows slight defect in the septum at the apical margin of the septal patch (arrow). Left panel shows microbubbles passing from the left ventricle through the defect at the distal end of the patch into the right ventricle (arrows), confirming the presence of a residual ventricular septal defect following surgery.

21]. Although it is possible to identify the coronary sinus by M-mode echocardiography with the benefit of contrast techniques, 2-D echo is superior because the spatial anatomic relationship of structures can be identified without contrast injections. The best 2-D echo views to use are parasternal long axis, parasternal right ventricular inflow, and apical four-chamber with posterior angulation (Fig. 13-4).

Two-dimensional echocardiography is a sensitive technique for detecting tricuspid regurgitation by visualizing microbubbles within the inferior vena cava following bolus injection of a liquid in a peripheral arm vein [22, 23]. Although M-mode echocardiography is superior to 2-D echo for critical timing of contrast appearance with the electrocardiogram, the utilization of 2-D imaging is essential for localizing the inferior vena cava and proper positioning of the M-mode cursor. Correlating the appearance of contrast within the inferior vena cava with the ECG serves as the basis for differentiating patients with tricuspid insufficiency (visualization of contrast after the QRS) from those with impaired right ventricular filling or high right atrial pressures (visualization of contrast before the QRS) or arrhythmia [23] (Fig. 13-5).

Contrast echocardiography has been used to explain the hemodynamic significance of early closure of the pulmonic valve in patients with pulmonary hypertension [24]. Meltzer and associates [24] showed that seven patients with pulmonary hypertension all demonstrated low flow velocity or retrograde flow during the second half of systole. They observed that early closure of the pulmonic valve occurred when antegrade flow ceased.

Aneurysms of the interatrial septum may be mistaken for atrial septal defects in the absence of contrast echocardiography to identify or exclude the presence of a shunt (Fig. 13-6).

A variety of experimental substances have been employed to create microbubbles but are not yet available for clinical use [25–27]. One of the more promising substances is gelatin-coated microbubbles that are uniform in diameter, produce contrast effect more consistently, and may be made small enough to pass through the lungs [25]. Pulmonary transmission and myocardial perfusion imaging are not

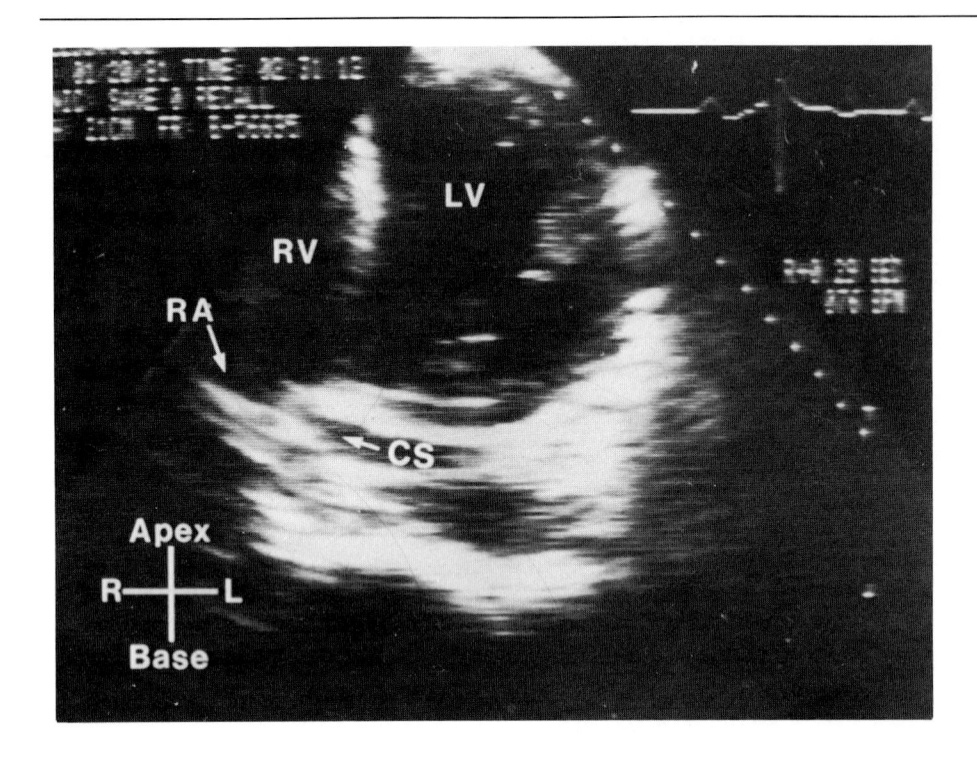

Fig. 13-4. Apical 4-chamber view with posterior angulation of the transducer to demonstrate the coronary sinus emptying into right atrium. Calibration dots are 1 cm apart.

available with standard contrast injections because high surface tension in blood causes a rapid collapse of the small (10 micron) microbubbles necessary for capillary transmission [26]. Bommer and colleagues [26] reported that various surfactants (such as lecithin and glycerin) stabilized these small microbubbles long enough to achieve pulmonary transmission and provide left heart and myocardial contrast images. The availability and convenience of such biocompatible surfactants offer promise in extending the usefulness of standard echo-contrast studies.

Meltzer and coworkers [28] have demonstrated that intravenous carbon dioxide can be used safely in patients as an echo contrast agent. These investigators employed 1 to 3 cc of medically pure CO_2 agitated with 5 to 8 ml of 5% dextrose in water and rapidly injected into an arm vein. They observed good contrast effect in all patients. To date carbon dioxide has not had significant clinical application in this country.

Although microbubbles produced by any clinically acceptable fluid are normally filtered by the pulmonary capillaries, injections made through an inflated balloon catheter in the wedge position may produce contrast effect in the left side of the heart [29]. Additional experience is needed to determine what risk, if any, is associated with this technique.

Shiina and associates [30] have used contrast echocardiography to estimate changes in flow velocity in the right side of the heart. Flow velocity at the tricuspid and pulmonic valve orifices was measured by means of an electromagnetic flow-velocity probe and simultaneous recording of the contrast echocardiogram. The investigators found the contrast flow velocity at the tricuspid valve orifice in 12 normal subjects to be 345 ± 30 mm/sec. The contrast flow velocity increased with inspiration and a 10 percent increase in heart rate resulted in a 45 percent average increase in contrast flow velocity.

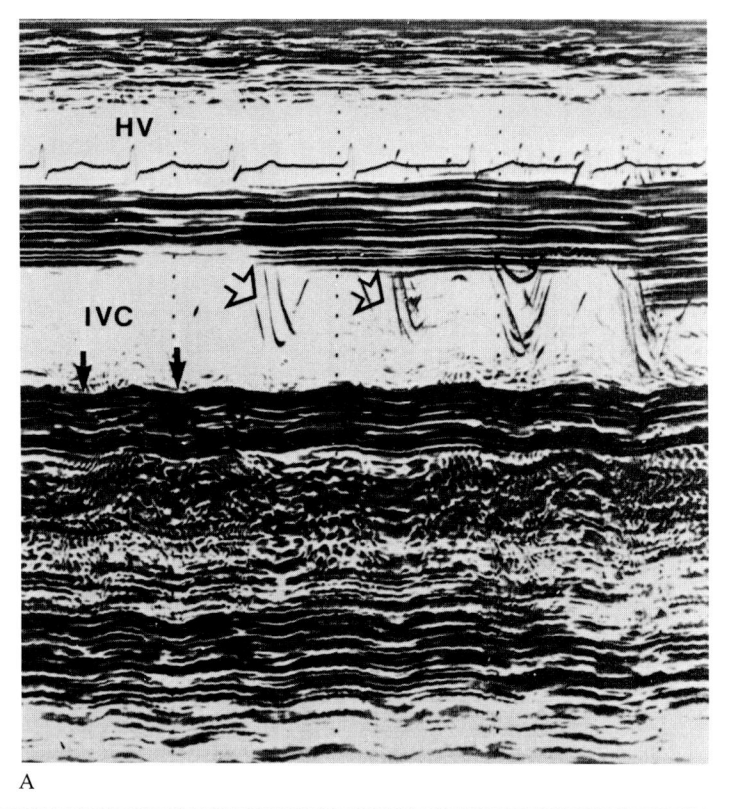

Fig. 13-5A. M-mode recording from subcostal position showing dilated hepatic vein (HV) and IVC; contrast echo injection demonstrates systolic reflux (open arrows) confirming the presence of tricuspid regurgitation. The solid arrows are pointing to V waves of the IVC. B. M-mode contrast echocardiogram of the IVC showing diastolic reflux following atrial contraction due to constrictive pericarditis. This should not be confused with systolic reflux due to tricuspid regurgitation. HV = hepatic vein. (From NK Wise et al, Contrast M-mode ultrasonography of the inferior vena cava. Circulation 63:1100, 1981, by permission of the American Heart Association, Inc.)

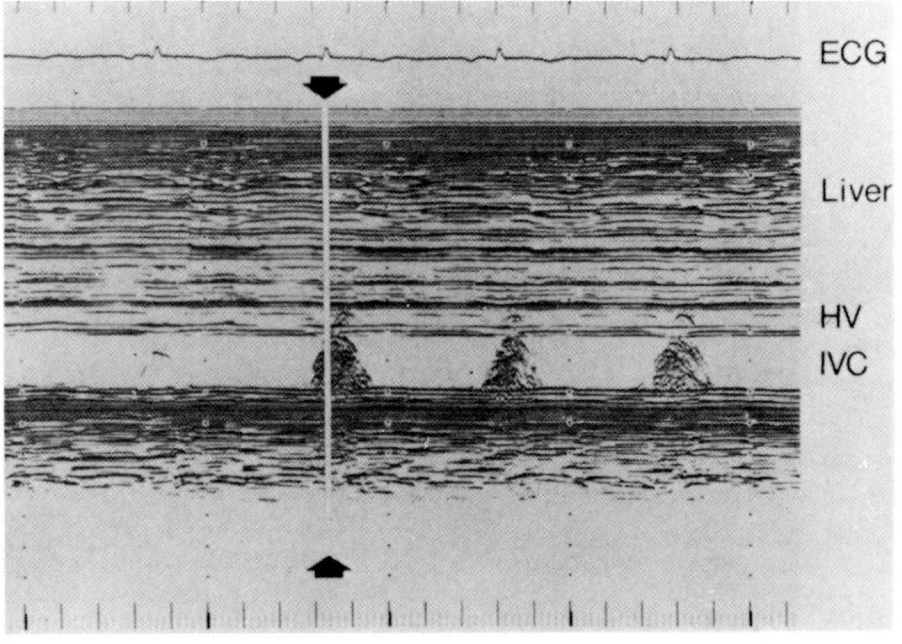

428   13. Interventional echocardiography

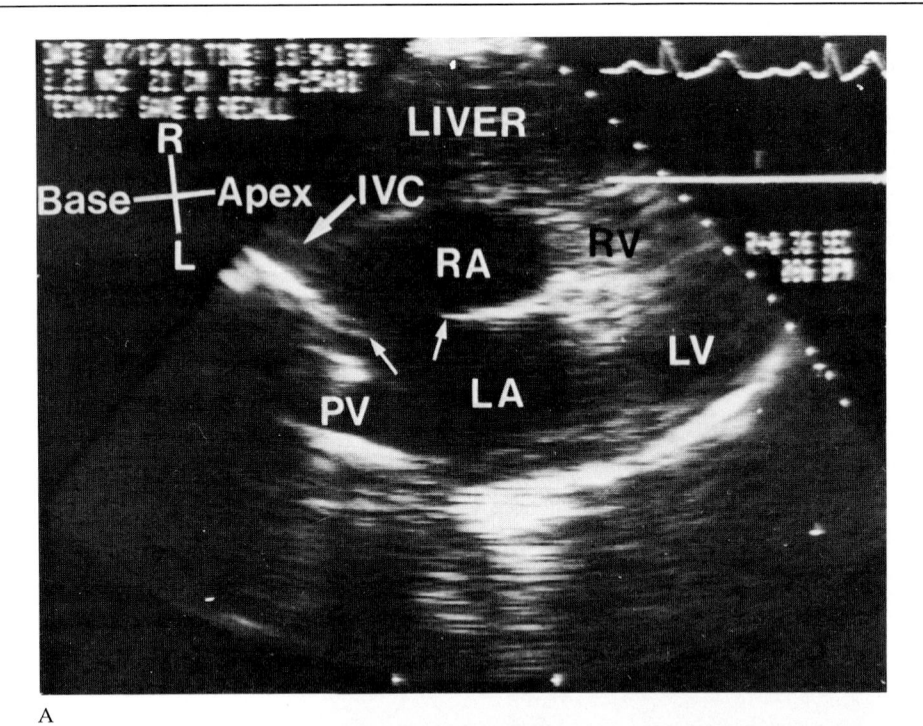

Fig. 13-6A. Subcostal 4-chamber view of an adult patient with a secundum atrial septal defect (arrows). B. Subcostal 4-chamber views of a patient with a large left atrium, thin wall in region of fossa ovalis (solid arrow, upper panel), and apparent atrial septal defect (open arrow, upper panel). Contrast echo study demonstrates an aneurysmal bulge of the interatrial septum (arrows) but no evidence of either atrial septal defect or patent fossa ovalis (lower panel). C. M-mode recording taken at same time as 2-D echo view shown in lower panel of B demonstrates a small RA and large LA without evidence of any shunt. The calibration dots are 1 cm apart. PV = pulmonary vein.

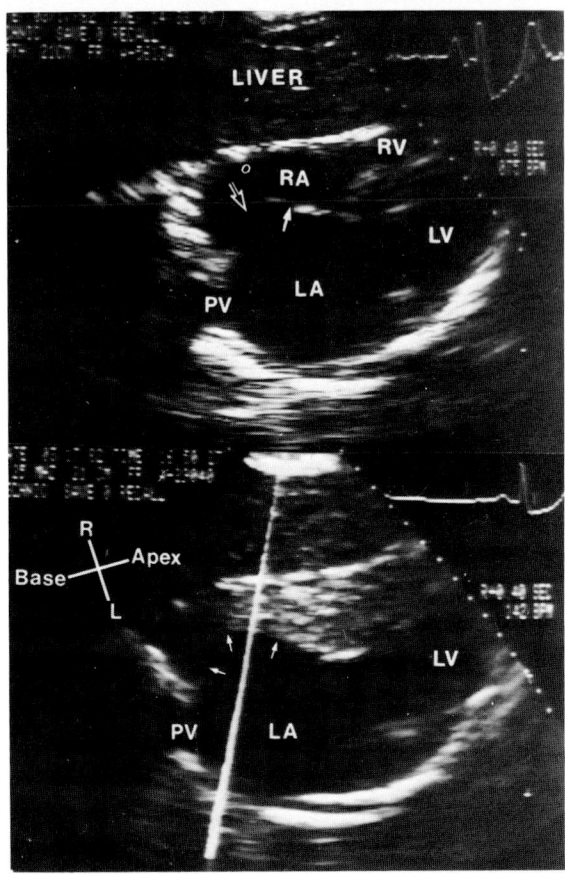

C

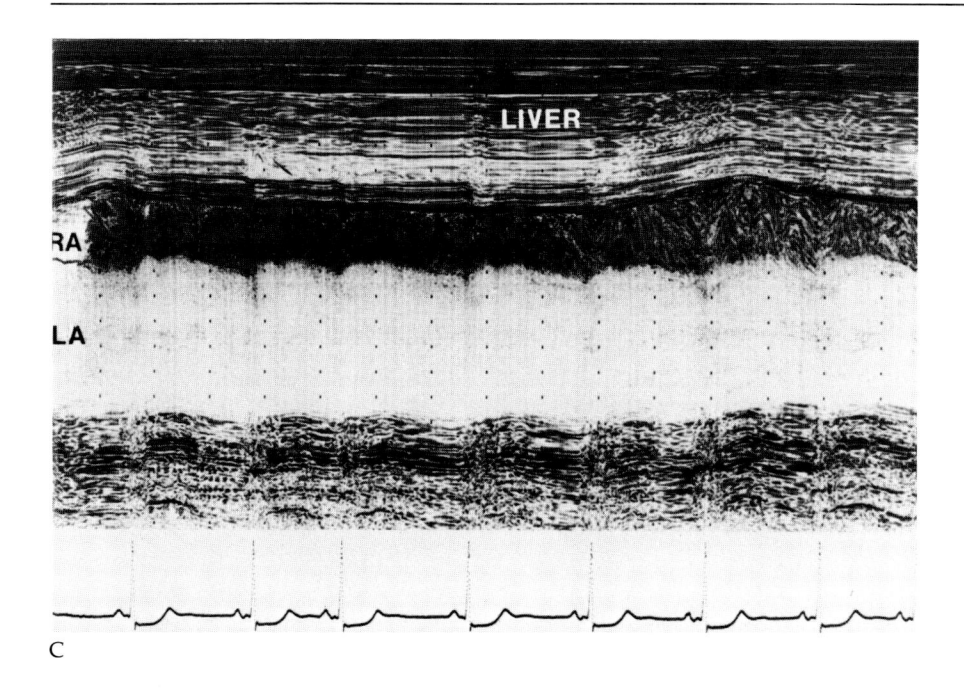

Pharmacologic and physiologic maneuvers. Echocardiography has the capability to measure the effects of physiologic interventions and drug-induced changes in heart size and left ventricular function. Although M-mode echocardiography has been utilized for many years as a potentially valuable noninvasive tool to monitor acute and chronic effects from cardiovascular drugs [31–39], it has had limited clinical application because of its inherent limitations in measuring global changes in a diseased left ventricle. The addition of two-dimensional echo has improved the echocardiographer's ability to assess the effects of cardiovascular drugs; this subject is discussed in more detail in Chapter 7.

The only drug we utilize in our laboratories as a diagnostic intervention for routine clinical purposes is inhaled amyl nitrite. Although it is administered infrequently, the two indications for its use are inducing mitral valve prolapse [40] and provoking systolic anterior motion of the mitral valve-chordal apparatus in patients with suspected hypertrophic cardiomyopathy. If physical findings and resting M-mode plus 2-D echo information are nondiagnostic in either of these two clinical conditions, and if inhalation of amyl nitrite is warranted in the overall clinical assessment of a given patient, administration is indicated in an attempt to induce an abnormality that is not present in the resting state (Fig. 13-7). The effects of amyl nitrite include drop in blood pressure, peripheral vasodilatation, transient decrease in venous return to the heart, and secondary tachycardia.

Patients must be carefully instructed regarding the transient symptoms they will experience, including pounding heart, lightheadedness, and sometimes a nervous, apprehensive feeling; they must remain supine until all symptoms abate and heart rate and blood pressure return to normal. After the patient is properly positioned to optimally image the anatomy and motion in question and baseline record-

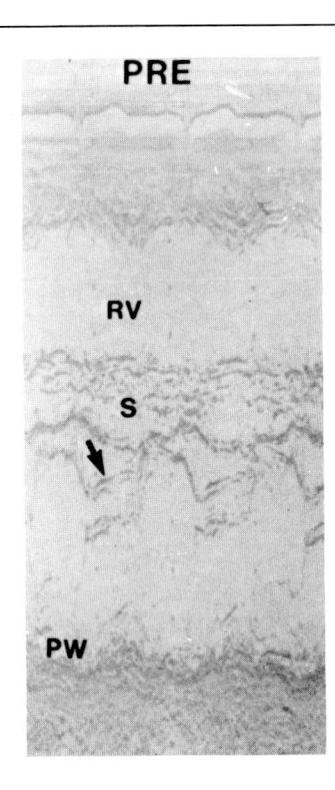

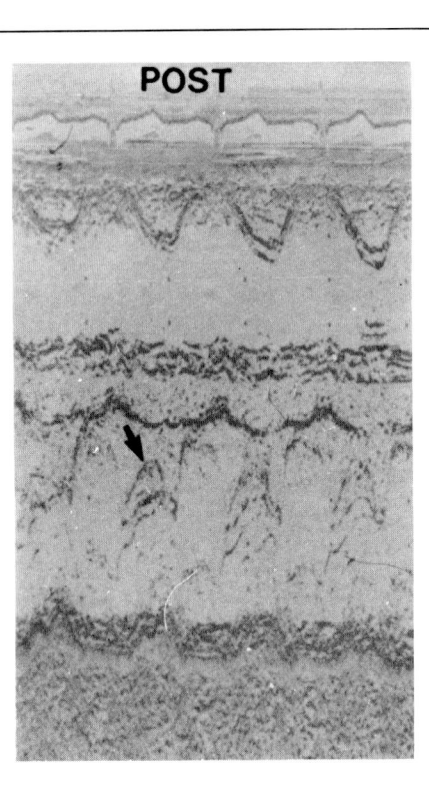

Fig. 13-7. Resting M-mode recording of a patient with hypertrophic cardiomyopathy but no systolic anterior motion (SAM) (arrow, left panel). Following amyl nitrite inhalation SAM developed (arrow, right panel).

ings (M-mode and 2-D) are obtained, an assistant breaks the ampul within a 4 × 4 gauze sponge close to the patient's nose, and the patient takes three deep breaths. The ampul is then quickly removed from the laboratory and deposited in water to minimize side effects on laboratory personnel. The echocardiographer should expect to observe an increase of 25 to 40 beats/min in the patient's heart rate if adequate inhalation and effect has occurred. The effect is very brief; the patient can expect to feel normal within five minutes.

Postural changes are useful tests for evaluation of systolic clicks and cardiac murmurs. Standing and squatting are widely used at the bedside during the examination of cardiac patients; however, because of technical difficulties such maneuvers are usually not performed during the course of the echocardiographic examination. Lewis and colleagues [41] have evaluated the effects of standing and Ssquatting on echocardiographic left ventricular function. As expected, these investigators found the ventricular end-diastolic diameter decreased by 13 ± 5 percent on changing from the supine to the standing position. Squatting was accompanied by an increase in left ventricular cavity dimension, while heart rate fell slightly and cardiac index increased. There was no significant change in global function (percent fractional shortening or mean Vcf with either standing or squatting.

The Valsalva maneuver, raising intrathoracic pressure against a closed glottis (forced expiration), and the Müller maneuver, reducing intrathoracic pressure behind a closed glottis (forced inspiration), are frequently used to evaluate cardiac murmurs, cardiovascular hemodynamics, and autonomic nervous system function [42, 43] (Fig. 13-8). Both produce significant hemodynamic changes that result in

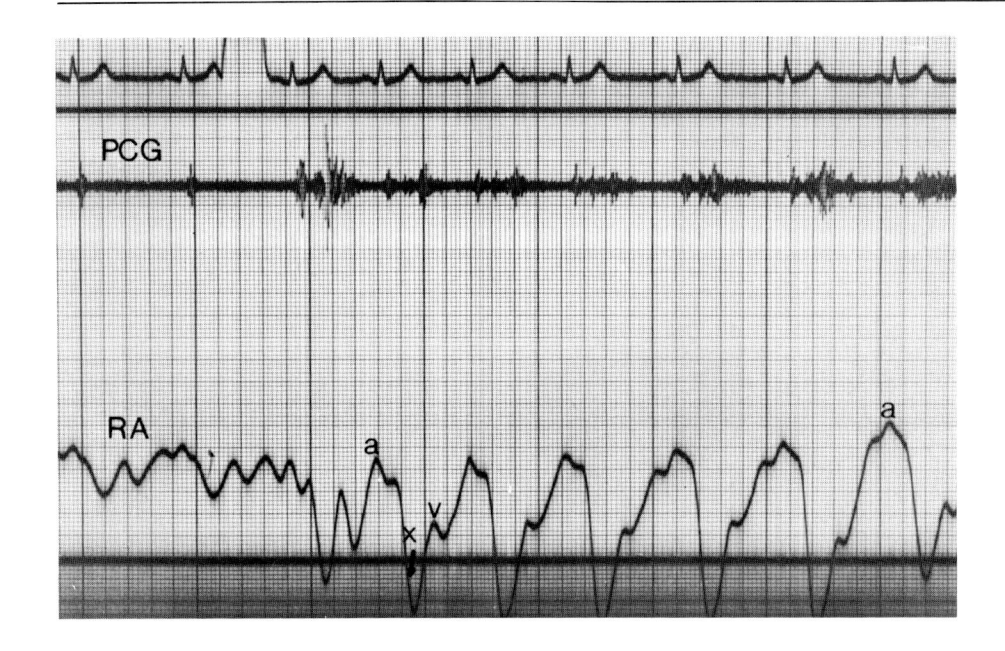

Fig. 13-8. Pressure recording of the right atrium at rest and no murmur on phonocardiogram (PCG) until onset of Müller maneuver, which causes a systolic murmur of tricuspid regurgitation as well as more prominent "A" waves and X descents.

widespread alterations in the central and peripheral circulation. The Valsalva maneuver is best understood in terms of its four phases [44]:

1. At onset of the maneuver, when intrathoracic and abdominal pressure rise suddenly, there is a corresponding transient increase in systemic blood pressure.
2. A fall in blood pressure and pulse pressure occurs accompanied by a reflux tachycardia.
3. On release of the raised intrathoracic pressure, systemic blood pressure falls.
4. A few seconds later increased venous return causes pulse pressure and mean blood pressure to rise to greater than control levels.

After seven seconds of the Valsalva maneuver at 40 mm Hg, the pulse pressure may be reduced 80 percent and 1500 ml of blood may pool into the periphery [42]. Angiographically estimated left ventricular size and stroke volume may decrease to 50 percent of control levels [45]. Robertson and colleagues [44] observed in 12 normal subjects that left ventricular end-diastolic dimension decreased 11.2 ± 1.5 percent, end-systolic dimension decreased 9.5 ± 1.3 percent, and stroke volume fell by 29 percent. The left atrial dimension decreased 30 percent in the normal subjects during Valsalva maneuver. These investigators noted that physiologic changes caused by the Valsalva maneuver were blunted or absent in patients with congestive heart failure and observed a diminished response related to the severity of the heart failure. Patients in New York Heart Association classes III and IV decreased left atrial dimension by only 3.8 percent with Valsalva maneuver, whereas patients in classes I and II had essentially normal responses.

Parisi and associates [46] also found that patients in heart failure did not diminish their left ventricular dimensions during Valsalva strain, and the same patients demonstrated a "square wave" in the arterial pressure elevation during strain without a overshoot in recovery. Patients with severely depressed ejection frac-

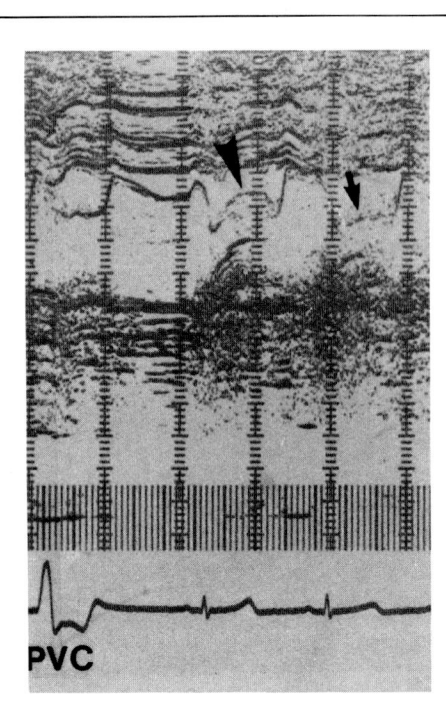

Fig. 13-9. M-mode recording of a patient with hypertrophic cardiomyopathy demonstrating normal aortic valve and mitral valve motion at rest. Following a premature ventricular contraction (PVC) mid-systolic closure of the aortic valve (large arrow, left panel) and systolic anterior motion (large arrow, right panel) of the mitral valve occur. This patient demonstrated no evidence of resting outflow obstruction except in the post-PVC beats.

tions, unlike those with normal ventricular function, are unable to alter stroke output in response to acutely increased intrathoracic pressure.

The augmentation of myocardial contractility that occurs in the normally conducted beat following a premature ventricular beat is referred to as post-extrasystolic potentiation (PESP). Cohn and colleagues [47] and Angoff and coworkers [48] have devised an external mechanical cardiac stimulator to induce ventricular premature contractions to evaluate the effect of PESP on ventricular function by echocardiography. The effect of PESP on ventricular contraction has demonstrated that areas of ventricular wall that exhibit absent or diminished motion during regular cardiac cycles often exhibit augmented contraction during the post-extrasystolic beat. In patients with coronary artery disease the degree of regional and global improvement of left ventricular function with PESP has proved useful in predicting: which areas of myocardium supplied by stenosed coronary arteries are reversibly rather than irreversibly damaged, hence suitable for myocardial revascularization [49, 50]; and which patients with depressed ventricular function have the greatest amount of contractile reserve, and thus are more likely to tolerate myocardial revascularization [51, 52]. Angoff and colleagues [48], in a study of 15 patients with idiopathic hypertrophic subaortic stenosis, after noninvasive induction of a ventricular extrasystole were able to show obstruction in the beat after the extrasystole in nine patients (Fig. 13-9).

Exercise echocardiography. There have been many studies in recent years to evaluate the clinical role of different methods of performing exercise echocardiography [53–63]. An advantage of echocardiography is its capability to measure left ventricular dimensions and function parameters intermittently or continuously before, during, and after an intervention without risk or discomfort to the patient and without affecting the normal response to the test conditions (see Chap. 6).

In evaluating handgrip and supine and upright bicycle exercise in normal subjects, Crawford and associates [56] concluded that: (1) end-diastolic left ventricular size is maintained during isometric exercise and moderate dynamic exercise, even in the upright position; (2) isometric exercise leads to a mild decrease in left ventricular shortening, whereas dynamic exercise results in marked increases in shortening (this difference may be related to the relatively greater increase in blood pressure than in heart rate during isometric exercise); and (3) M-mode echocardiography can be successfully accomplished in selected subjects during various forms of exercise.

Sugishita and Koseki [55] studied 46 healthy subjects and 47 cardiac patients with supine bicycle exercise with a special table upon which the subjects could be firmly attached at shoulder level to prevent bodily movements and minimize the disturbance of the echocardiographic recordings. In 83 percent of the subjects in whom a clear echocardiogram was obtained at rest, an adequate echocardiogram was also obtained during dynamic exercise. They found that changes in the mean velocity of left ventricular circumferential shortening during exercise differed in older and younger healthy men, and also in healthy subjects and those with left ventricular dysfunction.

Paulsen and coworkers [58] studied 20 normal subjects utilizing supine isometric handgrip and graded isotonic bicycle ergometer exercise. They observed that at the completion of isometric exercise there was no significant change in percentage of fractional shortening, while there was a small decrease in peak velocity of circumferential fiber shortening (peak Vcf); in contrast, isotonic exercise resulted in a significant increase in percent fractional shortening and peak Vcf. They concluded that isotonic exercise produces a much greater stimulus to left ventricular contractility than isometric exercise and is expected to provide a useful means of detecting latent left ventricular dysfunction by echocardiography.

Although it is feasible to detect wall motion abnormalities with M-mode echocardiography during exercise-induced ischemia, this method is fundamentally inadequate since the entire left ventricle must be evaluated when there is a question about the possibility of coronary artery disease. For that reason exercise stress tests for electrocardiographic and radionuclide assessment of coronary artery disease are still considered superior diagnostic tools compared to exercise echocardiography.

Although the technical quality of some of the early exercise 2-D echo studies was generally poor, recent improvements in 2-D echo equipment with better imaging ability of the left ventricle suggest that exercise 2-D echocardiography will have greater clinical application in the future [62, 63]. Some of this improvement in the clinical value of exercise 2-D echocardiography may occur as a result of new devices that stabilize the echo transducer on the chest during motion [61].

Gondi and Nanda [64] performed a cold pressor test by immersing the patient's right hand in ice water for 2 to 5 minutes during two-dimensional echocardiography in 14 patients. They found in 8 of 11 patients (72%) with coronary artery disease that the cold pressor test induced left ventricular wall motion abnormalities (dyskinesia in one, akinesia in two, and hypokinesia in five patients). These abnormal wall motions reverted to normal after the cold pressor test was stopped. The investigators found that the ejection fraction decreased during the cold pressor test by 8 to 37 percent (mean 20%) in all patients with coronary artery disease. This new technique may prove to be useful in identifying coronary artery disease patients with normal resting left ventricular wall motion.

Echophonocardiography. The combination of phonocardiograms together with echocardiograms provides valuable information for a better understanding of cardiac sounds and murmurs [65–73]. Millward and associates [65], by utilizing echophonocardiography, demonstrated the existence of a mitral valve opening snap in the following conditions: tricuspid atresia with a large atrial septal defect; idiopathic second- and third-degree heart block; ventricular septal defect; mitral regurgitation; thyrotoxicosis; and tetralogy of Fallot occurring after a Blalock-Taussig procedure. None of these patients had mitral stenosis; the sound coincided with the point of maximal opening (E point) of the anterior mitral leaflet and preceded the expected timing of a third heart sound which occurs with the rapid filling phase of the ventricle (Fig. 13-10).

Mills and coworkers [69] have shown that the two high-frequency components of S_1 are related to closure of the mitral and tricuspid valves. The same authors [70] have also shown that ejection sounds associated with semilunar valve stenosis or hypertension of the systemic or pulmonary circulation occur at the moment of complete opening of the aortic or pulmonic valve recorded echocardiographically. The ejection sound in the presence of stenotic valves occurs with checking of the opening motion of the thickened valve cusps. Although the hypertensive ejection sound also occurs at the precise moment of full opening of the valve, it is uncertain whether this relationship is causal or coincidental [70].

Echophonocardiography has proved useful in identifying the site of origin of systolic honks and musical murmurs [71–73]. In addition to the clinical value of the phonocardiogram in the assessment of other valvular abnormalities, it is particularly useful for the serial follow-up of valvular prostheses.

The performance of echophonocardiograms requires both clinical and technical skills. Simultaneous recording of ECG and phonocardiogram is essential, and concurrent pulse tracings are also helpful. Generally phonocardiograms are recorded from two locations simultaneously, such as the second left interspace and apex, in order to demonstrate transmission or lack of transmission of sounds and murmurs over the precordium. Mills and Craige [74] recommend a microphone that can be attached to the chest wall by a suction device and minimizing movement artifacts.

Esophageal echocardiography. Esophageal echocardiography has been developed for use in patients who are technically difficult to image from the chest wall or for continuous intraoperative monitoring of left ventricular performance [75, 76]. Measurements of left ventricular diameters with transesophageal technique correlate excellently with the corresponding measurements obtained with the standard parasternal method [76]. Matsumoto and associates [76] observed that pericardial and chest wall closures generally caused a significant decrease in cardiac output, and correlated with a decrease in diastolic diameter and an increase in the stiffness constant of the left ventricle. Thus the decrease in cardiac output may have been due to decreased distensibility of the ventricular cavity secondary to mechanical

435

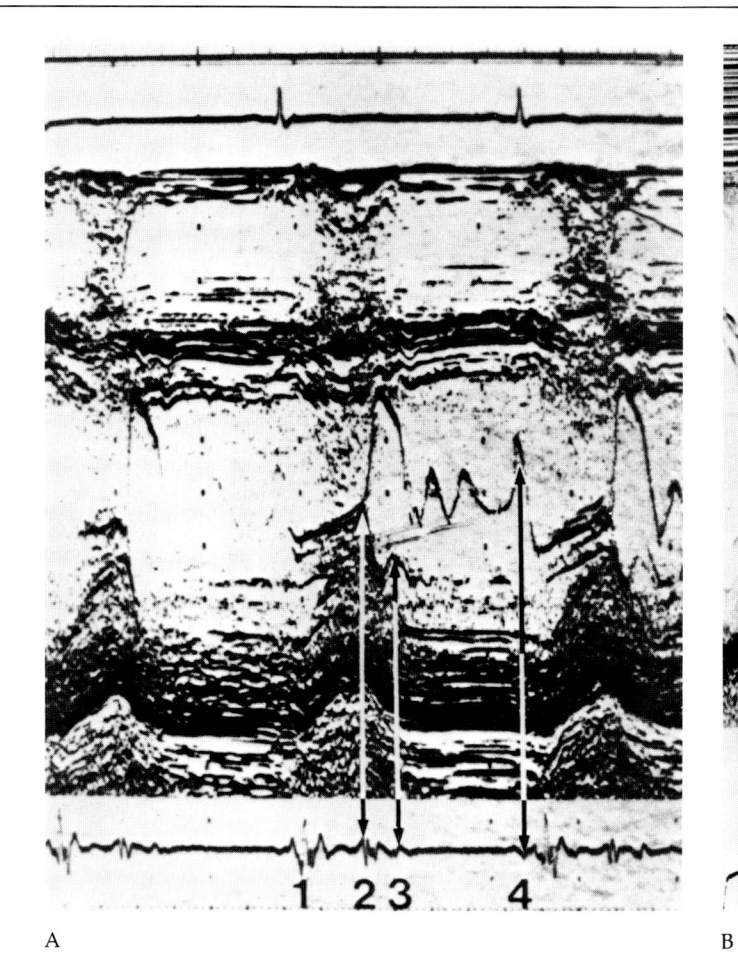

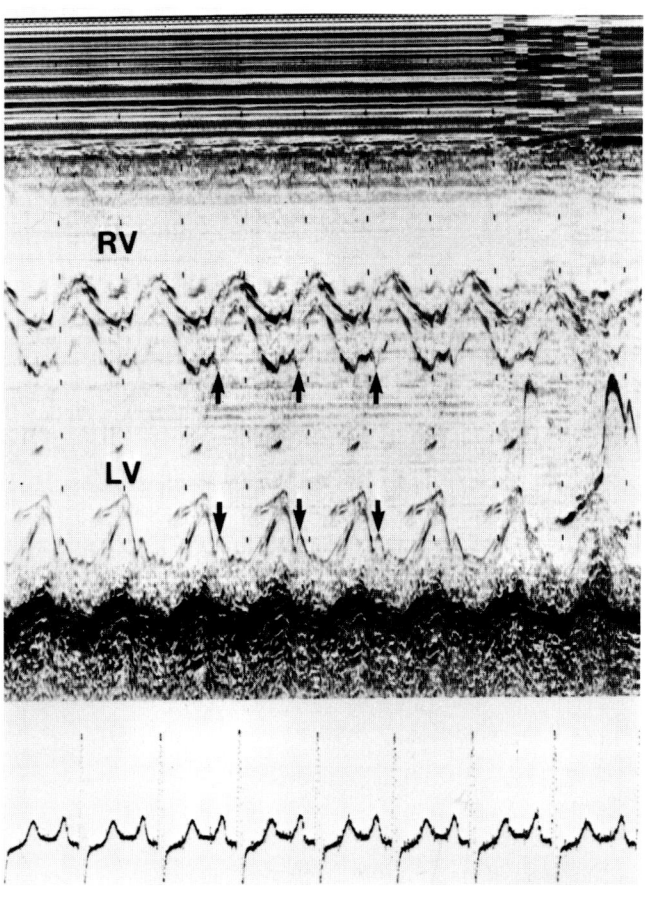

Fig. 13-10A. M-mode recording of a normal young male showing the timing relationship of the heart sounds (1, 2, 3, 4) on phonocardiogram with left ventricular and mitral valve motion. B. M-mode recording of a normal young female demonstrating prominent notches of septum and posterior wall of the left ventricle in the precise timing of the third heart sound, which was quite loud on auscultation. Although not seen commonly, this type of "rebound" motion following rapid filling appears to be a normal finding and related to a very compliant LV.

436   13. Interventional echocardiography

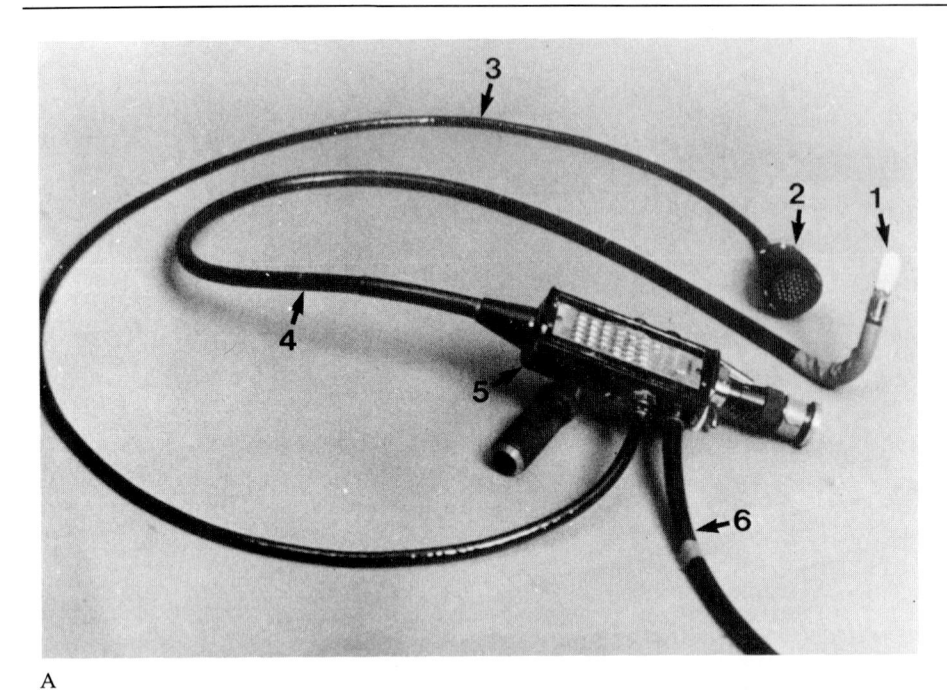

Fig. 13-11A. Esophageal transducer. 1 = 3.5 MHz phased array transducer; 2 = transducer connector; 3 = transducer cable; 4 = endoscope; 5 = control unit of endoscope; 6 = power supply of endoscope. (Prototype "Echoscope" from Diasonics Cardio/Imaging, Inc, Salt Lake City.) B. Close-up photograph of 3.5 MHz esophageal transducer tip. (Courtesy of Diasonics Cardio/Imaging, Inc, Salt Lake City.)

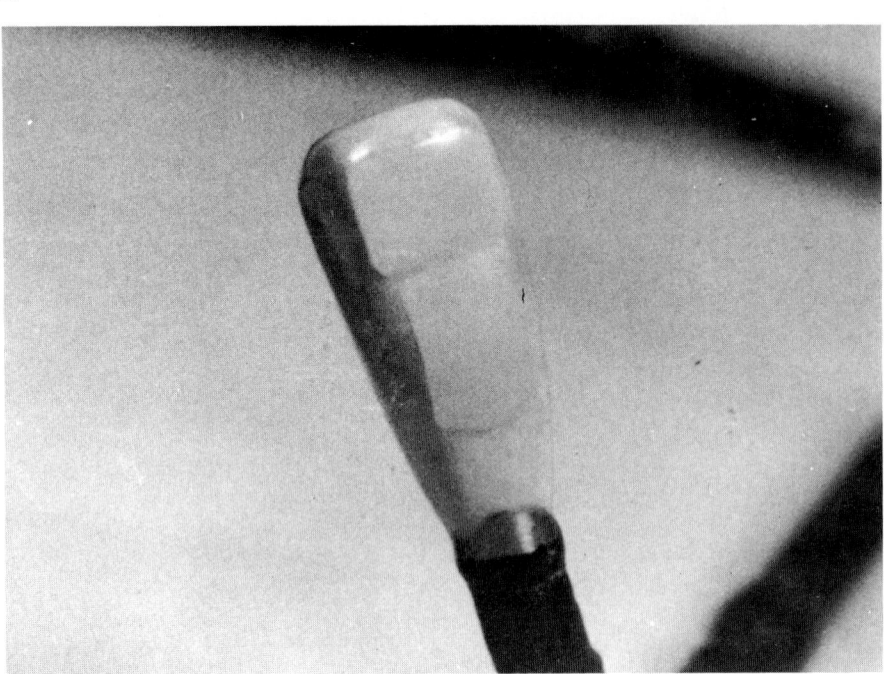

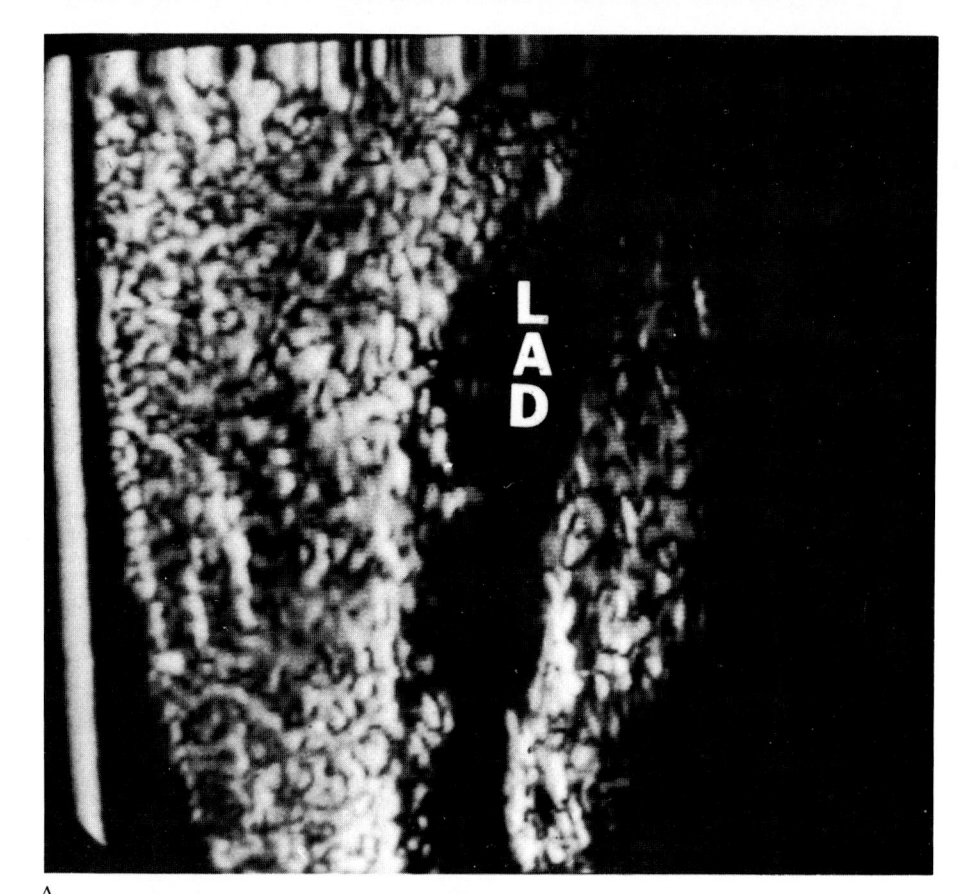

Fig. 13-12A. View of left anterior descending (LAD) coronary artery obtained with a 9 MHz vascular scanning probe applied directly to the epicardial surface by the surgeon at the time of open heart surgery. Mild endothelial irregularities due to plaque formation of atherosclerotic disease can be seen. B. Normal left anterior descending coronary artery obtained with a 12 MHz probe applied to the epicardial surface at the time of open heart surgery. (A and B courtesy of David J. Sahn, M.D.)

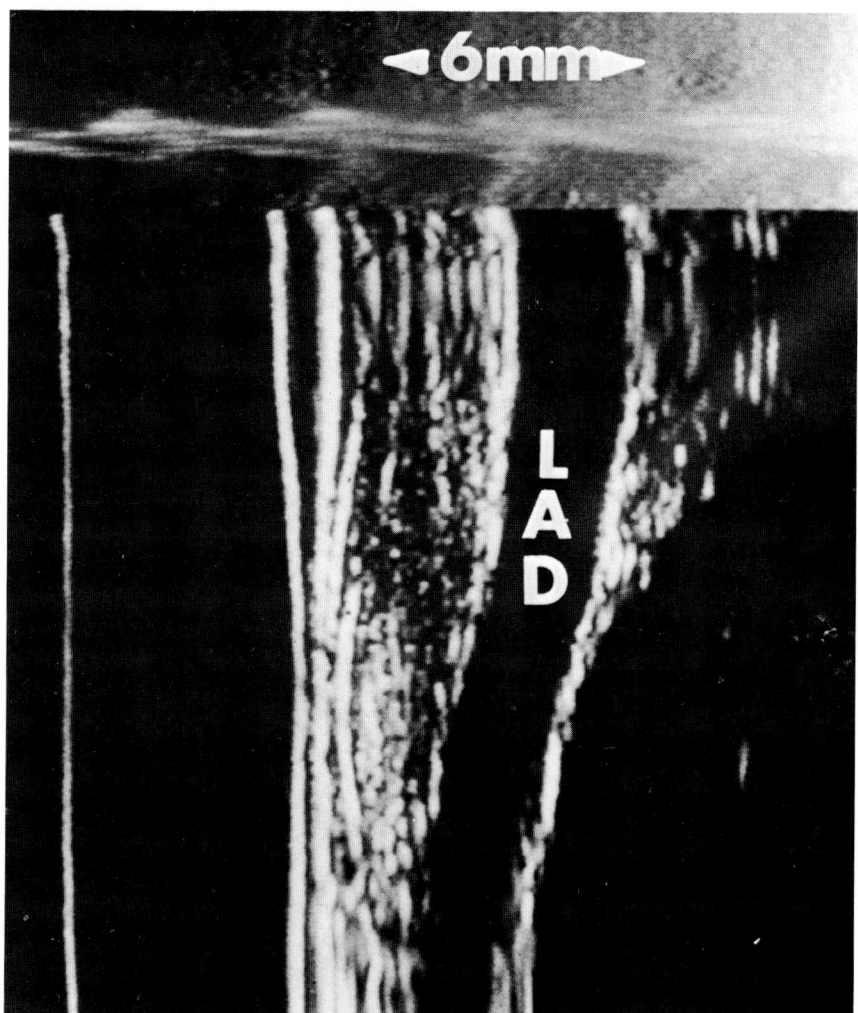

restriction by the pericardium and chest wall. They also noted that pericardial opening caused a significant delay in septal motion that was reversed by closing the pericardium.

Hisanaga and colleagues [77] have developed a transesophageal ultrasonic high-speed rotating scanner that rotates a single small transducer through a full 360 degrees in the esophagus. Before examination each patient received 0.5 mg atropine sulfate and 10 mg diazepam intramuscularly and 3 gm lidocaine jelly orally. The patient's throat was sprayed with 4% lidocaine liquid. Subjects usually swallowed the transducer in oil bag as easily as they would a commercially available gastrofiberscope. Although transesophageal cross-sectional echocardiography is largely investigational, there may be important areas of clinical application of this technique in the future, such as continuous monitoring during surgery or treatment interventions in acute care units (Fig. 13-11).

Intraoperative echocardiography. One of the promising new areas of future clinical application is intraoperative echocardiography [78–81]. Spotnitz [80] utilized a gas-sterilized phased-array transducer applied directly to the anterior surface of the heart and obtained high-quality images for qualitative and quantitative studies during cardiac operations in 74 patients. The techniques employed were successful in demonstrating alterations in cardiac anatomy associated with valve disease and cardiac tumors. Spotnitz also demonstrated continuous clouds of microbubbles ejected from the left ventricle immediately following cardiopulmonary bypass in 42 percent of 45 patients studied.

Reichek and coworkers [79] used a 7.5 MHz sterile fingertip transducer to perform epicardial echocardiographic mapping prebypass in 17 subjects with two- or three-vessel disease and in nine postbypass patients. Echo images were obtained in up to 54 sites on right and left ventricles. Unsuspected right ventricular dysfunction was found in six subjects. Postbypass maps showed improvement in akinetic and hypokinetic segments in six, worsening of prebypass hypokinesis in two, and a new segmental abnormality in one. These investigators also found that preoperative ventriculographic findings do not correlate well with intraoperative segmental myocardial performance.

Sahn and associates [81, 82] have used a 9 MHz high-resolution ultrasonic scanner for intraoperative verification and localization of coronary atherosclerotic lesions in patients undergoing bypass graft surgery. They found the correlation between angiographic and ultrasonic severity of obstruction was excellent, but the severity of mild atherosclerotic lesions was usually overestimated by echocardiography and endothelial irregularities had a more striking appearance on echo than on angiography (Fig. 13-12).

References

1. Gramiak R, Shah PM, Kramer DH: Ultrasound cardiography: Contrast studies in anatomy and function. *Radiology* 92:939, 1969.
2. Kerber RE, Kioschos JM, Lauer RM: Use of an ultrasonic contrast method in the diagnosis of valvular regurgitation and intracardiac shunts. *Am J Cardiol* 34:722, 1974
3. Seward JB, Tajik AJ, Spangler JG, Ritter DG: Echocardiographic contrast studies: Initial experience. *Mayo Clin Proc* 50:163, 1975
4. Seward JB, Tajik AJ, Hagler DJ, Ritter DG: Peripheral venous contrast echocardiography. *Am J Cardiol* 39:202, 1977
5. Weyman AE, Wann LS, Caldwell RL, Hurwitz RA, Dillon JC, Feigenbaum H: Negative contrast echocardiography: A new method for detecting left-to-right shunts. *Circulation* 59:498, 1979
6. Serwer GA, Armstrong BE, Anderson PAW, Sherman D, Benson DW Jr, Edwards SB: Use of contrast echocardiography for evaluation of right ventricular hemodynamics in the presence of ventricular septal defects. *Circulation* 58:327, 1978
7. Snider AR, Ports TA, Silverman NH: Venous anomalies of the coronary sinus: Detection by M-mode, two-dimensional and contrast echocardiography. *Circulation* 60:721, 1979
8. Fraker TD Jr, Harris PJ, Behar VS, Kisslo JA: Detection and exclusion of interatrial shunts by two-dimensional echocardiography and peripheral venous injection. *Circulation* 59:379, 1979
9. Danilowicz D, Kronzon I: Use of contrast echocardiography in the diagnosis of partial anomalous pulmonary venous connection. *Am J Cardiol* 43:248, 1979
10. Sahn DJ, Allen HD, George W, Mason M, Goldberg SJ: The utility of contrast echocardiographic techniques in the care of critically ill infants with cardiac and pulmonary diseases. *Circulation* 56:959, 1977
11. Shub C, Tajik AJ, Seward JB, Dines DE: Detecting intrapulmonary right-to-left shunt with contrast echocardiography: Observations in a patient with diffuse pulmonary arteriovenous fistulas. *Mayo Clin Proc* 51:81, 1976
12. Lieppe W, Scallion R, Behar VS, Kisslo JA: Two-dimensional echocardiographic findings in atrial septal defect. *Circulation* 56:447, 1977
13. Funabashi T, Yoshida H, Nakaya S, Maeda T, Taniguchi N: Echocardiographic visualization of ventricular septal defect in infants and assessment of hemodynamic status using a contrast technique: Comparison of M-mode and two-dimensional imaging. *Circulation* 64:1025, 1981
14. Gilbert BW, Drobac M, Rakowski H: Contrast two-dimensional echocardiography in inter-atrial shunts. *Am J Cardiol* 45:402, 1980 (Abstract)
15. Kronik G, Slany J, Moesslacher H: Contrast M-mode echocardiography in diagnosis of atrial septal defect in acyanotic patients. *Circulation* 59:372, 1979
16. Schiller NB: Personal communication, 1982
17. Valdez-Cruz LM, Pieroni DR, Roland JMA, Shematek JP: Recognition of residual postoperative shunts by contrast echocardiographic techniques. *Circulation* 55:148, 1977
18. Glover MU, Hagan AD, Evans M, Vieweg WVR: Use of two-dimensional, contrast echocardiography in the early postoperative assessment of septal defect repairs: Case Report. *Milit Med* 147:412, 1982
19. Orsmond GS, Ruttenberg HD, Bessinger FB, Moller JH: Echocardiographic features of total anomalous pulmonary venous connection to the coronary sinus. *Am J Cardiol* 41:597, 1978
20. Aziz KU, Paul MH, Bharati S, Lev M, Shannon K: Echocardiographic features of total anomalous pulmonary venous drainage into the coronary sinus. *Am J Cardiol* 42:108, 1978
21. Stewart JA, Fraker TD Jr, Slosky DA, Wise NK, Kisslo JA: Detection of persistent left superior vena cava by two-dimensional contrast echocardiography. *JCU* 7:357, 1979
22. Lieppe W, Behar VS, Scallion R, Kisslo JA: Detection of tricuspid regurgitation with two-dimensional echocardiography and peripheral vein injections. *Circulation* 57:128, 1978
23. Wise NK, Myers S, Fraker TD, Stewart JA, Kisslo JA: Contrast M-mode ultrasonography of the inferior vena cava. *Circulation* 63:1100, 1981
24. Meltzer RS, Valk NK, Vermeulen HWJ, Pierard LA, ten Cate FJ, Roelandt J: Contrast echocardiography to diagnose pulmonary hypertension and explain the hemodynamic significance of the early closure sign. *Circulation* 64(Suppl IV):IV-47, 1981

25. Bommer WJ, Mason DT, DeMaria AN: Studies in contrast echocardiography: Development of new agents with superior reproducibility and transmission through lungs. *Circulation* 60(Suppl II):II-17, 1979
26. Bommer WJ, Miller L, Takeda P, Mason DT, DeMaria AN: Contrast echocardiography: Pulmonary transmission and myocardial perfusion imaging using surfactant stabilized microbubbles. *Circulation* 64(Suppl IV):IV-203, 1981
27. Armstrong WF, Kinney EL, Mueller TM, Rasor J, Tickner EG, Dillon JC, Feigenbaum H: Contrast echocardiography for the detection of myocardial perfusion abnormalities. *Circulation* 64(Suppl IV): IV-204, 1981
28. Meltzer RS, Serruys PW, Hugenholtz PG, Roelandt J: Intravenous carbon dioxide as an echocardiographic contrast agent. *JCU* 9:127, 1981
29. Reale A: Contrast echocardiography: Transmission of echoes to the left heart across the pulmonary vascular bed. *Am J Cardiol* 45:401, 1980
30. Shiina A, Kondo K, Nakasone Y, Tsuchiya M, Yaginuma T, Hosoda S: Contrast echocardiographic evaluation of changes in flow velocity in the right side of the heart. *Circulation* 63:1408, 1981
31. Kraunz RF, Ryan TJ: Ultrasound measurements of ventricular wall motion following administration of vasoactive drugs. *Am J Cardiol* 27:464, 1971
32. Burggraf GW, Parker JO: Left ventricular volume changes after amyl nitrite and nitroglycerin in man as measured by ultrasound. *Circulation* 49:136, 1974
33. Redwood DR, Henry WL, Epstein SE: Evaluation of the ability of echocardiography to measure acute alterations in left ventricular volume. *Circulation* 50:901, 1974
34. Gibson DG: Estimation of left ventricular size by echocardiography. *Br Heart J* 35:128, 1973
35. Hirshleifer J, Crawford M, O'Rourke RA, Karliner JS: Influence of acute alterations in heart rate and systemic arterial pressure on echocardiographic measures of left ventricular performance in normal human subjects. *Circulation* 52:835, 1975
36. Mikulic E, Franciosa JA, Cohn JN: Comparative hemodynamic effects of chewable isosorbide dinitrate and nitroglycerin in patients with congestive heart failure. *Circulation* 52:477, 1975
37. Gomes JAC, Carambas CR, Moran HE, Dhatt MS, Calon AH, Caracta AR, Damato AN: The effect of isosorbide dinitrate on left ventricular size, wall stress and left ventricular function in chronic refractory heart failure: An echocardiographic study. *Am J Med* 65:794, 1978
38. Goldstein RE, Bennett ED, Leech GL: Effect of glyceryl trinitrate on echocardiographic left ventricular dimensions during exercise in the upright position. *Br Heart J* 42:245, 1979
39. Martin MA, Fieller NRJ: Echocardiography in cardiovascular drug assessment. *Br Heart J* 41:536, 1979
40. Winkle RA, Goodman DJ, Popp RL: Simultaneous echocardiographic-phonocardiographic recordings at rest and during amyl nitrite administration in patients with mitral valve prolapse. *Circulation* 51:522, 1975
41. Lewis BS, Lewis N, Gotsman MS: Effect of standing and squatting on echocardiographic left ventricular function. *Eur J Cardiol* 11:405, 1980
42. Sharpey-Schafer EP: Effect of respiratory acts on the circulation. In WF Hamilton, P Dow (eds), *Handbook of Physiology* (Vol. 3). Washington: American Physiological Society, 1965. P 1875
43. Thomson PD, Melmon KL: Clinical assessment of autonomic function. *Anesthesiology* 29:724, 1968
44. Robertson D, Stevens RM, Friesinger GC, Oates JA: The effect of the Valsalva maneuver on echocardiographic dimensions in man. *Circulation* 55:596, 1977
45. Brooker JZ, Alderman EL, Harrison DC: Alterations in left ventricular volumes induced by Valsalva maneuver. *Br Heart J* 36:713, 1974
46. Parisi AF, Harrington JJ, Askenazi J, Pratt RC, McIntyre KM: Echocardiographic evaluation of the Valsalva maneuver in healthy subjects and patients with and without heart failure. *Circulation* 54:921, 1976
47. Cohn PF, Angoff GH, Zoll PM, Sloss LJ, Markis JE, Graboys TB, Green LH, Braunwald E: A new, noninvasive technique for inducing post-extrasystolic potentiation during echocardiography. *Circulation* 56:598, 1977

48. Angoff GH, Wistran D, Sloss LJ, Markis JE, Come PC, Zoll PM, Cohn PF: Value of a noninvasively induced ventricular extrasystole during echocardiographic and phonocardiographic assessment of patients with idiopathic hypertrophic subaortic stenosis. *Am J Cardiol* 42:919, 1978
49. Hamby RI, Aintablian A, Wisoff BG, Hartstein ML: Response of the left ventricle in coronary artery disease to post-extrasystolic potentiation. *Circulation* 51:428, 1975
50. Popio KA, Gorlin R, Bechtel D, Levine JA: Postextrasystolic potentiation as a predictor of potential myocardial viability: Preoperative analyses compared with studies after coronary bypass surgery. *Am J Cardiol* 39:944, 1977
51. Cohn PF, Gorlin R, Herman MV, Sonnenblick EH, Horn HR, Cohn LH, Collins JJ Jr: Relation between contractile reserve and prognosis in patients with coronary artery disease and a depressed ejection fraction. *Circulation* 51:414, 1975
52. Cohn LH, Collins JJ Jr, Cohn PF: Use of the augmented ejection fraction to select patients with left ventricular dysfunction for coronary revascularization. *J Thorac Cardiovasc Surg* 72:835, 1976
53. Stein RA, Michielli D, Fox EL, Krasnow N: Continuous ventricular dimensions in man during supine exercise and recovery: An echocardiographic study. *Am J Cardiol* 41:655, 1978
54. Mason SJ, Weiss JL, Weisfeldt ML, Garrison JB, Fortuin NJ: Exercise echocardiography: Detection of wall motion abnormalities during ischemia. *Circulation* 59:50, 1979
55. Sugishita Y, Koseki S: Dynamic exercise echocardiography. *Circulation* 60:743, 1979
56. Crawford MH, White DH, Amon KW: Echocardiographic evaluation of left ventricular size and performance during handgrip and supine and upright bicycle exercise. *Circulation* 59:1188, 1979
57. Wann LS, Faris JV, Childress RH, Dillon JC, Weyman AE, Feigenbaum H: Exercise cross-sectional echocardiography in ischemic heart disease. *Circulation* 60:1300, 1979
58. Paulsen WJ, Boughner DR, Friesen A, Persaud JA: Ventricular response to isometric and isotonic exercise: Echocardiographic assessment. *Br Heart J* 42:521, 1979
59. Limacher MC, Pollner LR, Waggoner AD, Nelson JG, Miller RR, Quinones MA: Comparison of exercise two-dimensional echocardiography in the detection of coronary artery disease. *Circulation* 64(Suppl IV):IV-46, 1981
60. Ginzton LE, Conant R, Brizendine M, Lee F, Laks MM: Subcostal view maximal exercise two-dimensional echocardiography: An effective new method of segmental wall motion analysis. *Circulation* 64(Suppl IV):IV-92, 1981
61. Simard M, Heng MK, Udhoji VN, Weber L: Exercise 2-D echocardiography in diagnosis of coronary artery disease. *Circulation* 64(Suppl IV):IV-92, 1981
62. Rabinowitz AC, Amon KW, Crawford MH: Left ventricular size and performance during maximal exercise in trained athletes. *Circulation* 64(Suppl IV):IV-93, 1981
63. Crawford MH, Amon KW, Vance WS, Sorensen SG, Rabinowitz AC: Advantage of two-dimensional echo over radionuclide angiography for detecting acute changes in LV performance during exercise. *Circulation* 64(Suppl IV):IV-13, 1981
64. Gondi B, Nanda NC: Evaluation of coronary artery disease by cold pressor two-dimensional echocardiography. *Circulation* 64(Suppl IV):IV-14, 1981
65. Millward DK, McLaurin LP, Craige E: Echocardiographic studies to explain opening snaps in presence of nonstenotic mitral valves. *Am J Cardiol* 31:64, 1973
66. Fortuin NJ, Craige E: Echocardiographic studies of genesis of mitral diastolic murmurs. *Br Heart J* 35:75, 1973
67. Rothbaum DA, DeJoseph RL, Tavel M: Diastolic heart sound produced by mid-diastolic closure of the mitral valve. *Am J Cardiol* 34:367, 1974
68. Waider W, Craige E: First heart sound and ejection sounds. Echocardiographic and phonocardiographic correlation with valvular events. *Am J Cardiol* 35:346, 1975
69. Mills PG, Chamusco RF, Moos S, Craige E: Echophonocardiographic studies of the contribution of the atrioventricular valves to the first heart sound. *Circulation* 54:944, 1976
70. Mills PG, Brodie B, McLaurin L, Schall S, Craige E: Echocardiographic and hemodynamic relationships of ejection sounds. *Circulation* 56:430, 1977
71. Venkataraman K, Siegel R, Kim SJ, Allen JW: Musical murmurs: An echophonocardiographic study. *Am J Cardiol* 41:952, 1978

72. Doi YL, Sugiura T, Bishop RL, Paladino D, Moreau K, Spodick DH: High-speed Sechophonocardiographic detection of tricuspid valve prolapse in mitral valve prolapse with discrepancy in onset of systolic murmur. *Am Heart J* 103:301, 1982
73. Tei C, Shah PM, Tanaka H: Phonographic-echographic documentation of systolic honk in tricuspid prolapse. *Am Heart J* 103:294, 1982
74. Mills P, Craige E: Echophonocardiography. *Prog Cardiovasc Dis* 20:337, 1978
75. Frazin L, Talano JV, Stephanides L, Loeb HS, Kopel L, Gunnar RM: Esophageal echocardiography. *Circulation* 54:102, 1976
76. Matsumoto M, Oka Y, Strom J, Frishman W, Kadish A, Becker RM, Frater RWM, Sonnenblick EH: Application of transesophageal echocardiography to continuous intraoperative monitoring of left ventricular performance. *Am J Cardiol* 46:95, 1980
77. Hisanaga K, Hisanaga A, Hibi N, Nishimura K, Kambe T: High speed rotating scanner for transesophageal cross-sectional echocardiography. *Am J Cardiol* 46:837, 1980
78. Duff HJ, Buda AJ, Kramer R, Strauss HD, David TE, Berman ND: Detection of entrapped intracardiac air with intraoperative echocardiography. *Am J Cardiol* 46:255, 1980
79. Reichek N, Likoff M, St. John Sutton M, Plappert T, Harken A: Intraoperative echo analysis of segmental myocardial function in coronary disease. *Circulation* 64(Suppl IV):IV-94, 1981
80. Spotnitz HM: Two-dimensional ultrasound and cardiac operations. *J Thorac Cardiovasc Surg* 83:43, 1982
81. Sahn DJ, Barratt-Boyes B, Graham K, Kerr A, Agnew T, Roche A, Brandt P: Cross-sectional ultrasonic imaging of the coronary arteries in open chested humans; The evaluation of coronary atherosclerotic lesions at surgery. *Am J Cardiol* 47:403, 1981
82. Sahn DJ, Brandt PWT, Barratt-Boyes B, Graham K, Kerr A, Roche T, Hill D: Ultrasonic/angiographic correlations for imaging of coronary atherosclerotic lesions in open chested humans during surgery. *Circulation* 64(Suppl IV):IV-205, 1981

Acyanotic congenital heart disease with left-to-right shunt

Atrial septal defect: secundum type

CLINICAL FEATURES AND PHYSIOLOGY. Secundum atrial septal defect is a common form of congenital heart disease in children and adults [1, 2]. Although symptoms have been observed in infancy a majority of children are asymptomatic, and the presence of the defect is not detected until they are of school age. In contrast, adults with a secundum atrial defect may be impaired functionally. Saksena and associates reported 35 patients over age 35 with atrial septal defects. Of these 23 were functional class III or IV by the New York Heart Association classification before repair [3]. The difference between children and adults appears to be related to the development of pulmonary vascular disease or atrial fibrillation.

The physical, electrocardiographic, radiographic, and echocardiographic findings result from the large-volume left-to-right atrial shunt. In patients with uncomplicated atrial septal defect the jugular venous pulse may show the "A" and V waves to be equal because of the transmitted V wave from the left atrium. A prominent right ventricular heave is palpable along the left parasternal border. Characteristically the second heart sound is widely split and fixed. The former phenomenon is related to an increase in right ventricular volume and low pulmonary impedance producing prolonged right ventricular ejection and delayed pulmonic valve closure. The fixed splitting is related to the relative duration of right and left ventricular ejection, which remains constant. Typically the systolic murmur is diamond-shaped; it begins immediately after the first heart sound and ends well before the second heart sound. Since it is related to increased flow across the pulmonic valve, the murmur, which is usually soft, is best heard in the second left intercostal space. A diastolic murmur caused by increased flow across the tricuspid valve may be heard along the lower left sternal border.

The characteristic electrocardiographic findings include right axis deviation, right ventricular hypertrophy, and incomplete right bundle branch block. Only 25 percent of patients with atrial septal defect have electrocardiographic evidence of right atrial enlargement [1]. Chest radiographs will show mild cardiac enlargement, increased arterial markings, and a prominent main pulmonary artery segment.

ANATOMY. Anatomically the defect may occur at different positions in the atrial septum. It may be simply a widely patent foramen ovale (foramen ovale type, 6%), or it may occur in the central portion of the septum (fossa ovalis defect, 62%) (Fig. 14-1) [4]. Often when it extends to the inferior vena cava it is referred to as the inferior vena cava type (25%). Defects at the entrance of the superior vena cava are usually associated with anomalies of right-sided pulmonary venous return (sinus venosus type, 6%) [4]. Several effects of the atrial shunt are observed. The right atrium is dilated. The right ventricular cavity is enlarged, considerably larger than the left ventricle. The pulmonary artery is almost always larger than the aorta.

M-MODE ECHOCARDIOGRAPHY. Numerous reports describing the M-mode echocardiographic features of a secundum atrial septal defect emphasize enlargement of the right ventricular internal dimension and anterior systolic motion of the interventricular septum [5–8]. Other features include diastolic fluttering of the

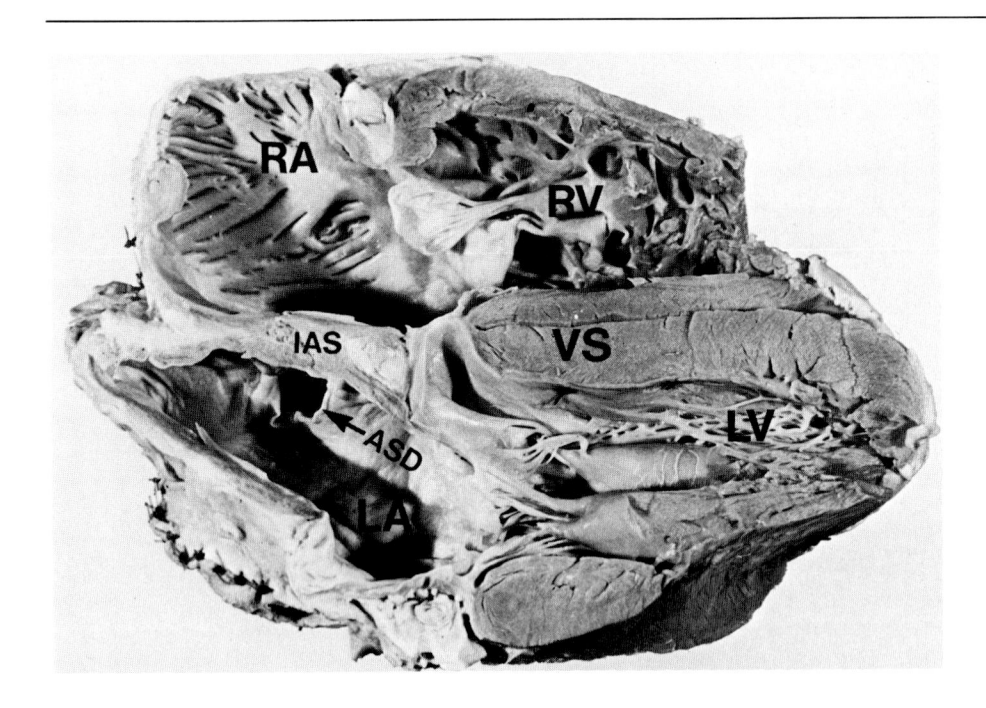

Fig. 14-1. Anatomic specimen cut in the plane of the subcostal 4-chamber view. A large fossa ovalis atrial septal defect exists in the central portion of the septum. IAS = interatrial septum; VS = ventricular septum.

tricuspid valve and an increase in tricuspid valve excursion caused by increased flow across the valve. These findings are not specific for secundum atrial septal defect but are also observed in patients with partial or total anomalous pulmonary venous return, tricuspid insufficiency, pulmonic insufficiency, and pulmonary hypertension. Visualization and measurement of the right atrium by M-mode echocardiography is impractical because of its inaccessible intrathoracic position.

TWO-DIMENSIONAL ECHOCARDIOGRAPHY. Cross-sectional imaging of the heart provides additional acoustic windows for examination of right-sided cardiac structures. From the apical window both the right atrium and right ventricle are imaged easily. Bommer and associates described a method for measuring the right atrium and right ventricle from the apical four-chamber view [9]. The right ventricular measurements were obtained at end diastole. The long axis was measured from the apex to the tricuspid valve–septal junction; the short axis was measured at the maximal diameter and at the midpoint of the long axis from the septal surface to the free wall. The right ventricular area was planimetered along the endocardial surface. The long axis, short axis, and planimetered area of right atrium were measured at end systole. These authors demonstrated that the short axis dimension and echo area of the right ventricle and right atrium more reliably separated adult patients with right atrial and right ventricular volume overload from normal subjects. We have demonstrated the same results in children with atrial septal defects (Fig. 14-2) [10, 11]. In addition, two-dimensional echocardiography allows direct imaging of the atrial septal defect. From the subcostal four-chamber echocardiographic view the ultrasonic beam is perpendicular to all portions of the interatrial septum. Since this plane is the optimal position for atrial septal visualization, areas of echo dropout in the septal image represent a defect in the interatrial septum (Fig. 14-3) [12, 13]. For this view the transducer is placed below the xiphisternal notch

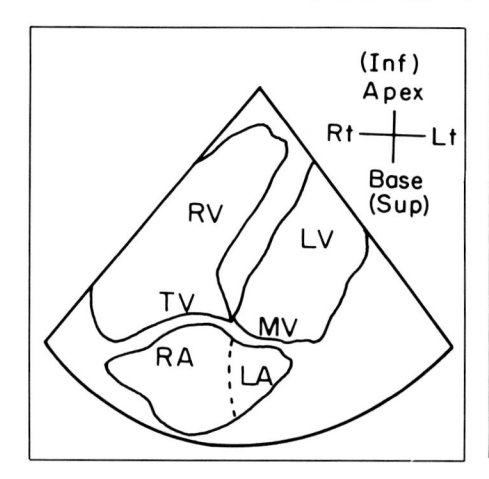

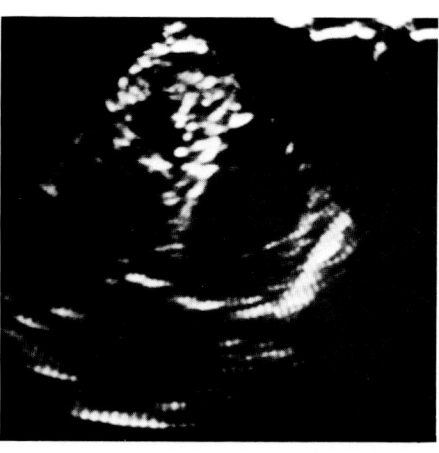

Fig. 14-2. Apical 4-chamber view recorded from a child with a secundum atrial septal defect. The right atrium and right ventricle are enlarged from volume overload. Dashed line = plane of atrial septum as observed in real time.

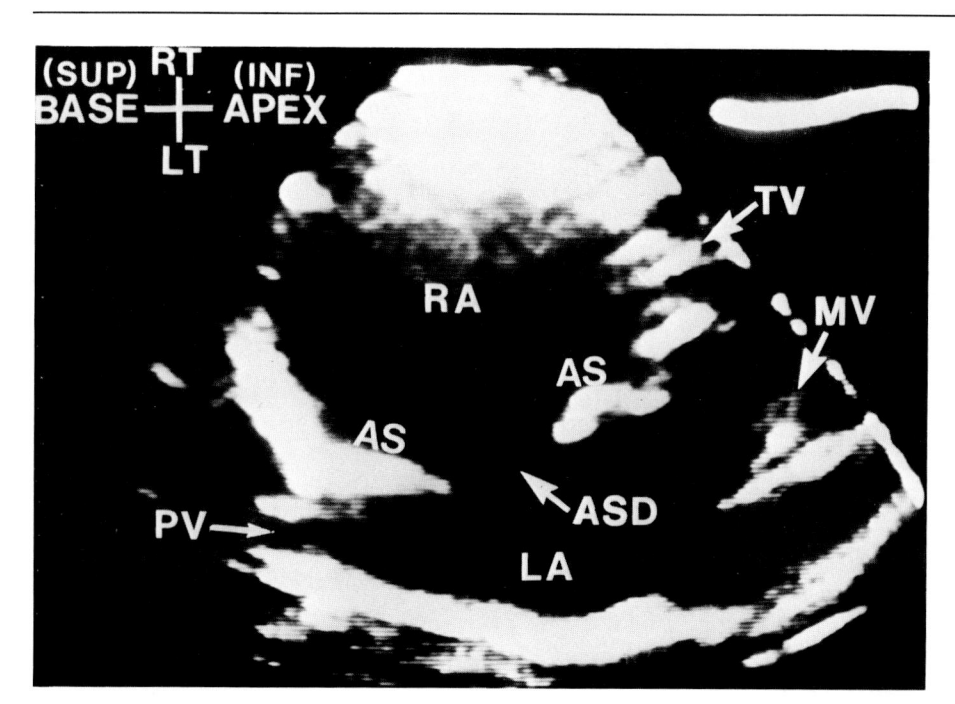

Fig. 14-3. Subcostal 4-chamber view recorded from a child with secundum atrial septal defect. The area of echo dropout in the region of the middle of the atrial septum (AS) is typical of a fossa ovalis defect. (Compare to Fig. 14-1.) PV = pulmonary vein.

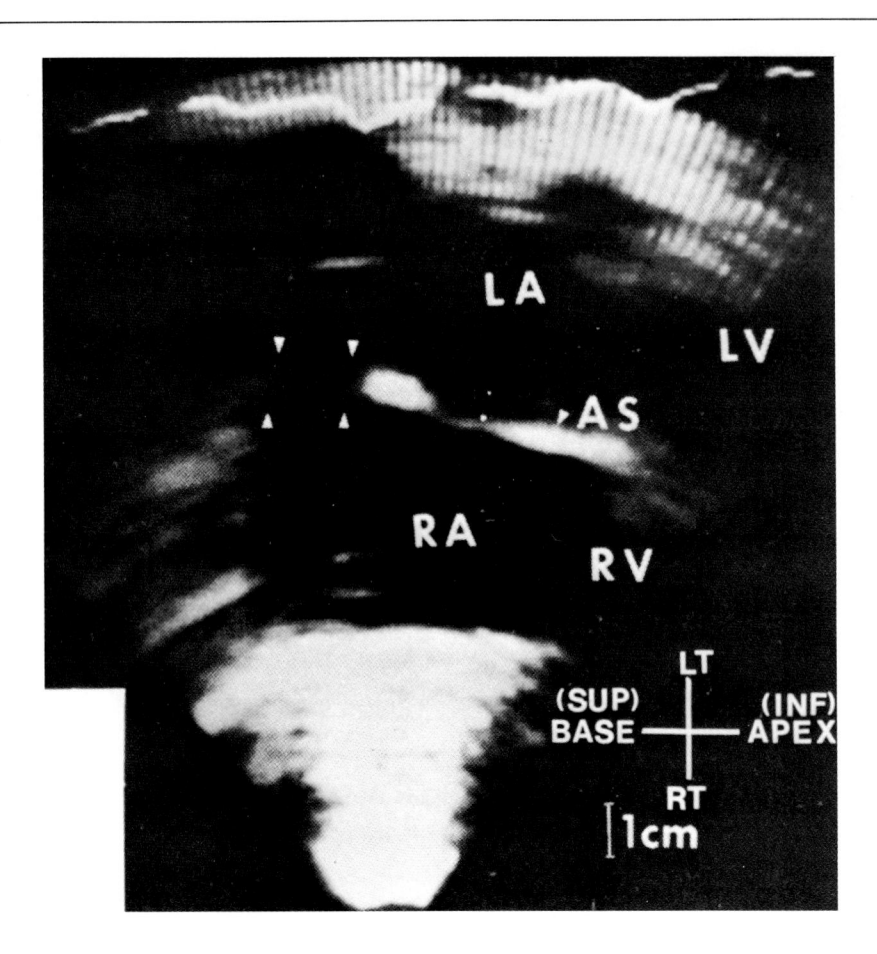

Fig. 14-4. Two-dimensional echocardiogram, subcostal view with the beam tilted anterosuperiorly to image a sinus venosus atrial septal defect (arrow). AS = atrial septum. (From FN Nasser et al, Mayo Clin Proc 56:568, 1981.)

and the plane of sector oriented from the left hip to the right shoulder. Fossa ovalis defects are imaged immediately as an area of echo dropout in the central portion of interatrial septum. In order to visualize the superior aspect of atrial septum the ultrasonic beam is tilted superiorly and rotated slightly clockwise until the orifice of the superior vena cava is imaged at its entry into the right atrium. This allows direct imaging of sinus venosus defects (Fig. 14-4) [14]. It must be remembered that the atrial septum in patients with right atrial volume overload will bow into the left atrium [15].

Numerous reports using systemic venous contrast echocardiography have demonstrated both right-to-left and left-to-right shunts through an atrial septal defect [16, 17]. Detection of right-to-left shunts by contrast echocardiography may be augmented by Valsalva maneuver; the shunt is more pronounced in patients with associated valvular pulmonic stenosis or pulmonary hypertension. Either M-mode or two-dimensional echocardiography may be used to detect microcavitations in the left side of the heart. The negative contrast effect of a left-to-right shunt may be imaged by two-dimensional techniques (Fig. 14-5).

Doppler echocardiography has been combined with two-dimensional imaging to detect the level of intracardiac shunts [18, 19]. In patients with atrial septal defects turbulent flow is detected when the Doppler sample volume is in the tricus-

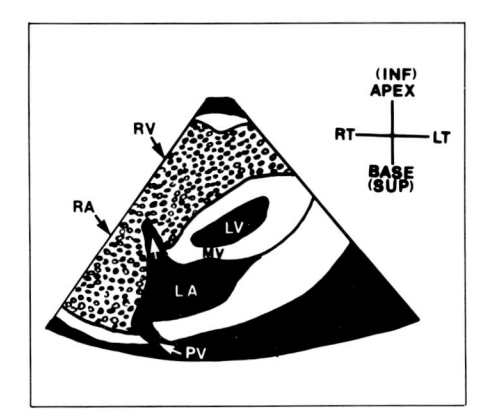

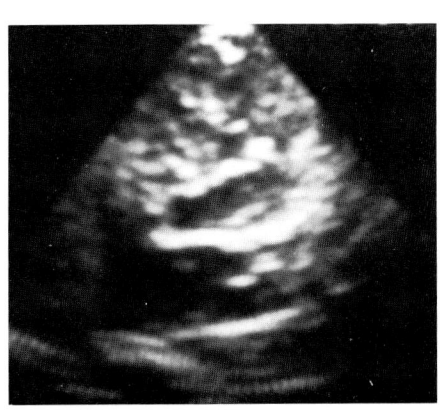

Fig. 14-5. Apical 4-chamber view. After peripheral venous injection of indocyanine green microcavitations appear in the right atrium. A negative filling defect is seen in the RA (arrow) from the left-to-right atrial shunt. PV = pulmonary vein.

pid valve orifice. Normal turbulence is observed when the sample volume is in the pulmonary trunk [18].

Atrial septal defect: primum type

CLINICAL FEATURES AND PHYSIOLOGY. Clinical symptoms depend upon the degree of mitral valve regurgitation from the associated mitral valve cleft. Infants and children with a primum atrial septal defect and a cleft but competent mitral valve will be relatively asymptomatic. Children with severe mitral regurgitation will manifest symptoms of congestive heart failure, fatigability, dyspnea, tachypnea, tachycardia, and failure to thrive.

Since patients with primum atrial septal defect also have abnormalities of the mitral valve and conduction system, the physical, electrocardiographic, radiographic, and echocardiographic examination will depend not only on the atrial shunt but also on the degree of hemodynamic derangement caused by the associated defects. Patients with a competent mitral valve will have findings on physical examination and chest radiograph indistinguishable from those of a secundum atrial septal defect. However, the electrocardiogram typically has left axis deviation with a counterclockwise superior frontal plane loop. Right ventricular hypertrophy and incomplete right bundle branch block are common. Patients with mitral regurgitation will have a prominent apical impulse, thrill, and apical holosystolic murmur in addition to the physical findings of the atrial septal defect. The electrocardiogram may show left atrial enlargement or left ventricular hypertrophy. Chest x-ray will also reflect the degree of mitral insufficiency in addition to the atrial shunt.

ANATOMY. In ostium primum atrial septal defect the deficiency is in the lower part of the atrial septum [20]. This form of atrial defect is associated invariably with anomalies of the atrioventricular valves. The most common form of atrioventricular valve anomaly is a cleft in the anterior leaflet of the mitral valve [4, 20]. Moreover, deficient development of the endocardial cushion portion of the ventricular septum without defect formation causes the mitral valve annulus to assume a more an-

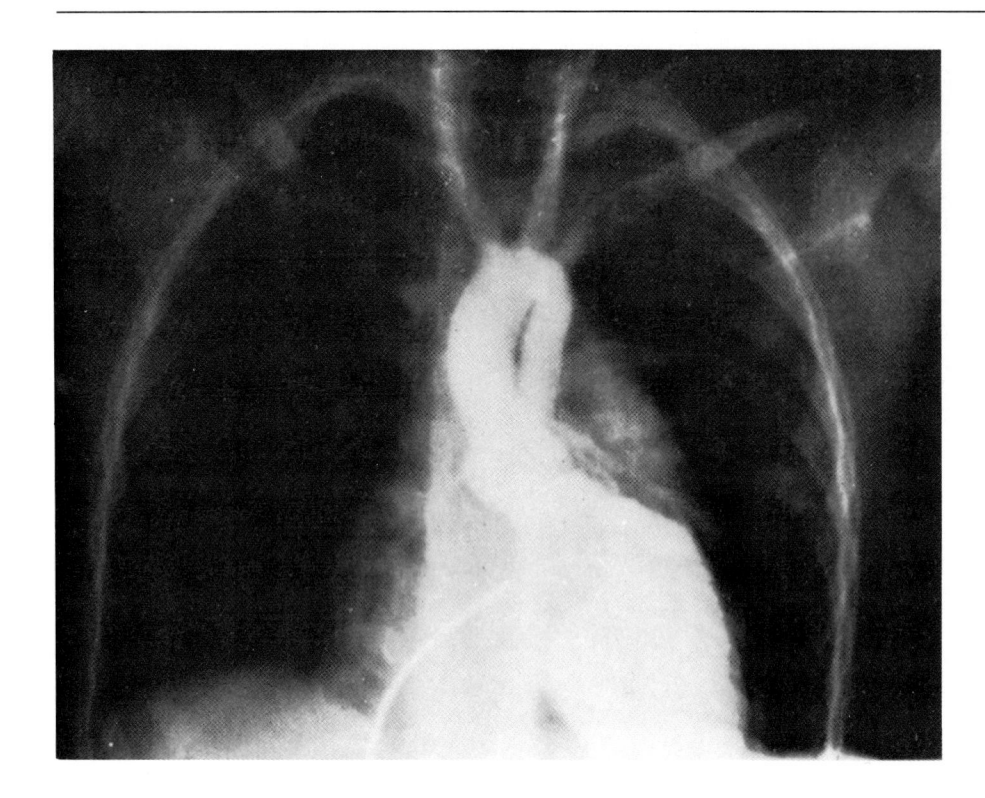

Fig. 14-6. Left ventricular cineangiocardiogram in a child with a primum atrial septal defect. The left ventricular outflow tract is elongated and narrowed due to the associated mitral valve abnormality. Presented here is the characteristic angiographic "goose neck" appearance that results from the anatomic deformity of the mitral valve. (From JK Perloff, The Clinical Recognition of Congenital Heart Disease. *Philadelphia: Saunders, 1978.*)

terosuperior position than usual [21]. Accessory chordae tendineae that spring from the margins of the cleft and insert directly into the ventricular septum are important anatomic features of this defect [22]. Thus in diastole the anterior leaflet of the mitral valve encroaches upon the left ventricular outflow tract (Fig. 14-6). On the right side the tricuspid valve is usually normal. Occasionally there is some shortening of the septal leaflet.

M-MODE ECHOCARDIOGRAPHY. The M-mode features of a primum atrial septal defect are those of right ventricular volume overload, plus those of the associated anomalies of the mitral valve apparatus. Right ventricular volume overload was discussed in the previous section on secundum atrial septal defects. In addition there is narrowing of the left ventricular outflow tract on the M-mode scan from the left ventricle to the aortic root. There is apparent motion of the mitral valve through the septum in diastole, and in systole the mitral valve generates multiple echo reflectances [23]. If significant mitral regurgitation is present the left atrium may also be enlarged.

TWO-DIMENSIONAL ECHOCARDIOGRAPHY. Two-dimensional imaging displays the complete spectrum of anatomic defects that occur with an ostium primum atrial septal defect. In the left parasternal long axis view the "goose neck" deformity produced by the abnormally positioned anterior mitral leaflet is imaged as narrowing of the left ventricular outflow tract in diastole (Fig. 14-7) [24]. In addition, the subcostal long axis image of the left ventricular outflow tract allows visualization of the goose neck deformity (Fig. 14-8) [25]. In the short axis view, accessory chordae

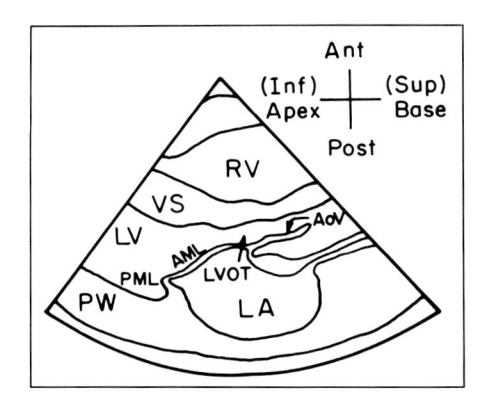

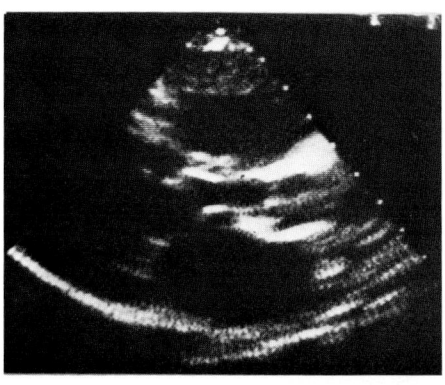

Fig. 14-7. Long axis scan from a patient with an ostium primum atrial septal defect. The right ventricle is enlarged. There is a narrow left ventricular outflow tract ("goose neck" deformity) due to the abnormal orientation of the mitral annulus and anterior mitral leaflet. The left atrium is enlarged from mitral insufficiency. AoV = aortic valve; PW = posterior wall; VS = ventricular septum.

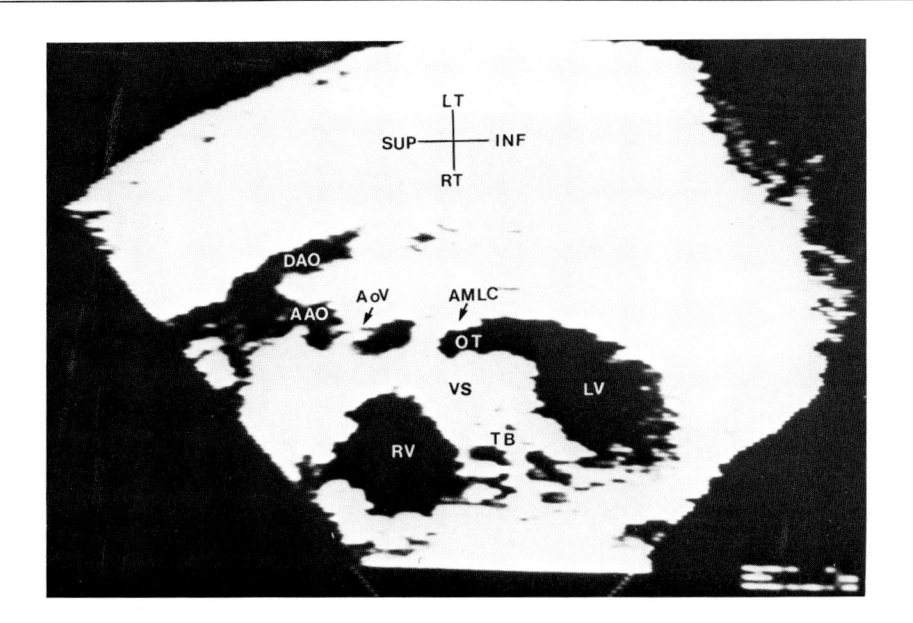

Fig. 14-8. Subcostal view demonstrating the "goose neck" deformity in a patient with an ostium primum atrial septal defect. In a diastolic frame accessory chords that arise from the anterior mitral leaflet (AMLC) are seen attaching to the ventricular septum (VS). These chords and the anterosuperior position of the mitral annulus cause the anterior mitral leaflet to encroach on the outflow tract (OT) and produce the echocardiographic "goose neck." The right ventricle is enlarged from the left-to-right shunt. AoV = aortic valve; OT = outflow tract; TB = trabeculations.

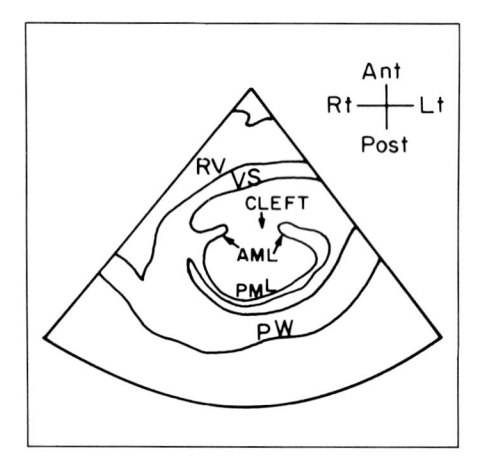

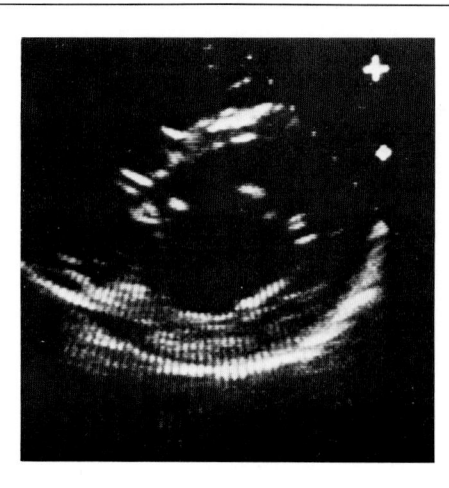

450   14. Acyanotic congenital heart disease with left-to-right shunt

Fig. 14-9. Left parasternal short axis view from a patient with an ostium primum atrial septal defect. There is diastolic separation of the anterior mitral leaflet secondary to a cleft. PW = posterior wall; VS = ventricular septum.

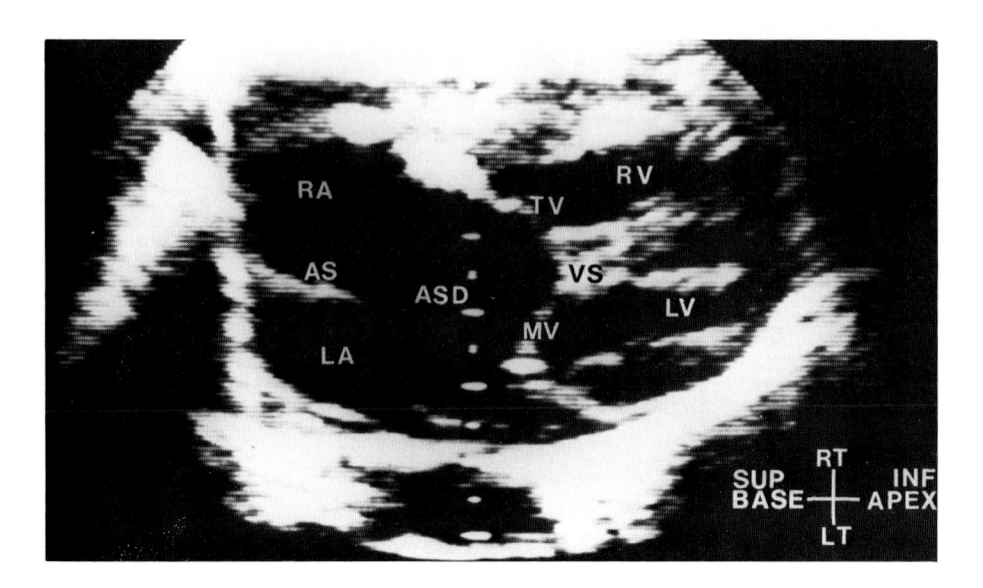

Fig. 14-10. Subcostal 4-chamber view from a patient with an ostium primum atrial septal defect. There is echo dropout in the inferior portion of the atrial septum (AS) from the defect. VS = ventricular septum.

of the mitral valve that attach to the ventricular septum are imaged, and the cleft in the anterior mitral leaflet is seen as diastolic separation of the leaflet (Fig. 14-9) [24, 26]. The defect in the atrial septum may be imaged directly from the apical four-chamber and subcostal four-chamber views [10, 12, 13, 24, 27]. In each view the defect is imaged as an area of echo dropout in the inferior portion of the atrial septum (Fig. 14-10).

The most severe form of ostium primum atrial septal defect is a common atrium. No evidence of an atrial septal remnant is visualized from either the apical four-chamber or subcostal four-chamber view in patients with this defect [24, 27].

Ventricular septal defect

CLINICAL FEATURES AND PHYSIOLOGY. The most common congenital cardiac anomaly is the ventricular septal defect. Clinical features of a ventricular septal defect depend upon the size and position of the communication. Children with a large defect are usually in congestive heart failure with dyspnea, tachypnea, tachycardia, and growth failure. The murmurs heard are a holosystolic murmur along the lower left sternal border often associated with a left parasternal thrill and a mitral diastolic rumble at the apex. The electrocardiogram in these patients may show left ventricular or biventricular hypertrophy. Chest radiography shows a large heart with increased pulmonary blood flow. In contrast, the patient with a small ventricular septal defect is asymptomatic and indistinguishable from a normal person. The murmur may be long or short and heard high or low along the left sternal border depending on the position of the defect. Chest x-ray and electrocardiogram are normal.

ANATOMY. An isolated defect in the ventricular septum can occur in four different positions (Fig. 14-11). These defects have been given various names, according to position, as follows:

Position 1	Outflow
	Supracristal
	Subpulmonic
	Bulbar
Position 2	Inflow
	Infracristal
	Subaortic
	Membranous
Position 3	Endocardial cushion
	Retrocristal
Position 4	Muscular

For the purposes of this text the terms *outflow* (position 1), *inflow* (position 2), *endocardial cushion* (position 3), and *muscular* (position 4) ventricular septal defects will be used. An inflow defect is the most common of ventricular septal defects. It usually involves the membranous portion and various amounts of the muscular portion of the ventricular septum. As visualized from the right ventricle, it lies immediately posterior and inferior to the crista supraventricularis and behind the left half of the anterior leaflet and anterior half of the septal leaflet of the tricuspid

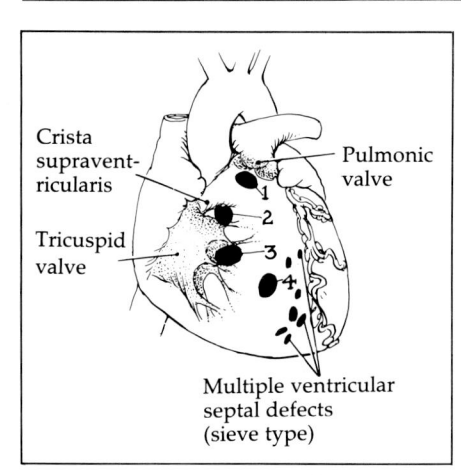

452 14. Acyanotic congenital heart disease with left-to-right shunt

Fig. 14-11. Composite locations of ventricular septal defects. 1 = outflow tract defect; 2 = inflow tract defect; 3 = endocardial cushion ventricular septal defect; 4 = muscular defect. (From WF Friedman et al, Multiple muscular ventricular septal defects. Circulation 32:35, 1965 by permission of the American Heart Association, Inc.)

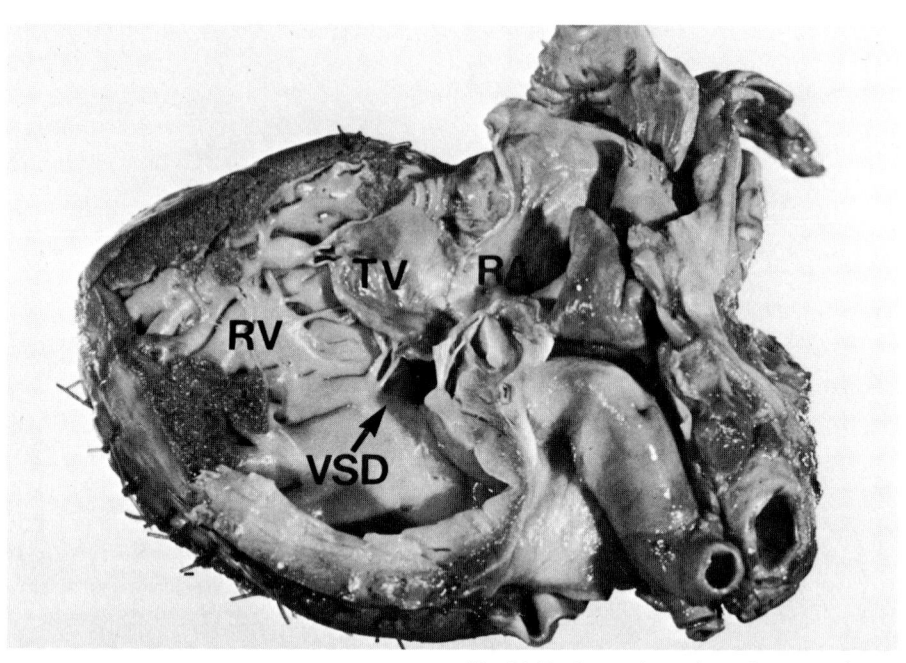

Fig. 14-12. Anatomic specimen demonstrating an inflow ventricular septal defect behind the septal leaflet of the tricuspid valve.

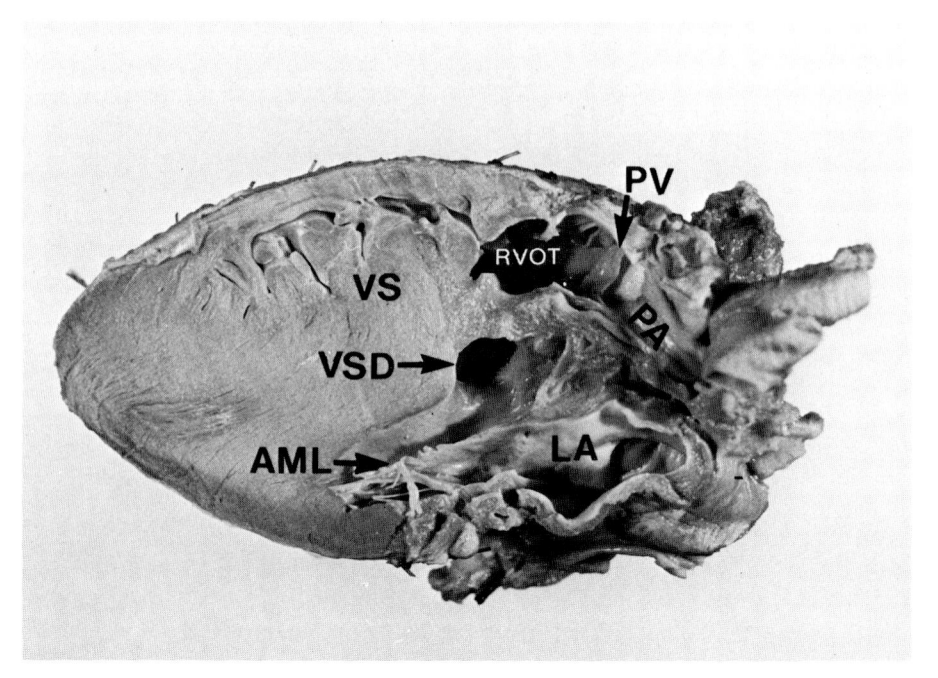

Fig. 14-13. Anatomic specimen cut in the plane of the outflow tract view to demonstrate an outflow tract ventricular septal defect. PV = pulmonic valve; RVOT = right ventricular outflow tract; VS = ventricular septum.

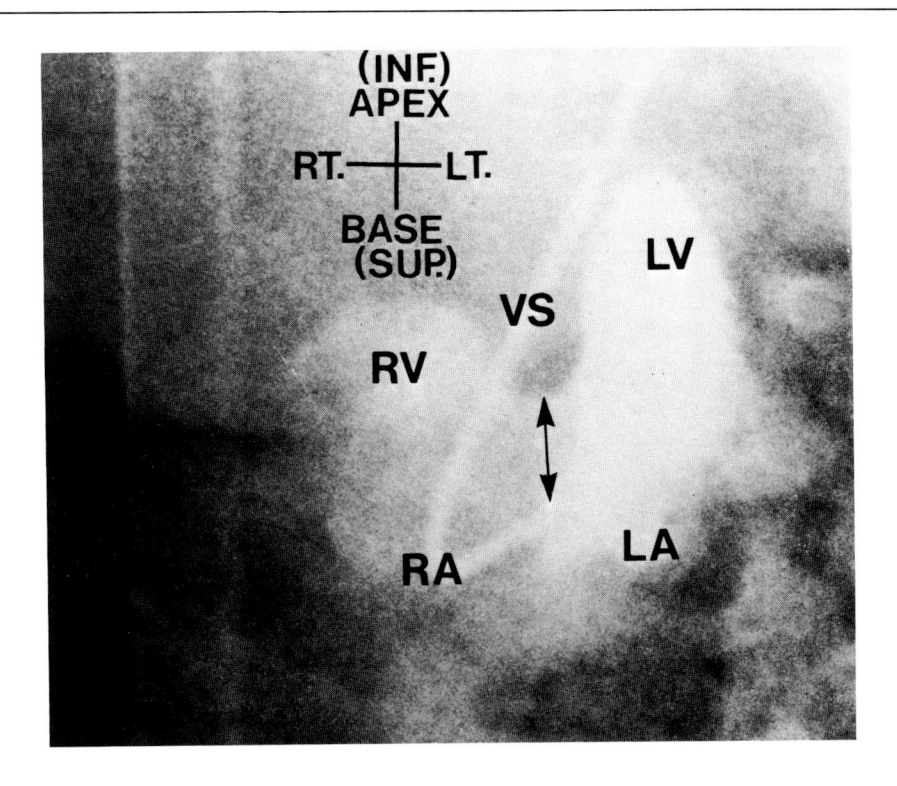

Fig. 14-14. Left ventricular cineangiocardiogram in the hepatoclavicular 4-chamber projection demonstrating an endocardial cushion ventricular septal defect (arrows). VS = ventricular septum.

valve (Fig. 14-12). The posterior boundary of the defect is the tricuspid ring [28]. Outflow defects exist in the area that extends from the crista supraventricularis to the annulus fibrosus of the pulmonic valve on the right side. The main characteristics of these defects are their close relationship to the pulmonic valve and their lack of extension below the crista supraventricularis (Fig. 14-13). An endocardial cushion ventricular septal defect is bounded anteriorly and superiorly by the membranous septum and posteriorly by the tricuspid ring [29]. This defect differs from an inflow defect in that the aortic valve does not form a boundary of the defect since the defect rests in the posterior portion of the septum (Fig. 14-14). Muscular defects may reside anywhere in the muscular septum.

M-MODE ECHOCARDIOGRAPHY. The M-mode features of a ventricular septal defect are those of left atrial and left ventricular enlargement from the large-volume left-to-right shunt. Direct imaging of the defect by M-mode technique is rare.

TWO-DIMENSIONAL ECHOCARDIOGRAPHY. In contrast to M-mode echocardiography, two-dimensional imaging allows the echocardiographer to scan the ventricular septum from multiple planes. With the transducer placed in the third or fourth left intercostal space and the plane of sector oriented from the left hip to the right shoulder, an image of the long axis of the left ventricle is achieved. Medial angulation and counterclockwise rotation from the left ventricular long axis permit an image of the right ventricle, tricuspid valve, and right atrium. This tomographic cross section allows visualization of the inlet portion of the ventricular septum. In a patient with an inflow ventricular septal defect, echo dropout will be observed in

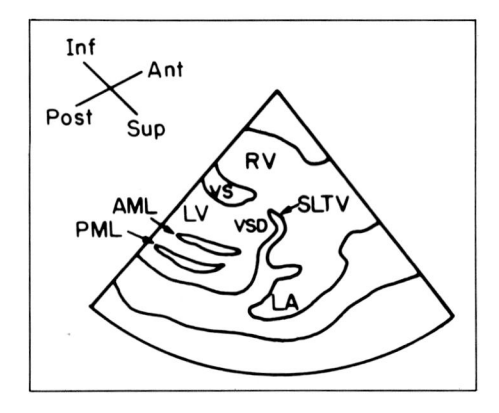

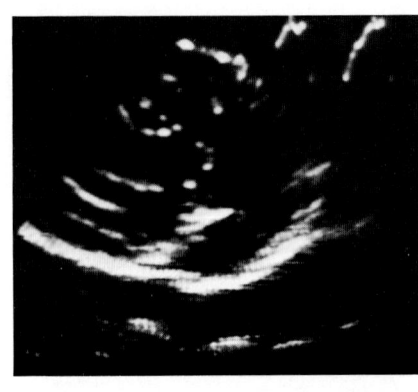

454   14. Acyanotic congenital heart disease with left-to-right shunt

Fig. 14-15. Inflow view of the right ventricle along the left parasternal border. There is echo dropout from a ventricular septal defect in the inlet portion of the ventricular septum (VS) behind the septal leaflet of the tricuspid valve (SLTV). (Compare with the anatomic specimen in Fig. 14-12.)

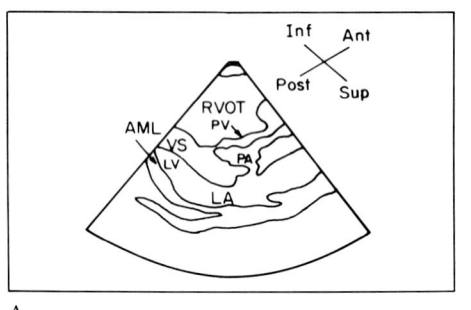

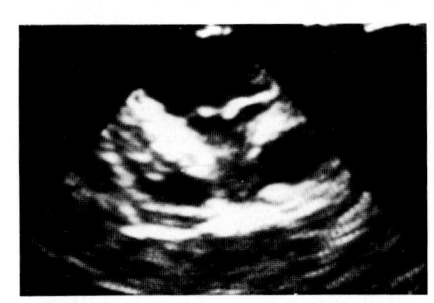

Fig. 14-16A. Normal outflow tract view of the right ventricle. B. There is echo dropout in the ventricular septum (VS) from an outflow ventricular septal defect. (Compare with the anatomic specimen in Fig. 14-13.) PA = pulmonary artery; PV = pulmonic valve; RVOT = right ventricular outflow tract.

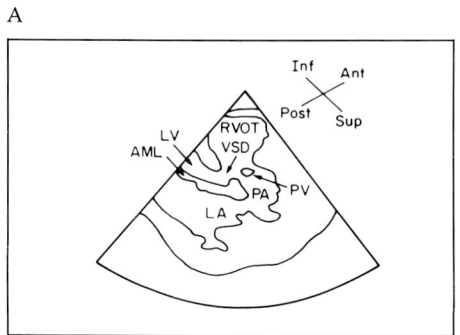

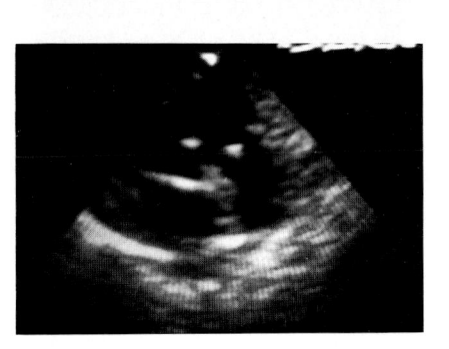

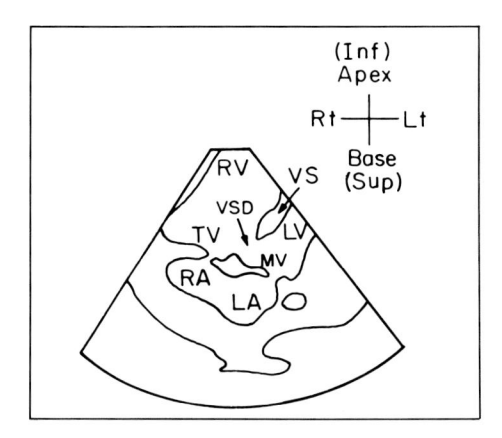

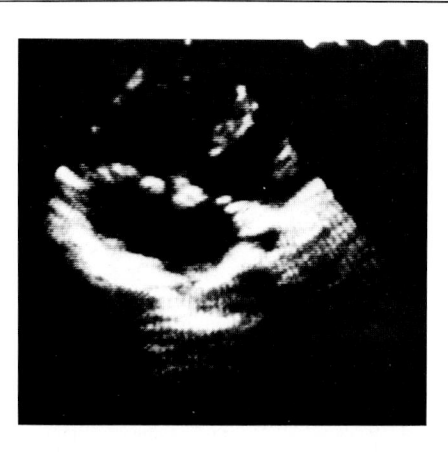

Fig. 14-17. Apical 4-chamber view demonstrating echo dropout in the superior portion of the ventricular septum (VS) from an isolated endocardial cushion ventricular septal defect. (Compare with the angiocardiographic image of this patient in Fig. 14-14.)

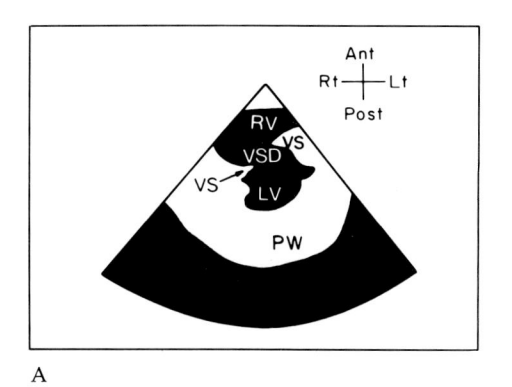

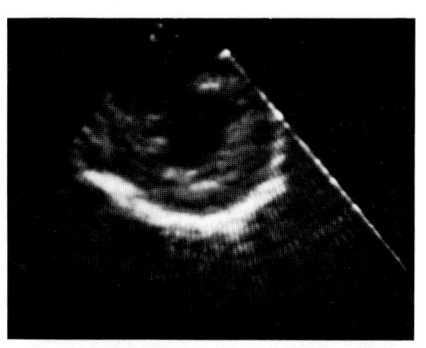

Fig. 14-18A. Short axis view showing echo dropout in the muscular ventricular septum (VS) from a ventricular septal defect. B. Apical 4-chamber view showing echo dropout in the inferior muscular portion of the ventricular septum (VS) from ventricular septal defect. PW = posterior wall; PV = pulmonary vein.

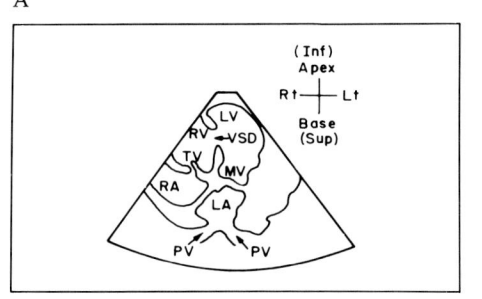

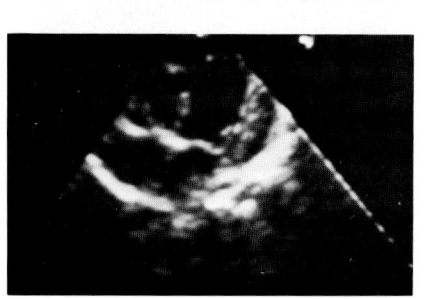

the area of the ventricular septum behind the septal leaflet of the tricuspid valve (Fig. 14-15). A lateral superior angulation from the left ventricular long axis images the right ventricular outflow tract, pulmonic valve, pulmonary artery, and outflow portion of the ventricular septum. An outflow defect is seen as an area of echo dropout in the ventricular septum in this view (Fig. 14-16). With the transducer placed at the patient's cardiac apex and the plane of sector oriented from the left hip to the right shoulder, the apical four-chamber view is achieved. In this view the posterior portion of the ventricular septum is seen. Echo dropout in the superior basilar portion of the septum in this view occurs with an isolated endocardial cushion ventricular septal defect (Fig. 14-17). In contrast to a complete atrioventricular canal there are two separate atrioventricular valves with this lesion. Muscular ventricular septal defects are the most difficult to image. These defects may be visualized by scanning the septum in the short axis view (Fig. 14-18A). They may also be observed as areas of echo dropout in the inferior portion of the septum in the apical four-chamber view (Fig. 14-18B) or subcostal four-chamber view. The subcostal window has been employed to distinguish the various positions of a ventricular septal defect in infants [30].

Defining a ventricular septal defect depends upon the resolution capabilities of the ultrasonic equipment and the size of the defect relative to the size of the ventricular septum. A rather large defect in a relatively small heart may be imaged easily. Very small defects in a large heart may be overlooked.

As mentioned previously, pulsed Doppler echocardiography has greatly facilitated the localization of intracardiac shunts. The presence and level of intracardiac shunting can be ascertained by recording turbulence distal to the lesion in question and then by "threading" the defect with the sample volume to show that there is flow within the defect itself. Turbulent flow may be recorded in the right ventricular outflow tract in patients with ventricular septal defect. Since this finding occurs also in patients with subpulmonic stenosis it is nonspecific. As previously mentioned the two-dimensional transducer can scan the septum and the sample volume can be placed in the defect to demonstrate actual flow through the ventricular septum [19, 31].

Complete endocardial cushion defect

CLINICAL FEATURES AND PHYSIOLOGY. Patients with a complete endocardial cushion defect are almost always in congestive heart failure. On physical examination there are biventricular overactivity and the holosystolic murmur of a ventricular septal defect. Electrocardiograms show left-axis deviation with a counterclockwise superior frontal plane loop and varying degrees of combined ventricular hypertrophy; chest radiographs show a large heart with torrential pulmonary blood flow.

ANATOMY. The principal features of complete atrioventricular canal include absence of the inferior segment of the atrial septum and posterosuperior segment of the ventricular septum, and a complex atrioventricular valve common to both ventricles. This valve is formed by an anterior and posterior leaflet related to the ventricular septum and two lateral leaflets, one related to the wall of each ventricle. Rastelli and associates described three types of complete atrioventricular canal [32]:

TYPE A. This most common type (70% of cases) has the anterior leaflet of the common atrioventricular valve divided at its midportion. Each half is usually triangular and well developed and is attached to the annulus fibrosus of the respective ventricle. The lateral margins are attached by normal chordae tendineae to an anterior papillary muscle in the corresponding ventricle. Medially the chordae tendineae insert onto the crest of the ventricular septum. On the right side these chordae insert into the body of the crista supraventricularis in part, and in part to the papillary muscle of the conus. On the left side these chordae attach to the interventricular septum in a fashion that results in elongation and narrowing of the left ventricular outflow tract.

The interventricular communication occurs between the anterior and posterior leaflets of the common atrioventricular valve. The membranous septum is well developed. The posterior leaflet of the common atrioventricular valve is usually irregular in shape and the leaflet tissue is deficient. The edges of the leaflet are curled and thickened. On the left side the chordae tendineae are normal and attach to the posterior papillary muscle in the left ventricle. On the right side the chordae attach to the right side of the septum or a posterior papillary muscle.

TYPE B. In this form (15% of cases) the anterior leaflet is divided but not attached to the ventricular septum. The lateral attachment of each leaflet is to a single papillary muscle in the right ventricle. The posterior leaflet has a morphology similar to that of type A.

TYPE C. In this form (15% of cases) the common anterior atrioventricular valve is undivided and rectangular or trapezoidal in shape. It is attached along its base to the annulus of both ventricles. Lateral attachments are to an anterior papillary muscle in each ventricle (Fig. 14-19). There are no medial attachments of the anterior leaflet. The posterior leaflet is similar to the previous two types. There is free interventricular communication beneath the anterior leaflet (Fig. 14-20).

Recently the common atrioventricular canal has been divided by Lev and associates into dominant right and dominant left forms [33]. In the former there is marked hypertrophy and dilatation of the right ventricle, and the left ventricle is smaller than normal. In the latter the left ventricle is hypertrophied and enlarged while the right ventricle is smaller than normal (see Fig. 14-19).

M-MODE ECHOCARDIOGRAPHY. The echocardiogram reflects the motion of the common atrioventricular valve. The common valve has an excursion that extends from the right ventricular anterior wall to the left ventricular posterior wall [23]. The anterior valve leaflet passes through the ventricular septal defect in diastole. In systole multiple redundant echoes are observed emanating from the common valve. M-mode echocardiography has also been able to separate dominant left ventricular from dominant right ventricular type of complete atrioventricular canal [34]. In patients with dominant left ventricular complete atrioventricular canal the left ventricular diastolic dimension is increased and the right ventricular diastolic dimension is small or normal. In patients with dominant right ventricular type the opposite occurs.

TWO-DIMENSIONAL ECHOCARDIOGRAPHY. Cross-sectional imaging allows a more precise differentiation of complete from partial atrioventricular canal. The

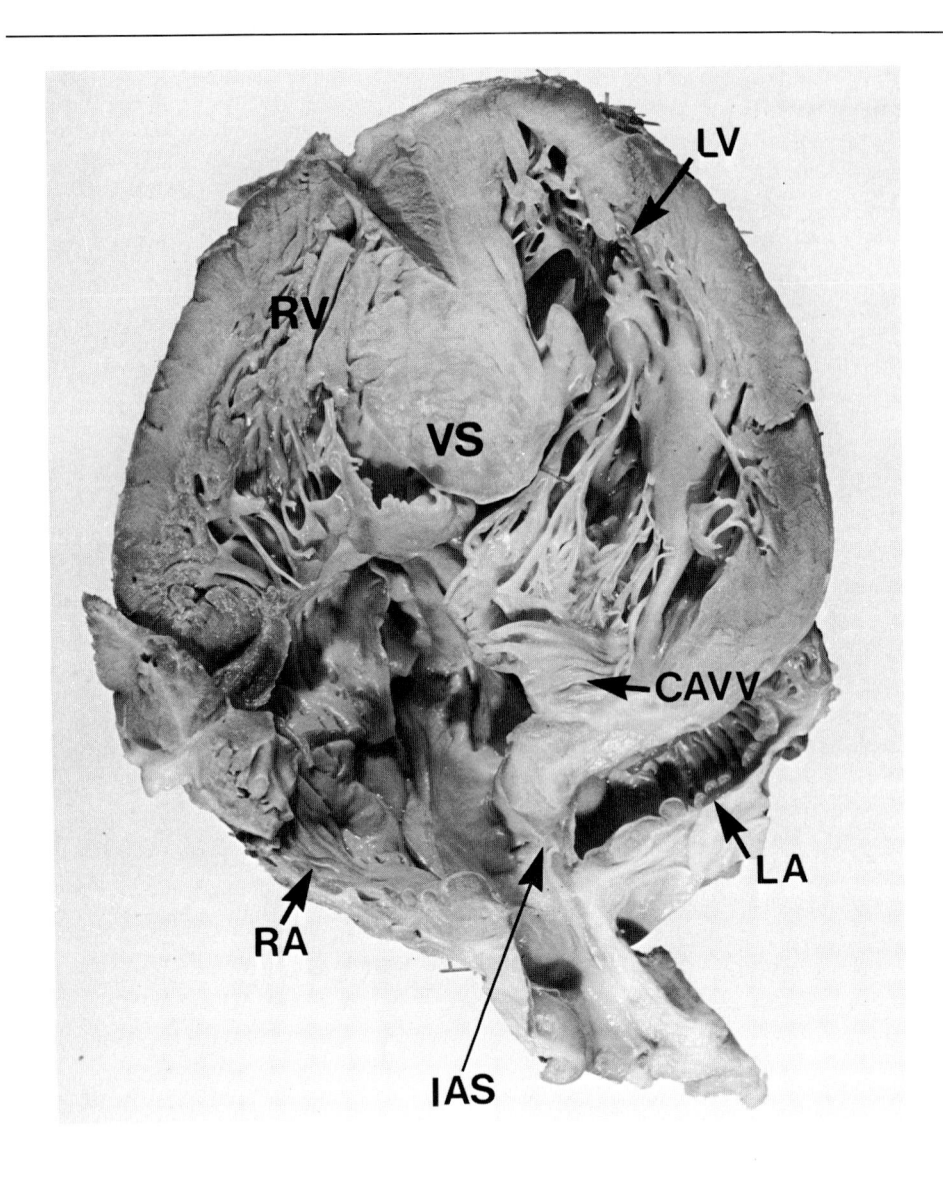

458   14. Acyanotic congenital heart disease with left-to-right shunt

Fig. 14-19. Anatomic specimen cut in the plane of the apical 4-chamber view. This is a Rastelli type C complete atrioventricular canal. Seen in this picture is the common undivided anterior leaflet (CAVV) and the lateral leaflet in the right ventricle. The chordae of the common anterior leaflet attach to an anterior papillary muscle in the left ventricle. This heart conforms to Lev's classification of left ventricular dominant type. The LV is dilated and hypertrophied. The RV is small. IAS = interatrial septum; VS = ventricular septum.

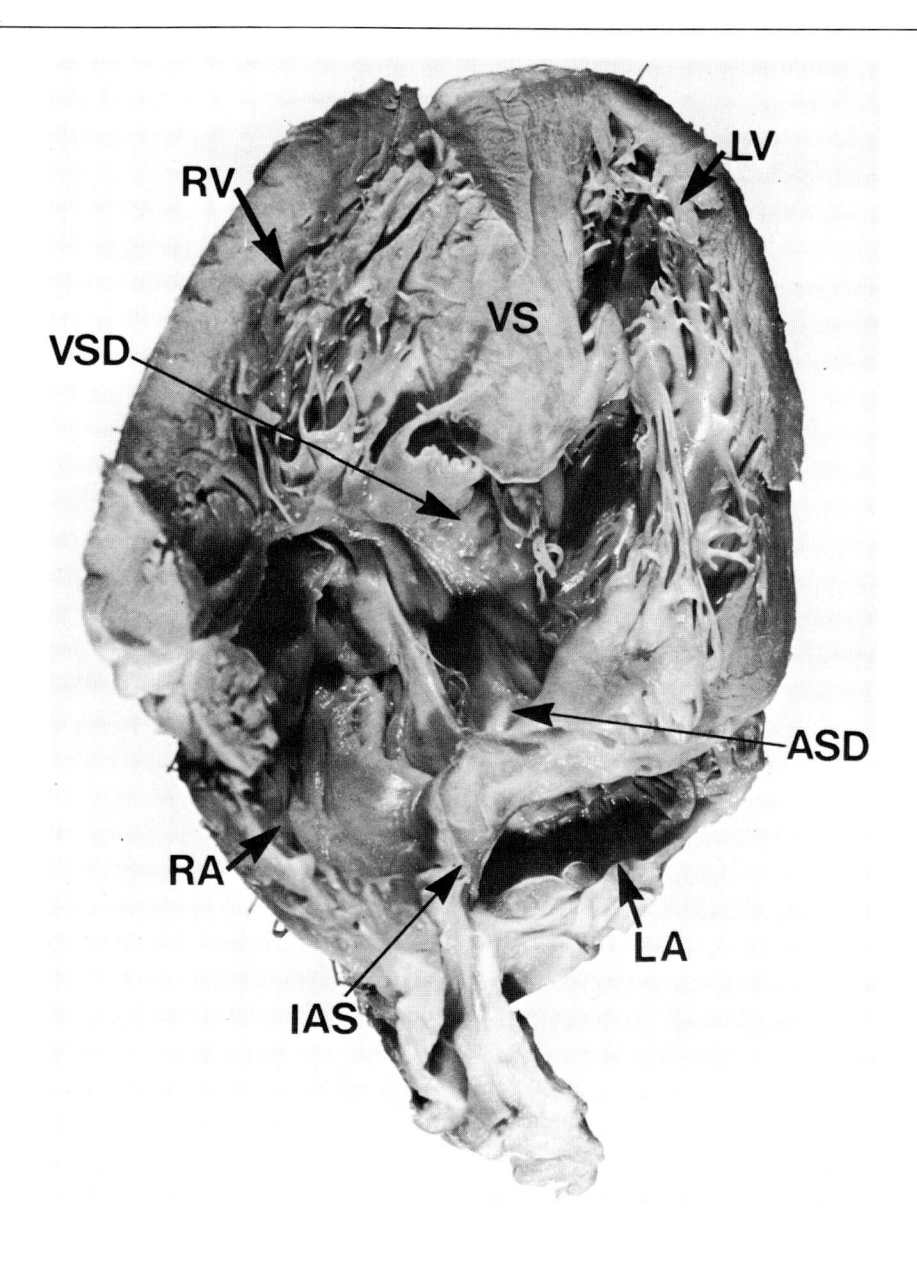

Fig. 14-20. Anatomic specimen (same as in Fig. 14-19). The common anterior leaflet has been retracted to demonstrate the scooped out ventricular septal defect, atrial septal defect, and common posterior leaflet. IAS = interatrial septum; VS = ventricular septum.

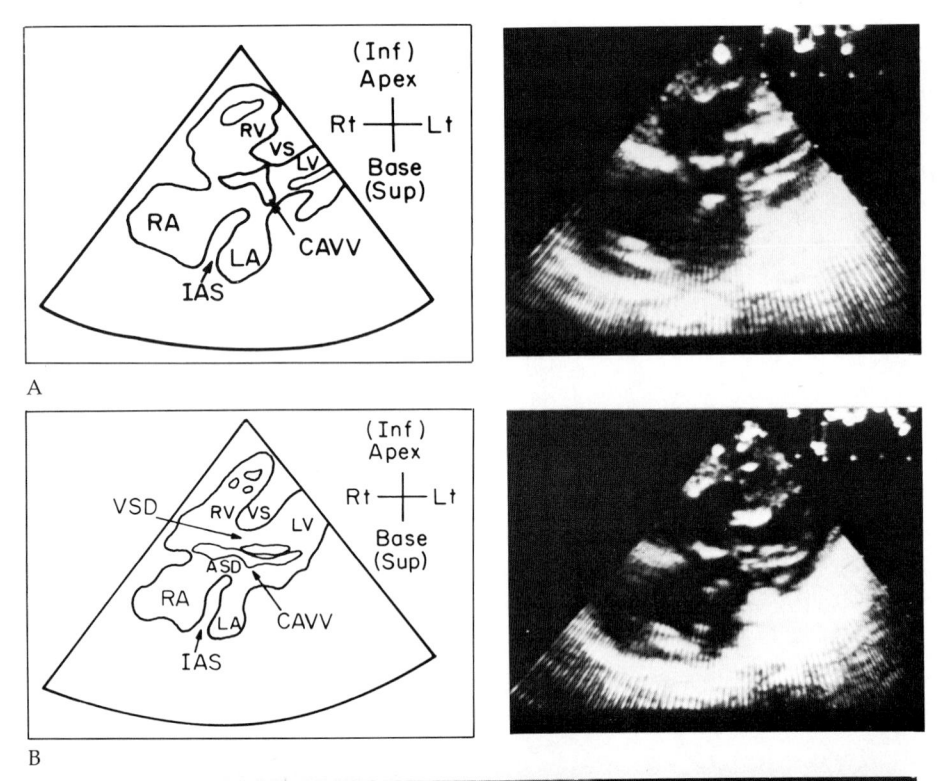

460 14. Acyanotic congenital heart disease with left-to-right shunt

Fig. 14-21A. Apical 4-chamber view in a patient with a Rastelli type A complete atrioventricular canal. Diastolic frame demonstrating the attachments of the common atrioventricular valve to the crest of the ventricular septum (VS). B. Systolic frame of same patient with common atrioventricular valve (CAVV) closed. There is echo dropout in the superior portion of the ventricular septum from a ventricular septal defect and in the inferior portion of the atrial septum from an atrial septal defect. C. Subcostal 4-chamber view from a patient with a Rastelli type B complete atrioventricular canal. The transducer is angled slightly to the right. The common atrioventricular valve (arrows) attaches to a large papillary muscle in the right ventricle. IAS = interatrial septum; VS = ventricular septum.

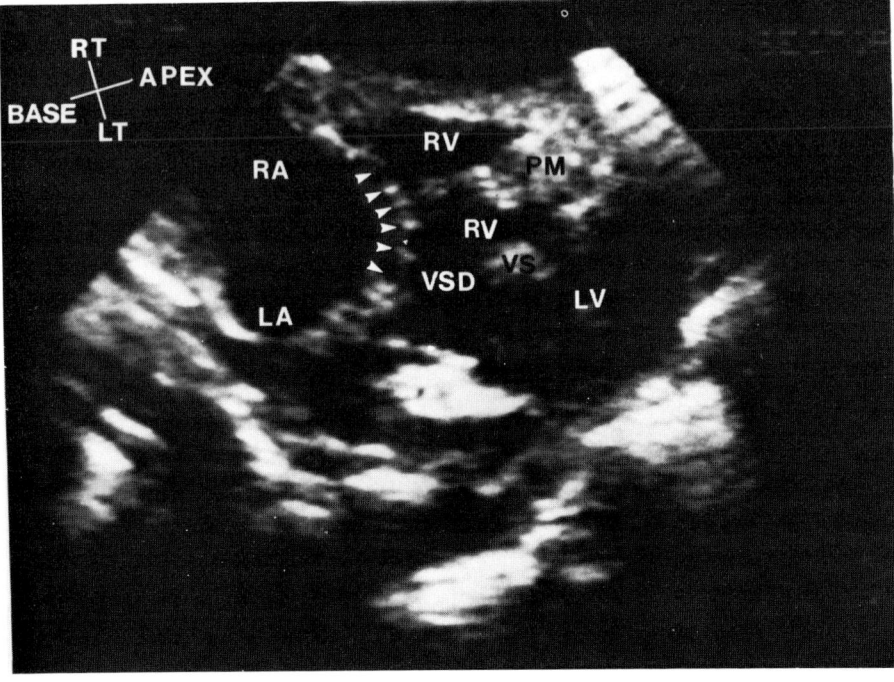

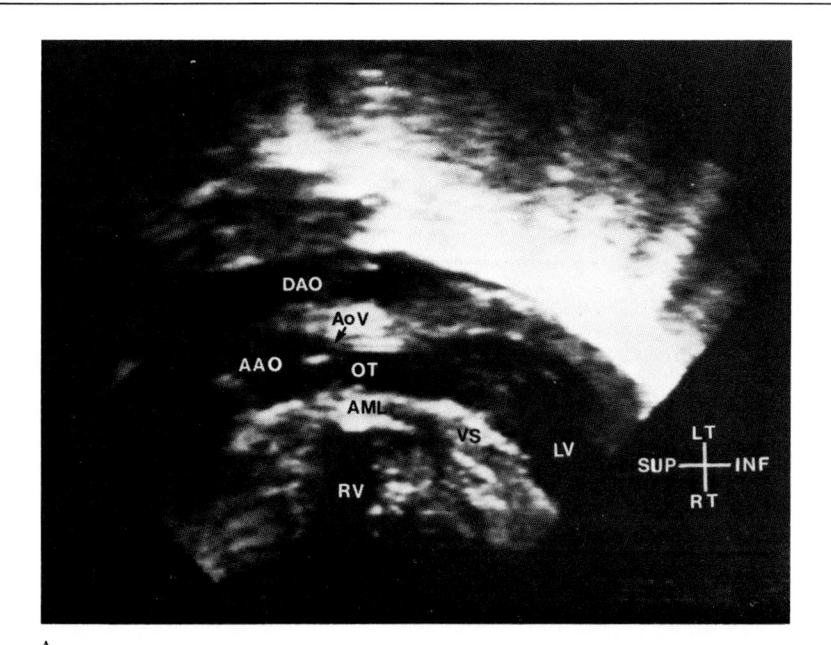

Fig. 14-22A. Subcostal long axis view of the left ventricle recorded from a patient with a complete endocardial cushion defect. There is a "goose neck" deformity of the outflow tract (OT) of the left ventricle produced by the abnormal anterior mitral leaflet. An early diastolic frame showing the OT to be narrow and clear of echo. The attachments of the anterior mitral leaflet to the ventricular septum (VS) are seen. B. Mid-diastolic frame shows the anterior mitral leaflet in the OT. The mitral valve movement into the OT reveals the ventricular septal defect. AoV = aortic valve.

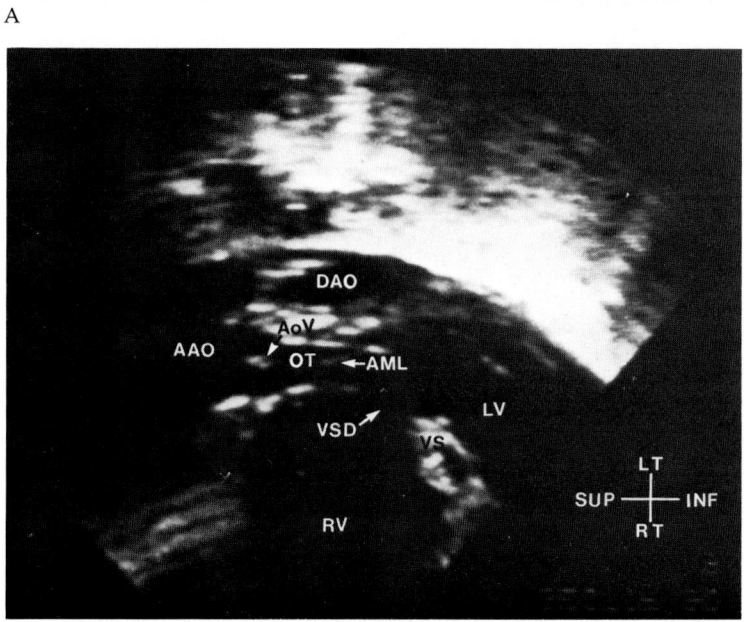

findings of partial atrioventricular canal were discussed in the section on primum atrial septal defects. Two-dimensional imaging allows the separation of complete atrioventricular canal into the three anatomic types described by Rastelli [32]. The apical four-chamber view permits visualization of the common atrioventricular valve and its relationship to the ventricular septal defect and ventricular septum. The chordal attachments of the common atrioventricular valve to the crest of the ventricular septum are imaged clearly in diastole in those patients with type A (Fig. 14-21). The chordal attachments of the left-sided portion of the common atrioventricular valve can be traced to a papillary muscle in the right ventricle in type B atrioventricular canal (Fig. 14-21C). In type C atrioventricular canal, a single (free-floating) anterior common leaflet is imaged. As with an ostium primum atrial septal defect, the goose neck deformity created by the abnormal mitral valve can be imaged from the subcostal window [25] (Fig. 14-22).

Patent ductus arteriosus

CLINICAL FEATURES AND PHYSIOLOGY. Patent ductus arteriosus is a clinical problem frequently found in the premature infant with hyaline membrane disease [35, 36]. Less frequently it is observed in children and adolescents. Its incidence in older children may increase with increased immigration from underdeveloped countries. The physical findings are typical of a run-off lesion. Bounding pulses are palpable. There is a prominent left ventricular impulse and a continuous murmur is heard in the second left intercostal space. Patients with large shunts develop congestive heart failure. However, most older patients have small shunts and are usually in good health. The chest radiograph and electrocardiogram reflect the magnitude of shunt.

M-MODE ECHOCARDIOGRAPHY. The M-mode features result from the left-to-right shunt. There is an increased left atrial dimension and left ventricular end-diastolic dimension [37, 38]. In newborn infants with an umbilical artery catheter positioned high in the thoracic aorta, contrast echocardiography has been used to establish a left-to-right ductal shunt [39, 40].

TWO-DIMENSIONAL ECHOCARDIOGRAPHY. Direct visualization of the ductus arteriosus by cross-sectional echocardiography is achieved by the short axis image at the base of the heart [41]. The transducer is tilted to image the main pulmonary artery and its bifurcation (Fig. 14-23). As the transducer is rotated superiorly from this position the ductus arteriosus is imaged as an area of echo dropout that produces a communication between the descending aorta and the pulmonary artery. Damping controls and overall gain settings must be adjusted to provide maximum background noise in order to achieve optimal imaging of ductal endothelium. In our experience there is variable echo dropout in the area of interest in normal subjects. This problem poses a considerable limitation to the accuracy of ductal imaging by two-dimensional echocardiography. We have, however, utilized suprasternal 2-D echo imaging in conjunction with contrast injections in the cardiac catheterization laboratory to reduce fluoroscopy time and in lieu of angiography (Fig. 14-24). Two-dimensional echocardiography also distinguishes patent ductus arteriosus from aortopulmonary window [42]. In the latter anomaly communication

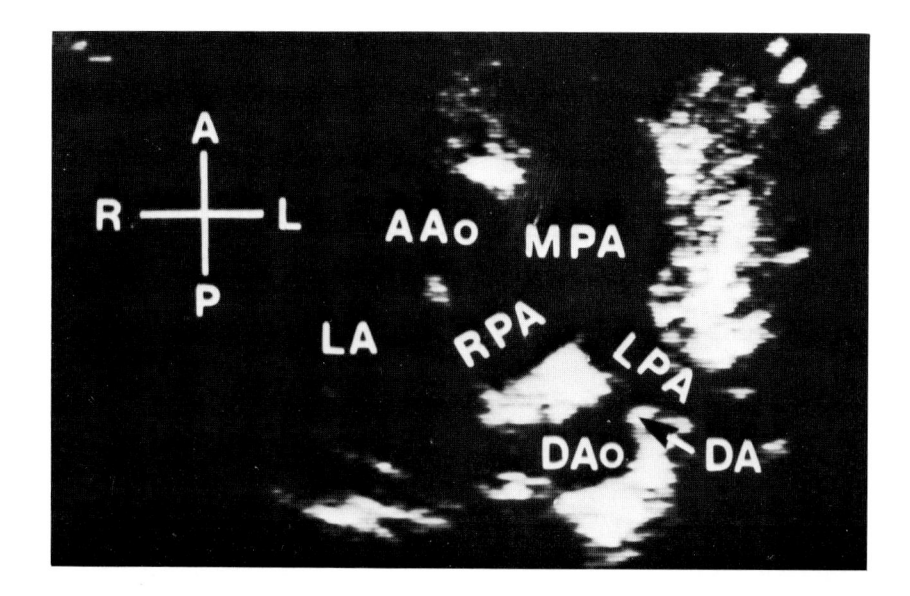

Fig. 14-23. Left parasternal short axis view at the cardiac base. With lateral angulation of the transducer both the right pulmonary artery (RPA) and left pulmonary artery (LPA) are imaged. In this plane a ductus arteriosus (DA) is seen as a communication between the LPA and descending aorta (DAo). AAo = ascending aorta; MPA = main pulmonary artery.

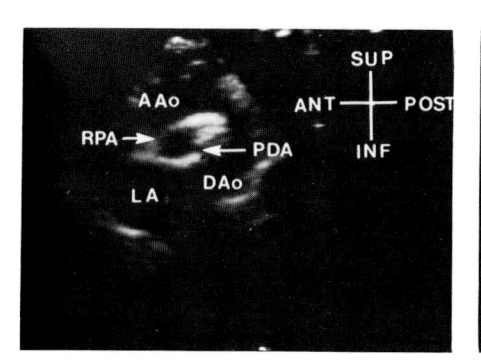

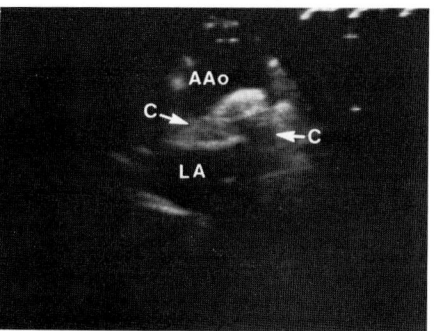

Fig. 14-24. Two-dimensional echocardiogram with a catheter in the descending aorta. After injection of indocyanine green dye, contrast (C) is seen crossing a patent ductus arteriosus (PDA) and filling the right pulmonary artery (RPA). In this patient the PDA is large and therefore appears to communicate directly with the RPA. Plane of sector is the suprasternal notch long axis.

between the aorta and pulmonary artery may be seen by utilizing a high parasternal short axis scan of the great arteries or by scanning anteriorly from the subcostal four-chamber view and imaging the ascending aorta [42].

References

1. Keith JD: Atrial Septal Defect: Ostium Secundum, Ostium Primum and Atrioventricular Communis. In JD Keith, RD Rowe, R Vlad (eds), *Heart Disease in Infancy and Childhood* (3rd ed). New York: Macmillan, 1978. Pp 380–404
2. Cooley DA, Hallman GL, Hammam AS: Congenital cardiovascular anomalies in adults: Results of surgical treatment in 167 patients over the age of 35. *Am J Cardiol* 17:303, 1966
3. Saksena FB, Aldridge HE: Atrial septal defect in the older patient: A clinical and hemodynamic study in patients operated on after age 35. *Circulation* 42:1009, 1970
4. Bedford DE, Sellors TH, Somerville W, Belcher JR, Besterman EMM: Atrial septal defect and its surgical treatment. *Lancet* 1:1255, 1957

5. Tajik AJ, Gau GT, Ritter DG, Schattenberg TT: Echocardiographic pattern of right ventricular diastolic volume overload in children. *Circulation* 46:36, 1972
6. Diamond MA, Dillon JC, Haine CL, Chang S, Feigenbaum H: Echocardiographic features of atrial septal defect. *Circulation* 43:129, 1971
7. Meyer RH, Schwartz DC, Benzing G, Kaplan S: Ventricular septum in right ventricular volume overload. *Am J Cardiol* 30:349, 1972
8. Hagan AD, Francis GS, Sahn DJ, Karliner JS, Friedman WF, O'Rourke RA: Ultrasound evaluation of systolic anterior motion in patients with and without right ventricular volume overload. *Circulation* 50:248, 1974
9. Bommer W, Weinert L, Neumann A, Neef J, Mason DT, DeMaria A: Determination of right atrial and right ventricular size by two-dimensional echocardiography. *Circulation* 60:91, 1979
10. DiSessa TG, Kirkman J, Hagan AD, Friedman WF: The Echocardiographic Evaluation of Patients with Atrial Septal Defects. In BL Tucker and GG Lindesmith (eds), *The Second Clinical Conference on Congenital Heart Disease*. New York: Grune & Stratton, 1982. Pp 31–47
11. Fontana GP, Kirkman JH, DiSessa TG, Hagan AD, Hiraishi S, Isabel-Jones J, Friedman WF: Evaluation of right ventricular and right atrial size in children with atrial septal defect using two-dimensional apex echocardiography. *JCU* 10:385, 1982
12. Bierman FZ, Williams RG: Subxiphoid two-dimensional imaging of the interatrial septum in infants and neonates with congenital heart disease. *Circulation* 60:80, 1979
13. Lange LW, Sahn DJ, Allen HD, Goldberg SJ: Subxiphoid cross-sectional echocardiography in infants and children with congenital heart disease. *Circulation* 59:513, 1979
14. Nasser FN, Tajik AJ, Seward JB, Hagler DJ: Diagnosis of sinus venosus atrial septal defect by two-dimensional echocardiography. *Mayo Clin Proc* 56:568, 1981
15. Tei C, Tanaka H, Kashima T, Yoshimura H, Minagoe S, Kanehisa T: Real-time cross-sectional echocardiographic evaluation of the interatrial septum by right atrium-interatrial septum-left atrium direction of the ultrasound beam. *Circulation* 60:539, 1979
16. Kronik G, Slany J, Moesslacher H: Contrast M-mode echocardiography in the diagnosis of atrial septal defect in acyanotic patients. *Circulation* 59:372, 1979
17. Fraker TD, Harris PJ, Behar VS, Kisslo JA: Detection and exclusion of interatrial shunts by two-dimensional echocardiography and peripheral venous injection. *Circulation* 59:379, 1979
18. Johnson SL, Baker DW, Lute RA, Dodge HT: Doppler echocardiography: The localization of cardiac murmurs. *Circulation* 48:810, 1973
19. Pearlman AS, Stenenson JG, Baker DW: Doppler echocardiography: Applications, limitations and future directions. *Am J Cardiol* 46:1256, 1980
20. Wakai CS, Edwards JE: Pathologic study of persistent common atrioventricular canal. *Am Heart J* 56:779, 1958
21. Steinfeld, L, Arnon R, Nazarian H: "Corrected" endocardial cushion defect. *Circulation* 62(Suppl III):III-73, 1980
22. Edwards JE: The problem of mitral insufficiency caused by accessory chordae tendineae in persistent common atrioventricular canal. *Proc Staff Meet Mayo Clin* 35:299, 1960
23. Williams RG, Rudd M: Echocardiographic features of endocardial cushion defects. *Circulation* 49:418, 1974
24. Hagler DJ, Tajik AJ, Seward JB, Mair DD, Ritter DG: Real-time wide-angle sector echocardiography: Atrioventricular canal defects. *Circulation* 59:140, 1979
25. Yoshida H, Funabashi T, Nakaya S, Maeda T, Taniguchi N: Subxiphoid cross-sectional echocardiographic imaging of the "goose neck" deformity in endocardial cushion defect. *Circulation* 62:1319, 1980
26. Beppu S, Nimura Y, Sakaibara H, Nagata S, Park YD, Baba K, Naito Y, Mitsushige O, Kamiya T, Koyanagi H, Fujita T: Mitral cleft in ostium primum atrial septal defect assessed by cross-sectional echocardiography. *Circulation* 62:1099, 1980
27. Silverman NH, Schiller NB: Apex echocardiography: A two-dimensional technique for evaluating congenital heart disease. *Circulation* 57:503, 1978
28. Becu LM, Fontana RS, DuShane JW, Kirklin JW, Burchell HB, Edwards JE: Anatomic and pathologic studies in ventricular septal defect. *Circulation* 14:349, 1956
29. Neufeld HN, Titus JL, DuShane JW, Burchell HB, Edwards JE: Isolated ventricular septal defect of the persistent common atrioventricular canal type. *Circulation* 23:685, 1961

30. Bierman FZ, Fellows K, Williams RG: Prospective identification of ventricular septal defects in infancy using subxiphoid two-dimensional echocardiography. *Circulation* 62:807, 1980
31. Stevenson JG, Kawabori L, Dooley T, Guntheroth WG: Diagnosis of ventricular septal defect by pulsed Doppler echocardiography—sensitivity, specificity and limitations. *Circulation* 58:322, 1978
32. Rastelli GC, Kirklin JW, Titus JL: Anatomic observations on complete form of persistent common atrioventricular canal with special reference to atrioventricular valves. *Mayo Clin Proc* 41:296, 1966
33. Bharati S, Lev M: The spectrum of common atrioventricular oriface (canal). *Am Heart J* 86:553, 1973
34. Mehta S, Hirschfeld S, Riggs T, Leibman J: Echocardiographic estimation of ventricular hypoplasia in complete atrioventricular canal. *Circulation* 59:888, 1979
35. Merritt TA, DiSessa TG, Feldman BH, Kirkpatrick SE, Gluck L, Friedman WF: Closure of the patent ductus arteriosus with ligation and indomethacin: A consecutive experience. *J Pediatr* 93:639, 1978
36. Jacob J, Gluck L, DiSessa TG, Edwards D, Kulovich M, Kurlinski J, Merritt TA, Friedman WF: Contribution of patent ductus arteriosus in the neonate with severe respiratory distress syndrome. *J Pediatr* 96:79, 1980
37. Baylen RB, Meyer RA, Kaplan S, Ringenburg WE, Korfhagan J: The critically ill premature infant with patent ductus arteriosus and pulmonary disease, and echocardiographic assessment. *J Pediatr* 86:423, 1975
38. Hirschklau MJ, DiSessa TG, Higgins CB, Friedman WF: Echocardiographic pitfalls in the premature infant with large patent ductus arteriosus. *J Pediatr* 92:474, 1978
39. Allen HD, Sahn DJ, Goldberg SJ: A new serial contrast technique for assessment of left-to-right shunting patent ductus arteriosus in the neonate. *Am J Cardiol* 41:288, 1978
40. Sahn DJ, Allen HD, Mason M, Goldberg SJ: The utility of contrast echocardiographic techniques in the care of critically ill infants with cardiac and pulmonary disease. *Circulation* 56:959, 1977
41. Sahn DJ, Allen HD: Real-time cross-sectional echocardiographic imaging and measurement of the patent ductus arteriosus in infants and children. *Circulation* 58:343, 1978
42. Rice MJ, Seward JB, Hagler DJ, Mair DD, Tajik AJ: Visualization of aortopulmonary window by two-dimensional echocardiography. *Mayo Clin Proc* 57:482, 1982

Congenital valvular, subvalvular, and supravalvular lesions

Ebstein's anomaly

CLINICAL FEATURES AND PHYSIOLOGY. Ebstein's anomaly is a congenital malformation of the tricuspid valve that is compatible with a long and relatively active life. Presence of cyanosis varies, but over 50 percent of patients will experience either persistent cyanosis or occasional episodes of arterial desaturation. When symptoms occur they are usually dyspnea, fatigue, and weakness. The patient may complain of palpitations secondary to an associated dysrhythmia. The auscultatory findings are quite characteristic. The first heart sound is widely split, and the second component has a clicking quality. The second heart sound is frequently single because of a soft pulmonic component. Third and fourth heart sounds are common and produce the classic triple and quadruple rhythm associated with Ebstein's anomaly [1, 2]. The murmur of tricuspid regurgitation may or may not be present. The electrocardiogram may reflect a right ventricular conduction delay, the various associated arrhythmias, or Wolff-Parkinson-White syndrome. The plain chest film may vary from near normal to massive cardiomegaly from an enlarged right atrium.

ANATOMY. The morphologic defect in Ebstein's anomaly consists of an inferior displacement of malformed portions of tricuspid valve tissue into the right ventricular cavity. The anterior leaflet is usually attached to the annulus fibrosus at its base. It attaches to the anterior and inferior walls of the right ventricle by means of chordae or papillary muscles, or in the form of a sheet. The leaflet is large and attached to one or more anterolateral papillary muscles. The base of the medial (septal) leaflet is displaced a varying distance downward into the right ventricle. The leaflet is relatively small and immobile. It is frequently hypoplastic or absent. The inferior (posterior) leaflet is displaced inferiorly into the ventricle and attaches to an aberrant inferior papillary muscle. This leaflet is often rudimentary and frequently absent [3–5]. The tricuspid valve deformity results in a large right-sided receiving chamber made up of an atrialized ventricle and true right atrium (Fig. 15-1).

M-MODE ECHOCARDIOGRAPHY. The M-mode features of Ebstein's anomaly are divided into those that are specific for the defect and those that are nonspecific. Nonspecific features include: (1) an increased excursion of the anterior leaflet of the tricuspid valve; (2) a reduced diastolic closure rate of the tricuspid valve; (3) abnormal anterior motion of the interventricular septum during systole; and (4) an increase in right ventricular dimension. Closure of the tricuspid valve more than 50 msec after mitral valve closure appears to be a specific characteristic of the anomaly [6–10].

TWO-DIMENSIONAL ECHOCARDIOGRAPHY. Two-dimensional echocardiography allows visualization of the specific morphologic defect in Ebstein's anomaly. In the left parasternal long axis view a large right ventricle is imaged. The anterior leaflet of the tricuspid valve appears elongated and thickened and it moves with a characteristic whipping motion [11]. The large "sail-like" anterior tricuspid leaflet can be seen also in the short axis view at the cardiac base. In this view its attachment to the

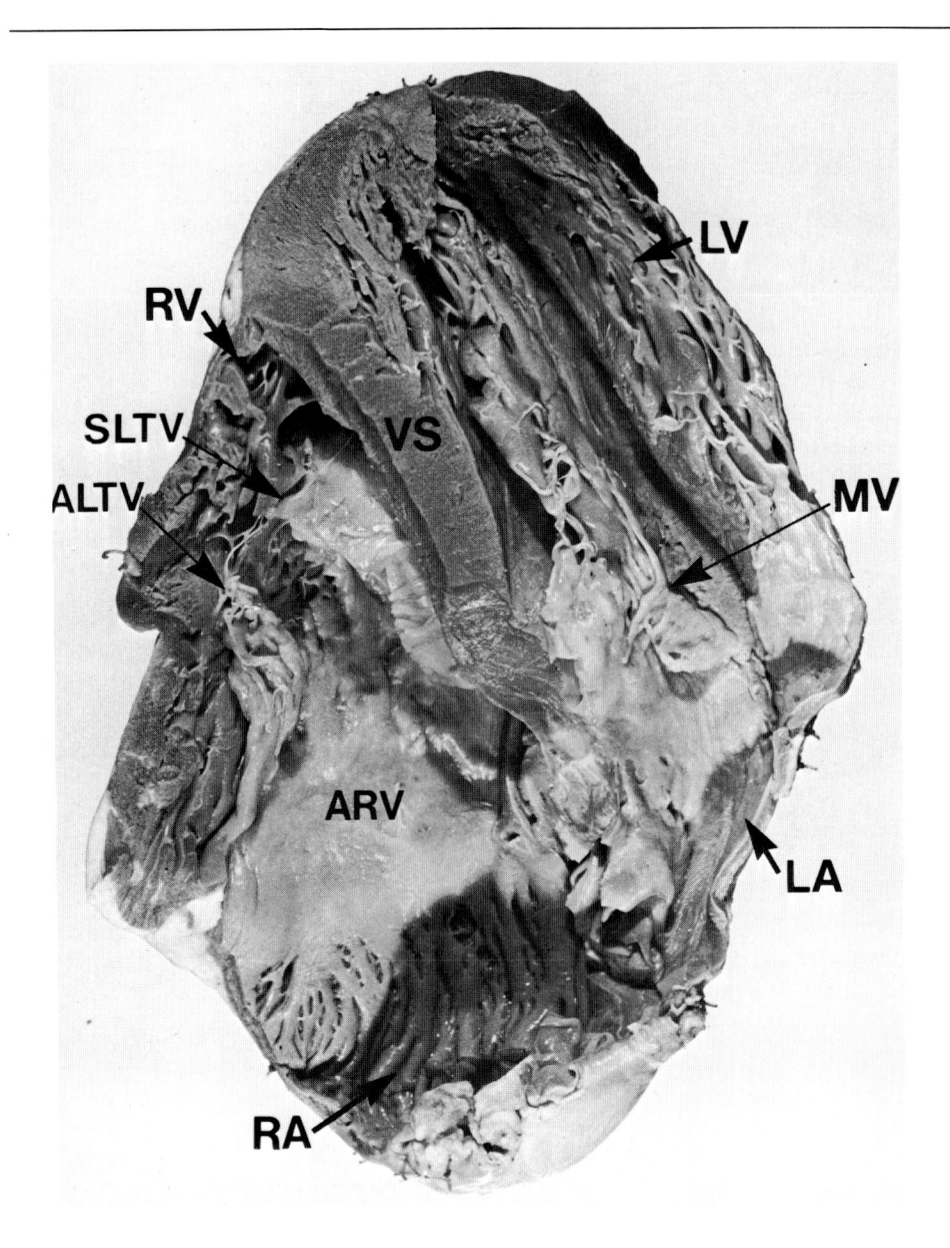

468   15. Congenital valvular, subvalvular, and supravalvular lesions

Fig. 15-1. Anatomic specimen of Ebstein's anomaly cut in the apical 4-chamber plane. The anterior leaflet of the tricuspid valve (ALTV) and septal leaflet of the tricuspid valve (SLTV) are displaced into the right ventricle. This displacement produces a small functional right ventricle and a large atrialized right ventricle (ARV). The pectinate muscles are seen in the right atrium. The left ventricle, left atrium, and mitral valve are normal. VS = ventricular septum.

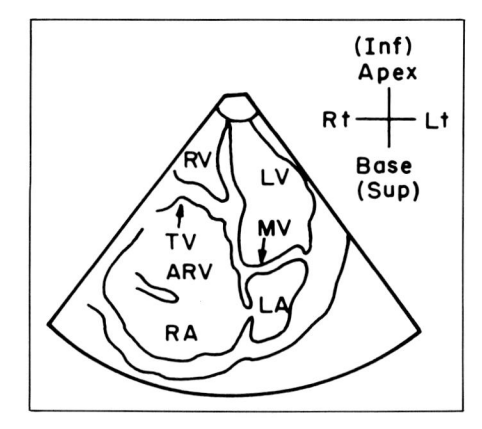

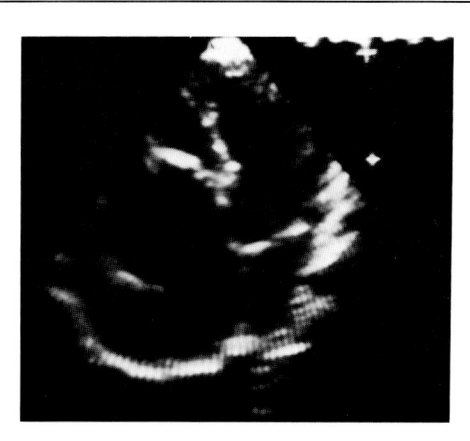

Fig. 15-2. Apical 4-chamber view recorded in a patient with Ebstein's anomaly. The tricuspid valve is seen displaced into the right ventricle. A large portion of the right ventricle is atrialized (ARV). The left ventricle, left atrium, and mitral valve are normal.

annulus fibrosus is difficult to define. However, the view aids in the estimation of right ventricular, right atrial, and pulmonary artery size. The apical four-chamber view best defines the anatomic features of the anomaly [12–15]. From this tomographic plane the tricuspid valve is seen displaced into the right ventricle. The relation of the tricuspid valve leaflets to the annulus of the valve is assessed easily. In a normal subject the tricuspid valve annulus is slightly inferior to the mitral valve ring in this view. The distance between the two annuli is approximately 5 mm. The septal and anterior tricuspid valve leaflets attach to the valve ring. In Ebstein's anomaly these leaflets can be seen displaced into the right ventricular cavity toward the apex. A clear image of the "atrialized" right ventricle is imaged between the valve leaflets and valve annulus (Fig. 15-2). The right atrium lies superior to the annulus fibrosus. Thus the size of the right ventricle, atrialized right ventricle, and right atrium may be assessed in the apical four-chamber view and the defect's degree of severity may be estimated [13]. The subcostal four-chamber view provides similar information. However, in patients with liver enlargement or tight abdominal muscles this cross-sectional plane may be difficult to image [14].

Isolated infundibular stenosis

CLINICAL FEATURES AND PHYSIOLOGY. Isolated infundibular stenosis is a rare congenital cardiac anomaly that produces obstruction to pulmonary blood flow without an associated ventricular septal defect [16]. Most patients are clinically in good health. In these patients a loud systolic murmur heard on routine examination is the first indication of heart disease. The murmur is usually associated with a right ventricular lift and a precordial thrill. The murmur is loud and heard well over the entire precordium. The electrocardiogram reveals right ventricular hypertrophy.

ANATOMY. The area of stenosis is composed of a ridge of fibrous tissue located in the infundibulum. In addition, a broad muscle band extends obliquely upward and across the lumen of the right ventricle [16].

M-MODE ECHOCARDIOGRAPHY. Characteristic changes in pulmonic valve motion have been described in patients with infundibular stenosis. These features are related to the turbulent flow across the pulmonic valve created by the infundibular obstruction. The depth of the "A" deflection remains normal. However, as the eddy currents pass across the valve in systole a characteristic chaotic motion is seen on the M-mode echocardiogram [17].

TWO-DIMENSIONAL ECHOCARDIOGRAPHY. The cross-sectional description of isolated infundibular stenosis has yet to be reported. The two-dimensional features of subpulmonic stenosis in tetralogy of Fallot are well described [18, 19]. The two cross-sectional views that best demonstrate the infundibular region are the short axis at the base with the beam directed toward the pulmonary artery and the right ventricular outflow view. The extent of narrowing may be better demonstrated by contrast echocardiography. The use of pulsed Doppler ultrasound in conjunction with two-dimensional imaging to detect the turbulent flow in the right ventricular outflow tract is discussed in Chapter 16.

Valvular pulmonic stenosis

CLINICAL FEATURES AND PHYSIOLOGY. The initial presentation of valvular pulmonic stenosis is the finding of a heart murmur on routine physical examination. In patients with mild stenosis the murmur begins after a pulmonic ejection sound, peaks in mid systole, and ends before the aortic component of the second heart sound. An increase in obstruction results in progressive lengthening of the murmur. In severe cases the murmur peaks in late systole and masks the aortic component of the second heart sound [20]. The murmur is best heard in the second left intercostal space along the parasternal border. Frequently a thrill may be palpated in the same area. The second heart sound is widely split. A prominent right ventricular impulse is always present. Right ventricular hypertrophy is usually present on the electrocardiogram, and chest radiography shows poststenotic dilatation of the pulmonary trunk.

ANATOMY. Characteristic changes in the pulmonic valve, seen at surgery or autopsy, include a dome shape, a narrow opening at the peak of the dome (Fig. 15-3), and commissural fusion. The valve tissue is usually thick and fibrous. Examination of the right ventricle reveals a concentric increase in wall thickness (Fig. 15-4). There is poststenotic dilatation of the pulmonary trunk [21].

M-MODE ECHOCARDIOGRAPHY. The traditional M-mode description of a stenotic pulmonic valve emphasizes an increased "A" deflection of the pulmonic valve echogram. An "A" wave depth of 7 to 10 mm has been measured in children and adults with moderate to severe stenosis [22, 23]. In patients with mild stenosis the pulmonic valve echo image is normal. The increase in "A" wave depth has been attributed to an increased force of right atrial contraction. This powerful right atrial impulse is transmitted through the right ventricle and produces the "A" deflection. The M-mode diagnosis of valvular pulmonic stenosis has a number of limitations, including difficulty in visualizing the diastolic motion of the pulmonic valve and the fact that the M-mode image does not allow direct visualization of the stenotic valve. M-mode information is only indirect evidence of a stenotic valve and is not specific for the anomaly [24].

471

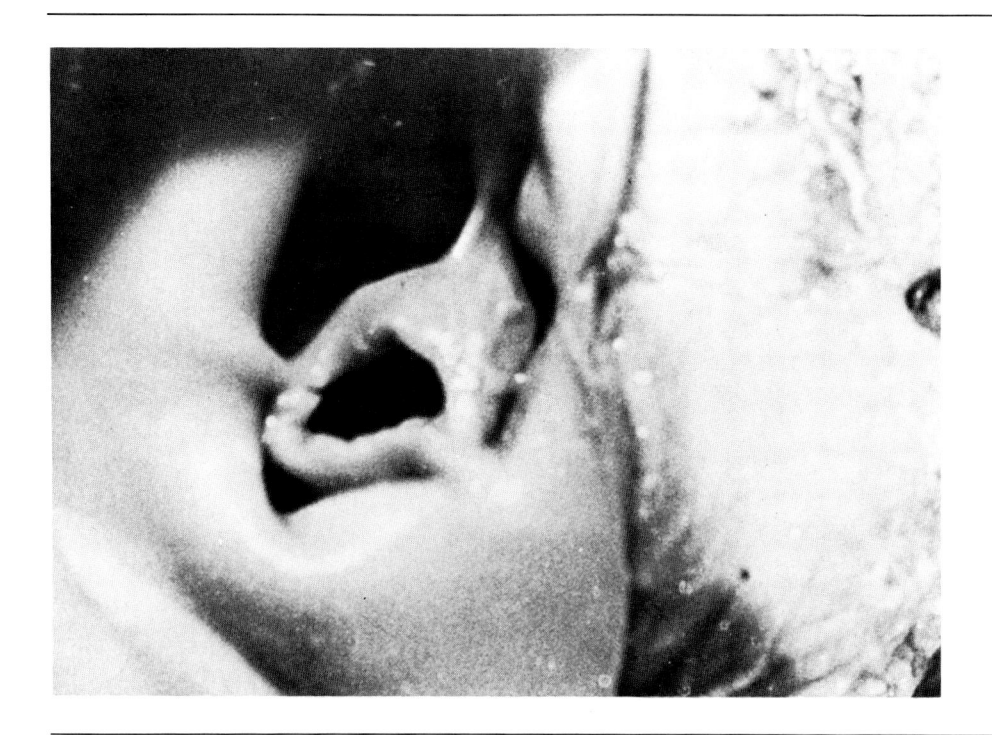

Fig. 15-3. Anatomic specimen of a stenotic pulmonic valve. The valve is dome-shaped. At the peak of the dome there is a narrow opening. Fusion of the three commissures is also visible.

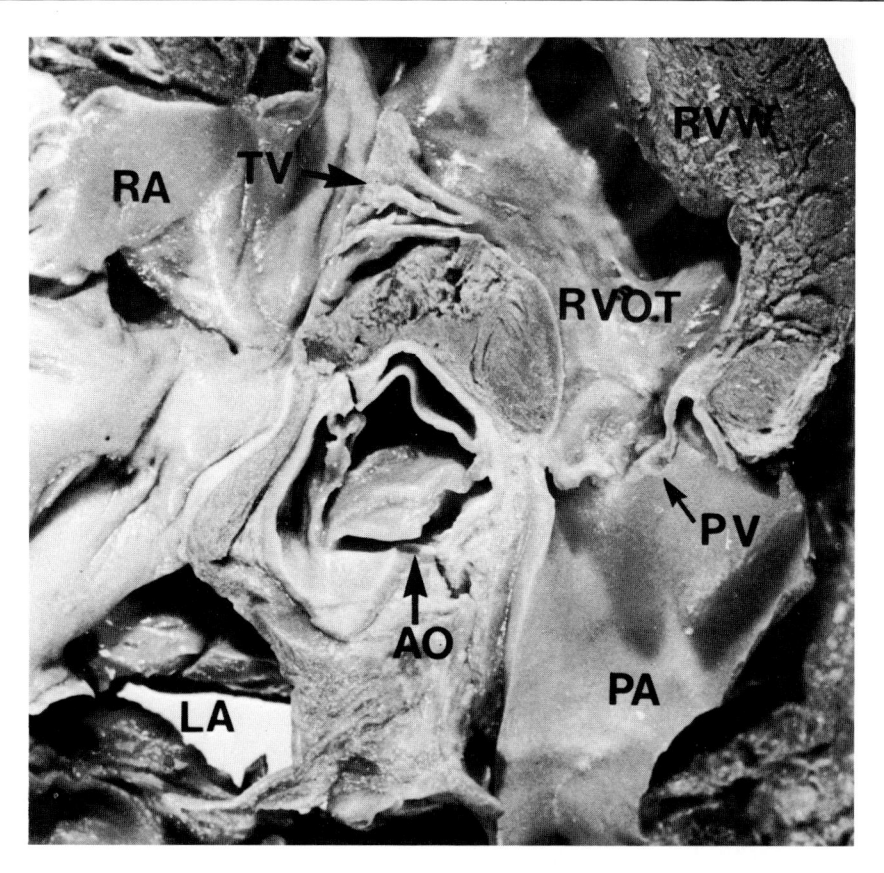

Fig. 15-4. Anatomic specimen of a stenotic pulmonic valve. The heart is cut in the short axis at the cardiac base. The pulmonic valve (PV) domes and is thickened. The right ventricular wall (RVW) is hypertrophied. PA = pulmonary artery.

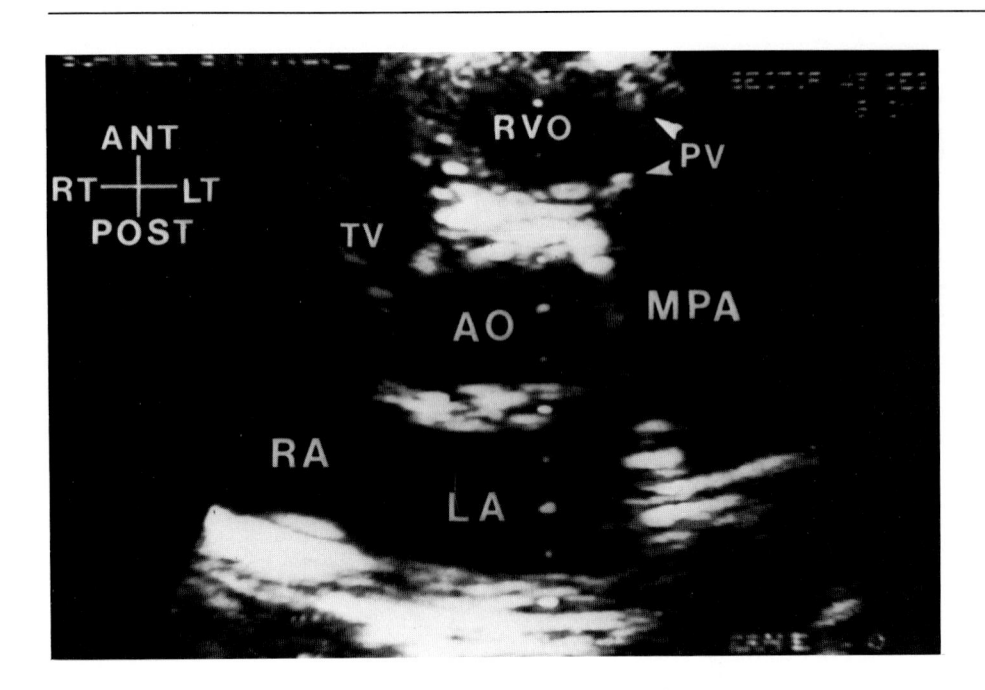

Fig. 15-5. *A two-dimensional echocardiogram during systole of a stenotic domed pulmonic valve (PV). Plane of sector is the short axis at the cardiac base.*

TWO-DIMENSIONAL ECHOCARDIOGRAPHY. The pulmonic valve may be imaged from three tomographic cross-sections, the left parasternal short axis at the cardiac base, the left parasternal long axis of the right ventricular outflow tract, and the subcostal long axis of the right ventricular outflow tract. Weyman and associates used a mechanical sector scanner and examined the pulmonic valve in the short axis at the cardiac base [24]. These authors found two-dimensional imaging of the pulmonic valve superior to M-mode techniques. The stenotic pulmonic valve produces a characteristic motion. The valve curves inward to the midportion of the main pulmonary artery in systole. This motion abnormality produces systolic doming of the stenotic valve (Fig. 15-5). The base of the pulmonic valve leaflet moves through a wide arc while the rim of the leaflets remain in close proximity. Diastolic motion of the stenotic valve is the same in normal subjects as in patients with valvular stenosis [24]. Using the subcostal window and a mechanical sector scanner, Sahn and colleagues have been able to differentiate infundibular from valvular pulmonic stenosis [18].

Range-gated pulsed Doppler ultrasound has been combined with the M-mode image to evaluate valvular pulmonic stenosis [25]. The M-mode image enables the operator to position the Doppler sample volume in the right ventricular outflow tract proximal to the pulmonic valve and in the pulmonary artery distal to the pulmonic valve. Turbulent flow recorded in the pulmonary artery and not in the outflow tract is evidence for pulmonic valve stenosis. Using this method, Goldberg and associates were able to detect turbulent flow in 13 of 14 children with pulmonic stenosis and 3 of 52 controls [25]. It appears, therefore, that range-gated pulsed Doppler ultrasound is an accurate method for detection of valvular pulmonic stenosis. To date, however, the stethoscope and phonocardiogram remain the best methods for evaluating the severity of stenosis [26].

Left ventricular inflow tract obstruction (cor triatriatum, supravalvular mitral ring, parachute mitral valve, and congenital mitral stenosis)

CLINICAL FEATURES AND PHYSIOLOGY. Patients with these conditions develop symptoms of congestive heart failure early in infancy. Obstruction to left ventricular inflow results in pulmonary venous hypertension, pulmonary edema, tachypnea, dyspnea, and tachycardia. Patients with severe obstruction may have episodes of syncope. A prominent right ventricular impulse may be felt on precordial palpation. In patients with cor triatriatum or an isolated supravalvular mitral ring a diastolic rumble similar to the rumble of mitral stenosis is heard. Children with a parachute mitral valve have both stenotic and regurgitant murmurs. Radiographic examination reveals cardiomegaly and pulmonary edema. Electrocardiography usually shows right ventricular hypertrophy. Frequently these anomalies appear together with membranous subaortic stenosis and coarctation of the aorta (Shone's complex) [26]. Congenital mitral stenosis is similar in presentation.

ANATOMY. In patients with cor triatriatum a thick fibrous diaphragm separates an accessory chamber from the left atrium. Communication with the left atrium is usually accomplished via a small hole in the diaphragm (Fig. 15-6). A supravalvular mitral ring is a rim of connective tissue that encircles the mitral valve orifice and prolapses into it. It originates on the left atrial wall above the mitral annulus [26–28]. The membrane may be obstructive or nonobstructive. The mitral valve leaflets and supporting apparatus of a parachute mitral valve constitute a complex anomaly. The leaflets and commissures of the mitral valve are normal. The chordae tendineae are shortened. They fuse and converge onto a solitary papillary muscle to form a funnel-shaped inflow to the left ventricle [26]. The mitral valve in congenital mitral stenosis is similar to the rheumatic mitral valve. The interchordal spaces are reduced, the leaflets are thickened and fibrotic, and the two papillary muscles are fibrosed [29, 30].

M-MODE ECHOCARDIOGRAPHY. All three forms of left ventricular inflow tract obstruction have similar M-mode echocardiographic findings, including diastolic flutter of the mitral valve, anterior motion of the posterior leaflet of the mitral valve in diastole, absent mitral valve "A" wave, reduced D–E excursion and E–F slope, and anomalous echoes in the mitral valve funnel [31–33].

TWO-DIMENSIONAL ECHOCARDIOGRAPHY. Snider and associates described the cross-sectional features of these inflow tract anomalies [33]. In patients with a supravalvular membrane in the left atrium the diaphragm is seen as a linear echo stretching obliquely across the left atrial cavity above the mitral valve in the left parasternal long axis view (Fig. 15-7). The membrane image moves toward the mitral valve in diastole and in superior direction in systole. In the apical four-chamber view the left atrial diaphragm is visualized stretching across the left atrium above the mitral valve (Fig. 15-8). The cross-sectional features of cor triatriatum are similar to those of a supravalvular mitral ring (Fig. 15-9). The mitral valve in patients with congenital mitral stenosis appears thickened in all tomographic views of examination. The valve moves poorly and has a diminished diastolic excursion. In the short axis view there are two distinct papillary muscles. In contrast the short

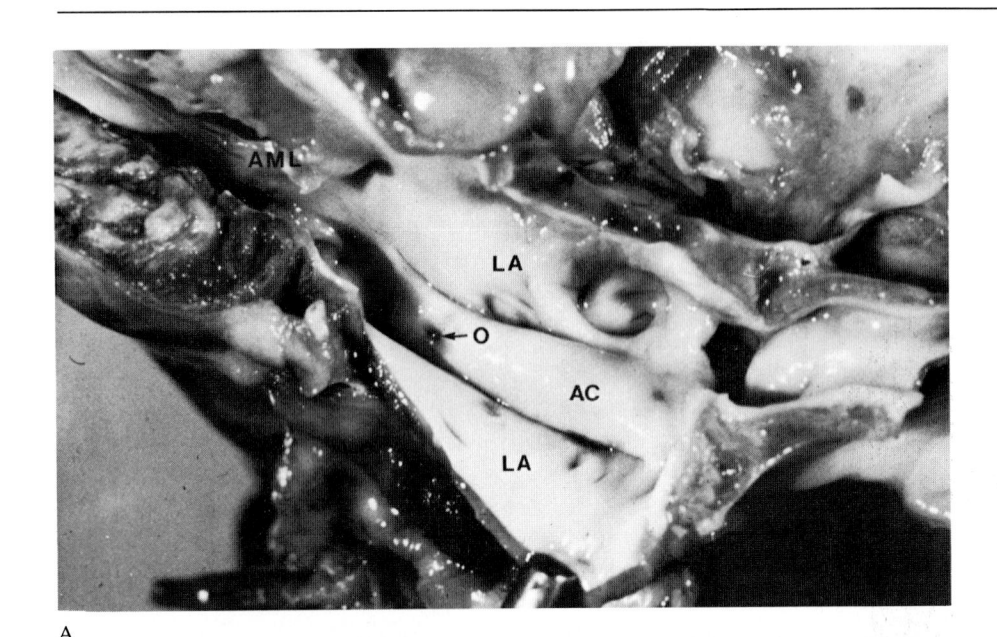

474   15. Congenital valvular, subvalvular, and supravalvular lesions

Fig. 15-6A. Anatomic specimen from a patient with cor triatriatum. An incision is made into the left atrial chamber. The accessory chamber (AC) communicates with the left atrium through a small orifice (O) in a thick fibrous diaphragm. B. In this view, the accessory chamber is opened. The pulmonary veins (PV) are seen draining into the accessory chamber. (From C Bloor, Cardiac Pathology. Philadelphia: Lippincott, 1978.)

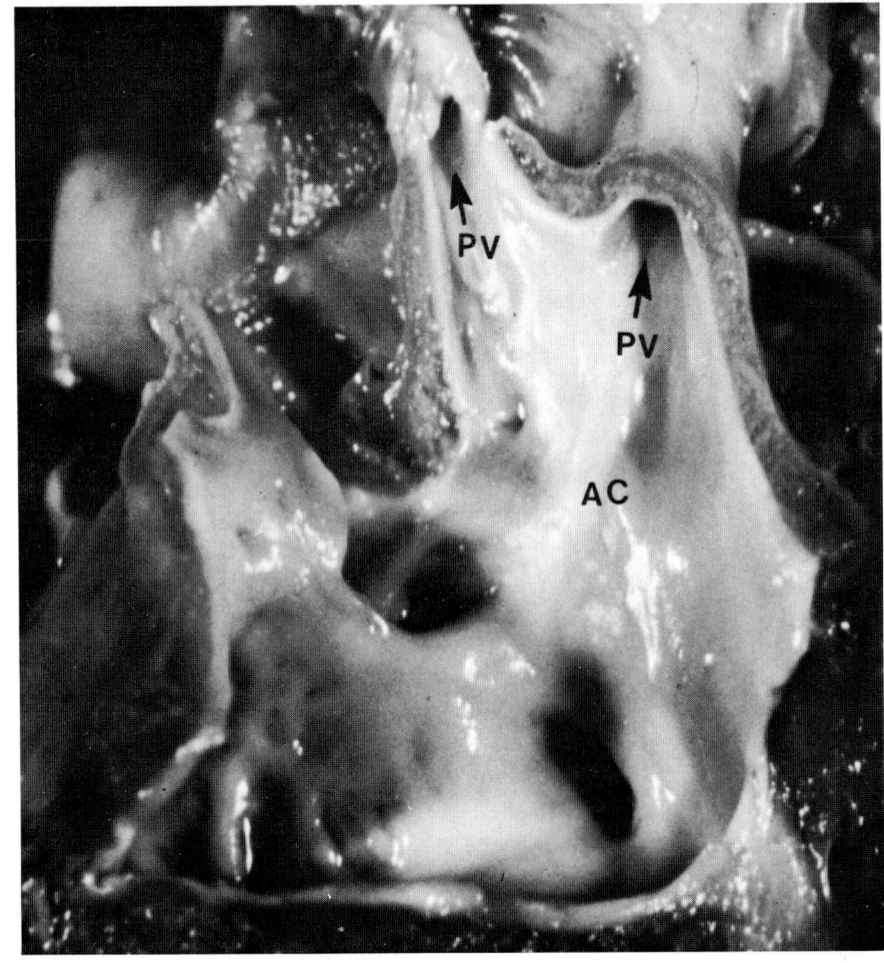

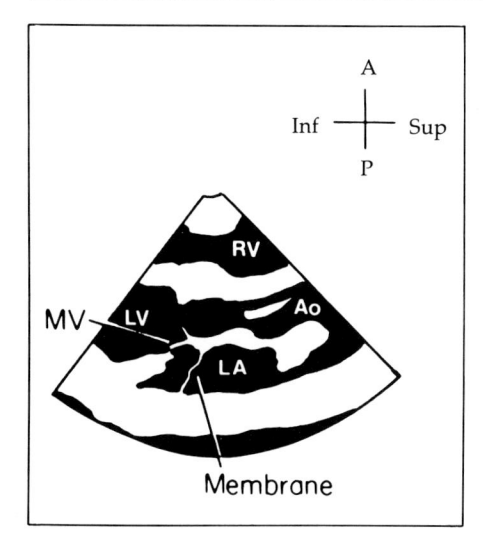

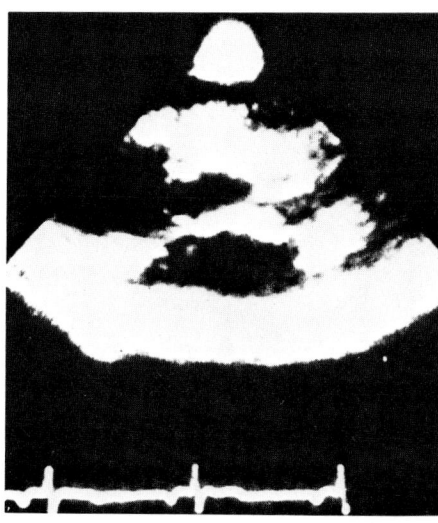

Fig. 15-7. Long axis view recorded from a patient with a supravalvular mitral ring. The membrane is imaged stretching above the mitral valve within the left atrium. (From R Snider et al, Congenital left ventricular inflow obstruction evaluated by two dimensional echocardiography. Circulation 61:848, 1980 by permission from the American Heart Association, Inc.)

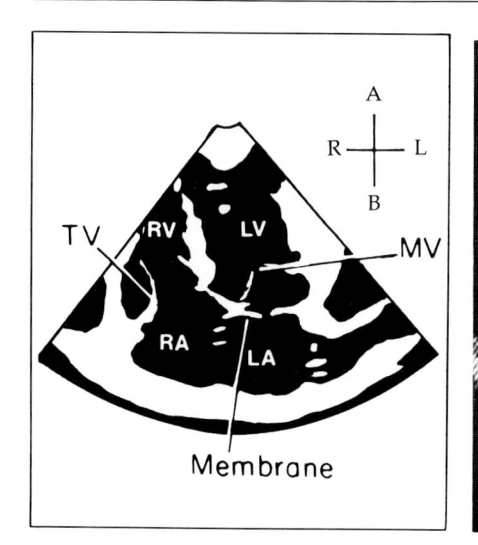

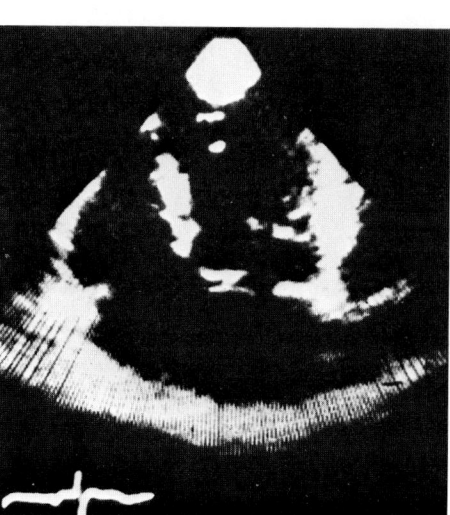

Fig. 15-8. Apical 4-chamber view recorded from a 14-year-old child with a supravalvular mitral ring. In this view the membrane is imaged above the mitral valve echo in the left atrium. A = apex; B = base. (From R Snider et al, Congenital left ventricular inflow obstruction evaluated by two dimensional echocardiography. Circulation 61:848, 1980 by permission from the American Heart Association, Inc.)

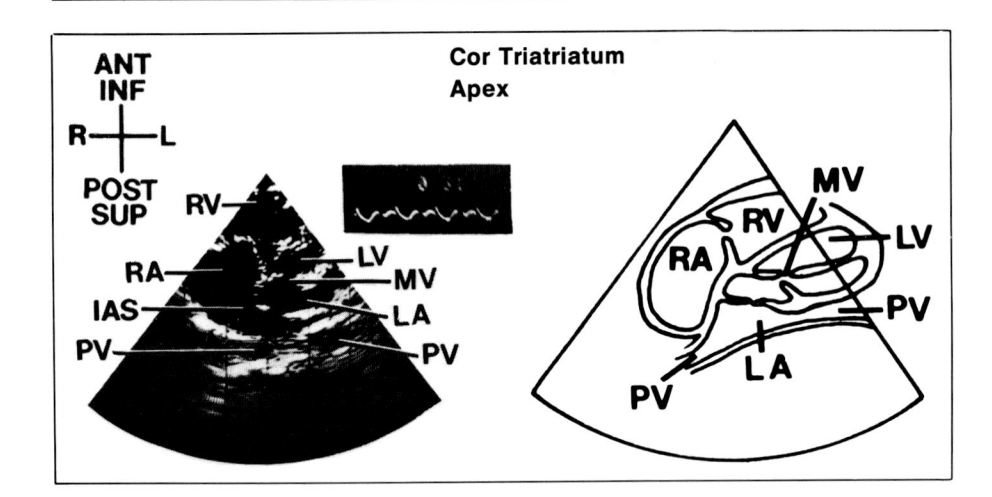

476   15. Congenital valvular, subvalvular, and supravalvular lesions

Fig. 15-9. Apical 4-chamber view recorded from a patient with cor triatriatum. A diaphragm is noted in the left atrium. This diaphragm separates the pulmonary veins (PV) from the LA. IAS = interatrial septum. (From D Sahn et al, Cross-sectional echocardiographic diagnosis of the sites of total anomalous pulmonary venous drainage. Circulation 60:1317, 1979 by permission of the American Heart Association, Inc.)

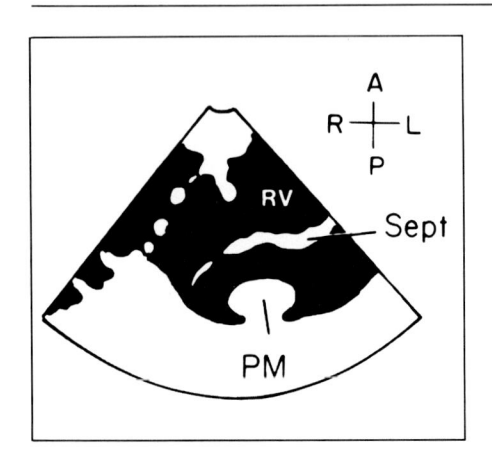

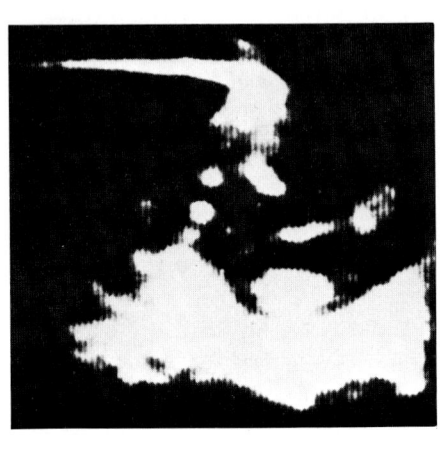

Fig. 15-10. Short axis view at the cardiac apex. A single large papillary muscle is seen in a patient with a parachute mitral valve. Sept = septum. (From R Snider et al, Congenital left ventricular inflow obstruction evaluated by two dimensional echocardiography. Circulation 61:848, 1980 by permission of the American Heart Association, Inc.)

axis image of a parachute mitral valve reveals only one large papillary muscle (Fig. 15-10). The parachute mitral valve moves in a fashion similar to that of the stenotic valve with two papillary muscles [33].

Discrete subaortic stenosis

CLINICAL FEATURES AND PHYSIOLOGY. Most children with this anomaly are asymptomatic and are referred for evaluation of a heart murmur [34]. There is a systolic crescendo-decrescendo murmur usually maximal at the midleft sternal border with radiation to the base. An aortic insufficiency murmur is audible in approximately 55 percent of cases. A palpable left ventricular heave is frequently present. On electrocardiogram there are changes consistent with left ventricular hypertrophy. Findings on chest x-ray depend upon the presence or absence of congestive heart failure and associated lesions.

ANATOMY. Fixed discrete subaortic stenosis is classified into three types. Obstruction may be membranous, in which a thin fibrous diaphragm encircles the left ventricular outflow tract below the aortic valve (Fig. 15-11). The membrane attaches to the ventricular septum and anterior leaflet of the mitral valve (Fig. 15-12). In patients with fibromuscular obstruction a muscular base to the fibrous membrane forms a collarlike obstruction to the left ventricular outflow tract (Fig. 15-11). The most severe form of subaortic obstruction is fibromuscular tunnel, in which there is diffuse narrowing of the left ventricular outflow tract [34-36].

M-MODE ECHOCARDIOGRAPHY. The M-mode echocardiographic features of discrete subaortic stenosis are useful in diagnosis, but considerable limitations exist. Motion abnormalities of the aortic valve such as brisk early closure of the aortic leaflets and systolic fluttering serve to distinguish valvular aortic stenosis from subvalvular obstruction [37-41]. The echocardiographic manifestations of aortic valve preclosure depend on beam angulation, stiffness of the aortic valve, and the direction of the jet as it crosses the aortic valve. A ratio of the left ventricular outflow tract dimension to aortic root dimension has been utilized to estimate the severity of obstruction [38, 40]. Narrowing of the left ventricular outflow tract observed on M-mode scan is highly dependent on scan speed. A fast scan may produce a normal outflow tract appearance, when, indeed, narrowing exists [42].

TWO-DIMENSIONAL ECHOCARDIOGRAPHY. The two-dimensional echocardiographic features of discrete subaortic stenosis have been well described [42-48]. The initial definition of the pathologic anatomy used a linear-array scanner [43]. The characteristics depicted were narrowing of the left ventricular outflow tract in all phases of the cardiac cycle. Subsequent studies using both mechanical and phased-array sector scanners have accurately differentiated the three anatomic types of discrete subaortic stenosis [42, 44-46]. It appears that cross-sectional echocardiography more accurately depicts the site and type of obstruction than angiocardiography [42, 45]. The left ventricular outflow tract may be examined from the left parasternal long axis or apical long axis view. From the left parasternal long axis view fibromembranous subaortic stenosis appears as a double linear echo in the left ventricular outflow tract beneath the aortic valve (Fig. 15-13). These

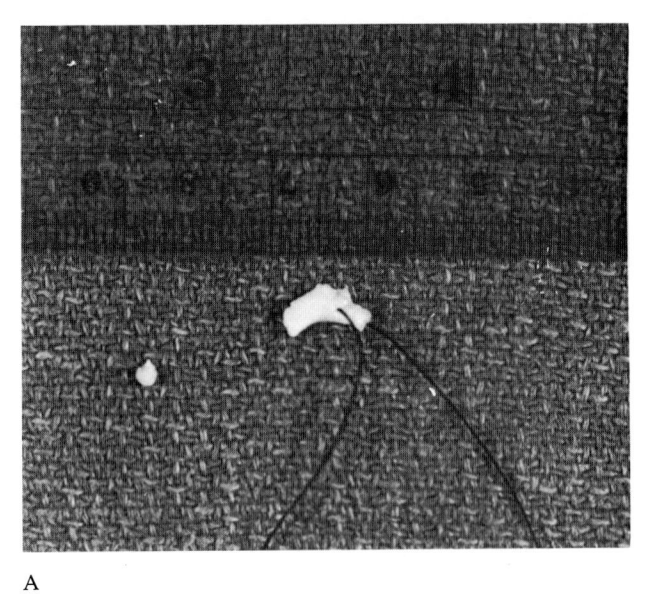

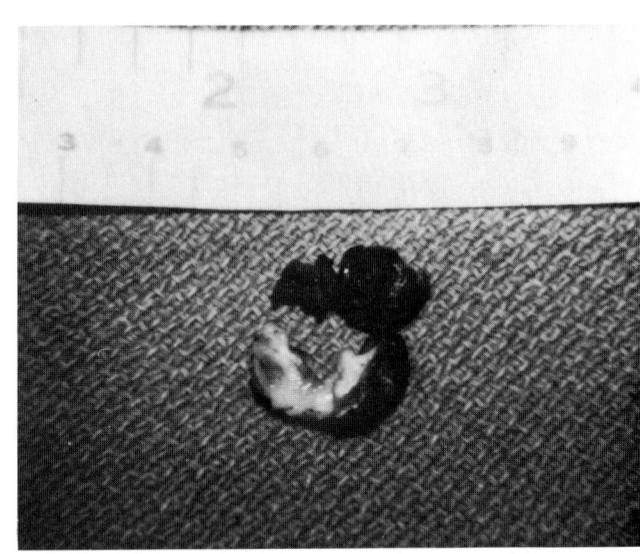

478 15. Congenital valvular, subvalvular, and supravalvular lesions

Fig. 15-11. Surgical specimen. A. Thick fibrous membrane removed from a patient with a discrete fibrous diaphragm beneath the aortic valve. B. Fibrous tissue and muscle base removed from a patient with fibromuscular subaortic stenosis. (From TG DiSessa et al, Am Heart J *101:774, 1981.)*

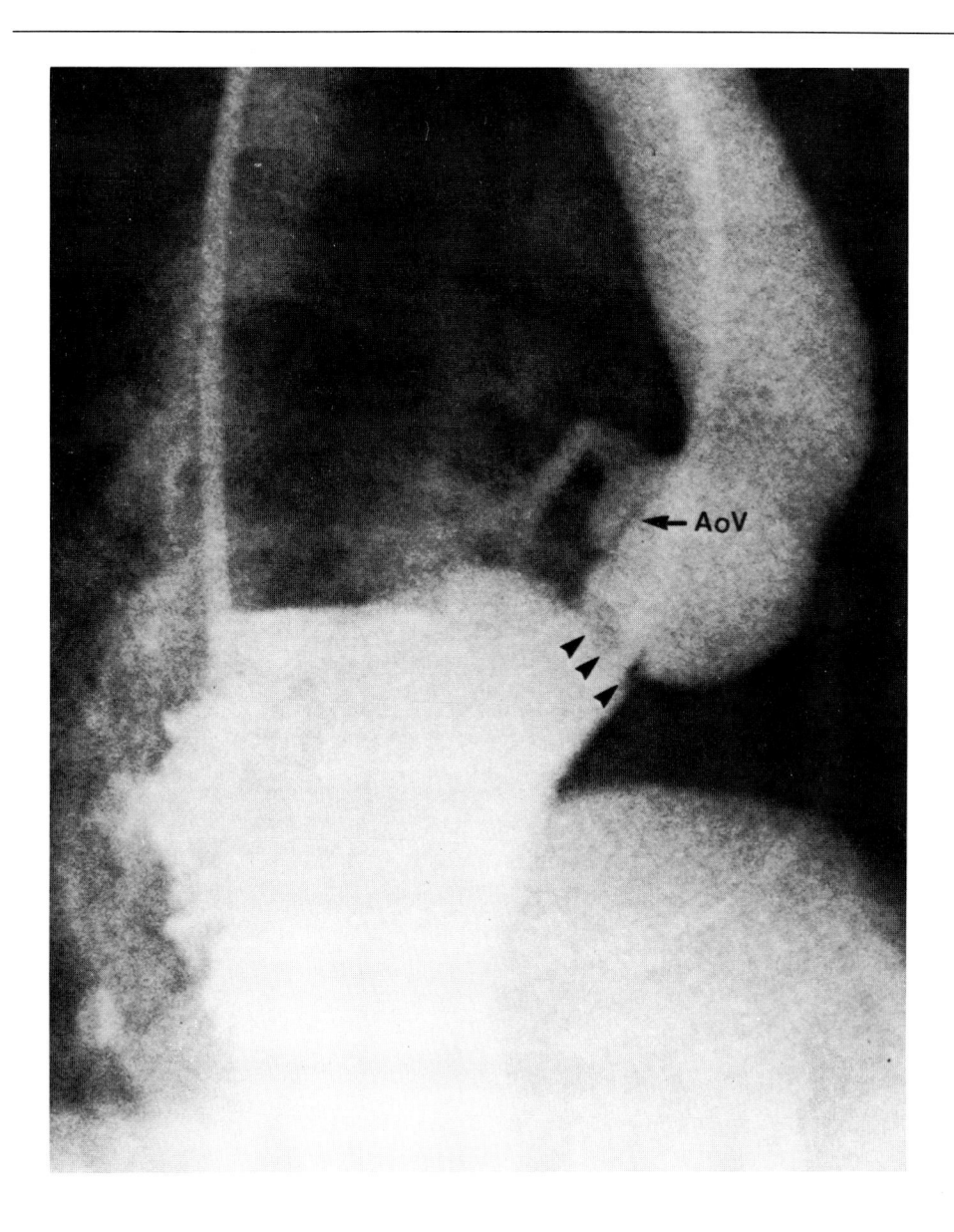

Fig. 15-12. *Left ventricular cineangiocardiogram obtained in the long axis oblique projection demonstrating the attachments of a fibrous subaortic diaphragm to the ventricular septum and the mitral valve* (arrows). AoV = *aortic valve.*

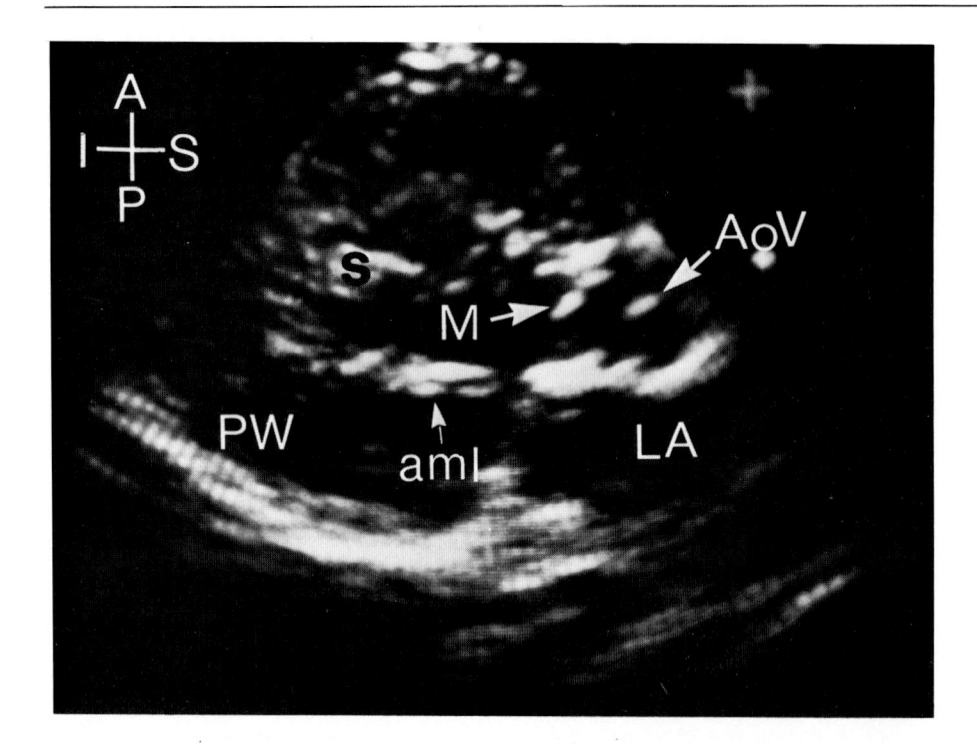

480   15. Congenital valvular, subvalvular, and supravalvular lesions

Fig. 15-13. Left parasternal long axis view recorded from a 23-year-old patient with a discrete subaortic fibrous diaphragm. The membrane (M) is imaged as a double linear echo beneath the aortic valve (AoV). These echoes are a result of a smear artifact from the blood tissue interface. PW = posterior wall; S = superior. (From TG DiSessa et al, Am Heart J 101:774, 1981.)

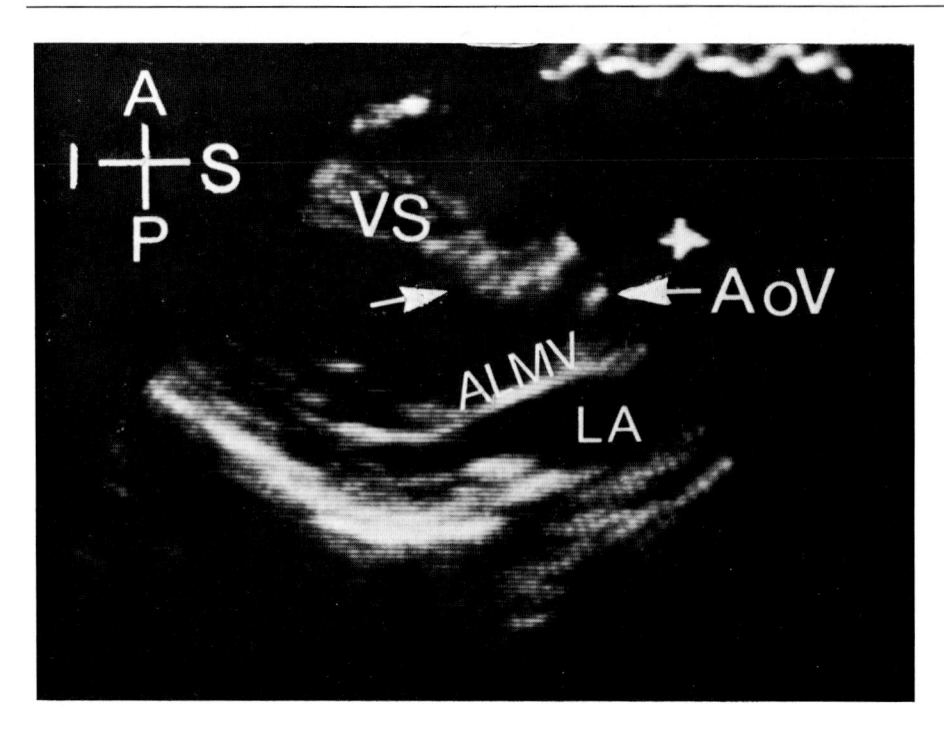

Fig. 15-14. Left parasternal long axis view recorded from a patient with discrete fibromuscular subaortic stenosis. A dense ridge of echoes (left arrow) is seen attached to the left side of the ventricular septum (VS). ALMV = anterior leaflet of the mitral valve; AoV = aortic valve; S = superior. (From TG DiSessa et al, Am Heart J 101:774, 1981.)

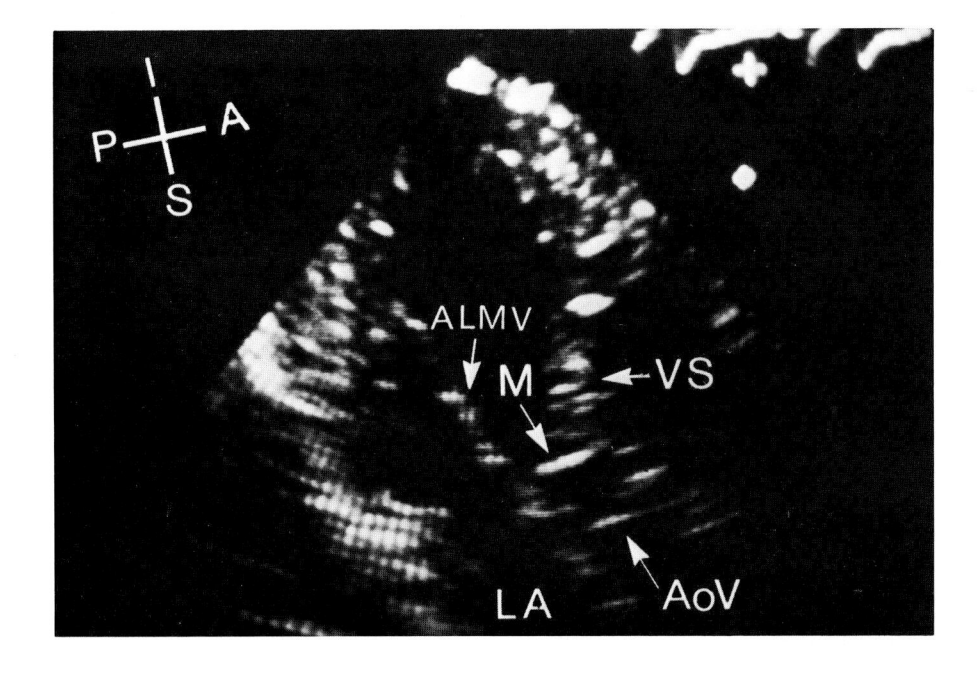

Fig. 15-15. Apical long axis view in discrete membranous subaortic stenosis. The fibrous membrane (M) is seen in the left ventricular outflow tract beneath and parallel to the aortic valve (AoV). The membrane extends from the ventricular septum (VS) to the anterior leaflet of the mitral valve (ALMV). S = superior. (From TG DiSessa et al, Am Heart J 101:774, 1981.)

echoes are parallel to the ventricular septum and are considered to result from a smear artifact that is produced by the "blood tissue interface at the inner margins of the fibrous membrane" [44]. Discrete fibromuscular obstruction produces a thick ridge of echoes that appear attached to the ventricular septum and extend into the left ventricular outflow tract below the aortic valve (Fig. 15-14). Tunnel obstruction produces diffuse narrowing of the left ventricular outflow tract. From the apical long axis view a fibrous diaphagm is imaged as a linear echo that extends across the left ventricular outflow tract from the ventricular septum to the mitral valve parallel to and beneath the aortic valve (Fig. 15-15). This difference in membrane imaging appears to be related to the more perpendicular relationship of the echo beam to all portions of the membrane from the apical long axis view [42]. Fibromuscular obstruction produces a thickened ridge on the ventricular septum when viewed from the typical long axis image.

Congenital aortic stenosis (bicuspid aortic valve)

CLINICAL FEATURES AND PHYSIOLOGY. Congenital aortic stenosis is a common anomaly that accounts for approximately 6 percent of all forms of congenital heart disease. The deformed aortic valve is most often bicuspid. Indeed the bicuspid nonstenotic aortic valve is probably the most common anomaly first diagnosed in adulthood. Patients with a stenotic aortic valve fall in three groups: infants presenting in congestive heart failure, the adolescent child who is commonly asymptomatic, and the adult in the fifth decade and beyond. We will confine our statements to the adolescent with bicuspid stenotic or nonstenotic aortic valve. It is not within the scope of this text to discuss the first group, and the third group is

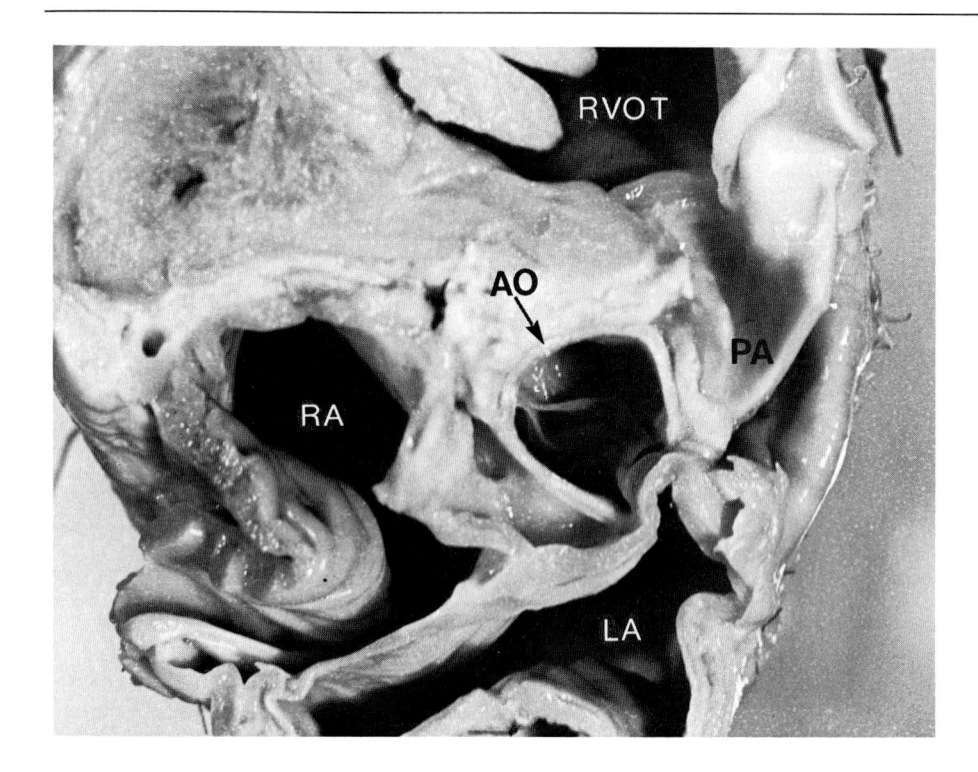

Fig. 15-16. Anatomic specimen of a bicuspid aortic valve cut in the short axis plane at the cardiac base. The aortic valve has a characteristic fishmouth appearance. PA = pulmonary artery.

discussed in detail in Chapter 4. Ninety-five percent of patients with coarctation of the aorta have a bicuspid aortic valve. We have studied 35 patients with Turner's syndrome and have found a 27 percent incidence of bicuspid nonstenotic aortic valve in this group of patients.

Most adolescents with aortic stenosis are asymptomatic and are referred for evaluation of a cardiac murmur. Because of the possibility of sudden death, it is important to select patients with severe stenosis for catheterization and surgery. Clinical findings that herald significant outlet obstruction include a left ventricular lift and a loud systolic murmur associated with a precordial thrill. Paradoxical splitting of the second heart sound usually signals severe obstruction. The electrocardiogram and vectorcardiogram may be normal in numerous children with severe stenosis. The chest x-ray is usually normal. Exercise-induced S–T segment changes indicate a left ventricular-to-aortic root pressure difference of at least 50 mm Hg [49]. A joint study on the natural history of congenital heart disease established a formula for the estimation of peak systolic pressure difference across the aortic valve in patients without changes indicative of myocardial ischemia on the electrocardiogram [50]:

$$\text{LV-Ao gradient (mm Hg)} = 13 \text{ (intensity of the systolic murmur)} + RV_6 - 6(QV_6) - 9 \quad (1)$$

Since this study echocardiography has provided additional useful information in the noninvasive detection and estimation of severity of congenital aortic stenosis.

ANATOMY. The bicuspid aortic valve is the most common anomaly that produces congenital aortic stenosis [51, 52]. The valve is made up of two cusps. The posterior cusp is usually larger than the anterior cusp [53] (Fig. 15-16) and the larger cusp usually has a median raphe. Obstruction depends upon commissural fusion, or gradual fibrous thickening and calcification. Other more uncommon forms of congenital aortic stenosis include the unicommissural valve, trileaflet aortic valve with a small annulus, and quadricuspid valve. Discussion will be confined to the bicuspid aortic valve.

M-MODE ECHOCARDIOGRAPHY. Recognition of a bicuspid aortic valve by M-mode echocardiography relies on visualization of eccentric diastolic motion of the valve within the aortic root [54, 55]. The diastolic eccentricity index of the aortic valve is defined by the equation: one-half the internal dimension of the aortic root measured at end systole divided by the minimum distance of the cusp echo to the nearest root wall [55]. In the absence of a ventricular septal defect, an index greater than 1.3 is suggestive evidence for a bicuspid valve. Eccentric systolic excursion of the anterior and posterior coronary cusps is another useful M-mode feature of bicuspid aortic valve. Recent information suggests that because of great variability in aortic valve imaging by M-mode echocardiography, the eccentricity index is not useful in the diagnosis of a bicuspid aortic valve [56]. Initially aortic valve cusp separation was used to predict severity of stenosis [57]. However, subsequent studies found this measurement to be a poor indicator of aortic valve gradient [58]. Bennett and colleagues were the first to employ a relative wall thickness formula to the preoperative noninvasive estimation of left ventricular peak systolic pressure and aortic valve pressure gradient [59]. The Bennett formula has been found to be extremely useful in children with aortic stenosis [60–63] but must be used with caution in adults. An in-depth discussion of the relative wall thickness formula in estimating the severity of aortic stenosis is included in Chapter 4. The use of this echocardiographic formula in the evaluation of the postoperative patient is discussed in Chapter 17.

TWO-DIMENSIONAL ECHOCARDIOGRAPHY. We use the M-mode echocardiogram to measure left ventricular wall thickness and cavity dimension. Frequently the M-mode tracing is derived from a two-dimensional image to ensure proper assessment of these variables. The two-dimensional image is used to define the anatomy of the valve. The aortic valve may be examined from the left parasternal long axis view and short axis view at the cardiac base, the apical four-chamber view, apical long axis view, and subcostal view. In the left parasternal long axis view the normal aortic valve has a central diastolic closure line and opens briskly in systole. The aortic valve cusps open parallel to the wall of the aortic root. In patients with a bicuspid aortic valve, the diastolic closure line is eccentric. In systole the base of the valve is fixed and the tips of the valve leaflets partially separate to produce a domed appearance (Fig. 15-17) [64–66]. In short axis at the cardiac base, the number of aortic valve cusps may be identified. The trileaflet aortic valve has a Y appearance. Using a phased-array sector scanner Bansal and colleagues [67] were able to identify a trileaflet aortic valve in 129 of 196 patients (66%). In 54 of these patients (28%) it was not possible to determine the number of aortic valve cusps, and in 13 patients (7%) the aortic valve was believed to be bicuspid [67]. The following problems prohibited cusp identification: inability to obtain an adequate view (12%), inadequate cusp visualization from an adequate view (12%), and a calcified valve (4%). There also appears to be a great deal of variability in aortic valve cusp visualization when viewed from the short axis. In this study 22 percent of patients had a com-

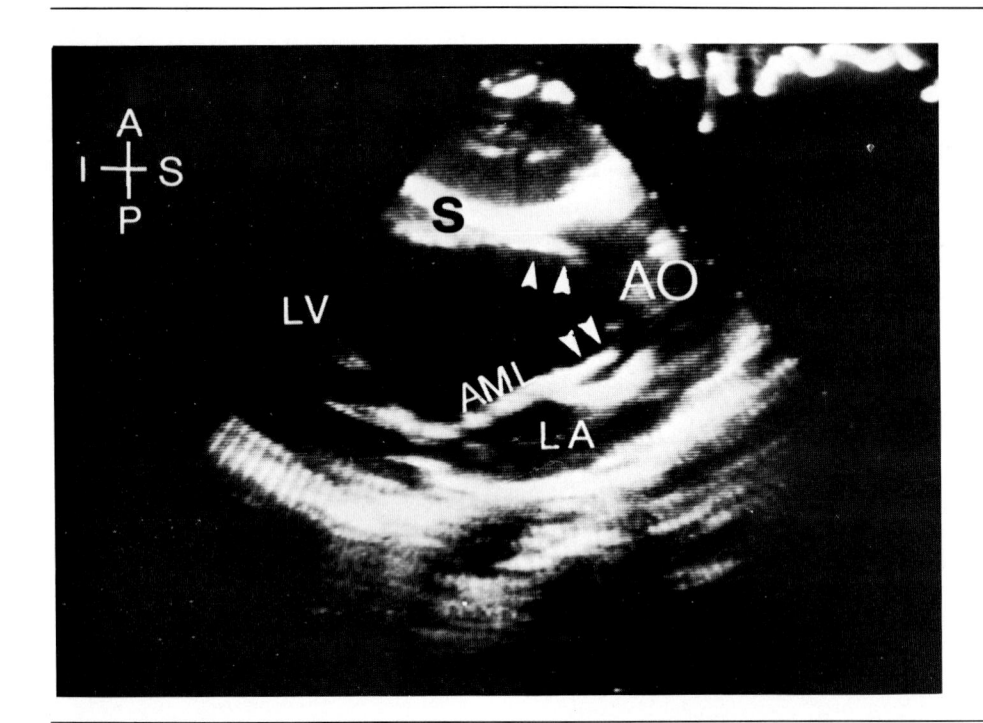

484   15. Congenital valvular, subvalvular, and supravalvular lesions

Fig. 15-17. Long axis view of a domed stenotic aortic valve (arrows). In this systolic frame the base of the valve is fixed and the leaflets (arrows) partially separate to produce a dome. S = superior. (From TG DiSessa et al, Cardiovasc Clin, in press.)

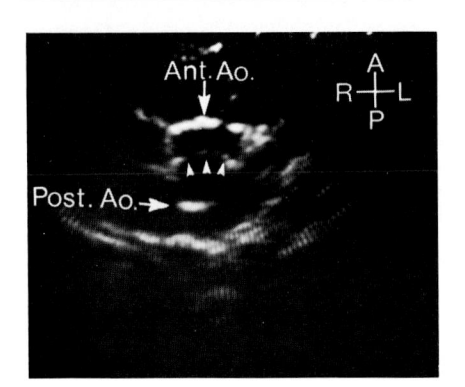

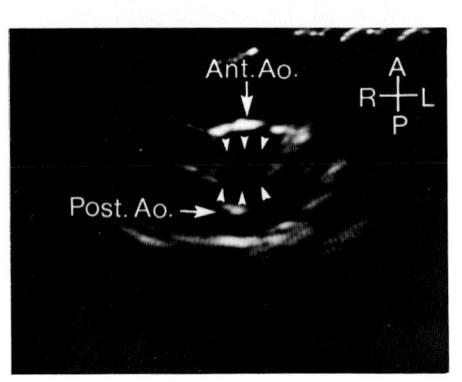

Fig. 15-18. Short axis view at the cardiac base of a biscuspid aortic valve. In the left panel the valve is imaged as a single diastolic echo (arrows) in the aortic root. In systole (right panel) the valve opens (arrows) into a typical fishmouth appearance. (Compare this echo with the anatomic specimen in Fig. 15-16). Ant Ao = anterior aorta; Post Ao = posterior aorta. (From TG DiSessa et al, Cardiovasc Clin, in press.)

plete Y configuration in diastole and visualization of three cusps in systole. In 50 percent of patients the three cusps could be identified in diastole only. In 28 percent of subjects an incomplete Y configuration was seen in diastole [67]. A bicuspid aortic valve has a single diastolic closure line and opens to a "fishmouth" appearance in systole [67] (Fig. 15-18). Weyman and associates measured maximum aortic valve separation in the parasternal long axis view and found a good correlation between this diameter and severity of stenosis [64, 65]. A subsequent study measured aortic cusp distance in the parasternal long axis view and found that the specificity of cross-sectional echocardiography for separating patients with aortic stenosis was limited [66]. A more elaborate discussion on the subject is conducted in Chapter 4.

Supravalvular aortic stenosis

CLINICAL FEATURES AND PHYSIOLOGY. Supravalvular aortic stenosis is a frequent congenital cardiac anomaly seen in children with William's syndrome [68]. These children, usually mentally retarded, have a small chin, large mouth, patulous lips, wide-set eyes, and malformed teeth (elfin facies). Pulses in the right arm are usually stronger than left arm pulses. Accordingly, right-arm blood pressure is greater than left-arm pressure [69, 70]. There may be a palpable thrill in the neck and prominent left ventricular impulse. The systolic murmur of supravalvular aortic stenosis is ejection in quality and best heard at the base of the heart. Radiation to the right neck is common. A murmur of aortic insufficiency is common. Electrocardiographic findings are indistinguishable from those of aortic stenosis. Chest radiograph shows a small ascending aorta rather than poststenotic dilatation.

ANATOMY. Supravalvular aortic stenosis has been categorized into three anatomic types: hourglass, membranous, and hypoplastic [71]. Localized segmental hourglass narrowing immediately distal to the aortic valve sinuses is the most common type [72] (Fig. 15-19). In this form of the anomaly there is marked thickening of the aortic media and fibrous internal proliferation. The next most common type is the membranous form. In this variety there is a localized fibrous membrane with a central opening. Finally, the hypoplastic variety is characterized by uniform underdevelopment of the ascending aorta.

M-MODE ECHOCARDIOGRAPHY. The diagnosis of supravalvular aortic stenosis by M-mode echocardiography involves scanning the aorta from the aortic valve level to high in the ascending portion. The diagnostic feature is narrowing of the aortic lumen above the level of the aortic valve echo [73–75]. The achievement of an adequate examination is beam-angle dependent.

TWO-DIMENSIONAL ECHOCARDIOGRAPHY. The additional dimension provided by cross-sectional examination allows a more precise characterization of the area of obstruction. The ascending aorta can be scanned easily from the left parasternal border and suprasternal notch. From the parasternal long axis view of the left ventricle, the transducer is tilted superiorly in order to image the ascending aorta distal to the aortic valve. In this tomographic plane, a decrease in luminal dimension of the aorta is imaged above the sinuses of Valsalva as well as the length of

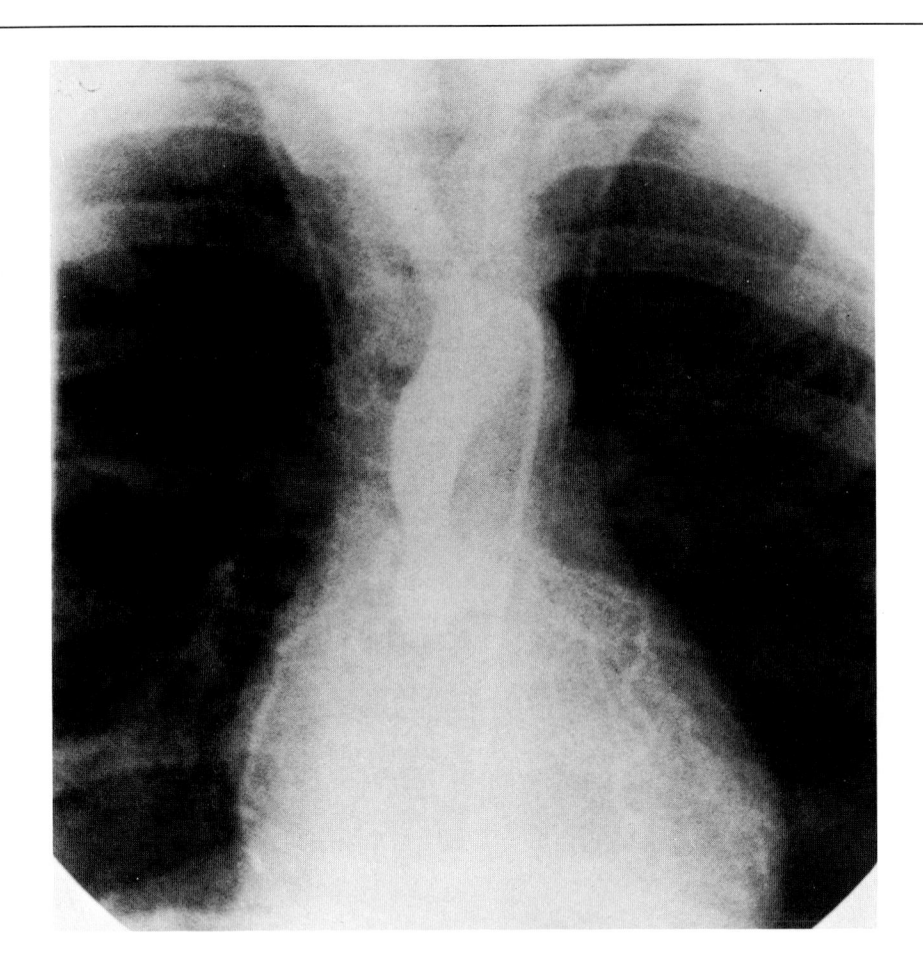

486   15. Congenital valvular, subvalvular, and supravalvular lesions

Fig. 15-19. Aortic root cineangiogram from a patient with supravalvular aortic stenosis. There is segmental hourglass narrowing above the aortic valve.

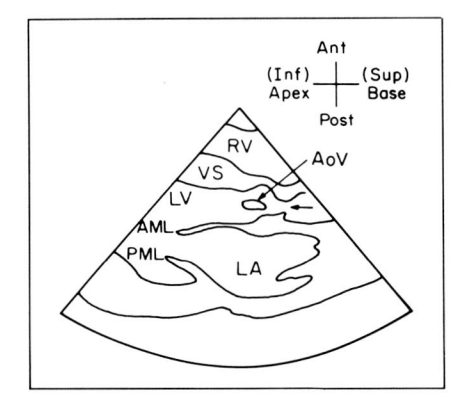

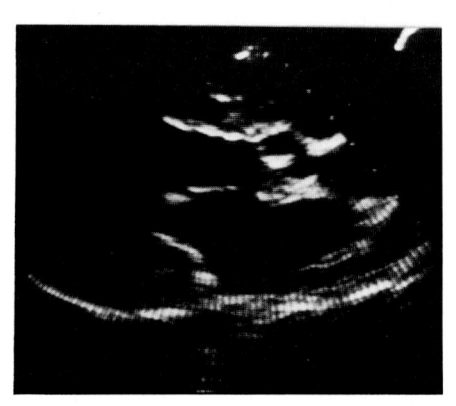

Fig. 15-20. Long axis view of the ascending aorta recorded from a patient with supravalvular aortic stenosis. The ascending aorta narrows (arrow) immediately above the aortic valve (AoV). VS = ventricular septum.

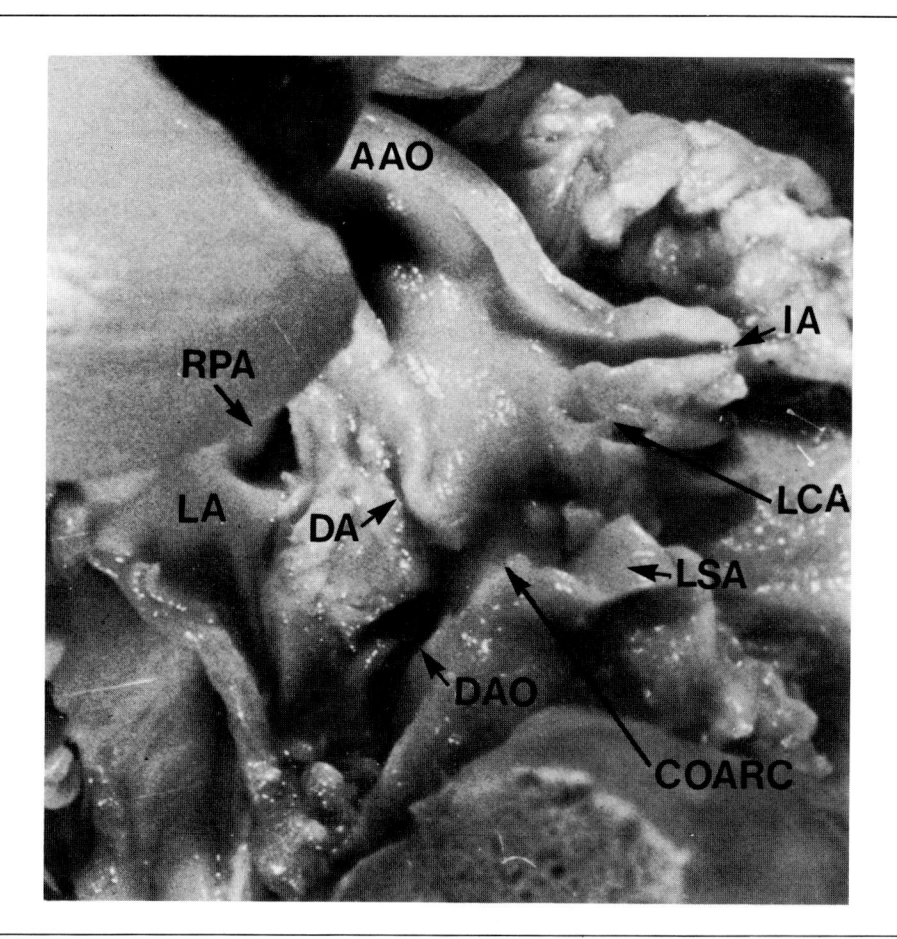

Fig. 15-21. Anatomic specimen cut in the suprasternal notch long axis plane from a patient with coarctation (COARC) of the aorta. There is discrete narrowing of the descending aorta due to coarctation. The ascending aorta is normal. DA = ductus arteriosus; IA = innominate artery; LCA = left carotid artery; LSA = left subclavian artery; RPA = right pulmonary artery.

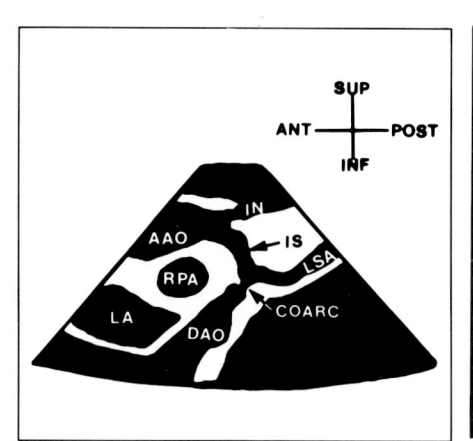

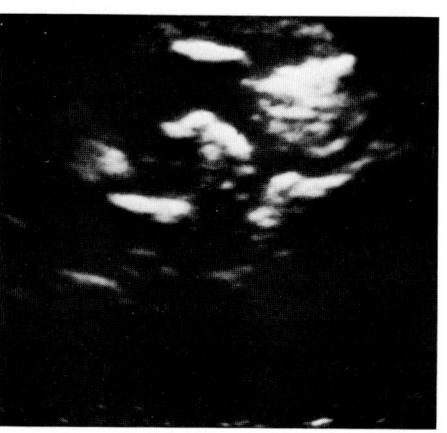

Fig. 15-22. Suprasternal notch echocardiogram recorded from a patient with coarctation (COARC) of the aorta. The aortic isthmus (IS) is also narrow. IN = innominate artery; LSA = left subclavian artery; RPA = right pulmonary artery.

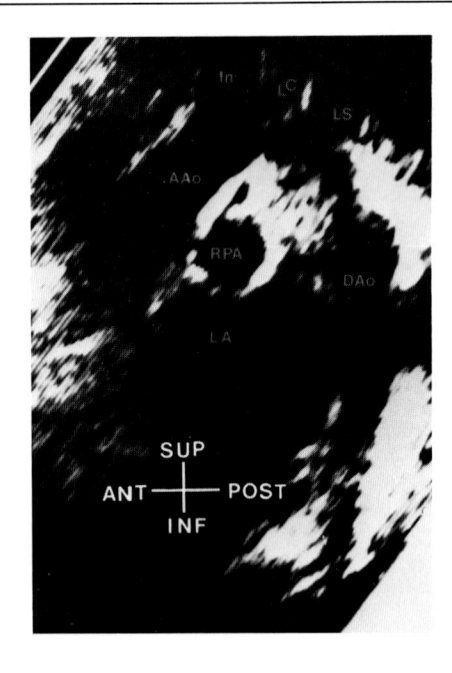

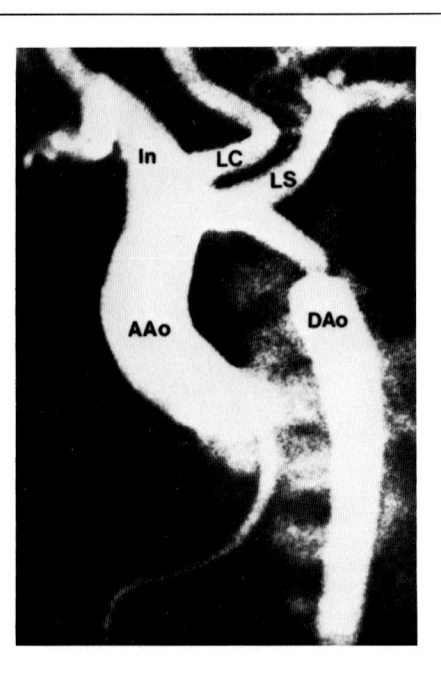

Fig. 15-23. *Suprasternal notch echocardiogram recorded from an infant with coarctation of the aorta* (left panel). *The ascending aorta (AAo) is of normal size. The aortic arch is hypoplastic and narrows to a discrete coarctation. There is poststenotic dilatation of the descending aorta (DAo). Compare this with the angiogram obtained from the same patient* (right panel). In = *innominate artery;* LC = *left carotid artery;* LS = *left subclavian artery;* RPA = *right pulmonary artery.*

narrowing [76] (Fig. 15-20). The image achieved is identical to the hourglass appearance of supravalvular aortic stenosis visualized by angiography. Moreover, measurement of the narrowed area correlates well with angiographic measurements of luminal diameter [76]. Scanning the ascending aorta with a moveable M-mode cursor enhances the capability of M-mode echocardiography to record the reduction in luminal diameter. The suprasternal notch image of the ascending aorta provides an additional approach for the evaluation of the ascending aorta [77].

Coarctation of the aorta

CLINICAL FEATURES AND PHYSIOLOGY. Clinical symptoms of the patient with coarctation of the aorta depend upon the age of the child. Infants less than 4 weeks old are almost always in congestive heart failure. Only 50 percent of infants between 4 weeks and 1 year of age are first seen in congestive heart failure. Children and adolescents are usually asymptomatic [78]. The discussion will deal with this latter group of patients. The principal findings on examination are a pulse discrepancy between upper and lower extremity; upper-extremity hypertension; and a systolic murmur best heard in the interscapular area. The electrocardiogram reflects the left ventricular strain. On plain chest film the heart size is usually normal. Rib notching is characteristic, and the poststenotic dilatation of the descending aorta produces the pathognomonic "three sign."

ANATOMY. Coarctation of the aorta is a localized narrowing located immediately distal to the origin of the left subclavian artery [78]. The zone of constriction may lie proximal, opposite, or distal to the site of entry of the ductus arteriosus (Fig. 15-21) [79]. Frequently there is diffuse narrowing of the transverse aortic arch proximal to the area of discrete constriction. Moreover, a significant number of patients have other associated intracardiac anomalies [79].

M-MODE ECHOCARDIOGRAPHY. The major role of M-mode echocardiography in the examination of patients with coarctation of the aorta is the evaluation of associated intracardiac anomalies such as a bicuspid aortic valve or parachute mitral valve.

TWO-DIMENSIONAL ECHOCARDIOGRAPHY. In children, adolescents, and adults, the most practical window for coarctation imaging is the suprasternal notch approach [77]. In infants the transverse and descending aorta may be imaged from the subcostal position or the second right intercostal space along the parasternal border [80]. The region of coarctation is visualized as an area of narrowing of the descending aorta when this structure is imaged in the suprasternal notch long axis view (Fig. 15-22) [77]. The poststenotic dilatation distal to the coarctation and long segment narrowing of the transverse aorta are also imaged in this view (Fig. 15-23).

References

1. Livesay WR: Clinical and physiologic studies in Ebstein's malformation. *Am Heart J* 57:701, 1959
2. Genton E, Blount SG: The spectrum of Ebstein's anomaly. *Am Heart J* 73:395, 1967
3. Lev M, Liberthson RR, Joseph RH, Seten CE, Kunske RD, Ockner FOA, Miller RA: The pathologic anatomy of Ebstein's disease. *Arch Pathol* 90:334, 1970
4. Edwards JE: Pathologic features of Ebstein's malformation of the tricuspid valve. *Proc Staff Mayo Clin* 28:89, 1953
5. Anderson KR, Lie JT: Pathologic anatomy of Ebstein's anomaly of the heart revisited. *Am J Cardiol* 41:739, 1978
6. Lundstrom NR: Echocardiography in the diagnosis of Ebstein's anomaly of the tricuspid valve. *Circulation* 48:597, 1973
7. Milner S, Meyer RA, Venables AW, Korfhagen J, Kaplan S: Mitral and tricuspid closure in congenital heart disease. *Circulation* 53:513, 1976
8. Farooki ZQ, Henry JG, Green EW: Echocardiographic spectrum of Ebstein's anomaly of the tricuspid valve. *Circulation* 53:63, 1976
9. Yuste P, Minguez I, Aza V, Senor J, Asin E, Martinez-Bordiu C: Echocardiography in the diagnosis of Ebstein's anomaly. *Chest* 66:273, 1974
10. Kotler MN: Tricuspid valve in Ebstein's anomaly. *Circulation* 49:194, 1974
11. Hirschklau MJ, Sahn DJ, Hagan AD, Williams DE, Friedman WF: Cross-sectional echocardiographic features of Ebstein's anomaly of the tricuspid valve. *Am J Cardiol* 40:400, 1977
12. Silverman NH, Schiller NB: Apex echocardiography: A new two-dimensional technique for evaluating congenital heart disease. *Circulation* 57:503, 1978
13. Ports TA, Silverman NH, Schiller NB: Two-dimensional echocardiographic assessment of Ebstein's anomaly. *Circulation* 58:336, 1978
14. Kambe T, Ishimiya S, Toguchi M, Hibi N, Fukui Y, Nishimura K, Sakamoto N, Hojo Y: Apex and subxiphoid approaches to Ebstein's anomaly using cross-sectional echocardiography. *Am Heart J* 100:53, 1980
15. Matsumoto M, Matsuo H, Nagata S, Hamanaka Y, Fujita T, Kawashima Y, Nimura Y, Abe H: Visualization of Ebstein's anomaly of the tricuspid valve by two-dimensional and standard echocardiography. *Circulation* 53:69, 1976
16. Blount SB, Vigoda PS, Swan H: Isolated infundibular stenosis. *Am Heart J* 57:684, 1959
17. Weyman AE, Dillon JC, Feigenbaum H, Chang S: Echocardiographic differentiation of infundibular from valvular pulmonary stenosis. *Am J Cardiol* 36:21, 1975
18. Lange LW, Sahn DJ, Allen HD, Goldberg SJ: Subxiphoid cross-sectional echocardiography in infants and children with congenital heart disease. *Circulation* 59:513, 1979
19. Caldwell RL, Weyman AE, Hurwitz RA, Girod DA, Feigenbaum H: Right ventricular outflow tract assessment by cross-sectional echocardiography in tetralogy of Fallot. *Circulation* 59:395, 1979
20. Vogelpoel L, Schrire V: Auscultatory and phonocardiographic assessment of pulmonary stenosis with intact ventricular septum. *Circulation* 22:55, 1960

21. Edwards JE: Pulmonary Stenosis with Intact Ventricular Septum. In SE Gould (ed) *Pathology of the Heart* (2nd ed). Springfield, Ill: Thomas, 1960. Pp 391–397
22. Weyman AE, Dillon JC, Feigenbaum H, Chang S: Echocardiographic patterns of pulmonary valve motion in valvular pulmonary stenosis. *Am J Cardiol* 34:644, 1974
23. Rey C, LaBlanche JM: Pulmonary valve motion in valvular pulmonary stenosis in childhood. *Acta Med Scand* (Suppl)627:185, 1979
24. Weyman AE, Hurwitz, RA, Girod DA, Dillon JC, Feigenbaum H, Green D: Cross-section echocardiographic visualization of the stenotic pulmonary valve. *Circulation* 56:769, 1977
25. Goldberg SJ, Areias JC, Spitaels SEC, de Villeneuve V: Echo-doppler detection of pulmonary stenosis by time-interval histogram analysis. *J Clin Ultrasound* 7:183, 1979
26. Shone JD, Sellers RD, Anderson RC, Adams P, Lillehei CW, Edwards JE: The developmental complex of "parachute mitral valve," supravalvular ring of left atrium, subaortic stenosis, and coarctation of aorta. *Am J Cardiol* 11:714, 1963
27. Mehrizi A, Hutchins GM, Wilson GF, Breckenbridge JC, Rowe RD: Supravalvular mitral stenosis. *J Pediatr* 67:1141, 1965
28. Rao BNS, Anderson RC, Lucas RV, Castaneda A, Ibarra-Perez C, Korns ME, Edwards JE: Supravalvular stenosing ring of the left atrium. *Am Heart J* 77:538, 1969
29. Bernstein A, Weiss F, Gilbert L: Uncomplicated congenital mitral stenosis. *Am J Cardiol* 2:102, 1958
30. Dauod G, Kaplan S, Perrin EV, Dorst JP, Edwards FK: Congenital mitral stenosis. *Circulation* 27:185, 1963
31. LaCorte M, Harada K, Williams RA: Echocardiographic features of congenital left ventricular inflow obstruction. *Circulation* 54:562, 1976
32. Driscoll DJ, Gutgesell HP, McNamara DG: Echocardiographic features of congenital mitral stenosis. *Am J Cardiol* 42:259, 1978
33. Snider AR, Roge CL, Schiller NB, Silverman NH: Congenital left ventricular inflow obstruction evaluated by two-dimensional echocardiography. *Circulation* 61:848, 1980
34. Newfeld EA, Muster AJ, Paul MH, Idriss FS, Riker WL: Discrete subvalvular aortic stenosis in childhood: Study of 51 patients. *Am J Cardiol* 38:53, 1976
35. Edwards JE: Pathology of left ventricular outflow tract obstruction. *Circulation* 31:586, 1965
36. Kelley DT, Wulfsberg E, Rowe RD: Discrete subaortic stenosis. *Circulation* 46:309, 1972
37. Davis RH, Feigenbaum H, Chang S, Konecke LL, Dillon JC: Echocardiographic manifestations of discrete subaortic stenosis. *Am J Cardiol* 33:277, 1974
38. Berry TE, Aziz KU, Paul MH: Echocardiographic assessment of discrete subaortic stenosis in childhood. *Am J Cardiol* 43:951, 1979
39. Gramiak R, Shah P: Echocardiography of the normal and diseased aortic valve. *Radiology* 96:1, 1970
40. Krueger SK, French JW, Forker AD, Caudill CC, Popp RL: Echocardiography in discrete subaortic stenosis. *Circulation* 59:506, 1976
41. Popp RL, Silverman JF, French JW, Stinson EB, Harrison DC: Echocardiographic findings in discrete subaortic stenosis. *Circulation* 49:226, 1974
42. DiSessa TG, Hagan AD, Isabel-Jones JB, Ti CC, Mercier JC, Friedman WF: Two-dimensional echocardiographic evaluation of discrete subaortic stenosis from the apical long axis view. *Am Heart J* 101:774, 1981
43. Williams DE, Sahn DJ, Friedman WF: Cross-sectional echocardiographic localization of sites of left ventricular outflow tract obstruction. *Am J Cardiol* 37:251, 1976
44. Weyman AE, Feigenbaum H, Hurwitz RA, Girod DA, Dillon JC, Chang S: Localization of left ventricular outflow tract obstruction by cross-sectional echocardiography. *Am J Med* 60:33, 1976
45. Wilcox WD, Seward JB, Haglar DJ, Mair DD, Tajik AJ: Discrete subaortic stenosis: Two-dimensional echocardiographic features with angiographic and surgical correlation. *Mayo Clin Proc* 55:425, 1980
46. Weyman AE, Feigenbaum H, Hurwitz RA, Girod DA, Dillon JC, Chang S: Cross-sectional echocardiography in evaluating patients with discrete subaortic stenosis. *Am J Cardiol* 37:358, 1976
47. Werner JC, Gewitz MH, Kleinman CS, Hellenbrand WE, Talner NS: Real-time echocardiography (RTE) in discrete membranous subaortic stenosis (DMSS). *Circulation* 57, 58(Suppl II):II-51, 1978 (Abstract)

48. Nanda NC, Gramiak R: Two-dimensional echocardiographic features of discrete subaortic stenosis. *Circulation* 59 (Suppl II):II-26, 1979
49. Halloran KH: The telemetered exercise electrocardiogram in congenital aortic stenosis. *Pediatrics* 47:31, 1971
50. Ellison RC, Wagner HR, Weidman WH, Miettinen HS: Congenital valvular aortic stenosis: Clinical detection of small pressure gradient. *Am J Cardiol* 37:757, 1976
51. Campbell M: Calcific aortic stenosis and congenital bicuspid aortic valves. *Br Heart J* 30:606, 1968
52. Fenoglio JJ, McAllister HA, DeCastro CM, Davia JE, Cheitlin MD: Congenital bicuspid aortic valve after age 20. *Am J Cardiol* 39:164, 1977
53. Walker BF, Carter JB, Williams HJ, Wang K, Edwards JE: Bicuspid aortic valve: Comparison of congenital and acquired types. *Circulation* 48:1140, 1973
54. Nanda NC, Gramiak R, Manning J, Mahoney EB, Lipchik EO, Dewese JA: Echocardiographic recognition of the congenital bicuspid aortic valve. *Circulation* 49:870, 1974
55. Radford DJ, Bloom KR, Izukawa T, Moes CAF, Rowe RD: Echocardiographic assessment of bicuspid aortic valves: Angiographic and pathological correlates. *Circulation* 53:80, 1976
56. Kececioglu-Drelos Z, Goldberg SJ: Role of M-mode echocardiography in congenital aortic stenosis. *Am J Cardiol* 47:1267, 1981
57. Yeh HC, Winsberg F, Mercer EN: Echocardiographic aortic valve orifice dimension: Its use in evaluating aortic stenosis and cardiac output. *J Clin Ultrasound* 1:182, 1973
58. Chang S, Clements S, Chang J: Aortic stenosis: Echocardiographic cusp separation and surgical description of the aortic valve in 22 patients. *Am J Cardiol* 39:499, 1977
59. Bennett DH, Evans DW, Raj MVJ: Echocardiographic left ventricular dimensions in pressure and volume overload: Their use in assessing aortic stenosis. *Br Heart J* 37:971, 1975
60. Johnson GL, Meyer RA, Schwartz DC, Korfhagen J, Kaplan S: Echocardiographic evaluation of fixed left ventricular outlet obstruction in children: Pre and post-operative assessment of ventricular systolic pressures. *Circulation* 56:299, 1977
61. Glanz S, Hellenbrand WE, Berman MA, Talner NS: Echocardiographic assessment of the severity of aortic stenosis in children and adolescents. *Am J Cardiol* 38:620, 1976
62. Blackwood RA, Bloom KR, Williams CM: Aortic stenosis in children: Experience with echocardiographic prediction of severity. *Circulation* 57:263, 1978
63. Hagan AD, DiSessa TG, Samtoy L, Friedman WF, Vieweg WVR: Reliability of echocardiography in diagnosing and quantitating valvular aortic stenosis. *J Cardiovasc Med* 5:391, 1980
64. Weyman AE, Feigenbaum H, Dillon JC, Chang S: Cross-sectional echocardiography in assessing the severity of valvular aortic stenosis. *Circulation* 52:828, 1975
65. Weyman AE, Feigenbaum H, Hurwitz RA, Girod DA, Dillon JC: Cross-sectional echocardiographic assessment of the severity of aortic stenosis in children. *Circulation* 55:773, 1977
66. DeMaria AN, Bommer W, Joye J, Lee G, Bouteller J, Mason DT: Value and limitations of cross-sectional echocardiography of the aortic valve in the diagnosis and quantification of valvular aortic stenosis. *Circulation* 62:304, 1980
67. Bansal RC, Tajik AJ, Seward JB, Offord KP: Feasibility of detailed two-dimensional echocardiographic examination in adults: Prospective study of 200 patients. *Mayo Clin Proc* 55:291, 1980
68. Beuren AJ, Apitz J, Harmjanz D: Supravalvular aortic stenosis in association with mental retardation and a certain facial appearance. *Circulation* 26:1235, 1962
69. French JW, Guntheroth WG: An explanation of asymmetric upper extremity blood pressures in supravalvular aortic stenosis: The Coanda effect. *Circulation* 42:31, 1970
70. Goldstein RE, Epstein SE: Mechanism of elevated innominate artery pressures in supravalvular aortic stenosis. *Circulation* 42:23, 1970
71. Blieden LC, Lucas RV, Carter JB, Miller K, Edwards JE: A developmental complex including supravalvular stenosis of the aorta and pulmonary trunk. *Circulation* 49:585, 1974
72. Roberts WC: Valvular, subvalvular and supravalvular aortic stenosis. *Cardiovasc Clin* 5:104, 1973
73. Nasrallah AT, Nihill M: Supravalvular aortic stenosis: Echocardiographic features. *Br Heart J* 37:662, 1975
74. Dolen JL, Popp RL, French JW: Echocardiographic features of supravalvular aortic stenosis. *Circulation* 52:817, 1975

75. Usher BW, Goulden D, Murgo JP: Echocardiographic detection of supravalvular aortic stenosis. *Circulation* 49:1257, 1975
76. Weyman AE, Caldwell RL, Hurwitz RA, Girod DA, Dillon JC, Feigenbaum H, Green D: Cross-sectional echocardiographic characterization of aortic obstruction I. Supravalvular aortic stenosis and aortic hypoplasia. *Circulation* 57:491, 1978
77. Snider AR, Silverman NH: Suprasternal notch echocardiography: A two-dimensional technique for evaluating congenital heart disease. *Circulation* 63:165, 1981
78. Shinebourne EA, Tam ESY, Elseed AM, Paneth M, Lennox SC, Cleland WP, Lincoln C, Joseph MC, Anderson RH: Coarctation of the aorta in infancy and childhood. *Br Heart J* 38:375, 1978
79. Becker AE, Becker MJ, Edwards JE: Anomalies associated with coarctation of aorta: Particular reference to infancy. *Circulation* 41:1067, 1970
80. George L, Waldman JD, Kirkpatrick SE, Turner SW, Pappelbaum SJ: Two-dimensional echocardiographic visualization of the aortic arch by right parasternal scanning in neonates and infants. *Pediatr Cardiol* 2:277, 1982

Cyanotic congenital heart disease

16

Tetralogy of Fallot. Tetralogy of Fallot is a type of cyanotic congenital heart disease first described by Stensen in 1671 [1]. Over 200 years later, in 1888, Etienne-Louis Arthur Fallot reported a cardiac malformation that included (1) stenosis of the pulmonary artery; (2) a ventricular septal defect; (3) deviation of the aorta to the right; and (4) hypertrophy of the right ventricle [2]. This cardiac malformation is the most common cause of cyanosis in children over 1 year of age and constitutes approximately 10 percent of all forms of congenital heart disease.

CLINICAL FEATURES AND PHYSIOLOGY. The hemodynamic derangement produced by a ventricular septal defect and pulmonary stenosis is responsible for the clinical manifestations of tetralogy of Fallot. Since the ventricular defect is large, there is equal pressure in the ventricles. The severity of the pulmonary stenosis governs the magnitude and direction of intracardiac shunt and ultimately the degree of cyanosis. In patients with mild stenosis the dominant shunt is left-to-right and the patient is not cyanotic (acyanotic tetralogy of Fallot). These patients have a loud crescendo-decrescendo murmur that begins after the first heart sound and peaks late in systole; it is heard best in the pulmonic area [3]. Such patients develop progressive infundibular obstruction and the typical clinical features of tetralogy of Fallot. With progressive stenosis the murmur becomes shorter and peaks earlier in systole. Concurrently cyanosis appears, becomes progressive, and digital clubbing occurs. The disappearance of the murmur signifies total occlusion of the right ventricular outflow tract. When this occurs acutely in the older child it produces hyperpnea and severe cyanosis, which may be relieved by squatting or progress to syncope.

The chest radiograph and electrocardiogram reflect the amount of right ventricular hypertrophy and pulmonary blood flow. On electrocardiogram the typical tall R wave in V1 and deep S wave in V6 are usually observed. In adolescents and adults tall peaked P waves of right atrial enlargement may appear. The chest radiograph usually shows an uptilted cardiac apex with a concave main pulmonary artery segment ("cor en sabot"). Pulmonary vascular markings depend upon the degree of outflow tract obstruction. With mild obstruction pulmonary vascular markings are normal to increased. With severe obstruction pulmonary markings are reduced. The aortic arch will be on the right in 20 percent of cases.

ANATOMY. From an anatomic point of view this anomaly consists of a ventricular septal defect and right ventricular outflow tract obstruction. The ventricular septal defect is positioned in the anterior portion of the muscular septum, anterior to the membranous septum. The defect is situated beneath the posterior portion of the right and the anterior portion of the posterior aortic cusp. In this position it is confluent with the orifice of the aorta. In all tetralogies the aorta overrides the ventricular septal defect and emerges from both ventricles (Fig. 16-1). The degree of override is variable. The structure of the right ventricular outflow tract in this anomaly is complex. The parietal band is displaced superiorly away from the tricuspid valve onto the anterior wall of the right ventricle. Thus the infundibulum of the right ventricle becomes narrowed [4]. In a majority of patients valvular pulmonic stenosis occurs in conjunction with the infundibular obstruction [5]. The right ventricle is hypertrophied but usually not dilated. There is fibrous continuity between the anterior leaflet of the mitral valve and the aortic valve.

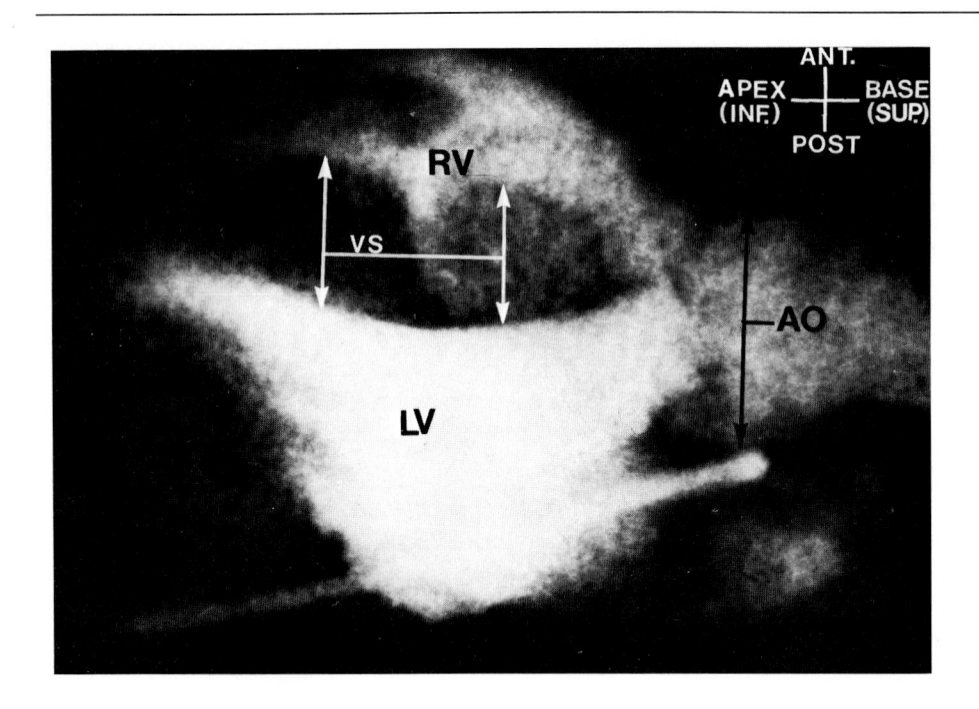

Fig. 16-1. Left ventricular cineangiocardiogram demonstrates the pathologic anatomy of tetralogy of Fallot. In this long axis oblique view the aorta (AO) is seen emerging from the right ventricle and left ventricle and overriding the ventricular septum (VS).

M-MODE ECHOCARDIOGRAPHY. The principal M-mode feature is an image of enlarged aortic root that overrides the ventricular septum [6, 7]. Visualization of the pulmonic valve varies, and inability to observe the valve does not imply its absence. In patients with pure infundibular stenosis, chaotic systolic motion of the pulmonic valve may be seen [8]. Demonstrable continuity between the anterior leaflet of the mitral valve and aortic valve is variable due to the dextraposed aortic root [9]. Peripheral venous contrast echocardiography has been used to demonstrate the right-to-left intracardiac shunt in patients with tetralogy of Fallot [10]. After a peripheral venous injection of a contrast solution (i.e., indocyanine green dye) microcavitations will appear first in the right ventricle, and on the next beat in the left ventricle anterior to the mitral valve prior to the E point.

TWO-DIMENSIONAL ECHOCARDIOGRAPHY. Sahn and colleagues were the first to describe the two-dimensional echocardiographic features of tetralogy of Fallot using a linear-array system [11]. The most important feature in their description was disruption of ventricular septal–aortic root continuity with the preservation of mitral valve–aortic valve continuity when viewing the heart in the sagittal long axis plane. In addition, they described an enlarged aortic root that originated from both ventricles. We subsequently described similar findings using a sector scan system [12]. In the left parasternal or subcostal long axis view an enlarged aortic root that overrides the ventricular septum is imaged (Figs. 16-2, 16-3). In these tomographic planes tetralogy of Fallot is indistinguishable from pulmonary atresia and truncus arteriosus. Visualization of a pulmonic valve and hypoplastic right ventricular outflow tract in the short axis or right ventricular outflow view, along the left parasternal border, or subcostal right ventricular outflow tract view allows distinction of patients with tetralogy of Fallot from those with truncus arteriosus and pulmonary atresia [13, 14]. Measurement of the right ventricular outflow tract

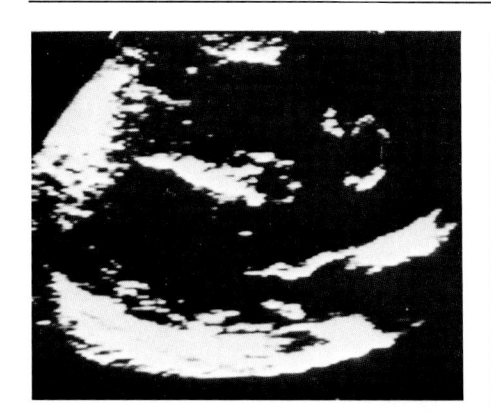

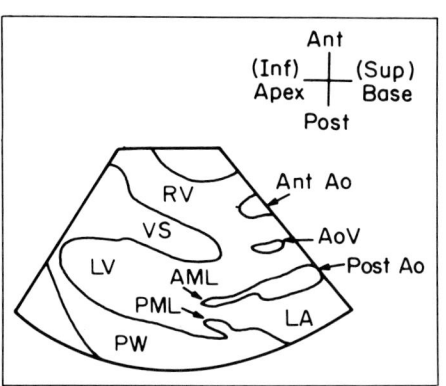

Fig. 16-2. Left parasternal long axis view in a patient with tetralogy of Fallot. The aortic root is enlarged and overrides the ventricular septum (VS). The anterior leaflet of the mitral valve is in continuity with the aortic valve (AoV). ANT Ao = anterior aorta; POST Ao = posterior aorta; PW = posterior wall.

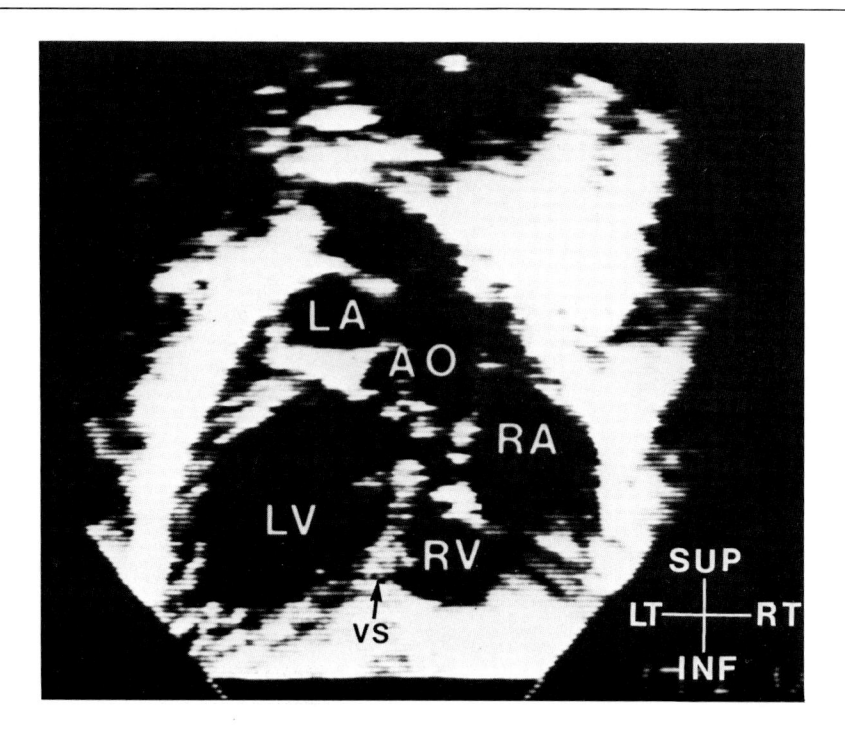

Fig. 16-3. Subcostal long axis view in a patient with tetralogy of Fallot. The aorta (AO) is enlarged and overrides the ventricular septum (VS).

A   B   C

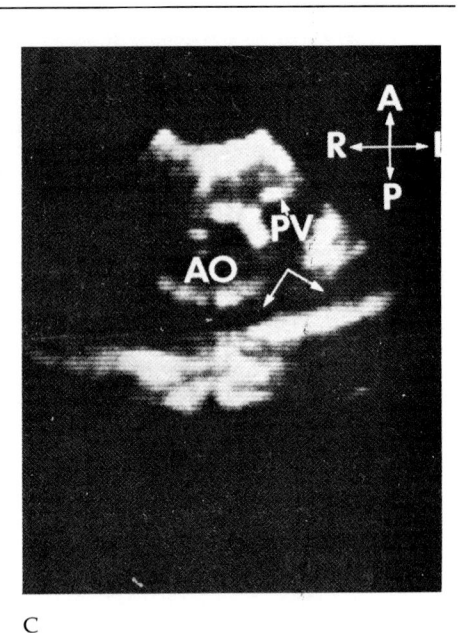

Fig. 16-4. Two-dimensional images in the short axis at the cardiac base. A. Truncus arteriosus shows a dilated truncal root (Tr) with no image of a right ventricular outflow tract or pulmonic valve. B. Pulmonary atresia with ventricular septal defect. The right ventricular outflow tract ends blindly (arrow) and the pulmonic valve is not seen. C. Tetralogy of Fallot. The right ventricular outflow tract is hypoplastic and the pulmonic valve (PV) is small. (From DJ Hagler et al, Mayo Clin Proc 55:73, 1980.)

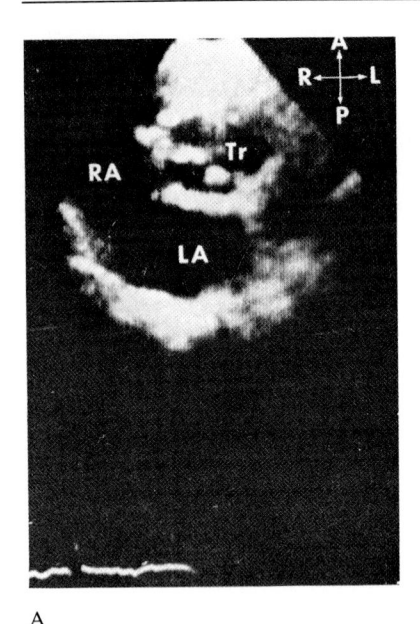

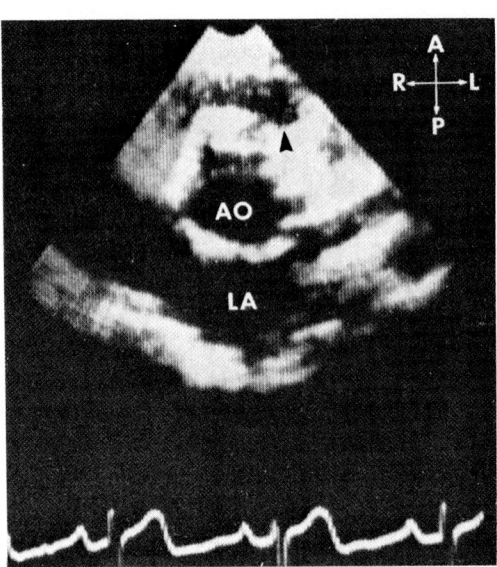

diameter at both end systole and end diastole from two-dimensional images has been shown to correlate well with angiocardiographic dimensions [14]. These measurements are made in a plane of sector 60 degrees from the left parasternal long axis view in order to align the ultrasound beam parallel to the long axis of the right ventricular outflow tract. Thus cross-sectional imaging is superior to the M-mode echocardiogram in the evaluation of the right ventricular outflow tract [14] (Fig. 16-4). Lange and associates [15] claim that the subcostal image of the right ventricular outflow tract is superior to left parasternal images that are too close to the transducer to permit an adequate view of the outflow tract. In order to achieve the subcostal long axis image of the right ventricular outflow tract the transducer is rotated clockwise approximately 90 degrees from the subcostal four-chamber view and scanned superiorly [16]. From this view both subvalvular (infundibular) and valvular obstruction are imaged clearly [15, 17] (Fig. 16-5). In our experience the subcostal window is more advantageous in infants and children. However, in adolescents and adults the left parasternal views are usually superior for imaging the right ventricular outflow tract.

Transposition of the great arteries

CLINICAL FEATURES AND PHYSIOLOGY. Transposition of the great arteries is a common form of cyanotic congenital heart disease in infancy. With the introduction of the intraatrial baffle in 1964 (Mustard's procedure) 95 percent of these children are surviving into adolescence and adulthood; they are acyanotic and have near normal exercise tolerance [18]. The clinical presentation of the infant will depend upon the number and size of intracardiac communications. In patients with an intact atrial and ventricular septum cyanosis occurs within hours of birth. In infants

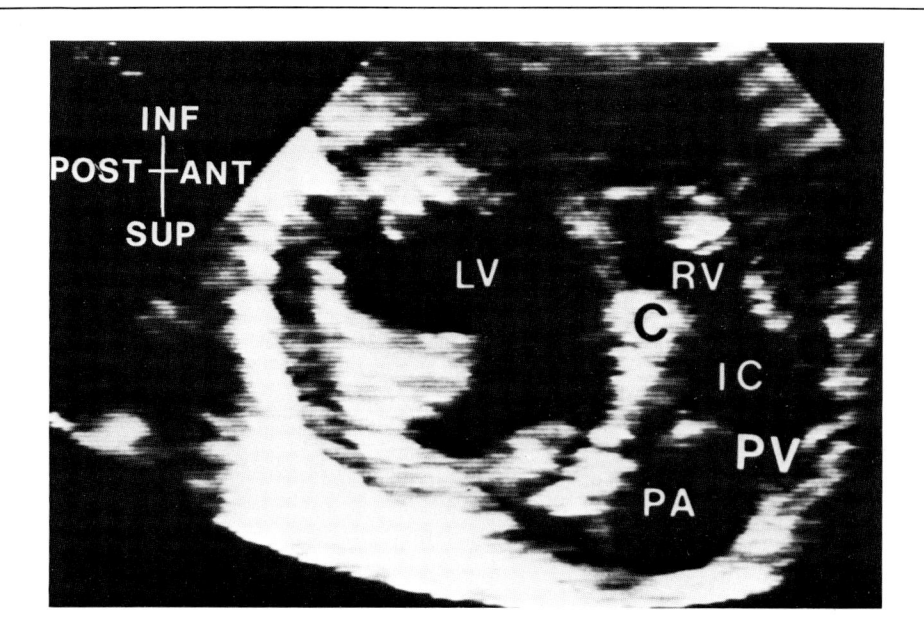

Fig. 16-5. Subcostal image of the right ventricular outflow tract in a patient with tetralogy of Fallot. There is hypertrophy of the crista supraventricularis (C) producing infundibular stenosis and an infundibular chamber (IC) between the body of the right ventricle and pulmonary valve (PV).

with a large ventricular septal defect cyanosis is less prominent. In these latter patients congestive heart failure is the dominant symptom complex. There is cardiomegaly with increased pulmonary blood flow on chest radiograph in both groups. Despite the pattern of torrential pulmonary blood flow, the main pulmonary artery segment is absent, since it is transposed posteriorly and medially. Since the right ventricle sees systemic pressure, the electrocardiogram shows right ventricular hypertrophy.

ANATOMY. In patients with complete transposition of the great arteries the atria and the ventricles are in the normal position. The anatomic right atrium communicates with the anatomic right ventricle, and the anatomic left atrium communicates with the anatomic left ventricle. The architecture of the ventricles is normal. The aorta springs from the morphologic right ventricle and the pulmonary artery emerges from the morphologic left ventricle. The mitral valve is in fibrous continuity with the pulmonic valve. Thus complete transposition may be defined as the displacement of both great arteries across the ventricular septum [19]. The aorta is usually situated to the right and anteriorly and the pulmonary artery is situated to the left and posteriorly (Fig. 16-6). The aorta may be either directly anterior to the pulmonary artery or, in a small number of cases, anterior and to the left of the pulmonary artery (Fig. 16-7). The coronary ostia are either in the posterior sinuses of Valsalva or posterior and left anterior sinus of Valsalva. The right ventricle is larger and thicker than the left [19].

Those patients with a ventricular septal defect have the same features mentioned above. The defect may assume four positions: (1) in the outflow tract of the right ventricle; (2) in the inflow tract of the right ventricle (membranous); (3) in the posterior septum; and (4) in the muscular septum [19]. Left ventricular outflow tract obstruction may occur and it may be either membranous (characterized by a fibrous membrane beneath the pulmonic valve), fibromuscular, tunnel, hypertrophic, or valvular [20, 21] (Fig. 16-8).

498   16. Cyanotic congenital heart disease

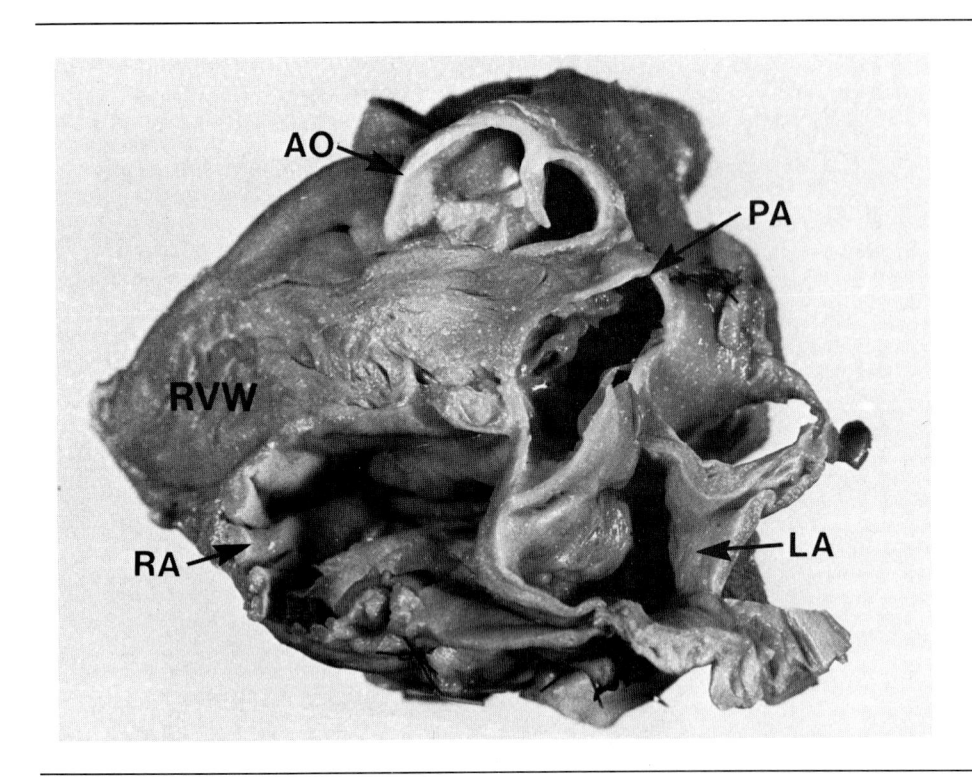

Fig. 16-6. Anatomic specimen cut in the plane of the short axis at the base of the heart in a patient with complete transposition of the great arteries. The aorta is anterior and to the right of the pulmonary artery (PA).

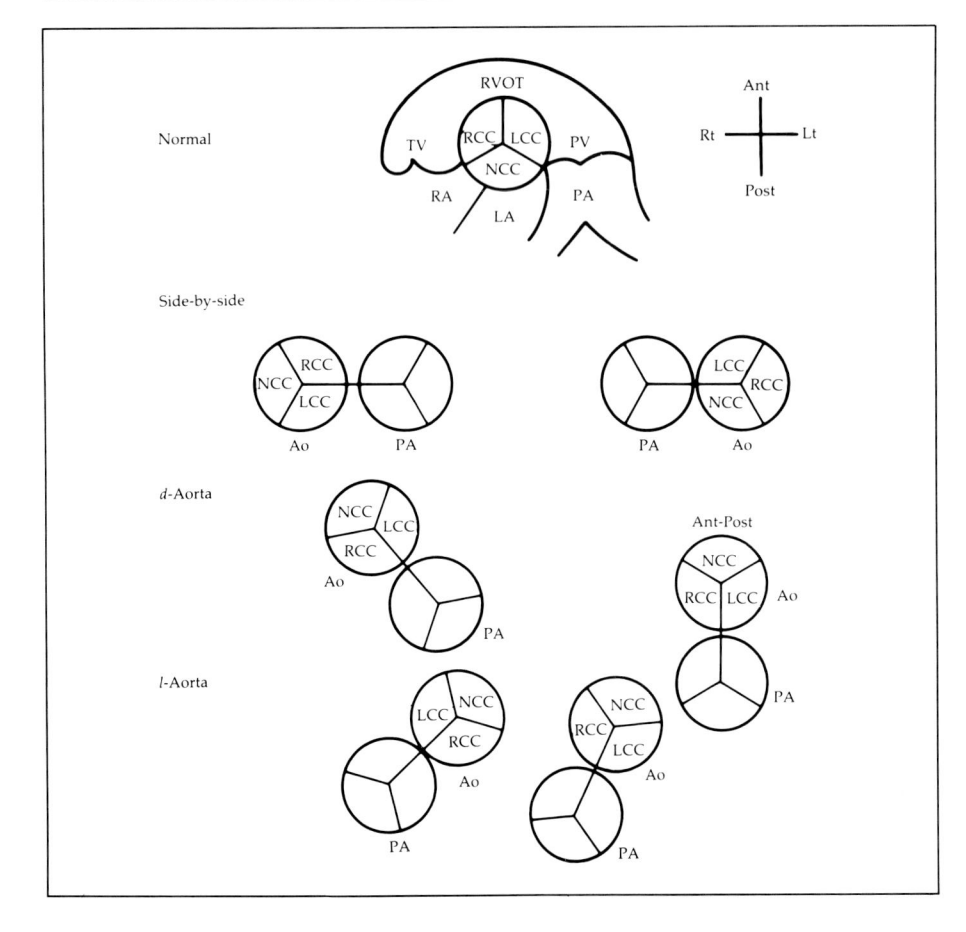

Fig. 16-7. Relationship of the great arteries to each other as visualized in short axis at the cardiac base. LCC = left coronary cusp; NCC = noncoronary cusp; PA = pulmonary artery; PV = pulmonic valve; RCC = right coronary cusp.

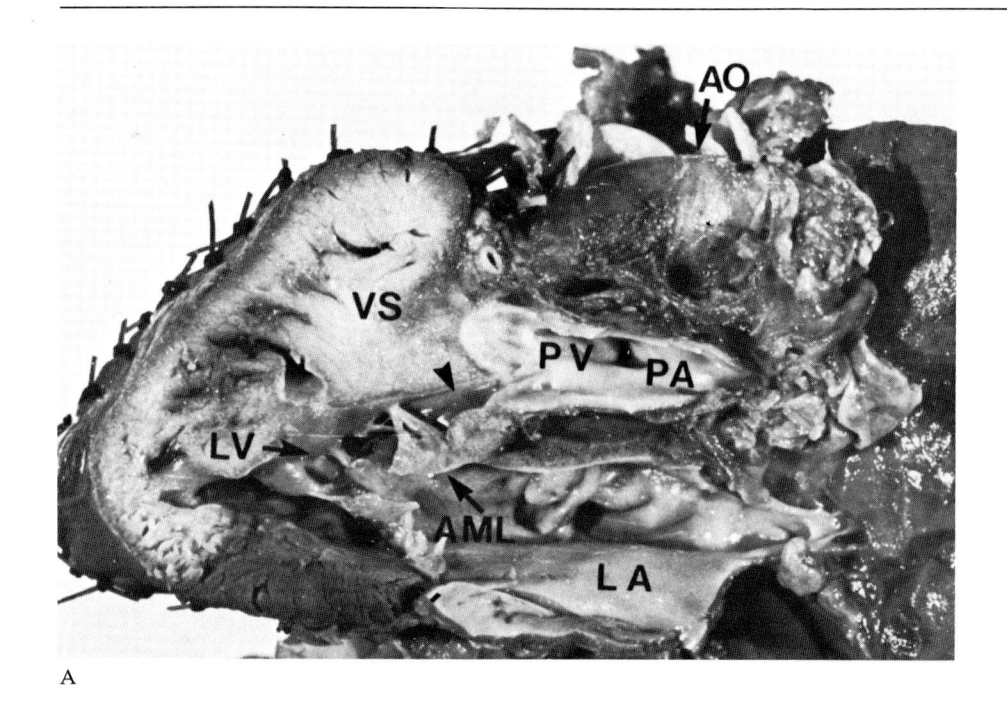

Fig. 16-8A. Anatomic specimen cut in the plane of the long axis. In this heart with complete transposition, the pulmonary artery (PA) is seen emerging from the left ventricle. There is tunnel left ventricular outflow tract obstruction (arrowhead). B. Left ventricular cineangiocardiogram in the long axial oblique view in a patient with complete transposition and left ventricular outflow tract obstruction. A diastolic frame shows marked narrowing of the outflow tract (arrows). The pulmonary artery emerges from the left ventricle and courses in a posterior direction. PV = pulmonic valve; VS = ventricular septum.

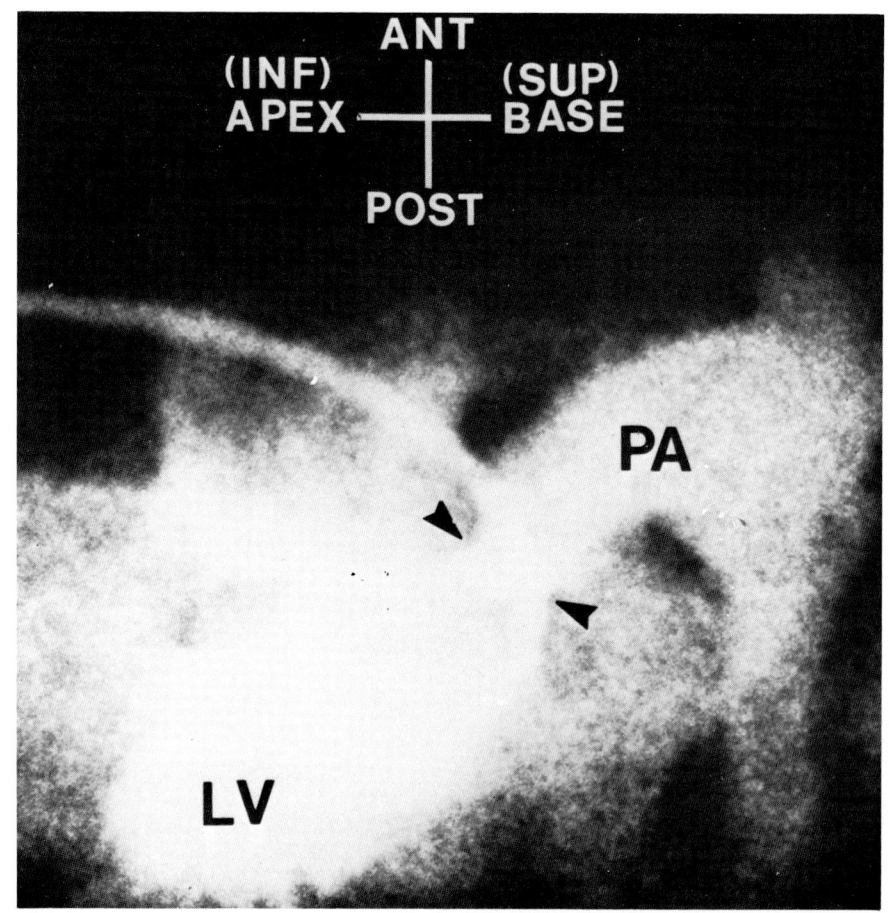

M-MODE ECHOCARDIOGRAPHY. The M-mode echocardiographic features of complete transposition include a normal long axis sweep with both atrioventricular valve (mitral valve)–semilunar valve (pulmonic valve) and septal–great artery continuity; an increased right ventricular dimension; simultaneous imaging of both semilunar valves; reversal of the systolic time intervals so that the anterior (aortic) semilunar valve opens after and closes before the posterior (pulmonic) semilunar valve; and a retrosternal anterior (aortic) semilunar valve [11, 22]. The appearance of these features is variable, and built-in limitations exist. As infants advance in age, a certain subset develop signs of left ventricular outflow tract obstruction. There occurs a characteristic systolic anterior motion of the mitral valve associated with dynamic outflow tract obstruction [23]. The pulmonic valve may exhibit early systolic closure followed by high frequency vibrations throughout the remainder of systole in patients with membranous subpulmonic obstruction [24]. Moreover, the stenotic pulmonic valve produces multiple diastolic reflectances.

TWO-DIMENSIONAL ECHOCARDIOGRAPHY. The two-dimensional features of complete transposition are very specific [25]. The position of the great arteries in relation to each other and to the ventricular septum is established from a short axis scan [26, 27] (Figs. 16-7, 16-9). In the normal subject the right ventricular outflow tract is observed wrapping around the aorta in a clockwise fashion when viewed from the short axis at the cardiac base (Fig. 16-10). In contrast this wraparound effect is absent in patients with transposition. Instead, the two great arteries are imaged as separate circles with the anterior great artery (aorta) either to the right, directly anterior, or to the left of the posterior great artery (pulmonary artery) (Fig. 16-10). On short axis scan the aorta will emerge from the heart anterior to the ventricular septum, and the pulmonary artery will emerge from the heart posterior to the ventricular septum. In long axis the great artery that springs from the left ventricle will travel in a posterior direction toward the lungs. This feature identifies the artery as the pulmonary artery [26] (Fig. 16-11). In addition, mitral valve–pulmonic valve continuity is identified in this view. Other features include an increase in right ventricular wall thickness, right ventricular cavity size, and abnormal septal motion [24].

Congenitally corrected transposition of the great arteries

CLINICAL FEATURES AND PHYSIOLOGY. The clinical features of this anomaly are related to the associated lesions. Those few individuals without other defects live a normal life. The vast majority of patients have other severe defects. The most common lesion is a ventricular septal defect with or without associated obstruction to pulmonary blood flow. The dominant symptoms in subjects with isolated ventricular septal defect are those of congestive heart failure. When the ventricular septal defect is associated with pulmonic stenosis, cyanosis (44%) is the dominant clinical problem. The electrocardiogram shows a reversal of septal depolarization caused by ventricular inversion (Q waves in the right precordial leads and absence of the Q wave in V6). Selective chamber hypertrophy depends upon associated defects. The characteristic radiographic feature is a straight left-heart border caused by the leftward position of the ascending aorta. The pulmonary artery segment is not seen because of its posterior rightward position. Pulmonary vascular markings depend upon the degree of pulmonary stenosis.

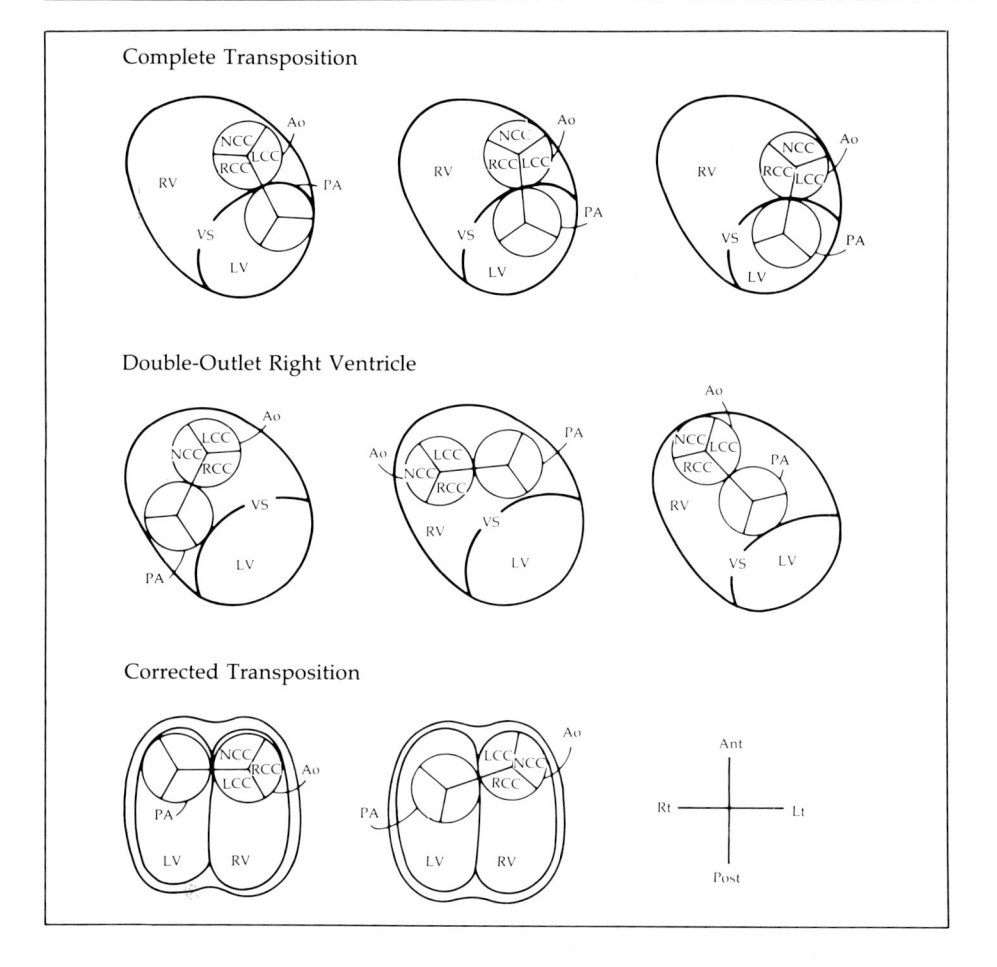

Fig. 16-9. Relationship of the great arteries to the ventricular septum (VS).

502 16. Cyanotic congenital heart disease

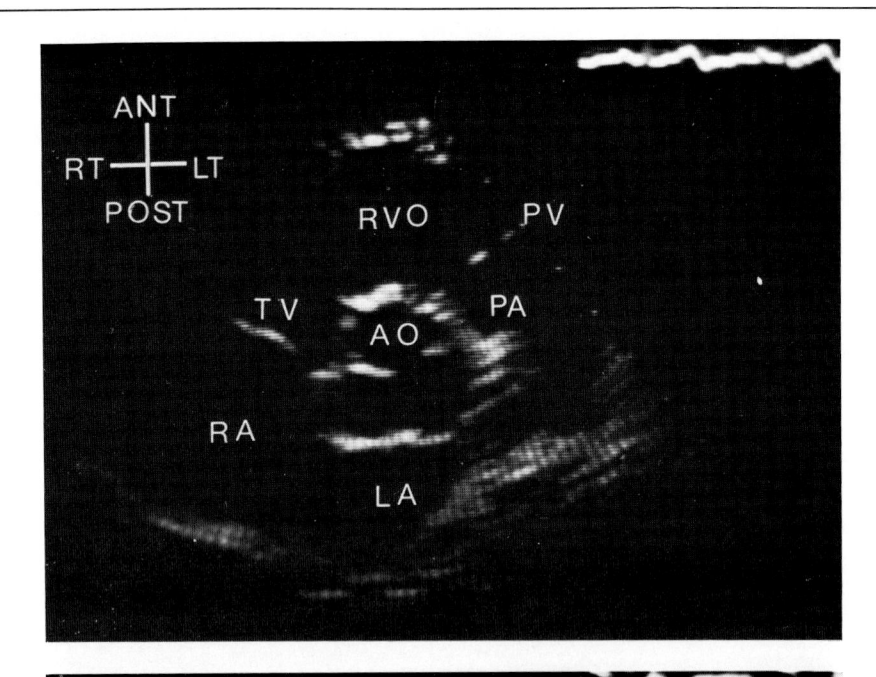

Fig. 16-10. Short axis view. Normal great arteries (top panel). The right ventricular outflow wraps around the aorta anteriorly. The pulmonic valve (PV) is anterior and to the left of the aortic valve. Transposition of the great arteries (bottom panel). The aorta is anterior to the pulmonary artery (PA). There is no right ventricular outflow tract, and both great arteries are seen as circles en face. (Compare with Fig. 1-8B and Fig. 16-6.)

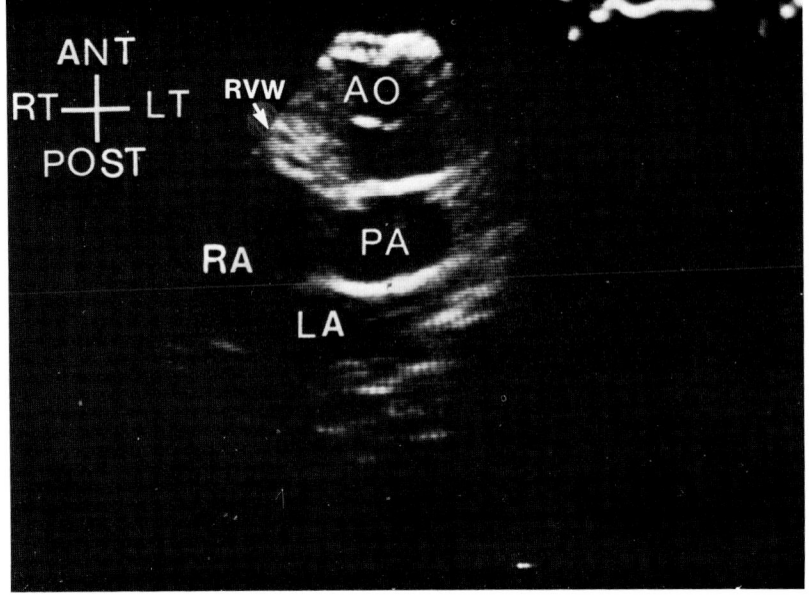

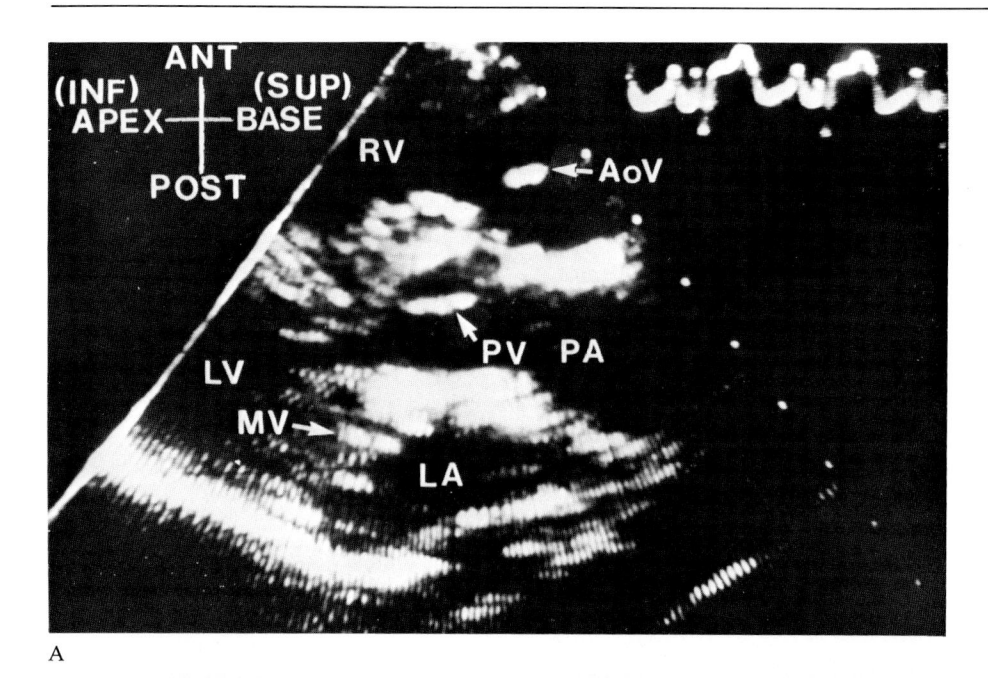

Fig. 16-11A. Transposition of the great arteries, long axis views along the left parasternal border. The pulmonary artery (PA) is imaged exiting the left ventricle and turning posteriorly toward the lungs. The aortic valve (AoV) is seen anterior to the pulmonic valve (PV). The aorta exits the right ventricle. The aorta and pulmonary artery emerge from the heart and are oriented parallel to each other. There is mitral valve to pulmonic valve continuity. (Compare this image with the left ventricular cineangiocardiogram from the same patient in Fig. 16-8.) B. Subcostal long axis view in a child with complete transposition of the great arteries. In this view the main pulmonary artery is visualized exiting the left ventricle. The main pulmonary artery bifurcates into a left pulmonary artery (LPA) and a right pulmonary artery (RPA). To achieve this view, the transducer is tilted anteriorly from the subcostal 4-chamber view. (Compare this image with the same view recorded in a patient with normally related great arteries, Fig. 14-8.) PV = pulmonic valve; VS = ventricular septum.

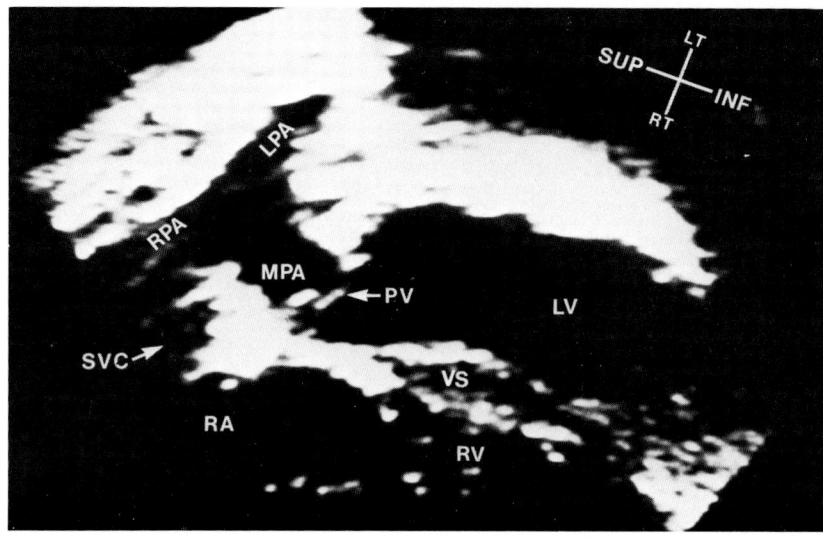

ANATOMY. The atria are in the normal position. The ventricles and atrioventricular valves are inverted. The right atrium empties into a right-sided anatomic left ventricle via the mitral valve. The left atrium empties into a left-sided morphologic right ventricle via a tricuspid valve. In other words, when ventricular inversion occurs, the mitral and tricuspid valves travel with their respective left and right ventricles. The aorta emerges from the anatomic right ventricle and the pulmonary artery springs from the anatomic left ventricle. Thus there is tricuspid valve–aortic valve discontinuity because of an interposed right ventricular infundibulum. The aortic valve is anterior, superior, and to the left of the pulmonic valve. In a few cases the great vessels may be side-by-side. The ventricular septum is rotated into the sagittal plane [28–30]. Since the interatrial septum and interventricular septum are malaligned, the membranous portion of the ventricular septum is much larger than in normal hearts [30]. The vast majority of ventricular defects occur in the membranous septum as a result of this phenomenon. Obstruction to pulmonary blood flow may be due to pulmonic valvular stenosis or subpulmonary membranous stenosis [30]. An Ebstein-like abnormality of the left atrioventricular valve (tricuspid valve) occurs frequently [30–32]. The anomaly has both the anatomic deformity of the leaflets and "atrialized" portion of the right ventricle of a right-sided Ebstein's anomaly.

M-MODE ECHOCARDIOGRAPHY. The sagittal, rather than perpendicular plane of the interventricular septum to the left precordium, may create problems in septal imaging. It is, therefore, important to locate the optimal transducer position for septal imaging; however, this is often difficult. A frequent pitfall is failure to identify ventricular septal echoes because of the tangential angle of the beam toward the septum. Thus a false diagnosis of single ventricle is entertained. Attention should be paid to the left-sided atrioventricular valve. If a scan from lateral to medial identifies chordal attachments of the left atrioventricular valve to the ventricular septum, there is suggestive evidence that the left-sided atrioventricular valve is the tricuspid valve. It must, however, be remembered that the mitral valve in an endocardial cushion defect attaches abnormally to the ventricular septum. A long axis scan from the left-sided ventricle (anatomic right ventricle) to the aortic root fails to demonstrate atrioventricular valve–semilunar valve continuity. This latter feature is also found in double-outlet right ventricle [33]. The M-mode features of corrected transposition, therefore, are nonspecific and further anatomic definition is needed.

TWO-DIMENSIONAL ECHOCARDIOGRAPHY. The position of the great arteries in corrected transposition was first described by Henry and associates [27]. The aorta and pulmonary artery are imaged as two circles either side-by-side, aorta on the left (Fig. 16-12), or the aorta anterior and to the left of the pulmonary artery (Fig. 16-13) in the short axis at the cardiac base. The criteria for identification of ventricular morphology by two-dimensional echocardiography have been defined [34, 35]. The anatomic right ventricle has (1) a more inferior atrioventricular valve attachment to the annulus when the atrioventricular valves are assessed from the apical four-chamber view (Fig. 16-14); (2) a multiple irregular papillary muscle arrangement when viewed from the apex or short axis; (3) prominent reflectances from right ventricular trabeculations and a characteristic bright reflectance from the moderator band in the apical four-chamber view; and (4) a trileaflet atrioventricular valve imaged on short axis (Fig. 16-15A). Since the plane of the tricuspid valve in short

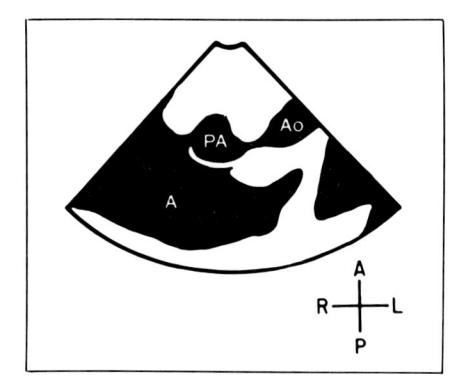

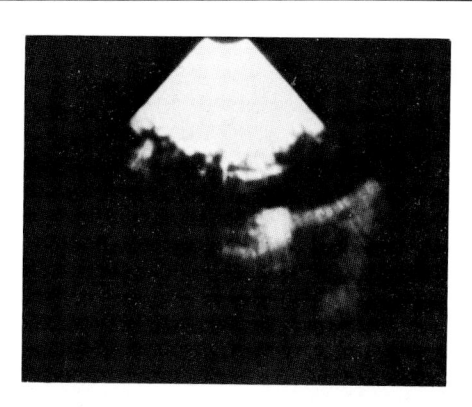

Fig. 16-12. Short axis view at the base of the heart in a patient with corrected transposition. The great arteries are seen as two circles side-by-side with the aorta to the left of the pulmonary artery (PA). A = atrium.

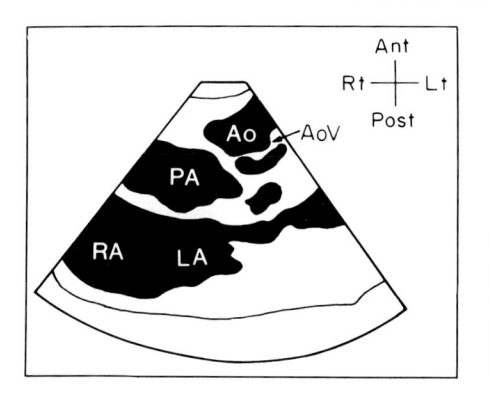

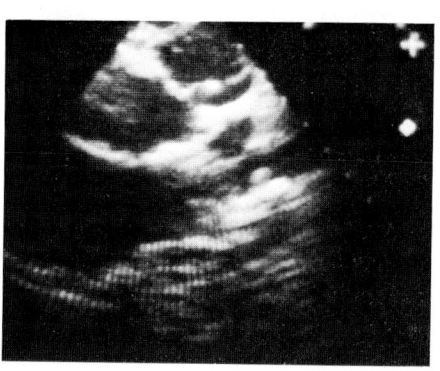

Fig. 16-13. Short axis view at the base of the heart in a patient with corrected transposition and an anterior leftward aorta. AoV = aortic valve; PA = pulmonary artery.

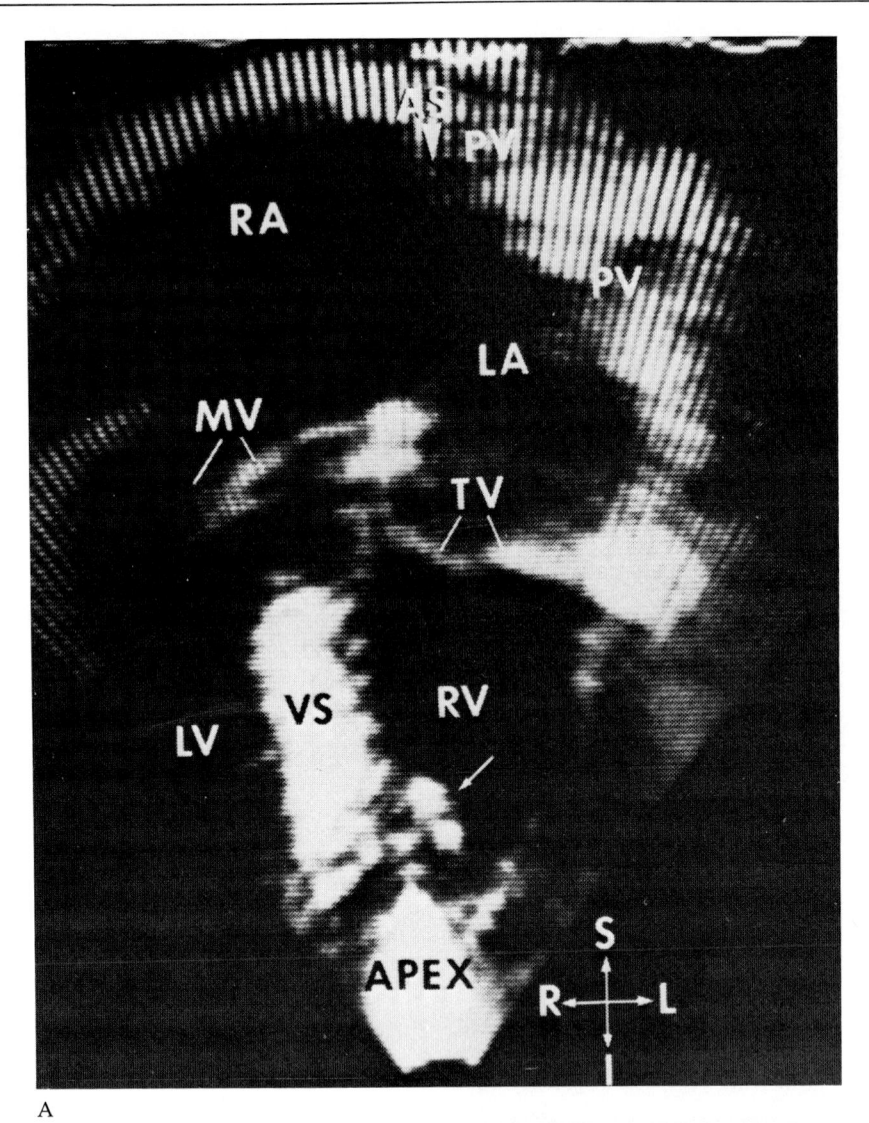

Fig. 16-14A. Apical 4-chamber view in corrected transposition. The atrioventricular valve on the left has a more inferior attachment to its annulus than the atrioventricular valve on the right. This feature identifies it as the tricuspid valve and diagnoses ventricular inversion. Thus, the right ventricle is on the left and the mitral valve and left ventricle are on the right. The right atrium and left atrium are in the normal position. (From DJ Hagler et al, Mayo Clin Proc 56:591, 1981.) *B.* Apical 4-chamber view in a patient with corrected transposition and Ebstein's anomaly. The left-sided tricuspid valve is displaced into the right ventricle. VS = ventricular septum.

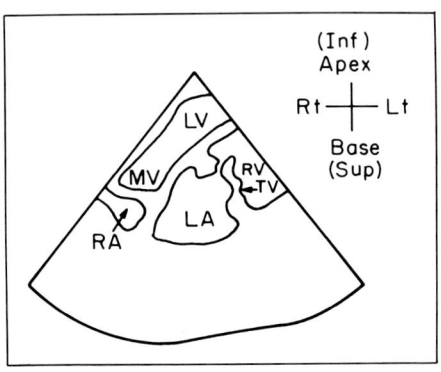

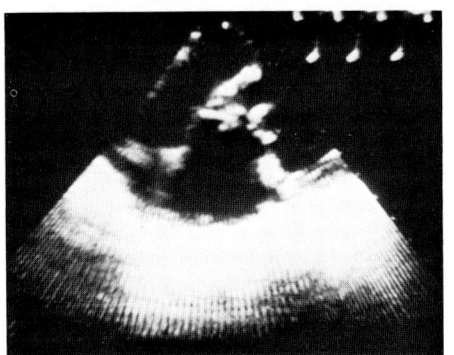

507

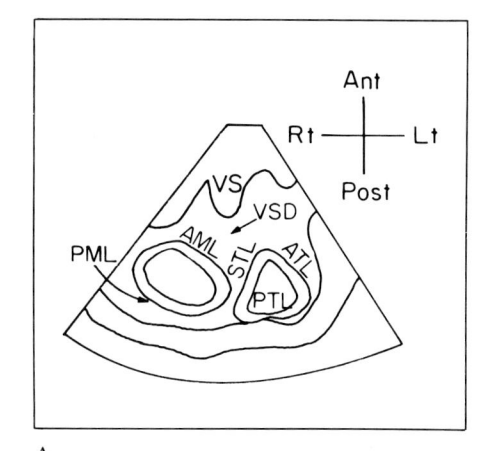

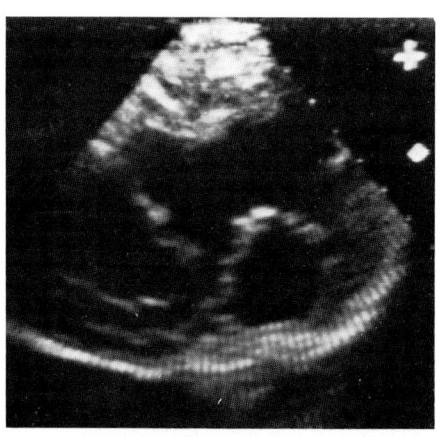

Fig. 16-15A. Short axis view at the atrioventricular valve level. The ventricular septum (VS) is in the sagittal plane. A fishmouth bileaflet mitral valve is seen on the right. A trileaflet tricuspid valve is seen on the left. B. Short axis view at the ventricular level recorded from a patient with congenitally corrected transposition. The ventricular septum is oriented vertically due to its sagittal plane. ATL = anterior tricuspid leaflet; PTL = posterior tricuspid leaflet.

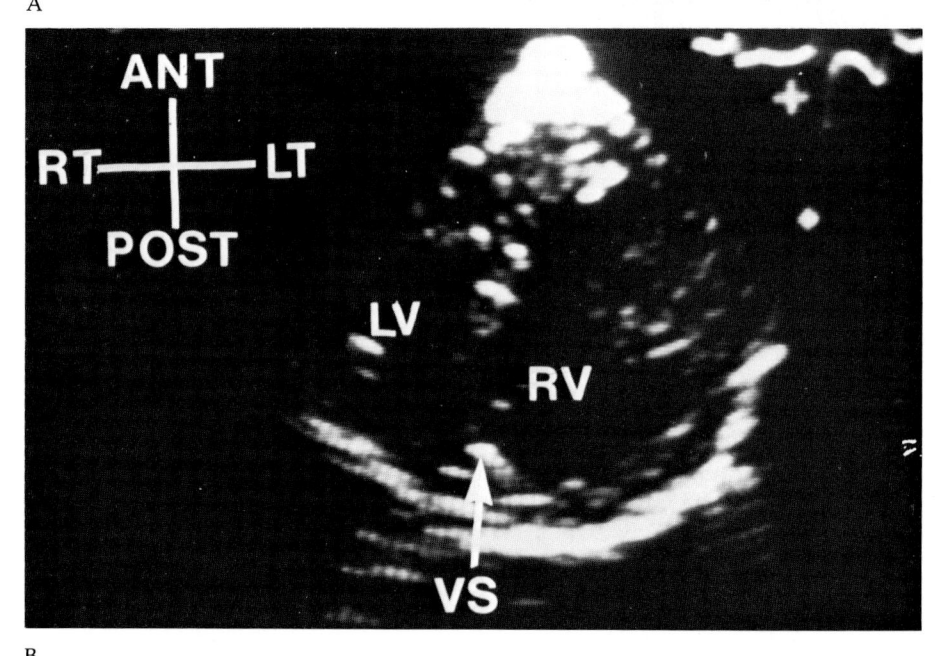

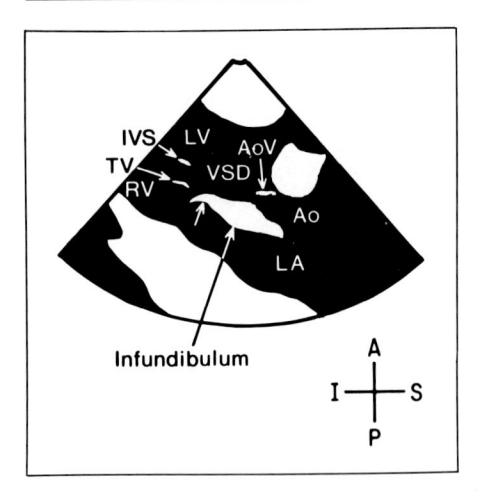

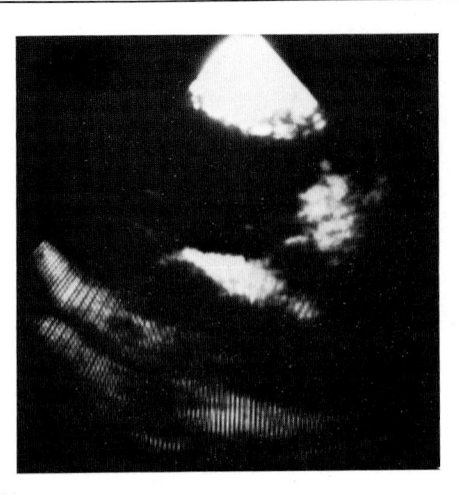

Fig. 16-16. Long axis view in a patient with corrected transposition. There is an area of increased echo denseness between the tricuspid valve and aortic valve (AoV). This atrioventricular valve to semilunar valve discontinuity is produced by a right ventricular infundibulum. (From TG DiSessa et al, Am J Cardiol 44:1146, 1979.)

axis is perpendicular to the echo beam in patients with ventricular inversion the three leaflets of the valve are seen easily. The anatomic left ventricle has (1) a more superior atrioventricular valve attachment to the annulus in the apical four-chamber view; (2) two discrete papillary muscles in short axis; and (3) a bileaflet (fishmouth) mitral valve in short axis (Fig. 16-15A). In patients with corrected transposition the plane of septum in short axis may be identified in the sagittal position because of ventricular inversion (Fig. 16-15B). Short axis scan identifies the aorta emerging from the left-sided anatomic right ventricle and the pulmonary artery emerging from the right-sided anatomic left ventricle [12]. In long axis discontinuity between the left-sided atrioventricular valve (the tricuspid valve) and the leftward semilunar valve (aortic valve) is established [12]. There is an area of increased echo denseness between the hinge point of the tricuspid valve and the leftward aortic root which represents the infundibulum of the right ventricle [12] (Fig. 16-16). Because of the sagittal position of the ventricular septum septal imaging is difficult in long axis, producing the false impression of a ventricular septal defect. In patients with Ebstein's anomaly of the left-sided atrioventricular valve the position of the ventricles is assessed easily. The echocardiographic features of a left-sided Ebstein's malformation, which are similar to those of the right-sided anomaly, include a displaced septal leaflet, enlarged anterior leaflet of the tricuspid valve, and atrialized right ventricle when the plane of sector is the apical four-chamber view [36, 37] (Fig. 16-14). Atrial position can be determined by imaging the drainage of the inferior vena cava. The inferior vena cava will always drain into the anatomic right atrium. Peripheral venous contrast injection may also be useful in determining the systemic venous (right) atrium.

Truncus arteriosus

CLINICAL FEATURES AND PHYSIOLOGY. The clinical presentation and physical findings in patients with truncus arteriosus depend on the volume of pulmonary blood flow. In infancy, when pulmonary flow is increased, the dominant picture is that of congestive heart failure and mild cyanosis. As the child grows older pulmonary vascular resistance increases and pulmonary blood flow becomes reduced.

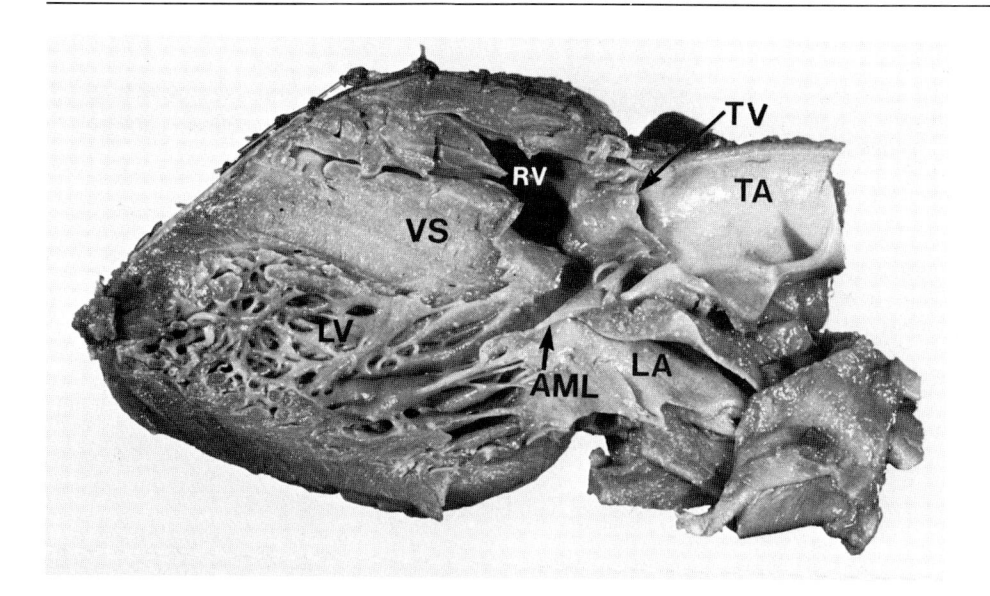

Fig. 16-17. Anatomic specimen cut in the long axis tomographic plane in a patient with truncus arteriosus. A large truncal artery (TA) is seen overriding the ventricular septum (VS). There is fibrous continuity between the anterior mitral leaflet and the truncal valve (TV).

Congestive heart failure gives way to progressive cyanosis. The patient with truncus arteriosus who survives to adolescence and adulthood is usually severely cyanotic from Eisenmenger's syndrome. Chest radiograph initially shows cardiomegaly with an increase in pulmonary vascular markings. As the patient grows, the cardiomegaly resolves. The main pulmonary artery segment is absent. Combined ventricular hypertrophy is most often seen on electrocardiogram.

ANATOMY. Truncus arteriosus is characterized by a single great vessel that arises from the base of the heart giving rise to the pulmonary, coronary, and systemic arteries. A large ventricular septal defect lies beneath the common trunk. Thus there is biventricular origin of the trunk [38, 39] (Fig. 16-17). The pulmonary arteries may arise from a short main pulmonary artery that originates from the common trunk (type 1), or directly from the lateral or posterior walls of the trunk (types 2 and 3) [40]. The mitral valve is in fibrous continuity with the truncal valve.

M-MODE ECHOCARDIOGRAPHY. The M-mode echocardiographic features of truncus arteriosus are indistinguishable from those of tetralogy of Fallot and pulmonary atresia [41]. A large truncal artery that overrides the ventricular septum is recorded. In order to separate truncus arteriosus from tetralogy of Fallot an image of the pulmonic valve must be recorded in the latter anomaly. However, it has been shown that M-mode echocardiography is successful in recording the pulmonic valve in only 25 percent of patients with tetralogy of Fallot [14].

TWO-DIMENSIONAL ECHOCARDIOGRAPHY. In the standard left parasternal long axis view a large ventricular septal defect, dilated truncal root overriding the ventricular septum, and mitral valve–truncal valve continuity are imaged (Fig. 16-18) [11–14]. Visualization of the pulmonic valve and hypoplastic right ventricular outflow tract allows the distinction of tetralogy of Fallot from truncus arteriosus and

510   16. Cyanotic congenital heart disease

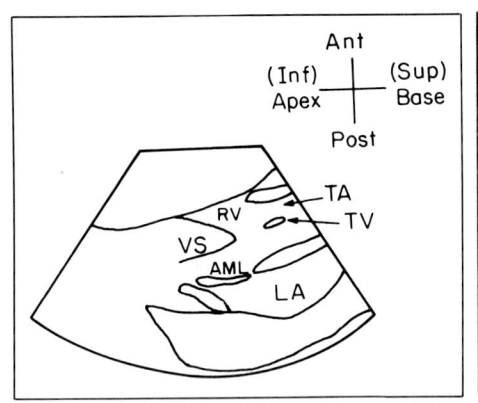

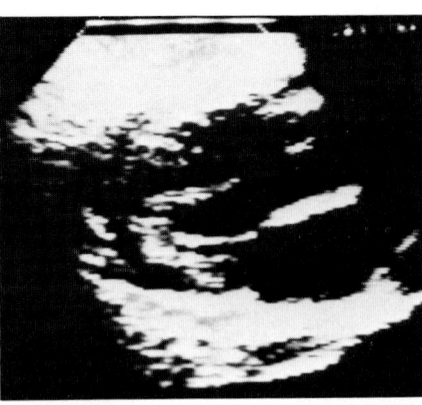

Fig. 16-18. Long axis view in a patient with truncus arteriosus. The truncal artery (TA) is enlarged and overrides the ventricular septum (VS). There is fibrous continuity between the anterior mitral leaflet and the truncal valve (TV). (Compare this echo image with the anatomic specimen in Fig. 16-17 and echocardiogram in Fig. 16-2.)

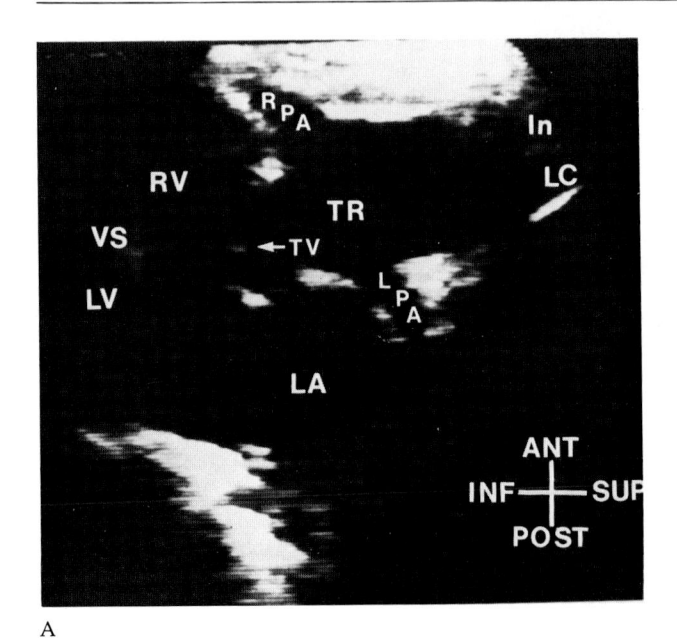

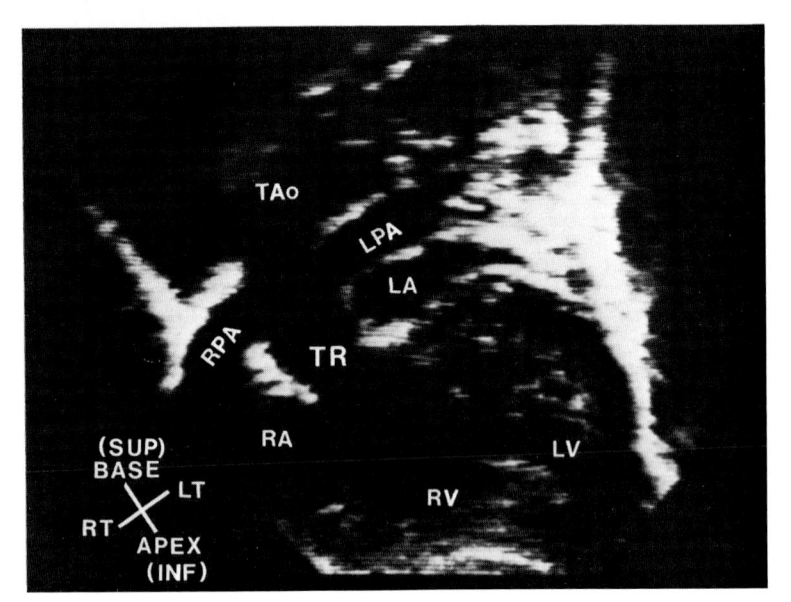

A

B

Fig. 16-19A. High left parasternal scan in a patient with truncus arteriosis type II. A large truncal root (TR) is imaged exiting both the right ventricle and left ventricle. The right pulmonary artery (RPA) and left pulmonary artery (LPA) are seen arising from the truncal root. B. Subcostal long axis scan in the same patient. The truncal root is imaged overriding the ventricular septum. The left (LPA) and right (RPA) pulmonary arteries arise from the truncal root. In = innominate artery, LC = left carotid, TV = truncal valve.

pulmonary atresia [12–14]. When imaging the short axis at the base of the heart in patients with truncus arteriosus, absence of the right ventricular outflow tract is observed; in patients with pulmonary atresia the right ventricular outflow tract ends blindly; and in patients with tetralogy of Fallot the right ventricular outflow tract is small and the pulmonic valve is imaged [13] (see Fig. 16-4). It must be reemphasized that two-dimensional echocardiography is far superior to M-mode techniques in defining the size and anatomy of the right ventricular outflow tract and presence of the pulmonic valve [13, 14]. The origin of the pulmonary arteries from the truncal root can be determined from a high parasternal long axis scan, short axis scan, subcostal long axis scan, or suprasternal notch scan of the truncal root (Fig. 16-19).

Double-outlet right ventricle

CLINICAL FEATURES AND PHYSIOLOGY. Patients with double-outlet right ventricle can be separated into four groups. The largest group of patients have a subaortic ventricular septal defect and pulmonic stenosis, and clinically appear like patients with tetralogy of Fallot. The next largest subset of patients have a subpulmonary ventricular septal defect with no pulmonic stenosis, and clinically mimic children with complete transposition of the great arteries and ventricular septal defect. These children have early onset of congestive heart failure and mild cyanosis. Patients with a subaortic ventricular septal defect and no pulmonic stenosis have a presentation similar to those with a ventricular septal defect and pulmonary hypertension. Finally, patients with an uncommitted ventricular septal defect resemble the patients in the third group [43]. The findings on chest radiograph depend upon the degree of obstruction to pulmonary blood flow. Patients without pulmonic stenosis have cardiomegaly with increased pulmonary blood flow and absence of the main pulmonary artery segment. Patients with pulmonic stenosis have a normal heart size with reduced pulmonary vascularity. The electrocardiogram usually shows right ventricular hypertrophy. A counterclockwise frontal plane loop is frequently found in patients with pulmonic stenosis [44]. These patients, therefore, may appear to have an endocardial cushion defect with pulmonic stenosis.

ANATOMY. Double-outlet right ventricle appears to result from a lack of conotruncal inversion, a failure of leftward conoventricular shift, and persistence of a subaortic conus [45, 46]. The anomaly was initially classified into two categories, one associated with pulmonic stenosis and one without pulmonic stenosis [47, 48]. Obstruction to pulmonary blood flow may be either valvular, subvalvular, supravalvular, or combinations of these [49]. The great arteries may either be side-by-side, *d*-malposed, *l*-malposed, or normally related [50]. Since only one great artery is displaced across the septum, the term *malposition* of the great arteries is used in patients with double-outlet right ventricle instead of *transposition*, which implies that both great arteries are displaced across the septum. The persistence of a subaortic conus prevents the normal leftward shift of the aorta and aortic valve. Thus the aorta remains to the right of the pulmonary artery, and muscle tissue (bilateral conus) separates the mitral valve from the aortic valve and the pulmonic valve (Figs. 16-20, 16-21) [47, 48]. The ventricular septal defect may be (1) related to the aortic valve (subaortic); (2) related to the pulmonic valve (subpulmonic) (Taussig-Bing anomaly); (3) related to both semilunar valves (doubly committed); or (4) related to neither semilunar valve (remote) [49].

512 16. Cyanotic congenital heart disease

Fig. 16-20. Anatomic specimen of a heart with double-outlet right ventricle is cut in the long axis plane. Conus (C) is seen between the anterior mitral leaflet and pulmonic valve (PV). The pulmonary artery (PA) courses in a posterior direction toward the lungs.

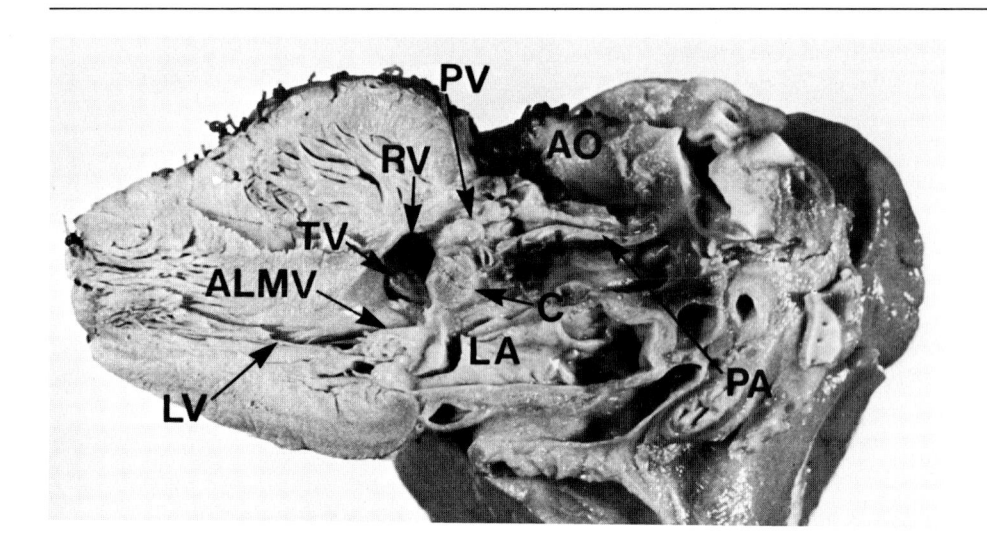

Fig. 16-21. Anatomic specimen of a heart with double-outlet right ventricle is cut in the long axis plane. There is discontinuity between the anterior leaflet of the mitral valve (ALMV) and pulmonic valve (PV) produced by conus (C). The pulmonary artery (PA) and aorta course in a parallel direction as they leave the heart. The tricuspid valve straddles the ventricular septum.

M-MODE ECHOCARDIOGRAPHY. The diagnosis by M-mode echocardiography relies principally on the establishment of mitral valve semilunar valve discontinuity and the inability to trace any great artery emerging from the left ventricle. However, recognition of such discontinuity may be difficult technically [9, 51].

TWO-DIMENSIONAL ECHOCARDIOGRAPHY. The initial cross-sectional echocardiographic description of double-outlet right ventricle used a linear-array scanner [11]. In the one patient studied both great arteries rose anteriorly in the transverse plane. Using a high-resolution sector scanner Henry and colleagues described both great arteries as anterior to the ventricular septum when scanning the heart in short axis along the left parasternal border [27]. We defined the complete anatomic spectrum of double-outlet right ventricle in 13 patients studied by two-dimensional echocardiography [12]. Hagler and associates subsequently reported similar findings in 36 patients [52]. The two-dimensional echocardiographic features reported in these 49 subjects included

In the left parasternal long axis view

1. Failure to identify any great artery emerging from the left ventricle
2. Identification of the outflow tract of the left ventricle as a ventricular septal defect
3. Lack of continuity between the anterior mitral valve leaflet and any semilunar valve produced by a muscular conus (Figs. 16-22, 16-23)
4. Parallel orientation and origin of both great arteries from the anterior right ventricle (Figs. 16-22, 16-24)

In the short axis view along the left parasternal border

1. Simultaneous imaging of both great arteries in an anterior location with the ventricular septum identified posteriorly on sweeping into the left ventricle (Fig. 16-25)
2. Lack of a counterclockwise wraparound of the aorta by the right ventricular outflow tract

These long axis and short axis features are specific for double-outlet right ventricle. In long axis the muscular conus is imaged as an area of increased echo denseness between the hinge point of the anterior mitral valve leaflet and the imaged semilunar valve (see Fig. 16-23). When the leftward great artery is the pulmonary artery it is seen coursing in a posterior direction toward the lungs. This image is similar to the long axis image of the pulmonary artery in complete transposition (see Figs. 16-20, 16-22). A short axis scan from the level of the ventricles superiorly shows both great arteries to be positioned anterior to the plane of the ventricular septum (see Figs. 16-7, 16-9). Thus the position of the great arteries to the ventricular septum is established (see Figs. 16-9, 16-25). From the short axis image at the cardiac base the position of the great arteries to each other is seen. In patients with double-outlet right ventricle the great arteries may be side-by-side (aorta on the right), *d*-malposed (aorta anterior and to the right of the pulmonary artery) (Figs. 16-25, 16-26A), or *l*-malposed (aorta anterior and to the left of the pulmonary artery) (Fig. 16-26B). Two-dimensional echocardiography may be useful in identification of the position of the ventricular septal defect [52]. In addition, it is useful in imaging associated malformations of the heart such as bicuspid stenotic pulmonic valve (Fig. 16-27), complete atrioventricular canal defect, straddling left and right atrio-

514   16. Cyanotic congenital heart disease

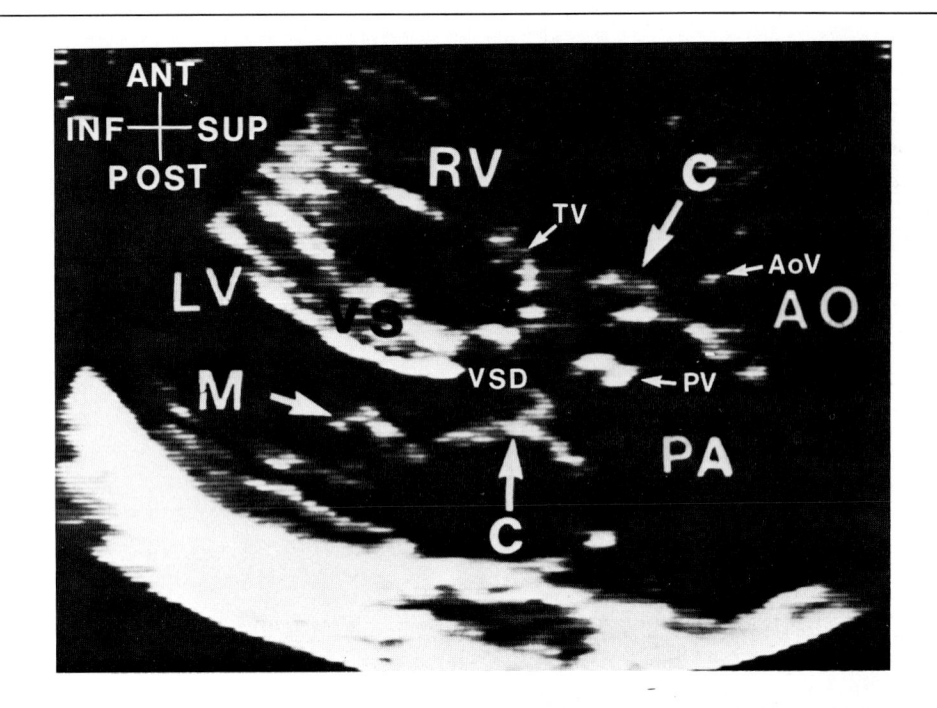

Fig. 16-22. Long axis scan in a patient with double-outlet right ventricle. The aorta and pulmonary artery (PA) originate entirely from the anterior right ventricle. A parallel orientation of both great arteries is imaged. The PA courses in a posterior direction toward the lungs. There is mitral valve (M) to pulmonic valve (PV) discontinuity produced by an area of increased echo denseness that originates from the muscular subpulmonic conus (C). The subaortic conus (C) is also imaged beneath the aortic valve (AoV). The only outlet of the left ventricle is through a subpulmonic ventricular septal defect (VSD). (Compare this image with the anatomic specimen in Fig. 16-21.)

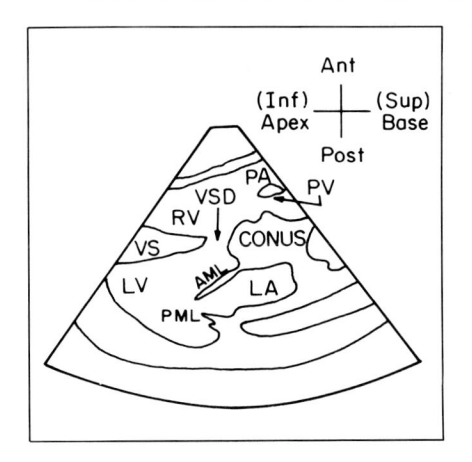

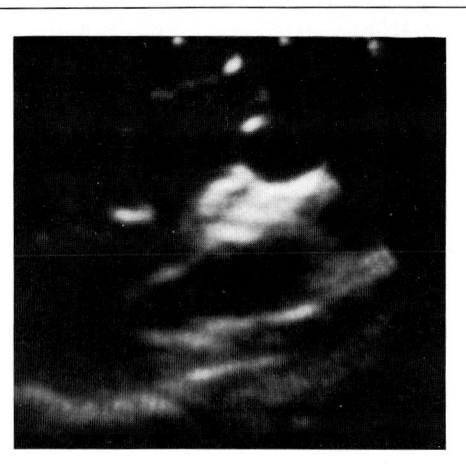

Fig. 16-23. Long axis scan in a patient with double-outlet right ventricle. There is no great artery seen arising from the left ventricle. The left ventricular outflow tract consists of the ventricular septal defect. There is discontinuity between the anterior mitral leaflet and the pulmonic valve (PV) produced by the muscular conus. This discontinuity is established by imaging the conus between the hinge point of the AML and the imaged semilunar valve (PV). PA = pulmonary artery; VS = ventricular septum.

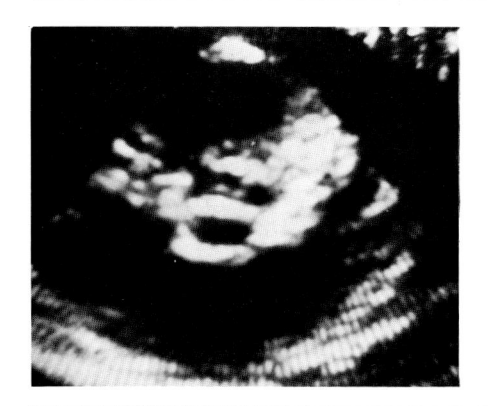

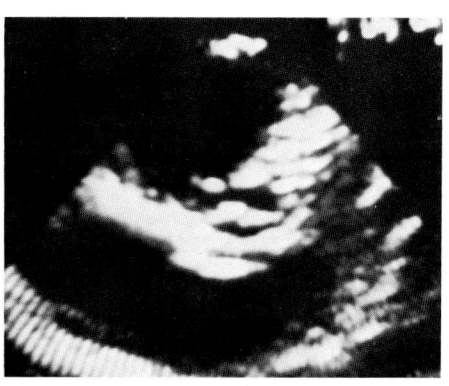

Fig. 16-27. Short axis at the cardiac base in a patient with double-outlet right ventricle and a bicuspid pulmonary valve. The plane of section is just below the aortic valve. Thus, the right ventricular outflow tract is seen anterior and to the right of the pulmonary artery (PA). The left panel shows a single diastolic closure line of the bicuspid pulmonic valve (arrows). The right panel shows the open pulmonic valve (PV), which has a fishmouth appearance. (Compare this image with the bicuspid aortic valve in Figs. 15-16 and 15-18.)

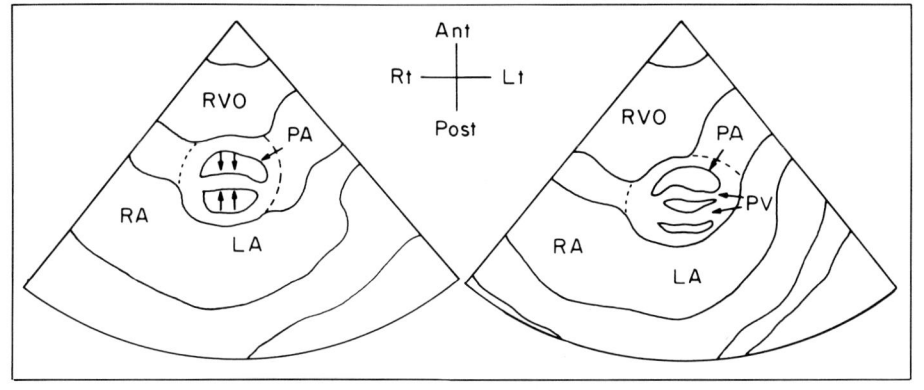

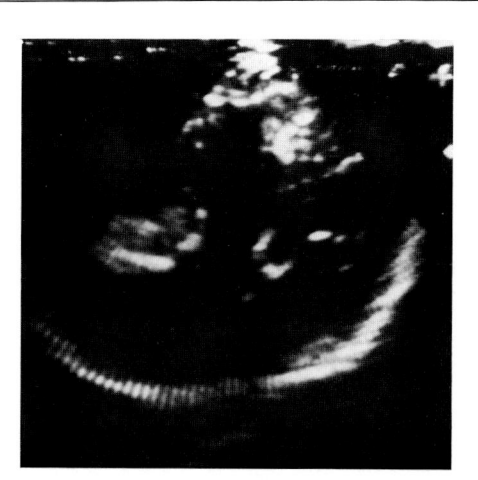

Fig. 16-28. Apical 4-chamber view in a patient with double-outlet right ventricle and a straddling tricuspid valve. The tricuspid valve annulus overrides the ventricular septal defect. VS = ventricular septum.

ventricular valves (Fig. 16-28), and isolated cleft in the anterior mitral valve leaflet [52].

Single ventricle (common ventricle)

CLINICAL FEATURES AND PHYSIOLOGY. Palliative surgery, and recently corrective surgery, has allowed long-term survival of patients with single ventricle into adolescence and adulthood. Discussion in this section will be confined to single ventricle of the left ventricular type with two atrioventricular valves in levocardia. Synonyms for this anomaly are: cor trioculare biatriatum, single ventricle, primitive ventricle, common ventricle, and double-inlet left ventricle. Clinical presentation depends upon the amount of pulmonary blood flow. If pulmonary flow is increased the patient has minimal cyanosis and congestive heart failure. If there is obstruction to pulmonary blood flow the patient is deeply cyanotic. The typical electrocardiogram shows equiphasic RS complexes from V2 to V6 on the precordial leads. Findings on chest radiograph depend on the degree of pulmonary blood flow.

ANATOMY. Single ventricle is an anomaly in which both atrioventricular valves enter a main ventricular chamber from which the arterial trunks emerge [53]. An outlet chamber may or may not be present [54]. The following types may be found: *d*-transposition of the great arteries (aorta anterior and to the right of the pulmonary artery); *l*-transposition of the great arteries (aorta anterior and to the left of the pulmonary artery) (Fig. 16-29A); and normal position of the arterial trunks. Lev and associates distinguish single ventricle from common ventricle, which they think is a heart with a large ventricular septal defect [53]. These authors also exclude straddling tricuspid valve, tricuspid atresia, and mitral atresia from the definition of single ventricle [53]. All types of single ventricle share the following features:

1. The mitral and tricuspid valves are not readily distinguishable. One atrioventricular valve is posteromedial and one is anterolateral. The anterior group of papillary muscles usually attaches to each valve (Fig. 16-29B).
2. The posterior wall of the common sinus is divided by a longitudinal ridge.
3. The posterior semilunar valve is in continuity with either or both atrioventricular valves.
4. The atrioventricular valves attach to the crux of the heart at the same level (Fig. 16-29C).

In single ventricle with *d*-transposition the outlet chamber is situated anterior and to the right of the main chamber. In hearts with *l*-transposition the outlet chamber is anterior and to the left of the main chamber (Fig. 16-29D). In these two types the pulmonic valve is continuous with the closest atrioventricular valve. In single ventricle with normally positioned arterial trunks the pulmonary artery springs from the outlet chamber and the aorta emerges from the main chamber and has fibrous continuity with an atrioventricular valve.

M-MODE ECHOCARDIOGRAPHY. The M-mode features of single ventricle include atrioventricular valve–semilunar valve continuity and simultaneous identification of both atrioventricular valves without an interposed ventricular septal echo [55]. Peripheral venous contrast echocardiography produces a distinctive flow pattern in single ventricle with two atrioventricular valves [56]. After injection of a contrast solution into a peripheral vein a cloud of echoes fills the main chamber through the anterior atrioventricular valve and anterior to the posterior atrioventricular valve after its E point. These features are nonspecific for single ventricle and may also be seen in patients with a straddling tricuspid valve [57]. In contrast to single ventricle ventricular septal echoes may be imaged at the apex of the heart in patients with straddling tricuspid valve.

TWO-DIMENSIONAL ECHOCARDIOGRAPHY. We have studied 13 patients with single ventricle. The features presented here are a composite of a few reports in the literature and our own experience. From the left parasternal long axis view a single posterior main chamber is imaged, and atrioventricular valve–semilunar valve continuity is established. In the short axis view two atrioventricular valves are imaged opening into a large main chamber (Fig. 16-30A); multiple papillary muscles and trabeculations are seen scattered irregularly around the main chamber (Fig. 16-30B); and the chordal attachments of each valve to a posterior group of papillary muscles is seen (Fig. 16-30A). Short axis scan from apex to base best identifies the position of the outflow chamber and the position of the great arteries (Fig. 16-30C) [58]. In the apical four-chamber view the two atrioventricular valves are seen to be attached to the crux of the heart at the same level (Fig. 16-31) [59, 60], with loss of the normal pattern of separated insertion.

Tricuspid atresia

CLINICAL FINDINGS AND PHYSIOLOGY. The clinical presentation of patients with tricuspid atresia occurs in infancy and depends upon anatomic type. In infants with marked obstruction to pulmonary blood flow intense cyanosis is the presenting symptom. Infants with little or no obstruction to pulmonary blood flow will be minimally cyanotic but in congestive heart failure. Electrocardiography typically shows left ventricular hypertrophy with a counterclockwise frontal plane loop in 80 percent of the cases [61]. Chest radiography reflects the degree of pulmonary blood flow.

ANATOMY. Hearts with tricuspid atresia have certain characteristics that are consistently present, including an atretic or imperforate tricuspid valve; hypoplasia of the anatomic right ventricle; an interatrial communication; a large anatomic left ventricle with a mitral valve; and a ventricular septal defect. Certain variable features included in the anomaly are the origin of the great arteries, and the presence or absence of obstruction to pulmonary blood flow [62]. Tricuspid valve leaflet tissue is not identifiable. Instead an imperforate dimple is found in the floor of the right atrium [63]. The interatrial communication is usually a patent foramen ovale, but occasionally there is a true atrial septal defect. The mitral valve is normal morphologically, and it empties into a true morphologic left ventricle. The great arteries exit from the left ventricle, one directly from the left ventricle, and one from a hypoplastic right ventricle, which communicates with the left ventricular chamber via a ventricular septal defect. Tricuspid atresia has been classified according to the position of the great arteries and presence of pulmonary outflow tract obstruction [64]. Type 1 tricuspid atresia has normally related great arteries. The aorta springs from the left ventricle and the aortic valve is in fibrous continuity with the mitral valve. The pulmonary artery emerges from the hypoplastic right ventricle. Type 2 tricuspid atresia has transposition of the great arteries. The pulmonary artery emerges from the left ventricle and the pulmonic valve is in fibrous continuity with

520   16. Cyanotic congenital heart disease

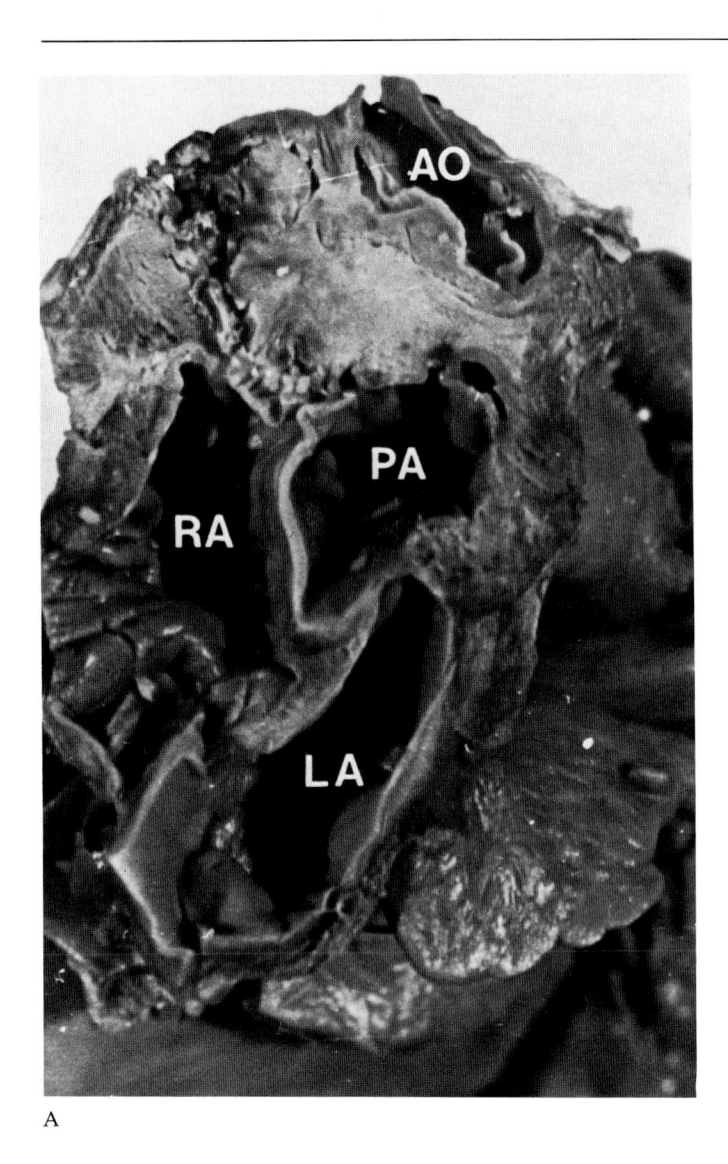

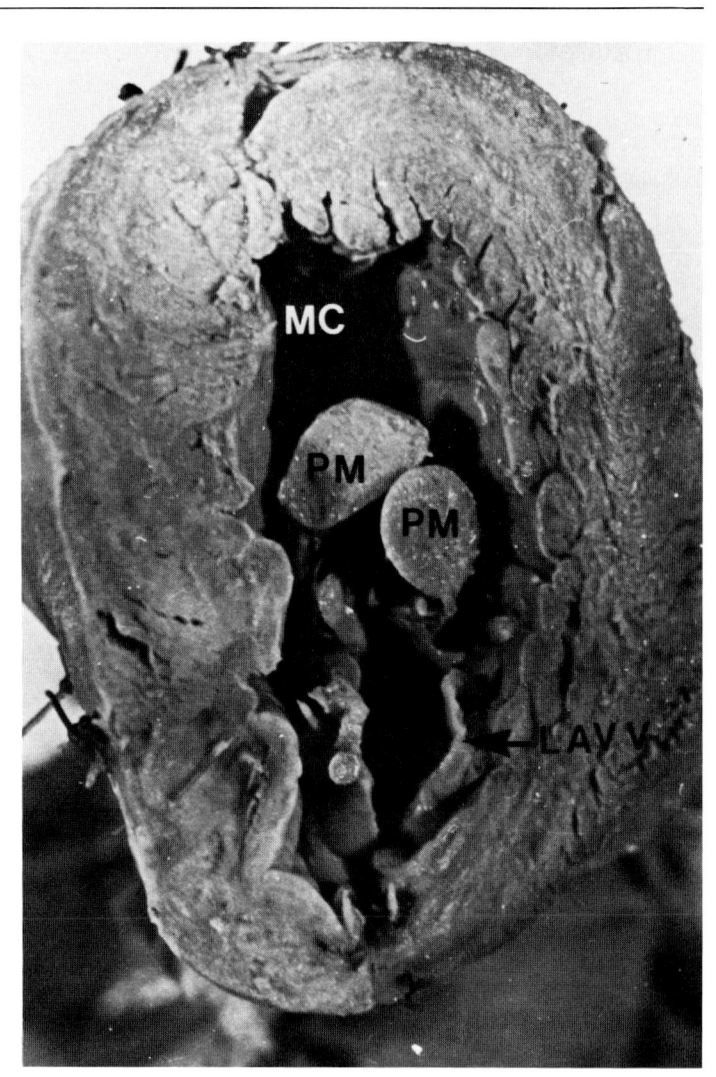

Fig. 16-29A. Anatomic specimen cut in the short axis plane at the cardiac base. The aorta emerges from the outlet chamber and is anterior and to the left of the pulmonary artery (PA). B. Anatomic specimen cut in the short axis plane at the cardiac apex. Two papillary muscles and the left atrioventricular valve (LAVV) are seen in a main chamber (MC). C. Anatomic specimen cut in the apical 4-chamber plane. A single main chamber (MC) is seen. Two atrioventricular valves enter the main chamber. These atrioventricular valves attach to the crux of the heart at the same level (arrow). D. Anatomic specimen cut in the short axis plane at the atrioventricular valve level. The left atrioventricular valve and right atrioventricular valve (RAVV) are seen entering a main chamber. The outflow chamber (OC) is anterior and to the left of the main chamber.

521

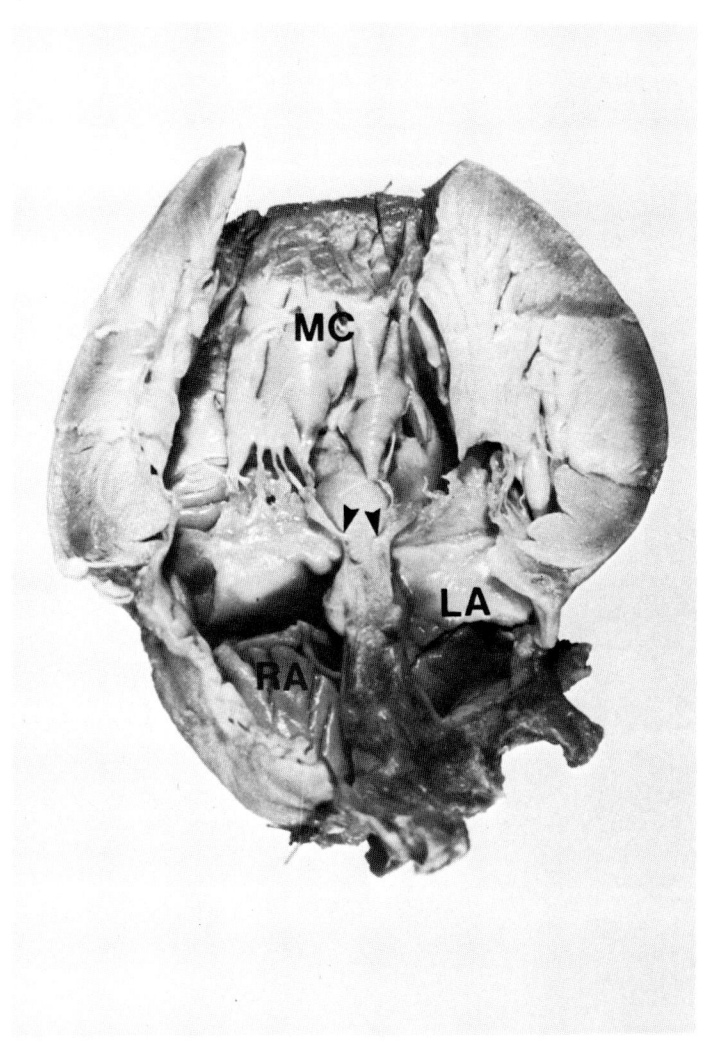

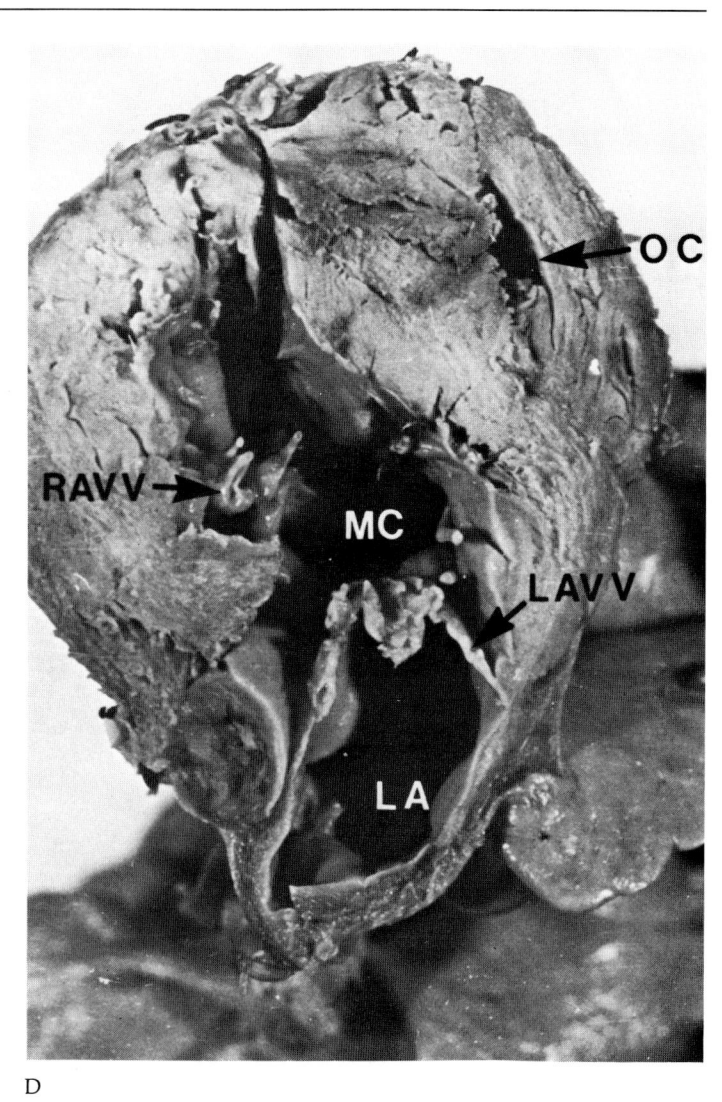

16. Cyanotic congenital heart disease

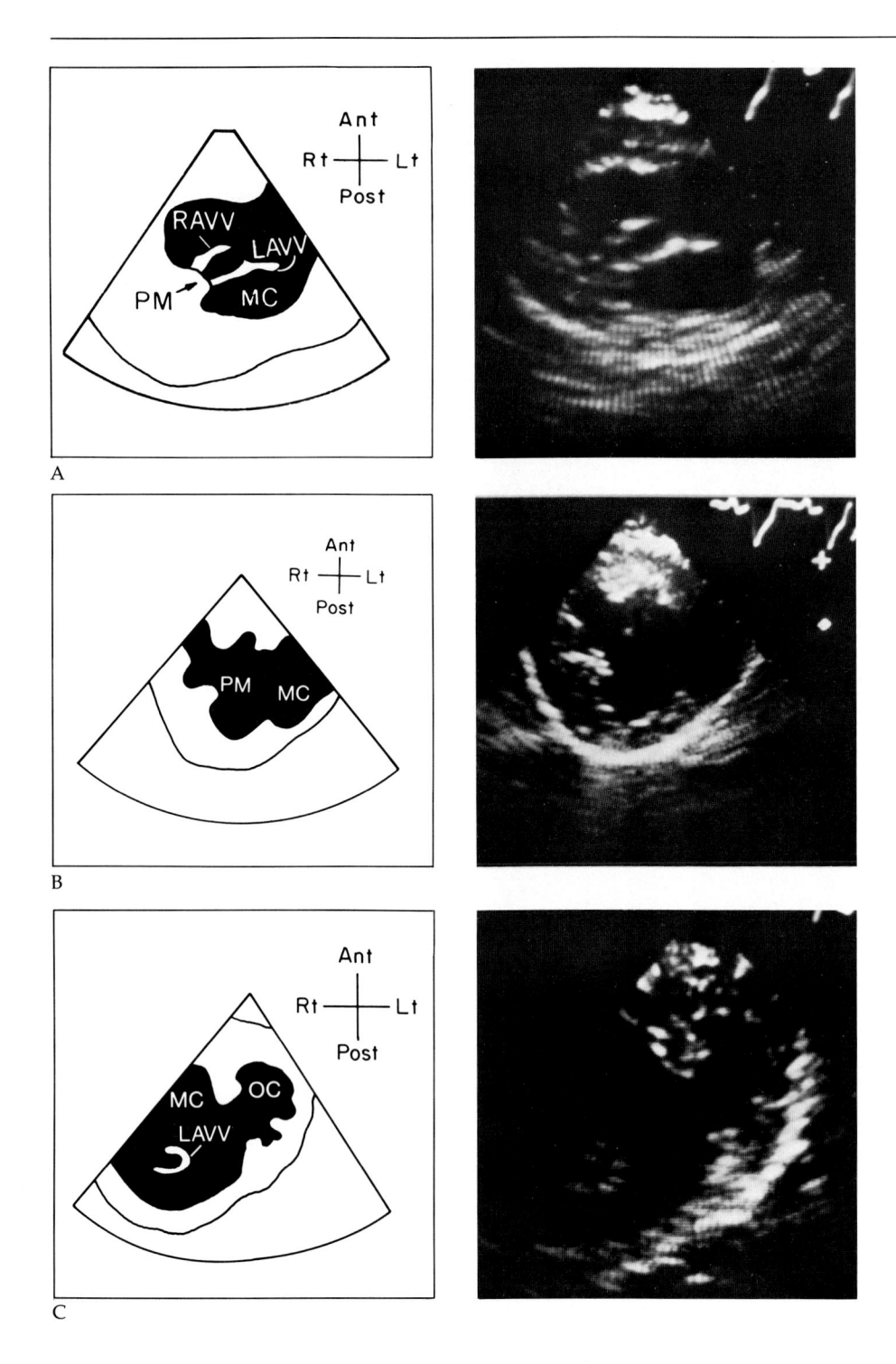

Fig. 16-30A. Short axis view in a patient with single ventricle. Two atrioventricular valves are imaged opening into a main chamber (MC). They are attached to a common posterior group of papillary muscles. The left atrioventricular valve (LAVV) is posteromedial and the right atrioventricular valve (RAVV) is anterolateral. B. Short axis view recorded through the cardiac apex. A single ventricular chamber is imaged. This main chamber has an irregular shape due to multiple papillary muscles scattered irregularly around it. C. Short axis view in a patient with single ventricle. At this level the outflow chamber (OC) is seen exiting the main chamber anterior and to the left of the main chamber.

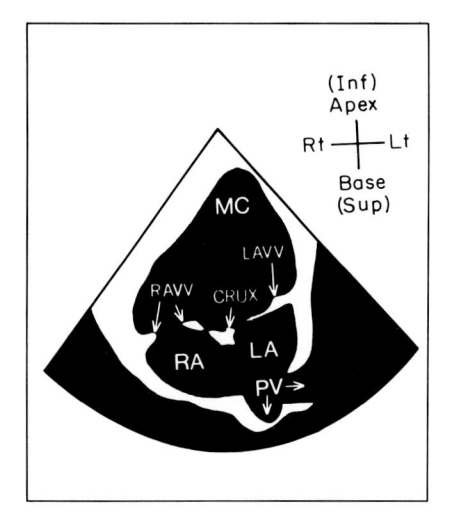

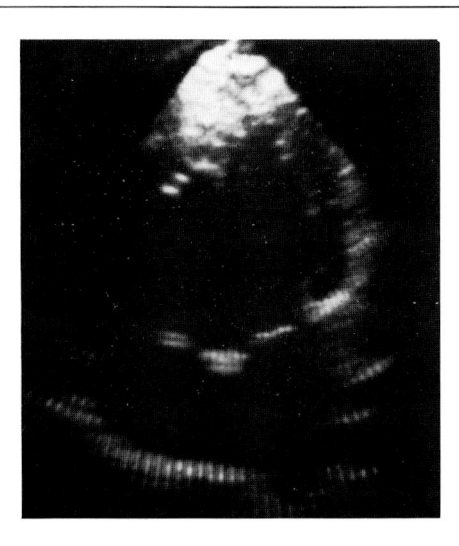

Fig. 16-31. Apical 4-chamber view in a patient with single ventricle. Two atrioventricular valves are imaged entering a single main chamber (MC). Both valves attach to the crux of the heart at the same level. (Compare this image with the anatomic specimen in Fig. 16-29C.) LAVV = left atrioventricular valve; PV = pulmonary vein; RAVV = right atrioventricular valve.

the mitral valve. The aorta emerges from the hypoplastic right ventricle, which communicates with the left ventricle via a ventricular septal defect. Each type is subdivided into three groups: group A patients have pulmonary atresia, group B patients have pulmonic stenosis, and group C patients do not have pulmonic stenosis.

M-MODE ECHOCARDIOGRAPHY. The M-mode features of tricuspid atresia are absence of the tricuspid valve echo in association with a right ventricular dimension that is less than normal [65]. There is mitral valve–semilunar valve continuity.

TWO-DIMENSIONAL ECHOCARDIOGRAPHY. We have examined 13 patients with tricuspid atresia. The features reported here are a synopsis of our experience and the sole report in the literature [66]. In the left parasternal long axis view a large posterior main chamber is imaged. There is mitral valve–semilunar valve continuity. In short axis the posterior ventricle has the circular shape of a morphologic left ventricle. There are an anterolateral and a posteromedial papillary muscle. Scan from apex to base identifies the position of the great arteries. The apical four-chamber view and subcostal four-chamber view identify an area of increased echo denseness in the area of the atretic tricuspid valve. In addition the hypoplastic right ventricle and ventricular septal defect may be seen in these views (Fig. 16-32). Colo and colleagues measured the diameter of the main pulmonary artery and aorta from the short axis view and found a good correlation between the aortic to pulmonary dimension ratio (Ao/Pa) by echocardiography with the same ratio measured by angiocardiography ($r = 0.91$) [66]. Moreover the pulmonary artery diameter corrected to body surface area correlated with pulmonary to systemic flow ratio ($\dot{Q}p/\dot{Q}s$) ($r = 0.80$). The authors were also able to accurately classify 10 of 13 patients, age 6 hours to 25 years, by two-dimensional imaging.

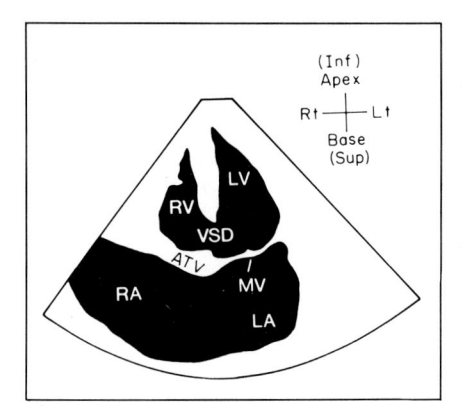

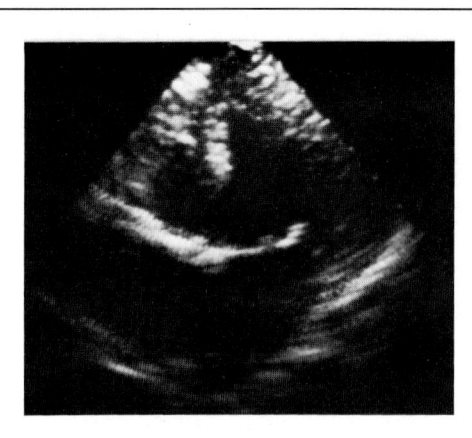

Fig. 16-32. Apical 4-chamber view recorded from a patient with tricuspid atresia. The right ventricle is hypoplastic. There is no communication between the right atrium and right ventricle. The atretic tricuspid valve (ATV) is seen as an area of increased echo denseness between the right atrium and right ventricle. VS = ventricular septum.

Total anomalous pulmonary venous return

CLINICAL FINDINGS AND PHYSIOLOGY. Although this cardiac anomaly is rarely found in adolescents and adults, its features should be mentioned for the sake of completeness. As with all the previously mentioned anomalies its clinical features depend upon the anatomic type that exists. Infants with severe pulmonary venous obstruction are intensely cyanotic and in severe congestive heart failure. On the other end of the spectrum is the infant with no pulmonary venous obstruction who is minimally cyanotic and not in congestive heart failure. Electrocardiography reflects the right-sided volume and pressure overload. Thus, peaked P waves of right atrial enlargement and precordial voltage, consistent with right ventricular hypertrophy, are present. Chest x-ray reflects the degree of pulmonary venous obstruction and pulmonary blood flow.

ANATOMY. Understanding the anatomy of total anomalous pulmonary venous return requires the clarification of the three major components of the anomaly: the pathway by which the pulmonary venous blood reaches the systemic atrium; the presence or absence of obstruction along the course of this pathway; and the status of the atrial septum. The anomaly has been divided into four types: supracardiac return, cardiac return, infracardiac return, and mixed [67]. Supracardiac connections are either to a confluence of pulmonary veins, left vertical vein, and persistent superior vena cava, or directly into the right superior vena cava or azygous vein. Cardiac connections are either directly to the right atrium or to the coronary sinus (Fig. 16-33). Infracardiac connections drain to the portal system, ductus venosus, or inferior vena cava. The overload to the right side of the heart produces right atrial and right ventricular dilatation.

M-MODE ECHOCARDIOGRAPHY. M-mode cardiac examination demonstrates an enlarged right ventricle, paradoxical septal motion, and an extra linear echo behind the aortic root in the left atrium [68].

TWO-DIMENSIONAL ECHOCARDIOGRAPHY. Two-dimensional imaging allows direct visualization of the pathways of pulmonary venous connection to the heart. From the apical four-chamber and subcostal four-chamber views, the right and left

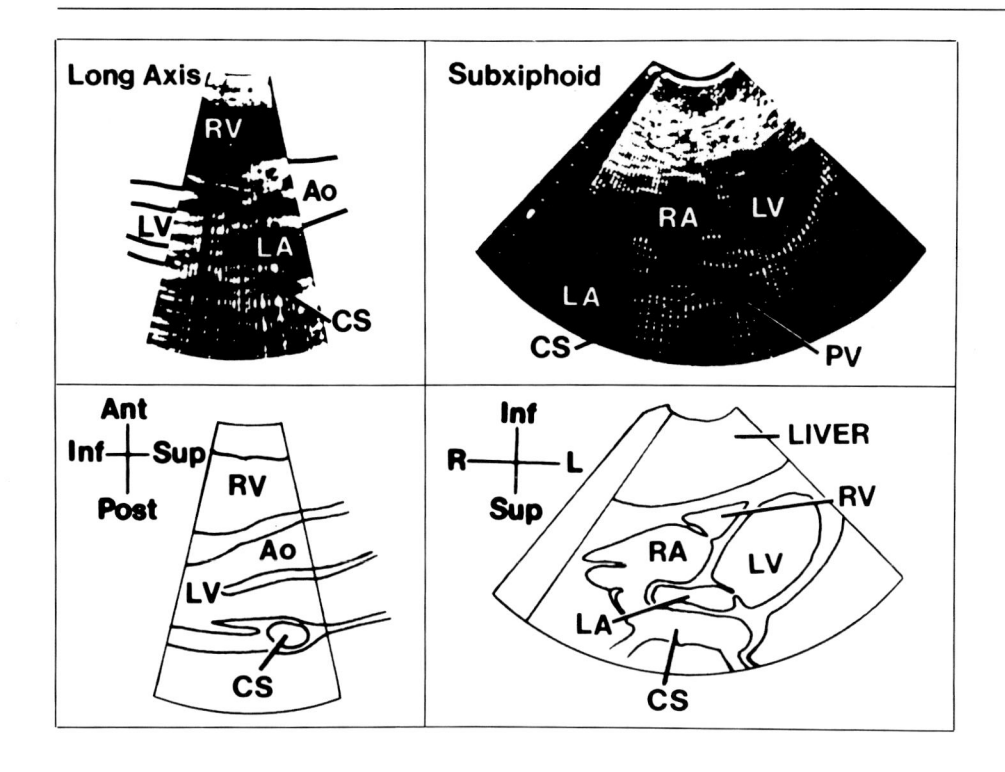

Fig. 16-33. *Left parasternal long axis view in a patient with total anomalous pulmonary venous return to the coronary sinus (left panel). The right ventricle is enlarged as is the coronary sinus. Subcostal view (right panel). The coronary sinus is enlarged and the pulmonary veins (PV) are imaged draining into it. (From DJ Sahn et al, Cross-sectional echocardiographic diagnosis of the sites of total anomalous pulmonary venous drainage. Circulation 60:1317, 1979 by permission of the American Heart Association, Inc.)*

upper pulmonary veins are imaged entering the left atrium. Identification of one pulmonary vein entering the left atrium excludes the diagnosis of total anomalous pulmonary venous connection [69]. From the subcostal window, the inferior vena cava is imaged, and from the suprasternal notch, the superior vena cava is seen. The coronary sinus is visualized in the atrioventricular groove on the left parasternal long axis image (Fig. 16-33). Enlargement of these structures is indirect evidence of anomalous connection to the structure [70]. Identification of the common pulmonary vein in total anomalous pulmonary venous connection below the diaphragm has been reported [71]. With the transducer in the subcostal position the descending aorta and spine are imaged. The common pulmonary vein is imaged parallel and anterior to the descending aorta and to the left of the inferior vena cava [71]. With a peripheral venous contrast injection below the diaphragm the inferior vena cava and aorta but not the common pulmonary vein fill with microcavitations [71].

References

1. Stensen N: Quoted by H.I. Goldstein. *Bull Hist Med* 22:526, 1948
2. Willius FA, Keys TE: *Classics of Cardiology*. New York: Dover, 1961
3. Vogelpoel L, Schrire V: Auscultatory and phonocardiographic assessment of Fallot's tetralogy. *Circulation* 22:73, 1960
4. Lev M, Eckner FOA: The pathologic anatomy of tetralogy of Fallot and its variations. *Dis Chest* 45:251, 1964
5. Guntheroth WG, Kawabori I: Tetrad of Fallot. In AJ Moss, FH Adams, G Emmanouilides, (eds), *Heart Disease in Infants, Children and Adolescents* (2nd ed). Baltimore: Williams and Wilkins, 1977. Pp 276–289
6. Morris DC, Felner JM, Schlant RC, Franch RH: Echocardiographic diagnosis of tetralogy of Fallot. *Am J Cardiol* 36:908, 1975
7. Tajik AJ, Gau GT, Ritter DG, Schattenberg TT: Echocardiogram in tetralogy of Fallot. *Chest* 64:107, 1973
8. Weyman AE, Dillon JC, Feigenbaum H, Chang S: Echocardiographic differentiation of infundibular from valvular pulmonary stenosis. *Am J Cardiol* 36:21, 1975
9. French JW, Popp R: Variability of echocardiographic discontinuity in double outlet right ventricle and truncus arteriosus. *Circulation* 51:848, 1975
10. Valdez-Cruz LM, Pieroni D, Roland JMA, Varghese PJ: Echocardiographic detection of intracardiac right-to-left shunt following peripheral vein injections. *Circulation* 54:558, 1976
11. Sahn DJ, Terry R, O'Rourke R, Leopold G, Friedman WF: Multiple crystal cross-sectional echocardiography in the diagnosis of cyanotic congenital heart disease. *Circulation* 50:230, 1974
12. DiSessa TG, Hagan AD, Pope C, Samtoy L, Friedman WF: Two-dimensional echocardiographic characteristics of double outlet right ventricle. *Am J Cardiol* 44:1146, 1979
13. Hagler DJ, Tajik AJ, Seward JB, Mair DD, Ritter DG: Wide-angle two-dimensional echocardiographic profiles of conotruncal abnormalities. *Mayo Clin Proc* 55:73, 1980
14. Caldwell RL, Weyman AE, Hurwitz RA, Girod DA, Fiegenbaum H: Right ventricular outflow tract assessment of cross-sectional echocardiography in tetralogy of Fallot. *Circulation* 59:395, 1979
15. Lange LW, Sahn DJ, Allen HD, Goldberg SJ: Subxiphoid cross-sectional echocardiography in infants and children with congenital heart disease. *Circulation* 59:513, 1979
16. Tajik AJ, Seward JB, Hagler DJ, Mair DD, Lie JT: Two-dimensional real-time ultrasonic imaging of the heart and great vessels: Technique, image orientation, structure identification and validation. *Mayo Clin Proc* 53:271, 1978
17. Sahn DJ, Sobol RG, Allen HD: Subxiphoid real-time cross-sectional echocardiography for imaging of the right ventricle (RV) and right ventricular outflow tract (RVOT). *Am J Cardiol* 41:354, 1978 (Abstract)
18. Mustard WT: Successful two-stage correction of transposition of the great vessels. *Surgery* 55:469, 1964
19. Lev M, Alcalde VM, Baffes TG: Pathologic anatomy of complete transposition of the arterial trunks. *Pediatrics* 28:293, 1961
20. Shaher RM, Puddu GC, Khoury G, Moes F, Mustard WT: Complete transposition of the great vessels with anatomic obstruction of the outflow tract of the left ventricle: Surgical implications and anatomic findings. *Am J Cardiol* 19:658, 1967
21. Shrivastava S, Tadavarthy SM, Fukuda T, Edwards JE: Anatomic causes of pulmonary stenosis in complete transposition. *Circulation* 54:154, 1976
22. Dillon JC, Feigenbaum H, Konecke L, Keutel J, Hurwitz RA, Davis RH, Chang S: Echocardiographic manifestations of d-transposition of the great vessels. *Am J Cardiol* 32:74, 1973
23. Aziz KU, Paul M, Muster AJ: Echocardiographic assessment of the left ventricular outflow tract in d-transposition of the great artery. *Am J Cardiol* 41:543, 1978
24. Silverman NH, Payot M, Stanger P, Rudolph AM: The echocardiographic profile of patients after Mustard's operation. *Circulation* 58:1083, 1978
25. Bierman FZ, Williams RG: Prospective diagnosis of d-transposition of the great arteries in neonates by subxiphoid, two-dimensional echocardiography. *Circulation* 60:1496, 1979
26. Henry W, Maron BJ, Griffith JM, Redwood DR, Epstein SE: Differential diagnosis of anomalies of the great arteries by real-time two-dimensional echocardiography. *Circulation* 51:283, 1975

27. Henry W, Maron BJ, Griffith JM: Cross-sectional echocardiography in the diagnosis of congenital heart disease: Identification of the relation of the ventricles and great arteries. *Circulation* 56:267, 1977
28. Berry WB, Roberts WC, Morrow AG, Braunwald E: Corrected transpositions of the aorta and pulmonary trunk; clinical, hemodynamic, and pathologic findings. *Am J Med* 36:35, 1964
29. Honey M: Anatomical and physiological features of corrected transposition of the great vessels. *Guy's Hosp Rep* 111:250, 1962
30. Allwork SP, Bentall HH, Becker AE, Cameron H, Gerlis LM, Wilkinson JL, Anderson RH: Congenitally corrected transposition of the great arteries: Morphologic study of 32 cases. *Am J Cardiol* 38:910, 1976
31. Dekker A, Mehrizi A, Vengsarker AS: Corrected transposition of the great vessels with Ebstein's malformation of the left atrioventricular valve. *Circulation* 31:119, 1965
32. Jaffe RB: Systemic atrioventricular valve regurgitation in corrected transposition of the great vessels. *Am J Cardiol* 37:395, 1976
33. Williams RG, Tucker CR: *Echocardiographic Diagnosis of Congenital Heart Disease* (1st ed). Boston: Little, Brown, 1977. P 257
34. Hagler DJ, Tajik AJ, Seward JB, Edwards D, Mair DD, Ritter DG: Atrioventricular and ventriculoarterial discordance (corrected transposition of the great arteries): Recognition by wide-angle two dimensional echocardiographic assessment of ventricular morphology. *Mayo Clin Proc* 56:591, 1981
35. Foale RA, Stenfanini L, Richards AF, Somerville J: Two-dimensional echocardiographic features of corrected transposition. *Am J Cardiol* 45:466, 1980 (Abstract)
36. Ports T, Silverman NH, Schiller NB: Two-dimensional echocardiographic assessment of Ebstein's anomaly. *Circulation* 58:336, 1978
37. Silverman NH, Schiller NB: Apex echocardiography: A two-dimensional technique for evaluating congenital heart disease. *Circulation* 57:503, 1978
38. Calder L, Van Praagh R, Van Praagh S, Seras WP, Corwin R, Levy A, Keith JD, Paul MH: Truncus arteriosus communis: Clinical, angiographic and pathologic findings in 100 patients. *Am Heart J* 92:23, 1976
39. Edwards JE: Persistent truncus arteriosus. *Am Heart J* 92:1, 1976
40. Collett RW, Edwards JE: Persistent truncus arteriosus: Classification according to anatomic types. *Surg Clin North Am* 29:1245, 1949
41. Chung KJ, Alexson CG, Manning JA, Gramiak R: Echocardiography in truncus arteriosus: The value of pulmonic valve detection. *Circulation* 48:281, 1973
42. Rice MJ, Seward JB, Hagler DJ, Mair DD, Rajik AJ: Definitive diagnosis of truncus arteriosus by two-dimensional echocardiography. *Mayo Clin Proc* 57:476, 1982
43. Sondheimer HM, Freedom RM, Olley PM: Double outlet right ventricle: Clinical spectrum and prognosis. *Am J Cardiol* 39:709, 1977
44. Krongrad E, Ritter DG, Weidman WH, DuShane JW: Hemodynamic and anatomic correlation of electrocardiogram in double outlet right ventricle. *Circulation* 46:995, 1972
45. Witham AC: Double outlet right ventricle: A partial transposition complex. *Am Heart J* 53:928, 1957
46. Goor DA, Edwards JE: The spectrum of transposition of the great arteries with specific reference to the developmental anatomy of the conus. *Circulation* 48:406, 1973
47. Neufeld HN, DuShane JW, Wood EH, Kirklin JW, Edwards JE: Origin of the great vessels from the right ventricle. I. Without pulmonic stenosis. *Circulation* 23:399, 1961
48. Neufeld HN, DuShane JW, Edwards JE: Origin of the great vessels from the right ventricle. II. With pulmonic stenosis. *Circulation* 23:603, 1961
49. Neufeld HN, Randall PA: Double Outlet Right Ventricle. In AJ Moss, FH Adams, G Emmanouilides (eds), *Heart Disease in Infants, Children and Adolescents* (2nd ed). Baltimore: Williams & Wilkins, 1977. Pp 355–366
50. Sridaromont S, Ritter EG, Feldt RH, Davis GD, Edwards JW: Double outlet right ventricle: Anatomic and angiocardiographic correlations. *Mayo Clin Proc* 53:555, 1978
51. Rosenquist GC, Clark EB, Sweeny LJ, McAllister HA: The normal spectrum of mitral-aortic valve discontinuity. *Circulation* 54:298, 1976
52. Hagler DJ, Tajik AJ, Seward JB, Mair DD, Ritter DG: Double outlet right ventricle: Wide-angle two-dimensional echocardiographic observations. *Circulation* 63:419, 1981

53. Lev M, Liberthson RR, Kirkpatrick JR, Eckner FAO, Arcilla RA: Single (primitive) ventricle. *Circulation* 39:577, 1969
54. Van Praagh R, Ongley PA, Swan HJC: Anatomic types of single or common ventricle in man: Morphologic and geometric aspects of 60 necropsied cases. *Am J Cardiol* 13:367, 1964
55. Felner JM, Brewer DB, Franch RH: Echocardiographic manifestations of single ventricle. *Am J Cardiol* 38:80, 1976
56. Seward JB, Tajik AJ, Hagler DJ, Ritter DG: Contrast echocardiography in single or common ventricle. *Circulation* 55:513, 1977
57. La Corte MA, Fellows KE, Williams RG: Overriding tricuspid valve: Echocardiographic and angiocardiographic features. *Am J Cardiol* 37:911, 1976
58. Rigby ML, Anderson RH, Gibson D, Jones ODH, Joseph MC, Shinebourne EA: Two-dimensional echocardiographic categorization of the univentricular heart. *Br Heart J* 46:603, 1981
59. Foale R, Donaldson R, Richards A, Somerville J: Double inlet ventricle: Two-dimensional echocardiographic (2DE) findings. *Circulation* 62(Suppl III):III-332, 1980
60. Sahn DJ, Harder JR, Freedom RM, Duncan WJ, Rowe RD, Allen HD, Yaides-Cruz L, Goldberg SJ: Cross-section echocardiographic diagnosis and subclassification of univentricular hearts: Imaging studies of atrioventricular valves, septal structures and rudimentary outflow chambers. *Circulation* 66:1070, 1982
61. Dick M, Fyler DC, Nadas AS: Tricuspid atresia: Clinical course in 101 patients. *Am J Cardiol* 36:327, 1975
62. Tandon R, Edwards JE: Tricuspid atresia: A reevaluation and classification. *J Thorac Cardiovasc Surg* 67:530, 1974
63. Rosenquist GC, Levy RJ, Rowe RD: Right atrial-left ventricular relationships in tricuspid atresia: Position of the presumed site of atretic valve as determined by transillumination. *Am Heart J* 80:493, 1970
64. Edwards JE, Burchell HB: Congenital tricuspid atresia: Classification. *Med Clin North Am* 33:1177, 1949
65. Meyer RA, Kaplan S: Echocardiography in the diagnosis of hypoplasia of the left or right ventricles in the neonate. *Circulation* 46:55, 1972
66. Colo J, Snider AR, Silverman NH: Evaluation of tricuspid atresia by two-dimensional echocardiography. *Am J Cardiol* 47:479, 1981 (Abstract)
67. Darling RC, Rothney WB, Craig JM: Total pulmonary venous drainage into the right side of the heart: Report of 17 autopsied cases not associated with other major cardiovascular anomalies. *Lab Invest* 6:44, 1951
68. Paquet M, Gutgesell H: Echocardiographic features of total anomalous pulmonary venous connection. *Circulation* 51:599, 1975
69. Sahn DJ, Allen HD, Lange LW, Goldberg SJ: Cross-sectional echocardiographic diagnosis of the sites of total anomalous pulmonary venous drainage. *Circulation* 60:1317, 1979
70. Bierman FZ, Williams RG: Subxiphoid two-dimensional echocardiographic diagnosis of total anomalous pulmonary venous return in infants. *Am J Cardiol* 43:401, 1979 (Abstract)
71. Snider AR, Silverman NH, Turley K, Ebert PA: Evaluation of infradiaphragmatic total anomalous pulmonary venous connection with two-dimensional echocardiography. *Circulation* 66:1129, 1982

Echocardiographic assessment of postoperative congenital heart disease   17

In the previous chapters we have shown that two-dimensional echocardiography is a valuable diagnostic tool in the preoperative evaluation of patients with congenital heart disease. However, few data exist on the postoperative echocardiographic assessment of congenital cardiac anomalies. The proper use of echocardiography in this setting requires knowledge not only of the preoperative disease but also of the anatomic and physiologic effects of surgical intervention. In addition, the ultrasonographer needs to recognize the extent of postoperative residua and sequelae. The echocardiographic features presented in this chapter are a composite of the few reports in the literature and our own experience. We studied 59 patients who had undergone surgical correction of congenital heart disease. Only those patients who had an intracardiac repair were considered. Excluded from analysis were patients with palliative procedures and patients with isolated aortic or mitral valve disease that required valve replacement. The latter patients are discussed in Chapter 12.

Tetralogy of Fallot

SURGICAL PROCEDURE. Surgical repair of tetralogy of Fallot requires closure of the ventricular septal defect and alleviation of the right ventricular outflow tract obstruction [1–3]. Surgical correction is performed through a right ventriculotomy. Thus resection of the infundibular tissue is accomplished. If a pulmonic valve and annulus fibrosus are involved, the incision is extended across the pulmonic valve ring. A synthetic patch is usually placed over the ventricular septal defect. Sutures are carried clockwise from the tricuspid annulus to the aortic annulus and up to the unresected crista supraventricularis. Continuity between the ventricular septum and the aortic root is accomplished by the ventricular septal defect patch (Fig. 17-1). The ventriculotomy is closed with a pericardial patch.

RESIDUA AND SEQUELAE. Surgical success depends on the absence of residual intracardiac shunt and the complete relief of right ventricular outflow tract obstruction. The patient with the most favorable preoperative anatomy has a subaortic ventricular septal defect and isolated infundibular stenosis. In this subject's repair the infundibular stenosis is relieved completely leaving a competent pulmonic valve. Closure of the ventricular septal defect leaves no residual shunt. Such a patient unfortunately is in the minority. The majority of patients with tetralogy of Fallot require a transannular patch in the reconstruction of the right ventricular outflow tract [1–3]. As a result varying degrees of pulmonary regurgitation and residual outflow tract obstruction exist postoperatively. A recent review of 233 adult and adolescent patients who had undergone surgery for tetralogy of Fallot revealed the following significant sequelae [1]:

1. Right ventricular pressure greater than 60 mm Hg, 32 percent
2. Radiographic evidence of cardiomegaly, 59 percent
3. Complete right bundle branch block, 88 percent
4. Left anterior hemiblock, 9 percent
5. Significant rhythm disturbances such as premature ventricular contractions, 11.2 percent

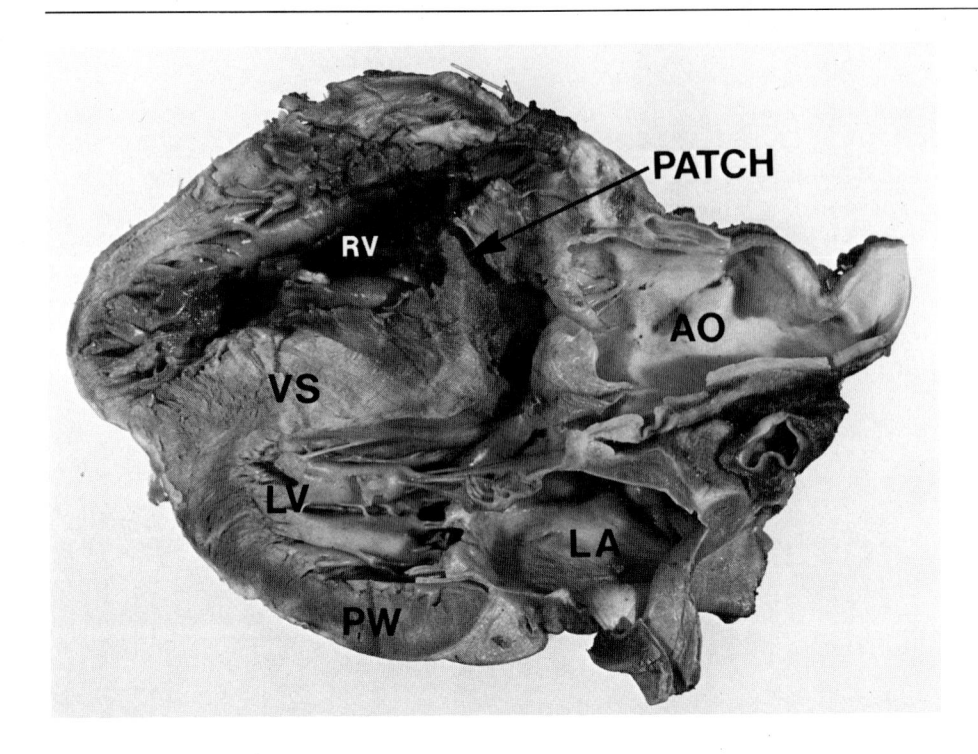

Fig. 17-1. Anatomic specimen cut in the long axis plane after surgical repair of tetralogy of Fallot. The patch is seen attached to the right side of the ventricular septum and the anterior aortic root. Thus the patch produces septal-aortic continuity. The aorta is enlarged. The native ventricular septum (VS) bulges into the left ventricular outflow tract.

6. Residual shunt, 15 percent
7. Pulmonary regurgitation, 85 percent

On physical examination nearly all patients have a systolic crescendo-decrescendo murmur in the third left intercostal space and approximately 85 percent of patients have a low-pitched early diastolic decrescendo murmur of pulmonary insufficiency. A prominent right ventricular impulse from the volume overloaded right ventricle is palpable.

M-MODE ECHOCARDIOGRAPHY. Patients with tetralogy of Fallot made up the largest population in our study group. In all subjects continuity between the ventricular septum and anterior aortic root was identified as an area of increased echo denseness that emanated from the ventricular septal patch. In 12 of 13 patients the right ventricular outflow tract diameter, right ventricular internal dimension (mean 30 mm, range 20–46 mm), and aortic root dimension (mean 30 mm, range 18–42 mm) were larger than norms. In six patients the pulmonic valve had been excised and therefore was not imaged. The right ventricular anterior wall was not consistently observed and determination of its thickness was difficult. In three patients a large right ventricular papillary muscle gave a false impression of asymmetric septal hypertrophy. Paradoxical septal motion was observed in eight patients, all of whom had a large right ventricle. Six patients had an increase in left atrial dimension (mean 34 mm, range 28–40 mm). In patients who had a right ventricular-to-left ventricular dimension ratio (RVDD/LVDD) greater than 0.9, a right ventricular pressure greater than 70 mm Hg in association with mild pulmonary regurgitation or severe pulmonic or tricuspid insufficiency were found at cardiac catheterization. In patients with an RVDD/LVDD less than 0.7, the right ventricular pressure was less than 50 mm Hg, and pulmonic insufficiency was mild. Paradoxical septal motion was found when the RVDD/LVDD ratio was greater than 0.7. Evidence for left atrial enlargement was found in patients with a left ventricular ejection fraction by angiography less than 60 percent. Thus the RVDD/LVDD ratio appears to be useful in identifying subjects with a right ventricular peak systolic pressure less than 45 mm Hg, mild pulmonic insufficiency, and no tricuspid regurgitation. In such patients this ratio is less than 0.65 to 0.7. Moreover, when the right ventricular peak systolic pressure is greater than 70 mm Hg in association with mild pulmonic insufficiency or there is severe pulmonic or tricuspid insufficiency, the RVDD/LVDD ratio is greater than 0.9 [4]. In these patients paradoxical septal motion is a consistent finding [4]. Systolic anterior septal motion disallows the use of shortening fraction as an index of left ventricular function. Left-sided systolic time intervals have been used to evaluate function in such patients [4]. Of greater utility is the estimation of left ventricular ejection fraction by two-dimensional echocardiography [5] or radionuclide angiography [6]. These techniques provide an accurate assessment of left ventricular function in children with abnormal septal motion [5, 6].

TWO-DIMENSIONAL ECHOCARDIOGRAPHY. The cross-sectional echocardiographic image of postoperative tetralogy of Fallot complements the M-mode findings. In the left parasternal long axis view, the ventricular septal patch is imaged as an area of increased echo denseness that produces septal-aortic continuity (Fig. 17-2). Continuity between the anterior leaflet of the mitral valve and aortic valve is also established in this view [7]. Since the ventricular septal defect patch is attached to the right side of the ventricular septum, a portion of the native septum may appear to project into the left ventricular outflow tract (see Figs. 17-1, 17-2). This cross-sectional image does not indicate subaortic obstruction. The aortic root is enlarged when imaged from the left parasternal long axis view and left parasternal short axis view. From the short axis at the base of the heart, qualitative estimation of the right ventricular outflow tract can be made. Moreover, in the short axis view the large septal papillary muscle that produces a false impression of increased septal thickness is identified easily (Fig. 17-3). The use of an M-mode cursor to scan the two-dimensional image aids in avoiding the potential errors in measuring septal thickness, for example, inclusion of the ventricular septal patch or inclusion of the septal papillary muscle in the measurement of septal thickness. The apical four-chamber view provides an added dimension to measurement of right ventricular size. In this view right atrial size is accurately determined. Twelve of thirteen patients in our study group had right atrial enlargement when this chamber was measured in the apical view.

Ventricular septal defect

SURGICAL PROCEDURE. Primary closure of a ventricular septal defect is accomplished either through the tricuspid valve or via a right ventriculotomy. Surgical approach depends on the site of the defect. A patch, usually of synthetic material, is sewn into position over the ventricular septal defect. After a period of time the surface of the patch becomes endothelialized.

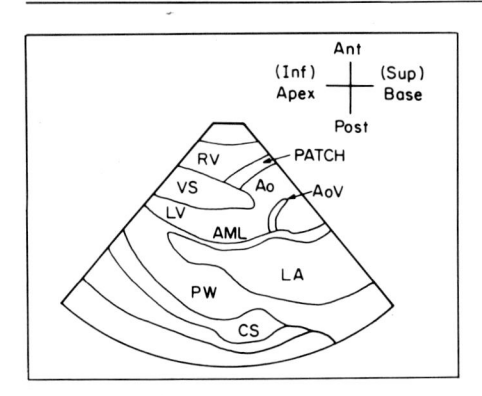

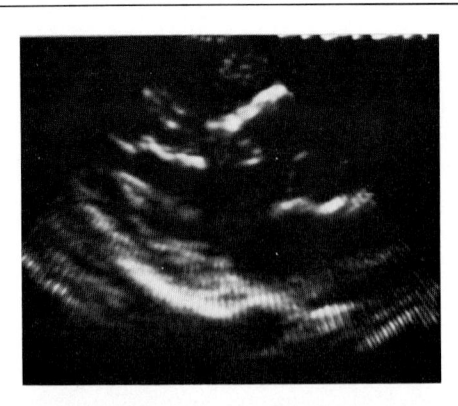

532   17. Echocardiographic assessment of postoperative congenital heart disease

Fig. 17-2. Long axis view in a patient after complete surgical repair of tetralogy of Fallot. The aorta is enlarged. Continuity between the aorta and the ventricular septum (VS) is produced by an area of increased echo denseness, the ventricular septal defect patch. The native ventricular septum bulges into the left ventricular outflow tract. (Compare this echo view with the pathological specimen in Fig. 17-1.) AoV = aortic valve.

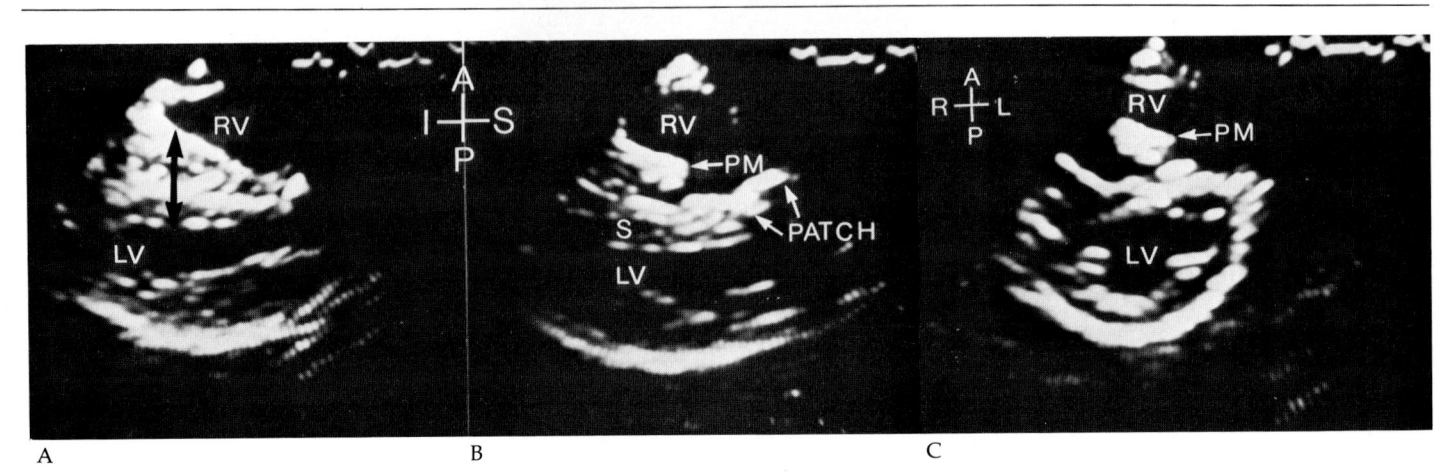

Fig. 17-3A. Long axis view after surgical repair of tetralogy of Fallot. The right ventricle is enlarged. The ventricular septum (arrows) appears thickened due to a large papillary muscle in the right ventricle. B. Long axis recorded from the same patient. With this slightly more medial angulation, the cause for the increase in septal thickness is noted. The papillary muscle in the right ventricle separates from the ventricular septum (S). The ventricular septal defect patch is also noted attached to the right side of the septum. The right ventricle is enlarged. C. Short axis view in the same patient. The right ventricle is enlarged. The large septal papillary muscle is imaged clearly.

RESIDUA AND SEQUELAE. Significant residua include persistent shunt, reduced left ventricular function, increased left ventricular mass, residual pulmonary hypertension, and aneurysm of the ventricular septal patch (Fig. 17-4). Surgical sequelae result from the right ventriculotomy and include conduction defects.

M-MODE ECHOCARDIOGRAPHY. In the immediate postoperative setting, M-mode echocardiography is of use in detecting residual intracardiac shunts, provided that the surgeon leaves a left atrial catheter in place [8]. An injection of a contrast agent into the left atrium will produce a cloud of echoes in the left atrium and simultaneously in the aortic root and right ventricular outflow tract. The contrast in the right ventricular outflow tract results from the residual intracardiac shunt. Late postoperative persistence of the left atrial or left ventricular enlargement may reflect the presence of a moderate-to-large-volume residual shunt. Small shunts, however, are not detected by measurement of left atrial dimensions. In the case of small shunts, radionuclide scintigraphy provides a sensitive indicator of left-to-right intracardiac shunt and complements echocardiographic information [9].

Of our eight postoperative patients three had left atrial enlargement that resulted from mitral regurgitation rather than from a shunt. The cause of left atrial enlargement was not defined by M-mode echocardiography. The differential diagnosis of left atrial enlargement in these patients may be solved by directional Doppler techniques [10]. The detection of turbulent flow in the right ventricular outflow tract provides evidence of a persistent ventricular septal defect. In contrast, turbulent flow in the left atrium indicates mitral insufficiency.

TWO-DIMENSIONAL ECHOCARDIOGRAPHY. Direct imaging of the patch by cross-sectional echocardiography identifies the position of the previous ventricular septal defect. The synthetic material produces a distinctive area of increased echo denseness. In four of our patients the patch was located in the inlet septum (Fig. 17-5), in two patients in the outlet septum, and in two patients in the posterior septum (Fig. 17-6). Two-dimensional imaging established a diagnosis of residual discrete subaortic stenosis in two patients and mitral valve prolapse in two cases.

Atrial septal defect: secundum type

SURGICAL PROCEDURE. An atrial septal defect may be closed either by direct suture or synthetic patch.

RESIDUA AND SEQUELAE. Postoperative residua of an isolated secundum atrial septal defect appear in a minority of cases. Selective residua are directly related to the age of the patient at operation. For example, pulmonary hypertension is frequently found in patients with atrial septal defect who are operated on at age 35 or older [11]. Atrial arrhythmias such as atrial fibrillation may persist or occur postoperatively. Preoperative increase in right ventricular muscle mass and left ventricular dysfunction will also remain in selected patients [11]. Physical examination, electrocardiogram, and chest x-ray depend upon the degree of postoperative residua.

M-MODE ECHOCARDIOGRAPHY. The findings on M-mode echocardiography primarily reflect the disturbances of cardiac conduction and the size of the right ventricle. Atrial fibrillation and atrial flutter produce fine and coarse diastolic undulations of the atrioventricular valves, high interventricular septum, aortic root, and aortic valve during diastole [12]. Some studies report a return to normal of right ventricular dimension postoperatively. We have made M-mode measurements of right ventricular dimension in six patients who had undergone repair of atrial septal defect. The mean right ventricular dimension was 27 mm with a range of 20 to 30 mm. These dimensions indicated a persistently enlarged right ventricle postoperatively. Paradoxical septal motion persisted in three, and two patients had residual mitral valve prolapse.

TWO-DIMENSIONAL ECHOCARDIOGRAPHY. Two-dimensional examination confirmed the diagnosis of mitral valve prolapse in the two patients mentioned. In contrast to the M-mode findings, the size of the right ventricle when measured from the apical four-chamber view was normal. The right atrial size was also within normal limits. These findings amplify the capability of two-dimensional imaging to more accurately assess the size of the right ventricle.

Atrial septal defect: primum type

SURGICAL PROCEDURE. As we stated in Chapter 14, a primum atrial septal defect is not an isolated anomaly. There are frequently associated deformities of the atrioventricular valves. The most common atrioventricular valve anomaly is a cleft in the anterior mitral leaflet. Surgical correction involves direct suturing of the cleft mitral valve in addition to patch closure of the atrial septal defect [13].

RESIDUA AND SEQUELAE. Once again, postoperative residua and sequelae depend upon the success of operative intervention. The abnormally rotated mitral annulus and abnormal attachments of the mitral valve to the ventricular outflow tract produced by the anterior mitral leaflet persist. Approximately 72 percent of patients will have a murmur of persistent mitral regurgitation postoperatively, and these subjects may have left atrial dilatation. A small percentage of patients will have a persistent atrial shunt and right atrial and right ventricular volume overload. Since the defect lies in close proximity to the atrioventricular node, disturbances in conduction are frequent findings after surgical repair [13]. In a small number of patients persistent pulmonary hypertension remains after surgical closure of the atrial defect. In the presence of persistent pulmonary hypertension, right ventricular enlargement and hypertrophy are present.

M-MODE ECHOCARDIOGRAPHY. Since the relationship of the mitral valve to the ventricular septum remains abnormal, the left ventricular outflow tract remains narrowed on long axis scan from apex to base. In addition, systolic reflections from the mitral valve remain postoperatively. Since mitral regurgitation frequently persists, left atrial enlargement is a common postoperative echocardiographic finding. Septal motion may remain paradoxical despite return to normal size of the right ventricular dimension. In patients with persistent shunts, right ventricular dimension may remain enlarged [14].

We have studied seven children who underwent repair of endocardial cushion defect. Of these, four children had a primum atrial septal defect. All patients had left atrial enlargement and two had left ventricular enlargement secondary to mitral

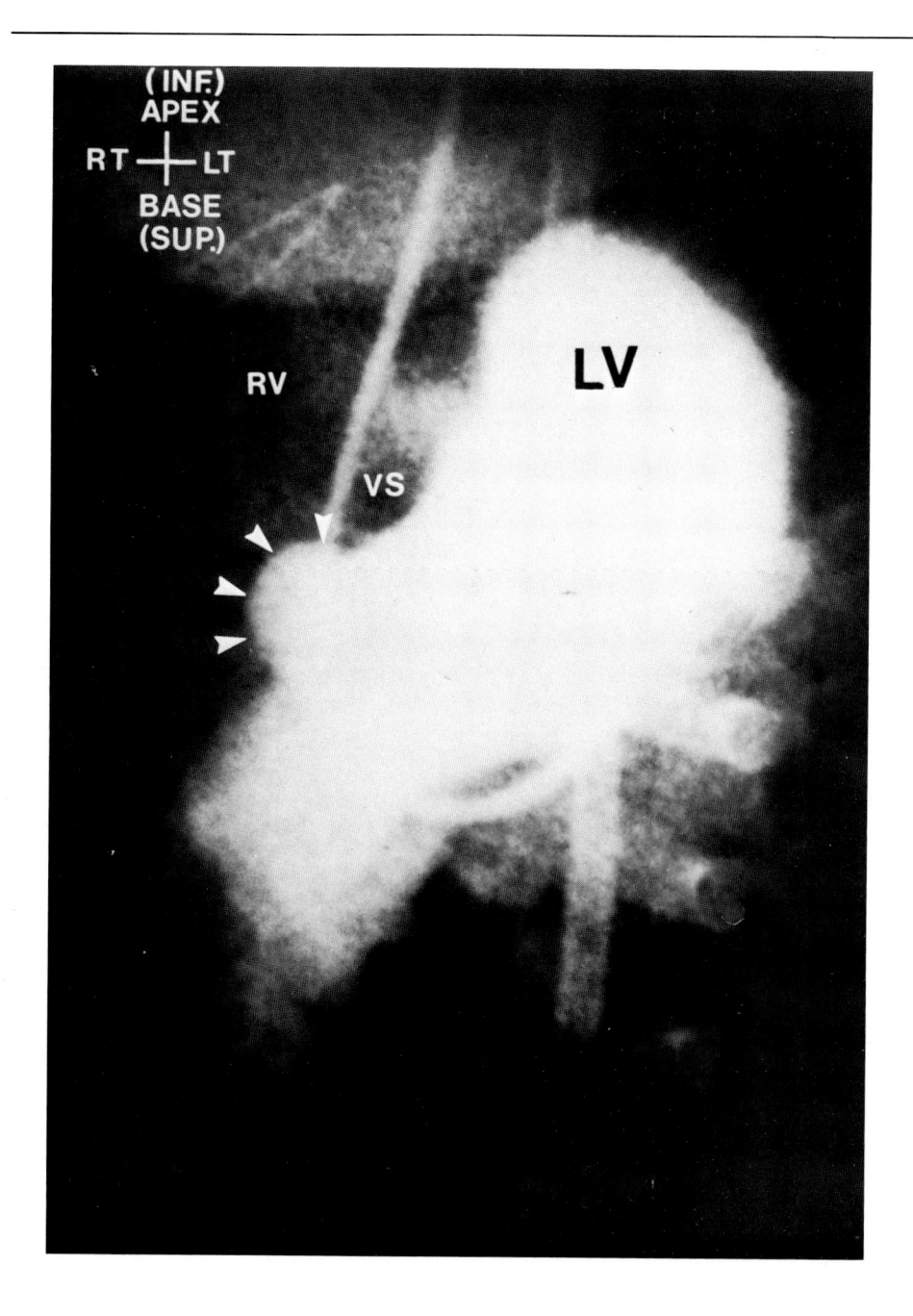

Fig. 17-4. Left ventricular cineangiocardiogram in postoperative ventricular septal defect. This patient's ventricular septal defect was in the endocardial cushion position (position 3). The left ventricular injection was performed in the hepatoclavicular view. The apex is placed at the top of the image similar to the echocardiographic apical 4-chamber view. A bulge (arrows) is noted in the ventricular septum (VS) due to an aneurysm of the defect patch.

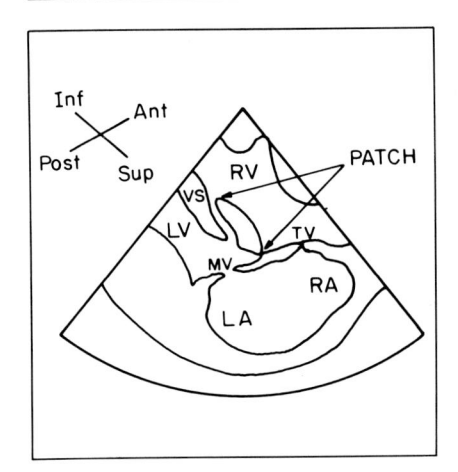

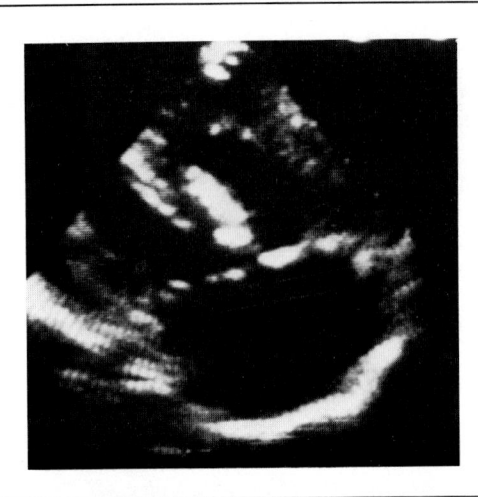

Fig. 17-5. Left parasternal inflow view of the right ventricle in a patient who has undergone repair of inflow ventricular septal defect. The synthetic patch material is imaged as an area of echo denseness in the inflow portion of the ventricular septum behind the septal leaflet of the tricuspid valve. VS = ventricular septum.

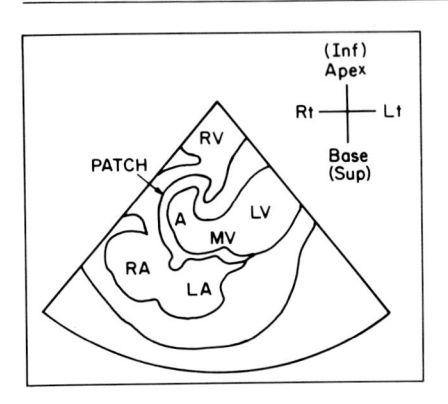

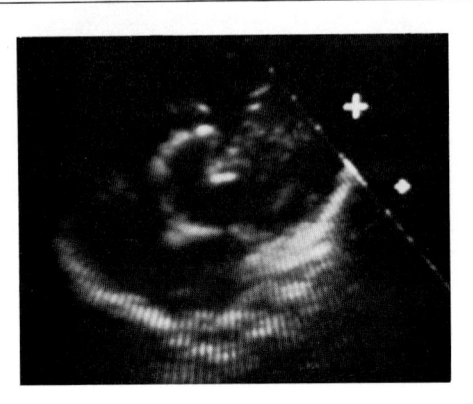

Fig. 17-6. Apical 4-chamber view in a patient who had patch repair of a ventricular septal defect located in the posterior portion of the ventricular septum. The synthetic material used to close the ventricular septal defect bulges into the right ventricle. This bulge is due to an aneurysm (A) of the patch.

regurgitation. The right atrium was enlarged in three subjects and the right ventricle in one. In these the right-sided chambers were enlarged secondary to global cardiac dysfunction in one subject and severe pulmonary hypertension in another. In one patient who had complete heart block, the motion disturbance related to the heart block was imaged easily by M-mode echocardiography [15].

TWO-DIMENSIONAL ECHOCARDIOGRAPHY. In the long axis view along the left parasternal border, narrowing of the left ventricular outflow tract persisted after operation in the seven patients mentioned previously (Fig. 17-7). This narrowing caused by an abnormally oriented anterior mitral leaflet did not prevent the ultrasonographer from diagnosing discrete membranous subaortic obstruction. In short axis, the repaired anterior leaflet of the mitral valve no longer separated into two components in diastole (Fig. 17-8). In the apical four-chamber and subcostal four-chamber views the synthetic material used to close the atrial septal defect is imaged as an area of increased echo denseness in the inferior portion of the interatrial septum (Fig. 17-9). In addition to identifying these anatomical residua, two-dimensional echocardiography also provides important information concerning cardiac chamber size.

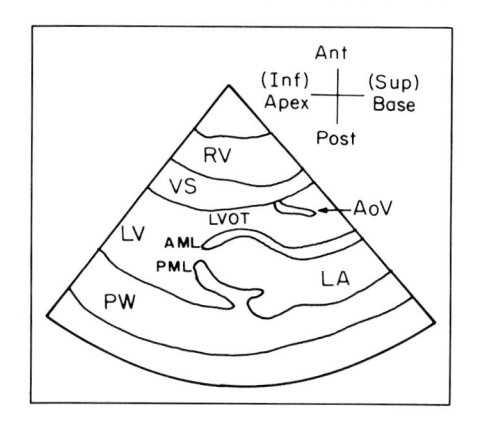

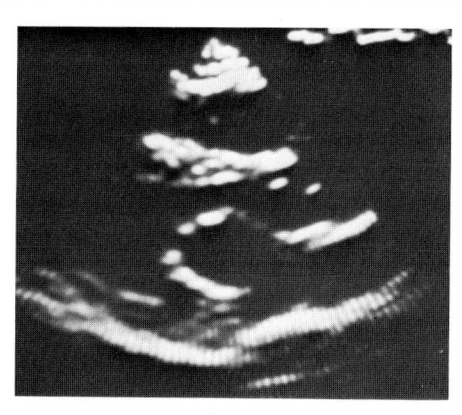

Fig. 17-7. Left parasternal long axis view in postoperative ostium primum atrial septal defect repair. The left ventricular outflow tract remains narrowed due to the abnormally displaced anterior mitral leaflet. The left atrium is enlarged secondary to mitral insufficiency. AoV = aortic valve; PW = posterior wall; VS = ventricular septum.

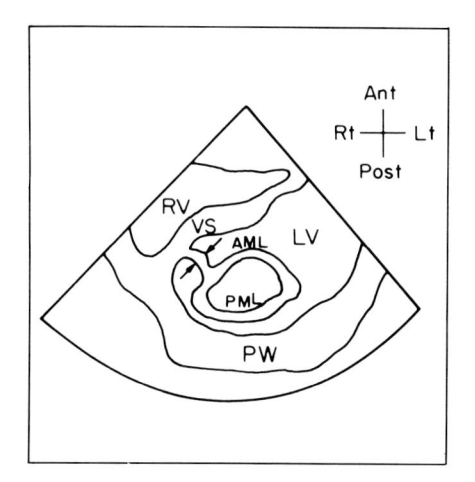

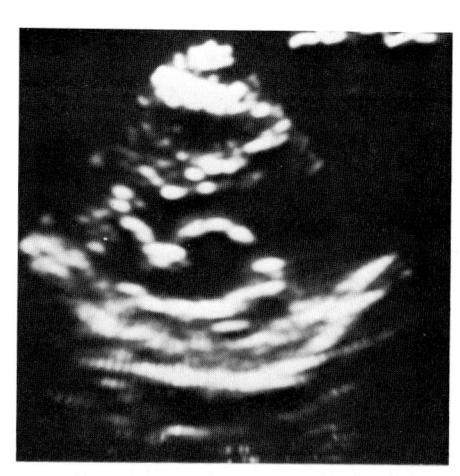

Fig. 17-8. Parasternal short axis view in a patient who had undergone repair of a primum atrial septal defect. The anterior leaflet of the mitral valve no longer demonstrates diastolic separation. There are still abnormal cordal attachments (arrows) of the mitral valve to the ventricular (VS). PW = posterior wall.

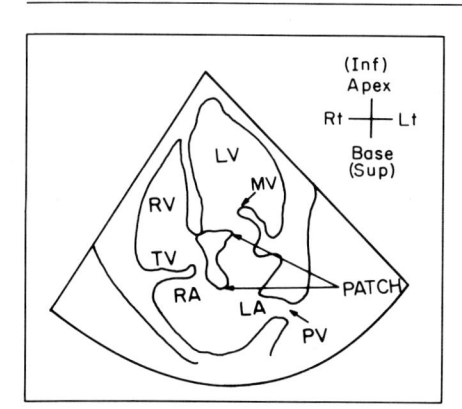

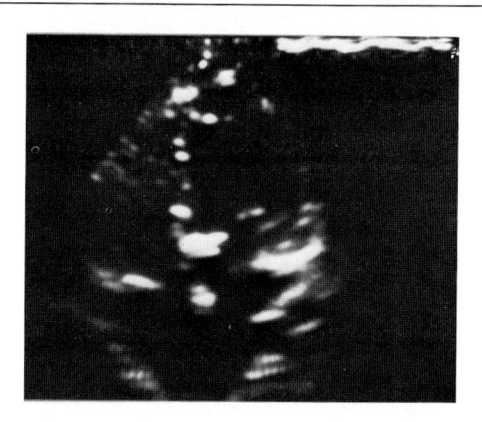

Fig. 17-9. Apical 4-chamber view in postoperative primum atrial septal defect. The right atrium and right ventricle have returned to normal size. The patch used to close the atrial defect is imaged in the inferior portion of the atrial septum. Significant echo dropout in the native portion of the atrial septum is a normal phenomenon. PV = pulmonary vein.

Complete endocardial cushion defect

SURGICAL PROCEDURE. Surgical repair requires division of the posterior common leaflet and reconstruction of the mitral valve. In addition, a semicircular patch is sutured to the crest of the ventricular septal defect. Sutures are continued to close the atrial septal defect. Prior to closure of the atrial septal defect, the anterior mitral leaflet is reconstructed by suturing the surgically divided posterior leaflet to the mitral component of the anterior common leaflet and to the patch. Surgical success depends upon the type of complete atrioventricular canal repaired. Type A complete atrioventricular canal has the best prognosis. The optimum surgical result is obliteration of intracardiac shunt with a competent mitral and tricuspid valve.

RESIDUA AND SEQUELAE. Postoperative sequelae include persistent intracardiac shunt, complete heart block, and atrioventricular valve regurgitation [13]. Patients who have undergone repair of complete atrioventricular canal are left with an abnormal mitral valve and synthetic material in the area occupied by the atrial and ventricular septal defect. The anterior leaflet of the mitral valve is now composed of the left-sided portion of the common anterior leaflet sutured to the surgically divided left-sided portion of the posterior common leaflet. The right ventricle and right atrium may remain enlarged and thickened in those patients with persistent shunt or persistent pulmonary hypertension after repair has been accomplished. The left atrium and left ventricle will be enlarged in patients with mitral regurgitation or stenosis.

TWO-DIMENSIONAL ECHOCARDIOGRAPHY. The two-dimensional image outlines the abnormal mitral apparatus and the position of the synthetic patch. In the left parasternal long axis view, the anterior mitral leaflet impinges upon the left ventricular outflow tract. The motion of the mitral leaflet is restricted. These same features are observed in the short axis view. Also in the short axis view, the abnormal attachments of the mitral valve to the ventricular septum are seen. An area of increased echo denseness in the anterior mitral leaflet indicates the suture site. The synthetic patch is best imaged from the apical four-chamber or subcostal four-chamber views. In these views an area of increased echo denseness is noted from the superior portion of the ventricular septum to the inferior portion of the atrial septum (Fig. 17-10). In our patients there was considerable echo dropout in the area of the native atrial septum. In addition to defining the residual abnormal anatomy, two-dimensional echocardiography provides a more accurate definition of chamber enlargement than M-mode echocardiography. Patients who have undergone repair of complete endocardial cushion defect usually have enlargement of all four cardiac chambers. The left-sided chambers are enlarged secondary to mitral valve regurgitation or stenosis. The right-sided chambers may be enlarged secondary to residual pulmonary hypertension or persistent shunt.

Transposition of the great arteries

SURGICAL PROCEDURE. Conventional surgery for correction of transposition of the great arteries involves redirection of systemic and pulmonary venous return at the atrial level (Mustard or Senning procedure) [18]. Such a repair requires the use of either a pericardial baffle or native atrial tissue to separate a newly created systemic venous atrium and pulmonary venous atrium.

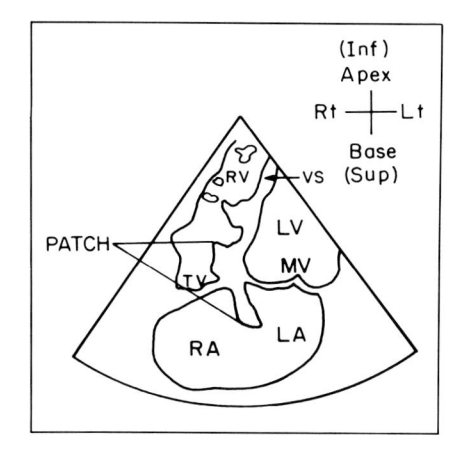

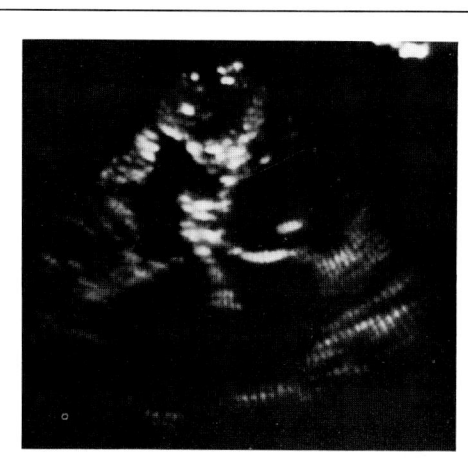

Fig. 17-10. Apical 4-chamber view in postoperative repair of complete atrioventricular canal. In this patient, the right ventricle and right atrium remain enlarged secondary to persistent pulmonary hypertension. The left atrium is enlarged secondary to severe mitral regurgitation. There is an area of increased echo denseness noted in the superior portion of the ventricular septum (VS) and inferior portion of the atrial septum secondary to the synthetic patch material. The notable echo dropout in the superior native portion of the interatrial septum is normal and does not reflect a residual defect.

RESIDUA AND SEQUELAE. Hemodynamic derangements that persist after Mustard operation include obstruction to systemic or to pulmonary venous return, tricuspid insufficiency, and right ventricular dysfunction [19–21]. A significant number of patients are left with conduction abnormalities [22, 23]. In addition to baffle obstruction, baffle leaks are common [24–26]. Despite these postoperative residua and sequelae, the majority of patients are asymptomatic and indistinguishable from normal persons except for the median sternotomy scar.

Surgical repair of complete transposition of the great arteries accomplishes redirection of pulmonary venous return to the anatomic right ventricle, which ejects this fully oxygenated blood into the aorta and systemic circulation. Systemic venous return is directed to the anatomic left ventricle, which ejects desaturated blood into the pulmonary circulation. The anatomic right ventricle remains the systemic ventricle and sees systemic pressure. After surgical repair right ventricular wall thickness remains hypertrophied and right ventricular size remains increased [27]. Mild to moderate left ventricular outflow tract obstruction is usually left untouched at operation, and the pathologic anatomy that produces obstruction to left ventricular outflow remains after repair. Obstruction to the superior vena cava may be either partial or complete. Whichever the case, venous drainage from the upper compartment of the body traverses the azygous vein to the inferior vena cava to the systemic venous atrium (Fig. 17-11).

M-MODE ECHOCARDIOGRAPHY. The M-mode echocardiographic features after Mustard repair have been well described [28–30]. There is high-frequency diastolic flutter on the anterior leaflet of both atrioventricular valves. This diastolic shutter is related to the high velocity of flow passing across the atrioventricular valves and the abnormal direction of this flow. The intraatrial baffle can be imaged behind the pulmonary artery and tricuspid valve echo. When imaged behind the pulmonary artery, the anterior echo-free space is the systemic venous atrium and the posterior echo-free space is the pulmonary venous atrium. Asymmetric septal hypertrophy and abnormal systolic anterior motion of the mitral valve that existed preoperatively persist after operation but do not herald significant left ventricular outflow tract obstruction. When compared to established norms, right ventricular wall thickness and cavity dimension are increased.

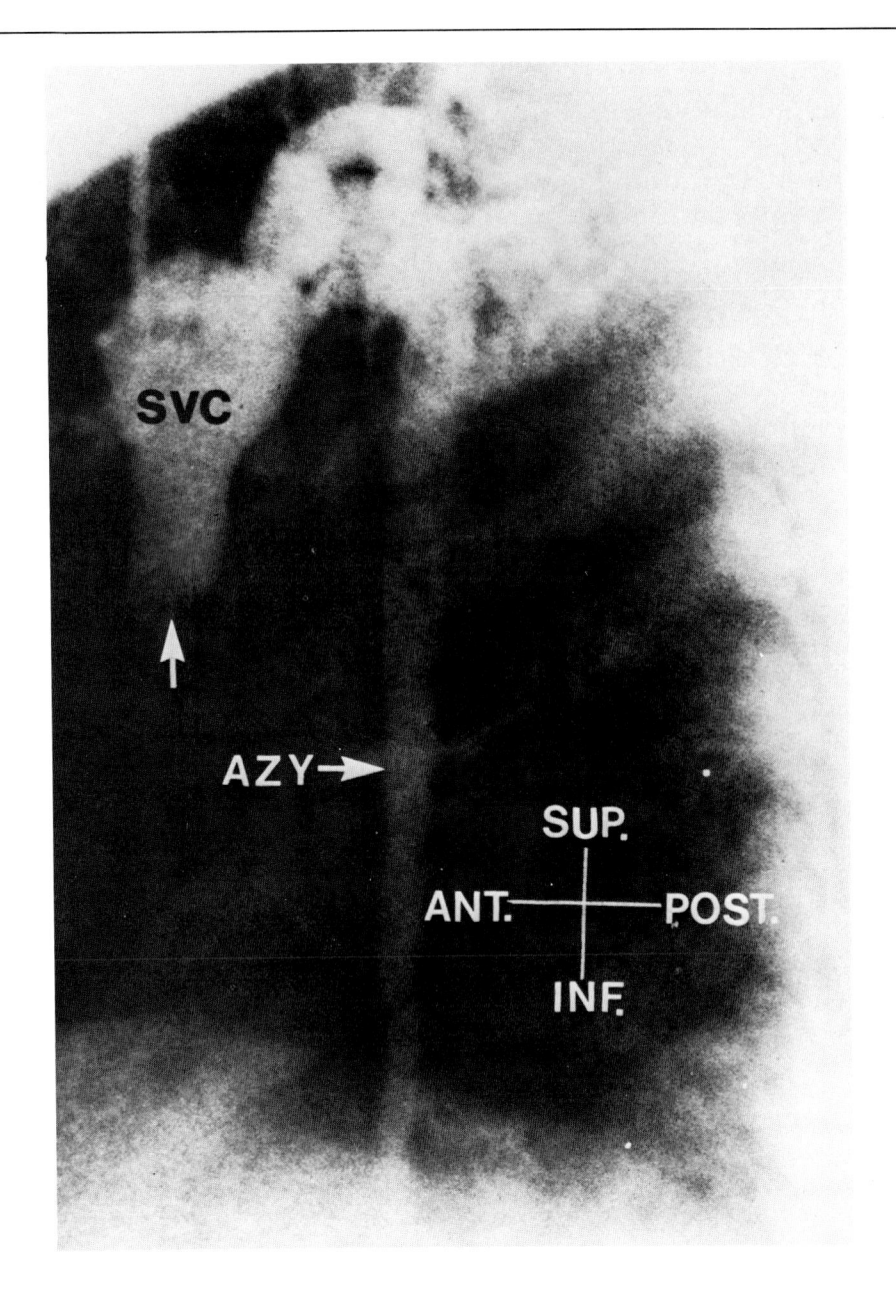

Fig. 17-11. Cineangiocardiogram in the lateral projection. The catheter is positioned in the superior vena cava and injection is made at the site. Superior vena cava fills with dye and is obstructed (arrow). Collateral flow is through the azygous vein (AZY) to the inferior vena cava.

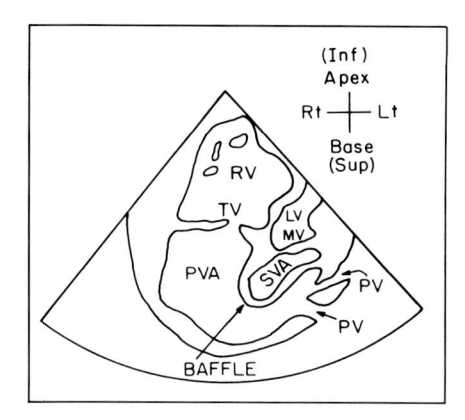

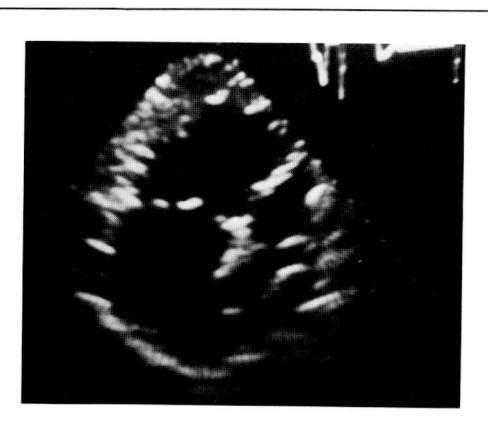

Fig. 17-12. Apical 4-chamber view. In this tomographic plane, the intraatrial baffle (arrows) is seen separating the systemic venous atrium (SVA) from the pulmonary venous atrium (PVA). The right ventricle is enlarged. PV = pulmonary veins.

TWO-DIMENSIONAL ECHOCARDIOGRAPHY. Cross-sectional imaging provides a relatively precise anatomic localization of the intraatrial baffle. The baffle may be imaged from the long axis and short axis views. However, the optimal tomographic planes for baffle imaging are the apical four-chamber and subcostal four-chamber views [26, 31] (Fig. 17-12). Contrast echocardiography has been combined with two-dimensional imaging for the detection of superior vena cava obstruction after Mustard repair [26]. In order to detect baffle obstruction, a contrast agent must be injected into an upper extremity vein. The heart should be imaged from the subcostal tomographic plane, which should include the inferior vena cava–systemic venous atrial junction. In a patient without baffle obstruction, microcavitations are imaged immediately in the systemic venous atrium. With atrial contraction there is reflux into the upper portion of the inferior vena cava (Fig. 17-13). With partial superior vena cava obstruction microcavitations are seen first in the systemic venous atrium. These contrast echoes originate from the superior vena cava. With subsequent cardiac cycles contrast echoes can be imaged flowing from the inferior vena cava into the systemic venous atrium. These microcavitations reach the inferior vena cava via the azygous collaterals (Fig. 17-14). With complete superior vena cava obstruction, flow into the systemic venous atrium is completely from the inferior vena cava. No contrast reaches the systemic venous atrium prior to flow from the inferior vena cava (Fig. 17-15) [26]. M-mode echocardiographic contrast techniques have detected baffle leaks in as many as 35 percent of patients. More recently two-dimensional echocardiography has detected baffle leaks in as many as 90 percent of patients [26]. It appears, therefore, that two-dimensional echocardiography is a more sensitive technique for detection of a baffle leak. Two-dimensional echocardiography also appears to be more sensitive in the detection of baffle obstruction than pulsed Doppler echocardiography [32].

Two-dimensional echocardiography provides the ultrasonographer with a method for evaluating right ventricular volumes and ejection fraction after Mustard's procedure [33]. Using the short axis view along the left parasternal border and the apical four-chamber view, right ventricular volume can be calculated by means of Simpson's rule. With this method a high correlation exists between volumes calculated by echocardiography and those obtained from angiography. Moreover, echocardiography accurately predicts right ventricular ejection fraction in these patients.

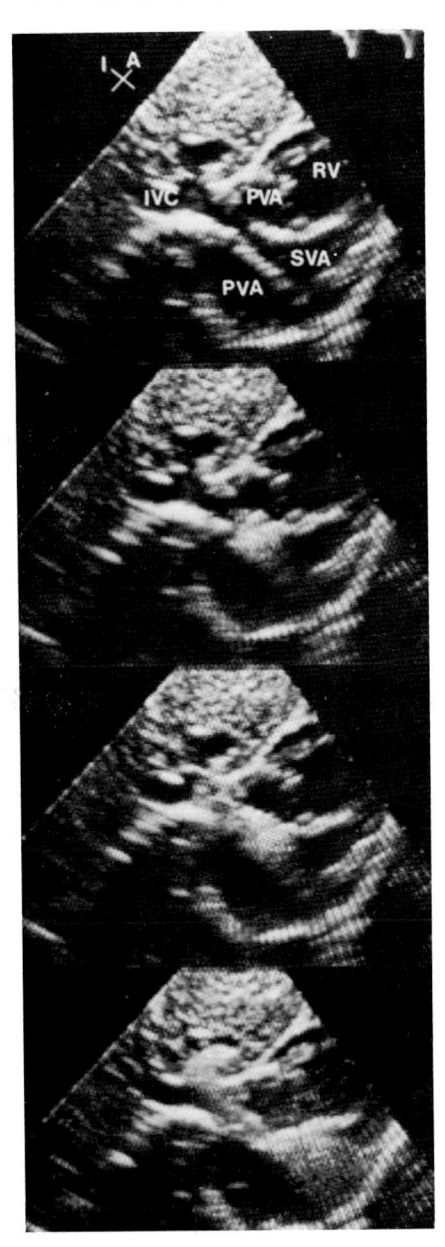

Fig. 17-13. Subcostal 4-chamber view recorded from a patient who underwent Mustard procedure for transposition of the great arteries. The inferior vena cava–systemic venous atrium (SVA) junction is imaged (first panel). After a peripheral venous injection of a contrast agent, contrast appears in the systemic venous atrium (second panel). Contrast echoes are refluxing into the inferior vena cava (third panel). Contrast can be seen in the pulmonary venous atrium secondary to a baffle leak (fourth panel). PVA = pulmonary venous atrium. (From NH Silverman et al, Superior vena cava obstruction after Mustard's operation. Circulation 64:392, 1981 by permission of the American Heart Association, Inc.)

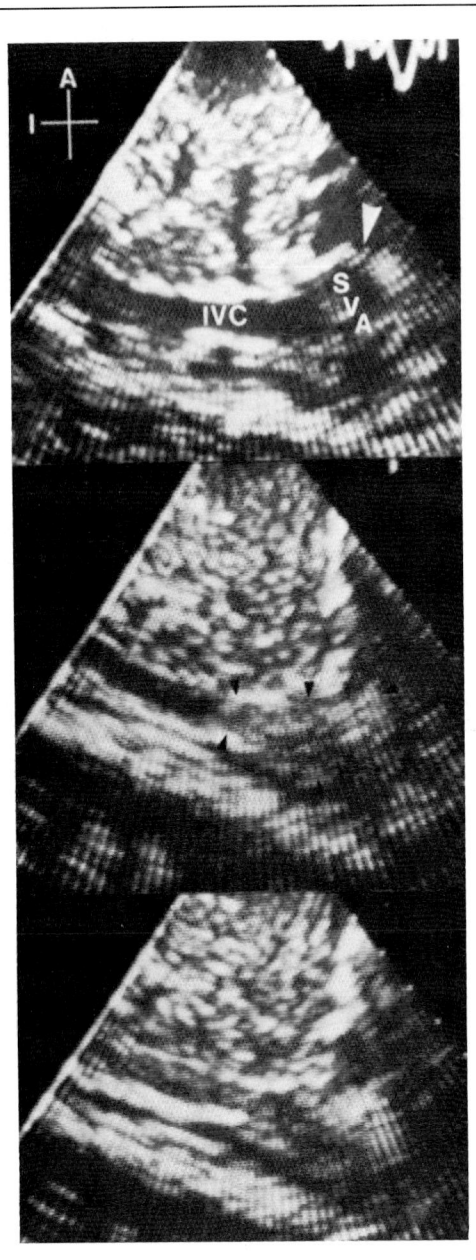

Fig. 17-14. Two-dimensional echocardiogram in a patient with partial superior vena cava obstruction. Prior to contrast injection the inferior vena cava–systemic venous atrium (SVA) junction is imaged (top panel). After injection of a contrast agent, microcavitations appear in the systemic venous atrium and upper inferior vena cava (black arrows, middle panel). In the bottom frame, microbubbles are visualized in the lower inferior vena cava traveling toward the systemic venous atrium. (From NH Silverman et al, Superior vena cava obstruction after Mustard's operation. Circulation 64:392, 1981 by permission of the American Heart Association, Inc.)

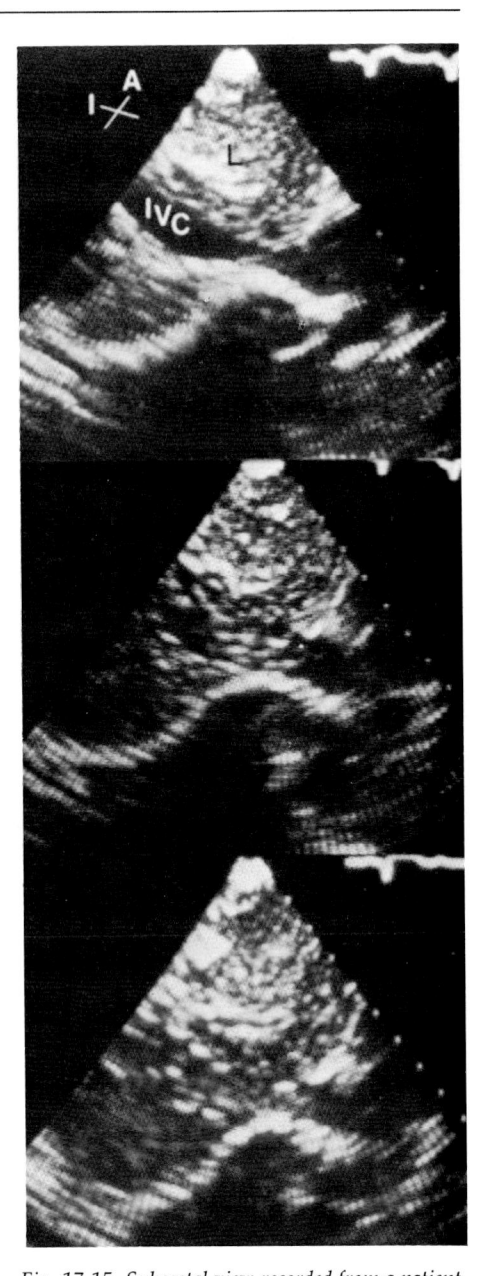

Fig. 17-15. Subcostal view recorded from a patient with complete superior vena cava obstruction. The inferior vena cava–systemic venous atrial junction recorded prior to contrast injection (top panel). After injection of a contrast agent, microcavitations are seen in the lower inferior vena cava traveling toward the heart (middle panel). The entire inferior vena cava is filled with microcavitations arriving via the azygous system (bottom panel). L = liver. (From NH Silverman et al, Superior vena cava obstruction after Mustard's operation. Circulation 64:392, 1981 by permission of the American Heart Association, Inc.)

Double-outlet right ventricle

SURGICAL PROCEDURE. The appropriate surgical approach to the correction of double-outlet right ventricle depends upon the anatomic type present. Repair of double-outlet right ventricle with a subaortic ventricular septal defect and pulmonic stenosis requires patch closure of the ventricular septal defect so that the aorta exits from the left ventricle, and reconstruction of the right ventricular outflow tract with relief of the pulmonic stenosis [34]. In double-outlet right ventricle with a subpulmonic ventricular septal defect and no pulmonic stenosis, the procedure of choice is closure of the ventricular septal defect so that the aorta exits from the right ventricle and the pulmonary artery exists from the left ventricle. This procedure is combined with an intraatrial baffle (Mustard procedure). Surgical correction of patients with doubly committed and remote ventricular septal defect carry a high mortality. In those patients with a subaortic ventricular septal defect and pulmonary atresia, the intracardiac repair can be accomplished by closure of the ventricular septal defect so that the aorta exits from the left ventricle; an external conduit is used to produce continuity between the right ventricle and pulmonary artery.

RESIDUA AND SEQUELAE. The residua and sequelae after surgical repair of double-outlet right ventricle depend upon the anatomic type and operative procedure performed. In patients with a subaortic ventricular septal defect repaired in the manner previously described, the left atrium communicates with the anatomic left ventricle. The morphologic left ventricle empties into the aorta. The subaortic conus persists, and there is discontinuity between the anterior mitral leaflet and the aortic valve. The ventricular septal defect patch produces continuity between the ventricular septum and the aortic root. The anatomic right ventricle empties into the pulmonary artery. Wall thickness and size of the cardiac chambers depend on the residual outlet obstruction or valve insufficiency. In patients with subpulmonic ventricular septal defect and no pulmonic stenosis repaired as described previously, the newly created pulmonary venous atrium communicates with the anatomic right ventricle from which emerges the aorta. The systemic venous atrium communicates with the anatomic left ventricle from which the pulmonary artery springs. In essence these patients are anatomically and physiologically similar to patients with complete transposition.

M-MODE ECHOCARDIOGRAPHY. To this author's knowledge, there are no data describing M-mode echocardiographic features of surgically corrected double-outlet right ventricle.

TWO-DIMENSIONAL ECHOCARDIOGRAPHY. The two-dimensional echocardiographic features of the surgically corrected heart with a subaortic ventricular septal defect and pulmonary stenosis are as follows:

1. In the long axis, the aorta springs from the anatomic left ventricle. Continuity between the anterior aortic root and ventricular septum is established by an area of increased echo denseness that emanates from the artificial patch.
2. There is an area of increased echo denseness between the hinge point of the anterior mitral leaflet and the aortic valve. This zone of echo denseness represents the subaortic conus [7]. The left ventricular outflow tract appears narrow

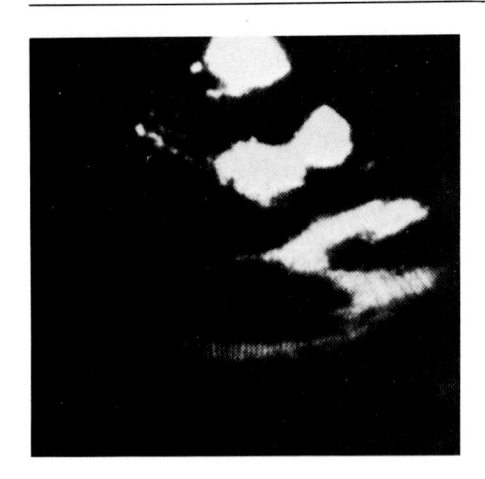

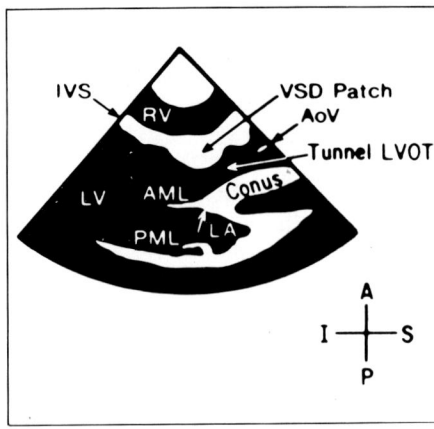

544   17. Echocardiographic assessment of postoperative congenital heart disease

Fig. 17-16. Long axis view in postoperative double-outlet right ventricle. The ventricular septal defect patch is imaged as an area of increased echo denseness between the interventricular septum and the aortic root. The conus rests between the hinge point (arrow) of the anterior mitral leaflet and the aortic valve (AoV). The left ventricular outflow tract appears tunnel-like. (From TG DiSessa et al, Am J Cardiol 44:1146, 1979.)

   because of the persistent subaortic conus and the ventricular septal patch (Fig. 17-16).
3. If a conduit is used in the surgical repair, it is imaged in the short axis at the base of the heart. The valve within the conduit is seen in the usual position of the normal pulmonic valve.

Truncus arteriosus

SURGICAL PROCEDURE. Recent advances in surgical techniques have provided a method for anatomic correction of the circulatory derangement in patients with type 1 truncus arteriosus. Through a right ventriculotomy patch closure of the ventricular septal defect is performed. Continuity between the right ventricle and the pulmonary artery is accomplished with a dacron conduit bearing a porcine semilunar valve.

RESIDUA AND SEQUELAE. Significant residua and sequelae include persistent left-to-right shunt and obstruction to pulmonary blood flow at multiple levels. Such obstruction can occur at the site of attachment of the external conduit to the heart, throughout the conduit, at the porcine valve, and at the site of attachment of the conduit to the pulmonary arteries [35]. In addition the truncal valve is frequently insufficient, and right bundle branch block results from the right ventriculotomy. The most significant anatomic residuum is a persistent increase in right ventricular wall thickness, secondary to right ventricular outflow tract obstruction. The ventricular septal defect patch is sewn so that it establishes continuity between the truncal artery root and the ventricular septum. The conduit rests on the anterior portion of the heart and circles the aorta to attach to the pulmonary artery.

M-MODE ECHOCARDIOGRAPHY. The M-mode echocardiographic appearance of surgically corrected truncus arteriosus is very similar to the echo appearance of surgically corrected tetralogy of Fallot. It is, however, exceptionally difficult to image the porcine valve using M-mode techniques.

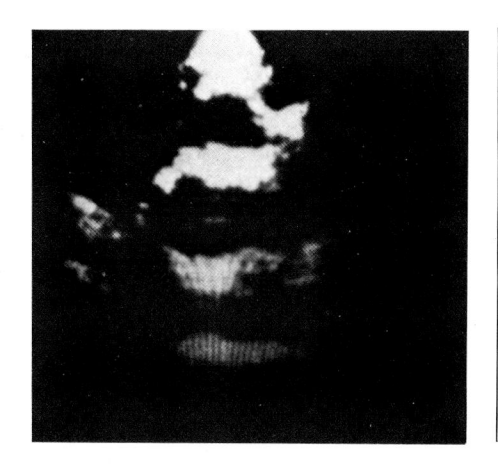

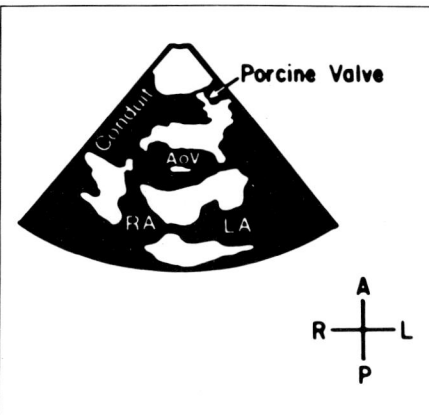

Fig. 17-17. Short axis view of a right ventricle to pulmonary artery conduit. The conduit is seen wrapping around the aorta. The porcine valve is imaged anterior and to the left of the aortic valve (AoV). (From TG DiSessa et al, Am J Cardiol 44:1146, 1979.)

TWO-DIMENSIONAL ECHOCARDIOGRAPHY. In the left parasternal long axis view, septal great artery continuity is produced by an area of increased echo denseness that emanates from the ventricular septal defect patch. The truncal root is dilated. There is mitral valve–semilunar valve continuity. The size of the right ventricle is variable. In short axis, at the cardiac base, the conduit is shown to be circling anterior to the truncal artery root, similar to a normal right ventricular outflow tract. The porcine valve is imaged in the area where the normal pulmonic valve would rest (Fig. 17-17).

Valvular pulmonic stenosis

SURGICAL PROCEDURE. Relief of obstruction is by pulmonary valvulotomy under direct vision while cardiopulmonary bypass is being performed. When this surgical technique is employed results are excellent [36].

RESIDUA AND SEQUELAE. Significant residua include leftover obstruction and pulmonary insufficiency. With significant residual obstruction, right ventricular muscle mass will remain increased, and with significant valve regurgitation the right ventricle will become enlarged.

M-MODE ECHOCARDIOGRAPHY. Since no data exist on the M-mode echocardiographic appearance of postoperative valvular pulmonic stenosis, we studied seven patients after pulmonary valvulotomy. Mean right ventricular pressure in these patients was 32 mm Hg with a range of 24 to 40 mm Hg. Mean right ventricular dimension measured by M-mode examination was 23 mm, with a range of 17 to 30 mm. Septal motion was paradoxical in two patients. Two patients had right ventricular wall thickness greater than 6 mm. The degree of right ventricular enlargement depended on the amount of pulmonic insufficiency. Thickness of the right ventricular wall appeared dependent on residual obstruction. The utility of M-mode echocardiography in the evaluation of right ventricular mass after relief of obstruction remains to be determined.

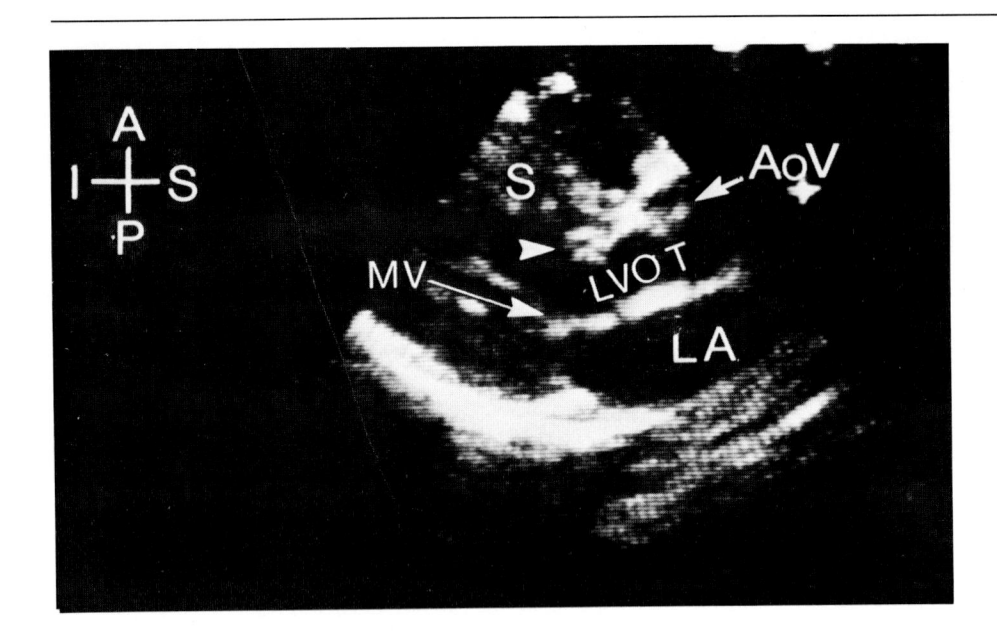

Fig. 17-18. Long axis view. Postoperative discrete subaortic stenosis. A ridge of tissue is noted on the left side of the septum (arrowhead) that produces narrowing of the left ventricular outflow tract. In this patient, a residual gradient was observed from the body of the left ventricle to the aorta. Ventricular septum and posterior wall are thickened. AoV = aortic valve.

TWO-DIMENSIONAL ECHOCARDIOGRAPHY. In addition to a more accurate assessment of right ventricular size, two-dimensional echocardiography aided in the evaluation of the size of the right ventricular outflow tract and right atrium. The right ventricular outflow tract was enlarged in three patients, and the right atrium was enlarged in two.

Discrete subaortic stenosis

SURGICAL PROCEDURE, RESIDUA, AND SEQUELAE. Surgical correction consists of excising the membrane or fibrous ridge, and may be expected to improve the hemodynamic state [37]. However, most patients with discrete subaortic stenosis have aortic valve insufficiency that remains postoperatively. In addition, the more diffuse the obstruction, the more likely will a residual gradient exist after surgical intervention.

M-MODE ECHOCARDIOGRAPHY. Few data exist regarding the echocardiographic features of postoperative discrete subaortic stenosis. It would be expected that with complete relief of obstruction, resolution of posterior wall thickness would occur. Moreover, aortic valve motion should return to normal, since turbulent flow no longer traverses the left ventricular outflow tract. We have studied serially three patients who have undergone resection of either membranous or fibromuscular subaortic stenosis. In two patients posterior wall thickness regressed to normal, and there was no residual postoperative gradient. Aortic valve motion was abnormal in the one patient in whom residual obstruction existed. In this patient the posterior wall remained persistently thickened.

TWO-DIMENSIONAL ECHOCARDIOGRAPHY. The two-dimensional echocardiogram specifically identified the presence or absence of residual obstruction. In the long axis view along the left parasternal border, residual tissue was imaged in the left ventricular outflow tract as an area of increased echo reflectance (Fig. 17-18). In the patients without residual obstruction, the left ventricular outflow tract was clear of extra echoes [38].

Valvular aortic stenosis

SURGICAL PROCEDURE. The most important decision concerns the advisability of surgical intervention. The factors influencing indications are the patient's age and the nature of the valvular deformity. At the present time operation is advised for any child with a peak systolic pressure gradient exceeding 75 mm Hg. The procedure of choice is commissurotomy.

RESIDUA AND SEQUELAE. The two major residua are leftover obstruction and aortic regurgitation. Postoperatively the valve leaflets remain thickened and deformed, and it is possible that further degenerative changes will lead to significant future stenosis.

M-MODE ECHOCARDIOGRAPHY. The use of M-mode echocardiography in the diagnosis and quantitation of valvular aortic stenosis was discussed in Chapters 4 and 15. Controversy exists concerning the utility of these M-mode criteria in the postoperative assessment of severity of residual obstruction. In an initial study left ventricular pressure fell to normal values within two months following surgery, and echocardiography provided an excellent indication of surgical relief of obstruction or persistence of left ventricular hypertension [39]. Gewitz and colleagues, however, report that left ventricular posterior wall thickness remained increased for as long as 122 months after surgery, so that echocardiography overestimated peak left ventricular systolic pressure [40].

TWO-DIMENSIONAL ECHOCARDIOGRAPHY. Cross-sectional imaging has been used to quantify left ventricular muscle mass. However, these techniques have not been serially employed to evaluate persistence or resolution of left ventricular muscle mass in the patient who had operative relief of aortic stenosis [41]. Perhaps further investigation using two-dimensional techniques to quantify left ventricular mass in the postoperative patient will increase our ability to assess residual obstruction.

References

1. Garson A, Nihill MR, McNamara DG, Cooley DA: Status of the adult adolescent after the repair of tetralogy of Fallot. *Circulation* 59:1232, 1979
2. Pacifico AD, Bargeron LM, Kirklin JW: Primary total correction of tetralogy of Fallot in children less than 4 years of age. *Circulation* 48:1085, 1973
3. Sunderland CO, Matarazzo RG, Lees MH, Menashe VD, Bonchek LI, Rosenberg JA, Starr A: Total correction of tetralogy of Fallot in infancy: Post-operative hemodynamic evaluation. *Circulation* 43:398, 1973
4. Vick GW, Serwer GA: Echocardiographic evaluation of the post-operative tetralogy of Fallot patient. *Circulation* 58:842, 1978
5. Mercier JC, DiSessa TG, Jarmakani JM, Nakanishi T, Hiraishi S, Isabel-Jones JB, Friedman WF: Two-dimensional echocardiographic assessment of left ventricular volumes and ejection fraction in children. *Circulation* 65:962, 1982

6. Folland ED, Parisi AF, Moynihan PF, Jones DR, Feldman CI, and Tow DE: Assessment of left ventricular ejection fraction and volumes by real-time two-dimensional echocardiography: A comparison of cineangiographic and radionuclide techniques. *Circulation* 60:760, 1979
7. DiSessa TG, Hagan AD, Pope C, Samtoy L, Friedman WF: Two-dimensional echocardiographic characteristics of double outlet right ventricle. *Am J Cardiol* 44:1146, 1979
8. Valdez-Cruz LM, Pieroni DR, Roland RMA, Shematek JP: Recognition of residual postoperative shunts by contrast echocardiographic techniques. *Circulation* 55:148, 1977
9. Botvinick EH, Schiller NB: The complementary roles of M-mode echocardiography and scintigraphy in the evaluation of adults with suspected left to right shunts. *Circulation* 60:1070, 1980
10. Baker DW, Rubinstein SA, Lorch GS: Doppler echocardiography principles and applications. *Am J Med* 63:69, 1977
11. Saksena SB, Aldridge HE: Atrial septal defect in the older patient: A clinical and hemodynamic study in patients operated on after age 35. *Circulation* 42:1009, 1970
12. Zoneraich S, Zoneraich O, Ree JJ: Echocardiographic findings in atrial flutter. *Circulation* 52:455, 1975
13. McCabe JC, Engle MA, Gay WA, Ebert PA: Surgical treatment of endocardial cushion defects. *Am J Cardiol* 39:72, 1977
14. Eshaghpour E, Turnoff HB, Kingsley B, Kawai N, Linhart JW: Echocardiography in endocardial cushion defects: A pre-operative and post-operative study. *Chest* 68:172, 1975
15. DiSessa TG, Hagen AD: Echocardiographic Manifestations of Normal Sinus Rhythm, Arrhythmias and Conduction Defects. In AS Abassi (ed), *Echocardiographic Interpretation*. Springfield, Ill: Thomas, 1981. Pp 342–365
16. Beppu S, Yasuharu N, Sakakibara H, Nagata S, Yung-dae P, Kiyoshi B, Naito Y, Mitsushige O, Kamiya T, Koyanagi H, Fujita T: Mitral cleft and ostium primum atrial septal defect assessed by cross-sectional echocardiography. *Circulation* 62:1099, 1980
17. Hagler DJ, Tajik AJ, Seward JB, Mair DD, Ritter DG: Real-time wide-angle sector echocardiography: Atrioventricular canal defects. *Circulation* 59:140, 1979
18. Mustard WT: Successful two-stage correction of transposition of the great vessels. *Surgery* 55:469, 1964
19. Hagler DJ, Ritter DG, Mair DD, Davis GD, McGoon DC: Clinical, angiographic, and hemodynamic assessment of late results after Mustard operation. *Circulation* 57:1214, 1978
20. Godman MJ, Friedli B, Pasternac A, Kidd BSO, Trusler GA, Mustard WT: Hemodynamic studies in children four to ten years after Mustard operation for transposition of the great arteries. *Circulation* 53:532, 1976
21. Takahashi M, Lindesmith GG, Lewis AB, Stiles Q, Stanton RE, Meyer DW, Lurie PR: Long-term results of Mustard procedure. *Circulation* 56(Suppl II):II-85, 1977
22. Gillette PC, El-Said GN, Sivarajan N, Mullins CE, Williams RL, McNamara DG: Electrophysiological abnormalities after Mustard's operation for transposition of the great arteries. *Br Heart J* 36:186, 1974
23. Sunderland CO, Henken DP, Nichols GM, Dhindsa DS, Bonchek LI, Menashe VD, Rahintoola SH, Starr A, Lees MH: Post-operative hemodynamic and electrophysiologic evaluation of the intra-atrial baffle procedure. *Am J Cardiol* 35:660, 1975
24. Rakowski H, Drobac N, Bonet J, Benson L, McLaughlin PR, Olley P, Rowe RD: Long-term follow-up of Mustard's operation. *Circulation* 59:429, 1979 (Abstract)
25. Pieroni D, Gingell RL, Zavanella C, Vlad T, Subramanian S: Echocardiographic assessment of atrial septum following Senning repair of transposition of the great arteries. *Am J Cardiol* 43:402, 1979 (Abstract)
26. Silverman NH, Snider AR, Colo J, Ebert PA, Turley K: Superior vena cava obstruction after Mustard's operation: Detection by two-dimensional contrast echocardiography. *Circulation* 64:392, 1981
27. Graham TP, Atwood GF, Boucek RJ, Boerth RC, Nelson JH: Right heart volume characteristics in transposition of the great arteries. *Circulation* 51:881, 1975
28. Silverman NH, Payot M, Stanger P, Rudolph AM: The echocardiographic profile of patients after Mustard's operation. *Circulation* 58:1083, 1978
29. Aziz KU, Paul MH, Muster AJ: Echocardiographic localization of intra-atrial baffle after Mustard operation for dextro-transposition of the great arteries. *Am J Cardiol* 38:67, 1976

30. Nanda NC, Stewart S, Gramiak R, Manning JA: Echocardiography of the intra-atrial baffle in dextro-transposition of the great vessels. *Circulation* 53:1130, 1975
31. Silverman NH, Schiller NB: Apex echocardiography: A two-dimensional technique for evaluating congenital heart disease. *Circulation* 57:503, 1978
32. Stevenson G, Kawabori I, Dooley T, Dillard D, Gunteroth W: Pulsed Doppler echocardiographic detection of obstruction of systemic venous return following repair of transposition of the great arteries. *Circulation* 58(Suppl II):II-51, 1978
33. Ninomiya K, Duncan WJ, Cook DH, Olley PM, Rowe RD: Right ventricular ejection fraction and volumes after Mustard repair: Correlation of two-dimensional echocardiograms and cineangiograms. *Am J Cardiol* 48:317, 1981
34. Stewart S: Double outlet right ventricle: A collective review with a surgical viewpoint. *J Thorac Cardiovasc Surg* 71:355, 1976
35. Marcelletti C, McGoon DC, Danielson GK, Wallace RB, Mair DD: Early and late results of surgical repair of truncus arteriosus. *Circulation* 55:636, 1977
36. Danielson GK, Exarhos MD, Weidman WH, McGoon DC: Pulmonic stenosis with intact ventricular septum. *J Thorac Cardiovasc Surg* 61:228, 1971
37. Champsaur G, Trusler GA, Mustard WT: Congenital discrete valvar aortic stenosis: Surgical experience and long-term follow-up in twenty pediatric patients. *Br Heart J* 35:443, 1973
38. Wilcox WD, Seward JG, Hagler DJ, Mair DD, Tajik AJ: Discrete subaortic stenosis: Two-dimensional echocardiographic features with angiographic and surgical correlation. *Mayo Clinic Proc* 55:425, 1980
39. Johnson GL, Meyer R, Schwartz DC, Korfahagen J, Kaplan S: Echocardiographic left ventricular outlet obstruction in children: Pre- and post-operative assessment of left ventricular systolic pressures. *Circulation* 56:299, 1977
40. Gewitz NH, Werner JC, Kleinman CS, Hellenbrand WE, Talner NS, Taunt RA: Role of echocardiography in aortic stenosis: Pre- and post-operative studies. *Am J Cardiol* 43:67, 1979
41. Wyatt HL, Heng MK, Meerbaum S, Hestenes JD, Cobo JM, Davidson RN, Corday E: Cross-sectional echocardiography I. Analysis of mathematic models for quantifying mass of the left ventricle in dogs. *Circulation* 60:1104, 1979

Appendix. Normal values of echocardiographic measurements

Values listed in the tables are derived from both M-mode and two-dimensional imaging methods.

Table A-1. Normal values in newborns measured by M-mode echocardiography

Value	Hagan et al[a]	Meyer, Kaplan[b]	Solinger et al[c]
Weight (kg)	2.7–4.5	2.3–4.9	2.2–4.5
RVDD (mm)	6.1–15	10–17	10.4–17.7
ST (mm)	1.8–4		2.1–4.5
PWT (mm)	1.8–3.7		2–4.6
LVEDD (mm)	12.2–23.3	12–20	16.1–24.1
LVESD (mm)	8–18.6		
AOD (mm)	8.1–12	7–12 (s)	9–13.6 (s)
LAD (mm)	5–10	6–13 (s)	6.8–13.5 (s)

RVDD = right ventricular diastolic dimension; ST = septal thickness; PWT = posterior wall thickness; LVEDD = left ventricular end diastolic dimension; LVESD = left ventricular end systolic dimension; AOD = aortic root diameter; LAD = left atrial dimension; s = systolic.
[a]AD Hagan et al, *Circulation* 48:1221, 1973.
[b]RH Meyer, S Kaplan, *Circulation* 46:55, 1972.
[c]R Solinger et al, *Circulation* 47:108, 1973.

Table A-2. Normal values of the right ventricle and right atrium in infants and children measured from the apical four-chamber view*

Index	Mean	SD
RVSA (cm/m^2)	3.3	0.8
RVA (cm^2/m^2)	10.8	2.3
RASA (cm/m^2)	3.2	0.6
RALA (cm/m^2)	3.6	0.9
RAA (cm^2/m^2)	7.6	1.4
RVA/LVA	0.68	0.2
RAA/LAA	0.98	0.1

*Body surface area = 0.32–1.38 m^2.
SD = standard deviation; RVSA = right ventricular short axis; RVA = right ventricular area; RASA = right atrial short axis; RALA = right atrial long axis; RAA = right atrial area; LVA = left ventricular area; LAA = left atrial area.
Source: From GP Fontana et al, *JCU* 10:385, 1982.

Table A-3. Normal values for children

Value	BSA (m^2)	Mean (mm)	Range (mm)
RVDD	≤ 0.5	9	4–15
	0.6–1.0	15	5–23
	1.1–1.5	17.5	8–24
	> 1.5	22.5	10–28
ST	≤ 0.5	4	2.5–6
	0.6–1	6	4–7
	1.1–1.5	7	4–8
	> 1.5	8	5–9
PWT	≤ 0.5	4	2.5–5
	0.6–1	5.5	3–7
	1.1–1.5	7	4–7.5
	> 1.5	8	5–9
LVEDD	≤ 0.5	20	9–30
	0.6–1.0	34	24–40
	1.1–1.5	40	35–45
	> 1.5	43	38–50
LVESD	≤ 0.5	12	5–20
	0.6–1.0	21	15–28
	1.1–1.5	25	15–30
	> 1.5	28	20–32
AOD (s)	≤ 0.5	12	8–18
	0.6–1.0	20	15–25
	1.1–1.5	25	20–30
	> 1.5	27	20–30
LAD	≤ 0.5	13	8–20
	0.6–1.0	22	18–27
	1.1–1.5	26	18–30
	> 1.5	27	20–33

BSA = body surface area; RVDD = right ventricular diastolic dimension; ST = septal thickness; PWT = posterior wall thickness; LVEDD = left ventricular end diastolic dimension; LVESD = left ventricular end systolic dimension; AOD (s) = aortic root diameter (systolic); LAD = left atrial dimension.
Source: Modified from CLL Rogé, NH Silverman, *Circulation* 57:285, 1978.

Table A-4. Normal values of left ventricular function in children

Index	Mean	SD
Shortening fraction	36%	± 4%
LVPEP/LVET	0.31	± 0.03
Vcf	1.075 − 0.005 (HR) − 0.02 (age)	

SD = standard deviation; LVPEP = left ventricular preejection period; LVET = left ventricular ejection time; Vcf = mean velocity of circumferential fiber shortening; HR = heart rate.
Source: Modified from HP Gutgesell et al, *Circulation* 56:457, 1977.

Table A-5. Normal adult criteria of right heart structures measured by two-dimensional echocardiography*

Structure	View	Mean	Two Standard Deviations	Number of Patients
RV area	Apical 4-chamber	21.3 cm^2	10.6	112
RV area index	Apical 4-chamber	11.5 cm^2/m^2	5.0	112
RV/LV area ratio	Apical 4-chamber	0.7	0.2	109
RV short axis dimension	Apical 4-chamber	35.8 mm	10.6	77
RV/LV short axis dimension ratio	Apical 4-chamber	0.8	0.2	113
RV wall thickness	Subcostal 4-chamber	4.0 mm	2.0	36
RA area	Apical 4-chamber	13.8 cm^2	5.6	112
RA area index	Apical 4-chamber	7.5 cm^2/m^2	2.6	112
RA/LA area ratio	Apical 4-chamber	1.0	0.2	108
RA inf/sup dimension	Apical 4-chamber	43.8 mm	12.2	115
PA diameter	Parasternal short axis at base	22.1 mm	7.0	74
Ao diameter	Parasternal short axis at base	23.5 mm	7.6	76
PA/Ao ratio	Parasternal short axis at base	1.0	0.2	73
IVC diameter	Subcostal IVC long and short axis	18.0 mm	9.8	38

*Body surface area = 1.3–2.2 m^2.
Source: AD Hagan, unpublished data.

Table A-6. Equations for predicting normal M-mode measurements from body surface area and age

Measurements*	Equation
LVEDD	45.3 (BSA) ⅓ − 0.03 (age) − 7.2 ± 12%
LVESD	28.8 (BSA) ⅓ − 0.03 (age) − 4.1 ± 18%
LVPWT	5.56 (BSA) ½ + 0.03 (age) + 1.1 ± 16%
LVST	5.44 (BSA) ½ + 0.03 (age) + 1.5 ± 18%
ARD	24.0 (BSA) ⅓ + 0.1 (age) − 4.3 ± 18%
LAD	28.5 (BSA) ⅓ + 0.08 (age) − 0.9 ± 18%

*Measurements were made according to standards recommended by the American Society of Echocardiography.
LVEDD = left ventricular end diastolic dimension; BSA = body surface area; LVESD = left ventricular end systolic dimension; LVPWT = left ventricular posterior wall thickness; LVST = left ventricular septal thickness; ARD = aortic root dimension; LAD = left atrial dimension.
Source: Modified from WL Henry et al, Circulation 62:1054, 1980.

554 Appendix. Normal values of echocardiographic measurements

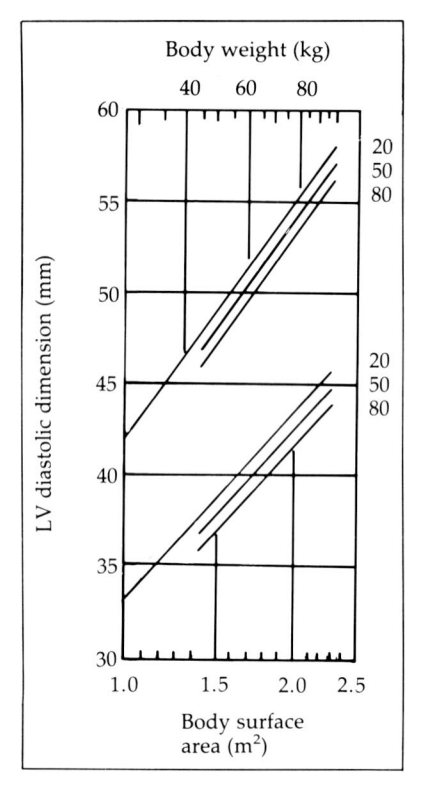

Fig. A-1. Left ventricular dimension at end-diastole (vertical axis) *plotted against body surface area (BSA)* (lower horizontal axis) *and body weight* (upper horizontal axis) *for normal adult subjects. The 95% prediction intervals for 20, 50, or 80 years of age are indicated by the solid lines extending from a BSA of 1.4 to 2.3 m^2.*

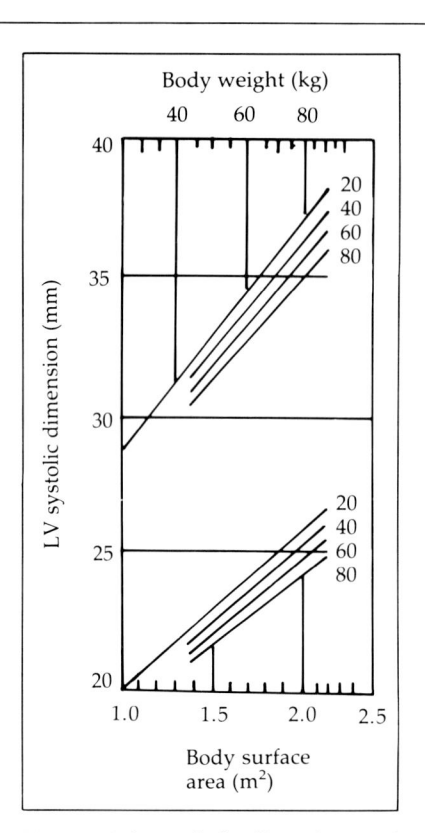

Fig. A-2. Left ventricular dimension at end-systole (vertical axis) *plotted against body surface area (BSA)* (lower horizontal axis) *and body weight* (upper horizontal axis) *for normal adult subjects. The 95% prediction intervals for 20, 40, 60, and 80 years of age are indicated by the solid lines extending from a BSA of 1.4 to 2.3 m^2.*

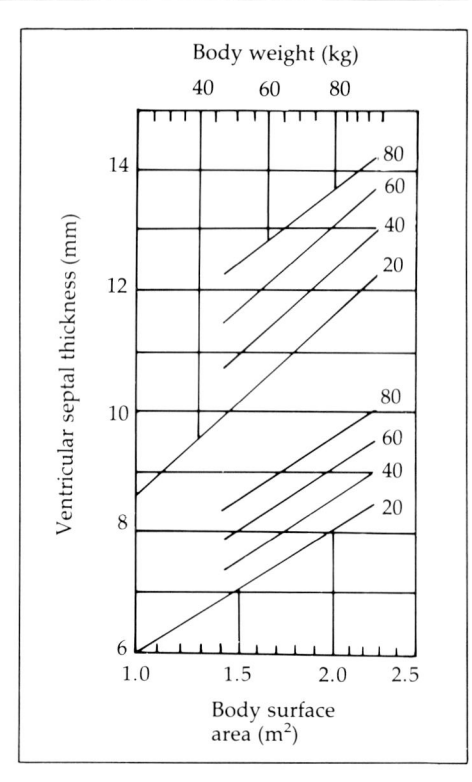

Fig. A-3. Ventricular septal thickness plotted against body surface area (BSA) (lower horizontal axis) *and body weight* (upper horizontal axis) *for normal adult subjects. The 95% prediction intervals for 20, 40, 60, and 80 years of age are indicated by the solid lines extending from a BSA of 1.4 to 2.3 m^2.*

The figures are modified from WL Henry et al, Echocardiographic measurements in normal subjects from infancy to old age. *Circulation* 62:1054, 1980. Measurements have been made according to standards recommended by the American Society of Echocardiography.

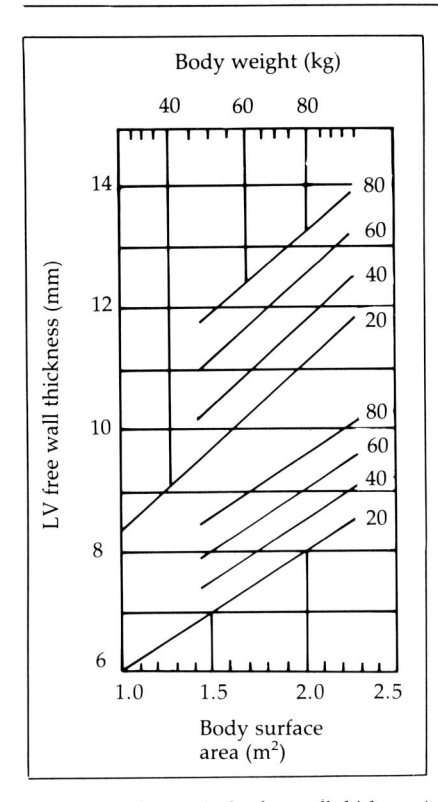

Fig. A-4. Left ventricular free wall thickness (vertical axis) plotted against body surface area (BSA) (lower horizontal axis) and body weight (upper horizontal axis) for normal adult subjects. The 95% prediction intervals for 20, 40, 60, and 80 years of age are indicated by the solid lines extending from a BSA of 1.4 to 2.3 m^2.

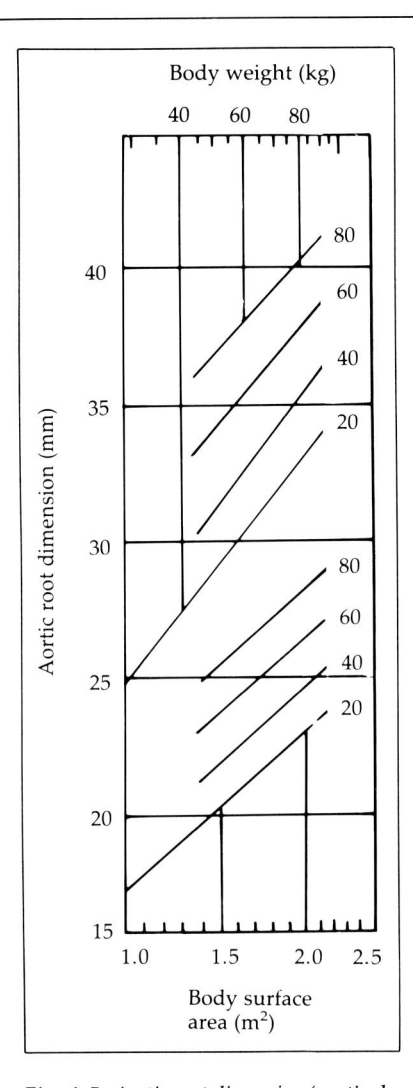

Fig. A-5. Aortic root dimension (vertical axis) plotted against body surface area (BSA) (lower horizontal axis) and body weight (upper horizontal axis) for normal adult subjects. The 95% prediction intervals for 20, 40, 60, and 80 years of age are indicated by the solid lines extending from a BSA of 1.4 to 2.3 m^2.

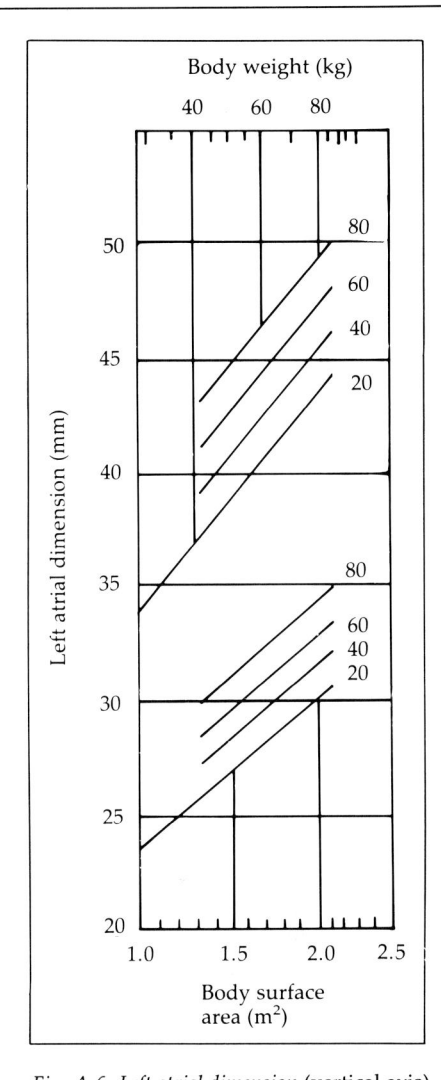

Fig. A-6. Left atrial dimension (vertical axis) plotted against body surface area (BSA) (lower horizontal axis) and body weight (upper horizontal axis) for normal adult subjects. The 95% prediction intervals for 20, 40, 60, and 80 years of age are indicated by the solid lines extending from a BSA of 1.4 to 2.3 m^2.

Index

Page numbers in *italics* indicate illustrations.

"A" wave
  in inferior vena cava, 269
  of pulmonic valve, 269, 276, 470
Afterload, and end-systolic meridional wall stress, 231–232
Aging, mitral valve effects of, 89
Alcohol, toxic effects on heart, 324
Alcoholism, congestive cardiomyopathy in, 324
Allied health personnel, and echocardiography, 3
Amyl nitrite
  and diagnostic intervention, 429–430
  in hypertrophic cardiomyopathy, 316, 317
Amyloid heart disease, 329–330
Aneurysm
  aortic, 135, *139*
  of interatrial septum, 268–269, *272*, 425, *428*
  sinus of Valsalva, 135
  ventricular, 189–191
Angiography. *See* Ventriculography
Aorta
  coarctation of, 488–489
    anatomy, 488
    clinical features and physiology, 488
    echocardiography of, 489
    suprasternal notch view of, 128, 135
  in complete transposition, 496–500
  in corrected transposition, 504
  diseases of, 134–139
  imaging techniques of, 111–115
  pericardial effusion and descending portion, 346
  pulmonary artery diameter compared with, 252
  suprasternal notch view of, *32–33*, 128, 135
  two-dimensional echocardiography of, *135–139*, 146
Aortic aneurysm, 135, *139*
Aortic annulus, 111, *112*
Aortic regurgitation, 128–134
  echocardiography
    aortic leaflet imaging, 131, 133
    findings, 129–134
    indications for, 129
    M-mode, 130–133
    two-dimensional, 133–134
  etiology, 128–129
  murmur in, 129
  premature closure of mitral valve in, 129, *130*
  timing for surgical valve replacement, 133–134
Aortic root
  in hypertrophic cardiomyopathy, 304
  stroke volume estimated using echo of, 238–239
Aortic root diameter, 134
Aortic stenosis
  calcification in, 116, *120–121*
  catheterization and M-mode echo findings, 117
  congenital, 481–485
    anatomy, 482–483
    clinical features and physiology, 481–482
    M-mode echocardiography in, 483
    two-dimensional echocardiography in, 483–485
  echocardiography in
    Doppler method, 124
    imaging techniques, 125–128
    M-mode, 116–117, *122*, 123
    in postoperative assessment, 124–125, 547
    two-dimensional, 124
  estimating severity of, 117, 123
  etiology, 116
  in left ventricular tumors, 371
  pathologic types, 116
  subaortic stenosis, 477–481, 546–547
  subvalvular, 128
  supravalvular, 128, 485, *486*, 488
    anatomy, 485
    clinical features and physiology, 485
    M-mode echocardiography in, 485
    two-dimensional echocardiography in, 485, 488
  surgical repair of, 547
    postoperative echocardiographic assessment, 547
    residua and sequelae, 547
Aortic valve. *See also* Aortic valve disease
  anatomy and physiology of, 111
  apical four-chamber view of, *24*
  apical long axis view of, *26*
  bicuspid, 116, *118–119*, 481–485
  cusp visualization on, 483, 485
  diastolic eccentricity index of, 483
  gradient across, method of calculating, 117, 123
  imaging techniques of, 111–115
  M-mode recording of, 113, 115
  and parasternal view, *37*
  preclosure, 477
  prolapse of, 133, *134*
  prosthesis
    measuring excursion of, 396
    qualitative assessment of, 396
  in subaortic stenosis, 477
Aortic valve disease, 115–139. *See also* Aortic valve; Rheumatic valvular disease
  aortic regurgitation, 128–134
  aortic stenosis, 115–128, 481–485
  clinical presentation, 115–116
  infective endocarditis, 147–151
  membranous subvalvular and supravalvular aortic stenosis, 128, 477–481, 485–488
  vegetations of, 147–155
Apical four-chamber view
  for aorta, 112–113
  for congestive cardiomyopathy, 325, 327
  end-diastolic planimetry of both ventricles, 266
  in hypertrophic cardiomyopathy, 302–303

Apical four-chamber view—*Continued*
  for mitral valve prolapse, 91, *93–94*
  for right heart structures, 253–254
    right atrium, 265–266
      right atrium and ventricle measurements in, 444
      right ventricular dilatation, 259, *262*, 264–266
Apical views, 22
  four-chamber plane, 22–24. *See also* Apical four-chamber view
  long axis plane, *25–26*
  oblique, *27*
  short axis plane, *21*
Asymmetric septal hypertrophy, 287. *See also* Cardiomyopathy, hypertrophic
Asynergy, in chronic ischemia, 173–174
Atherosclerosis. *See* Coronary artery disease
Atrial emptying index, in mitral stenosis, 50, 51
Atrial myxoma. *See* Left atrial myxoma; Right atrial myxoma
Atrial septal defect
  apical four-chamber view in, *262, 264,* 444
  contrast echocardiography in diagnosis of, 422, *423, 446, 447*
  mitral valve prolapse and, 89
  primum type, 447–451
    anatomy, 447–448
    clinical features and physiology, 447
    M-mode echocardiography, 448
    surgical repair of, 534, *536, 537*
      postoperative echocardiographic assessment, 534, 536
      residua and sequelae, 534
    two-dimensional echocardiography, 448–451
  secundum type, 443–447
    anatomy of, 443
    clinical features and physiology, 443
    echocardiography in
      M-mode, 443–444
      two-dimensional, 444–447
    surgical repair of, 533–534
      postoperative echocardiographic assessment, 533–534
      residua and sequelae, 533
  Valsalva maneuver enhancing echo result in, 424, 446
Atrial septum. *See* Interatrial septum
Atrioventricular canal. *See also* Endocardial cushion defect
  three types of, 456–457
Atrioventricular sulcus, parasternal view, *16*
Austin Flint murmur, 129
Axial resolution, 4
Azimuthal resolution, 4–5

Balloon counterpulsation, and segmental wall motion, 181
Bjork-Shiley tilting disc, 401

Calcification
  in aortic stenosis, 116, *120–121*
  of mitral annulus, 96–98

Carbon dioxide, as echocardiographic contrast agent, 426
Carcinoid heart disease, tricuspid valve abnormalities in, 279, *280*
Cardiac output, echocardiography and Doppler flowmeter estimates of, 238–239
Cardiac tamponade
  echocardiographic findings in, 346–347
  left and right diastolic pressures in, 343
  pulsus paradoxus in, 343
Cardiac tumors, 363–391
  left atrial myxoma, 363–370. *See also* Left atrial myxoma
  left ventricular, 370–374. *See also* Left ventricle, tumors and masses
  metastases, 375, 390
  right atrial, 374–375
  right ventricular, 375, *386,* 390
Cardiomyopathy, 287–330
  congestive, 323–328
    in alcoholism, 324
    clinical features, 325
    echocardiographic features, 323–328
    left ventricular hypertrophy-dilatation index in, 325
  endomyocardial fibrosis, 330
  hypertrophic, 287–322
    abnormal systolic motion of mitral valve in, 287, 289
    amyl nitrite use in diagnosis of, 429
    angiographic and hemodynamic findings in, 304
    apical, 309
    association with other cardiac disorders, 320–321
    catenoid shape of interventricular septum in, 294
    clinical features, 290, 294–297
    conditions mimicking, 309, 312–316
    disproportionate septal thickening in, 312
    echocardiographic imaging techniques in, 297–309
    echocardiographic subclassification, 290
    electrocardiogram in, 296
    genetics of, 289
    hallmarks of, 288
    hypertension associated with, 321–322
    in hypothyroidism, 322–323
    left ventricular function in, 321–322
    left ventricular outflow tract obstruction in, 288
      mechanism of, 290–292
      systolic anterior motion of mitral valve in, 289
    medical and surgical therapy assessment by echocardiography, 318–320
    mitral regurgitation in, 320–321
    mitral stenosis distinguished from, 52, 53
    pathophysiology, 287–290
    pharmacologic and maneuver interventions in, 316–317

regional myocardial function in, 292–294
in hypothyroidism, 322–323
restrictive, 328–330
  hemodynamic pattern of, 328
in scleroderma, 323
Cell disorganization in interventricular septum, 288–289
Chagas' heart disease, 330
Chest pain
  in mitral valve prolapse, 86
  two-dimensional echocardiography in, 163, 165
Chest x-ray, in interpreting echocardiogram, 2
Chiari's network, 375, *382–383*
Chordae tendineae
  ectopic, 198
  parasternal view of, *18*
    M-mode recordings and, *40*
  ruptured, 98–102
    anatomic features of, 102
    echocardiographic appearance, 100–102
  thickening in rheumatic valvular disease, 59–61
  of tricuspid valve, 276
Circumferential fiber shortening rate, 185
  in hypertrophic cardiomyopathy, 292
  left ventricular function assessed by, 235–236
Coarctation of aorta. *See* Aorta, coarctation of
Cold pressor test, as diagnostic intervention, 433–434
Common ventricle. *See* Single ventricle
Compliance, 241
Congenital heart disease
  acyanotic with left-to-right shunt, 443–463. *See also under specific disease*
    atrial septal defect
      primum type, 447–451
      secundum type, 443–447
    endocardial cushion defect, 456–462
    patent ductus arteriosus, 462–463
    ventricular septal defect, 451–456
  cyanotic, 493–525
    corrected transposition of great arteries, 500, 504–508
    double-outlet right ventricle, 511–518
    single ventricle, 518–519, *522–523*
    tetralogy of Fallot, 493–496
    total anomalous pulmonary venous return, 524–525
    transposition of great arteries, 496–503
    tricuspid atresia, 519, 523, *524*
    truncus arteriosus, 508–511
    with disproportionate septal thickening, 309, 312
  postoperative echocardiographic assessment, 529–547
    in aortic stenosis, 547
    in atrial septal defect
      primum type, 534, 536, *537*
      secundum type, 533–534
    in double-outlet right ventricle, 543–544
    in endocardial cushion defect, 538
    in pulmonic stenosis, 545–546
    in subaortic stenosis, 546–547
    in tetralogy of Fallot, 529–532
    in transposition of great arteries, 538–542
    in truncus arteriosus, 544–545
    in ventricular septal defect, 531, 533
  valvular, subvalvular and supravalvular lesions, 467–489
    aortic stenosis, 481–485
    coarctation of aorta, 488–489
    Ebstein's anomaly, 467–469
    isolated infundibular stenosis, 469–470
    left ventricular inflow tract obstruction, 473–477
    pulmonic stenosis, 470–472
    subaortic stenosis, 477–481
    supravalvular aortic stenosis, 485–488
Congestive cardiomyopathy. *See* Cardiomyopathy, congestive
Contrast echocardiography, 421–429
  in atrial septal defect, 422, *423*, 446, *447*
  carbon dioxide use in, 426
  for enlarged coronary sinus, 424–425
  and flow velocity in right side of heart, 425
  in postoperative assessment of transposition of great arteries, 541, *542*
  in pulmonary hypertension, 425
  in pulmonic insufficiency, 80
  for residual postoperative shunts, 424
  shunts determined by, 421, 446, *447*
  in single ventricle, 518–519
  technique, 421
  in tricuspid regurgitation, 76–78, 279, *281*, *425*, *427*
  in ventricular septal defect, 422, 424
Cor triatriatum, 473, *474*, *476*, 477
Cor trioculare biatriatum. *See* Single ventricle
Coronary arteries
  imaging techniques for orifice of, 112, *114–115*
  two-dimensional echocardiographic examination of, 214
Coronary artery bypass graft, postoperative assessment, *213*, 214
Coronary artery disease, 163–216. *See also* Myocardial infarction; Myocardial ischemia
  disproportionate septal thickening in, 313
  echocardiographic evaluation of, 214
  imaging techniques
    distinguishing ischemia from infarction, 172–176
    wall motion index, 175–176
  limitations of M-mode echocardiography in, 163
  pharmacologic agents in evaluation of, 180–181
  quantitation of infarct size and ischemia in, 186–188
  regional analysis in, 176–180
  two-dimensional echocardiography in, 163, 165–166, 170

Coronary artery disease—*Continued*
  two-dimensional imaging techniques in, 170–180
    exercise-induced wall motion abnormalities, 170–172
    technical problems with, 175
    uncomplicated myocardial infarction and left ventricular function in, 181–185
Coronary sinus, contrast echocardiography and, 424–425
Corrected transposition of great arteries, 500, 504–508
  anatomy, 504
  clinical features and physiology, 500
  M-mode echocardiography in, 504
  two-dimensional echocardiography in, 504, 508
Creatine kinase MB fraction, estimation of infarct size by, 172–173
Cross-sectional imaging. *See* Imaging techniques; Transducer, position of
Cysts, in heart, 374

Diastolic doming, 125, *126*
Diastolic pressure-volume relationship, 241
  pericardium effect on, 341–342
  M-mode echocardiography and, 243
Digoxin, left ventricular function, 241
Doppler echocardiography
  in aortic regurgitation, 133
  in aortic stenosis, 124
  cardiac output estimated by, 238–239
  in hypertrophic cardiomyopathy, 304
  in mitral regurgitation, 64
  for prosthetic mitral valve, 405
  in pulmonic stenosis, 472
  shunts determined by, 446–447
    in ventricular septal defect, 456
  in tricuspid regurgitation, 78
Doppler flowmeter, cardiac output determined by, 238–239
Doppler-phased array system, for cardiac output, 238
Double-outlet right ventricle. *See* Right ventricle, double-outlet
Dressler's syndrome, 209
Drug abuse, and right-sided infective endocarditis, 153
Dyssynergy, echocardiographic determination of, 176

E point-septal separation, 185
  left ventricular function and, 236, *237*
Ebstein's anomaly, 467–469
  anatomy, 467
  clinical features and physiology, 467
  in corrected transposition, 508
  M-mode echocardiography in, 467
  two-dimensional echocardiography in, 467–469
Eccentricity index, of aortic valve, 483
Echinococcosis cyst of myocardium, 374
Echo dropout, in ventricular septal defect, 453–456

Echophonocardiography
  applications of, 434
  for prosthetic valves, 395, 401, 405
E–F slope
  changes in mitral stenosis, 51, *52*
  diastolic filling evaluated by, 243
Ejection fraction
  algorithm for determination of, 232, *234*, 235
  two-dimensional echocardiography and, 184–185
Ejection phase indices, 166
Electrocardiogram
  in hypertrophic cardiomyopathy, 296
  importance in interpreting echocardiogram, 2
  limitations in evaluation of uncomplicated myocardial infarction, 181–182
  in mitral valve prolapse, 87
  in right ventricular infarction, 209
Endocardial cushion defect, 456–462
  anatomy, 456–457
  clinical features and physiology, 456
  M-mode echocardiography in, 457
  surgical repair of, 538
    postoperative echocardiographic assessment, 538
    residua and sequelae, 538
  two-dimensional echocardiography in, 457–462
Endocarditis
  infective, 145–159
    clinical features, 145–147
    echocardiographic features of vegetations, 147–159
      aortic valve, 147–151
      mitral valve, 151–155
      pulmonic valve, 158–159
      tricuspid valve, 153, 155–158
    gonococcal, 158–159
    left atrial myxoma mimicking, 364
    in neonatal period, 153
    of prosthetic valve, 416
    secondary to instrumentation or catheters, 159
Endocardium, border recognition of, 186, 187
Endomyocardial fibrosis, 330
Epicardium, border recognition of, 186, 187
Equipment, 4
Esophageal echocardiography, 434, *436*, 438
Eustachian valves, 375, *384–385*
Exercise
  as diagnostic intervention, 432–434
  left ventricular dimensions and mass related to, 230–232
  wall motion abnormalities induced by, 170–172

Fibromuscular subaortic obstruction, 477, 481
Flail mitral leaflet, echocardiography for, 98, *99*, 101–102
Fossa ovalis, aneurysm of, 272
Four-chamber plane, 6, 7, *9*. *See also* Apical four-chamber view

apical views, 22–24
M-mode recordings and, 40
subcostal views, 28–29

Gallium scan, in infective endocarditis, 146–147
Gonococcal endocarditis, 158–159
Goose neck deformity, 448, 449, 461

Heart, echinococcosis cyst of, 374
Heart failure, pericardium and, 342–343
Heart sounds
  in Ebstein's anomaly, 467
  first, 434
    wide splitting of, 158
  fourth, in hypertrophic cardiomyopathy, 296
  mitral valve opening snap, 434
  second, 111
    fixed splitting in atrial septal defect, 443
Hemodialysis, 241
Heterotopic tissue tumors and cysts, 374
Hydatid cyst, 374
Hypertension
  disproportionate septal thickening due to, 312–313
  ejection sounds in, 434
  hypertrophic cardiomyopathy distinguished from, 321–322
  pulmonary. See Pulmonary hypertension
  rapid filling of left ventricle in, 243
Hypertrophic cardiomyopathy. See Cardiomyopathy, hypertrophic
Hypothyroidism, cardiomyopathy of, 322–323

Idiopathic hypertrophic subaortic stenosis. See Cardiomyopathy, hypertrophic
Imaging
  planes, 5–6
  systems, 4–5
  techniques, 22, 34. See also Transducer, position of
Indocyanine green dye, 421
Infants, bacterial endocarditis in, 153
Infarct expansion, 182
Infective endocarditis. See Endocarditis, infective
Inferior vena cava
  dimensions of, 269
  enlargement in constrictive pericarditis, 358, 360
  parasternal short axis view of, 38
  in pericardial effusion, 347
  subcostal view of, 30, 41, 254, 268, 269, 273–275
Infundibular stenosis, 469–470
Integration of two-dimensional and M-mode recordings, 34–42
Interatrial septum
  aneurysm of, 268–269, 272, 425, 428
  echocardiographic features of, 268–271
  subcostal view of, 29
Interventional echocardiography, 421–438
  contrast, 421–429. See also Contrast echocardiography

echophonocardiography, 434, 435
esophageal, 434, 436, 438
exercise, 432–434. See also Exercise
in hypertrophic cardiomyopathy, 316–317
intraoperative, 437, 438
in mitral valve prolapse, 94
pharmacologic and physiologic maneuvers, 429–432
Interventricular septum
  abnormal motion
    in aortic regurgitation, 129–132
    in coronary artery disease, 177, 179
    in right ventricle volume overload, 257–258
  catenoid shape of, 294
  cell disorganization in, 288–289
  conditions causing paradoxical motion of, 257
  defect of. See Ventricular septal defect
  diastolic bulging of, 244
  disproportionate thickening of, 288
    in coronary artery disease, 313
    distinguishing hypertrophic cardiomyopathy from secondary form, 289–290
    hypertension causing, 312–313
    in hypertrophic cardiomyopathy, 312
    nongenetically transmitted, 309, 312–314
  in hypertrophic cardiomyopathy, 292
  membranous, 111
  ratio of posterior wall thickness to, 314
  rupture of, 204–206
  tumors in, 374
Intraaortic balloon counterpulsation. See Balloon counterpulsation
Intraoperative echocardiography, 438
Intramural fibrous tumors of heart, 374
Ischemia. See Myocardial ischemia
Isosorbide dinitrate, 240

Kussmaul's sign of inferior vena cava, 347

Lateral resolution, 4–5
Left anterior descending artery, lesions of, 179–180
Left atrial appendage, visualization in mitral disease, 68–71
Left atrial myxoma, 363–370
  auscultatory findings, 363
  differential diagnosis, 364
  echocardiography for, 363–370
  hemodynamic abnormalities, 363
  mitral vegetation distinguished from, 364
  pathologic appearance, 364
  signs and symptoms, 363, 364
Left atrium
  echocardiographic measurements of, 42
  pseudomass in, 370
  tumors of. See Left atrial myxoma
  visualization in rheumatic mitral disease, 68–70
Left ventricle
  alcohol, toxic effects on, 324
  anatomic divisions for echocardiography, 167, 170

Left ventricle—*Continued*
  aortic stenosis and wall stress of, 116–117, 123
  apical views of, 21–27
  congenital inflow tract obstruction, 473–477
    anatomy, 473
    clinical features and physiology, 473
    M-mode echocardiography in, 473
    two-dimensional echocardiography in, 473, 475–477
  diastolic filling in restrictive cardiomyopathy, 329
  diastolic thickness, 241
  double-inlet. *See* Single ventricle
  echinococcosis cyst of, 374
  echocardiographic measurements of, 42, 44
  ejection phase indices, 166
  in hypertrophic cardiomyopathy, 288, 289
  imaging techniques for, 168–170
  interdependence of right ventricle and, 243–244
  internal dimensions of, 227–230
  long axis view of, *8*
  muscle mass of
    M-mode determination of, 228, 230
    two-dimensional echocardiographic determination of, 230
  outflow tract assessment for mitral valve prosthesis, 395
  parasternal long axis view, 10, *11*
  pericardial effusion, and disease of, 343
  pericardium role in diastolic properties of, 341–342
  pressure and volume in diastole, 243
  regional analysis of, 176–180
  right ventricle dysfunction and, 342–343
  right ventricle interdependence of, 255
  short axis view of, *8*
  subcostal view, *31*
  techniques for segmental wall motion of, 174
  thrombus of, 193–201
  tumors and masses, 370–374
    in children, 371
    echinococcosis cysts, 374
    heterotopic tumors and cysts, 374
    incidence, 370
    intramural fibrous tumors, 374
    primary versus metastatic, 371, *373*
    rhabdomyosarcoma, 371
    signs and symptoms, 371
  volume of, 227–228
    algorithm for determination of, 232, *234*, 235
    echocardiographic determination of, 183–184
    performance related to, 232, 234–237
    respiration effects on, 227–228
  wall motion abnormalities induced by exercise, 170–172
  wall stress of, 230–232
    determinations of, 230–231
    and diagnosis of aortic stenosis, 116–117, 123
    end-systolic meridional, 231–232
    formulas for, 231
  wall thickening in hypertrophic cardiomyopathy, 292
  wall thickness variation in ischemia, 182–183
Left ventricular function, 227–244. *See also* Wall motion studies
  alcohol effects on, 324
  cardiovascular drugs and exercise influence on, 240–241
  circumferential fiber shortening rate and, 235–236
  in constrictive pericarditis, 347
  determinants of, 227
  diastolic filling and compliance, 241, 243
  E point–septal separation and, 236, *237*
  echocardiography in determination of, 166
  exercise, effect on, 433
  global function indices in assessment of, 235–236
  in hypertrophic cardiomyopathy, 292–294, 321–322
  inflow tract obstruction, 473, 475–477
  left ventricular volume related to, 232, 234–237
  in mitral valve prolapse, 88–89
  normal echocardiographic values in children, 552
  percent fractional shortening and, 236
  pharmacologic agents and echocardiography in evaluation of, 180–181
  postextrasystolic potentiation effects on, 432
  quantification of regional function, 181
  segmental wall motion abnormalities and, 172
  Valsalva maneuver and, 431–432
  wall stress and, 230–232
  wall thickening as measure of, 183
Left ventricular hypertrophy. *See also* Cardiomyopathy, hypertrophic
  dilatation index in congestive cardiomyopathy, 325
  in hypothyroidism, 323
  muscle mass determinations for, 228, 230
  patterns of distribution, 304
  wall stress in, 232
Linear-array scanners, 4
Long axis plane, 5–8
  apical views, 25–26
  parasternal views, 10–13
Lymphoma, disproportionate septal thickening in, 314

Mean circumferential fiber shortening rate. *See* Circumferential fiber shortening rate
Mechanical scanners, 4
Mediastinal tumor, cardiac tamponade due to, 391
Metastases, cardiac, 371, *373*
  antemortem diagnosis of, 375, 390
  incidence, 390
Microbubbles, 421, 425–426. *See also* Contrast echocardiography

Mitral annulus calcification, 96–98
  clinical entities associated with, 96
  two-dimensional echocardiography in, 96–98
Mitral E point–septal separation. *See* E point–septal separation
Mitral regurgitation
  in alcoholic congestive cardiomyopathy, 324
  congenital, 106
  echocardiography in, 64, *66–67*
  in hypertrophic cardiomyopathy, 320–321
  mitral annulus calcification causing, 96–98
  in mitral valve prolapse, 96
  papillary muscle dysfunction causing, 103, 106, 207
  pathophysiology of, 83
  in primum atrial septal defect, 447
  two-dimensional echocardiography for, 96
Mitral stenosis
  anatomic types, 59, 61
  clinical features, 51
  congenital, 473
  echocardiography in, 50–69
    measuring mitral orifice, 55, *57*, 63
    M-mode, 50–54
    qualitative changes seen by, 58
    severity determined by, 61, 63
    two-dimensional, 54–58
    valve contour and, 64, 68
  negative intraventricular diastolic pressure in, 64, 68
  parasternal long axis view in, 55, *56*
  posterior leaflet movement in, 52–53
  prosthetic valve sticking causing, 403
  pulmonary hypertension in, 79
Mitral valve. *See also* Mitral valve disease
  abnormal M-mode recordings in, 53–54
  in atrial septal defect on primum type, 447
  aging effects on, 89
  anatomy of, 47–50
    differences from tricuspid valve, 276
  annulus, 49–50
  causes of abnormal M-mode recording of, 53–54
  cleft in anterior leaflet, 447–448, 451
  flail, 207
  leaflets of, 47, 49
  measuring orifice of, 55, *57*
  normal echocardiographic appearance, 47–50
  opening snap of, 434
  parachute, 473, *476*, 477
  parasternal view of, 17
    M-mode recordings integrated with, *39*
  premature closure in aortic insufficiency, 129, *130*
  prosthesis
    assessment of left ventricular outflow tract for, 395
    imaging views for, 401, 403
    intermittent sticking, 401, 403
    interval between aortic second sound and mitral opening and, 403
    measuring excursion of, 396

porcine heterografts, 405, 408
velocity measurements, 401
stroke volume estimated using echo of, 239, *240*
structures determining normal function of, 49
supravalvular ring, 473, *475*
systolic anterior motion of, 287, 289
  in complete transposition of great arteries, 500
  differential diagnosis, 314–316
  mechanism of, 291–292
  pseudo, 314
  role in left ventricular obstruction, 290–291
Mitral valve area, 63
Mitral valve disease, 83–106. *See also* Mitral regurgitation; Mitral stenosis; Mitral valve; Mitral valve prolapse; Rheumatic valvular disease
  annulus calcification, 96–98
  flail valve due to ruptured papillary muscle, 207
  history of echocardiography for, 47
  infective endocarditis, 151–155
  left atrium visualization in, 68–71
  myxomatous degeneration causing, 83–85
  papillary muscle dysfunction, 102–106
  rheumatic, 51–69
  ruptured chordae tendineae, 98–102
  tricuspid regurgitation after surgery for, 75
Mitral valve E–F slope. *See* E–F slope
Mitral valve prolapse, 83–96
  amyl nitrite use in diagnosis of, 429
  angiographic-echocardiographic correlations in, 89–91
  atrial septal defect and, 89
  clinical manifestations of, 85–89
    electrocardiogram, 87
    left ventricular contraction abnormalities, 88–89
    natural history, 85–86
    physical examination, 86–87
    prevalence, 85
    symptoms, 86
  echocardiography in, 91–96
    in mitral regurgitation, 96
  fibrosis and calcification of chordae tendineae and papillary muscles in, 102–103
  M-mode echocardiography in, 91–95
  myxomatous degeneration causing, 83–85
  pathologic changes in, *84*, 85
  physiologic interventions to induce, 94
  serious conditions related to, 83
  systolic bulging of anterior leaflet distinguished from, 68
  tricuspid valve prolapse concomitant with, 279
  vegetations distinguished from, 151, *152*
M-mode echocardiography. *See under specific entity*
Müller maneuver, as diagnostic intervention, 430
Multiscan, 4

Murmur
  in aortic regurgitation, 129
  in aortic stenosis, 115–116
  in atrial septal defect, 443
  Austin Flint, 129
  in mitral valve prolapse, 86–87
  in pulmonic stenosis, 470
  in tetralogy of Fallot, 493, 530
  in ventricular septal defect, 451
Muscle bridging, 198, *202–203*
Mustard procedure, 538
Myocardial contractility
  in hypertrophic cardiomyopathy, 292–294
  in mitral valve prolapse, 88–89
Myocardial infarction. *See also* Coronary artery disease
  complications of, 189–214
    flail mitral valve, 207
    left ventricular thrombus, 193–201
    muscle bridges, 198, 202–203
    postinfarction pericarditis, 209, *210*
    pseudoaneurysm, 189, *192*, 193
    ventricular aneurysm, 189–191
    ventricular septal rupture, 204–206
  echocardiography in, 166, 170
    to distinguish ischemia from, 172–175
    infarct expansion detected by, 182
    in quantitation of, 186–187
    in uncomplicated attack, 181–185
  limitation of electrocardiogram in uncomplicated attack, 181–182
  regional abnormalities in, 176–180
  right ventricular, 209, 211, *212*, 214
  right ventricular dysfunction after, 255
  sequential changes after, 182
Myocardial ischemia
  distinguishing infarction from, 172–175
  quantitation of, 186–187
  ventricular asynergy in, 173–174
  wall thickness variation during, 182–183
Myocardial regions, 176
  abnormalities in, 176–180
  echocardiography and, 180–181
Myxedema. *See* Hypothyroidism
Myxoma
  left atrial, 363–370. *See also* Left atrial myxoma
  left ventricular, 371
Myxomatous degeneration
  of aortic valve, 133
  of cardiac valves, 83–85
  definition, 83, 85

Negative contrast effect, 421–423
  in atrial septal defect, 446, *447*
Neoplasms
  cardiac, 363–391. *See also* Cardiac tumors
  extracardiac, 390–391
Newborn, normal echocardiographic values in, 551
Nitroglycerin, in evaluation of myocardial function, 180, 240
Nitroprusside
  in evaluation of left ventricular obstruction in hypertrophic cardiomyopathy, 317
  in evaluation of myocardial function, 180, 183, *184*
  pericardium role in fall of diastolic pressure due to, 342
Normal echocardiographic values, 551–555

Oblique sinus, 344–345
Opening snap, of mitral valve, 434
Orthogonal planes, 5–6
Oxygen consumption, left ventricular mass and wall stress related to, 232

Papillary muscle dysfunction, 102–106
  causes of, 103
  two-dimensional echocardiography in, 103–106
Papillary muscle rupture, 207
  flail mitral valve due, 207
Papillary muscles
  apical oblique view of, 27
  in parachute mitral valve, 473
  parasternal short axis view of, *19, 20*
  of right ventricle, 276
Parasternal views, 7, 10–20, 22
  of aorta, 111, 135, *137–139*
  in aortic stenosis, 125–128
  in hypertrophic cardiomyopathy, 297–301
  long axis, 10–13
  for mitral valve prolapse, 91, *92*, 94
  M-mode recordings integrated with, *35–40*
  of right heart structures, 253
  for right volume overload, 257–261
  short axis, 10, *14–21*
Patent ductus arteriosus, 462–463
  clinical features and physiology, 462
  diastolic fluttering of pulmonic valve in, 276
  M-mode echocardiography in, 462
  two-dimensional echocardiography in, 462–463
Patient
  history, 1–2
  positioning, 22, 34
Percent fractional shortening, 185
  left ventricular function assessed by, 236
Pericardial disease, 341–360
Pericardial effusion
  echocardiographic diagnosis of, 343–347
  and primary left ventricular disease, 343
  structures mimicking, 345
Pericardial thickening, 347, 354–360
Pericarditis
  constrictive, echocardiography in, 347, 354–360
  postinfarction, 209, *210*
Pericardium
  anatomy and function of, 341
  esophageal echocardiography in evaluation of, 434, 438
  measurement of thickness of, 358
  and pathophysiology of cardiac failure, 342–343
  role in diastolic properties of ventricles, 341–342

Personnel, requirements in echocardiography, 2–4
Phased-array echocardiography, 346
Phased-array scanners, 4–5
  for cardiac output, 238
Phenylephrine, effect on left ventricular function, 240
Phonocardiography, and prosthetic valves, 395, 401, 405
Planimetry
  apical four-chamber view for both ventricles, *265, 266*
  of mitral valve orifice, 63–64
Positive expiratory pressure, effects on left ventricular function, 244
Post-extrasystolic potentiation
  as diagnostic intervention, 432
  echocardiography and, 431–432
  in hypertrophic cardiomyopathy, 316–317
PR–AC interval, and left ventricular end-diastolic pressure, 243
Preload. *See* Left ventricle, volume of
Primitive ventricle. *See* Single ventricle
Propranolol
  effect on left ventricular function, 240–241
  in hypertrophic cardiomyopathy, 317
Prosthetic valves, 395–416
  clinical questions in evaluation of, 411
  differential diagnosis of dysfunction, 395
  endocarditis risk after replacement, 145–146
  evaluation of function with two prostheses, 405
  imaging techniques for, 395–401, 403
  infective endocarditis of, 416
  with metallic components, 403
  porcine heterografts, 395
  preoperative assessment of left ventricular outflow tract and, 395
  St. Jude Medical cardiac valve, 403, 405
  simultaneous phonocardiography and echocardiography for 395, 401, 405
  in truncus arteriosus, 544–545
  two-dimensional echocardiographic imaging of, 405, 408–411
  types of, 395, *414–415*
  vegetations on, 147, 416
Pseudoaneurysm, 189, *192*, 193
Pulmonary artery
  aorta diameter compared with, 252
  in complete transposition, 496–500
  in corrected transposition, 504
  echocardiographic imaging techniques for, 253
  parasternal view of, 10, *15*
    M-mode recordings integrated with, *38*
  in right ventricular volume overload, 266
  transducer position for, 79–80
Pulmonary hypertension
  contrast echocardiography in, 425
  in mitral stenosis, 79
  pulmonic valve motion in, 255–257
  and right ventricular function, 254–257
Pulmonary veins, total anomalous return, 524–525

Pulmonic regurgitation, pseudotumor in right ventricle due to, 390
Pulmonic stenosis
  congenital, 470–472
    anatomy, 470
    clinical features and physiology, 470
    M-mode echocardiography in, 470
    two-dimensional echocardiography in, 472
  in corrected transposition, 500
  in double-outlet right ventricle, 511
  echocardiographic diagnosis of, 276, 470, 472
  in hypertrophic cardiomyopathy, 321
  isolated infundibular stenosis, 469–470
  surgical repair of, 545–546
  in tetralogy of Fallot, 493
Pulmonic valve
  "A" wave of, 269, 276
  diastolic fluttering of, 276
  echocardiographic imaging techniques for, 253, 472
  infective endocarditis involving, 158–159
  in infundibular stenosis, 469–470
  motion caused by pulmonary hypertension, 255–257
  parasternal view of, and M-mode recordings, *38*
  and pulmonary artery pressure, 269
  rheumatic disease of, 78–80
    associated valvular lesions in, 79
  transducer position for, 79–80
  vegetations of, 158–159
Pulsus paradoxus, absence in cardiac tamponade, 343

Radionuclide ventriculography, in segmental wall motion, 174
Resolution in echocardiography, 4–5
Respiration, and left ventricular volume, 227–228
Rhabdomyosarcoma, cardiac, 371
  metastases of, 390
Rheumatic valvular disease, 47–80. *See also* Prosthetic valves
  aortic regurgitation, 128–129
  of mitral valve, 51–69
    clinical manifestations, 51
    echocardiographic features, 50–69
    pathological features of different stages and severity, 58–71
    mitral regurgitation, 64
    mitral stenosis, 59, 61
    thickening of valve surfaces, 59–61
    verrucae, 58–59
  of pulmonic valve, 78–80
  of tricuspid valve, 69, 72–78
  valves involved in, 47
  vegetations, 147
Right atrial myxoma, 374–375
  conditions mimicking, 374–375
Right atrium
  dimensions of, 251–252
  imaging techniques, 253
  measurements of, 42

Right atrium, measurements of—*Continued*
    from apical four-chamber view, 444
    normal values in children, 551
  parasternal short axis view of, *38*
  subcostal view of, *30, 41*
Right heart disease, 251–283
  limitation of M-mode echocardiography in, 251
Right heart structures. *See also* Right atrium; Right ventricle
  imaging techniques for, 252–254
  normal criteria for dimensions of, 251–252
  normal measurements, 553
Right ventricle
  abscess of, 390
  dimensions of, 251, 252
  double outlet, 511–518
    anatomy, 511, *512*
    clinical features and physiology, 511
    echocardiographic features, 513–518
    surgical repair of, 543–544
      postoperative echocardiographic assessment, 543–544
      residua and sequelae, 543
  imaging techniques for, 253–254
  interdependence of left ventricle and, 243–244
  left ventricle dysfunction causing failure of, 342–343
  left ventricle interdependence of, 255
  measurements of, *42*
    from apical four-chamber view, 444
    normal values in children, 551
  parasternal inflow plane of, 10, *12*
  parasternal outflow view, 10, *13, 15*
  pericardium role in diastolic properties of, 341–342
  subcostal four-channel view of, and M-mode recordings, *40–41*
  tumors of, 375, *386*, 390
    pulmonic regurgitation simulating, 390
    sarcomas, 390
  volume overload, 257–266
Right ventricular function
  poor compliance, 255
  and pulmonary hypertension, 254–257
Right ventricular infarction, 209, 211, *212*, 214
  bedside diagnosis of, 209
  clinical features of, 209, 211
Ring abscess, clues suggestive of, 146

St. Jude Medical cardiac valve, 403, 405
Sarcoma, cardiac
  disproportionate septal thickening in, 314
  in left ventricle, 371
  of right ventricle, 390
Scleroderma heart disease, 323
Segmental wall motion abnormalities. *See* Wall motion studies
Senning procedure, 538
Septum
  interatrial. *See* Interatrial septum
  interventricular. *See* Interventricular septum
  ventricular. *See* Interventricular septum

Shone's complex, 473
Short axis plane, 6, *8*
Shunting
  contrast echocardiography and, 446, *447*
  Doppler echocardiography in determination of, 446–447
  left-to-right. *See also* Congenital heart disease, acyanotic with left-to-right shunt
  postoperative, 424
  right-to-left, 421
    contrast echocardiography in diagnosis of, 421
Single ventricle, 518–519, *522–523*
  anatomy, 518
  clinical features and physiology, 518
  M-mode echocardiography in, 518–519
  two-dimensional echocardiography in, 519
Sinus of Valsalva
  aneurysm of, 135
  imaging techniques for, 111
Sinus venosus, congenital remnants of, 375
Smearing effect, 5
  in mitral annulus calcification, 98
Squatting, left ventricular function effects of, 430
Staphylococci, in prosthetic valve endocarditis, 416
Standard views and recording sequence, 34, *39*
Streptococci, in prosthetic valve endocarditis, 416
Stroke volume, echocardiographic estimates of, 238–239
Subaortic stenosis, 477–481
  anatomy, 477
  clinical features and physiology, 477
  M-mode echocardiography in, 477
  surgical repair of, 546–547
  two-dimensional echocardiography in, 477, 481
Subcostal views, 22
  atrial septal defect detected in, 444, 446
  four-chamber plane, *28–29, 41*
  of inferior vena cava, *30, 41*, 268, 269, 273–275
  of left ventricle, *31*
  in pericardial effusion, 347, *353*
  for right heart structures, 254, 266, *267*
Subpulmonic view, 10, *13*
  M-mode recordings and, *36*
Superior vena cava, echocardiographic imaging of, 269
Suprasternal notch view, 22, *32–33*, 135–137
  for superior vena cava, 269
  in supravalvular aortic stenosis, *487*, 488
Supravalvular aortic stenosis. *See* Aortic stenosis, supravalvular
Surgery
  indications in infective endocarditis, 146
  postoperative echocardiographic assessment, 529–547
    in aortic stenosis, 547
    in atrial septal defect

primum type, 534, 536, *537*
secundum type, 533–534
in double-outlet right ventricle, 543–544
in endocardial cushion defect, 538
in pulmonic stenosis, 545–546
in subaortic stenosis, 546–547
in tetralogy of Fallot, 529–532
in transposition of great arteries, 538–542
in truncus arteriosus, 544–545
in ventricular septal defect, 531, 533
Systolic anterior motion. *See* Mitral valve, systolic anterior motion of
Systolic doming, 125, *126*
Systolic thickening, 174–175

T artifact, *262*
Technologist, requirements in echocardiography, 2–4
Terminology, for transducer location and imaging planes, 5–10
Tetralogy of Fallot, 493–496
  anatomy, 493, *494*
  clinical features and physiology, 493
  M-mode echocardiography in, 494
  surgical repair of, 529, *530*
    postoperative echocardiographic assessment, 530–531
    residua and sequelae, 529–530
  truncus arteriosus distinguished from, 509, 511
  two-dimensional echocardiography in, 494–496
Thebesian valves, 375, *384*
Thrombus
  left atrial myxoma distinguished from, 370
  left ventricular, 193–201
  left ventricular tumor differentiated from, 371
  on prosthetic valve, 395
Total anomalous pulmonary venous return, 524–525
  anatomy, 524
  clinical features and physiology, 524
  echocardiography in, 524–525
Training, of nonphysician echocardiographer, 3
Transducer
  in esophageal echocardiography, 438
  index mark placement on, 10
  intraoperative, 438
  position of, 5–22
    for aorta, 111–115, 135–139
    in aortic stenosis, 125–128
    apical, 21–27
    in atrial septal defect of secundum type, 444–446
    in congenital aortic stenosis, 483–485
    in corrected transposition, 504, 508
    in double-outlet right ventricle, 513–518
    in hypertrophic cardiomyopathy, 297–309
    for inferior vena cava, *268*, 269
    for left atrial mass, 370
    for left ventricle, 170
    for left ventricular dimensions, 227
    for left ventricular volume, 232
    for mitral stenosis, 54–55
    parasternal, 10–20, 22
    in patent ductus arteriosus, 462
    for prosthetic valves, 396–401
    for pulmonary artery, 79–80
    for pulmonic valve, 472
    for right atrial masses, 375
    for right heart structures, 252–254
    in right ventricular volume overload, 257–259, 265–266
    subcostal, 22, *28–29*, *41*
    for superior vena cava, 269
    suprasternal notch, 22, *32–33*
    in supravalvular aortic stenosis, 485–488
    terminology, 5–10
    in tetralogy of Fallot, 496
    in ventricular septal defect, 422, 424, 453–456
  in two-dimensional imaging systems, 4–5
Transposition of great arteries, 496–503
  anatomy, 497–499
  clinical features and physiology, 496–497
  corrected. *See* Corrected transposition of great arteries
  echocardiographic features, 500
  malposition distinguished from, 511
  surgical repair of, 538–542
    postoperative echocardiographic assessment, 539, 541, *542*
    residua and sequelae, 539
Transverse sinus, 345
Tricuspid atresia, 519, 523, *524*
  anatomy, 519, 523
  clinical features and physiology, 519
  echocardiography in, 523
Tricuspid regurgitation
  associated valvular lesions in rheumatic disease, 75–76
  causes of, 75
  echocardiography for, 76–78
    with contrast, 279, *281*, 425, *427*
  false positive diagnosis of, 76, 78
  after mitral surgery, 75
  prominent V waves in, 78
  right ventricular infarction and, 211, 214
Tricuspid stenosis
  appropriate echocardiographic views in, 73–75
  echocardiographic features of, 276, *278*, 279
Tricuspid valve
  abnormal motion in secundum atrial septal defect, 443–444
  anatomic differences from mitral valve, 276
  atresia of, 519, 523, *524*
  chordae tendineae of, 276
  contrast flow velocity in, 426
  Ebstein's anomaly of, 467–469
  echocardiography of, 69, 72–73
    imaging techniques, 253
  infective endocarditis involving, 153, 155–158
  prolapse of, 94, *95*

Tricuspid valve—*Continued*
  rheumatic disease of, 69, 72–78
  secondary motion abnormalities of, 283
  vegetations of, 153, 155–158
Tricuspid valve prolapse, 94, *95*
  mitral valve prolapse concomitant with, 279
Truncus arteriosus, 508–511
  anatomy, 509
  clinical features and physiology, 508–509
  M-mode echocardiography in, 509
  surgical repair of, 544–545
    postoperative echocardiographic assessment, 544–545
    residua and sequelae, 544
  two-dimensional echocardiography in, 509–511
Tumors, cardiac. *See* Cardiac tumors
Two-dimensional echocardiography. *See specific entity*

V wave
  in inferior vena cava, 269
  in tricuspid regurgitation, 78
Valsalva, sinuses of. *See* Sinuses of Valsalva
Valsalva maneuver
  as diagnostic intervention, 430–432
  in atrial septal defect, 424
  four phases of, 431
  in hypertrophic cardiomyopathy, 316
Valve ring abscess, and endocarditis, 146
Valvular heart disease. *See also* Prosthetic valves; Rheumatic valvular disease; *and under specific valves*
  echophonocardiography in, 434
  infective endocarditis, 145–159. *See also* Endocarditis, infective
  vegetations, 147–159
Vegetations
  of aortic valve, 147–151
  echocardiographic features of valvular lesions, 147
  of mitral valve, 151–155
  of prosthetic valve, 416
  of pulmonic valve, 158–159
  of tricuspid valve, 153, 155–158
  valvular lesions in endocarditis, 146
Ventricle, single. *See* Single ventricle

Ventricles. *See* Left ventricle; Right ventricle
Ventricular aneurysm, 189–191
Ventricular septal defect, 451–456
  anatomy, 451–453
  clinical features and physiology, 451
  contrast echocardiography in diagnosis of, 422, 424
  in corrected transposition, 500
  in double-outlet right ventricle, 511
  echocardiography in, 453–456
  endocardial cushion defect, 453, *455*, 456
  importance of resolution in echocardiography of, 5
  inflow defect, 451, 453, *454*, 456
  muscular defect, 453, *455*, 456
  outflow defect, 453, *454*, 456
  surgical repair of, 531, 533
    in double-outlet right ventricle, 543
    postoperative echocardiographic assessment, 533
    residua and sequelae, 533
    in tetralogy of Fallot, 529, *530*
  systolic fluttering of tricuspid valve in, *281*, 283
  in tetralogy of Fallot, 493
  in transposition of great arteries, 497
Ventricular septum. *See* Interventricular septum
Ventriculography, mitral valve prolapse identified by, 89–91
Verrucae, on valve leaflets or cusps, 58–59

Wall motion abnormalities, echocardiography for, 165
Wall motion index, 175–176
Wall motion studies
  in coronary artery disease, 170–172
  in left ventricular thrombus, 195
  most commonly used techniques, 174
  and enzymatic estimate of infarct size, 172–173
  regional abnormalities in myocardial infarction, 172–174
  in right ventricular infarction, 211
Wall stress. *See* Left ventricle, wall stress of
William's syndrome, 485

X-ray, chest. *See* Chest x-ray